REVIEW OF ORTHOPAEDICS

SECOND EDITION

Mark D. Miller, M.D.
Major USAF MC
Clinical Assistant Professor of Surgery
Uniformed Services University of Health Sciences
Bethesda, Maryland
Assistant Clinical Professor of Orthopaedic Surgery
University of Colorado Health Sciences Center
Associate Team Physician
Department of Orthopaedic Surgery
US Air Force Academy Hospital/SGOSO
USAF Academy, Colorado

W.B. SAUNDERS COMPANY
A Division of Harcourt Brace & Company
Philadelphia London Toronto Montreal Sydney Tokyo

W.B. SAUNDERS COMPANY
A Division of Harcourt Brace & Company

The Curtis Center
Independence Square West
Philadelphia, Pennsylvania 19106

Library of Congress Cataloging-in-Publication Data

Review of orthopaedics / [edited by] Mark D. Miller.—2nd ed.
p. cm.
Includes bibliographical references and index.
ISBN 0-7216-5901-2
1. Orthopedics.
[DNLM: 1. Bone Diseases—outlines. 2. Joint Diseases—outlines.
WE 18.2 R454 1996]
RD731.R44 1996
617.3—dc20
DNLM/DLC 95-24469

REVIEW OF ORTHOPAEDICS, 2nd edition ISBN 0-7216-5901-2

Printed in the United States of America

Last digit is the print number: 9 8 7 6 5 4 3 2

This book is dedicated to the families of the contributing authors. I sincerely appreciate the sacrifices they made to make the second edition a source of pride for us all.

Contributors

MARK R. BRINKER, M.D.
Clinical Assistant Professor of Orthopaedic Surgery, Tulane University School of Medicine, New Orleans, Louisiana; Director of Orthopaedic Research, Department of Orthopaedic Surgery and Residency Training Program, St. Luke's Medical Center, Cleveland, Ohio; Orthopaedic Surgeon, Fondren Orthopedic Group, L.L.P., Texas Orthopaedic Hospital, Houston, Texas
Basic Sciences

JAMES F. BRUCE, M.D.
Orthopedic Surgeon, Southern Center for Orthopedics Sports Medicine and Rehabilitation, La Grange, Georgia
Hand

CHARLES A. ENGH, M.D.
Clinical Assistant Professor, University of Maryland, College Park, Maryland; Clinical Assistant Professor, Georgetown University, Washington, D.C.
Adult Reconstruction

JOHN FERNANDEZ, M.D.
Department of Orthopaedic Surgery, University of Pittsburgh, Pittsburgh, Pennsylvania
Adult Reconstruction

FRANK J. FRASSICA, M.D.
Associate Professor, Orthopaedic Oncology, The Johns Hopkins University; Chief, Division of Adult Orthopaedics and Reconstructive Surgery, The Johns Hopkins Hospital, Baltimore, Maryland
Orthopaedic Pathology

BEN A. GOMEZ, M.D.
Associate Professor, Orthopaedics, Wright State University, Dayton, Ohio; Instructor in Surgery, Uniformed Services University, Bethesda, Maryland; Orthopaedic Surgeon, Wright Patterson Medical Center, Wright Patterson Air Force Base, Ohio
Anatomy

WILLIAM C. LAUERMAN, M.D.
Associate Professor, Department of Orthopaedic Surgery, Georgetown University School of Medicine; Chief, Division of Spine Surgery, Georgetown University, Washington, D.C.
Spine

EDWARD F. McCARTHY, JR, M.D.
Associate Professor, Pathology and Orthopaedic Surgery, The Johns Hopkins University; Director, Bone and Joint Laboratories, The Johns Hopkins Hospital, Baltimore, Maryland
Orthopaedic Pathology

MARK D. MILLER, M.D.
Clinical Assistant Professor of Surgery, Uniformed Services University of the Health Sciences, Bethesda, Maryland; Assistant Clinical Professor of Orthopaedic Surgery, University of Colorado Health Sciences Center; Assistant Chief, Sports Medicine, Associate Team Physician, Department of Orthopaedic Surgery, US Air Force Academy Hospital/SGHST, USAF Academy, Colorado
Basic Sciences; Sports Medicine

MARK S. MIZEL, M.D.
Assistant Professor of Orthopaedic Surgery, The Johns Hopkins University, Baltimore, Maryland
Disorders of the Foot and Ankle

MICHAEL S. PINZUR, M.D.
Professor of Orthopaedic Surgery, Loyola University Medical School; Director, Gait Analysis Laboratory, Loyola University Medical Center, Maywood, Illinois
Rehabilitation

MICHAEL REGAN, M.D.
Orthopaedic Surgeon, Maine Medical Center, Portland, Maine
Spine

THOMAS E. SHULER, M.D.
Assistant Professor of Clinical Orthopedic Surgery, University of Virginia, Charlottesville, Virginia; Director, Orthopedic Trauma, Co-Director, Orthopedic Education, Roanoke Memorial Hospitals, Roanoke, Virginia
Trauma

MARK SOBEL, M.D.
Director, Orthopaedic Foot and Ankle Service, Beth Israel Medical Center—North Division, New York, New York
Disorders of the Foot and Ankle

NICHOLAS G. SOTEREANOS, M.D.
Assistant Clinical Professor, University of Pittsburgh, Pittsburgh, Pennsylvania
Adult Reconstruction

RAYMOND M. STEFKO, M.D.
Chief, Pediatric Orthopaedics, Wilford Hall USAF Medical Center, Lackland Air Force Base, San Antonio, Texas
Pediatric Orthopaedics

DENNIS R. WENGER, M.D.
Clinical Professor, Orthopedic Surgery, University of California—San Diego; Director, Pediatric Orthopedics, Children's Hospital, San Diego, California
Pediatric Orthopaedics

Foreword

It is with great pleasure that I write this foreword for Dr. Mark Miller, an active-duty Air Force officer in Colorado Springs who trained as a fellow in our Sports Medicine Program within the University of Pittsburgh Medical Center. Dr. Mark Miller is known for his balance, energy, and dedication to orthopaedic education. The first edition of *Review of Orthopaedics* has proved to be a tremendous success for all of those students studying for the in-training and board examinations. Reflecting on the increased specialization within the field, Dr. Miller invited the fellowship training experts to write each individual chapter for the second edition. In addition, the new edition has greatly increased coverage of reconstruction and sports medicine. The contributors also updated and expanded the selected bibliography for each chapter to include a wide range of both contemporary and classic information. All of this information has been carefully edited by Dr. Miller to ensure that it remains clear and useful. I am sure that this second edition will be of great value for educating orthopaedic residents and fellows as well as for practicing surgeons. It is a pleasure for me to have worked with Dr. Miller and to see his tremendous contribution to the field within such a short period of time.

FREDDIE H. FU, M.D.
PITTSBURGH, PA

Preface
to the Second Edition

Thank you for making the first edition of this book such a success. This project originally began as a self-study tool, and eventually became an orthopaedic "best seller". I would be naive to think that this was all because of my work. This text is nothing more than a synopsis of other people's work. To them we all are indebted. The true credit belongs to those who have been bold enough to challenge conventional teaching, and those who have challenged us to be bold enough to teach.

The second edition of this text is not just a "repackaged" version of the first edition. I invited young fellowship-trained orthopaedic surgeons from around the country to re-write each chapter of this book. I challenged them to expand each section with the latest in their field. Each author reviewed the latest In-Training and Self Assessment examinations, specialty journals, review courses and fellowship training information and integrated these into their chapters. We have expanded the "Selected Bibliography" in each chapter and have organized the references into major categories. Two new chapters have been added. Because the American Board of Orthopaedic Surgeons has expanded Part I of their examination to include more basic science questions, we placed special emphasis on updating this chapter, and have made it the first chapter in the book.

Despite our best efforts, there may be some errors or omissions in this edition. I remain totally committed to correcting these inaccuracies, and making subsequent printings and editions even better. Please feel free to drop me a line with your comments and suggestions. After all, this is your book!

Mark D. Miller, M.D.

Preface
to the First Edition

The writer does the most, who gives the reader the most knowledge and takes from him the least time.

C.C. Colton *Lacon*, Preface

This book was created to fill an important void in the existing orthopaedic literature. Although there exists a large number of quality texts of operative orthopaedics, musculoskeletal basic science, and the various sub-specialties, nowhere is there an essential "core" of orthopaedic knowledge. This book attempts to provide this core by distilling the existing orthopaedic textbooks, journal articles, review courses, intraining examinations, self assessment guides, and specialty examinations into one resource.

REVIEW OF ORTHOPAEDICS has been extensively edited by two groups of consultants: First by a cadre of younger orthopaedic surgeons who have recently finished residency and fellowship training and successfully completed their boards, and second by an impressive assemblage of senior surgeons who have added a vital element of experience to the text.

It is my intention that this book will serve as a review for intraining and board examinations, and also as a curriculum guide for orthopaedic residency training programs.

Mark D. Miller, M.D.

Contents

1

BASIC SCIENCES

MARK R. BRINKER and MARK D. MILLER

The fund of knowledge and discovery in orthopaedic basic science continues to expand at an almost logarithmic pace. Areas of study virtually unknown to the musculoskeletal scientific community only 10 years ago have now moved to the forefront and are the major focus of research in centers throughout the world. Examples of such areas of recent rapid advancement are molecular biology, biochemistry, immunology, and cellular mechanics. The rapid expansion of knowledge is exemplified by the annual Orthopaedic Research Society meeting where more than 800 original scientific works are presented each year by musculoskeletal scientists from around the globe.

It is difficult if not impossible for the young orthopaedic surgeon to keep pace with the explosion of information on the musculoskeletal basic sciences. Keeping current and up to date in this rapidly expanding field may be likened to trying to take a sip of water from a fire hydrant opened full-blast. It is therefore the intent of this chapter, entitled Basic Sciences, to act as a life preserver so that the young orthopaedic surgeon in training should not drown in the turbulent waters of musculoskeletal scientific discovery. Staying afloat will become particularly important in the coming years, as the American Board of Orthopaedic Surgeons has elected to increase the emphasis on basic science testing with a proposed additional *100 questions—all basic science—for the Part I written examination.*

When compiling information for this chapter a number of basic science resources were reviewed. *Orthopaedic Basic Science,* edited by Sheldon R. Simon and published by the American Academy of Orthopaedic Surgeons, is an exceptional textbook that should serve as a reference text for more in-depth knowledge on material covered in this chapter. Basic science test questions from the Orthopaedic In-Training Examinations (OITE) from 1991 to 1994 and Orthopaedic Self Assessment Examinations (OSAE) from 1991 to 1995 have been reviewed and collated into a wide variety of topical categories. Table 1–1 summarizes these basic science test questions. Specific information regarding these questions has been summarized in greater detail within each of the eight sections of this chapter. Furthermore, information specifically tested on the OITE and OSAE is denoted by an *asterisk in parentheses* (*). Information specifically tested more than once on the OITE (1991–1994) and OSAE (1991–1995) is denoted by a number of asterisks in parentheses corresponding to the number of times the information has been tested. Finally, included within each of the eight sections of this chapter are detailed summaries of test questions (denoted by specific test and question number) in topical categories covered in the specific section.

SECTION 1
Bone

I. Histology of Bone

A. Types—Normal bone is lamellar and can be cortical or cancellous. Immature or pathologic bone is woven, is more random with more osteocytes than lamellar bone, has increased turnover, and is weaker and more flexible than lamellar bone. Lamellar bone is stress-oriented; woven bone is not stress-oriented.

1. Cortical Bone (Compact Bone) (Figs. 1–1, 1–2, 1–3)—Makes up 80% of the skeleton and is composed of tightly packed osteons or haversian systems that are connected by haversian (or Volkmann's) canals. These canals contain arterioles, venules, capillaries, nerves, and possibly lymphatic channels. Interstitial lamellae lie between the osteons. Fibrils frequently connect lamellae but do not cross cement lines (where bone resorption has stopped and new bone formation has begun). Cement lines define the outer border of an osteon. Nutrition is via the intraosseous circulation (canals and canaliculi [cell processes of osteocytes]). Cortical bone is characterized by a slow turnover rate, a relatively high Young's modulus (E), and a high resistance to torsion and bending.
2. Cancellous Bone (Spongy or Trabecular Bone) (Figs. 1–2, 1–3)—Less dense and undergoes more remodeling according to lines of stress (Wolff's law). It has a higher turnover rate, has a smaller Young's modulus, and is more elastic than cortical bone.

B. Cellular Biology

1. Osteoblasts—Form bone. Derived from undifferentiated mesenchymal cells (stimulated by immo-

TABLE 1–1. TOTAL NUMBER OF BASIC SCIENCE TEST QUESTIONS: OITE 1991–1994 AND OSAE 1991–1995

TEST	BONE	JOINTS	NEURO-MUSCULAR & CONNECTIVE TISSUES	CELL & MOLEC. BIOLOGY, IMMUNOLOGY, GENETICS	INFECTIONS & MICROBIOLOGY	PERIOPERATIVE PROBLEMS	IMAGING & SPECIAL STUDIES	BIOMATERIALS & BIOMECHANICS
1995 OSAE—Adult Recon Hip/Knee	3	4	2	0	3	0	3	14
1995 OSAE—Pediatric Ortho	4	2	2	2	4	0	1	0
1995 OSAE—Sports Medicine	0	1	19	0	0	0	3	4
1994 OITE	2	6	3	0	7	5	0	17
1994 OSAE—Adult Spine	1	0	3	0	5	1	9	4
1994 OSAE—Foot & Ankle	3	7	2	0	4	2	6	2
1994 OSAE—M/S Trauma	3	1	1	0	5	10	0	3
1993 OITE	7	6	2	1	4	6	2	20
1993 OSAE—M/S Tumors & Diseases	11	9	1	0	5	0	1	0
1993 OSAE—Shoulder & Elbow	1	1	0	0	0	0	1	2
1992 OITE	15	3	1	0	9	3	5	14
1992 OSAE—Adult Recon Hip/Knee	4	2	0	0	5	0	4	20
1992 OSAE—Pediatric Ortho	5	0	0	0	3	0	1	0
1992 OSAE—Sports Medicine	2	2	23	0	1	1	2	3
1991 OITE	13	4	1	2	14	13	1	9
1991 OSAE—Adult Spine	3	3	3	1	1	0	4	6
1991 OSAE—Anatomy-Imaging	0	0	1	0	0	0	0	0
1991 OSAE—Foot & Ankle	2	5	1	1	7	3	3	2
1991 OSAE—M/S Trauma	2	0	0	0	11	20	5	4
Totals	81	56	65	7	88	64	51	124

bilization). These cells have more endoplasmic reticulum, Golgi apparatus, and mitochondria than other cells (to fulfill the cell's role in the synthesis and secretion of matrix). More differentiated, metabolically active cells line bone surfaces, and less active cells in "resting regions" or entrapped cells maintain the ionic milieu of bone. Disruption of the lining cell layer activates these cells. Osteoblast differentiation in vivo is effected by the interleukins, platelet-derived growth factor (PDGF), and insulin-derived growth factor (IDGF). Osteoblasts produce type I collagen, respond to parathyroid hormone (PTH), and produce osteocalcin (stimulated by 1,25-dihydroxyvitamin D). Osteoblasts have receptor-effector interactions for: (1) PTH; (2) 1,25-dihydroxyvitamin D; (3) glucocorticoids; (4) prostaglandins; and (5) estrogen. Osteoblastic activity is inhibited by calcitonin.

2. Osteocytes—Make up 90% of the cells in the mature skeleton and serve to maintain bone. These cells represent former osteoblasts that have been trapped within newly formed matrix (which they help preserve). Osteocytes have an increased nucleus/cytoplasm ratio with long interconnecting cytoplasmic processes and are not as active in matrix production as osteoblasts. Osteocytes have an important role in controlling the extracellular concentration of calcium and phosphorus; they are directly stimulated by calcitonin and inhibited by PTH.
3. Osteoclasts—Resorb bone. These multinucleated, irregularly shaped giant cells originate from hematopoietic tissues (monocyte progenitors form giant cells by fusion), and possess a ruffled ("brush") border (plasma membrane enfoldings that increase surface area and are important in bone resorption) and a surrounding clear zone. Bone resorption occurs in depressions known as Howship's lacunae and occurs more rapidly than bone formation; bone formation and resorption are linked ("coupled"). Osteoclasts bind to bone surfaces via cell attachment (anchoring) proteins (**integrins**). Osteoclasts produce hydrogen ions (via carbonic anhydrase) to lower the pH, which increases the solubility of hydroxyapatite crystals, and the organic matrix is removed by proteolytic digestion. Osteoclasts have specific **receptors for calcitonin** to allow them to directly regulate bone resorption (*).
4. Osteoprogenitor Cells—Become osteoblasts. These local mesenchymal cells line haversian canals, endosteum, and periosteum, awaiting the stimulus to differentiate into osteoblasts.
5. Lining Cells—Narrow, flattened cells that form an "envelope around bone."

C. Matrix—Composed of organic components (40%) and inorganic components (60%).

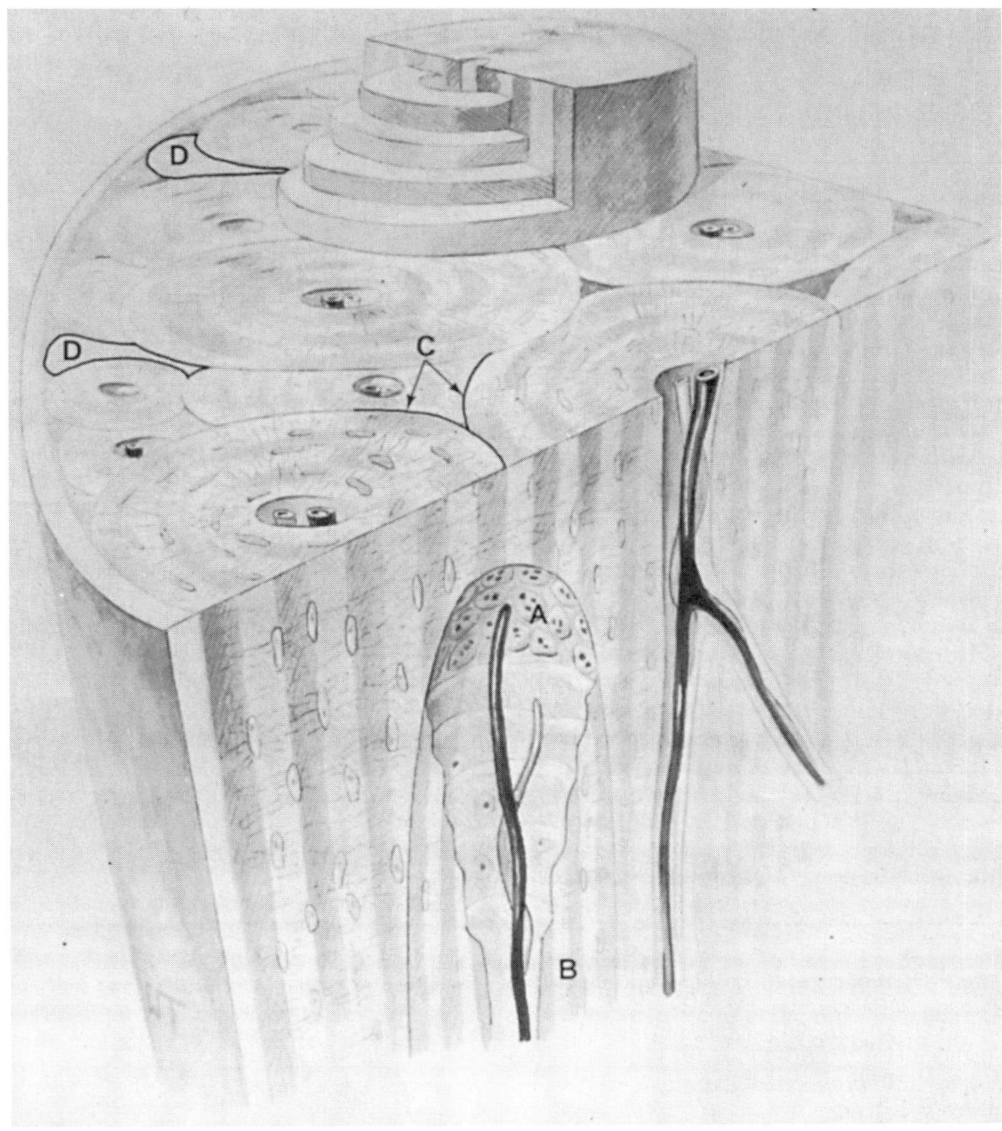

FIGURE 1–1. Architecture of cortical bone. *A*, Cutting cone of osteoclasts. *B*, Osteoblasts lay down new osteones. *C*, Cement lines. *D*, Interstitial lamellae. (From Owen, R., Goodfellow, J., and Bullough P.: Scientific Foundations of Orthopaedics and Traumatology, p. 6. Philadelphia, WB Saunders, 1981; reprinted by permission.)

1. Organic Components—Make up 40% of the dry weight of bone. Organic components include collagen, proteoglycans, noncollagenous matrix proteins (glycoproteins, phospholipids, phosphoproteins), and growth factors and cytokines.
   a. Collagen—Responsible for tensile strength of bone. Makes up 90% of the matrix of bone and is composed primarily of type I collagen (the word "b**one**" contains the word "one" as its terminal three letters, so it is easy to remember that bone is comprised primarily of type I collagen). Collagen structure consists of a triple helix of tropocollagen (two α_1 and one α_2 chains) that is quarter-staggered to produce a collagen fibril. **Hole zones** (gaps) exist within the collagen fibril between the **ends** of molecules. **Pores** exist between the **sides** of parallel molecules. Mineral deposition (calcification) occurs within these hole zones and pores (Fig. 1–4). Cross-linking decreases solubility and increases the tensile strength of collagen.
   b. Proteoglycans—Partially responsible for the compressive strength of bone, they inhibit mineralization. Composed of glycosaminoglycan (GAG)–protein complexes (discussed below in Section 2: Joints).
   c. Matrix Proteins (Noncollagenous)—Promote mineralization and bone formation. Matrix proteins include osteocalcin (bone γ-carboxyglutamic acid-containing protein [bone Gla protein]), osteonectin (SPARC), osteopontin, and others. **Osteocalcin** (produced by osteoblasts) attracts osteoclasts and is directly

TYPES OF BONE

MICROSCOPIC | STRUCTURAL

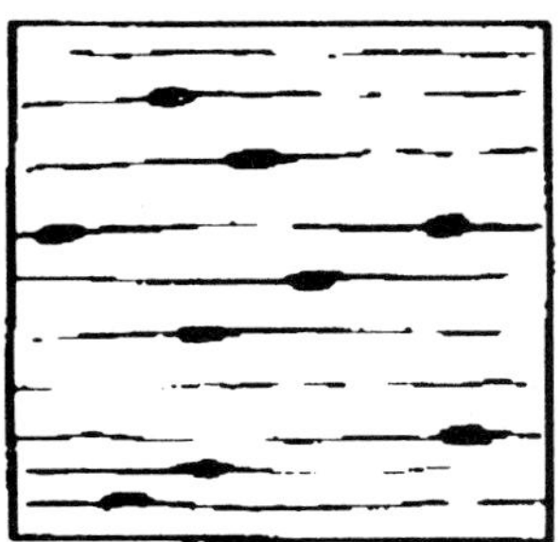

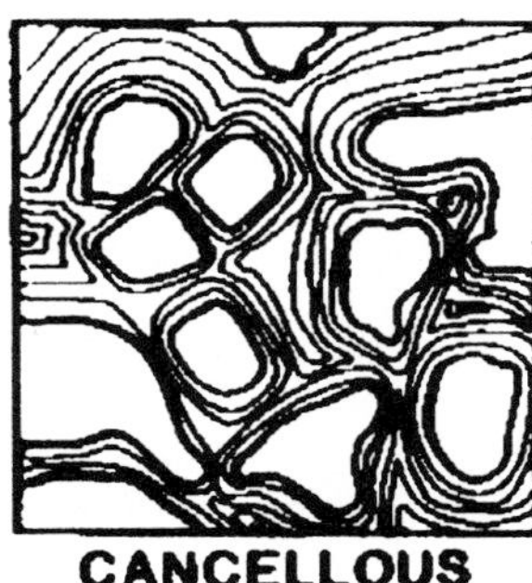

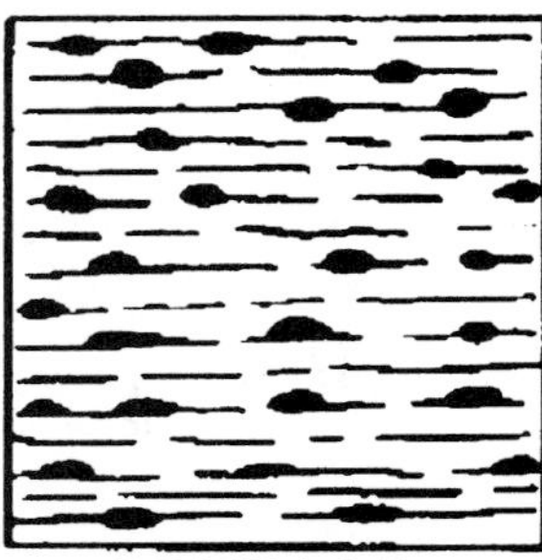

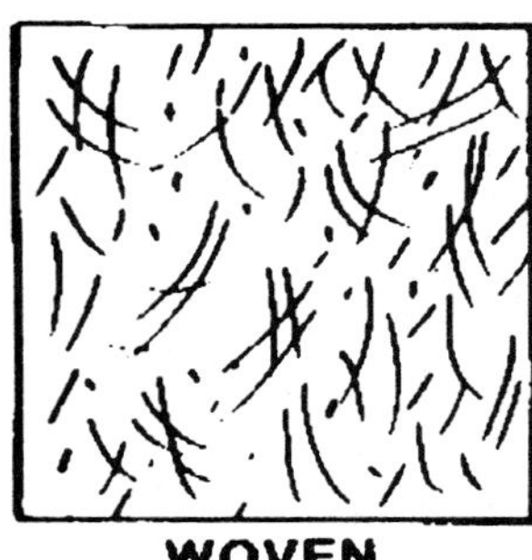

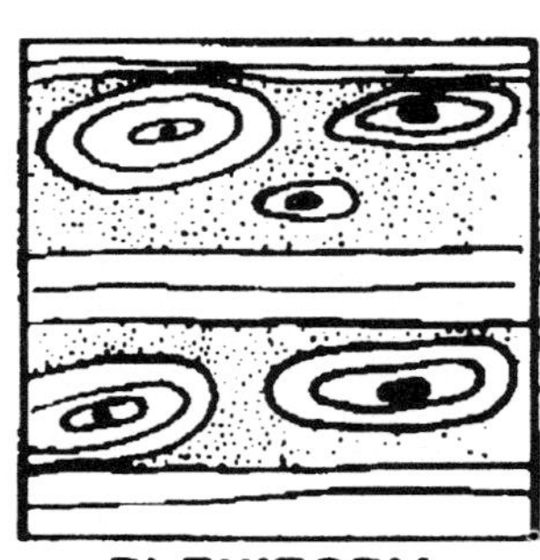

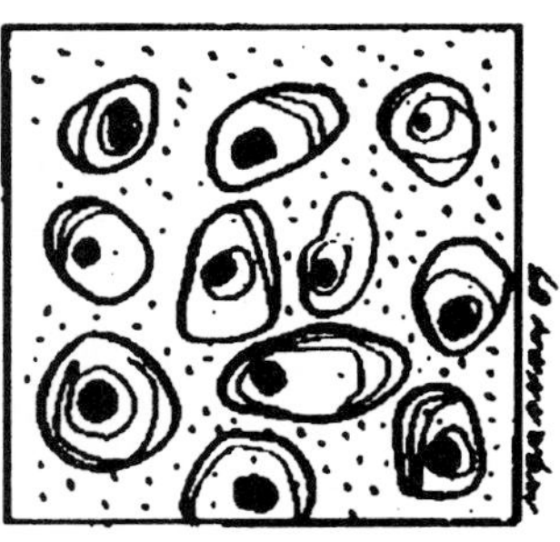

FIGURE 1–2. Types of bone. (From Simon, S.R., ed: Orthopaedic Basic Science, 2nd ed., p. 129. Rosemont, IL, American Academy of Orthopaedic Surgeons, 1994; reprinted by permission.)

related to the regulation of bone density. Osteocalcin accounts for 10–20% of the noncollagenous protein of bone. The synthesis of osteocalcin is inhibited by PTH and stimulated by 1,25-dihydroxyvitamin D. Osteocalcin levels in urine and serum are elevated in Paget's disease, renal osteodystrophy, and hyperparathyroidism. **Osteonectin** (secreted by platelets and osteoblasts) is postulated to play a role in the regulation of calcium or the organization of mineral within the matrix. **Osteopontin** is a cell-binding protein (similar to an integrin).

d. Growth Factors and Cytokines—Present in small amounts in bone matrix. They include (1) transforming growth factor-beta (TGF-β); (2) insulin-like growth factor (IGF); (3) interleukins (IL-1, IL-6); and (4) bone morphogenic proteins (BMP_{1-6}). These proteins aid in bone cell differentiation, activation, growth, and turnover.

2. Inorganic (Mineral) Components—Make up 60% of the dry weight of bone.
   a. Calcium Hydroxyapatite [$Ca_{10}(PO_4)_6(OH)_2$]—Responsible for the compressive strength of bone. Makes up most of the inorganic matrix and is responsible for mineralization of the matrix. Primary mineralization occurs in gaps in the collagen; secondary mineralization occurs on the periphery.
   b. Osteocalcium Phosphate (Brushite)—Makes up remaining inorganic matrix.

D. Bone Remodeling—Affected by mechanical function according to Wolff's law. Removal of external stresses can lead to significant bone loss; but this situation can be reversed to varying degrees upon remobilization.
   1. General—Bone remodels in response to stress and responds to piezoelectric charges (compression side is electronegative, stimulating osteoblasts [bone formation]; tension side is electropositive, stimulating osteoclasts [bone resorption]). Both cortical and cancellous bone are continuously being remodeled by osteoclastic and osteoblastic activity (Fig. 1–5). Bone remodeling occurs throughout life. Bone mass peaks at 16–25 years of age.
   2. Cortical Bone—Remodels by osteoclastic tunneling (cutting cones) (Fig. 1–6) followed by layering of osteoblasts and successive deposition of layers of lamellae (after the cement line has been laid down) until the tunnel size has narrowed to the diameter of the osteonal central canal. The head of the cutting cone is made up of osteoclasts, which bore holes through hard cortical bone. Behind the osteoclast front are capillaries, followed by osteoblasts, which lay down osteoid to fill the resorption cavity.
   3. Cancellous Bone—Remodels by osteoclastic resorption, followed by osteoblasts, which lay down new bone.

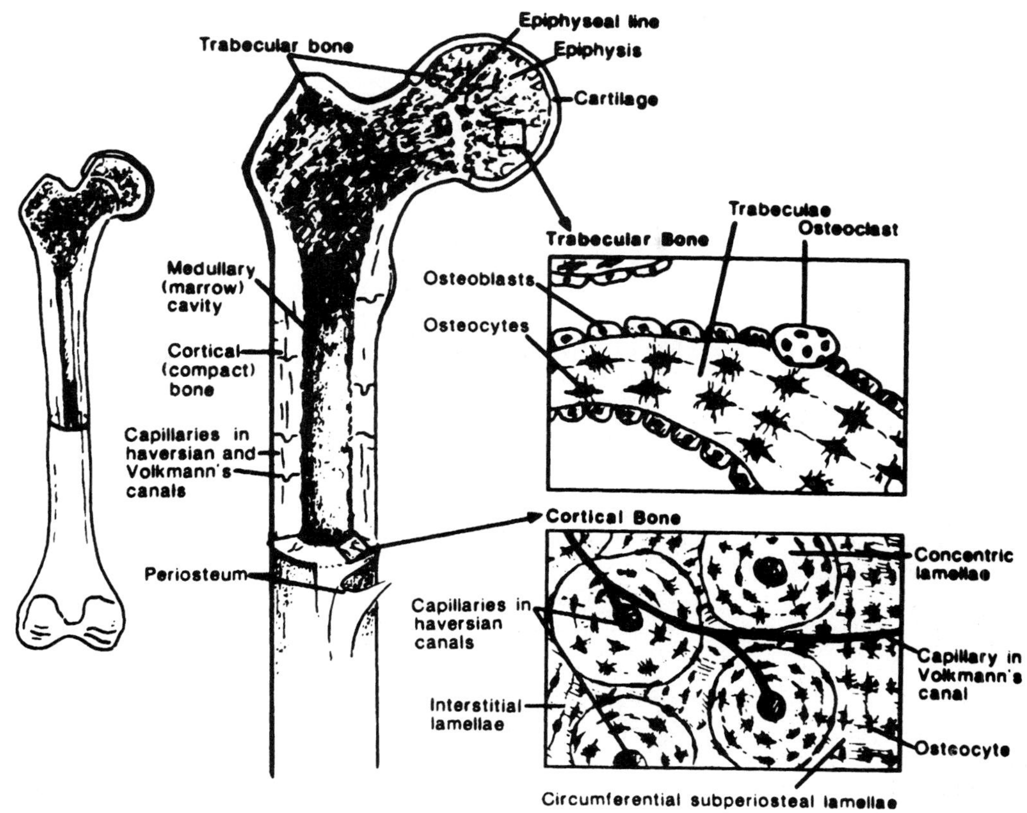

FIGURE 1–3. Cortical and trabecular bone demonstrating the various microstructures. (From Keaveny, T.M., and Hayes, W.C.: Mechanical properties of cortical and trabecular bone. Bone 7:285–344, 1993; reprinted by permission.)

MINERAL ACCRETION: ***BIOLOGICAL CONSIDERATIONS***

HETEROGENEITY WITHIN A COLLAGEN FIBRIL

PROGRESSIVELY INCREASING MINERAL MASS DUE TO:

1. INCREASED NUMBER OF NEW MINERAL PHASE PARTICLES (NUCLEATION)
   a. HETEROGENEOUS NUCLEATION BY MATRIX IN COLLAGEN HOLES (? PORES)
   b. 2° CRYSTAL INDUCED NUCLEATION IN HOLES AND PORES
2. INITIAL GROWTH OF PARTICLES TO ~ 400Å x 15–30Å x 50–75Å

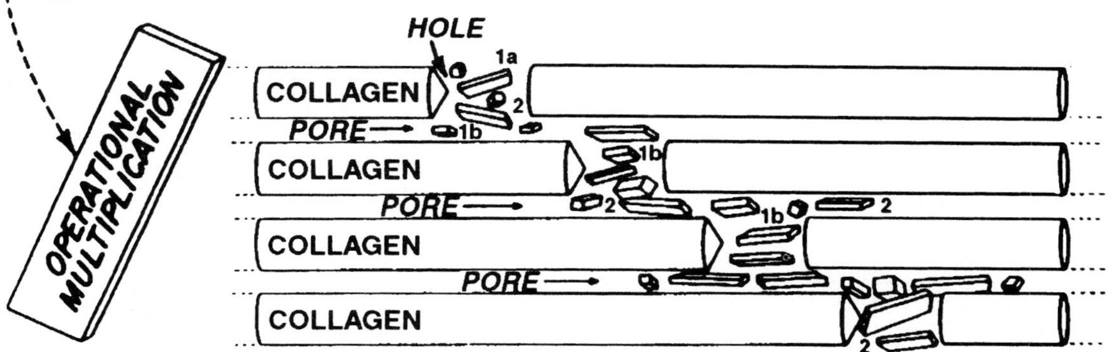

FIGURE 1–4. Mineral accretion. (From Simon, S.R., ed: Orthopaedic Basic Science, 2nd ed., p. 139. Rosemont, IL, American Academy of Orthopaedic Surgeons, 1994; reprinted by permission.)

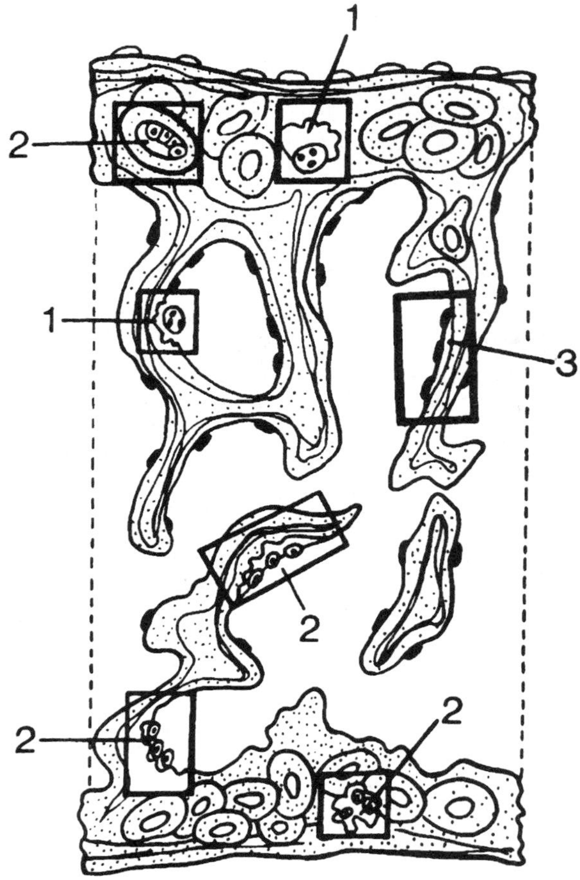

FIGURE 1–5. Bone remodeling. *1,* Bone resorbed by osteoclastic activity in the cortex and trabeculae. *2,* Osteoblasts form new bone at the site of prior bone resorption. *3,* Osteoblasts become incorporated into bone as osteocytes. (From Simon, S.R., ed.: Orthopaedic Basic Science, 2nd ed., p. 141. Rosemont, IL, American Academy of Orthopaedic Surgeons, 1994; reprinted by permission.)

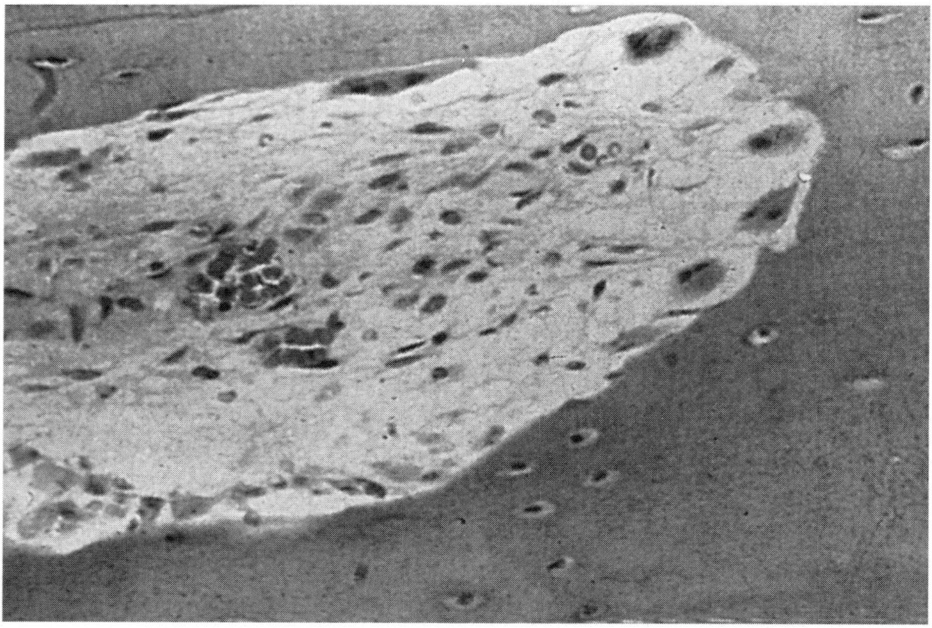

FIGURE 1–6. Mechanism of cortical bone remodeling via cutting cones. (From Simon, S.R., ed.: Orthopaedic Basic Science, 2nd ed., p. 142. Rosemont, IL, American Academy of Orthopaedic Surgeons, 1994; reprinted by permission.)

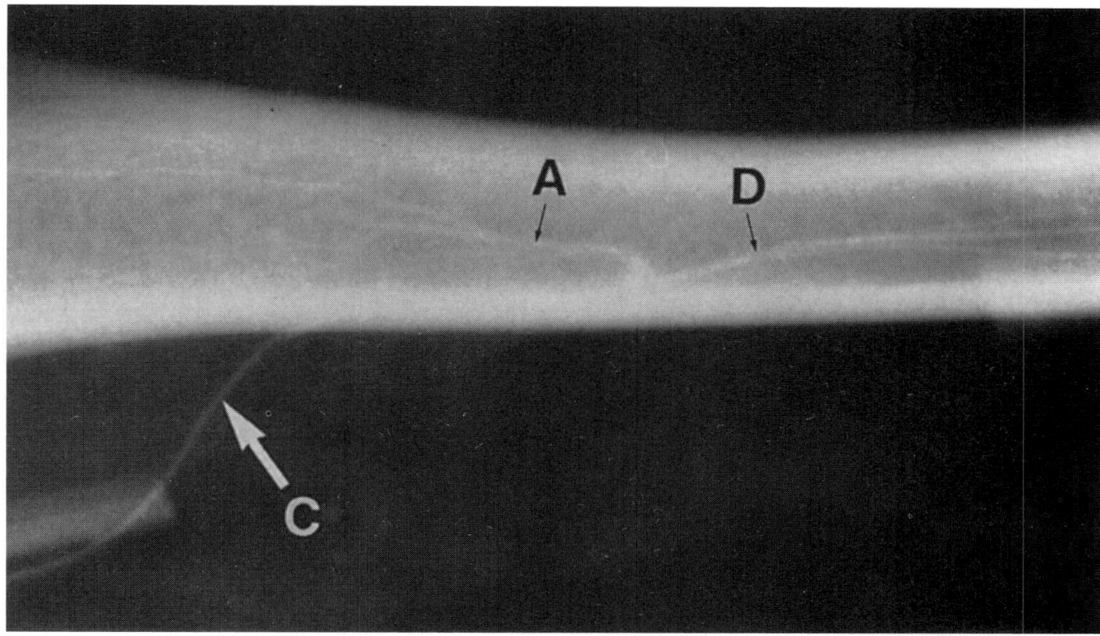

FIGURE 1–7. Intraoperative arteriogram (canine tibia) demonstrating ascending (A) and descending (D) branches of the nutrient artery. C, cannula. (From Brinker, M.R., Lippton, H.L., Cook, S.D., and Hyman, A.L.: Pharmacological regulation of the circulation of bone. J. Bone Joint Surg. [Am.] 72:964–975, 1990; reprinted by permission.)

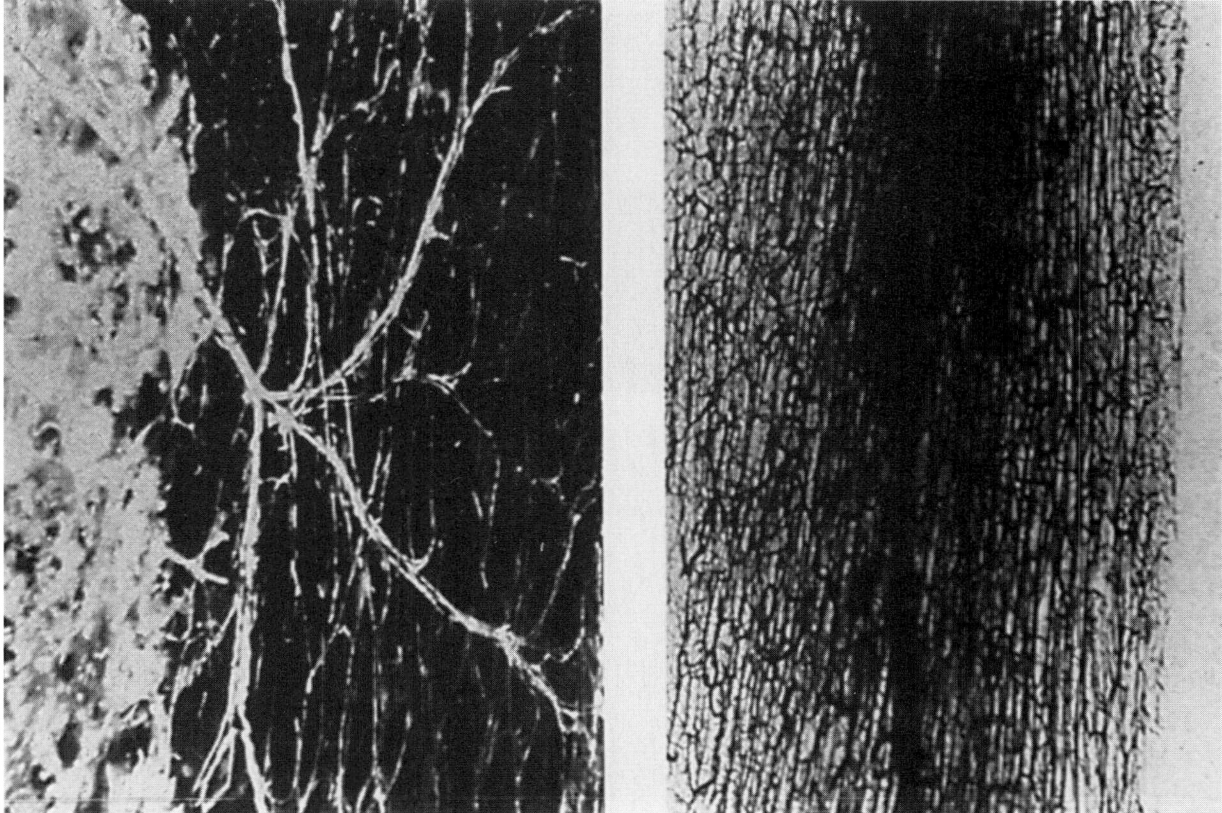

FIGURE 1–8. Vasculature of cortical bone. (From Simon, S.R., ed.: Orthopaedic Basic Science, 2nd ed., p. 131. Rosemont, IL, American Academy of Orthopaedic Surgeons, 1994; reprinted by permission.)

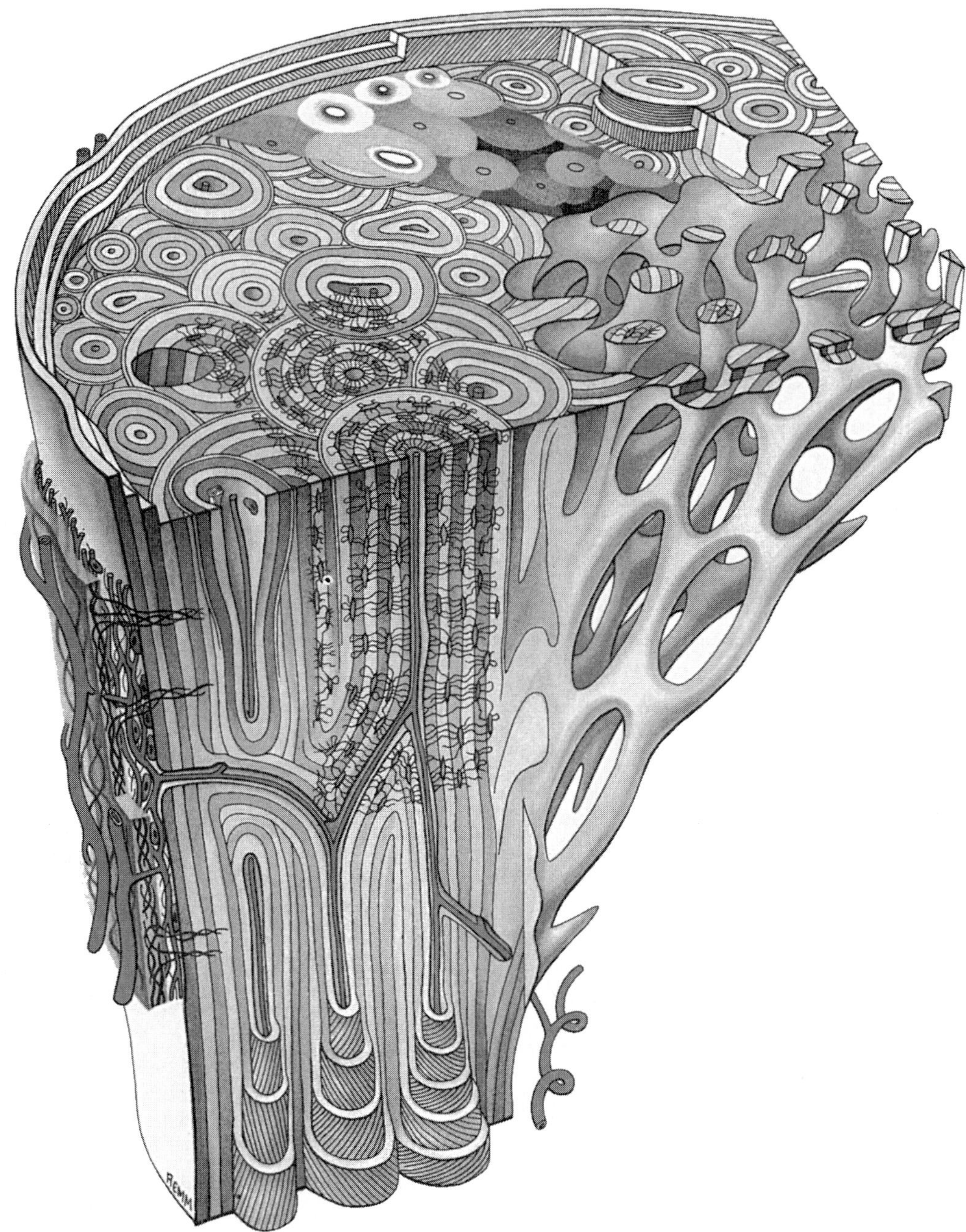

FIGURE 1–9. Mature bone demonstrating bone circulation and haversian systems. (From Gray's Anatomy, 38th British ed., p. 254. New York, Churchill Livingstone, 1995; reprinted by permission.)

E. Bone Circulation

1. Anatomy—As an organ, bone receives 5–10% of the cardiac output. The long bones receive blood from three sources: (1) nutrient artery system; (2) metaphyseal-epiphyseal system; and (3) periosteal system. Bones with a tenuous blood supply include the scaphoid, talus, femoral head, and odontoid (*).
   a. Nutrient Artery System—The nutrient artery(s) originate as branches from major arteries of the systemic circulation. The nutrient artery enters the diaphyseal cortex (outer and inner tables) through the nutrient foramen to enter the medullary canal. Once in the medullary canal the nutrient artery branches into ascending and descending small arteries (Fig. 1–7), which branch into arterioles that penetrate the endosteal cortex to supply at least the inner two-thirds of mature diaphyseal cortex via vessels that traverse the haversian system (Figs. 1–8, 1–9). The nutrient artery system is a **high pressure** system.

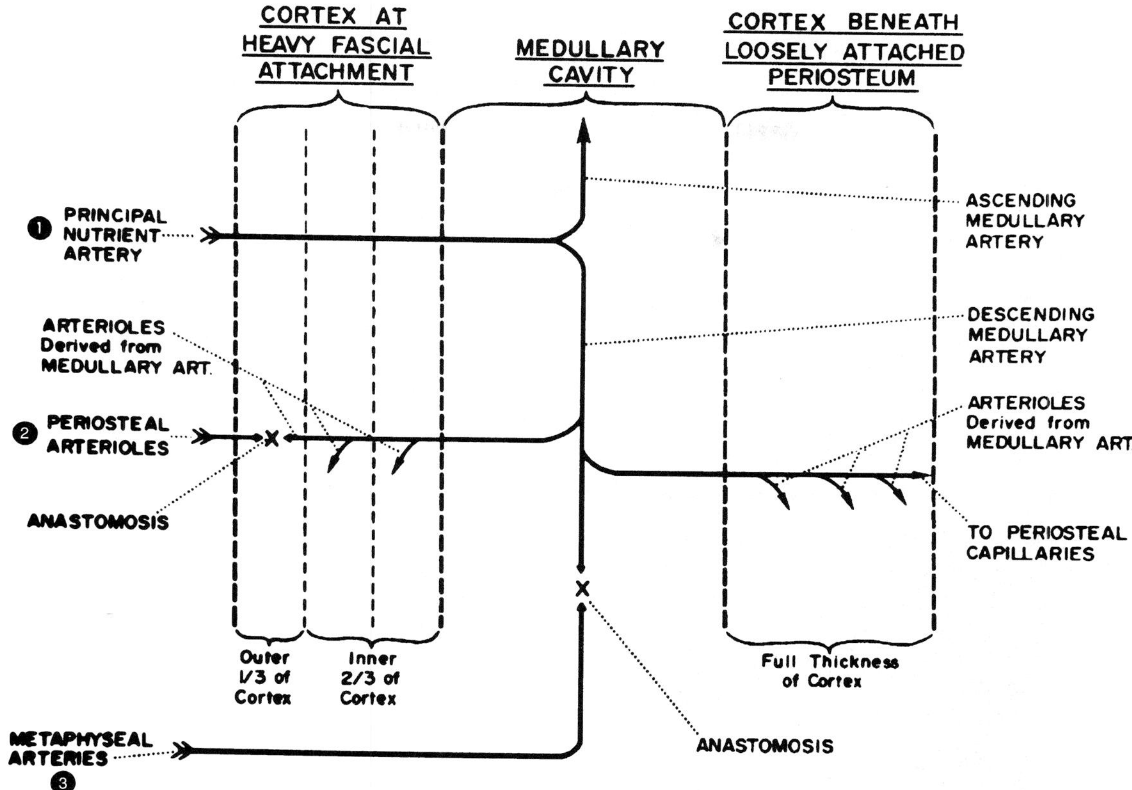

FIGURE 1–10. Major components of the afferent vascular system of long bone. Components 1, 2, and 3 constitute the total nutrient supply to the diaphysis. Arrows indicate the direction of blood flow. (From Rhinelander, F.W.: Circulation in bone. In The Biochemistry and Physiology of Bone, 2nd ed., vol. 2, Bourne, G., ed. Orlando, FL, Academic Press, 1972; reprinted by permission.)

b. Metaphyseal-Epiphyseal System—Arises from the periarticular vascular plexus (i.e., geniculate arteries).
c. Periosteal System—Comprised primarily of capillaries that supply the outer one-third (at most) of the mature diaphyseal cortex. The periosteal system is a **low pressure** system.

2. Physiology
   a. Direction of Flow (Fig. 1–10)
      1. Arterial flow in mature bone is centrifugal (inside to outside), a result of the net effect of the high pressure nutrient arterial system (endosteal system) and the low pressure periosteal system.
      2. In the case of a completely displaced fracture with complete disruption of the endosteal (nutrient) system, the pressure head is reversed, the periosteal system predominates, and blood flow is centripetal (outside to inside).
      3. Arterial flow in immature developing bone is centripetal, as the periosteum is highly vascularized and is the predominant component of bone blood flow.
      4. Venous flow in mature bone is centripetal; cortical capillaries drain to venous sinusoids, which drain in turn to the emissary venous system.
   5. Fluid Compartments of Bone

Extravascular	65%
Haversian	6%
Lacunar	6%
RBCs	3%
Other	20%

TABLE 1–2. TECHNIQUES USED TO STUDY BONE CIRCULATION

DIRECT METHODS
Vital microscopy
Electromagnetic flow probes
Laser-Doppler flowmetry
Pulsed ultrasound Doppler velocimetry
INDIRECT METHODS
Effluent collection
Ex vivo perfusion
Extracorporeal circulation
Radioactive isotope clearance
Radioactive isotope injection with radiologic detection
Cr-labeled RBCs
Intraosseous pressure measurement
Heated thermocouples
Hydrogen or oxygen washout
Venous plethysmography
Radioactive microspheres

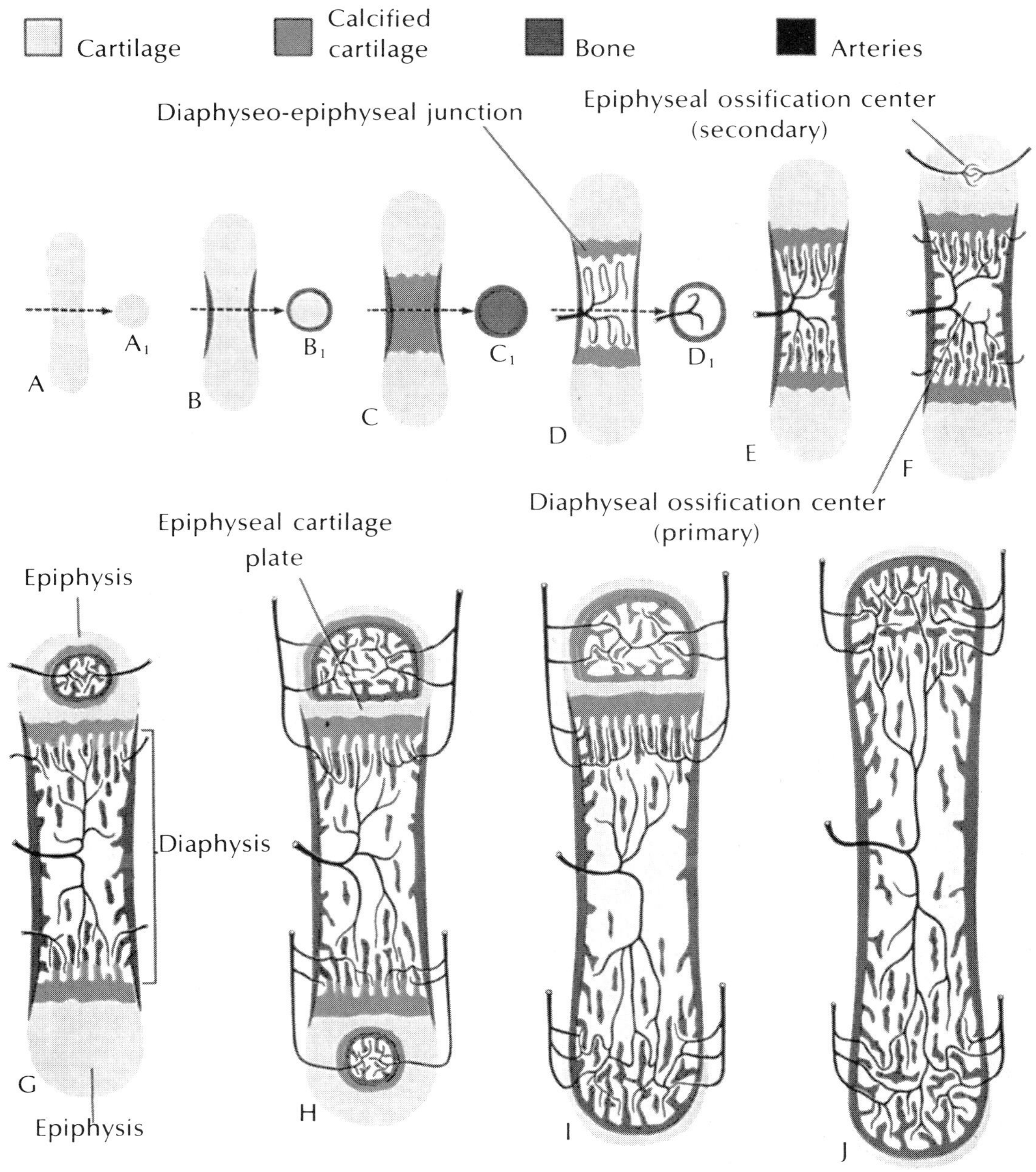

1F11

FIGURE 1–11. Enchondral ossification of long bones. Note that phases F–J often occur after birth. (From Moore, K.L.: The Developing Human, p. 346. Philadelphia: WB Saunders, 1982; reprinted by permission.)

b. Physiologic States' Effect on Blood Flow
   1. Hypoxia—increases flow
   2. Hypercapnia—increases flow
   3. Sympathectomy—increases flow

3. Fracture Healing—Bone blood flow is responsible for the delivery of nutrients to the site of bony injury. The **initial response** of bone blood flow to a fracture is **decreased flow** secondary to disruption of the vascular anatomy at the fracture site. **Within hours to days bone blood flow increases** (as part of the **regional acceleratory phenomenon**) and **peaks at approximately 2 weeks.** Blood flow **returns to normal** between **3 and 5 months.** Bone blood flow is the **major determinant** of fracture healing. The major advantage of using unreamed intramedullary (IM) nails is the preservation of endosteal blood supply (*); reaming devascularizes the inner 50–80% of cortex (**) and is the type of fixation associated with the greatest delay in revascularization (*).
4. Regulation—Bone blood flow is under the control of metabolic, humeral, and autonomic inputs. The arterial system of bone has great potential for vasoconstriction (from the resting state) and much less potential for vasodilation. The vessels within bone possess a variety of vasoactive receptors (α-adrenergic, muscarinic, thromboxane/prostaglandin) that may be useful in the future

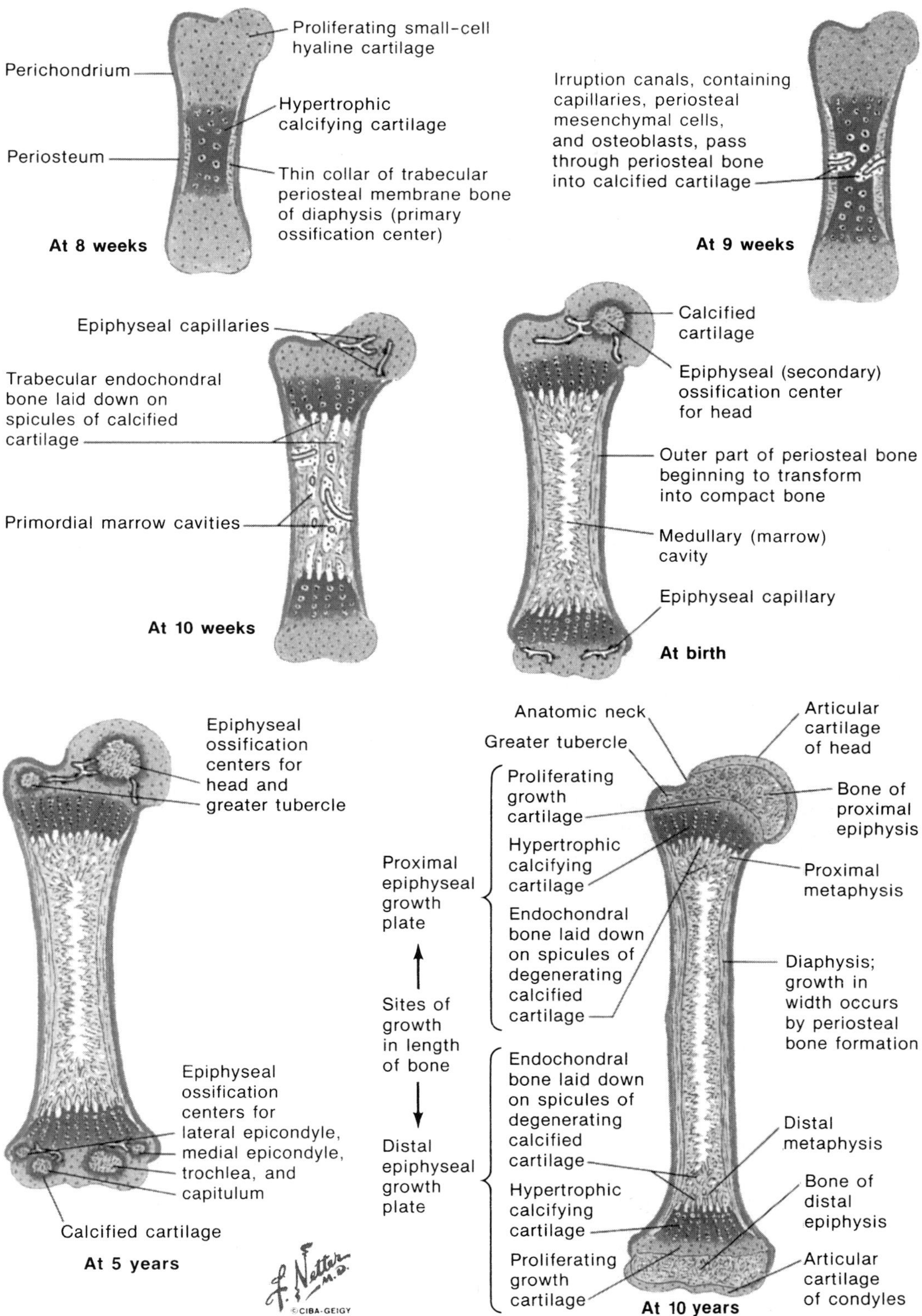

FIGURE 1–12. Development of a typical long bone: formation of the growth plate and secondary centers of ossification. (From The Ciba Collection of Medical Illustrations, vol. 8, part I, p. 136, 1987. Illustrated by Frank H. Netter. Reprinted by permission.)

for pharmacologic treatment of bone diseases related to aberrant circulation (e.g., osteonecrosis, fracture nonunions).

5. Techniques for Studying Bone Circulation (Table 1–2)

F. Tissues Surrounding Bone

1. Periosteum—Connective tissue membrane that covers bone. It is more highly developed in children because of its role in the deposition of cortical bone, which is responsible for growth in bone diameter. The inner, or cambium, layer of periosteum is loose, more vascular, and osteogenic; the outer, fibrous layer is less cellular and is contiguous with joint capsules.
2. Bone Marrow—Source of progenitor cells; controls inner diameter of bone.
   a. Red Marrow—Hematopoietic (40% water, 40% fat, 20% protein). Red marrow slowly changes to yellow marrow with age, beginning in the appendicular skeleton and later the axial skeleton.
   b. Yellow Marrow—Inactive (15% water, 80% fat, 5% protein).

G. Enchondral Bone Formation/Mineralization

1. Cartilage Model (Figs. 1–11, 1–12)—Formed from mesenchymal anlage, usually at 6 weeks. Vascular buds invade this model, bringing in osteoprogenitor cells that differentiate into osteoblasts and form the primary centers of ossification at approximately 8 weeks. The cartilage model grows through appositional (width) and interstitial (length) growth. **Remember: Bone replaces the cartilage model; cartilage is not converted to bone.** The marrow is formed by resorption of the central cancellous bone and invasion of myeloid precursor cells brought in by the capillary buds. Secondary centers of ossification develop at the bone ends, forming epiphyseal centers of ossification (growth plates), which are responsible for longitudinal growth of immature bones. During this developmental stage there is a rich arterial supply composed of an epiphyseal artery (which terminates in the proliferative zone), metaphyseal arteries, nutrient arteries, and perichondrial arteries (Fig. 1–13).

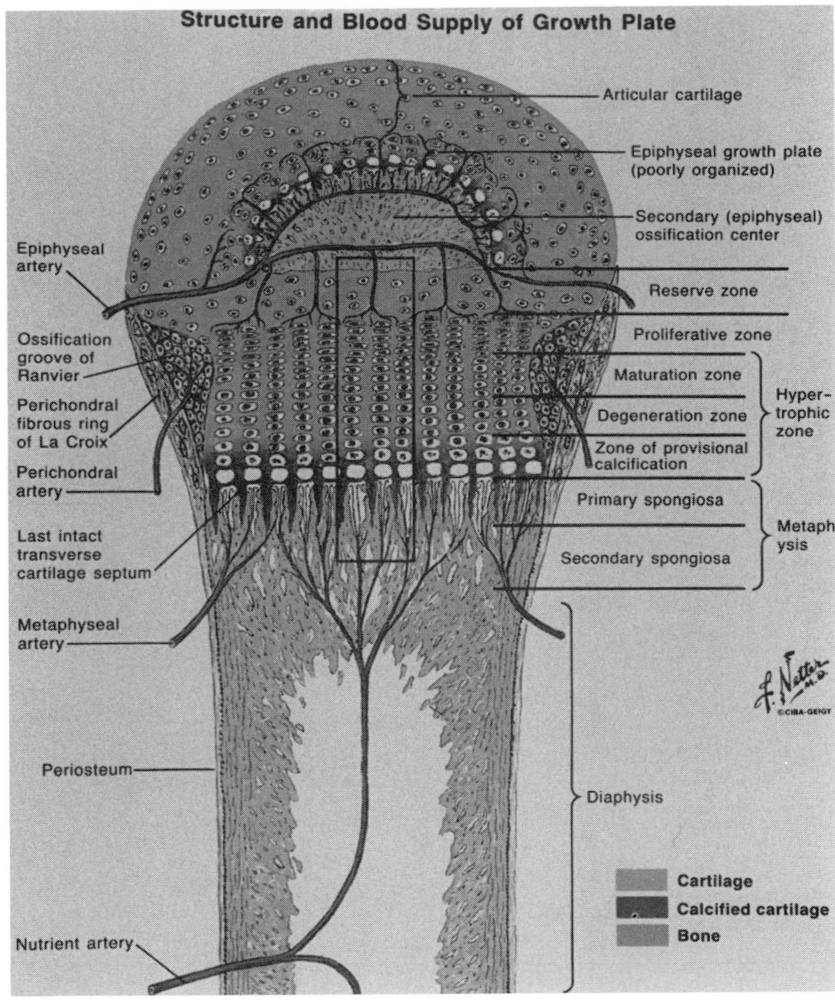

FIGURE 1–13. Structure and blood supply of a typical growth plate. (From The Ciba Collection of Medical Illustrations, vol. 8, part I, p. 166, 1987. Illustrated by Frank H. Netter. Reprinted by permission.)

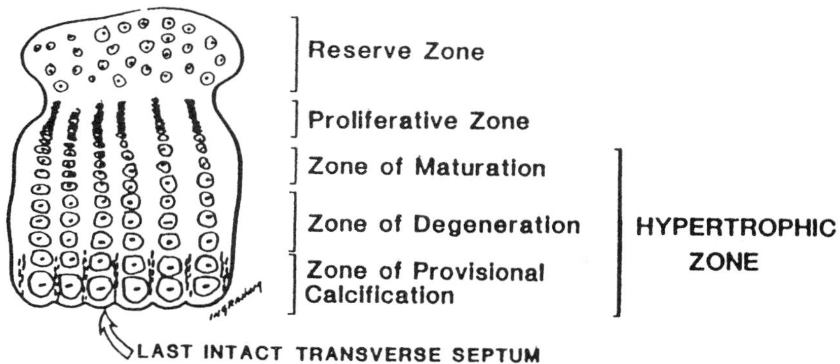

FIGURE 1–14. Physeal layers. (From Orthopaedic Science Syllabus, p. 11. Park Ridge, IL, American Academy of Orthopaedic Surgeons, 1986; reprinted by permission.)

Zones Structures	Histology	Functions	Blood supply	Po_2	Cell (chondrocyte) health	Cell respiration	Cell glycogen
Secondary bony epiphysis	Epiphyseal artery						
Reserve zone		Matrix production Storage	Vessels pass through, do not supply this zone	Poor (lōw)	Good, active. Much endoplasmic reticulum, vacuoles, mitochondria	Anaerobic	High concentration
Proliferative zone		Matrix production Cellular proliferation (longitudinal growth)	Excellent	Excellent Fair	Excellent. Much endoplasmic reticulum, ribosomes, mitochondria. Intact cell membrane	Aerobic Progressive change to anaerobic	High concentration (less than in above)
Hypertrophic zone – **Maturation zone**		Preparation of matrix for calcification	Progressive decrease	Poor (low) Progressive decrease	Still good		Glycogen consumed until depleted
Hypertrophic zone – **Degenerative zone**					Progressive deterioration	Anaerobic glycolysis	
Hypertrophic zone – **Zone of provisional calcification**		Calcification of matrix	Nil	Poor (very low)	Cell death	Anaerobic glycolysis	Nil
Metaphysis – Last intact transverse septum **Primary spongiosa**		Vascular invasion and resorption of transverse septa Bone formation	Closed capillary loops Good	Poor Good		Progressive reversion to aerobic	?
Metaphysis – **Secondary spongiosa** Branches of metaphyseal and nutrient arteries		Remodeling Internal: removal of cartilage bars, replacement of fiber bone with lamellar bone External: funnelization	Excellent	Excellent		Aerobic	?

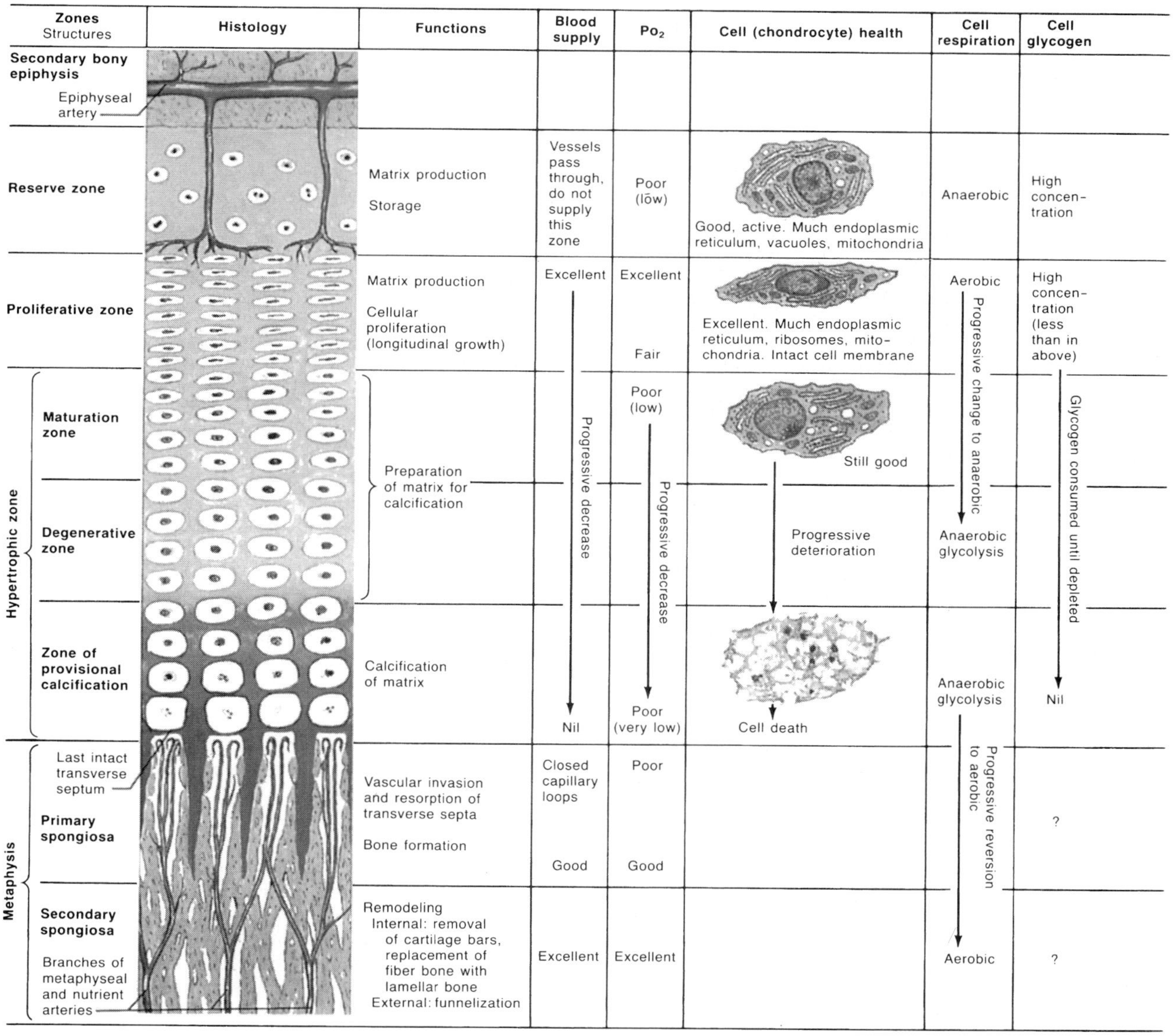

FIGURE 1–15. Zonal structure function, and physiology of the growth plate. (From The Ciba Collection of Medical Illustrations, vol. 8, part I, p. 164, 1987. Illustrated by Frank H. Netter. Reprinted by permission.)

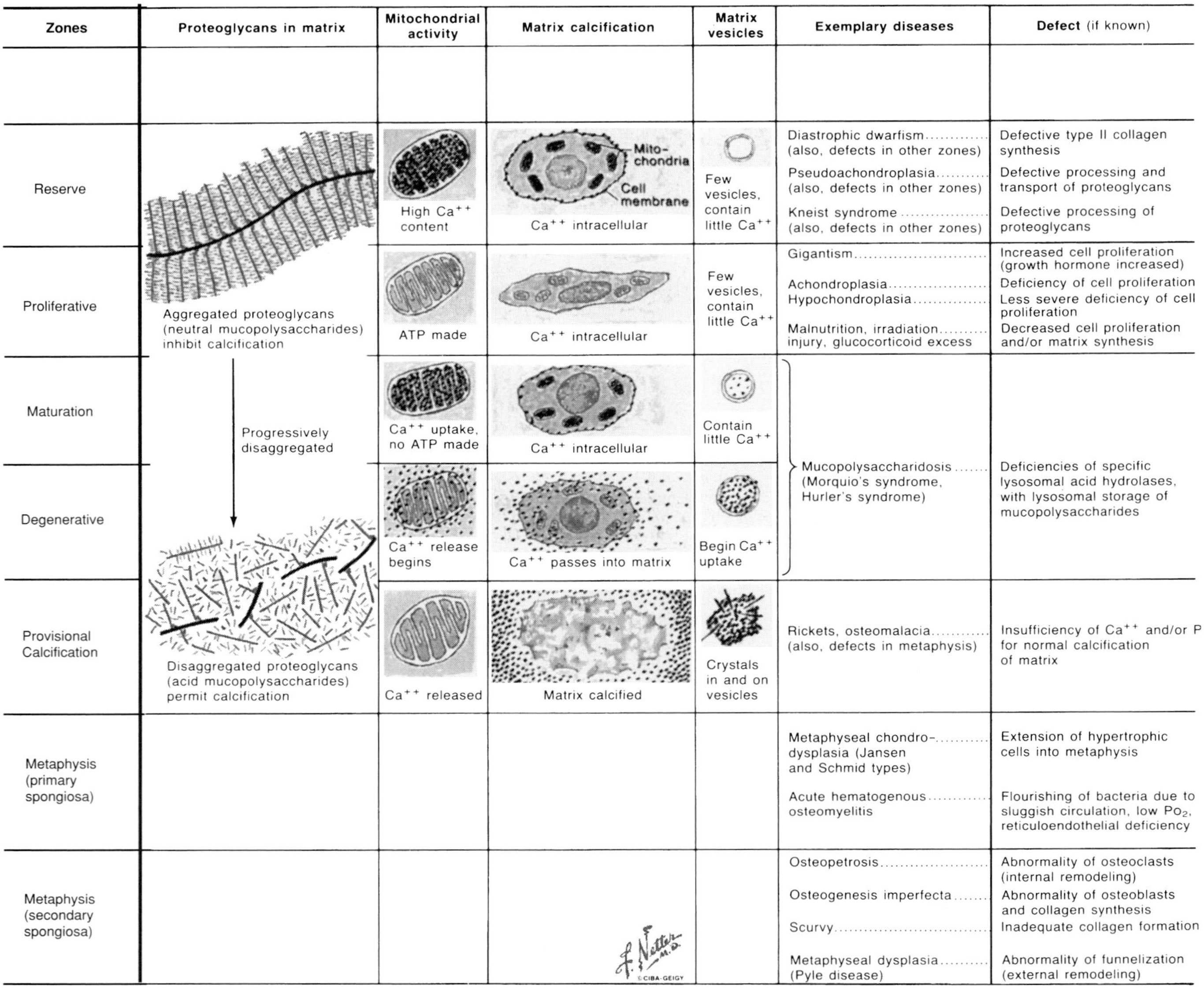

Zones	Proteoglycans in matrix	Mitochondrial activity	Matrix calcification	Matrix vesicles	Exemplary diseases	Defect (if known)
Reserve		High Ca^{++} content	Mito-chondria; Cell membrane; Ca^{++} intracellular	Few vesicles, contain little Ca^{++}	Diastrophic dwarfism (also, defects in other zones) Pseudoachondroplasia (also, defects in other zones) Kneist syndrome (also, defects in other zones)	Defective type II collagen synthesis Defective processing and transport of proteoglycans Defective processing of proteoglycans
Proliferative	Aggregated proteoglycans (neutral mucopolysaccharides) inhibit calcification	ATP made	Ca^{++} intracellular	Few vesicles, contain little Ca^{++}	Gigantism Achondroplasia Hypochondroplasia Malnutrition, irradiation injury, glucocorticoid excess	Increased cell proliferation (growth hormone increased) Deficiency of cell proliferation Less severe deficiency of cell proliferation Decreased cell proliferation and/or matrix synthesis
Maturation	Progressively disaggregated	Ca^{++} uptake, no ATP made	Ca^{++} intracellular	Contain little Ca^{++}	Mucopolysaccharidosis (Morquio's syndrome, Hurler's syndrome)	Deficiencies of specific lysosomal acid hydrolases, with lysosomal storage of mucopolysaccharides
Degenerative		Ca^{++} release begins	Ca^{++} passes into matrix	Begin Ca^{++} uptake		
Provisional Calcification	Disaggregated proteoglycans (acid mucopolysaccharides) permit calcification	Ca^{++} released	Matrix calcified	Crystals in and on vesicles	Rickets, osteomalacia (also, defects in metaphysis)	Insufficiency of Ca^{++} and/or P for normal calcification of matrix
Metaphysis (primary spongiosa)					Metaphyseal chondro-dysplasia (Jansen and Schmid types) Acute hematogenous osteomyelitis	Extension of hypertrophic cells into metaphysis Flourishing of bacteria due to sluggish circulation, low Po_2, reticuloendothelial deficiency
Metaphysis (secondary spongiosa)					Osteopetrosis Osteogenesis imperfecta Scurvy Metaphyseal dysplasia (Pyle disease)	Abnormality of osteoclasts (internal remodeling) Abnormality of osteoblasts and collagen synthesis Inadequate collagen formation Abnormality of funnelization (external remodeling)

F. Netter M.D. ©CIBA-GEIGY

FIGURE 1–16. Zonal structure, function, and intracellular calcium transfer in the growth plate. (Adapted from The Ciba Collection of Medical Illustrations, vol. 8, part I, p. 165, 1987. Illustrated by Frank H. Netter. Reprinted by permission.)

2. Physis—Two growth plates exist in immature long bones: (1) a **horizontal** growth plate (the physis); and (2) a **spherical** growth plate that allows growth of the epiphysis. The spherical growth plate has the same arrangement as the physis but is less organized. Acromegaly and spondyloepiphyseal dysplasia affect physeal growth; multiple epiphyseal dysplasia adversely affects growth of the epiphysis. Physeal cartilage is divided into zones based on growth (Fig. 1–14) and function (Fig. 1–15, 1–16).
   a. Reserve Zone—Cells store lipids, glycogen, and proteoglycan aggregates for later growth. Decreased oxygen tension occurs in this zone. **Lysosomal storage diseases (Gaucher's)** and other diseases can affect this zone, which is involved in matrix production.
   b. Proliferative Zone—Longitudinal growth occurs with stacking of chondrocytes (top cell is the dividing "mother" cell). There is increased oxygen tension; and increased proteoglycan in surrounding matrix which inhibits calcification (Fig. 1–17). This zone functions in cellular proliferation and matrix production. Defects in this zone (chondrocyte proliferation and column formation) are seen in **achondroplasia** (Fig. 1–18) (does not affect intramembranous bone [width]).
   c. Hypertrophic Zone—Sometimes subdivided into three zones: **maturation, degeneration,**

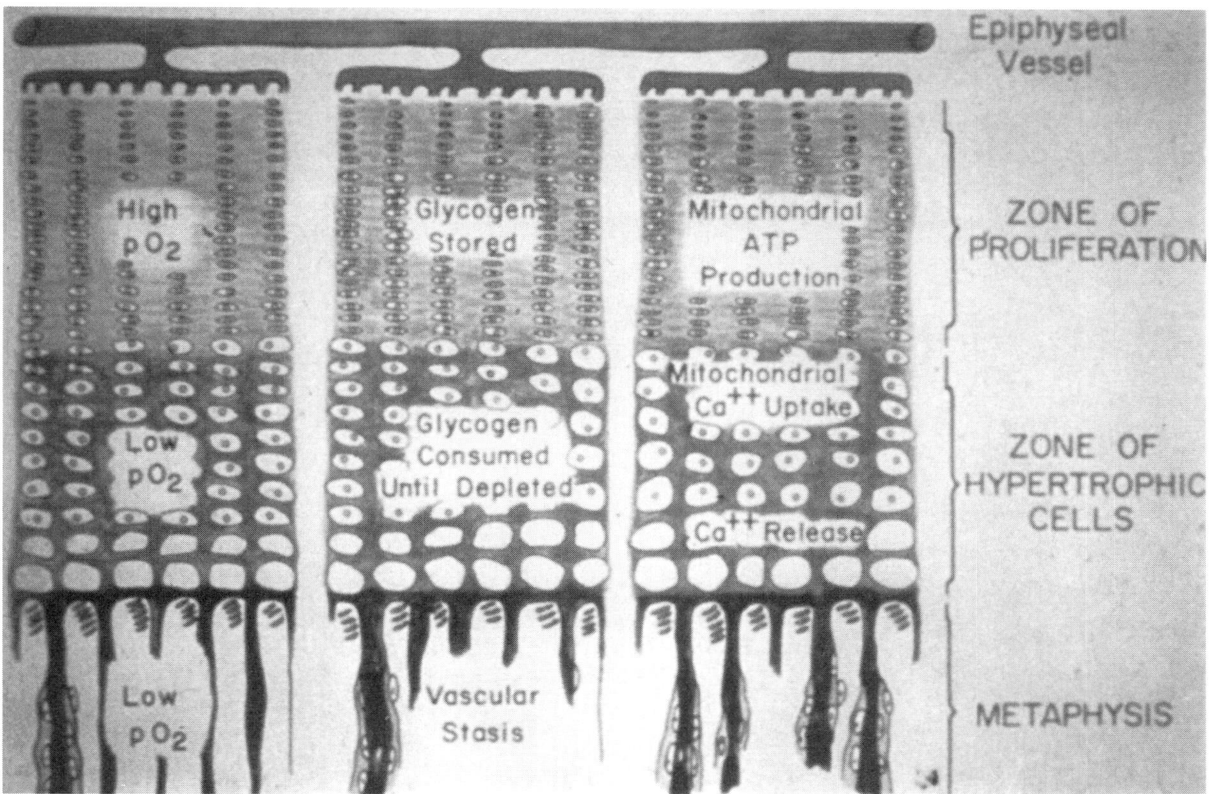

FIGURE 1–17. Metabolic events in the growth plate. (From Simon, S.R., ed.: Orthopaedic Basic Science, 2nd ed., p. 194. Rosemont, IL, American Academy of Orthopaedic Surgeons, 1994; reprinted by permission.)

and **provisional calcification.** In the hypertrophic zone, cells increase five times in size, accumulate calcium in their mitochondria, and then die (releasing calcium from matrix vesicles). Osteoblasts, which migrate from sinusoidal vessels, use cartilage as a scaffolding for bone formation. Low oxygen tension and decreased proteoglycan aggregates aid in this process (Fig. 1–17). **This zone is widened in rickets** (Fig. 1–18), where little or no provisional calcification occurs. **Enchondromas** also originate in this zone. **Mucopolysaccharidic diseases** (Fig. 1–18) also affect the zone, leading to chondrocyte degeneration (swollen, abnormal chondrocytes). **Physeal fractures are classically believed to occur through the zone of provisional calcification** (within the hypertrophic zone), but they probably traverse several zones depending on the type of loading (Fig. 1–19). The hypertrophic zone is also believed to be involved in slipped capital femoral epiphysis.

3. Metaphysis—Adjacent to the physis, the metaphysis expands with skeletal growth. Osteoblasts from osteoprogenitor cells line up on cartilage bars produced by physeal expansion. Primary spongiosa (calcified cartilage bars) is mineralized to form woven bone and is remodeled to form secondary spongiosa and a "cutback zone" at the metaphysis. Cortical bone is made by remodeling of physeal (enchondral) and intramembranous bone in response to stress along the periphery of growing long bones.
4. Periphery of the Physis—Composed of two elements.
   a. Groove of Ranvier—Supplies chondrocytes to the periphery of the growth plate for lateral growth (width).
   b. Perichondrial Ring of LaCroix—Dense fibrous tissue anchors and supports the physis.
5. Mineralization—Consists of seeding of collagen hole zones with calcium hydroxyapatite crystals through branching and accretion (crystal growth).
6. Effect of Hormones and Growth Factors on the Growth Plate—Several hormones and growth factors have both direct and indirect effects on the developing growth plate. Some factors are produced and act within the growth plate (paracrine or autocrine), and others are produced at a site distant from the growth plate (endocrine). The actions of hormones and growth factors are via their effect on chondrocytes and matrix mineralization (summarized in Figure 1–20 and Table 1–3).

H. Intramembranous Ossification—Occurs without a cartilage model during embryonic life, usually in the flat bones (and clavicle). This process also provides for growth in the width of long bones. It is heralded by aggregation of mesenchymal cells into condensed layers or membranes. Cells adjacent to capillaries differentiate into osteoblasts and set up a center of

Zones Structures	Histology	Functions	Exemplary diseases	Defect (if known)
Secondary bony epiphysis Epiphyseal artery	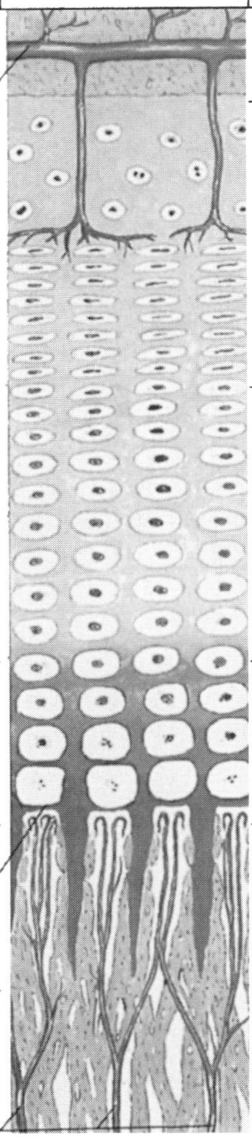			
Reserve zone		Matrix production Storage	Diastrophic dwarfism (also, defects in other zones)	Defective type II collagen synthesis
			Pseudoachondroplasia (also, defects in other zones)	Defective processing and transport of proteoglycans
			Kneist syndrome (also, defects in other zones)	Defective processing of proteoglycans
Proliferative zone		Matrix production Cellular proliferation (longitudinal growth)	Gigantism	Increased cell proliferation (growth hormone increased)
			Achondroplasia	Deficiency of cell proliferation
			Hypochondroplasia	Less severe deficiency of cell proliferation
			Malnutrition, irradiation injury, glucocorticoid excess	Decreased cell proliferation and/or matrix synthesis
Hypertrophic zone: Maturation zone		Preparation of matrix for calcification	Mucopolysaccharidosis (Morquio's syndrome, Hurler's syndrome)	Deficiencies of specific lysosomal acid hydrolases, with lysosomal storage of mucopolysaccharides
Hypertrophic zone: Degenerative zone				
Hypertrophic zone: Zone of provisional calcification		Calcification of matrix	Rickets, osteomalacia (also, defects in metaphysis)	Insufficiency of Ca^{++} and/or P for normal calcification of matrix
Metaphysis: Last intact transverse septum Primary spongiosa		Vascular invasion and resorption of transverse septa Bone formation	Metaphyseal chondrodysplasia (Jansen and Schmid types)	Extension of hypertrophic cells into metaphysis
			Acute hematogenous osteomyelitis	Flourishing of bacteria due to sluggish circulation, low PO_2, reticuloendothelial deficiency
Metaphysis: Secondary spongiosa Branches of metaphyseal and nutrient arteries		Remodeling Internal: removal of cartilage bars, replacement of fiber bone with lamellar bone External: funnelization	Osteopetrosis	Abnormality of osteoclasts (internal remodeling)
			Osteogenesis imperfecta	Abnormality of osteoblasts and collagen synthesis
			Scurvy	Inadequate collagen formation
			Metaphyseal dysplasia (Pyle disease)	Abnormality of funnelization (external remodeling)

FIGURE 1–18. Zonal structure and pathologic defects of cellular metabolism. (Adapted from The Ciba Collection of Medical Illustrations, vol. 8, part I, p. 165, 1987. Illustrated by Frank H. Netter. Reprinted by permission.)

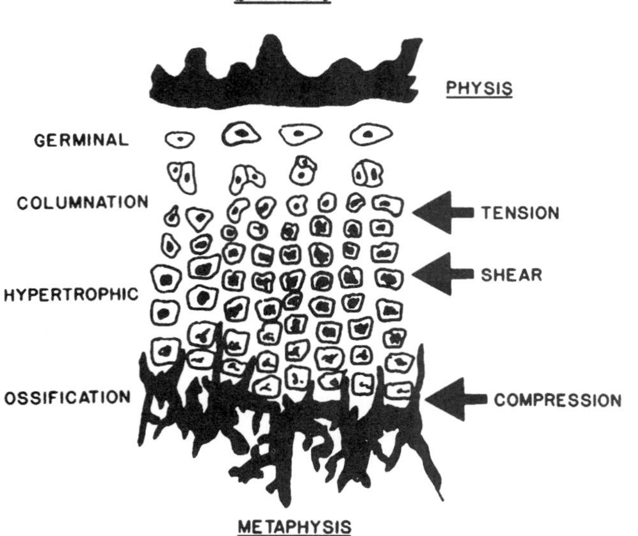

ossification, which expands by appositional growth. Blastema bone is membranous bone formation (appositional bone growth) that occurs in young children with amputations/resections (*).

FIGURE 1–19. Histologic zone of failure varies with the type of loading applied to a specimen. (From Moen, C.T., and Pelker, R.R.: Biomechanical and histological correlations in growth plate failure. J Pediatr Orthop 4:180–184, 1984; reprinted by permission.)

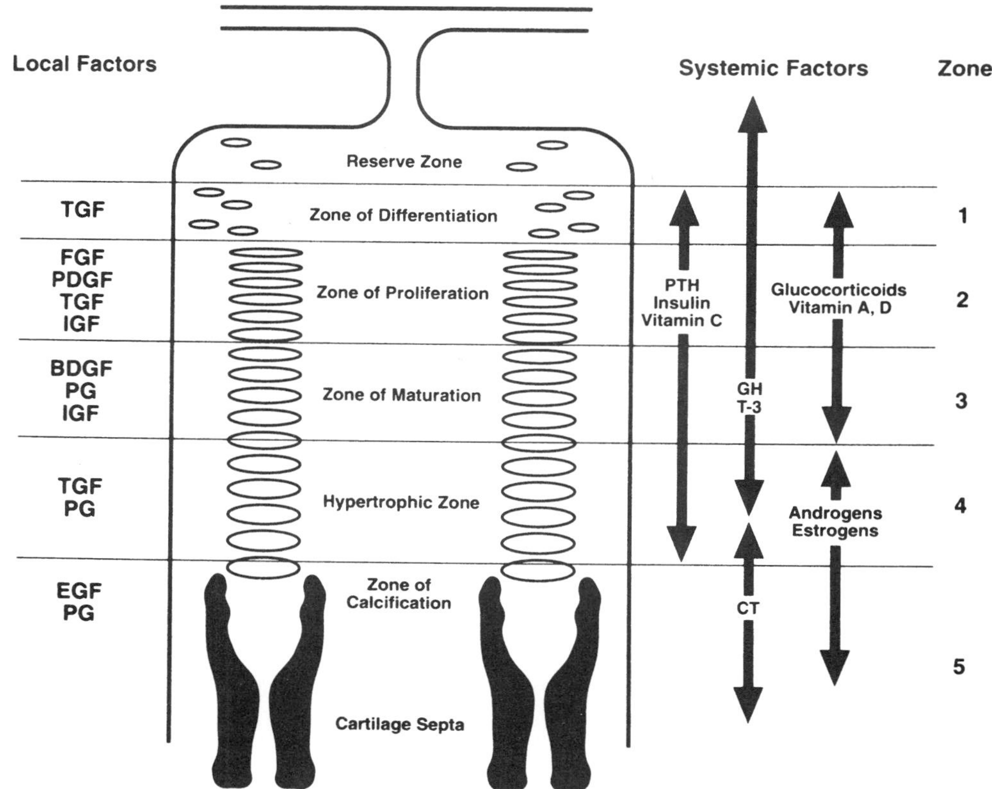

FIGURE 1–20. Growth plate, demonstrating the proposed sites of action of hormones, growth factors, and vitamins. (From Simon, S.R., ed.: Orthopaedic Basic Science, 2nd ed., p. 197. Rosemont, IL, American Academy of Orthopaedic Surgeons, 1994; reprinted by permission.)

TABLE 1–3. EFFECTS OF HORMONES AND GROWTH FACTORS ON THE GROWTH PLATE

HORMONE/ FACTOR	SYSTEMIC/ LOCAL DERIVATION	BIOLOGIC EFFECT: PROLIFERATION	MACROMOLECULE BIOSYNTHESIS	MATURATION DEGRADATION	MATRIX CALCIFICATION	ZONE PRIMARILY AFFECTED
Thyroxine	Systemic (thyroid)	+ (T_3 with IGF-I)	0	+ (T_3 alone)	0	Proliferative zone and upper hypertrophic zone
Parathyroid	Systemic (parathyroid)	+	+ + (Proteoglycan)	0	0	Entire growth plate
Calcitonin	Systemic (thyroid)	0	0	+	+	Hypertrophic zone and metaphysis
Excess corticosteroids	Systemic (adrenals)	–	–	–	0	Entire growth plate
Growth hormone	Systemic (pituitary)	+ (through IGF-I locally)	+ (Slight)	0	0	Proliferative zone
Somatomedins	Systemic Local paracrine (liver, chondrocytes)	+	+ (Slight)	0	0	Proliferative zone
Insulin	Systemic (pancreas)	+ (through IGF-1 receptor)	0	0	0	Proliferative zone
1,25-$(OH)_2D_3$	Systemic (liver, kidney)	0	0	+ (Indirect effect serum [Ca] × [PO])		Hypertrophic zone
24,25-$(OH)_2D_3$	Systemic (liver, kidney)	+	+ (Collagen II)	0	0	Proliferative zone and hypertrophic zone
Vitamin A	Systemic (diet)	0	0	–	0	Hypertrophic zone
Vitamin C	Systemic (diet)	0	+ (Collagen)	0	+ (Matrix vesicles)	Proliferative zone and hypertrophic zone

Table continued on following page

TABLE 1–3. *Continued*

HORMONE/ FACTOR	SYSTEMIC/ LOCAL DERIVATION	Biologic Effect: PROLIFER-TION	MACRO-MOLECULE BIO-SYNTHESIS	MATURATION DEGRADATION	MATRIX CALCIFICATION	ZONE PRIMARILY AFFECTED
EGF	Local paracrine (endothelial cells)	+	− (Collagen)	0	0	Metaphysis
FGF	Local paracrine (endothelial cells)	+	0	0	0	Proliferative zone
PDGF	Local paracrine (platelets)	+	+ (Noncollagenous proteins)	0	0	Proliferative zone
TGF-β	Local paracrine (platelets, chondrocytes)	±	±	0	0	Proliferative zone and hypertrophic zone
BDGF	Local paracrine (bone matrix)	0	+ (Collagen)	0	0	Upper hypertrophic zone
IL-1	Local paracrine (inflammatory cells, synoviocytes)	0	−	+ + Activates tissue metalloproteinases	0	Entire growth plate
Prostaglandin	Local autocrine	±	+ (Proteoglycan) − (Collagen and alkaline phosphatase)	0	Bone resorption with osteoclasts	Hypertrophic zone and metaphysis

From Simon, S.R.: Orthopaedic Basic Science, 2nd ed., p. 196. Rosemont, IL, American Academy of Orthopaedic Surgeons, 1994; reprinted by permission.
+, increase stimulation; 0, no known effect; −, inhibitory; ±, depending on the local hormonal milieu.
EGF, epidermal growth factor; FGF, fibroblast growth factor; PDGF, platelet-derived growth factor; TGF-β, transforming growth factor-beta; BDGF, bone-derived growth factor; IL-1, interleukin-1, IGF-I, Insulin-like growth factor I.

TEST QUESTIONS ON HISTOLOGY OF BONE

TEST	QUESTION NUMBERS
1995 OSAE—Adult Reconstruction Hip/Knee	
1995 OSAE—Pediatric Orthopaedics	
1995 OSAE—Sports Medicine	
1994 OITE	
1994 OSAE—Adult Spine	
1994 OSAE—Foot and Ankle	
1994 OSAE—M/S Trauma	99
1993 OITE	
1993 OSAE—M/S Tumors and Diseases	
1993 OSAE—Shoulder and Elbow	
1992 OITE	85, 138, 139, 183
1992 OSAE—Adult Reconstruction Hip/Knee	
1992 OSAE—Pediatric Orthopaedics	55
1992 OSAE—Sports Medicine	
1991 OITE	22
1991 OSAE—Adult Spine	
1991 OSAE—Anatomy and Imaging	
1991 OSAE—Foot and Ankle	
1991 OSAE—M/S Trauma	24, 96

TABLE 1–4. FACTORS INFLUENCING FRACTURE HEALING

SYSTEMIC FACTORS	LOCAL FACTORS
Age	Degree of local trauma
Hormones	Vascular injury
Functional activity	Type of bone affected
Nerve functions	Degree of bone loss
Nutrition	Degree of immobilization
	Infection
	Local pathologic conditions

Adapted from Simon, S.R.: Orthopaedic Basic Science, 2nd ed., p. 311. Rosemont, IL, American Academy of Orthopaedic Surgeons, 1994, reprinted by permission.

II. Bone Injury and Repair

A. General Principles—The response of bone to injury can be thought of as a continuum of processes, beginning with **inflammation,** proceeding through **repair** (soft callus followed by hard callus), and finally ending in **remodeling.** Fracture healing may be influenced by a variety of systemic and local factors (Table 1–4).

1. Inflammation—Bleeding from the fracture site and surrounding soft tissues creates a hematoma (and fibrin clot), which provides a source of hematopoietic cells capable of secreting growth factors (*). Subsequently fibroblasts, mesenchymal cells, and osteoprogenitor cells are present at the fracture site; and granulation tissue forms around the fracture ends. Osteoblasts, from surrounding osteogenic precursor cells, fibroblasts, or both proliferate. **Endosteal bone erosion (osteolysis;** aggressive granulomatous lesions) surrounding an uninfected femoral stem after total hip arthroplasty (THA) is associated with **monocytes–macrophages** (*).
2. Repair—Primary callus response occurs within 2 weeks. If the bone ends are not in continuity, **bridging (soft) callus** occurs (enchondral ossification). Another type of callus, **medullary (hard) callus,** supplements the bridging callus, although it forms more slowly and occurs later (Fig. 1–21). The amount of callus formation is indirectly proportional to the amount of immobilization of the fracture. Primary cortical healing, which resembles normal remodeling, occurs with rigid immobilization and anatomic (or near-anatomic) reduction. Fracture healing varies with the method of treatment. With closed treatment, "enchondral healing" with periosteal bridging callus occurs. With rigidly fixed fractures, direct osteonal or primary bone healing occurs without visible callus. The initial histologic change observed in hypertrophic nonunions treated with plate stabilization is fibrocartilage mineralization (*).
3. Remodeling—This process begins during the middle of the repair phase and continues long after the fracture has clinically healed (up to 7 years). Remodeling allows the bone to assume its normal configuration and shape based on the stresses to which it is exposed (Wolff's law). Throughout the process, woven bone formed during the repair phase is replaced with lamellar bone. Fracture healing is complete when there is repopulation of the marrow space.

B. Biochemistry of Fracture Healing—Four biochemical steps of fracture healing have been described (Table 1–5).

TABLE 1–5. BIOCHEMICAL STEPS OF FRACTURE HEALING

STEP	COLLAGEN TYPE
Mesenchymal	I, II, (III, V)
Chondroid	II, IX
Chondroid-osteoid	I, II, X
Osteogenic	I

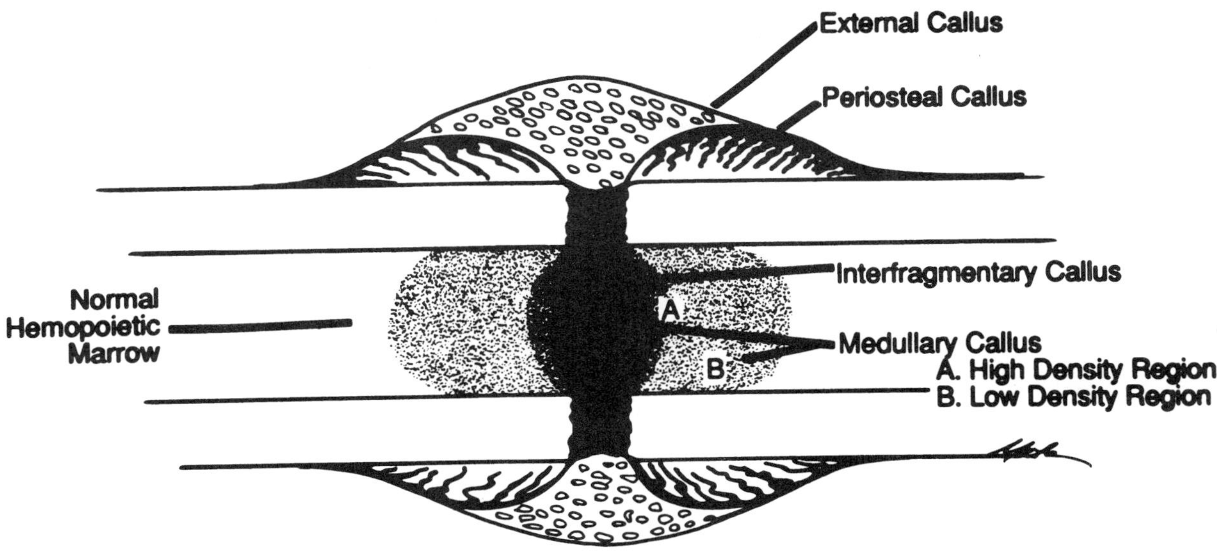

FIGURE 1–21. Histology of typical fracture healing. (From Brighton, C.T., and Hunt, R.M.: Early histological and ultrastructural changes in medullary fracture callus. J. Bone Joint Surg. [Am.] 73:832–847, 1991; reprinted by permission.)

TABLE 1–6. ENDOCRINE EFFECTS ON FRACTURE HEALING

HORMONE	EFFECT	MECHANISM
Cortisone	−	Decreased callus proliferation
Calcitonin	+?	Unknown
TH/PTH	+	Bone remodeling
Growth hormone	+	Increased callus volume

TH/PTH, thyroid hormone/parathyroid hormone.

C. Growth Factors of Bone
   1. Bone Morphogenic Protein (BMP)—Osteoinductive; induces metaplasia of mesenchymal cells into osteoblasts. **The target cell for BMP is the undifferentiated perivascular mesenchymal cell** (*).
   2. Transforming Growth Factor-Beta (TGF-β)—Induces mesenchymal cells to produce type II collagen and proteoglycans. Also induces osteoblasts to synthesize collagen. TGF-β is found in fracture hematomas and is believed to **regulate cartilage and bone formation in fracture callus.**
   3. Insulin-Like Growth Factor II (IGF-II)—Stimulates type I collagen, cellular proliferation, and cartilage matrix synthesis.
   4. Platelet-Derived Growth Factor (PDGF)—Released from platelets; attracts inflammatory cells to the fracture site (chemotactic).

D. Hormonal Effects on Fracture Healing (Table 1–6)

E. Electricity and Fracture Healing
   1. Definitions
      a. Stress-Generated Potentials—Serve as signals that modulate cellular activity. Piezoelectric effect and streaming potentials are examples of stress-generated potentials.
      b. Piezoelectric Effect—Charges in tissues are displaced secondary to mechanical forces.
      c. Streaming Potentials—Occur when electrically charged fluid is forced over a tissue (cell membrane) with a fixed charge.
      d. Transmembrane Potentials—Generated by cellular metabolism.
   2. Fracture Healing—Electrical properties of cartilage and bone are dependent on their charged molecules. Devices intended to stimulate fracture repair by altering a variety of cellular activities have been introduced.
   3. Types of Electrical Stimulation
      a. Direct Current (DC)—Stimulates an inflammatory-like response (stage I).
      b. Alternating Current (AC)—"Capacity coupled generators." Affects cyclic AMP, collagen synthesis, and calcification during the repair stage.
      c. Pulsed Electromagnetic Fields (PEMF)—Initiate calcification of fibrocartilage (cannot induce calcification of fibrous tissue).

F. Bone Grafting—Allows a template (osteoconduction) for host osteoblasts and osteoclasts to function and may influence its own incorporation (osteoinduction). Commonly, autografts (from same person) or allografts (from another person) are used. Cancellous bone is commonly used for grafting nonunions or cavitary defects because it is quickly remodeled and incorporated (via creeping substitution). Cortical bone is slower to turn over than cancellous bone and is used for structural defects. Osteoarticular (osteochondral) allografts are being used with increasing frequency for tumor surgery. These grafts are immunogenic (cartilage is vulnerable to inflammatory mediators of immune response [cytotoxic injury from antibodies and lymphocytes]); cryogenically preserved grafts leave few viable chondrocytes. Tissue-matched fresh osteochondral grafts produce minimal immunogenic effect and incorporate well (*). Vascularized bone grafts, though technically difficult, allow more rapid union with preservation of most cells. Vascularized grafts are best employed for irradiated tissues or when large tissue defects exist. (However, there may be donor site morbidity with the vascularized grafts [i.e., fibula]). Nonvascular

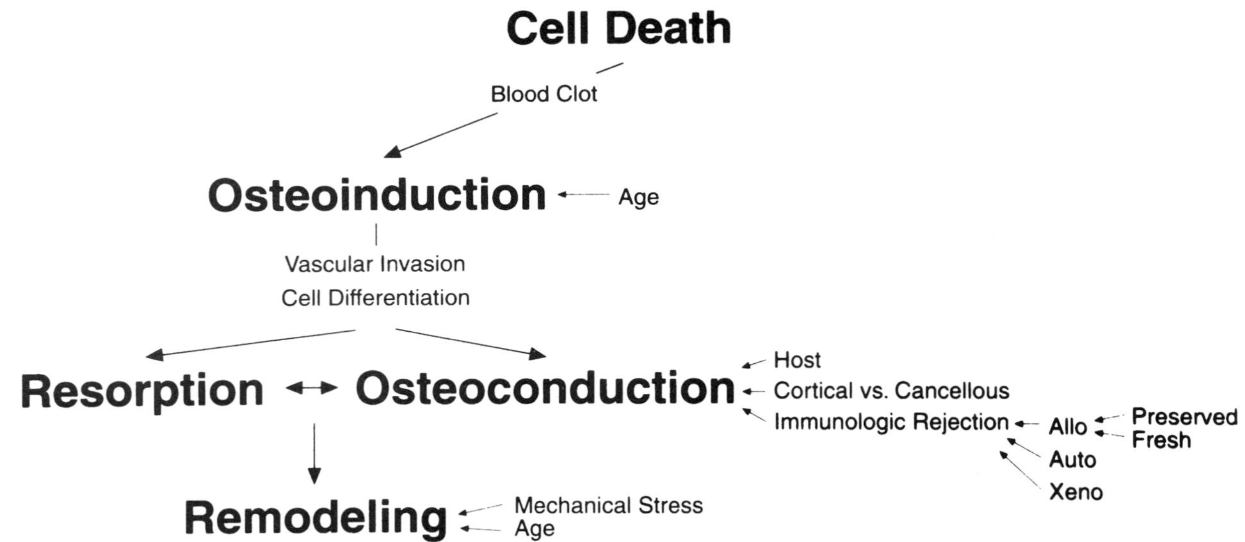

FIGURE 1–22. Major factors influencing bone graft incorporation. (From Simon, S.R., ed.: Orthopaedic Basic Science, 2nd ed., p. 284. Rosemont, IL, American Academy of Orthopaedic Surgeons, 1994; reprinted by permission.)

TABLE 1–7. STAGES OF GRAFT HEALING

STAGE	ACTIVITY
1—Inflammation	Chemotaxis stimulated by necrotic debris
2—Osteoblast differentiation	From precursors
3—Osteoinduction	Osteoblast and osteoclasts function
4—Osteoconduction	New bone forming over scaffold
5—Remodeling	Process continues for years

bone grafts are used more commonly than vascularized grafts. Bone grafts can be (1) fresh (increased antigenicity); (2) fresh frozen—less immunogenic than fresh (*), preserves bone morphogenic protein (BMP), a 17,500 dalton (molecular weight) protein that promotes osteoinduction and preserves articular cartilage (40–50% of chondrocytes) with glycerol or dimethylsulfoxide (DMSO) preservation; (3) freeze-dried (lyophilized)—loses structural integrity and depletes BMP, **least immunogenic** (*), commonly known as "croutons"; and (4) in bone matrix gelatin (BMG digested source of BMP). Five stages of graft healing have been recognized (Urist) (Table 1–7).

1. Cortical Bone Grafts—Incorporate through slow remodeling of existing haversian systems via a process of resorption (which weakens the graft) followed by deposition of the new bone (restoring its strength). Resorption is confined to the osteon borders, and interstitial lamellae are preserved.
2. Cancellous Grafts—Revascularized more quickly; osteoblasts lay down new bone on old trabeculae, which are later remodeled ("creeping substitution"). All allografts must be harvested with sterile technique, and donors must be screened for potential transmissible diseases. The major factors influencing bone graft incorporation are shown in Figure 1–22.
3. Synthetic Bone Grafts—Composed of calcium, silicon, or aluminum.
   a. Silicate-Based Grafts—Incorporate the element silicon (Si) in the form of silicate (silicon dioxide).
      1. Bioactive Glasses
      2. Glass–Ionomer Cement
   b. Calcium Phosphate-Based Grafts—Capable of osseoconduction and osseointegration. Many are prepared as ceramics (apatite crystals are heated to fuse the crystals [sintered]).
      1. Tricalcium Phosphate
      2. Hydroxyapatite (example: Collagraft Bone Graft Matrix [Zimmer, Inc., Warsaw, IN]; purified bovine dermal fibrillar collagen plus ceramic hydroxyapatite granules and β-tricalcium phosphate granules).
   c. Calcium Sulfate—Plaster of Paris.
   d. Calcium Carbonate (chemically unaltered marine coral)—Is resorbed and replaced by bone (osteoconductive). (example: Biocora; Inoteb, France.)
   e. Corralline Hydroxyapatite—Calcium carbonate skeleton is converted to calcium phosphate via a thermoexchange process. (example: Interpore 200 and 500; Interpore Orthopaedics, Irvine, CA.)
   f. Other Materials
      1. Aluminum Oxide—Alumina ceramic bonds to bone in response to stress and strain between implant and bone.
      2. Hard Tissue—Replacement polymer.

TEST QUESTIONS ON BONE INJURY AND REPAIR

TEST	QUESTION NUMBERS
1995 OSAE—Adult Reconstruction Hip/Knee	30
1995 OSAE—Pediatric Orthopaedics	
1995 OSAE—Sports Medicine	
1994 OITE	
1994 OSAE—Adult Spine	
1994 OSAE—Foot and Ankle	
1994 OSAE—M/S Trauma	
1993 OITE	125, 146
1993 OSAE—M/S Tumors and Diseases	14
1993 OSAE—Shoulder and Elbow	
1992 OITE	88
1992 OSAE—Adult Reconstruction Hip/Knee	44
1992 OSAE—Pediatric Orthopaedics	
1992 OSAE—Sports Medicine	
1991 OITE	23, 105
1991 OSAE—Adult Spine	
1991 OSAE—Anatomy and Imaging	
1991 OSAE—Foot and Ankle	
1991 OSAE—M/S Trauma	

III. Conditions of Bone Mineralization, Bone Mineral Density, and Bone Viability

A. Normal Bone Metabolism

1. Calcium—Bone serves as a reservoir for more than 99% of the body's calcium. Calcium is also important in muscle and nerve function, the clotting mechanism, and many other areas. Plasma calcium (less than 1% of total body calcium) is about equally free and bound (usually to albumin). It is absorbed from the gut (duodenum) by active transport (ATP and calcium-binding protein required), which is regulated by 1,25-$(OH)_2$-vitamin D_3 and by passive diffusion (jejunum). It is 98% reabsorbed by the kidney (60% in the proximal tubule). The dietary requirement of **elemental calcium** is approximately 600 mg/day for children, increasing to about 1300 mg/day for adolescents and young adults (growth spurt [age 10–25 years]). The requirement for adult men and women (age 25–65 years) is 750 mg/day. Pregnant women require 1500 mg/day, and **lactating women require 2000 mg/day.** Postmenopausal women and patients with a healing long bone fracture require 1500 mg/day. Most people have a positive calcium balance during their first three decades of life and a negative balance after the fourth decade. About 400 mg of calcium is released from bone on a daily basis. Calcium may be excreted in stool. **Hypercalcemia** can lead to **hyperreflexia** and **convulsions. Hypocalcemia** leads to **somnolence** and **areflexia.**
2. Phosphate—In addition to being a key component of bone mineral, phosphate has an important role in enzyme systems and molecular interactions (metabolite and buffer). Approximately 85% of the body's phosphate stores are in bone. Plasma phosphate is mostly in the unbound form and is reabsorbed by the kidney (in the proximal tubule). Dietary intake of phosphate is usually adequate; the daily requirement is 1000–1500 mg/day. Phosphate may be excreted in urine.
3. Parathyroid Hormone (PTH)—An 84-amino-acid peptide synthesized in and secreted from the chief cells of the (four) parathyroid glands. PTH helps regulate plasma calcium. It probably acts via a β_2-receptor in the parathyroid gland. PTH directly activates osteoblasts and modulates renal phosphate filtration (*). Decreased calcium levels in the extracellular fluid stimulate release of PTH, which acts at the intestine, kidney, and bone (Table 1–8). PTH may also have a role in bone loss in the elderly.
4. Vitamin D_3—Naturally occurring steroid that is activated by UV irradiation from sunlight or utilized from dietary intake (vitamin D_2) (Fig. 1–23). It is hydroxylated to the 25-(OH)-vitamin D_3 form in the liver and is hydroxylated a second time in the kidney. Conversion to the 1,25-$(OH)_2$-vitamin D_3 form activates the hormone, whereas conversion to the 24,25-$(OH)_2$-vitamin D_3 form inactivates it (Fig. 1–24). The active form works at the intestine, kidney, and bone (Table 1–8). Phenytoin (Dilantin) causes impaired metabolism of vitamin D (*).
5. Calcitonin—A 32-amino-acid peptide hormone made by clear cells in parafollicles of the thyroid

TABLE 1–8. REGULATION OF CALCIUM AND PHOSPHATE METABOLISM

PARAMETER	PARATHYROID HORMONE (PTH) (PEPTIDE)	1,25-$(OH)_2$D (STEROID)	CALCITONIN (PEPTIDE)
Origin	Chief cells of parathyroid glands	Proximal tubule of kidney	Parafollicular cells of thyroid gland
Factors stimulating production	Decreased serum Ca^{2+}	Elevated PTH Decreased serum Ca^{2+} Decreased serum P_i	Elevated serum Ca^{2+}
Factors inhibiting production	Elevated serum Ca^{2+} Elevated 1,25$(OH)_2$D	Decreased PTH Elevated serum Ca^{2+} Elevated serum P_i	Decreased serum Ca^{2+}
Effect on end-organs for hormone action			
Intestine	No direct effect Acts indirectly on bowel by stimulating production of 1,25-$(OH)_2$D in kidney	Strongly stimulates intestinal absorption of Ca^{2+} and P_i	?
Kidney	Stimulates 25-(OH)D-1α-OH_{ase} in mitochondria of proximal tubular cells to convert 25-(OH)D to 1,25-$(OH)_2$D Increases fractional resorption of filtered Ca^{2+} Promotes urinary excretion of P_i	?	?
Bone	Stimulates osteoclastic resorption of bone Stimulates recruitment of preosteoclasts	Strongly stimulates osteoclastic resorption of bone	Inhibits osteoclastic resorption of bone ? Role in normal human physiology
Net effect on Ca^{2+} and P_i concentrations in extracellular fluid and serum	Increased serum Ca^{2+} Decreased serum P_i	Increased serum Ca^{2+} Increased serum P_i	Decreased serum Ca^{2+} (transient)

Adapted from an original figure by Frank H. Netter. From *The Ciba Collection of Medical Illustrations,* vol. 8, part I, p. 179. Copyright by Ciba-Geigy Corporation; reprinted by permission.
1,25-$(OH)_2$D, 1,25-dihydroxyvitamin D; PTH, parathyroid hormone; 25-(OH)D, 25-hydroxyvitamin D.

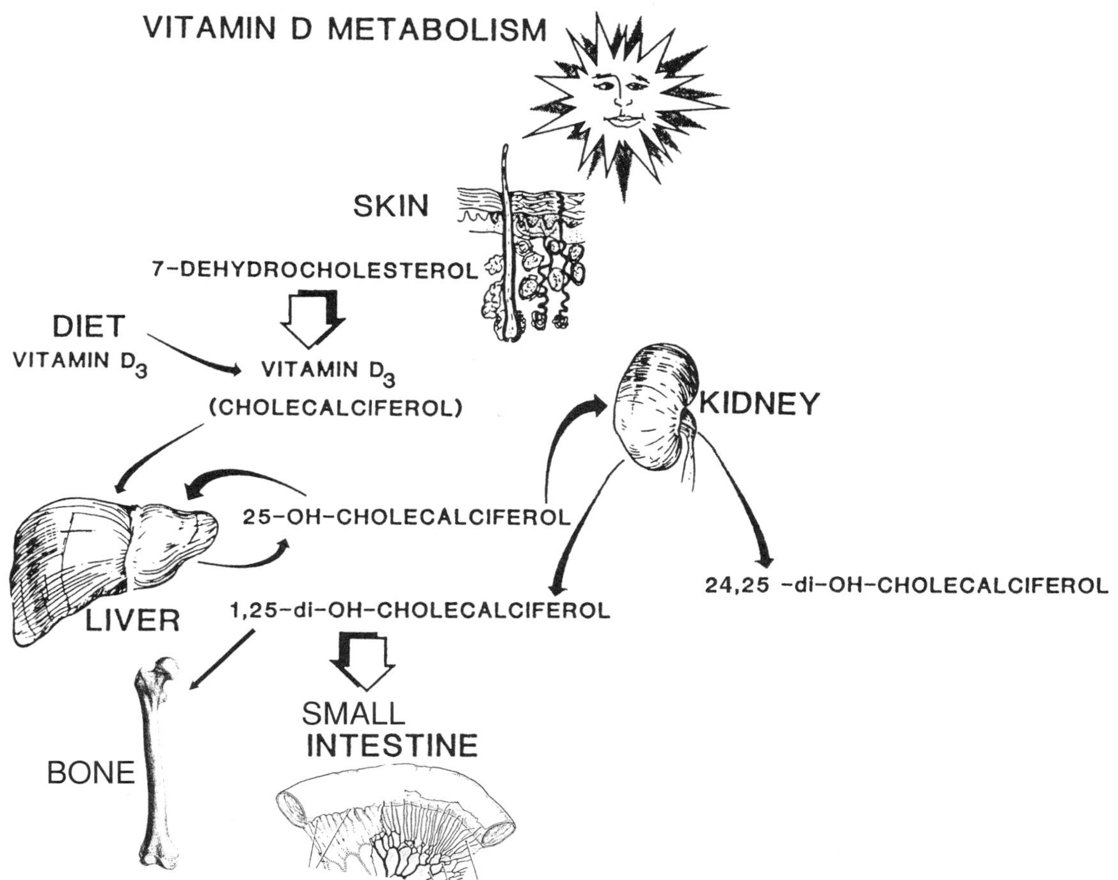

FIGURE 1–23. Vitamin D metabolism. (Modified from Orthopaedic Science Syllabus, p. 11. Park Ridge, IL, American Academy of Orthopaedic Surgeons, 1986; reprinted by permission.)

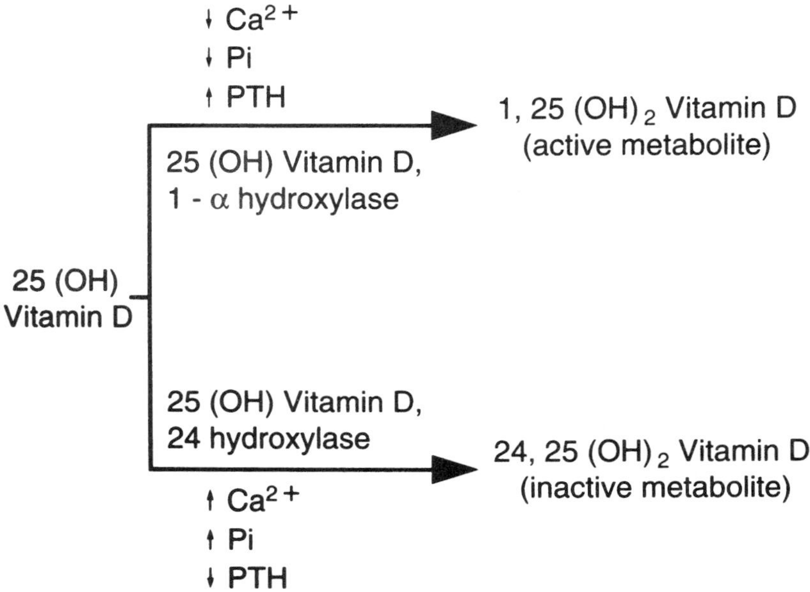

FIGURE 1–24. Vitamin D metabolism in the renal tubular cell. (From Simon, S.R., ed.: Orthopaedic Basic Science, 2nd ed., p. 165. Rosemont, IL, American Academy of Orthopaedic Surgeons, 1994; reprinted by permission.)

gland; this hormone also has a limited role in calcium regulation. Increased calcium levels in the extracellular milieu cause secretion of calcitonin. Like PTH, calcitonin secretion is controlled by a β_2 receptor. Its role (still not fully known) is to decrease plasma calcium by working at the intestine, kidney, and bone (Table 1–8). Calcitonin may also have a physiologic role in fracture healing and treatment of osteoporosis.

6. Other Hormones—The following hormones also have an effect on bone metabolism.
   a. Estrogen—**Prevents bone loss** by inhibiting resorption (may be related to calcitonin). Supplementation is helpful in postmenopausal women but only if it is started within the first 5–10 years after the onset of menopause. The risk of endometrial cancer for patients taking estrogen is reduced when it is combined with cyclic progestin therapy.
   b. Corticosteroids—**Increase bone loss** (decrease gut absorption by decreasing binding proteins and decrease bone formation [cancellous bone more affected than cortical bone] through inhibition of collagen synthesis). Adverse effects may be reduced with alternate-day therapy.
   c. Thyroid Hormones—Affect bone resorption more than bone formation, **leading to osteoporosis** (large [thyroid-suppressive] doses of thyroxine can lead to osteoporosis).
   d. Growth Hormone—**Causes a positive calcium balance** by increasing gut absorption more than its increase in urinary excretion. Insulin and somatomedins participate in this effect.
   e. Growth Factors—TGF-β, PDGF, and mono/lymphokines have a role in bone and cartilage repair (discussed elsewhere within this chapter).
7. Interaction—Calcium and phosphate metabolism is affected by an elaborate interplay of hormones and even the levels of the metabolites themselves. Feedback mechanisms play an important role in the regulation of plasma levels of calcium and phosphate. It is now believed that peak bone mass usually occurs between 16 and 25 years of age and is greater in men and African-Americans. After this peak, bone loss occurs at a rate of 0.3–0.5% per year (2–3% per year for untreated women during the sixth through tenth years after menopause).

B. Conditions of Bone Mineralization (Tables 1–9, 1–10)
   1. Hypercalcemia—Can present as polyuria, constipation, lethargy, and disorientation. Hyperreflexia, kidney stones, excessive bony resorption ± fibrotic tissue replacement (osteitis fibrosa cystica), weakness, and CNS and GI effects are also common.
      a. Primary Hyperparathyroidism—Caused by overproduction of PTH, usually as a result of a parathyroid adenoma (which generally affects only one parathyroid gland). Excessive PTH causes a net **increase in plasma calcium** (from all three sources) and a **decrease in plasma phosphate** (due to enhanced urinary excretion). It results in **increased osteoclastic resorption** and failure of repair attempts (poor mineralization due to low phosphate). Diagnosis is based on signs and symptoms of hypercalcemia (described above), and characteristic laboratory results (increased serum calcium, PTH, urinary phosphate; decreased serum phosphate). Bony changes include osteopenia, osteitis fibrosa cystica (fibrous replacement of marrow), "**brown tumors**" (increased giant

TABLE 1–9. OVERVIEW OF CLINICAL AND RADIOGRAPHIC ASPECTS OF METABOLIC BONE DISEASES

DISEASE	ETIOLOGY	CLINICAL FINDINGS	RADIOGRAPHIC FINDINGS
HYPERCALCEMIA			
Hyperparathyroidism	PTH overproduction—adenoma	Kidney stone, hyperreflexia	Osteopenia, osteitis fibrosa cystica
Familial syndromes	PTH overproduction—MEN/renal	Endocrine/renal abnormalities	Osteopenia
HYPOCALCEMIA			
Hypoparathyroidism	PTH underproduction—idiopathic	Neuromuscular irritability, eye	Calcified basal ganglia
PHP/Albright	PTH receptor abnormality	Short MC/MT, obesity	Brachydactyly, exostosis
Renal osteodystrophy	CRF—↓ phosphate excretion	Renal abnormalities	"Rugger jersey" spine
Rickets (osteomalacia)			
Vit. D—deficient	↓ Vit. D diet; malabsorption	Bone deformities, hypotonia	"Rachitic rosary," wide growth plates, fxs
Vit. D—dependent	Def. 1-Hydroxylation in kidney	Total baldness	Poor mineralization
Vit. D—resistant (hypophosphatemic)	↓ Renal tubular phosphate resorption	Bone deformities, hypotonia	Poor mineralization
Hypophosphatasia	↓ Alkaline phosphatase	Bone deformities, hypotonia	Poor mineralization
OSTEOPENIA			
Osteoporosis	↓ Estrogen—↓ bone mass	Kyphosis, fractures	Compression vertebral fx, hip fx
Scurvy	Vit. C deficiency—defective collagen	Fatigue, bleeding, effusions	Thin cortices, corner sign
OSTEODENSE			
Paget's disease	Osteoclastic abn.—↑ bone turnover	Deformities, pain, CHF, fxs	Coarse trabeculae, "picture frame" vertebrae
Osteopetrosis	Osteoclastic abn.—unclear	Hepatosplenomegaly, anemia	Bone within bone

↓, decreased; ↑, increased; Def., defective; abn., abnormality; PTH, parathyroid hormone; CRF, chronic renal failure; CHF, congestive heart failure; fxs, fractures; PHP, pseudohypoparathyroidism; MEN, multiple endocrine neoplasia.

TABLE 1–10. SERUM AND URINE FINDINGS IN VARIOUS METABOLIC BONE DISEASES

DISORDER	[Ca]	[P_i]	AP	PTH	25-(OH) VITAMIN D	1,25-$(OH)_2$ VITAMIN D	URINARY CALCIUM	BONE BIOPSY FINDINGS	ASSOCIATED FINDINGS
Postmenopausal osteoporosis (type I)	N	N	N	N, ↓	N	N	↑, N	Variable	Osteopenia
Age-related osteoporosis (type II)	N	N	N	↑, N	N	N	N	Variable	Osteopenia
Chronic glucocorticoid-associated osteoporosis	N	N	N	↑, N	N	N	↑, N	Inactive turnover	Severe osteopenia
Primary hyperparathyroidism	↑	N, ↓	N, ↑	↑	N	↑, N	↑	Active turnover; peritrabecular fibrosis	Variable, depending on degree of hypercalcemia
Cancer with bony metastases	↑	↑, N	↑, N	N, ↓	N	N, ↓	↑↑	Tumor	History of primary tumor; bony destruction; + bone scan
Multiple myeloma; lymphoma	↑	↑, N	↑, N	N, ↓	N	N, ↓	↑↑	Confirmatory for tumor	Destructive lesions on radiographs; abnormal protein electrophoresis
Primary carcinoma not involving bone	↑	↓	↑, N	↓	N	↓	↑↑	Variable	Osteopenia, ↑ PTH-related peptide
Sarcoidosis	↑	↑, N	↑, N	N, ↓	N	↑	↑	Active turnover	Hilar adenopathy
Hyperthyroidism	↑	N	N	N, ↓	N	N	↑	Active turnover	↑ FTI; ↓ TSH; Osteopenia; tachycardia, tremor, systemic hyperthyroid changes
Vitamin D intoxication	↑	↑, N	↑, N	N, ↓	↑↑↑	N	↑	Active turnover	History of excessive vitamin D intake
Milk-alkali syndrome	↑	↑, N	↑, N	N, ↓	N	N, ↓	↑	Variable	History of excessive calcium and alkalai ingestion (antacids)
Severe generalized immobilization	↑	↑, N	↑, N	N, ↓	N	N, ↓	↑↑	Active turnover	Osteopenia; multiple fractures; neurologic dysfunction
Vitamin D deficiency (dietary; gastrointestinal)	N, ↓	↓	↑	↑	↓	↓	↓	Osteomalacia	
Dietary phosphate deficiency (rare)	N	↓	↑	N	N	↑	N	Osteomalacia; absence of hyperparathyroid changes	Phosphate-binding antacid abuse with normal renal function
Mesenchymal tumor producing phosphaturic factor	N	↓	↑	N	N	N	N	Osteomalacia; absence of hyperparathyroid changes	Normal 1,25-$(OH)_2$ vitamin D level but inappropriately low considering degree of phosphaturia
Vitamin D resistance (X-linked dominant—Albright's syndrome)	N	↓	↑	N	N	N	N	Osteomalacia; absence of hyperparathyroid changes	Normal 1,25-$(OH)_2$ vitamin D level but inappropriately low considering degree of phosphaturia
Fanconi type II	N	↓	↑	N	N	N	N	Osteomalacia; absence of hyperparathyroid changes	Normal 1,25-$(OH)_2$ vitamin D level but inappropriately low considering degree of phosphaturia; glycosuria
Fanconi type III	N	↓	↑	N	N	N	N	Osteomalacia; absence of hyperparathyroid changes	Normal 1,25-$(OH)_2$ vitamin D level but inappropriately low considering degree of phosphaturia; aminoaciduria
Vitamin D-dependent rickets type I (rare)	↓	↓	↑	↑	N	↓↓	↓	Osteomalacia; hyperparathyroid changes	Defect in renal converting enzyme from 25-(OH) vitamin D to 1,25-$(OH)_2$ vitamin D
Vitamin D-dependent rickets type II (rare)	↓	↓	↑	↑	N	↑↑	↓	Osteomalacia; hyperparathyroid changes	Probable 1,25-$(OH)_2$ vitamin D receptor defect
Renal tubular acidosis	↓	↓	↑	↑	N	↑, N	↑	Osteomalacia; hyperparathyroid changes	Elevated BUN and creatinine
Renal osteodystrophy (mixed)	N, ↓	↑↑	↑	↑↑	N	↓↓	—	Pure osteomalacia; aluminum at mineralization front	Elevated BUN and creatinine
Renal osteodystrophy (predominant aluminum-associated osteomalacia)	↑, N	↑, N	↑	↑	N	↓↓	—	Pure osteomalacia; aluminum at mineralization front	Elevated BUN and creatinine
Hypophosphatasia	↑	↑	↓↓	N	N	N	↑	Pure osteomalacia	Elevated urinary phosphoethanolamine; early loss of teeth

Adapted from Simon, S.R.: Orthopaedic Basic Science, 2nd ed., p. 170. Rosemont, IL, American Academy of Orthopaedic Surgeons, 1994, reprinted by permission.

Ca, calcium; P_i, phosphate; AP, alkaline phosphatase; PTH, parathyroid hormone; 25-(OH) vitamin D, 25-hydroxyvitamin D; 1,25-$(OH)_2$ vitamin D, 1,25-dihydroxyvitamin D; FTI, free thyroxin index; TSH, thyroid stimulating hormone; BUN, blood urea nitrogen; ↑, increased; ↓ decreased.

cells, extravasation of RBCs, hemosiderin staining, fibrous tissue hemosiderin), and chondrocalcinosis. Radiographs may demonstrate deformed, osteopenic bones, fractures, "shaggy" trabeculae, areas of radiolucency (phalanges, distal clavicle, skull), and calcification of the soft tissues. Histologic changes include osteoblasts and osteoclasts active on both sides of trabeculae (as seen in Paget's disease), areas of destruction, and wide osteoid seams. Surgical parathyroidectomy is curative.

b. Other Causes of Hypercalcemia
   1. Familial Syndromes—Hypercalcemia can result from pituitary adenomas associated with multiple endocrine neoplasia (MEN) types I and II and from familial hypocalciuric hypercalcemia (which is caused by poor renal clearance of calcium).
   2. Other causes of hypercalcemia—Include malignancy (most common), hyperthyroidism, Addison's disease, steroid administration, peptic ulcer disease, kidney disease, and sarcoidosis.

2. Hypocalcemia—Low plasma calcium can result from low PTH or vitamin D_3. Hypocalcemia leads to increased neuromuscular irritability (tetany, seizures, Chvostek's sign), cataracts, fungal infections of the nails, EKG changes (prolonged QT interval), and other signs and symptoms.
   a. Primary Hypoparathyroidism—Decreased PTH causes diminished plasma calcium and increased plasma phosphate (urinary excretion not enhanced due to lack of PTH). Common findings include fungal infections of the nails, hair loss, and blotchy skin due to pigment loss (vitiligo). Skull radiographs may show basal ganglion calcification. Iatrogenic hypoparathyroidism can follow thyroidectomy.
   b. Pseudohypoparathyroidism (PHP)—A rare genetic disorder that causes a lack of effect of PTH at the target cells. PTH level is normal or even high, but PTH action at the cellular level is blocked by an abnormality at the receptor, the cAMP system, or by a lack of required cofactors (e.g., Mg^{2+}). **Albright hereditary osteodystrophy,** a form of PHP, is associated with short first, fourth, and fifth MCs and MTs, brachydactyly, exostoses, obesity, and diminished intelligence.
   c. Renal Osteodystrophy (Fig. 1–25)—**Chronic renal failure (CRF) leads to an inability to excrete phosphate.** Often considered a form of osteomalacia, it is commonly associated with **long-term hemodialysis.** High levels of plasma phosphate lead to a decrease in plasma calcium, which is ordinarily adjusted by PTH, which increases urinary excretion of phosphate. The latter often leads to hyperplasia of the parathyroid chief cells, resulting in **secondary hyperparathyroidism.** In CRF the phosphate cannot be secreted, however, and symptoms similar to hypoparathyroidism re-

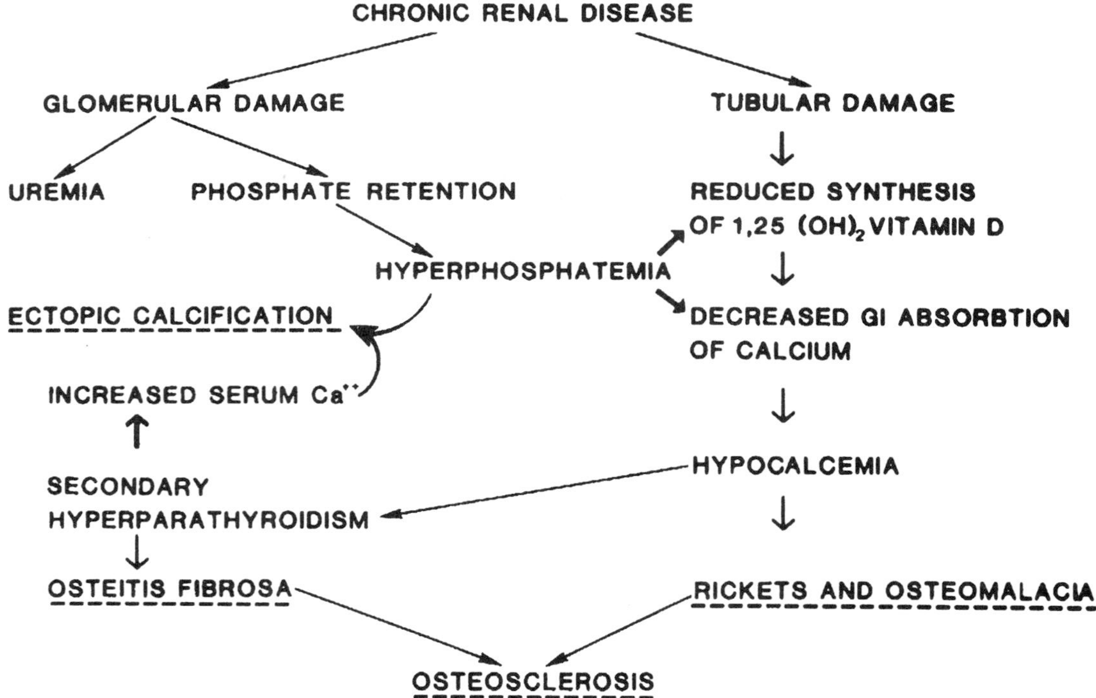

FIGURE 1–25. Pathogenesis of bone changes in renal osteodystrophy. (From Simon, S.R., ed.: Orthopaedic Basic Science, 2nd ed., p. 171. Rosemont, IL, American Academy of Orthopaedic Surgeons, 1994; reprinted by permission.)

sult. Radiographs may demonstrate a "rugger jersey" spine, like that in childhood osteopetrosis, and soft tissue calcification. An additional complication of chronic dialysis is **amyloidosis,** which may be associated with carpal tunnel syndrome, arthropathy, and pathologic fractures. Laboratory tests show an abnormal glomerular filtration rate (GFR); increased alkaline phosphatase, BUN, and creatinine; and decreased venous bicarbonate. **Treatment** should be directed at relieving the urologic obstruction or kidney disease.

d. Rickets (Osteomalacia in Adults)—**Failure of mineralization** leading to changes in the physis (increased width and disorientation) and bone (cortical thinning, bowing). The causes of rickets and osteomalacia are summarized in Table 1–11.

1. Vitamin D Deficiency Rickets (Fig. 1–26)—Almost eliminated after addition of vitamin D to milk in the United States; the disease is still seen in Asian immigrants, patients with dietary peculiarities, premature infants, and those with malabsorption (sprue) or chronic parenteral nutrition. Decreased absorption of calcium and phosphate leads to secondary hyperparathyroidism (PTH continues to be produced because of low plasma calcium). **Laboratory studies** show **low normal calcium** (maintained by high PTH), **low phosphate** (excreted because of the effect of PTH), **increased PTH,** and **low levels of vitamin D.** Enlargement of the costochondral junction ("**rachitic rosary**"), bony deformities (**bowing of the knees,** "codfish" vertebrae), retarded bone growth (defect in hypotrophic zone with widened osteoid seams and physeal cupping), muscle hypotonia, dental disease, pathologic fractures (Looser's zones [pseudofracture on compression side of bone]), **milkman's fracture** [pseudofracture in adults]), a waddling gait, and other problems may result. Treatment with vitamin D (5000 U daily) and calcium (up to 3 g daily) resolves most deformities. Characteristic radiographic changes seen in rickets include physeal widening, physeal cupping, and coxa vara (*).
2. Hereditary Vitamin D-Dependent Rickets—Rare autosomal recessive (AR) disorder that may represent a defect in 1-hydroxylation of vitamin D_3 in the kidney, leading to low levels of or defective 1,25-$(OH)_2$-vitamin D_3 (or both). The disease features are similar to those of vitamin D-deficient rickets, except that they **may be worse** and include total baldness. High levels of vitamin D are required to treat this form of rickets (on the order of 20,000–100,000 units per day followed by maintenance dosage of a vitamin D_3 analogue).
3. Familial Hypophosphatemic Rickets (Vitamin D-Resistant Rickets; a.k.a. "Phosphate Diabetes")—X-linked dominant disorder that is a result of **impaired renal tubular reabsorption of phosphate.** Affected patients have a normal GFR and an impaired vitamin D_3 response. Phosphate replacement (1–4 g daily) with vitamin D_3 can correct the effects of the disorder, which are similar to those of the other forms of rickets.
4. Hypophosphatasia—AR disorder caused by **low levels of alkaline phosphatase,** which is required for the synthesis of inorganic phosphate, important in bone matrix formation. Features are similar to those of rickets, and treatment may include phos-

TABLE 1–11. CAUSES OF RICKETS AND OSTEOMALACIA

NUTRITIONAL DEFICIENCY
- Vitamin D deficiency
- Dietary chelators (rare) of calcium
  - Phytates
  - Oxalates (spinach)
- Phosphorus deficiency (unusual)
  - Antacid (aluminum-containing) abuse leading to severe dietary phosphate binding

GASTROINTESTINAL ABSORPTION DEFECTS
- Postgastrectomy (rare today)
- Biliary disease (interference with absorption of fat-soluble vitamin D)
- Enteric absorption defects
  - Short bowel syndrome
  - Rapid-transit (gluten-sensitive enteropathy) syndromes
  - Inflammatory bowel disease
    - Crohn's disease
    - Celiac disease

RENAL TUBULAR DEFECTS (RENAL PHOSPHATE LEAK)
- X-linked dominant hypophosphatemic vitamin D-resistant rickets (VDRR) or osteomalacia
- Classic Albright syndrome or Fanconi syndrome type I
- Fanconi syndrome type II
- Phosphaturia and glycosuria
- Fanconi syndrome type III
- Phosphaturia, glycosuria, aminoaciduria
- Vitamin D-dependent rickets (or osteomalacia) type I (A genetic or acquired deficiency of renal tubular 25-hydroxyvitamin D; 1-alpha hydroxylase enzyme prevents conversion of 25-hydroxyvitamin D to active polar metabolite 1,25-dihydroxyvitamin D.)
- Vitamin D-dependent rickets (or osteomalacia) type II (This entity represents enteric end-organ insensitivity to 1,25-dihydroxyvitamin D and is probably caused by an abnormality in the 1,25-dihydroxyvitamin D nuclear receptor.)
- Renal tubular acidosis
  - Acquired—associated with many systemic diseases
  - Genetic
    - Debre-De Toni-Fanconi syndrome
    - Lignac-Fanconi syndrome (cysteinosis)
    - Lowe syndrome

RENAL OSTEODYSTROPHY

MISCELLANEOUS CAUSES
- Soft tissue tumors secreting putative factors
  - Fibrous dysplasia
  - Neurofibromatosis
  - Other soft tissue and vascular mesenchymal tumors
- Anticonvulsant medication (Induction of hepatic P450 microsomal enzyme system by some anticonvulsants—phenytoin, phenobarbital, mysoline—causes increased degradation of vitamin D metabolites.)
- Heavy metal intoxication
- Hypophosphatasia
- High dose diphosphonates
- Sodium fluoride

Adapted from Simon, S.R.: Orthopaedic Basic Science, 2nd ed., p. 169. Rosemont, IL, American Academy of Orthopaedic Surgeons, 1994; reprinted by permission.

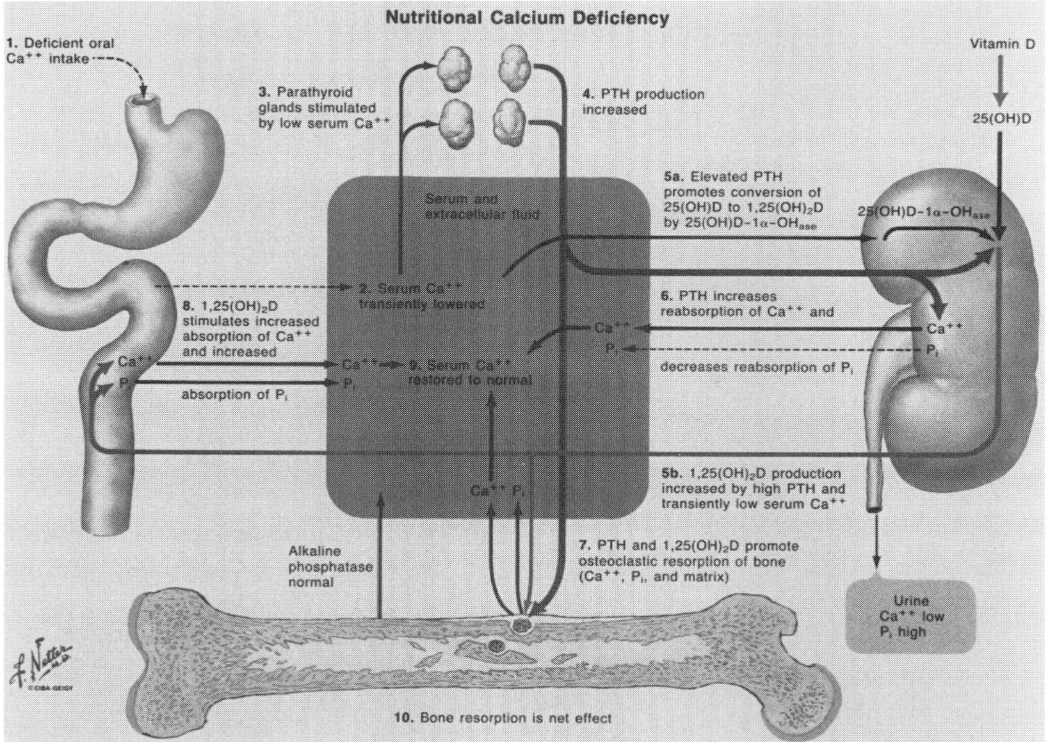

FIGURE 1–26. Nutritional calcium deficiency. (From The Ciba Collection of Medical Illustrations, vol. 8, part I, p. 184, 1987. Illustrated by Frank H. Netter. Reprinted by permission.)

phate therapy. **Increased urinary phosphoethanolamine is diagnostic.**

C. Conditions of Bone Mineral Density—Bone mass is regulated by the relative rates of deposition and withdrawal (Fig. 1–27).

1. Osteopenia

a. Osteoporosis—Age-related decrease in bone mass usually associated with loss of estrogen in postmenopausal women (Fig. 1–28). Osteoporosis is responsible for more than 1 million fractures per year (vertebral body most common) (*). It is a quantitative, not a qualitative, defect in bone. Sedentary, **thin Caucasian women of northern European descent,** particularly **smokers,** heavy **drinkers,** and patients on **phenytoin** (impairs vitamin D metabolism), with low calcium and low vitamin D diets who **breast-fed their infants,** are at greatest risk. Cancellous bone is most markedly affected. Clinical features include kyphosis and vertebral fractures (compression fractures of T11–L1 [creating an anterior wedge-shaped defect or resulting in a centrally depressed "codfish" vertebrae]), hip fractures, and distal radius fractures. Two types of osteoporosis have been characterized: type I (postmenopausal) and type II (age-related).

1. Type I Osteoporosis (Postmenopausal)—Affects trabecular bone primarily; vertebral and distal radius fractures are common.
2. Type II Osteoporosis (Age-Related)—Seen in patients older than 75 years of age; affects both trabecular and cortical bone; is related to poor calcium absorption; hip and pelvic fractures are common.

Laboratory studies, including urinary calcium and hydroxyproline and serum alkaline phosphatase, are helpful for evaluating osteopenic conditions. Results of these **laboratory studies** are usually **unremarkable** in osteoporosis; but hyperthyroidism, hyperparathyroidism, Cushing syndrome, hematologic disorders, and malignancy should be ruled out. Plain **radiographs** are usually not helpful unless >30% bone loss is present. Special studies used for the work-up of osteoporosis include single-photon (appendicular) and double-photon (axial) absorptiometry, quantitative CT, and dual-energy x-ray absorptiometry (DEXA). **DEXA is most accurate with less radiation.** Biopsy (after tetracycline labeling) may be used to evaluate the severity of osteoporosis and to identify osteomalacia. **Histologic changes in osteoporosis are thinning of trabeculae, decreased size of osteons, and enlargement of haversian and marrow spaces.** Physical activity, calcium supplements (more effective in type II [age-related] osteoporosis), estrogen–progesterone therapy (in type I [postmenopausal] osteoporosis; best when initiated within 6 years of menopause), and fluoride (inhibits bone resorption, but bone is more brittle) have a role in the treatment of osteoporosis. Other drugs, such as intramuscular calcitonin, may also be helpful but are expen-

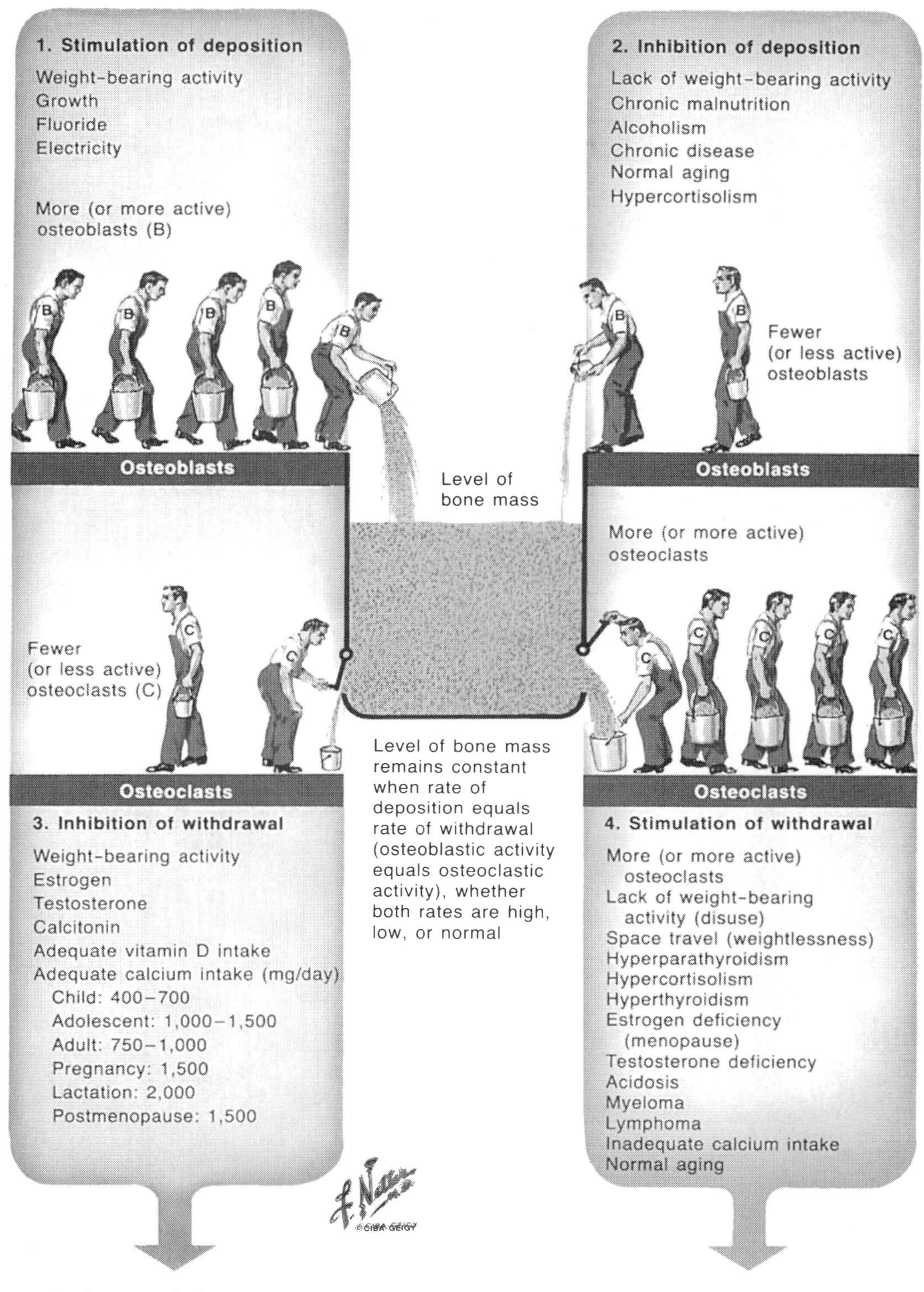

FIGURE 1–27. Four mechanisms of bone mass regulation. (From The Ciba Collection of Medical Illustrations, vol. 8, part I, p. 181, 1987. Illustrated by Frank H. Netter. Reprinted by permission.)

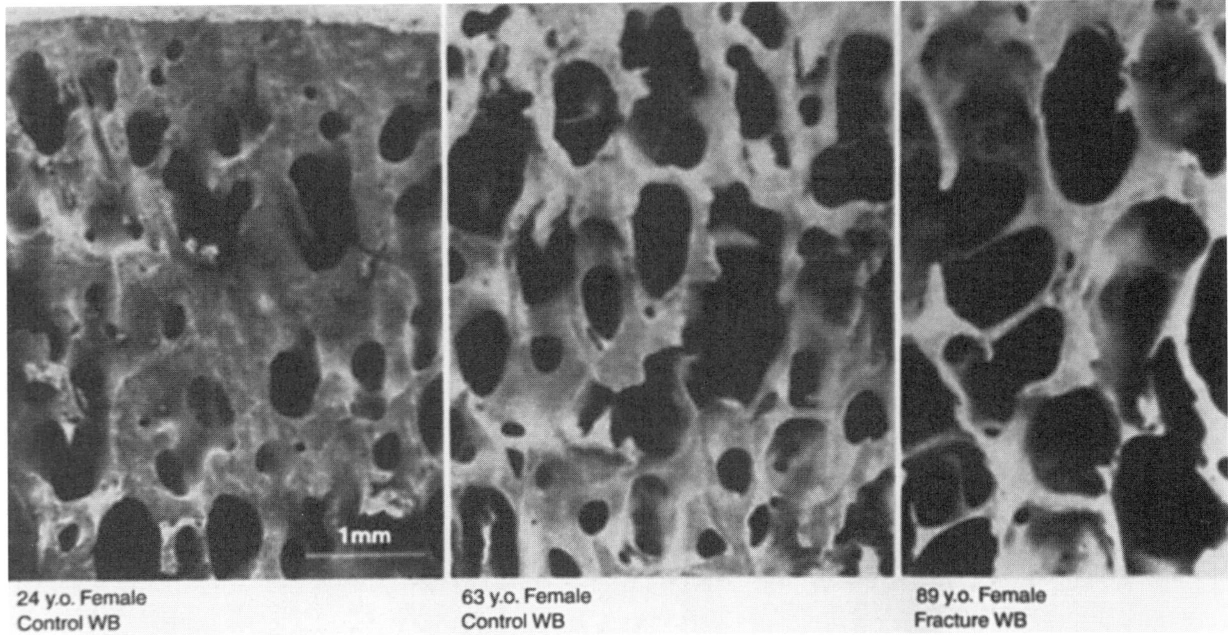

FIGURE 1–28. Age-related changes in density and architecture of human trabecular bone from the lumbar spine. (From Keaveney, T.M., and Hayes, W.C.: Mechanical properties of cortical and trabecular bone. Bone 7:285–344, 1993; reprinted by permission.)

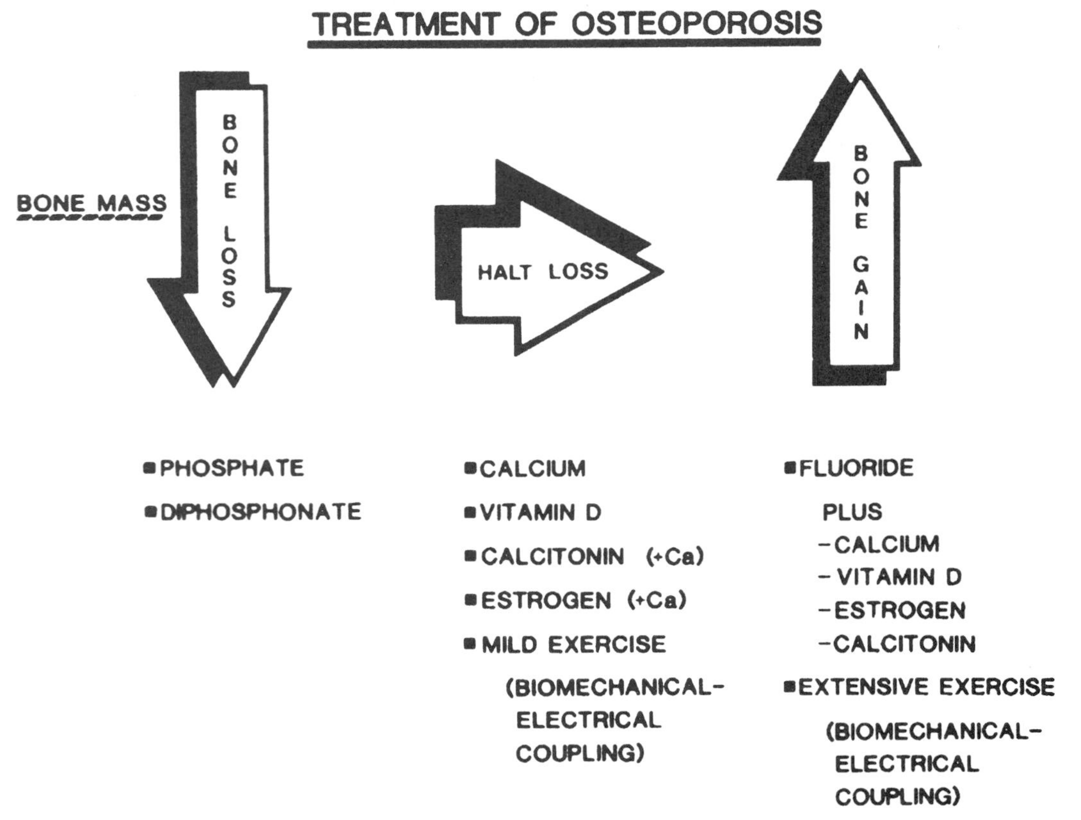

FIGURE 1–29. Treatment options for osteoporosis. (From Simon, S.R., ed.: Orthopaedic Basic Science, 2nd ed., p. 174. Rosemont, IL, American Academy of Orthopaedic Surgeons, 1994; reprinted by permission.)

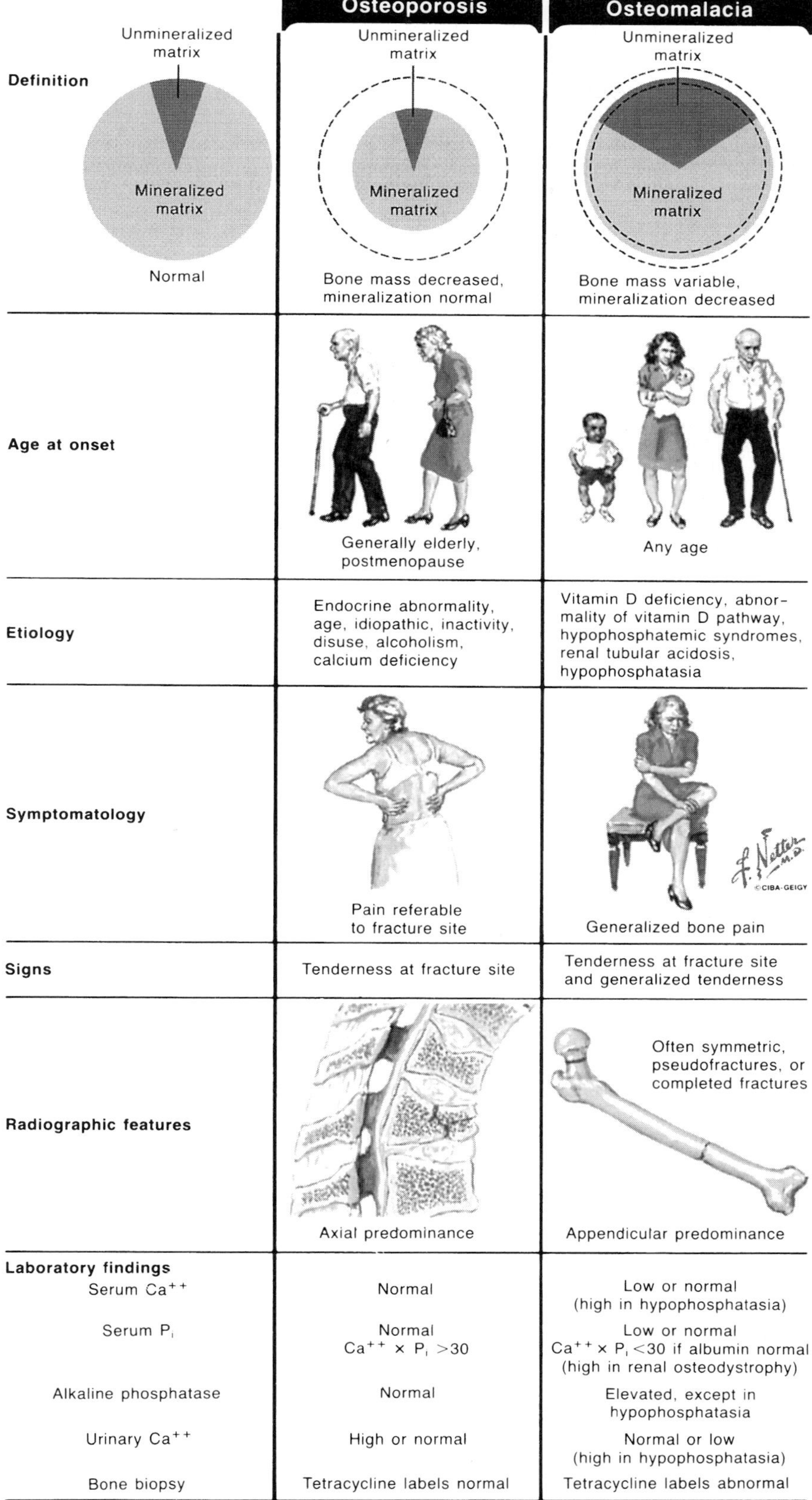

Comparison of Osteoporosis and Osteomalacia

	Osteoporosis	Osteomalacia
Definition Unmineralized matrix Mineralized matrix Normal	Unmineralized matrix Mineralized matrix Bone mass decreased, mineralization normal	Unmineralized matrix Mineralized matrix Bone mass variable, mineralization decreased
Age at onset	Generally elderly, postmenopause	Any age
Etiology	Endocrine abnormality, age, idiopathic, inactivity, disuse, alcoholism, calcium deficiency	Vitamin D deficiency, abnormality of vitamin D pathway, hypophosphatemic syndromes, renal tubular acidosis, hypophosphatasia
Symptomatology	Pain referable to fracture site	Generalized bone pain
Signs	Tenderness at fracture site	Tenderness at fracture site and generalized tenderness
Radiographic features	Axial predominance	Often symmetric, pseudofractures, or completed fractures Appendicular predominance
Laboratory findings		
Serum Ca^{++}	Normal	Low or normal (high in hypophosphatasia)
Serum P_i	Normal $Ca^{++} \times P_i > 30$	Low or normal $Ca^{++} \times P_i < 30$ if albumin normal (high in renal osteodystrophy)
Alkaline phosphatase	Normal	Elevated, except in hypophosphatasia
Urinary Ca^{++}	High or normal	Normal or low (high in hypophosphatasia)
Bone biopsy	Tetracycline labels normal	Tetracycline labels abnormal

FIGURE 1–30. Osteoporosis versus osteomalacia. (From The Ciba Collection of Medical Illustrations, vol. 8, part I, p. 228, 1987. Illustrated by Frank H. Netter. Reprinted by permission.)

sive and may cause hypersensitivity reactions. The future of bone augmentation with PTH, growth factors, prostaglandin inhibitors, and other modes of therapy remains to be determined. An overview of recommended treatment for osteoporosis is shown in Figure 1–29. The best prophylaxis for patients at risk of developing osteoporosis comprises (*): (1) diet with adequate calcium intake; (2) weight-bearing exercise program; and (3) estrogen therapy evaluation at menopause.

3. Idiopathic Transient Osteoporosis (**) of the Hip—Uncommon; diagnosis of exclusion; most common during third trimester of pregnancy. Presents with groin pain, limited ROM, and localized osteopenia. Treatment includes limited weight-bearing and analgesics; spontaneous recovery is typical but stress fractures can occur.

b. Osteomalacia—Discussed with rickets. **Defect in mineralization** results in a large amount of **unmineralized osteoid** (qualitative defect). Osteomalacia is caused by vitamin D-deficient diets, GI disorders, renal osteodystrophy, and certain drugs (aluminum-containing phosphate-binding antacids [aluminum deposition in bone prevents mineralization] and phenytoin [Dilantin]). It is commonly associated with Looser's zones (microscopic stress fractures), other fractures, biconcave vertebral bodies, and trefoil pelvis seen on plain radiographs. Biopsy (transiliac) is required for diagnosis (histologically, widened osteoid seams are seen). Femoral neck fractures are common in patients with osteomalacia. Treatment usually includes large doses of vitamin D. Osteoporosis and osteomalacia are compared in Figure 1–30.

c. Scurvy—**Vitamin C (ascorbic acid) deficiency leads to defective collagen growth and repair and impaired intracellular hydroxylation of collagen peptides** (*). Clinical features include fatigue, gum bleeding, ecchymosis, joint effusions, and iron deficiency. Radiographic changes may include thin cortices and trabeculae and metaphyseal clefts (corner sign). Laboratory studies are normal. Histologic changes include replacement of primary trabeculae with granulation tissue, areas of hemorrhage, and widening of the zone of provisional calcification in the physis.

d. Marrow Packing Disorders—Myeloma, leukemia, and other disorders can cause osteopenia (see Chapter 8, Orthopaedic Pathology).

e. Osteogeneis Imperfecta (see Chapter 2, Pediatric Orthopaedics)—Caused by abnormal collagen synthesis (failure of cross-linking) (**). Abnormality is primarily due to a mutation in the genes that produce type I collagen (*).

2. Increased Osteodensity

a. Paget's Disease—Discussed in Chapter 8, Orthopaedic Pathology.

b. Osteopetrosis (Marble Bone Disease)—A group of bone disorders that lead to increased sclerosis and obliteration of the medullary canal due to **decreased osteoclast (and chondroclast) function** (a failure of bone resorption). The disorder may result from an abnormality of the immune system (thymic defect).

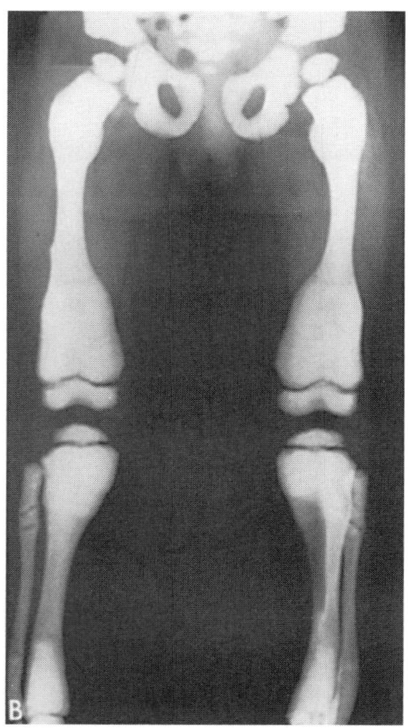

FIGURE 1–31. Typical "marble bone" appearance in osteopetrosis. (From Tachdijian, M.O.: Pediatric Orthopaedics, 2nd ed., p. 795. Philadelphia: WB Saunders, 1990; reprinted by permission.)

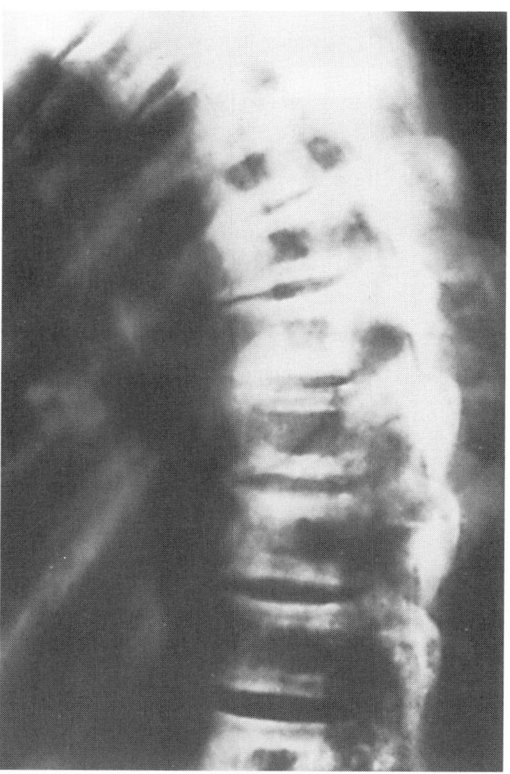

FIGURE 1–32. Typical "rugger Jersey" spine seen in osteopetrosis. (From Tachdijian, M.O.: Pediatric Orthopaedics, 2nd ed., p. 797. Philadelphia, WB Saunders, 1990; reprinted by permission.)

Histologically, osteoclasts lack the normal ruffled border and clear zone. The marrow spaces become filled with **necrotic calcified cartilage,** and cartilage may be trapped within osteoid. Empty lacunae and plugging of haversian canals is also seen. The most severe juvenile autosomal recessive (AR) "malignant" form leads to a "bone within a bone" appearance on radiographs, hepatosplenomegaly, and aplastic anemia. **Bone marrow transplantation** (***) (of osteoclast precursors) can be lifesaving during childhood. High doses of calcitriol ± steroids may also be helpful. The autosomal dominant (AD) "tarda" form (**Albers-Schönberg disease**) demonstrates generalized osteosclerosis (including the typical **"rugger jersey" spine**), usually without other anomalies (Figs. 1–31, 1–32). Pathologic fractures through abnormal (brittle) bone are common.

c. Osteopoikilosis ("Spotted Bone Disease")—Islands of deep cortical bone appear within the medullary cavity and cancellous bone of long bones (especially in the hands and feet). These areas are usually asymptomatic, and there is no known incidence of malignant degeneration.

D. Conditions of Bone Viability

1. Osteonecrosis—Osteonecrosis (ON) represents death of bony tissue (usually adjacent to a joint surface) from causes other than infection. It is usually caused by loss of blood supply due to trauma or other etiology [e.g., following a slipped capital femoral epiphysis (**)]. Osteonecrosis

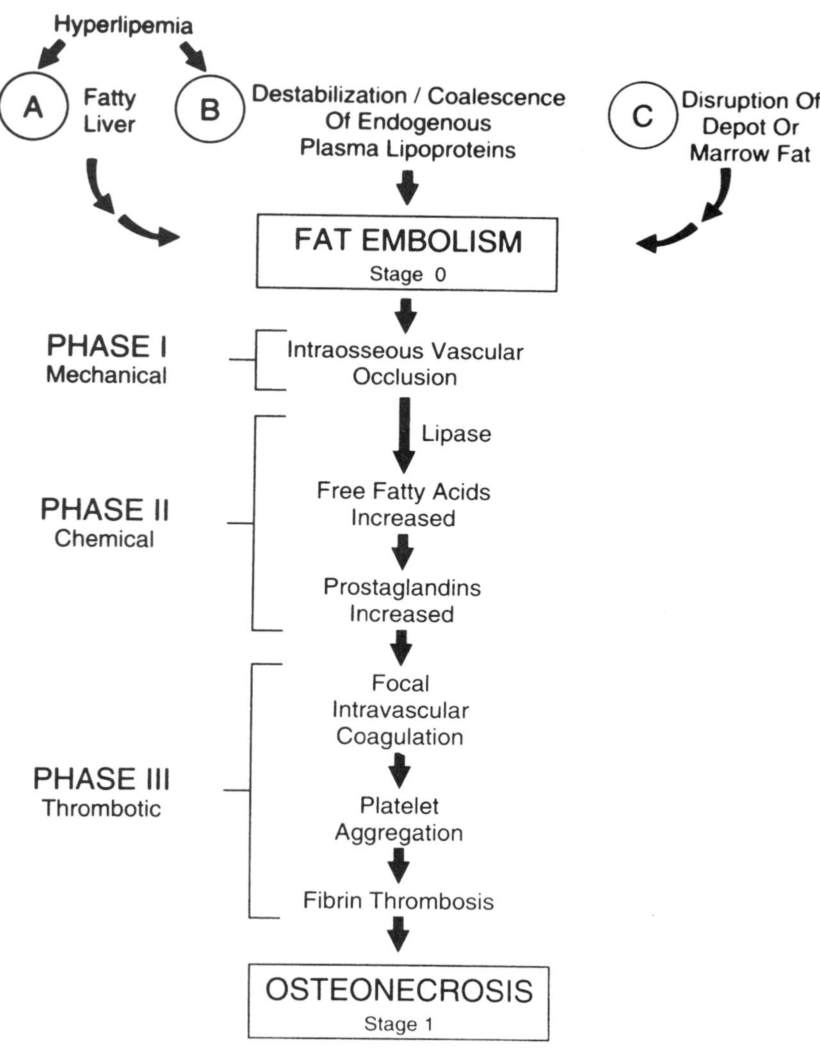

FIGURE 1–33. Possible mechanisms of intraosseous fat embolism leading to focal intravascular coagulation and osteonecrosis. (From Jones, J.P., Jr.: Fat embolism and osteonecrosis. Clin. Orthop. 16:595–633, 1985; reprinted by permission.)

TABLE 1–12. ENNEKING'S STAGES OF OSTEONECROSIS

STAGE	PAIN	RADIOGRAPHS	PATHOLOGY	TREATMENT
I	None	Slight ↑ density	Creeping substitution	Observation
II	None	Reactive rim	Rim, reinfarction	Core decompression(?)
III	Occasional	Crescent sign	Fracture	Core decompression(?)
IV	Limp	Step-off, flattening	Loose fragments	?
V	Continuous	Collapse	Cartilage flap	Hemiarthroplasty
VI	Severe	Deformed	Advanced arthritis	THA/Girdlestone

Adapted from Enneking, W.F.: Clinical Musculoskeletal Pathology, 3rd revised ed., pp. 144–155. Gainsville, University of Florida Press, 1990.
THA, total hip arthroplasty.

commonly affects the hip joint, leading to eventual collapse and flattening of the femoral head. The condition is associated with steroid and heavy alcohol use; it is also associated with blood dyscrasias (e.g., sickle cell disease), dysbaric (Caisson disease), excessive radiation therapy, and Gaucher's disease.

a. Etiology—Theories regarding the etiology of ON vary (Fig. 1–33). It may be related to enlargement of space-occupying marrow fat cells, which leads to ischemia of adjacent tissues. Vascular insults and other factors may also be significant. Idiopathic ON (Chandler's disease) is diagnosed when no other cause can be identified. Idiopathic/alcohol and dysbaric ON are associated with multiple insults and have been classified by Enneking as described in Table 1–12. The incidence of ON of the fem-

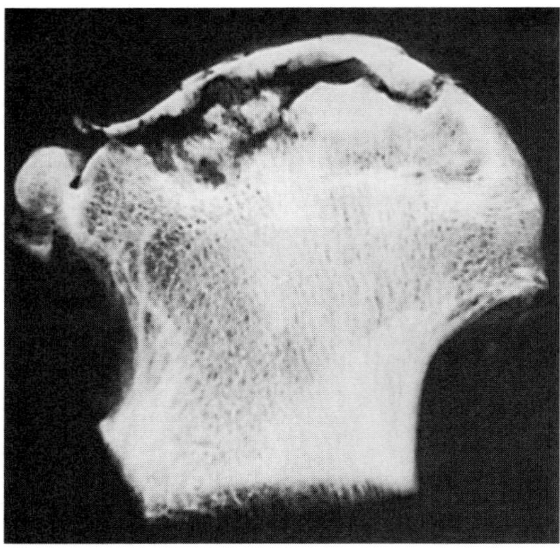

FIGURE 1–34. Fine-grain radiograph demonstrating space between the articular surface and subchondral bone: "crescent sign" of osteonecrosis. (From Steinberg, M.E.: The Hip and Its Disorders, p. 630. Philadelphia, WB Saunders, 1991; reprinted by permission.)

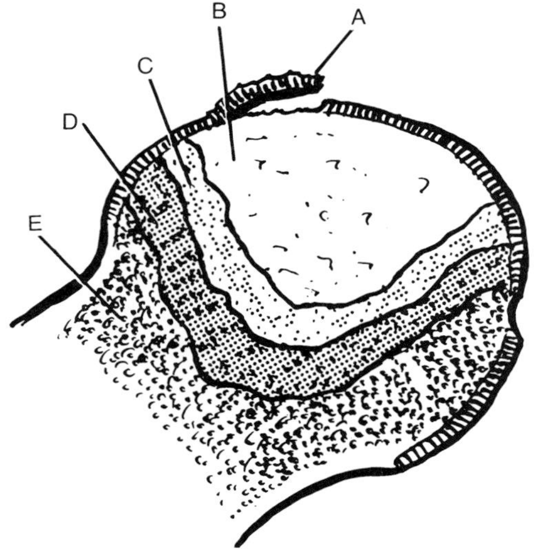

FIGURE 1–35. Pathology of avascular necrosis. *A*, Articular cartilage. *B*, Necrotic bone. *C*, Reactive fibrous tissue. *D*, Hypertrophic bone. *E*, Normal trabeculae. (From Steinberg, M.E.: The Hip and Its Disorders, p. 630. Philadelphia: WB Saunders, 1991; reprinted by permission.)

TABLE 1–13. FICAT'S STAGES OF OSTEONECROSIS

STAGE	PAIN	PHYSICAL EXAMINATION	RADIOGRAPHS	BONE SCAN	MRI	IOP	TREATMENT
0	None	Normal	Normal	Normal	Normal	↑	None
I	Minimal	↓ Int. rot.	Normal	Nondiagnostic	Early changes	↑	Core decompression(?)
II	Moderate	↓ ROM	Porosis/sclerosis	Positive	Positive	↑	Strut graft
III	Advanced	↓ ROM	Flat/crescent sign	Positive	Positive	↑	Hemiarthroplasty
IV	Severe	Pain	Acetabular changes	Positive	Positive	↑	THA

IOP, intraosseous pressure; ↑, increased; ↓, decreased; ROM, range of motion; Int. rot., internal rotation; THA, total hip arthroplasty.

TABLE 1–14. COMMON OSTEOCHONDROSES

DISORDER	SITE	AGE (YEARS)
Van Neck's disease	Ischiopubic synchrondrosis	4–11
Legg-Calvé-Perthes disease	Femoral head	4–8
Osgood-Schlatter disease	Tibial tuberosity	11–15
Sinding-Larsen-Johansson syndrome	Inferior patella	10–14
Blount's disease (infant)	Proximal tibial epiphysis	1–3
Blount's disease (adolescent)	Proximal tibial epiphysis	8–15
Sever's disease	Calcaneus	9–11
Köhler's disease	Tarsal navicular	3–7
Freiberg's infraction	Metatarsal head	13–18
Scheuermann's disease	Discovertebral junction	13–17
Panner's disease	Capitellum of humerus	5–10
Thiemann's disease	Phalanges of hand	11–19
Kienböck's disease	Carpal lunate	20–40

oral head in renal transplant patients has been reduced by the use of cyclosporine (*).

b. Pathologic Changes—Grossly necrotic bone, fibrous tissue, and subchondral collapse may be seen (Figs. 1–34, 1–35). Histologically, early changes involve autolysis of osteocytes (14–21 days) and necrotic marrow, followed by inflammation with invasion of buds of primitive mesenchymal tissue and capillaries. Later, **new woven bone is laid down on top of dead trabecular bone.** This stage is followed by resorption of the dead trabeculae and remodeling during a process of "creeping substitution." It is during this process that the bone is weakest, and collapse (crescent sign, seen on radiographs) and fragmentation can occur.

c. Evaluation—Careful history-taking (risk factors) and physical examination (e.g., decreased ROM, limp) should precede additional studies. Evaluation of other joints (especially the contralateral hip) is important in order to identify the disease process early. The process is bilateral in 50% of cases of idiopathic ON and up to 80% of steroid-induced ON. MRI and bone scanning are helpful for making an early diagnosis. Femoral head pressure measurement is possible but invasive. Pressure >30 mm Hg or increased >10 mm Hg with injection of 5 ml of saline (stress test) is considered abnormal (but these values have varied widely from one investigation to another).

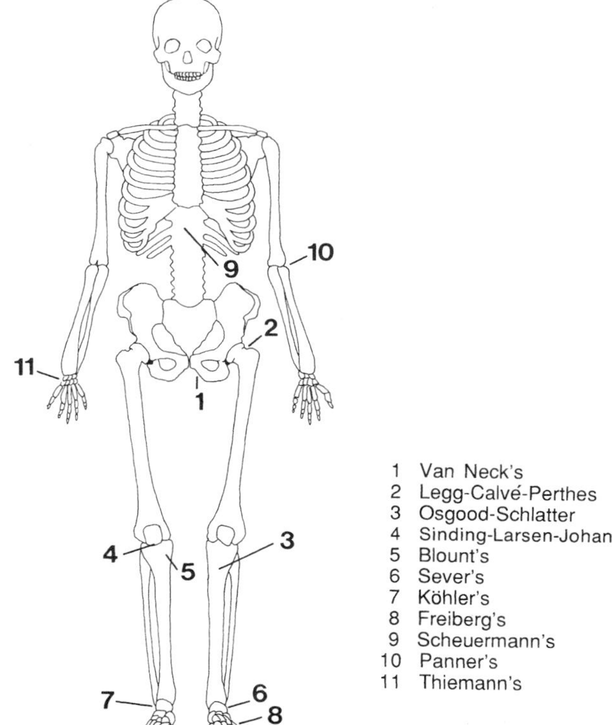

FIGURE 1–36. Location of common osteochondroses.

d. Treatment—Replacement arthroplasty of the hip is associated with increased loosening. Nontraumatic ON of the femoral condyle and proximal humerus may improve spontaneously without surgical correction. The precise role of core decompression remains unresolved, but results are best for Ficat stage I (*).

e. Classification—ON of the hip has been classified by Ficat, and Table 1–13 highlights important features of the disease process.

2. Osteochondrosis—Can occur at traction apophyses in children and may or may not be associated with trauma, inflammation of the joint capsule, or vascular insult/secondary thrombosis. The pathology is similar to that described for ON in the adult. Table 1–14 shows the common osteochondroses (*know them!*) (**). Most are discussed separately in the chapters covering the respective sites of disease (Fig. 1–36; Table 1–14).

Test Questions continued on following page

TEST QUESTIONS ON CONDITIONS OF BONE MINERALIZATION, BONE MINERAL DENSITY, AND BONE VIABILITY

TEST	QUESTION NUMBERS
1995 OSAE—Adult Reconstruction Hip/Knee	43, 56
1995 OSAE—Pediatric Orthopaedics	10, 39, 53, 56
1995 OSAE—Sports Medicine	
1994 OITE	158, 206
1994 OSAE—Adult Spine	9
1994 OSAE—Foot and Ankle	7, 55, 102
1994 OSAE—M/S Trauma	6, 100
1993 OITE	27, 54, 66, 85, 194
1993 OSAE—M/S Tumors and Diseases	6, 10, 15, 17, 18, 20, 31, 41, 76, 81
1993 OSAE—Shoulder and Elbow	36
1992 OITE	25, 37, 43, 89, 90, 140, 141, 196, 200, 207
1992 OSAE—Adult Reconstruction Hip/Knee	7, 8, 96
1992 OSAE—Pediatric Orthopaedics	23, 48, 52, 99
1992 OSAE—Sports Medicine	14, 64
1991 OITE	7, 95, 100, 103, 104, 107, 110, 128, 132, 244
1991 OSAE—Adult Spine	49, 92, 98
1991 OSAE—Anatomy and Imaging	
1991 OSAE—Foot and Ankle	2
1991 OSAE—M/S Trauma	

SECTION 2
Joints

I. Articular Tissues

A. Cartilage—There are several types of cartilage. **Growth plate (physeal) cartilage** has been previously discussed; **fibrocartilage** is important for tendon and ligament insertion into bone (and for healing of articular cartilage); **elastic cartilage** is seen in tissues such as the trachea; **fibroelastic cartilage** makes up menisci; and finally, **articular cartilage** is critical to the function of joints and is the focus of this section. Articular cartilage functions in decreasing friction and in load distribution. Classically, mature articular cartilage has been described as avascular, aneural, and alymphatic. Chondrocytes receive nutrients and oxygen from synovial fluid via diffusion through the cartilage matrix. The pH of cartilage is 7.4; changes in pH can disrupt the structure of cartilage.

1. Articular Cartilage Composition
   a. Water (65–80% of wet weight)—Allows for deformation of the cartilage surface in response to stress by shifting in and out of cartilage. Water is not distributed homogeneously throughout cartilage (65% at deep zone, 80% at surface). Water content increases (90%) in osteoarthritis. Water is also responsible for nutrition and lubrication. Increased water content leads to increased permeability, decreased strength, and decreased Young's modulus (E).
   b. Collagen (10–20% of wet weight; >50% of dry weight) (Fig. 1–37)—Type II collagen represents approximately 90–95% of the total collagen content of articular cartilage and allows for a cartilaginous framework and **tensile strength.** Increased amounts of Gly, Lys-OH, Pro-OH, and hydrogen bonding are responsible for its unique characteristics. Small amounts of types V, VI, IX, X, and XI collagen are present in the matrix of articular cartilage. An overview of collagen types for all tissues is shown in Table 1–15. **Collagen type X is associated with calcification of cartilage** (**).

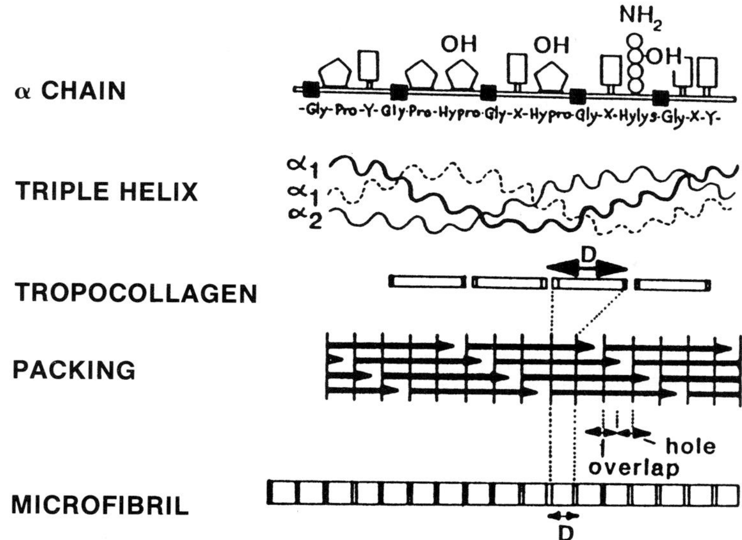

FIGURE 1–37. Collagen microstructure. (From Orthopaedic Science Syllabus, p. 73. Park Ridge, IL, American Academy of Orthopaedic Surgery, 1986; reprinted by permission.)

c. Proteoglycans (10–15% of wet weight) —Protein polysaccharides responsible for the **compressive strength** of cartilage. Proteoglycans are produced by chondrocytes, are secreted into the extracellular matrix, and are composed of subunits known as **glycosaminoglycans** (GAGs, disaccharide polymers). These GAGs include **chondroitin-4-sulfate** (decreases with age), **chondroitin-6-sulfate,** and **keratin sulfate** (increases with age). GAGs are bound to a protein core by sugar bonds to form a proteoglycan aggrecan molecule. Link proteins stabilize aggrecan molecules to hyaluronic acid to form a proteoglycan aggregate. Proteoglycans have a half-life of 3 months, are responsible for the porous structure of cartilage, and serve to trap and hold water (**regulate matrix hydration**) (*). A proteoglycan aggrecan molecule is shown in Figure 1–38 and a proteoglycan aggregate is represented in Figure 1–39.

TABLE 1–15. TYPES OF COLLAGEN

TYPE	LOCATION
I	Bone Tendon Meniscus Annulus of intervertebral disc Skin
II	Articular cartilage Nucleus pulposus of intervertebral disc
III	Skin Blood vessels
IV	Basement membrane (basal lamina)
V	Articular cartilage (in small amounts)
VI	Articular cartilage (in small amounts) Tethers the chondrocyte to its pericellular matrix
VII	Basement membrane (epithelial)
VIII	Basement membrane (epithelial)
IX	Articular cartilage (in small amounts)
X	Hypertrophic cartilage Associated with calcification of cartilage (matrix mineralization)
XI	Articular cartilage (in small amounts)
XII	Tendon
XIII	Endothelial cells

d. Chondrocytes (5% of wet weight)—Active in protein synthesis and possess a double effusion barrier; produce collagen, proteoglycans, and some enzymes for cartilage metabolism; less active in the calcified zone. Deeper zones of cartilage have chondrocytes with decreased rough endoplasmic reticulum (RER) and increased intraplasmic filaments (degenerative products). Chondroblasts, which are derived from undifferentiated mesenchymal cells (stimulated by motion), are later trapped in lacunae to become chondrocytes.

e. Other Matrix Components
   1. Adhesives (fibronectin, chondronectin, anchorin CII)—Involved in interactions between chondrocytes and fibrils. Fibronectin may be associated with osteoarthritis.
   2. Lipids—Unknown function.

2. Articular Cartilage Layers—The various layers of articular cartilage are described in Table 1–16 and are illustrated in Figure 1–40. The tangential zone has a high concentration of collagen fibers arranged at right angles to each other (and parallel to the articular surface) (*).
3. Articular Cartilage Metabolism
   a. Collagen Synthesis—The events and sites involved in collagen synthesis are shown in Figure 1–41.
   b. Collagen Catabolism—Little is known of the exact mechanism. Enzymatic processes have been proposed such that metalloproteinase collagenase cleaves the triple helix. Mechanical factors may also play a role.
   c. Proteoglycan Synthesis (Fig. 1–42)—A series of molecular events beginning with proteoglycan gene expression and transcription of messenger

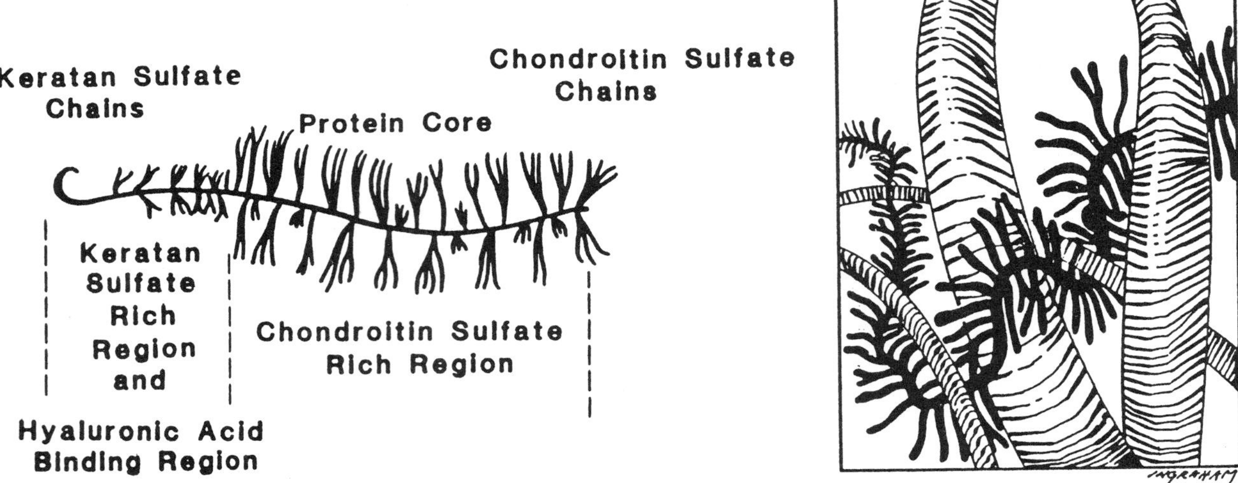

FIGURE 1–38. Collagen microstructure; proteoglycan aggrecan molecule. Note the proteoglycans interspersed with collagen fibrils (*inset*). (From Orthopaedic Science Syllabus, p. 22. Park Ridge, IL, American Academy of Orthopaedic Surgery, 1986; reprinted by permission.)

RNA and concluding with proteoglycan aggregate formation in the extracellular matrix.

d. Proteoglycan Catabolism (Fig. 1–43)

4. Articular Cartilage Growth Factors—Regulate cartilage synthesis; may have a role in osteoarthritis.
   a. Platelet-Derived Growth Factor (PDGF)—May play a role in healing in cartilage lacerations (and perhaps osteoarthritis).
   b. Transforming Growth Factor-Beta (TGF-β)—**Stimulates proteoglycan synthesis** while **suppressing synthesis of type II collagen.** Stimulates the formation of plasminogen activator inhibitor-1 and tissue inhibitor of metalloproteinase (TIMP), which prevent the degradative action of plasmin and stromelysin.
   c. Fibroblast Growth Factor (Basic) (b-FGF)—Sti-

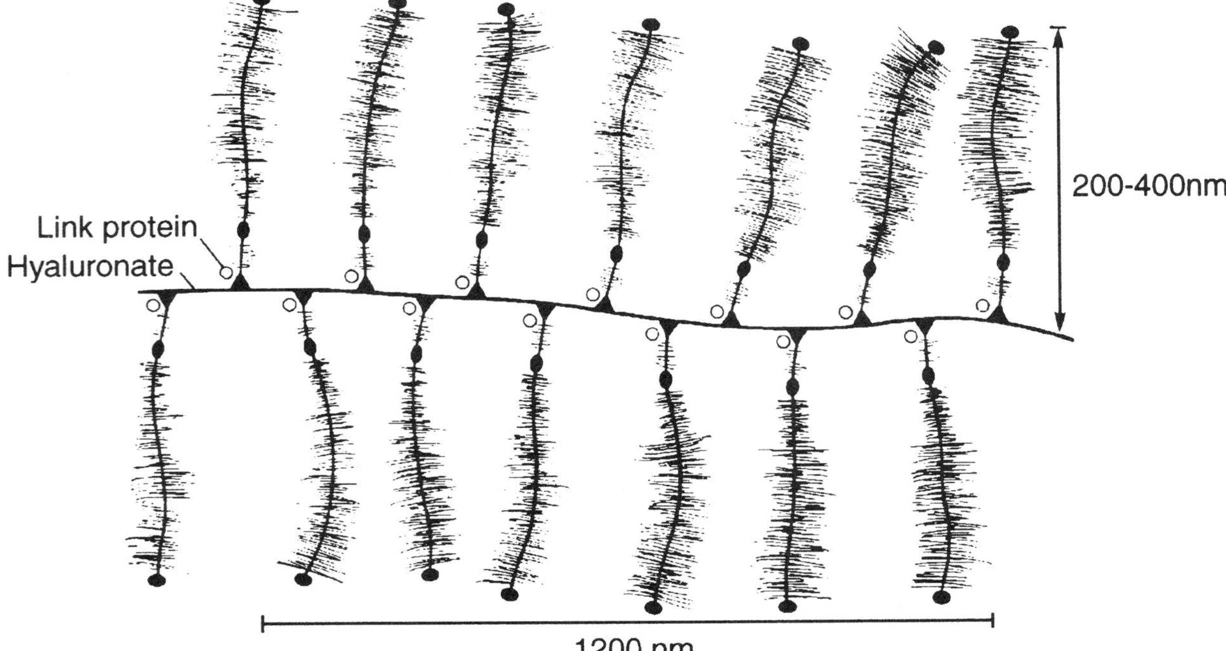

FIGURE 1–39. Proteoglycan aggregate. Sugar bonds attach sulfates to the protein core. (Modified from Simon, S.R., ed.: Orthopaedic Basic Science, 2nd ed., p. 10. Rosemont, IL, American Academy of Orthopaedic Surgeons, 1994; reprinted by permission.)

TABLE 1–16. ARTICULAR CARTILAGE LAYERS

LAYER	WIDTH (μm)	CHARACTERISTIC	ORIENTATION	FUNCTION
Gliding zone	40	↓ Metabolic activity	Tangential	vs. Shear
Transitional zone	500	↑ Metabolic activity	Oblique	vs. Compression
Radial zone	1000	↑ Collagen size	Vertical	vs. Compression
Tidemark	5	Undulating barrier	Tangential	vs. Shear
Calcified zone	300	Hydroxyapatite crystals		Anchor

↑, increased; ↓, decreased.

mulates DNA synthesis in adult articular chondrocytes; may play a role in the cartilage repair process.

d. Insulin-Like Growth Factor-I (IGF-I)—Previously known as somatomedin C. Stimulates DNA and cartilage matrix synthesis in adult articular cartilage and immature cartilage of the growth plate.

5. Biomechanics and Lubrication of Articular Cartilage (Figs. 1–44, 1–45, 1–46)
6. Articular Cartilage Aging—With aging, chondrocytes become larger, acquire increased lysosomal enzymes, and no longer reproduce (so cartilage becomes relatively **hypocellular**). **Cartilage has increased stiffness and decreased solubility with aging.** With aging, cartilage proteoglycans decrease in mass and size (decreased length of chondroitin sulfate chains) and change in proportion (decreased chondroitin sulfate and **increased keratin sulfate**). Protein content increases with aging, and **water content decreases.** These changes decrease the elasticity of cartilage.
7. Articular Cartilage Healing—**Deep lacerations** extending below the tidemark that penetrate the underlying bone may heal with fibrocartilage (or with tissue whose structure is intermediate between hyaline and fibrocartilage); fibrocartilage is not as durable as hyaline cartilage). Blunt trauma may induce changes in cartilage similar to those seen with osteoarthritis. **Superficial articular cartilage** lacerations that do not cross the tidemark cause chondrocytes to proliferate but do not heal. Continuous passive motion is believed to have a beneficial effect on cartilage healing; immobilization of a joint leads to atrophy or cartilage degeneration.

B. Synovium—Synovium mediates the exchange of nutrients between blood and joint (synovial) fluid. Synovial tissues are composed of vascularized connective tissue that lacks a basement membrane. Two cell types are present in synovium: **type A cells,** which are important in **phagocytosis;** and **type B cells (fibroblast-like cells),** which produce synovial fluid (**B**roth). Other undifferentiated cells have a reparative role. A third type of cell, type C, may exist as an intermediate

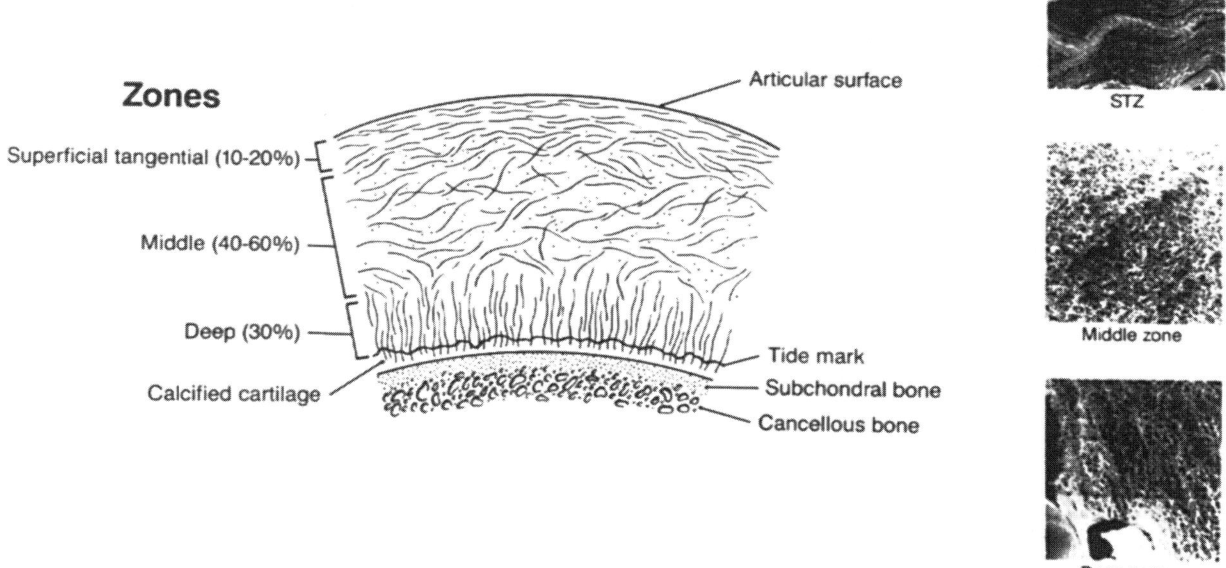

FIGURE 1–40. Articular cartilage zones. Scanning electron micrographs demonstrate collagen arrangement within these zones (*right*). (From Mow, V.C., Proctor, C.S., and Kelly, M.A.: Biomechanics of articular cartilage. In Basic Biomechanics of the Musculoskeletal System, Nordin, M., Franke, V.H., eds., 2nd ed., pp. 31–57. Philadelphia, Lea & Febiger, 1989; reprinted by permission.)

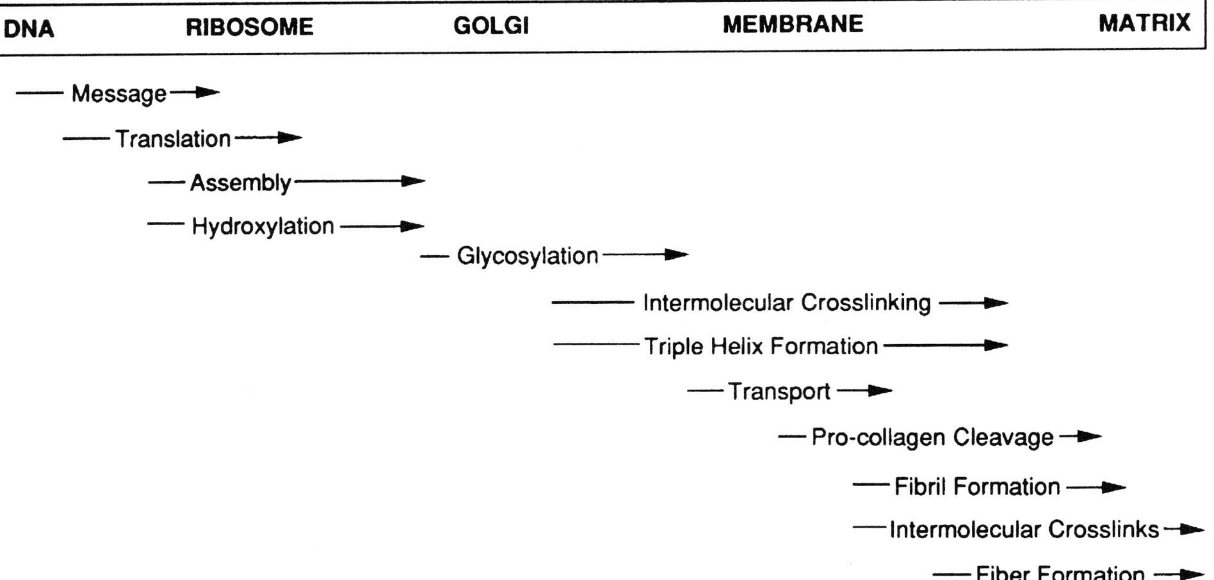

FIGURE 1–41. Collagen synthesis is accomplished at various intracellular sites. (From Mankin, H.J., and Brandt, K.D.: Biochemistry and metabolism of articular cartilage in osteoarthritis. In Osteoarthritis: Diagnosis and Medical/Surgical Management, Moskowitz, R.W., Howell, D.S., Goldberg, V.M., et al., eds., pp. 109–154. Philadelphia, WB Saunders, 1992; reprinted by permission.)

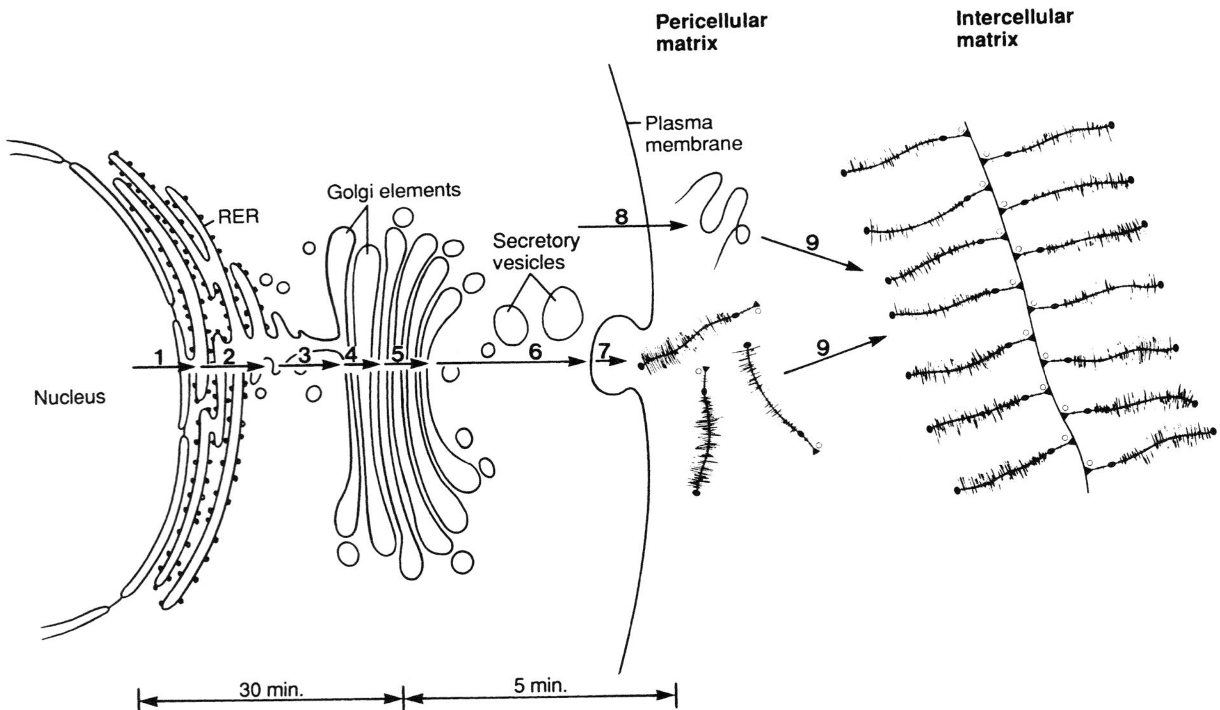

FIGURE 1–42. Synthesis and secretion of proteoglycan aggrecan molecules and link protein by a chondrocyte. *1*, Transcription of aggrecan and link protein genes to mRNA. *2*, Translation of mRNA to form protein core. *3*, Transportation. *4*, *5*, *cis* and medial *trans* Golgi compartments, respectively, where glycosaminoglycan chains are added to the protein core. *6*, Transportation to the secretory vesicles. *7*, Release into the extracellular matrix. *8*, *9*, Hyaluronate from the plasma membrane binds with the aggrecan and link proteins to form aggregates in the extracellular matrix. RER, rough endoplasmic reticulum. (From Simon, S.R., ed.: Orthopaedic Basic Science, 2nd ed., p. 13. Rosemont, IL, American Academy of Orthopaedic Surgeons, 1994; reprinted by permission.)

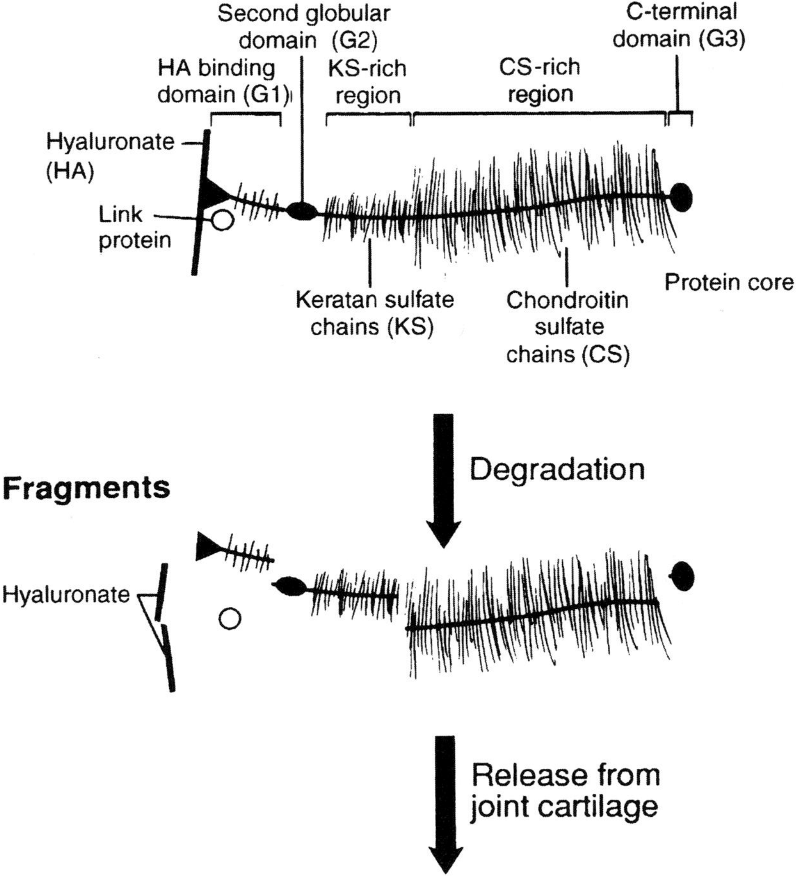

FIGURE 1–43. Proteoglycan degradation in articular cartilage. Cleavage of the G1 and G2 domains make the fragments nonaggregating. (From Simon, S.R., ed.: Orthopaedic Basic Science, 2nd ed., p. 14. Rosemont, IL, American Academy of Orthopaedic Surgeons, 1994; reprinted by permission.)

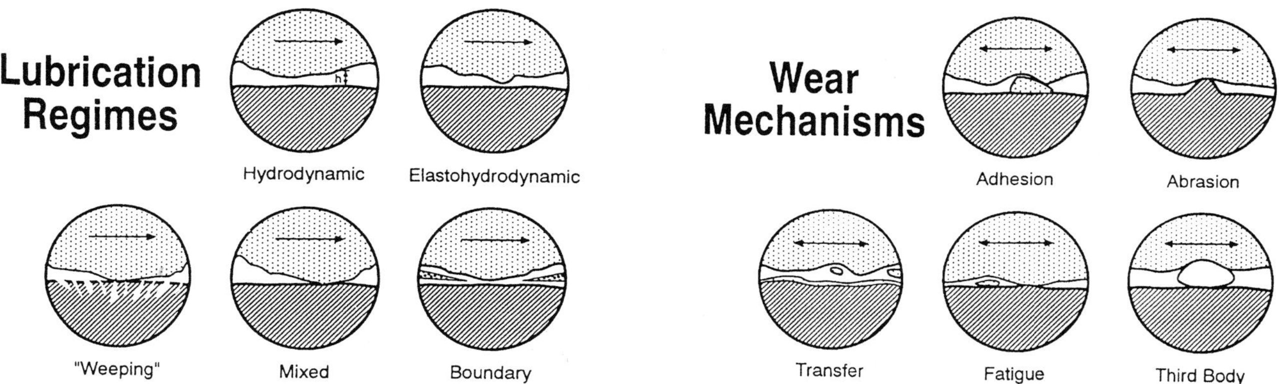

FIGURE 1–44. Types of lubrication. (From Simon, S.R., ed.: Orthopaedic Basic Science, 2nd ed., p. 465. Rosemont, IL, American Academy of Orthopaedic Surgeons, 1994; reprinted by permission.)

FIGURE 1–45. Wear mechanisms. (From Simon, S.R., ed.: Orthopaedic Basic Science, 2nd ed., p. 466. Rosemont, IL, American Academy of Orthopaedic Surgeons, 1994; reprinted by permission.)

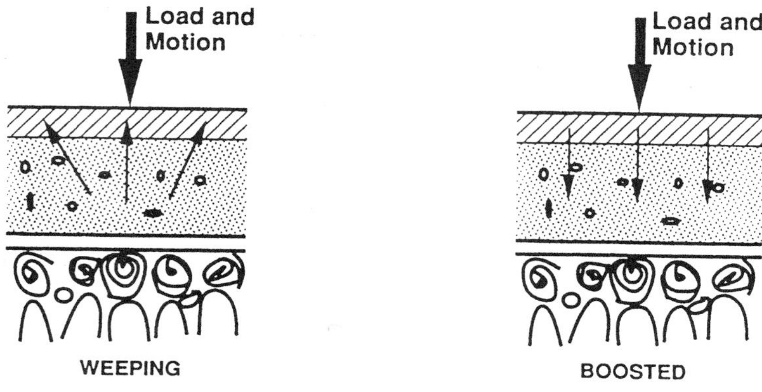

FIGURE 1–46. Fluid film lubrication models include Hydrodynamic, Squeeze-Film, Weeping, and Boosted. (From Mow, V.C., and Soslowsky, L.J.: Friction, lubrication, and wear of diarthrodial joints. In Basic Orthopaedic Biomechanics, Mow, V.C., and Hayes, W.C., eds., pp. 245–292. New York, Raven Press, 1991; reprinted by permission.)

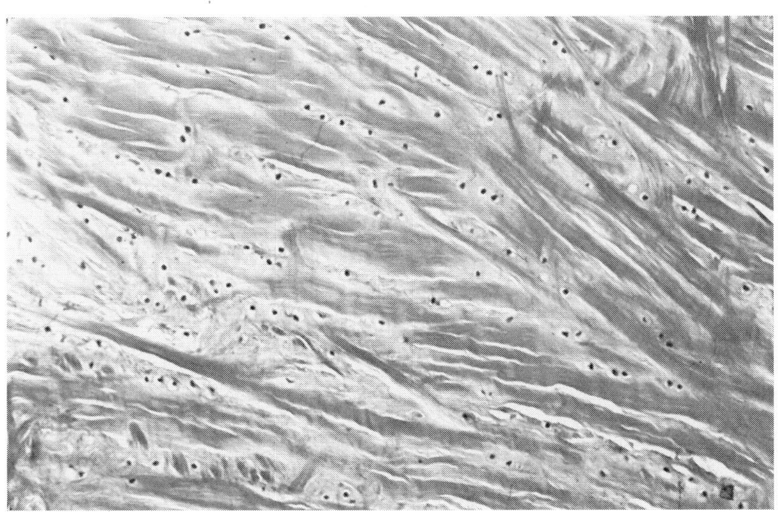

FIGURE 1–47. Histology of menisci.

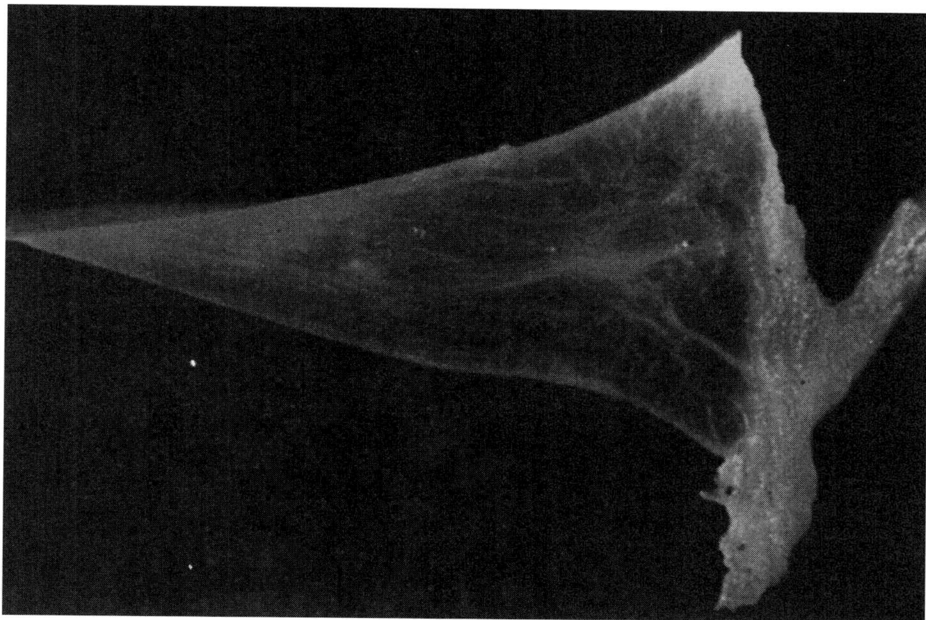

FIGURE 1–48. Meniscal cross section demonstrating radial orientation of fibrous ties within the meniscus. (From Arnoczky, S.P., and Torzelli, P.A.: The biology of cartilage. In Rehabilitation of the Injured Knee, Hunter, L.Y., and Funk, J.Y., Jr., eds., pp. 148–209. St. Louis, CV Mosby, 1984; reprinted by permission.)

cell type. **Synovial fluid** is made up of proteinase, collagenases, hyaluronic acid, and prostaglandins. It is an ultrafiltrate (dialysate) of blood plasma added to fluid produced by the synovial membrane; it contains no RBCs, clotting factors, or hemoglobin. It **nourishes articular cartilage through diffusion** and **lubricates via hydrodynamic** (fluid separates the surfaces under load), **boundary** (slippery surfaces), **weeping** (fluid shift to loaded areas), and **boosted** (fluid entrapment) mechanisms (Fig. 1–46). Synovial fluid exhibits **non-newtonian flow characteristics** (the viscosity coefficient μ is not a constant; the fluid is not linearly viscous), and its viscosity increases as the shear rate increases (*). **Lubricin,** a **glycoprotein,** is the key lubricating component of synovial fluid. **Hyaluronan molecules** in the knee become entangled and behave like an elastic solid during high strain activities (running, jumping) (*). Analysis of synovial fluid in disease processes is important and is discussed later in this section under Arthroses.

TABLE 1–17. HISTOLOGIC FEATURES OF MENISCUS

EXTRACELLULAR MATRIX

Collagen—**primarily type I collagen** (55–65% of dry weight)
- Also types II, III, V, and VI (5–10% of dry weight)
  - *Superficial layer*—mesh-like fibers oriented primarily radially
  - *Surface layer*—(deep to superficial layer) irregularly aligned collagen bundles
  - *Middle layer*—(deep) parallel circumferential fibers

Elastin (0.6% of dry weight)

Proteoglycans, Glycoproteins } (1–3% of dry weight)

Adhesive glycoproteins (fibronectin, thrombospondin)

CELLULAR COMPONENTS—synthesize and maintain extracellular matrix
—anaerobic metabolism (few mitochondria)

Chondrocytes, Fibroblasts } **Fibrochondrocytes:**

Fusiform cells
- Found in superficial layer
- Resemble fibroblasts and chondrocytes
- Found in lacunae
- Contain abundant endoplasmic reticulum (ER) and Golgi

Ovoid cells
- Found in surface and middle layer
- Contain abundant ER and Golgi

C. Meniscus—Functions to deepen the articular surface of a variety of synovial joints (acromioclavicular [AC], sternoclavicular [SC], glenohumeral, hip, knee) and thereby broaden the contact area to distribute the load such as on the tibial plateau (*). The meniscus of the knee is the focus of this section.
   1. Anatomy—Triangular semilunar structure. Peripheral border is attached to the joint capsule. Medial meniscus is semicircular; lateral meniscus is circular.
   2. Histology—Meniscus is composed of **fibrocartilage** (Fig. 1–47). There is an interlacing network of collagen fibers (Fig. 1–48), proteoglycans, glycoproteins, and cellular elements (Table 1–17).
   3. Innervation and Blood Supply—The peripheral two-thirds of the menisci is innervated by type I and type II nerve endings (concentrated in the anterior and posterior horns with few fibers in the meniscal body). **Menisci obtain blood supply from the geniculate arteries.** Vessels branch to form a circumferentially arranged plexus that supplies the **peripheral 25% of the meniscus** (*); the remaining portion of the meniscus receives its nutrition via diffusion. Peripheral meniscal tears in the vascularized region ("red zone") can heal via fibrovascular scar formation; more central tears in the avascular region ("white zone") cannot. The cell responsible for healing a meniscal tear is the **fibrochondrocyte** (*).

TEST QUESTIONS ON ARTICULAR TISSUES

TEST	QUESTION NUMBERS
1995 OSAE—Adult Reconstruction Hip/Knee	13
1995 OSAE—Pediatric Orthopaedics	
1995 OSAE—Sports Medicine	69
1994 OITE	176
1994 OSAE—Adult Spine	
1994 OSAE—Foot and Ankle	
1994 OSAE—M/S Trauma	
1993 OITE	1, 61
1993 OSAE—M/S Tumors and Diseases	
1993 OSAE—Shoulder and Elbow	
1992 OITE	
1992 OSAE—Adult Reconstruction Hip/Knee	
1992 OSAE—Pediatric Orthopaedics	
1992 OSAE—Sports Medicine	24, 110
1991 OITE	43
1991 OSAE—Adult Spine	
1991 OSAE—Anatomy and Imaging	
1991 OSAE—Foot and Ankle	
1991 OSAE—M/S Trauma	

II. Arthroses

A. Introduction—Arthroses can be classified into four basic groups based on their common characteristics. The arthritides are summarized in Table 1–18.
   1. Noninflammatory Arthritides—Include osteoarthritis, neuropathic arthropathy, acute rheumatic fever, and a variety of other entities (osteonecrosis, osteochondritis dissecans, osteochondromatosis).
   2. Inflammatory Arthritides—Include a wide range of rheumatologic disorders: rheumatoid arthritis, systemic lupus erythematosus, the spondyloarthropathies, and crystalline arthropathies. These disorders may be associated with an HLA complex region.
   3. Infectious Arthritides—Include pyogenic arthritis, tuberculous arthritis, fungal arthritis, and Lyme disease.
   4. Hemorrhagic Arthritides—include hemophilic arthropathy, sickle cell joint destruction, and pigmented villonodular synovitis.

B. Joint Fluid Analysis
   1. Noninflammatory Arthritides—200 WBCs with 25% PMNs; glucose and protein equal serum values; normal viscosity (high), straw color, firm mucin clot.
   2. Inflammatory Arthritides—2,000–75,000 WBCs with 50% PMNs; moderately decreased glucose (25 mg/dl lower than serum glucose); low viscosity, yellow-green, friable mucin clot. **Synovial**

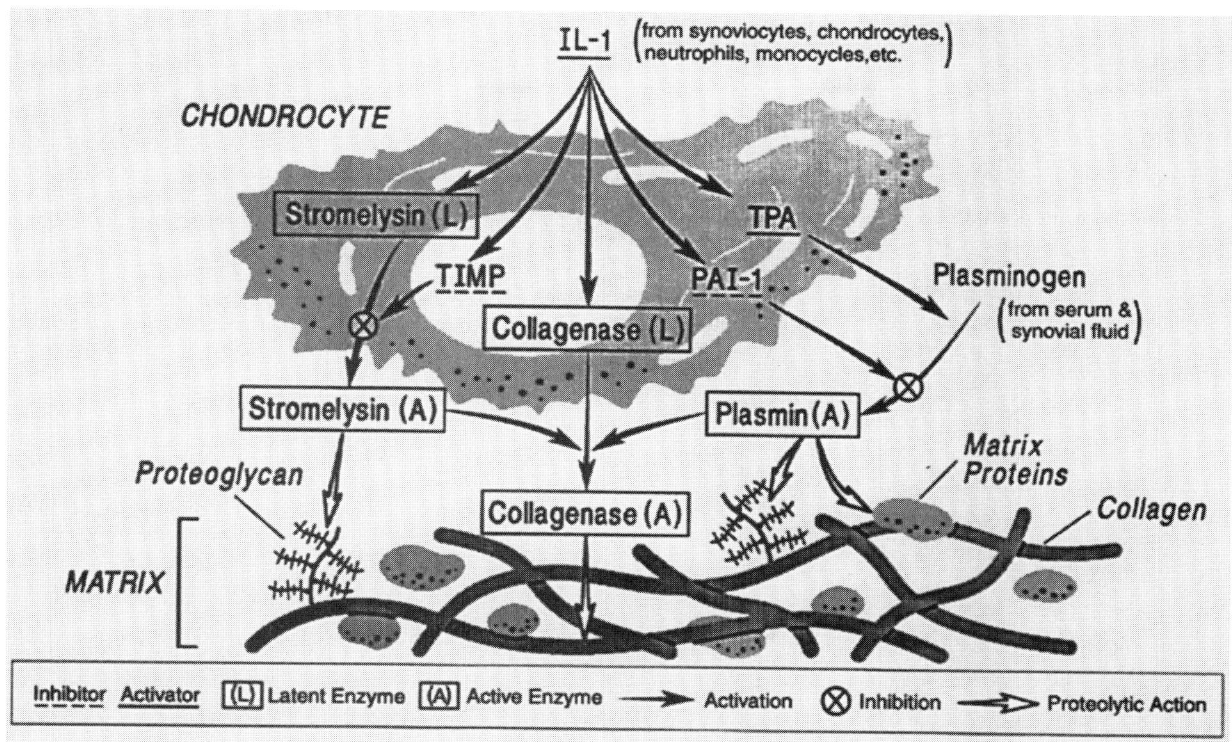

FIGURE 1–49. Enzyme cascade of interleukin-1-stimulated degradation of articular cartilage. (From Simon, S.R., ed.: Orthopaedic Basic Science, 2nd ed., p. 40. Rosemont, IL, American Academy of Orthopaedic Surgeons, 1994; reprinted by permission.)

fluid complement is decreased in rheumatoid arthritis and normal in ankylosing spondylitis.

3. Infectious Arthritides—More than 80,000 WBCs (*) with ≥75% PMNs, a positive gram stain (also positive cultures later), low glucose (more than 25 mg/dl **less** than serum values), opaque fluid, increased synovial lactate.

C. Noninflammatory Arthritides

1. Osteoarthritis (Degenerative Joint Disease) (see Table 1–18)—Although it is the **most common form** of arthritis, little is known about this disease.
   a. Etiology—On a cellular level, osteoarthritis (OA) may be a result of a failed attempt of chondrocytes to repair damaged cartilage. Osteoarthritic cartilage is characterized by **increased water content** (*) (in contrast to the decreased water content seen with aging), **alterations in proteoglycans** (shorter chains and decreased chondroitin/keratin sulfate ratio), **collagen abnormalities** (disrupted by collagenase), and **binding of proteoglycans to hyaluronic acid** (caused by the action of proteolytic enzymes from increased prostaglandin E (PGE) and decreased numbers of link proteins). In addition, the **rate of synthesis** of DNA, collagen, and proteoglycans is **increased in OA** (*). Levels of cathepsins B and D and the **metalloproteinases** (collagenase, gelatinase, stromelysin) are **increased in OA** cartilage. **Interleukin-1** (IL-1) enhances enzyme synthesis and may have a **catabolic effect** leading to cartilage degeneration; GAGs and polysulfuric acid may have a protective effect. The cascade of enzymes involved in the degradation of articular cartilage is shown in Figure 1–49. Cartilage degeneration is encouraged by shear stress and is prevented with normal compressive forces. Excessive stresses and inadequate chondrocyte response lead to degeneration. Genetic predisposition may be an important factor in OA. **Rapidly destructive OA** occurs most commonly in the hip and may mimic septic arthritis, rheumatoid arthritis, or ON (*).
   b. General Characteristics—From a larger perspective, OA can be primary (from an intrinsic defect, e.g., mechanical, immune, vascular, cartilage) or secondary (e.g., from trauma, infection, congenital disorders). Changes that occur in OA begin with deterioration and loss of the bearing surface, followed by development of osteophytes and breakdown of the osteochondral junction. Later, disintegration of the cartilage with subchondral microfractures exposes the bony surface. **Subchondral cysts** (from microfractures) and **osteophytes,** which are part of this process, along with "**joint space narrowing**" and eburnation of bone are demonstrated on radiographs. Microscopic changes include loss of superficial chondrocytes, **chondrocyte cloning** (>1 chondrocyte per lacunae), replication and breakdown of the tidemark, fissuring, cartilage destruction with eburnation of subchondral "pagetoid" bone, and other changes (Figs. 1–50, 1–51). Notable features on physical examination include decreased ROM and crepitus. **The knee is the most common joint af-**

TABLE 1–18. COMPARISON OF COMMON ARTHRITIDES

ARTHRITIS	AGE	SEX	SYM?	JOINTS	PHYSICAL EXAM
Noninflammatory					
Osteoarthritis	Old	M > F	Asym	Hip, knee, CMC	↓ROM, crepitus
Neuropathic	Old	M > F	Asym	Foot, ankle, LE	Effusion, unstable
ARF	Child	M = F	Asym	Mig; lg joints	Red tender joint, rash
Ochronosis	Adult	M = F	Asym	Lg joints/spine	↓ROM, locking
Inflammatory					
Rheumatoid	Young	F > M	Sym	Hands, feet	Ulnar dev, claw toes
SLE	Young	F > M	Sym	PIP, MCP, knee	Red swollen joint, rash
JRA	Child	F > M	Sym	Knee, multiple	Swollen joint, normal color
Relapsing polychondritis	Old	M = F	Sym	All joints	Eye, ear involved
Spondyloarthropathies					
AS	Young	M > F	Sym	SI, spine, hip	Rigid spine "chin on chest"
Reiter's syndrome	Young	M > F	Asym	Wt-bearing	Urethral D/C, conjunctivitis
Psoriatic	Young	M = F	Asym	DIP, small joints	Rash, sausage digit, pitting
Entereopathic	Young	M > F	Asym	Wt-bearing	Synovitis, GI manifestations
Crystal Deposition Disease					
Gout	Young	M > F	Asym	Great toe, LE	Tophi, red, swollen
Chondrocalcinosis	Old	M = F	Asym	Knee, LE	Acute swelling
Infectious					
Pyogenic	Any	M = F	Asym	Any joint	Red, hot, swollen
Tuberculous	Old	M > F	Asym	Spine, LE	Indolent, swelling
Lyme disease	Young	M = F	Asym	Any joint	Acute effusion
Fungal	Any	M > F	Asym	Any joint	Indolent
Hemorrhagic					
Hemophilic	Young	M	Asym	Knee, UE (elbow, shoulder)	↓ROM, swelling
Sickle cell	Young	M = F	Asym	Hip, any bone	Pain, ↓ROM
PVNS	Young	M = F	Asym	Knee, LE	Pain, synovitis

ARF, acute rheumatic fever; SLE, systemic lupus erythematosus; JRA, juvenile rheumatoid arthritis; AS, ankylosing spondylitis; PVNS, pigmented villonodular synovitis; Asym, asymmetric; Sym, symmetric; CMC, carpometacarpal; LE, lower extremity; Mig, migratory; Lg, large; PIP, proximal interphalangeal; MCP, metacarpophalangeal; SI, sacroiliac; DIP, distal interphalangeal; UE, upper extremity; ↓ROM, decreased range of motion; D/C, discharge; GI, gastrointestinal. ASO, antistreptolysin O; ESR, erythrocyte sedimentation rate; CRP, C-reactive protein; RF, rheumatoid factor; ANA, antinuclear antibody; alk. phos, alkaline phosphatase; CPK, creatine phosphokinase; B27, HLA (human leukocyte antigen) B27; Birefr., birefringent; WBC, white blood cells; PPD, purified protein

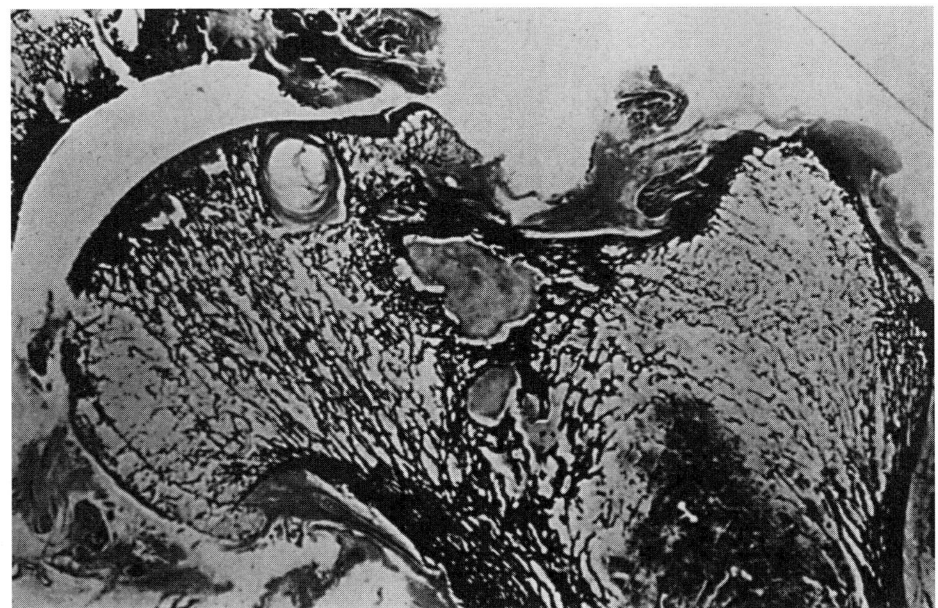

FIGURE 1–50. Macro section of osteoarthric human femoral head demonstrating subarticular cysts, sclerotic bone formation, and inferior femoral head osteophyte. (From Simon, S.R., ed.: Orthopaedic Basic Science, 2nd ed., p. 35. Rosemont, IL, American Academy of Orthopaedic Surgeons, 1994; reprinted by permission.)

LAB TESTS	RADIOGRAPHY	SYSTEMIC	TREATMENT
Nonspecific	Asym. narrowing, eburnation, cysts, osteophytes	None	NSAID, arthrodesis, osteotomy, TJA
For underlying disease	Destruction/heterotopic bone	None	Brace, **TJA contraindicated**
ASO titer	Usually normal	Eryth. marg, nodules, carditis	Symptomatic
Urine homogentisic acid	Destruction, disc calcification	Spondylosis	Supportive
ESR, CRP, RF	Sym. narrow, periart. resorp.	Pericard. & pulm. disease	Pyramid Tx, synovitis, reconstr. surg.
ANA	Less destruction	Cardiac, renal, pancytopenia	Drug therapy like RA
RF/ANA	Juxta-art. late, osteopenia	Iridocyclitis, rash	ASA; 75% remission
ESR	Normal	Ear, cardiac	Supportive, dapsone?
ESR, alk. phos., CPK, B27	SI arth, bamboo spine	Uveitis	PT, NSAID, osteotomy
ESR, WBC, B27	MT head erosion, periostitis	Urethritis, conjunctivitis, ulcer	PT, NSAID, sulfa?
ESR, B27	DIP—pencil in cup	Rash, conjunctivitis	Drug therapy as for RA
ESR, B27	Normal	Eryth. nodosum, pyoderma	Tx bowel disease, symptomatic
Uric acid; − Birefr. crystals	Soft tissue swell, erosions	Tophi, renal stones	Colchicine, indomethacin
+ Birefr. rod-shaped crystals	Art, fibrocart. calcified	Ochronosis, hyperparathyroidism, hypopthyroidism	Symptomatic, avoid surgery
WBC, ESR, bacteria	Joint narrowing (late)	Fever, chills, infection	I&D, IV antibiotics
PPD, AFB, cultures	Both sides, cysts	Lung, multiorgan	Antibiotics ± I&D
Culture, ELISA	Usually normal	ECM rash, neuro., cardiac	Penicillin, tetracycline
Special studies/cultures	Minimal changes	Immunocompromised	5-FU, amphotericin
PTT, factor VIII	Squared-off patella	Soft tissue bleeding	Support, synovectomy, TJA (unless + inhibitor)
Sickle prep.	Osteonecrosis	Infarcts, osteonecrosis	
Aspirate, biopsy	Juxtacortical erosion	None	Surgical excision

derivative; AFB, acid fact bacilli; ELISA, enzyme linked immunosorbent assay; PTT, partial thromboplastin time; resorp., resorption; arth, arthritis; MT, metatarsal; DIP, distal interphalangeal; Art, articular; fibrocart, fibrocartilage; Eryth. marg, erythema marginatum; Pericard., pericardial; Pulm, pulmonary; Eryth., erythema; ECM, erythema chronicum migrans; Neuro., neurologic; NSAID, nonsteroidal anti-inflammatory drugs; TJA, total joint arthroplasty; Tx, treat/treatment; reconstr. surg., reconstructive surgery; RA, rheumatoid arthritis; ASA, acetylsalicylic acid; PT, physical therapy; I&D, incise and drain; IV, intravenous; 5-Fu, 5-Fluorouracil.

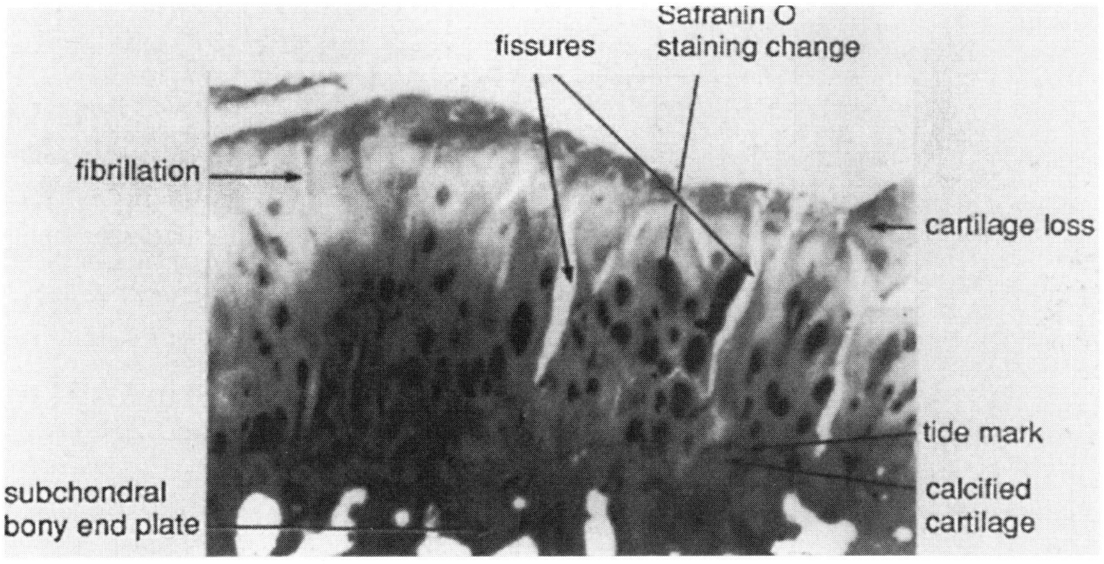

FIGURE 1–51. Low-power micrograph of osteoarthritis demonstrating fibrillation, fissures, and cartilage loss. (From Simon, S.R., ed.: Orthopaedic Basic Science, 2nd ed., p. 34. Rosemont, IL, American Academy of Orthopaedic Surgeons, 1994; reprinted by permission.)

fected. Treatment begins with supportive measures (e.g., activity modification, cane) and includes nonsteroidal anti-inflammatory drugs (NSAIDs; misoprostol [Cytotec] may lower GI complications via a prostaglandin effect). A variety of surgical procedures ranging from arthroscopic débridement to total joint arthroplasties (TJAs) may be useful in advanced cases that are resistant to nonoperative treatment.

c. Radiographic Characteristics—Osteophytes and "joint space" narrowing. Subchondral cysts from microfractures/bone repair.
   1. Hand—DIP, PIP, CMC.
   2. Hip—Superolateral involvement.
   3. Knee—Asymmetric involvement.

2. Neuropathic Arthropathy (Charcot Joint) (see Table 1–18)—An extreme form of OA caused by a disturbance in the sensory innervation of a joint. Causes include diabetes (foot), tabes dorsalis (lower extremity), **syringomyelia (most common cause of upper extremity neuropathic arthropathy** [most commonly in the shoulder and elbow]), Hansen's disease (second most common cause of neuropathic joints in the upper extremity), myelomeningocele (ankle and foot), congenital insensitivity to pain (ankle and foot), and other neurologic problems. A Charcot joint develops in 25% of patients with syringomyelia (80% of them involve the upper extremity). Typically seen in an older patient with an unstable, painless, swollen joint, who may present with hemarthrosis. These conditions may be confused with infection. Radiographs show advanced destructive changes on both sides of the joint, scattered "chunks" of bone embedded in fibrous tissue, joint distention by fluid, and heterotopic ossification. Treatment is focused on limitation of activity and appropriate bracing or casting (best indicator for discontinuation of cast is the skin temperature of the involved side compared to the uninvolved side) (*). **A Charcot joint is usually a contraindication for total joint arthroplasty and other orthopaedic hardware.**

3. Acute Rheumatic Fever (see Table 1–18) (sometimes included in the inflammatory group)—Formerly the most common cause of childhood arthritis, acute rheumatic fever has rarely been seen since the advent of antibiotics. Arthritis and arthralgias can follow untreated group A β-hemolytic strep infections and can present with acute onset of red, tender, extremely painful joint effusions. Systemic manifestations include carditis, erythema marginatum (painless macules with red margins usually involving the abdomen but never seen on the face), subcutaneous nodules (extensor surfaces of upper extremities), and chorea. The arthritis is **migratory** and typically involves **multiple large joints.** Diagnosis is based on **Jones criteria** (preceding strep infection with two major criteria [carditis, polyarthritis, chorea, erythema marginatum, subcutaneous nodules] or one major and two minor criteria [fever, arthralgia, prior rheumatic fever, elevated ESR, prolonged PR interval on EKG]). **Antistreptolysin O titers are elevated in 80% of affected patients.** Treatment includes penicillin and acetylsalicylic acid.

4. Ochronosis (see Table 1–18)—Degenerative arthritis resulting from **alkaptonuria,** a rare inborn defect of the **homogentisic acid oxidase enzyme system** (tyrosine and phenylalanine catabolism). Excess homogentisic acid is deposited in joints and then polymerizes (turns black) and leads to early degenerative changes. Homogentisic acid can also deposit in other tissues (e.g., the heart valves). These patients may also present with **black urine. Ochronotic spondylitis,** which usually occurs during the fourth decade of life, includes progressive degenerative changes and **disc space narrowing** and **calcification.**

5. Secondary Pulmonary Hypertrophic Osteoarthropathy—A clinical diagnosis. Involves a lung tumor mass, joint pain and stiffness, periostitis of long bones, and clubbing of fingers (*).

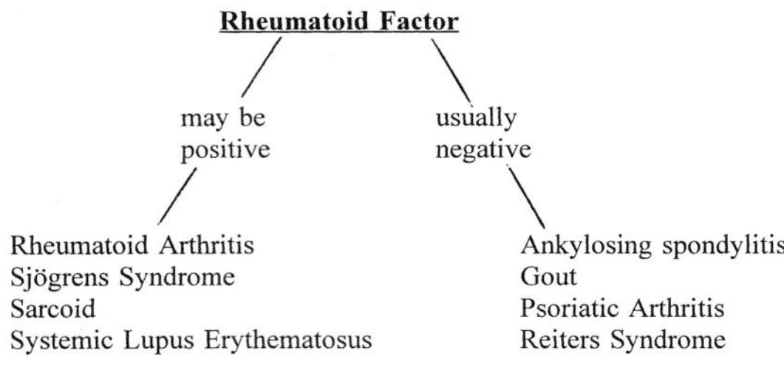

HLA - B27 +

Ankylosing Spondylitis
Reiters Syndrome
Psoriatic Arthritis
Inflammatory Bowel Disease with Spondylitis

ANA +

Systemic Lupus Erythematosus
Sjögrens Syndrome
Scleraderma

FIGURE 1–52. Commonly confused laboratory findings.

D. Inflammatory Arthritides—An overview of commonly confused laboratory findings in inflammatory and rheumatoid conditions is shown in Figure 1–52 and Table 1–19. As a general rule, inflammatory arthritides produce radiographic evidence of destruction on both sides of a joint.

1. Rheumatoid Arthritis (RA) (see Table 1–18)—The most common form of inflammatory arthritis, RA affects 3% of women and 1% of men. Several of the following diagnostic criteria, developed by the American Rheumatism Association, are required: morning stiffness, swelling, nodules, positive laboratory tests, and radiographic findings.
   a. Etiology—Unclear, but probably related to a cell-mediated immune response (T cell) that incites an inflammatory response initially against soft tissues and later against cartilage (chondrolysis) and bone (periarticular bone resorption). May be associated with an infectious etiology or an HLA focus (**HLA-DR4 and DW4**). Lymphokines and other inflammatory mediators initiate a destructive cascade that leads to joint destruction. RA cartilage is sensitive to PMN degradation and IL-1 effects (phospholipase A_2, PGE_2, and plasminogen activators). **Class II molecules** are involved in antigen–T lymphocyte interaction.
   b. General Characteristics—Usually an insidious onset of morning stiffness and polyarthritis.

TABLE 1–19. ASSOCIATIONS BETWEEN HUMAN LEUKOCYTE ANTIGEN ALLELES AND SUSCEPTIBILITY TO SOME RHEUMATIC DISEASES

DISEASE	HLA MARKER	FREQUENCY (%) IN PATIENTS (WHITES)	FREQUENCY (%) IN CONTROLS (WHITES)	RELATIVE RISK
Ankylosing spondylitis	B27	90	9	87
Reiter's syndrome	B27	79	9	37
Psoriatic arthritis	B27	48	9	10
Inflammatory bowel disease with spondylitis	B27	52	9	10
Adult rheumatoid arthritis	DR4	70	30	6
Polyarticular juvenile rheumatoid arthritis	DR4	75	30	7
Pauciarticular juvenile rheumatoid arthritis	DR8	30	5	5
	DR5	50	20	4.5
	DR2.1	55	20	4
Systemic lupus erythematosus	DR2	46	22	3.5
	DR3	50	25	3
Sjögren syndrome	DR3	70	25	6

From Nepom, B.S., and Nepom, G.T.: Immunogenetics and the rheumatic diseases. In Arthritis and Allied Conditions: A Textbook of Rheumatology, 12th ed., McCarty, D.J., ed. Philadelphia, Lea & Febiger, 1993, reprinted by permission.

Most commonly the hands (ulnar deviation and subluxation of MCPs) and feet (MTPs, claw toes, and hallux valgus) are affected early; but involvement of knees, elbows, shoulders, ankles, and neck is also common. **Subcutaneous nodules** are seen in 20% of RA patients (over their lifetime) and are strongly associated with positive serum rheumatoid factor (RF). Synovium and soft tissues are affected first, and only later are joints significantly involved. Pannus ingrowth denudes articular cartilage and leads to chondrocyte death. Laboratory findings include **elevated ESR and C-reactive protein** and a **positive RF titer (immunoglobulin M, IgM)** in most patients (at least 80%). Joint fluid assays can also demonstrate RF, decreased complement levels, and other helpful findings. Systemic manifestations can include rheumatoid vasculitis, pericarditis, and pulmonary disease (pleurisy, nodules, fibrosis). Popliteal cysts in rheumatoid patients (confirmed by ultrasonography) can mimic thrombophlebitis. **Felty syndrome is RA with splenomegaly and leukopenia. Still's disease is acute-onset RA with fever, rash, and splenomegaly. Sjögren syndrome** is an autoimmune exocrinopathy often associated with RA. Symptoms include **decreased salivary and lacrimal gland secretion** (keratoconjunctivitis sicca complex) and lymphoid proliferation. Treatment is aimed at controlling synovitis and pain, maintaining joint function, and preventing deformities. A multidisciplinary approach involving therapeutic drugs, physical therapy, and sometimes surgery is necessary to achieve these goals. A "pyramid" approach to drug therapy for rheumatoid patients involves beginning with NSAIDs and slowly progressing to antimalarials, remittive agents (methotrexate, suphasalazine, gold and penicillamine), steroids, cytotoxic drugs, and finally experimental drugs. This pyramidal approach has been challenged in recent years and a more aggressive approach (beginning with remittive agents [single or in combination]) has been advocated. Surgery includes synovectomy (rarely indicated—only if aggressive drug therapy fails), soft tissue realignment procedures (usually not favored because the deformity progresses), and various reconstructive procedures (at increased risk of infection following TJA) (**). Chemical and radiation synovectomy (dysprosium 165) can be successful if it is done early. Arthroscopic synovectomy, especially in the knee, has proved efficacy. After all forms of synovectomy, the synovium initially regenerates normally, but with time it degenerates back to rheumatoid synovial tissue. **Evaluation of the cervical (C-) spine with preoperative radiographs is important.**

c. Radiographic Characteristics—Include **periarticular erosions** and **osteopenia.** Areas commonly affected are the hand, wrist, and C-spine. In the hand and wrist the MCPs, PIPs, and carpal bones are commonly involved. In the knee, osteoporosis and erosions may be seen in all three compartments. **Protrusio acetabuli** is also common (*).

2. Systemic Lupus Erythematosus (SLE) (see Tables 1–18, 1–19)—Chronic inflammatory disease of unknown origin usually affecting women (especially African-Americans). Probably immune complex-related. Manifestations include fever, butterfly malar rash, pancytopenia, pericarditis, nephritis, and polyarthritis. **Joint involvement is the most common feature,** affecting more than 75% of SLE patients. Arthritis typically presents as acute, red, tender swelling of PIPs, MCPs, and the carpus, as well as the knees and other joints. **SLE is typically not as destructive as RA.** Treatment for SLE arthritis usually includes the same medications described for RA. Mortality due to SLE is usually related to renal disease. Differential diagnosis of SLE includes polymyositis and dermatomyositis, which also present with symmetric weakness ± a characteristic "heliotropic" rash of the upper eyelids. These patients are typically positive for antinuclear antibody (ANA) and HLA-DR3, and may be positive for RF.
3. Polymyalgia Rheumatica—A common disease of the elderly. Aching and stiffness of the shoulder

and pelvic girdle, associated with malaise, headaches, and anorexia, are common symptoms. Physical examination is usually unremarkable. Laboratory studies are notable for a markedly increased ESR, anemia, increased alkaline phosphatase, and increased immune complexes. This disorder, which **may be associated with temporal arteritis** (*) (often requiring biopsy for definitive diagnosis), is usually treated symptomatically, with steroid use for refractory cases.

4. Juvenile Rheumatoid Arthritis (JRA) (see Tables 1–18, 1–19)—JRA is also discussed in Chapter 2, Pediatric Orthopaedics. Three major types are recognized: systemic (20%), polyarticular (50%), and pauciarticular (30%). **Seronegative polyarticular JRA** is characterized by five or more joints being involved and is seen more frequently in girls. **Seropositive polyarticular JRA** also involves five or more joints, is seen more frequently in girls, exhibits a **positive RF** and **destructive degenerative joint disease (DJD),** and frequently **develops into adult RA** (*). **Early-onset pauciarticular JRA** involves four or fewer joints, is seen more frequently in girls, and is associated with **iridiocyclitis** (***). **Late-onset pauciarticular JRA** involves four or fewer joints and is seen in **boys** more commonly than girls. JRA may also be associated with an HLA focus (HLA-DR2, HLA-DR4, HLA-DR5, HLA-DR8, and HLA-B27 in boys). Treatment includes high-dose aspirin, only occasionally gold or remittive agents (refractory polyarticular), and frequent ophthalmologic examinations (with a slit lamp) for asymptomatic ocular involvement. The **most common joint affected in JRA is the knee** (66%) (*), followed by the ankle (25%), finger/wrist (33%), hip and C-spine (3%).
5. Relapsing Polychondritis (see Table 1–18)—Rare disorder associated with **episodic inflammation, diffuse self-limited arthritis,** and progressive cartilage destruction ± systemic vasculitis. The disorder typically involves the **ears** (thickening of the auricle); also seen are inflammatory eye disorders, tracheal involvement, hearing disorders, and sometimes cardiac involvement. It may be an autoimmune disorder (type II collagen affected). Treatment is supportive, although dapsone may have a role in the future.
6. Spondyloarthropathies/Enthesopathies (occur at ligament insertions into bone)—Characterized by **positive HLA-B27** (sixth chromosome, "D" focus) and a **negative RF** titer.
   a. Ankylosing Spondylitis (AS) (see Tables 1–18, 1–19)—Bilateral sacroiliitis ± acute anterior uveitis in an HLA-B27-positive man is diagnostic of this disease. There is insidious onset of back and hip pain during the third to fourth decade. The disease progresses for approximately 20 years (progressive **spinal flexion deformities**). Radiographic changes in the spine include **squaring of the vertebra, vertical syndesmophytes,** obliteration of sacroiliac (SI) joints, and "whiskering" of the enthesis. Ascending ankylosis of the spine usually begins in the thoracolumbar (TL-) spine, often causing the entire spine to become rigid. Spinal manifestations include the "chin on chest" deformity (which may require corrective osteotomy of the cervicothoracic junction), difficult **cervical fractures (associated with epidural hemorrhage [high mortality rate]),** and severe kyphotic deformities (corrected via posterior closing wedge osteotomy). Lower spinal deformities with hip flexion deformities and pain (plus **morning stiffness**) are often helped with bilateral total hip arthroplasty (THA). Protrusio acetabuli (medial displacement of the acetabulum beyond the radiographic teardrop) is also associated with AS and requires special THA techniques. The need for prophylaxis for heterotopic bone formation has been questioned in patients undergoing routine primary, noncemented THA. Initial treatment with physical therapy (PT) and NSAIDs (phenylbutazone is best but can cause bone marrow depression) may be helpful. AS is often associated with heart disease and pulmonary fibrosis. Other extraskeletal manifestations include: iritis; aortitis, colitis, arachnoiditis, amyloidosis, and sarcoidosis. Pulmonary involvement (restriction of chest excursion), hip involvement, and young age at onset of disease are prognostic indicators of poor outcomes in patients with AS.
   b. Reiter's Syndrome (see Tables 1–18, 1–19)—Classic presentation is a young man with the triad **urethritis, conjunctivitis,** and **oligoarticular arthritis.** Painless **oral ulcers, penile lesions,** and ulcers on the extremities, **palms,** and **soles** (**keratoderma blennorrhagicum**) (*), as well as plantar heel pain (**), are also common. The arthritis usually has an abrupt onset of asymmetric swelling and pain in weight-bearing joints. Recurrence is common and can lead to erosions of MT heads and calcaneal periostitis. Approximately **80% of patients are HLA-B27-positive** (**), and 60% with chronic disease have **sacroiliitis.** Treatment includes NSAIDs, PT, and possibly sulfa drugs in the future.
   c. Psoriatic Arthropathy (see Tables 1–18, 1–19)—Affects approximately 5–10% of patients with psoriasis. Many HLA loci may be involved, but HLA-B27 is found in 50% of patients with psoriatic arthritis. Many forms exist; most patients have the oligoarticular form, which (asymmetrically) affects the small joints of the hands and feet. **Nail pitting** (also fragmentation and discoloration), **"sausage" digits,** and **"pencil in cup" deformity** (*) (with **DIP** involvement) (**) are well recognized, which may progress to fusion. Treatment is similar to that for RA.
   d. Enteropathic Arthritis (see Tables 1–18, 1–19)—Approximately 10–20% of Crohn's disease and ulcerative colitis patients develop peripheral joint arthritis, and 5% or more develop axial disease. The arthritis is nondeforming and occurs more commonly in the large, weight-bearing joints. It usually presents as an acute monarticular synovitis that may precede any bowel symptoms. Enteropathic arthritis is HLA-B27-positive in approximately half of all affected individuals and is associated with AS in 10–15% of cases.
7. Crystal Deposition Disease
   a. Gout (see Table 1–18)—**Disorder of nucleic acid metabolism causing hyperuricemia, which leads to monosodium urate (MSU) crystal deposition in joints.** Inflammatory mediators (proteases, chemotactic factors, prostaglandins, leukotriene B_4, and free oxygen radicals) are activated by the crystals (**inhibited by colchicine**). Crystals also activate platelets, phago-

cytosis (**inhibited by phenylbutazone and indomethacin [Indocin]**), IL-1, and the complement system. Local polypeptides may inhibit the crystal inflammatory response via glycoprotein "coating." Recurrent attacks of arthritis, especially in men 40–60 years of age (usually in the lower extremity, **especially the great toe [podagra]**), crystal deposition in **tophi** (ear helix, eyelid, olecranon, Achilles; usually seen in chronic form), and renal disease/stones (2% Ca^{2+} versus normal 0.2%) are characteristic. The kidneys are the second most commonly affected organ. **Gout may be precipitated by chemotherapy for myeloproliferative disorders.** Radiographs may show soft tissue changes and **"punched-out" periarticular erosions** with **sclerotic overhanging borders. An elevated serum uric acid level is not diagnostic of gout; the demonstration of MSU crystals is mandatory for the diagnosis.** Demonstration of **thin, tapered intracellular crystals that are strongly negatively birefringent** (Fig. 1–53) in joint aspirate is essential for the diagnosis. **Initial treatment with indomethacin** (75 mg tid) is indicated followed by a rheumatology consult (patients with GI symptoms or a history of peptic ulcer disease should receive intravenous colchicine for acute attacks) (*). **Allopurinol** is used to lower serum uric acid levels in hyperuricemic patients with **chronic gout** and is given prior to chemotherapy for myeloproliferative disorders. **Colchicine** can be used for **prophylaxis following recurrent attacks.**

b. Chondrocalcinosis (see Table 1–18)—Caused by several disorders, including calcium pyrophosphate deposition disease (CPPD), ochronosis, **hyperparathyroidism,** hypothyroidism, and **hemochromatosis,** which lead to increased calcium ± pyrophosphate crystal deposition. **CPPD (a.k.a. pseudogout)** is a common disorder of pyrophosphate metabolism that occurs in older patients and occasionally causes acute attacks (again usually in the lower extremities, especially the **knee**). An amplification-loop hypothesis has been proposed. Chondrocalcinosis of knee menisci is often related to a previous knee injury (*). **Short, blunt (rhomboid-shaped) rods that are weakly positively birefringent** (Fig. 1–54) are demonstrated following aspiration (*). Radiographs show fine linear calcification in hyaline cartilage and more diffuse calcification of **menisci** (Fig. 1–55) **and other fibrocartilage** (acetabular labrum, triangular fibrocartilage complex). NSAIDs are often helpful. Intra-articular yttrium 90 injections have also been successful in chronic cases.

c. Calcium Hydroxyapatite Crystal Deposition Disease—Also associated with chondrocalcinosis and DJD. It is a **destructive arthropathy** commonly seen in the shoulder (causing cuff arthropathy, the "**Milwaukee shoulder**") and in the knee. Treatment is usually supportive. These crystals are too small to see with light microscopy.

d. Birefringence
   1. Positive—long axis of crystal is parallel to compensator (of microscope) and crystal is blue.
   2. Negative—long axis of crystal is parallel to compensator and crystal is yellow.

   (Note: when long axis of crystal is perpendicular to compensator, the rules of color are reversed).

E. Infectious Arthritides
   1. Pyogenic Arthritis (see Table 1–18)—Results from hematogenous spread or by extension of osteo-

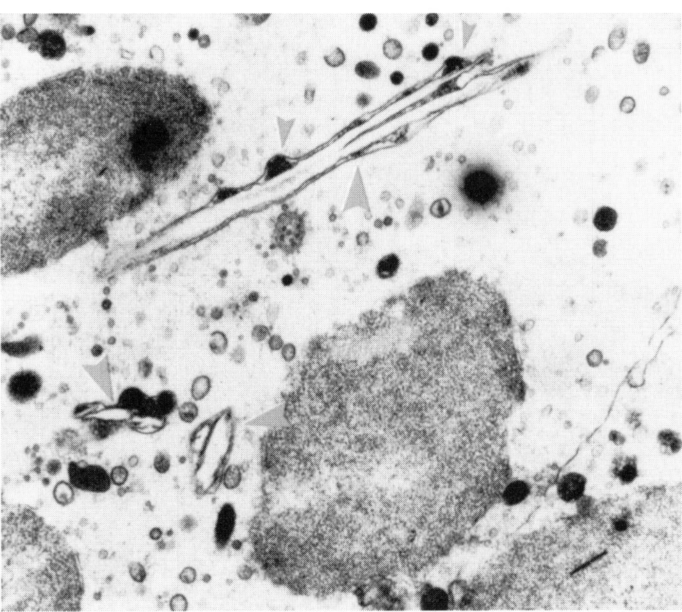

FIGURE 1–53. A neutrophil has phagocytosed a number of MSU crystals (large arrows). Although the crystals have almost completely dissolved, the outlines of the vacuoles remain, one still needle-shaped. Lysosomes discharge their contents directly into the phagosomes (small arrows). (Magnification, ×22,000; original magnification, ×31,250.) (From Krey, P.R. and Lazaro, D.M.: Analysis of Synovial Fluid. Summit, NJ, Ciba-Geigy, 1992, with permission.)

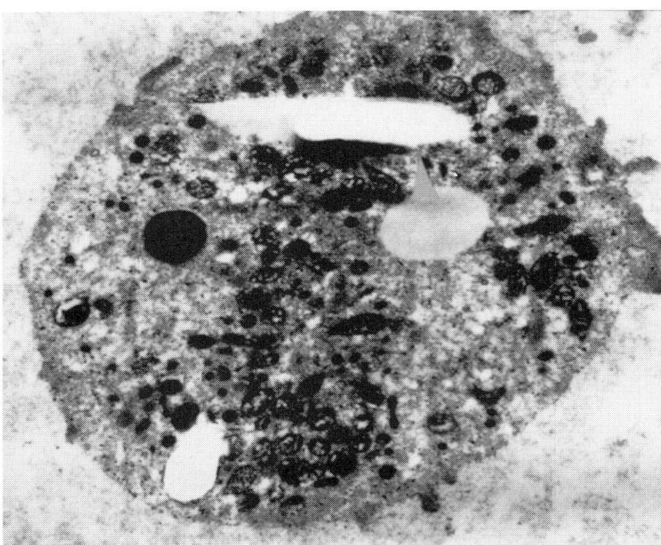

FIGURE 1–54. A synovial fluid leukocyte showing the outline of a phagocytosed CPPD crystal that has dissolved (arrow). (Magnification, ×14,000; original magnification, ×17,000.) (From Krey, P.R. and Lazaro, D.M.: Analysis of Synovial Fluid. Summit, NJ, Ciba-Geigy, 1992, with permission.)

myelitis. Commonly occurs in children and is discussed in detail in Chapter 2, Pediatric Orthopaedics. In adult patients, pyogenic arthritis occurs more commonly in individuals who are at risk, including IV drug abusers (especially SC and SI joints), sexually active young adults (gonococcal [intracellular diplococci], especially if seen with skin papules), diabetics (feet and lower extremities), and RA patients; it is also seen following trauma (fight bites, open injuries) or surgery (iatrogenic). Histology may demonstrate synovial hyperplasia, numerous PMNs, and cartilage destruction. Destruction of cartilage can be direct (proteolytic enzymes) or indirect (caused by pressure and lack of nutrition). Treatment includes I&D(s) and up to several weeks of antibiotics.

2. Tuberculous Arthritis (see Table 1–18)—The chronic granulomatous infection caused by *Mycobacterium tuberculosis* usually involves joints by **hematogenous spread.** The spine and lower extremities are most often involved, typically in Mexicans and Asians. It is 80% monarticular. Radiographically, tuberculous arthritis causes changes on both sides of the joint. Diagnosis is helped with a **positive PPD,** demonstration of **acid-fast bacilli** and **"rice bodies" (fibrin globules) in joint fluid,** positive cultures (may take several weeks), and characteristic radiographs (subchondral osteoporosis, cystic changes, notch-like bony destruction at the edge of the joint, and joint space narrowing with osteolytic changes on both sides of the joint). Histology may demonstrate **characteristic granulomas with Langerhans giant cells.** Treatment includes I&D and long-term antibiotics.
3. Fungal Arthritis (see Table 1–18)—More common in neonates, **AIDS patients,** and drug users. Pathogens include *Candida albicans.* KOH preparations

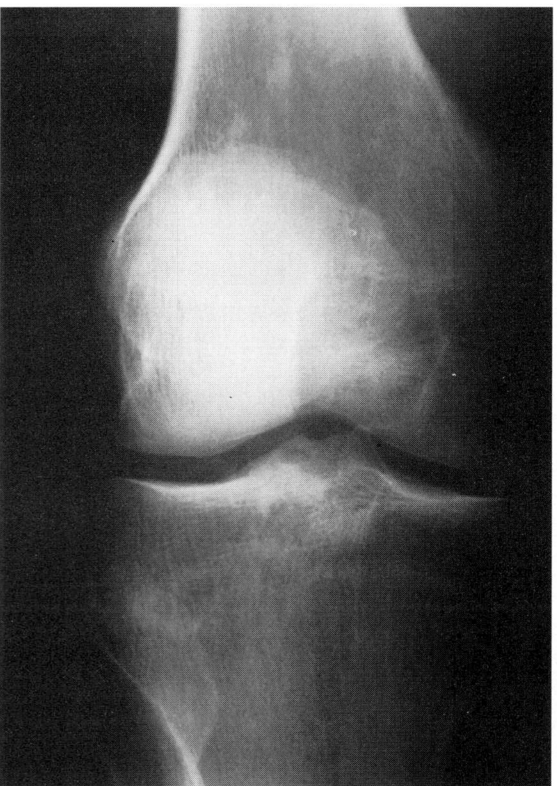

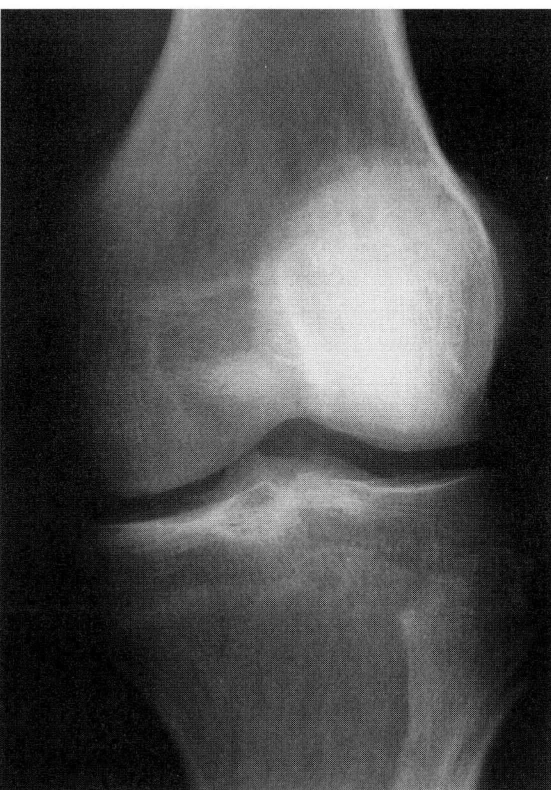

FIGURE 1–55. Knee radiographs demonstrating calcium pyrophosphate deposition (pseudogout) in a meniscus. (Courtesy of G. William Woods, M.D. Fondren Orthopedic Group L.L.P. Texas Orthopedic Hospital, Houston, Texas.)

of synovial fluid are helpful, as cultures require prolonged incubation. Arthritis can be treated with 5-flucytosine. Blastomycosis, coccal infections and other fungal infections often require treatment with amphotericin (this treatment is sometimes administered intraarticularly with fewer side effects).

4. Lyme Disease (see Table 1–18)—Acute, self-limited joint effusions (especially in the shoulder and knee) that recur at frequent intervals. It is caused by the **spirochete *Borrelia burgdorferi*** (*Borrelia garinii* in Europe), which is transmitted by tick bites (*Ioxodes*) endemic in half of the United States. Transmission of *B. burgdorferi* occurs in approximately 10% of bites by infected ticks. Sometimes called the "great mimicker." Systemic signs may include a characteristic "bull's-eye" rash (**erythema chronicum migrans**) and neurologic (Bell's palsy is common) or cardiac symptoms. The disease occurs in three stages (I—rash, II—neurologic symptoms, III—arthritis). **Immune complexes and cryoglobulins accumulate in the synovial fluid** of affected individuals. Diagnosis is confirmed by **ELISA testing,** which should be sought in endemic areas after a gram stain and joint cultures of an infectious aspirate show no organisms. Treatment is with tetracycline/doxycycline, amoxicillin, or cefuroxime.

F. Hemorrhagic Effusions

1. Hemophilic Arthropathy (see Table 1–18)—**X-linked recessive, factor VIII deficiency** (hemophilia A—classic or factor IX deficiency; hemophilia B—Christmas disease) associated with repeated hemarthrosis due to minor trauma, leading to synovitis, cartilage destruction (enzymatic processes), and joint deformity. Severity of disease is related to the degree of factor deficiency (mild, 5–25% levels; moderate, 1–5% levels; severe, 0–1% levels). Repeated episodes of hemarthrosis lead to replacement of the normal joint capsule with dense scar tissue. The **knee is most commonly involved,** followed by the elbow, ankle, shoulder, and spine. Joint swelling, decreased ROM, and pain are characteristic. **A joint aspirate should be obtained to rule out a concomitant infection.** Radiographs later in the disease process may demonstrate a **"squared off" patella (Jordan's sign** [also seen in JRA]), widening of the intercondylar notch, and enlarged femoral condyles that appear to "fall off" the tibia. Ultrasonography can be used to diagnose and follow intramuscular bleeding episodes. **Iliacus hematomas can cause femoral nerve palsies.** Management includes correction of factor levels, splints, compressive dressings, bracing, and analgesics. Occasionally, steroids are helpful. Surgical management includes synovectomy (for recurrent hemarthroses and synovial hypertrophy refractory to conservative treatment), TJA (for end-stage arthropathy), or arthrodesis (especially for the ankle). Synovectomy has been shown to reduce the incidence of recurrent hemarthroses (less pain and swelling) (*). **The presence of an inhibitor (15% incidence in hemophiliacs) is a relative contraindication to any elective surgical procedure.** Factor levels should be maintained near 100% during the first postoperative week and at 50–75% during the second week. There is a high incidence of HIV positivity in hemophiliacs (up to 90%).

2. Sickle Cell Disease—Hemoglobin SS is found in 1% of North American blacks and leads to local infarction due to capillary stasis. **Dactylitis** with MC/MT periosteal new bone formation, bone infarcts, osteomyelitis (***Salmonella* and *Staphylococcus* are most common**) (*). ESR is usually falsely low. ON (especially of the femoral head, which leads to joint destruction and may require THA) is common in sickle cell patients. Results of TJA are poor owing to ongoing negative bone remodeling. *Salmonella* spread can come from a gallbladder infection.

3. Pigmented Villonodular Synovitis (PVNS) (see Table 1–18)—Synovial disease with **exuberant proliferation of villi and nodules.** Pain, swelling, synovitis, and a **rust-colored effusion** are common. The **knee is the most frequent site of PVNS,** with occasional involvement of the hip and ankle. Radiographs show juxtacortical erosions. Histologic features include pigmented histiocytes, foam cells (lipid-laden histiocytes), and multinucleated giant cells. Treatment is surgical excision of the affected synovium.

Test Questions continued on following page

TEST QUESTIONS ON ARTHROSES

TEST	QUESTION NUMBERS
1995 OSAE—Adult Reconstruction Hip/Knee	11, 17, 80
1995 OSAE—Pediatric Orthopaedics	31, 52
1995 OSAE—Sports Medicine	
1994 OITE	12, 52, 109, 113, 124
1994 OSAE—Adult Spine	
1994 OSAE—Foot and Ankle	30, 64, 71, 72, 100, 101, 125
1994 OSAE—M/S Trauma	32
1993 OITE	71, 114, 174, 209
1993 OSAE—M/S Tumors and Diseases	13, 49, 51, 55, 56, 70, 85, 96, 97
1993 OSAE—Shoulder and Elbow	93
1992 OITE	133, 230, 232
1992 OSAE—Adult Reconstruction Hip/Knee	11, 20
1992 OSAE—Pediatric Orthopaedics	
1992 OSAE—Sports Medicine	
1991 OITE	61, 64, 246
1991 OSAE—Adult Spine	40, 78, 87
1991 OSAE—Anatomy and Imaging	
1991 OSAE—Foot and Ankle	1, 7, 35, 64, 80
1991 OSAE—M/S Trauma	

SECTION 3

Neuromuscular and Connective Tissues

I. Skeletal Muscle and Athletics

A. Noncontractile Elements (Fig. 1–56)
1. Muscle Body Epimysium—Surrounds individual muscle bundles; **perimysium** surrounds muscle fascicles, and **endomysium** surrounds individual fibers.
2. Myotendon Junction—The weak link in the muscle, **often the site of tears,** especially with eccentric contraction. Sarcolemma filaments interdigitate with basement membrane (type IV collagen) and tendon tissue (type I collagen). Involution of muscle cells in this region gives maximum surface area for attachment. Linking proteins and specialized membrane protein (vetroneotin) are also present.
3. Sarcoplasmic Reticulum—Stores calcium in intracellular membrane-bound channels, including T-tubules (which go to each myofibril) and cisternae (small storage areas) (Fig. 1–57).

B. Contractile Elements (Fig. 1–58)—Derived from myoblasts. Each **muscle** is composed of several muscle **bundles,** which in turn contain muscle **fibers** (the basic unit of contraction); fibers are composed of **myofibrils** (1–3 μm in diameter and 1–2 cm long), a collection of **sarcomeres.** A muscle fiber is an elongated cell. Fibers are most commonly arranged in parallel bundles but can run oblique to one another, as in a bipennate muscle. The architectural arrangement of muscle fibers is specific for the specific function required. **Maximal force production is related to the physiologic cross-sectional area of a muscle.**
1. Sarcomere—Composed of thick and thin filaments in an intricate arrangement that allows fibers to slide past each other. Thick filaments are composed of **myosin** and thin filaments are com-

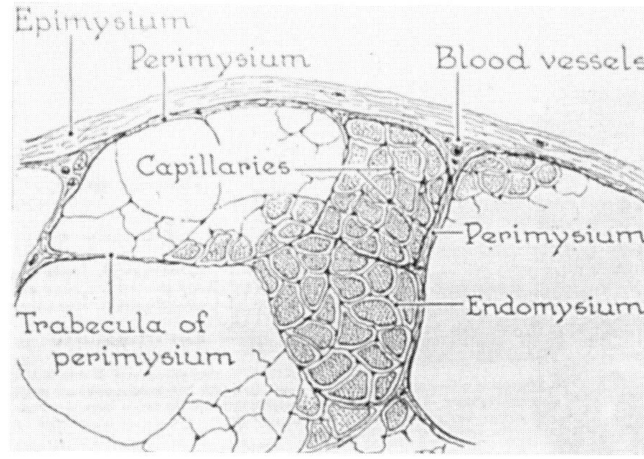

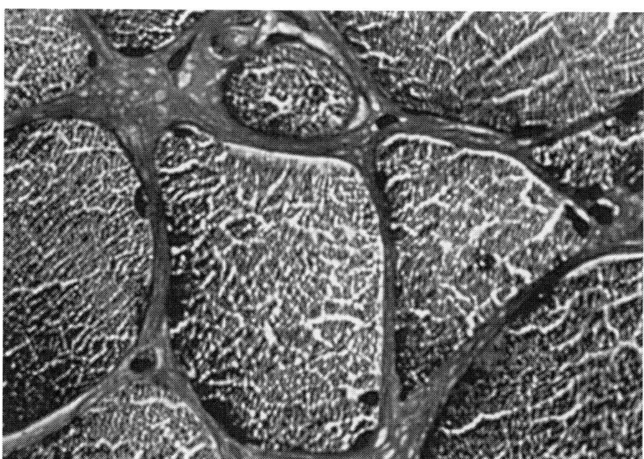

FIGURE 1–56. Muscle; noncontractile elements. (From Orthopaedic Science Syllabus, p. 27. Park Ridge, IL, American Academy of Orthopaedic Surgery, 1986; reprinted by permission.)

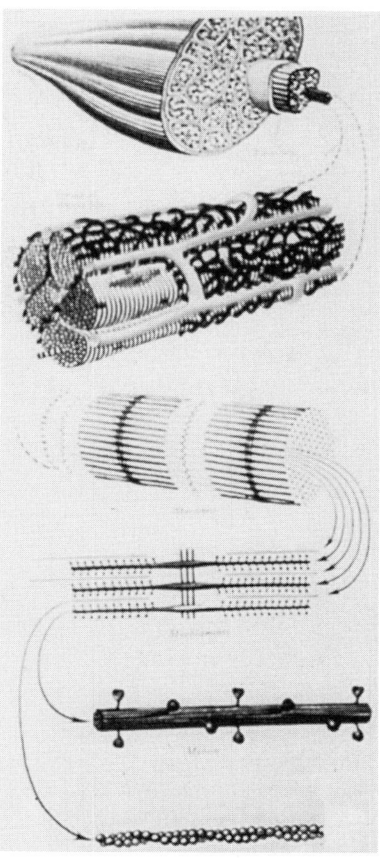

FIGURE 1–58. Muscle microstructure. (From Orthopaedic Science Syllabus, p. 27. Park Ridge, IL, American Academy of Orthopaedic Surgery, 1986; reprinted by permission.)

posed of **actin.** The thin filaments also have **troponin (C)** and **tropomycin** on their surface. The sarcomere is arranged into bands and zones, as shown in Figures 1–59 and 1–60. The **H zone** contains only thick (myosin) filaments, and the **I band is composed solely of thin (actin) filaments.** Thin filaments are attached to the **Z line** and extend across I bands, partially into the A band.

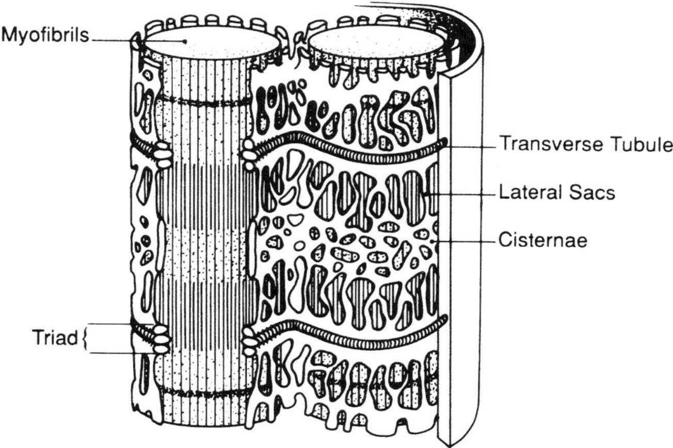

FIGURE 1–57. Sarcoplasmic reticulum. Action potentials travel down the transverse tubules causing calcium release from the outer vesicles. (From Simon, S.R., ed.: Orthopaedic Basic Science, 2nd ed., p. 94. Rosemont, IL, American Academy of Orthopaedic Surgeons, 1994; reprinted by permission.)

C. Action—Stimulus for a muscle contraction originates in the cell body of a nerve and is carried toward the neuromuscular junction via an electrical impulse that is propagated down the entire length of the axon (from the spinal cord to skeletal muscle). Once the impulse reaches the **motor end plate** (a specialized synapse formed between muscle and nerve) (Fig. 1–61), acetylcholine (stored in presynaptic vesicles) is released. Acetylcholine then diffuses across the **synaptic cleft** (50 nm) to bind a specific receptor on the muscle membrane (myasthenia gravis is a shortage of acetylcholine receptors). This binding triggers depolarization of the sarcoplasmic reticulum, releasing calcium. Calcium binds to troponin (on the thin filaments), causing them to change the position of tropomycin (also on the thin filaments) and exposing the actin filament. Actin–myosin crossbridges form; and with the breakdown of ATP, the thick and thin filaments slide past one another, contracting the muscle (Fig. 1–62). Table 1–20 shows the effects of some commonly used agents that affect impulse transmission.

D. Types of Muscle Contraction—An **isotonic contraction (dynamic strength)** allows constant tension (re-

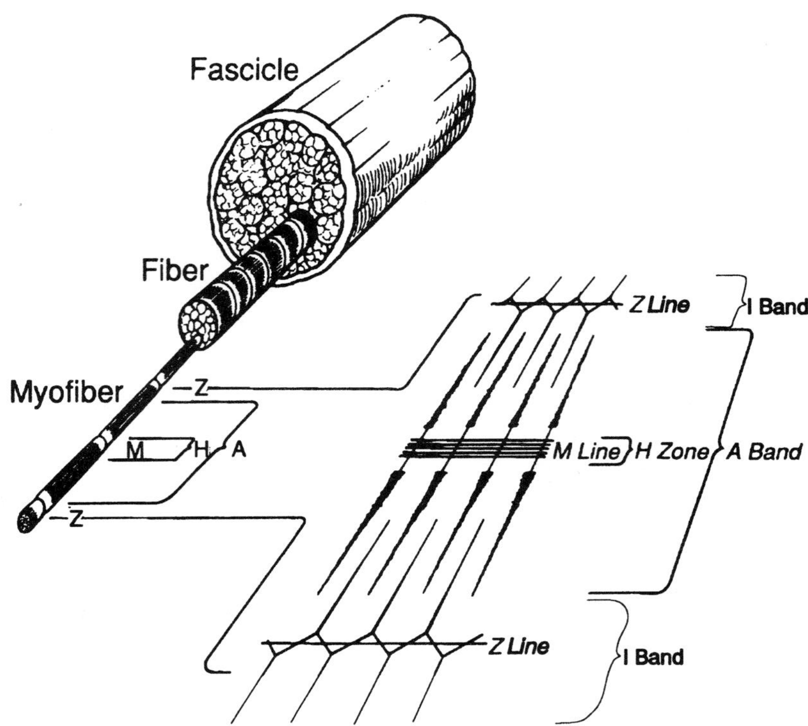

FIGURE 1–59. Muscle structure. (From Simon, S.R., ed.: Orthopaedic Basic Science, 2nd ed., p. 91. Rosemont, IL, American Academy of Orthopaedic Surgeons, 1994; reprinted by permission.)

sistance) through a range of motion (using free weights). During a **concentric contraction,** the muscle shortens, and its tension is proportional to the externally applied load (*). During an **eccentric contraction,** the muscle lengthens (**), and the internal force is less than the external force (**); eccentric contractions have the **greatest potential for high muscle tension** (*) **and muscle injury** (*). During an **isometric contraction (static strength),** tension is generated, but the muscle does not shorten. **Isokinetic contractions** (dynamic strength) occur when maximal tension is generated in a muscle contracting at a **constant speed** over the full range of motion (not eccentric) (*). Isokinetic exercises require special equipment.

E. Types of Muscle Fiber—Include fast and slow twitch; comprise individual motor units (motor nerve and fibers innervated). Table 1–21 shows the characteristics of type I and type II muscle fibers.
   1. Slow Twitch (ST) (Type I; Oxidative) Fibers—**Aerobic** and therefore have **more mitochondria,** enzymes, and triglycerides (energy source). They have low concentrations of glycogen and glycolytic enzymes (ATPase). A helpful

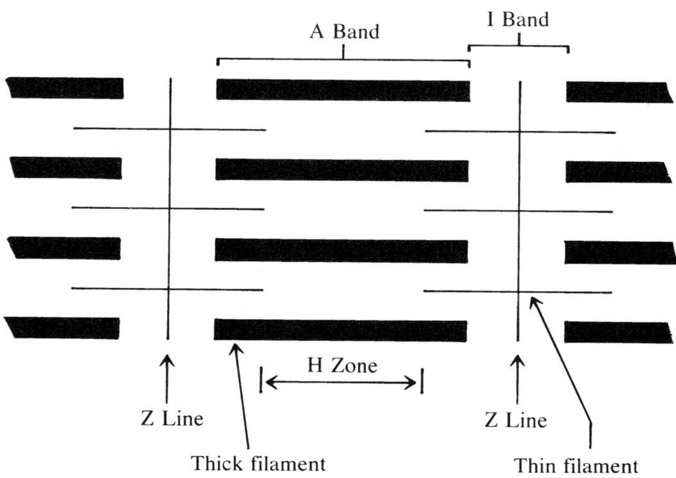

FIGURE 1–60. Sarcomere nomenclature.

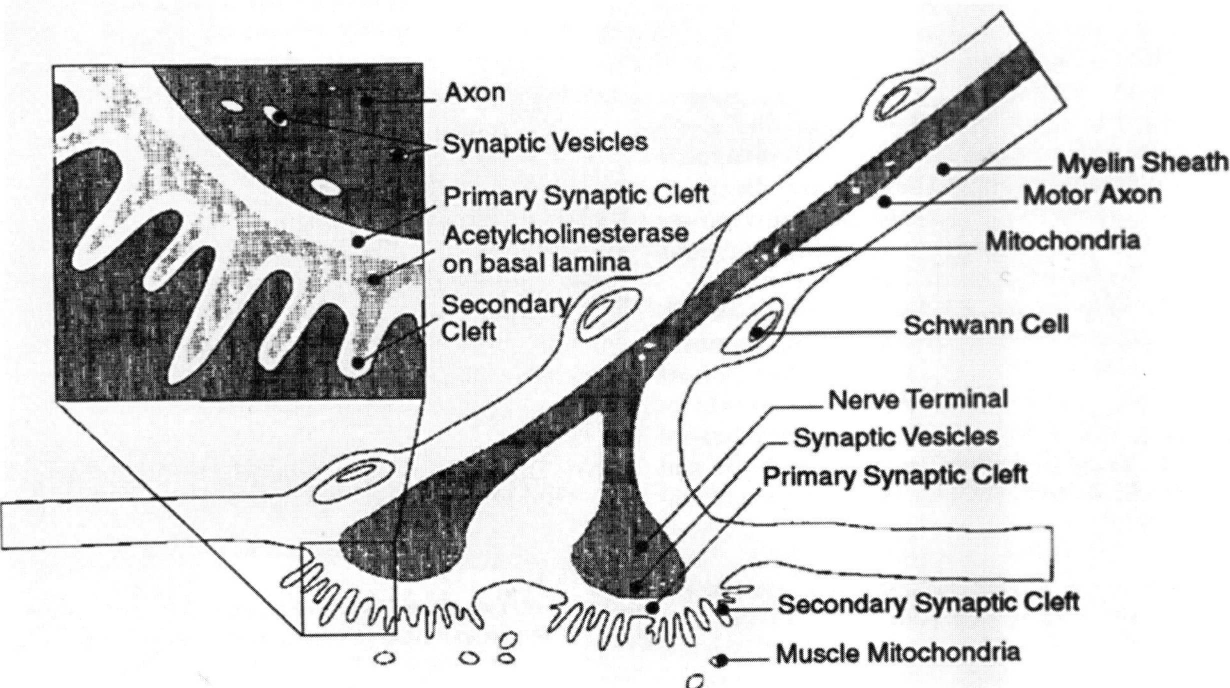

FIGURE 1–61. Motor end plate. (From Simon, S.R., ed.: Orthopaedic Basic Science, 2nd ed., p. 93. Rosemont, IL, American Academy of Orthopaedic Surgeons, 1994; reprinted by permission.)

way to remember: "**slow red ox**" (slow twitch fibers are slower, are typically more vascularized, and undergo aerobic oxidations). Type I fibers specialize in **endurance activities.** Slow twitch fibers are the first lost without rehabilitation.

2. Fast Twitch (FT) (Type II; Glycolytic ["White"(*)]) Fibers—Contract more quickly, and their motor units are larger and stronger than ST fibers (increased ATPase). However, they do it at the expense of efficiency and are **anaerobic.** Type IIA and IIB fibers are associated with sprinting (ATP-CP system) (**). These fibers are specialized for fine motor skills. Subtypes of type II fibers are based on myosin heavy chains.

F. Metabolism—Figures 1–63 and 1–64 illustrate the aerobic system (for glycolysis, fatty acid oxidation, and Krebs cycle) and provide a summary of ATP production via anaerobic and aerobic mechanisms.

G. Athletes and Training—The distribution of FT versus ST fibers is genetically determined; however, different types of training can selectively improve these fibers. **Endurance athletes typically have a higher percentage of ST fibers,** whereas **athletes participating in "strength"-type sports (and sprinters) have more FT fibers. Training for endurance** sports consists in decreased tension and increased repetitions, which help increase the efficiency of the ST fibers and increase the number of mitochondria, capillary density, and oxidative capacity. **Training for strength** consists in increasing tension and decreasing repetition, which leads to an increased number of myofibrils/fibers and hypertrophy (increased cross-sectional area) (*) of fast twitch (type II) fibers. Either form of training slows the increase of lactate in response to exercise. Isokinetic exercises produce more strength gains than do isometric exercises. Iso-

TABLE 1–20. AGENTS THAT AFFECT NEUROMUSCULAR IMPULSE TRANSMISSION

AGENT	SITE OF ACTION	MECHANISM	EFFECT
Nondepolarizing drugs (curare, pancuronium, vecuronium)	Neuromuscular junction	Competitively binds to acetylcholine receptor to block impulse transmission	Paralytic agent (long term)
Depolarizing drugs (succinylcholine)	Neuromuscular junction	Binds to acetylcholine receptor to cause temporary depolarization of muscle membrane	Paralytic agent (short term)
Anticholinesterases (neostigmine, edrophonium)	Autonomic ganglia	Prevents breakdown of acetylcholine to enhance its effect	Reverses effect of nondepolarizing drugs; muscarinic effects (bronchospasm, bronchorrhea, bradycardia)

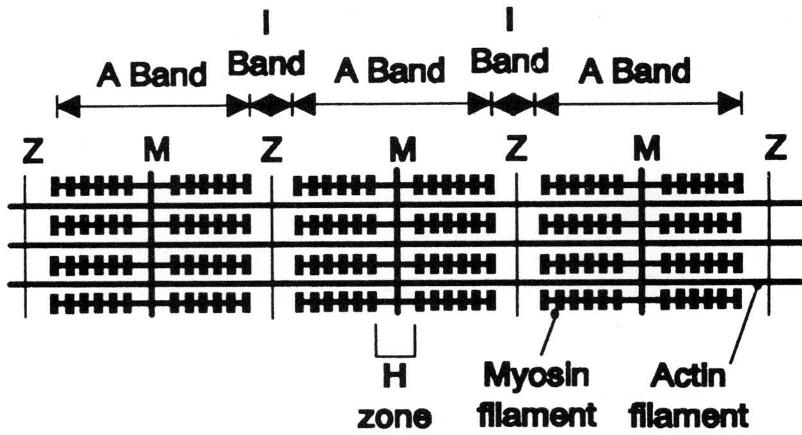

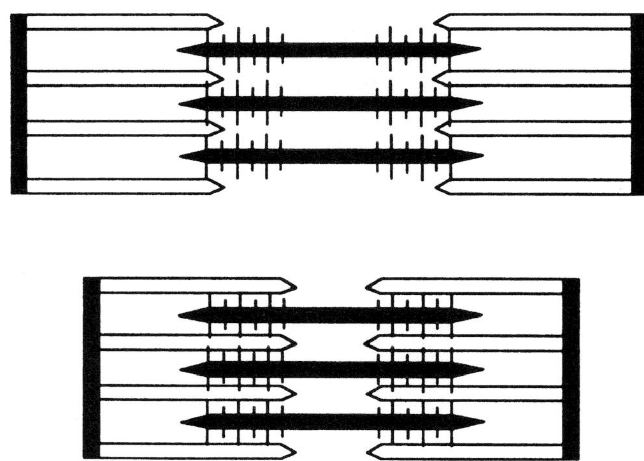

FIGURE 1–62. Sliding of the thick and thin filaments occurs when a muscle is stretched. (Adapted from Carlson, F.D., and Wilkie, D.R.: Muscle Physiology. Englewood Cliffs, NJ, Prentice-Hall, 1974.)

tonic exercises produce a uniform increase in strength throughout the ROM of a joint. Oxygen consumption (VO_2) is an important consideration in athletic training. **Closed chain rehabilitation exercise** is defined as extremity loading with the most distal part of the extremity stabilized or not moving (*); it places less stress on the anterior cruciate ligament (ACL) (*). **Weight reduction** with fluid and food restriction (wrestler, boxers, and jockeys trying to "make weight") is associated with reduced cardiac output (*). **Anabolic steroids** (******) cause increased muscle strength, testicular atrophy, oligospermia, azoospermia, gynecomastia, striae, cystic acne, alopecia (irreversible), liver tumors, increased LDL, decreased HDL, and abnormal liver isoenzymes (LDH). **Aerobic conditioning (cardiorespiratory fit-**

TABLE 1–21. CHARACTERISTICS OF HUMAN SKELETAL MUSCLE FIBER TYPES

CHARACTERISTIC	TYPE I	TYPE IIA	TYPE IIB
Other names	Red, slow twitch (ST) Slow oxidative (SO)	White, fast twitch (FT) Fast oxidative glycolytic (FOG)	Fast glycolytic (FG)
Speed of contraction	Slow	Fast	Fast
Strength of contraction	Low	High	High
Fatigability	Fatigue-resistant	Fatigable	Most fatigable
Aerobic capacity	High	Medium	Low
Anaerobic capacity	Low	Medium	High
Motor unit size	Small	Larger	Largest
Capillary density	High	High	Low

From Simon, S.R.: Orthopaedic Basic Science, 2nd ed., p. 100. Rosemont, IL, American Academy of Orthopaedic Surgeons, 1994; reprinted by permission.

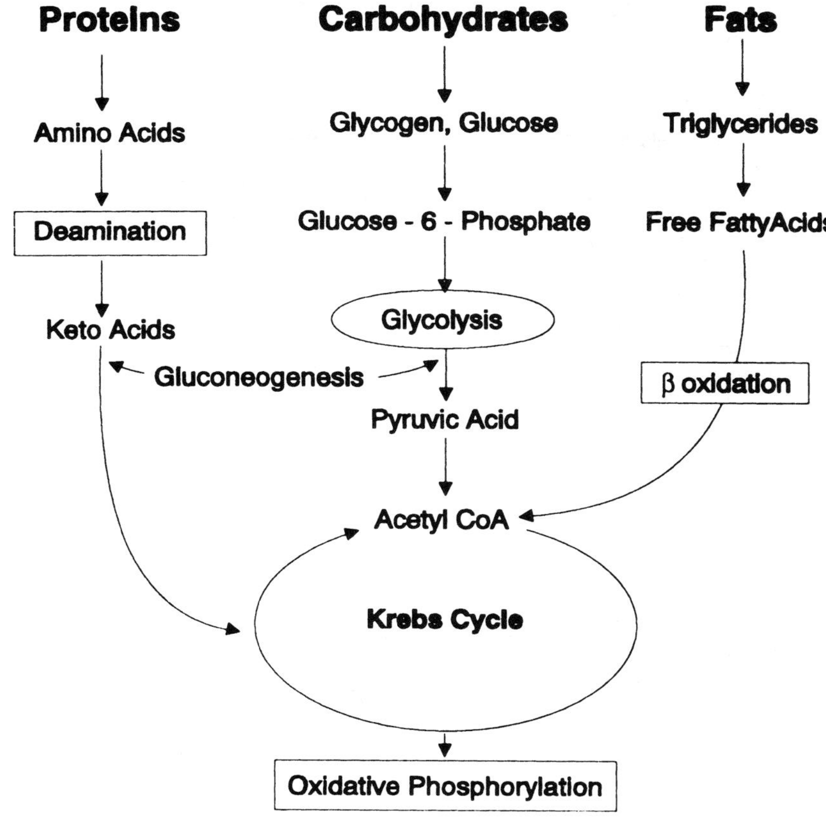

FIGURE 1–63. Aerobic system for ATP (energy) production of skeletal muscle. (From Simon, S.R., ed.: Orthopaedic Basic Science, 2nd ed., p. 103. Rosemont, IL, American Academy of Orthopaedic Surgeons, 1994; reprinted by permission.)

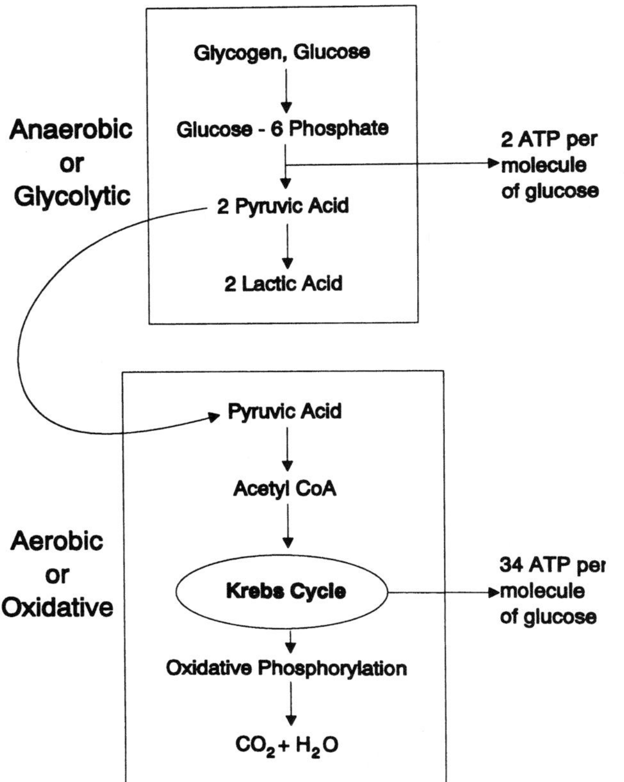

FIGURE 1–64. ATP production via anaerobic and aerobic breakdown of carbohydrates: Glycolysis and anaerobic metabolism occurs in the cytoplasm; oxidative phosphorylation occurs in the mitochondria. (From Simon, S.R., ed.: Orthopaedic Basic Science, 2nd ed., p. 104. Rosemont, IL, American Academy of Orthopaedic Surgeons, 1994; reprinted by permission.)

ness) in a healthy adult is recommended 3–5 days per week for 20–60 minutes per session, (training at 60–90% of maximum heart rate). Aerobic conditioning has proved effective in lowering the incidence of back injury in workers (*). A significant decline in aerobic fitness occurs after just 2 weeks of no training ("detraining") (*). The most common cause of **sudden death** in young athletes is hypertrophic obstructive cardiomyopathy (**). Abdominal injuries in athletes most commonly affect the kidney (*). Wrap-around polycarbonate glasses should be worn to protect the eyes in racquet sports (*). **Carbohydrate loading** involves increasing carbohydrates 3 days prior to an event (marathon) and decreasing physical activity (*). The best **fluid replacement** regimen for a competitive athlete is to replace enough water to maintain prepractice weight and maintain a normal diet (*). Treatment of heat cramps includes passive stretching, cooling, and fluid/electrolyte replacement (*).

1. Female Athletes—Three common problems are amenorrhea, osteoporosis, and anorexia (***). Amenorrhea results from a decrease in percent body fat, increased training, hormonal changes, competitive running before menarche (*), and changes in the hypothalamic–pituitary axis. Initial management includes increasing weight, decreasing exercise, and possibly administration of cyclic estrogens or progesterones.

H. Muscle Injury—As noted earlier, most muscle strains (the most common sports injury) occur at the myotendinous junction. These injuries occur most commonly in muscles that cross two joints (hamstring, gastrocnemius), with increased type II fibers. Initially there is inflammation and later fibrosis. Muscle activation (via stretching) allows twice the energy absorption prior to failure; "bouncing" types of stretching are deleterious. Muscle soreness may result from eccentric muscle contractions and may be associated with changes in the I-band of the sarcomere. Tears in muscle typically heal with dense scarring. Surgical repair of clean lacerations in the midbelly of skeletal muscle usually results in minimal regeneration of muscle fibers distally, scar formation at the laceration, and recovery of about one-half of muscle strength. Denervation causes muscle atrophy and increased sensitivity to acetylcholine, causing spontaneous fibrillations at 2–4 weeks after damage to the motor axon. Muscle strength gains during the first 10 days of rehabilitation after injury are due to improved neural firing patterns (*). Trunk extensors are stronger than trunk flexors (*).

I. Immobilization—Causes changes in the number of sarcomeres at the musculotendinous junction and acceleration of granulation tissue response in the injured muscle. Immobilization in lengthened positions decreases contractures and increases strength. Atrophy can result from disuse or altered nervous system recruitment. Electrical stimulation can help offset these effects.

TEST QUESTIONS ON SKELETAL MUSCLE AND ATHLETICS

TEST	QUESTION NUMBERS
1995 OSAE—Adult Reconstruction Hip/Knee	
1995 OSAE—Pediatric Orthopaedics	
1995 OSAE—Sports Medicine	32, 49, 50, 54, 57, 67, 68, 72, 74, 82, 83, 92, 97, 108, 109
1994 OITE	136, 141, 172
1994 OSAE—Adult Spine	6, 100
1994 OSAE—Foot and Ankle	
1994 OSAE—M/S Trauma	16
1993 OITE	
1993 OSAE—M/S Tumors and Diseases	
1993 OSAE—Shoulder and Elbow	
1992 OITE	21
1992 OSAE—Adult Reconstruction Hip/Knee	
1992 OSAE—Pediatric Orthopaedics	
1992 OSAE—Sports Medicine	11, 16, 28, 33, 35, 42, 51, 63, 70, 78, 95, 100, 108, 109, 113, 119, 121
1991 OITE	120
1991 OSAE—Adult Spine	41
1991 OSAE—Anatomy and Imaging	
1991 OSAE—Foot and Ankle	
1991 OSAE—M/S Trauma	

II. Nervous System

A. Organization

1. Central Nervous System (CNS)

Stroke patients may continue to improve up to 6 months after their vascular event (*). **Traumatic brain injury** patients may improve for up to 18 months. **Spinal cord injury** patients have the best chance for optimizing their neurologic outcome if given a methylprednisone bolus (30 mg/kg) within 8 hours of injury followed by methylprednisone infusion (5.4 mg/kg) for 23 hours (**). **Concussion** (*) is a jarring injury to the brain that results in disturbance (to some degree) of cerebral function. Grade I injuries are mild, and the athlete may return to play if he or she becomes asymptomatic. Grade II injuries are moderate and are characterized by retrograde amnesia (which persists several minutes after the injury) despite the resolution of confusion and disorientation. A first time grade II concussion allows return to play after a week without symptoms. Long periods without play (months) are required for a second grade II or a grade III (severe) concussion.

2. Peripheral Nervous System (PNS)

a. Nerves—Bundles of axons enclosed in a connective tissue sheath.

b. Nerve fiber—Axon plus surrounding Schwann cell sheath.

1. Myelinated Fibers—An axon is considered myelinated once it reaches a diameter of 1–2 μm. One myelinated axon is associated with one Schwann cell. Conduction velocity is faster than in unmyelinated fibers.

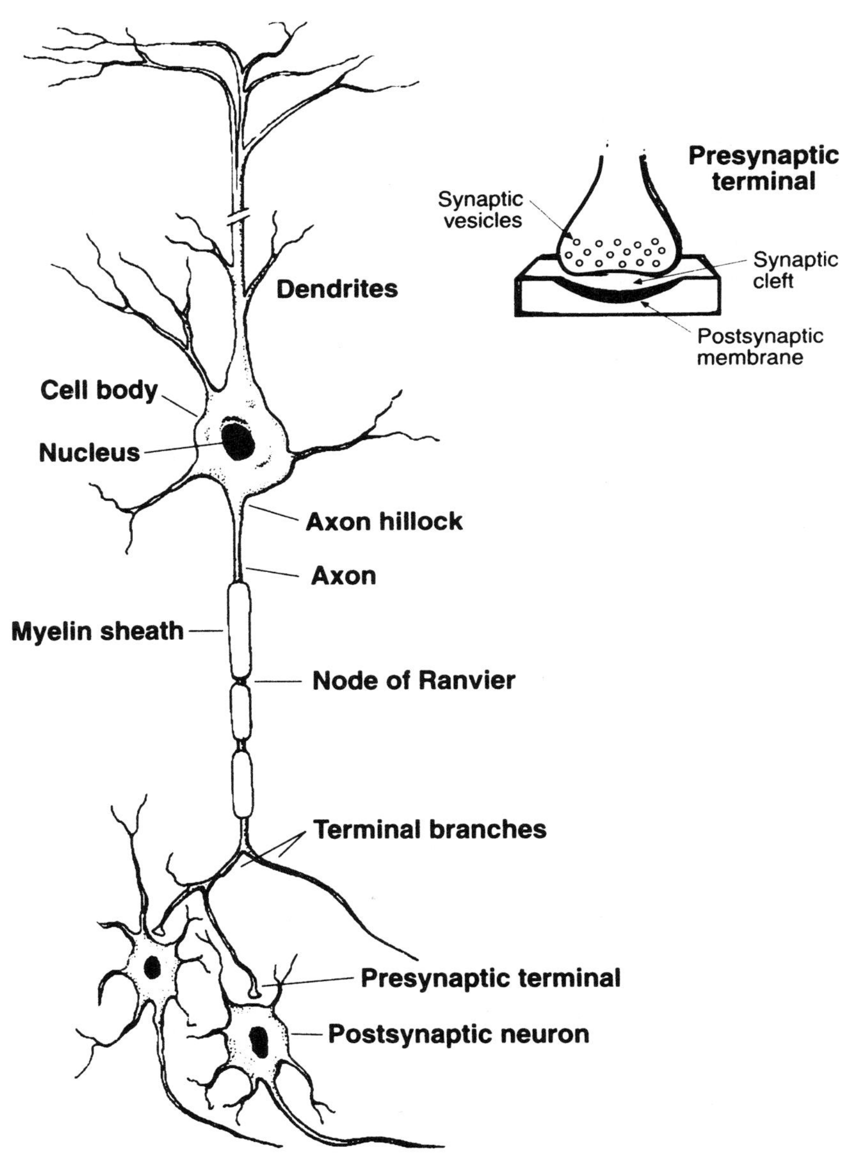

FIGURE 1–65. Typical neuron with a presynaptic terminal–postsynaptic receptor shown at upper right. (From Simon, S.R., ed.: Orthopaedic Basic Science, 2nd ed., p. 327. Rosemont, IL, American Academy of Orthopaedic Surgeons, 1994; reprinted by permission.)

2. Unmyelinated fibers—One Schwann cell surrounds several axons. Conduction velocity is relatively slow.

3. Nerve Fibers
   a. Afferents—Transmit information from sensory receptors to the CNS.
      1. Somatic Afferents—Afferent fibers originate in receptors in muscle, skin, and sensory organs of the head (vision, hearing, taste, smell).
      2. Visceral Afferents—Afferent fibers originate in viscera.
   b. Efferents—Transmit information from CNS to periphery. Motor efferents are those that innervate skeletal muscle fibers.
      1. Somatic Nerves—Innervate skin, skeletal muscle, and joints.
      2. Autonomic Nerves (Splanchnics)—Innervate viscera.

B. Histology and Signal Generation
   1. Neuron (Fig. 1–65)—Composed of four regions: cell body, axon, dendrites, and presynaptic terminal.
      a. Cell Body—Neurons' metabolic center; comprises less than 10% of the size of the neuron; gives rise to a single axon.
      b. Axon—Primary conducting vehicle of the neuron; conveys electrical signals (over long distances) via action potentials.
      c. Dendrites—Thin processes that branch from the cell body to receive input (synaptic) from surrounding nerve cells.
      d. Presynaptic Terminals—Transmit information from one neuron to another (to the cell body or dendrites of the "receiving" neuron).
   2. Glial Cells (Fig. 1–66)—Three basic types have been described: Schwann cells, oligodendrocytes, and astrocytes.
      a. Schwann cells—Responsible for myelinating **peripheral nerve axons** (forms an elongated double-membrane structure). Loss of the myelin sheath (demyelination) causes disruption in the conduction of action potentials along the axon. Myelin = lipid (70%) and protein (30%).
      b. Oligodendrocytes—Found only in the **CNS;** responsible for the formation of myelin.
      c. Astrocytes—Most common of the glial cells. Found only in the CNS. Glial cells have many functions but serve primarily as a supporting structure of the brain.

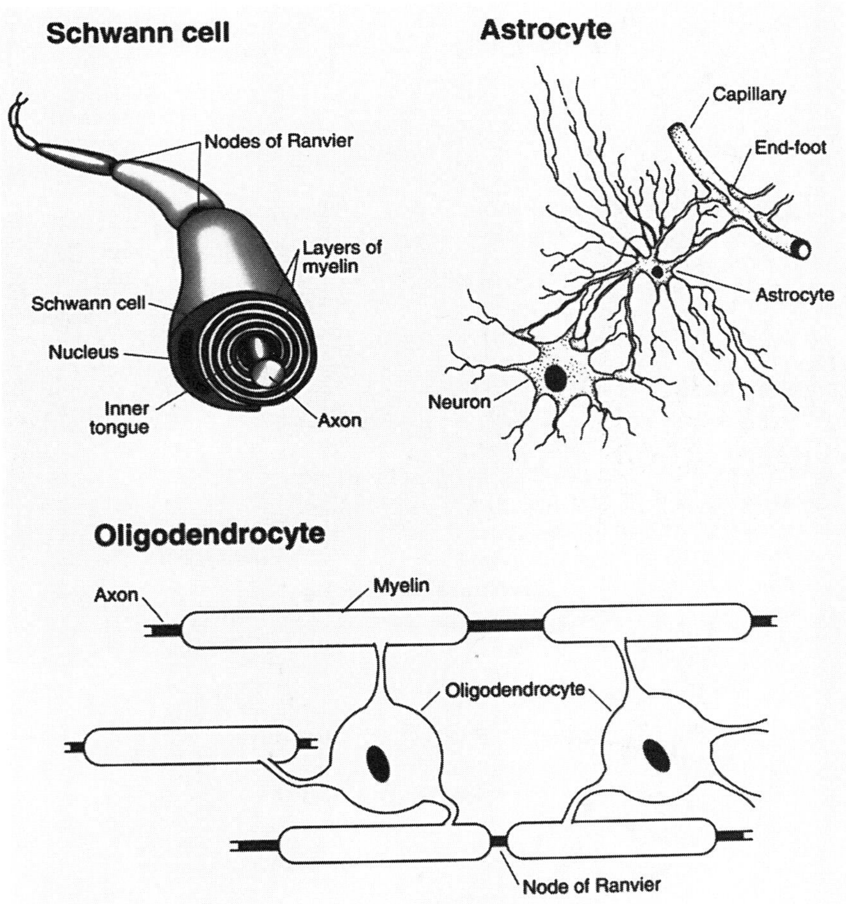

FIGURE 1–66. Glial cells include the Schwann cell, astrocytes, and oligodendrocytes. (From Simon, S.R., ed.: Orthopaedic Basic Science, 2nd ed., p. 320. Rosemont, IL, American Academy of Orthopaedic Surgeons, 1994; reprinted by permission.)

3. Resting and Action Potentials
   a. Resting Potential—Results from unequal distribution of ions on either side of the neuronal cell membrane (lipid bilayer). The four most plentiful ions about the cell membrane are Na^+, K^+, Cl^-, and a group of other organic ions (A^-). The resting potential of a neuron is −50 to −80 mV (Fig. 1–67).
   b. Action Potential—Transmits signals rapidly via electrical impulses to other neurons or effector organs (e.g., muscle). Depolarization and the action potential result from an increase in cell membrane permeability to Na^+ in response to a stimulus. This process is related to gated ion channels (Fig. 1–68), which are of three types: voltage-gated channels, mechanical gated channels, and chemical-transmitter gated channels. Action potentials propagate via both passive current flow and active membrane changes (Fig. 1–69).

C. Sensory System—Receives messages from the environment and other parts of the body via transmission from **sensory receptors** (located peripherally) to the CNS. The four attributes of a stimulus are quality, intensity, duration, and location. Sensory receptor types include photoreceptors (vision), mechanoreceptors (hearing, balance, mechanical stimuli), thermoreceptors (temperature), chemoreceptors (taste, smell), and nociceptors (pain). Neurogenic pain (and inflammatory) mediators are identifiable within the dorsal roof ganglia of the lumbar spine (*). The pain associated with an osteoid osteoma comes from prostaglandins secreted by the tumor itself (*).
   1. Somatosensory System—Conveys three modalities: mechanical, pain, and thermal. Each of these three somatic modalities is mediated by a specific class of sensory receptor (Table 1–22). Somatosensory input from each of these three modalities is transmitted to the spinal cord (or brain stem) via the **dorsal root ganglia** (Fig. 1–70).

D. Motor System—Organized into four areas: spinal cord, brain stem, motor cortex, and premotor cortical areas (basal ganglia and cerebellum).
   1. Spinal Cord (Fig. 1–71)—Contains white matter and gray matter.
      a. White Matter—Ascending and descending fiber tracts of myelinated and unmyelinated axons.

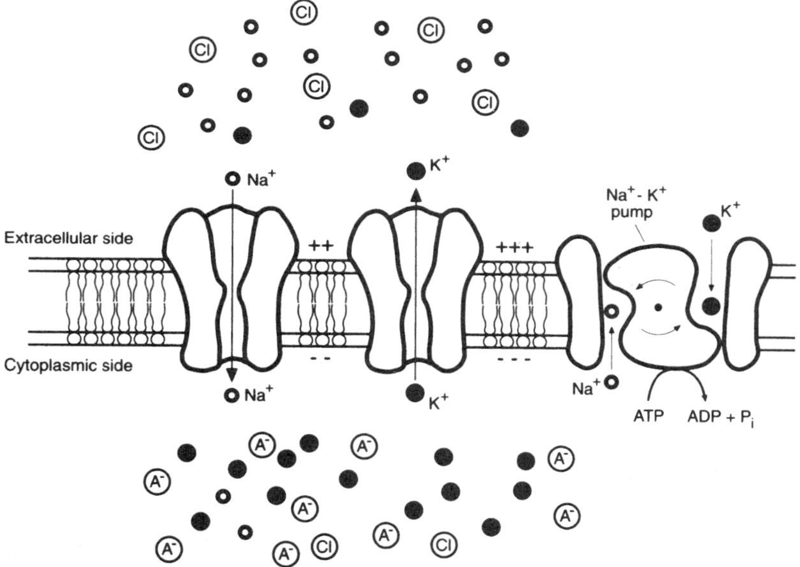

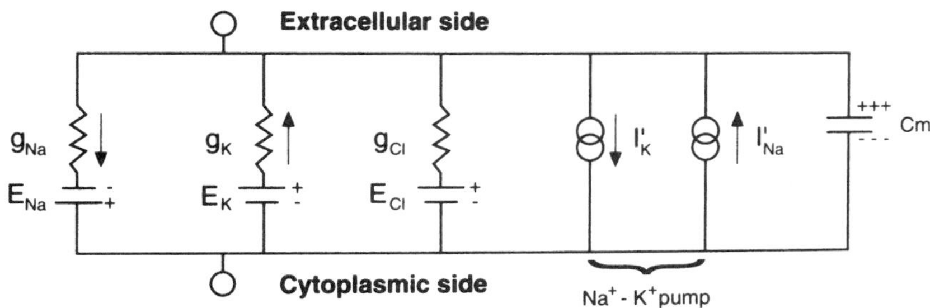

FIGURE 1–67. Electrolyte transport across cell walls. *Top*, Passive fluxes of Na^+ and K^+ into and out of the cell are balanced by the energy-dependent sodium–potassium pump. *Bottom*, Electrical circuit model of a neuron at rest. (From Simon, S.R., ed.: Orthopaedic Basic Science, 2nd ed., p. 332. Rosemont, IL, American Academy of Orthopaedic Surgeons, 1994; reprinted by permission.)

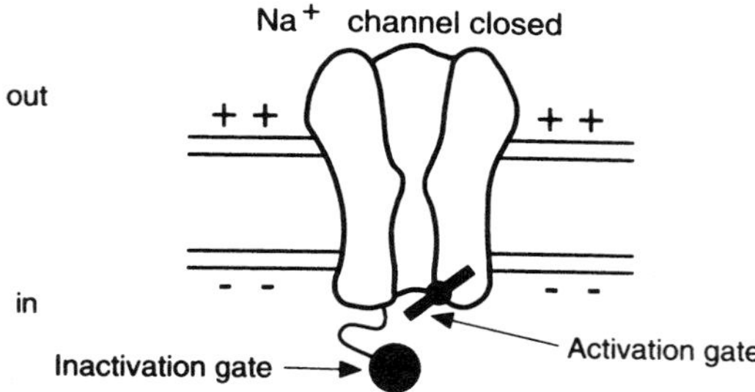

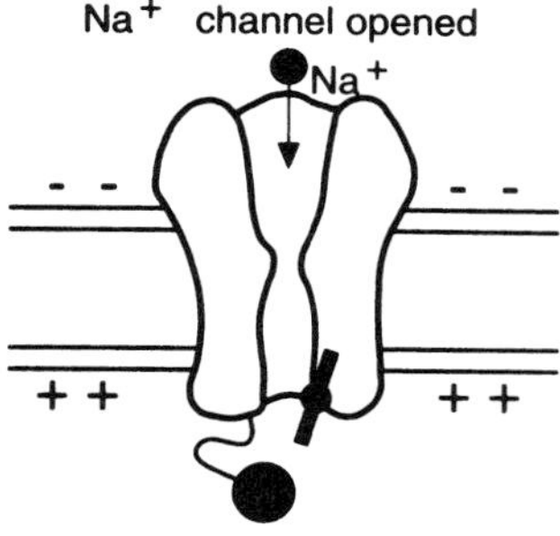

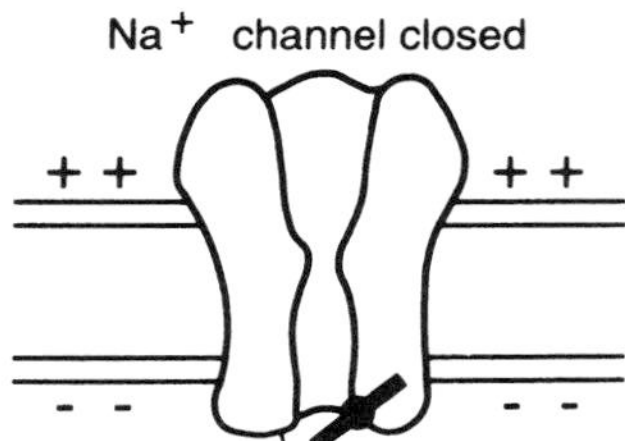

FIGURE 1–68. Gated sodium channel response during an action potential. *Top to bottom*: rest, depolarization, maintenance of depolarization, repolarization. (From Kandel, E.R., Schwartz, J.H., and Jessel, T.M.: Principles of Neural Science, 3rd ed., p. 14. Norwalk, CT, Appleton & Lange, 1991; reprinted by permission.)

b. Gray Matter—Contains neuronal cell bodies, glial cells, dendrites, and axons (myelinated and unmyelinated). Three types of neuron are found in spinal cord gray matter.
   1. Motoneurons (α and γ)—Axons exit the CNS via ventral roots.
   2. Interneurons—Axons remain in spinal cord.
   3. Tract Cells—Send axons that ascend to supraspinal centers.

c. Spinal Cord Reflexes (Table 1–23)—A reflex is a "stereotyped response" to a specific sensory stimulus. The pathway of a reflex involves a sensory organ (receptor), an interneuron, and a motoneuron.
   1. Monosynaptic Reflex—Only one synapse involved (between receptor and effector).
   2. Polysynaptic Reflex—Involves one or more interneurons. **Most human reflexes are polysynaptic.**

2. Motor Unit—Comprised of an α motoneuron and the muscle fibers it innervates. Motor units are of four types based on the physiologic demands of the motor unit: type S (slow, fatigue-resistant); type FR (fast, fatigue-resistant); type FI (fast, fatigue-intermediate); and type FF (fast-fatigue). Table 1–24 shows an overview of the motor unit subtypes.
3. Upper and Lower Motoneurons
   a. Upper Motoneurons—Located in descending pathways of the cortex, brain stem, and spinal cord.
   b. Lower Motoneurons—Located in ventral gray matter of the spinal cord.
   c. Motoneuron Lesions—Synopsis of findings in patients with upper and lower motoneuron lesions is shown in Table 1–25. **Spasticity** is a common finding in patients with a **lower motoneuron** lesion.

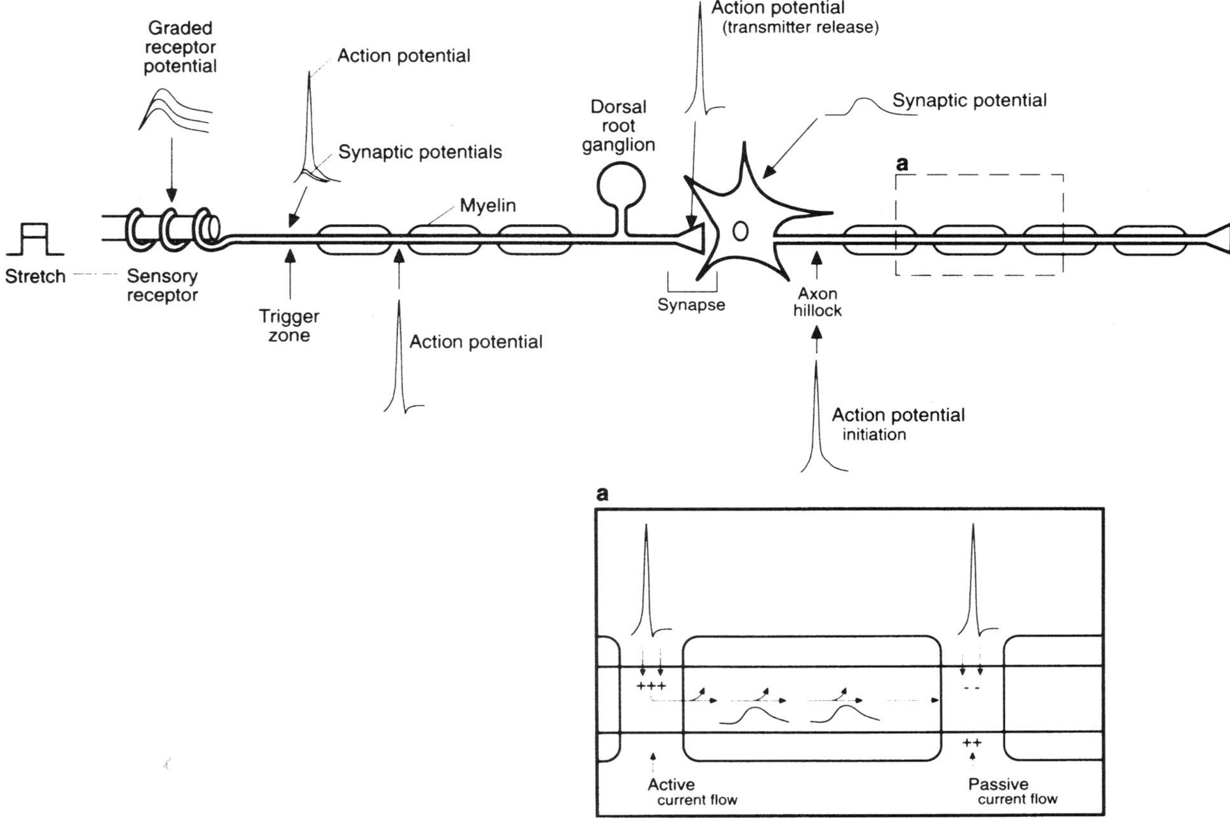

FIGURE 1–69. Action potential is propagated to the terminal region, where it triggers the release of transmitter, which initiates a synaptic potential in the motoneuron. Action potential propagation results from the spread of local passive depolarizing currents between the nodes of Ranvier (*inset*). At the nodes, voltage-gated channels open, producing an action potential. (From Simon, S.R., ed.: Orthopaedic Basic Science, 2nd ed., p. 337. Rosemont, IL, American Academy of Orthopaedic Surgeons, 1994; reprinted by permission.)

TABLE 1–22. RECEPTOR TYPES

RECEPTOR TYPE	FIBER TYPE	QUALITY
Nociceptors		
Mechanical	Aδ	Sharp, pricking pain
Thermal and mechanothermal	Aγ	Sharp, pricking pain
Thermal and mechanothermal	C	Slow, burning pain
Polymodal	C	Slow, burning pain
Cutaneous and Subcutaneous Mechanoreceptors		
Meissner's corpuscle	Aβ	Touch
Pacini's corpuscle	Aβ	Flutter
Ruffini's corpuscle	Aβ	Vibration
Merkel's receptor	Aβ	Steady skin indentation
Hair-guard, hair-tylotrich	Aβ	Steady skin indentation
Hair-down	Aβ	Flutter
Muscle and Skeletal Mechanoreceptors		
Muscle spindle primary	Aα	Limb proprioception
Muscle spindle secondary	Aβ	Limb proprioception
Golgi tendon organ	Aα	Limb proprioception
Joint capsule mechanoreceptor	Aβ	Limb proprioception

From Kandel, E.R., Schwartz, J.H., and Jessel, T.M. (eds): Principles of Neural Science, 3rd ed., p. 342. Norwalk, CT, Appleton & Lange, 1991; reprinted by permission.

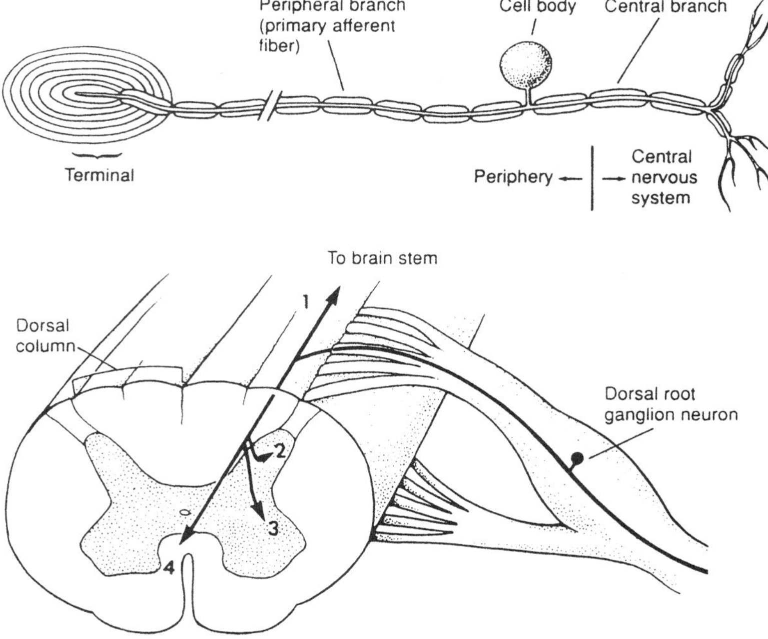

FIGURE 1–70. Morphology of dorsal root ganglion cells. The cell body lies in a ganglion in the dorsal root of a spinal nerve. *Bottom,* Dorsal root ganglion cells that mediate pressure, touch, and proprioception have central branches that ascend to the brain stem (1) and terminate in the spinal cord at the entry level (2, 3) or descend a few segments (4). Branches 2, 3, and 4 participate in local spinal reflexes. (From local spinal reflexes. (From Kandel, E.R., Schwartz, J.H., and Jessell, T.M.: Principles of Neural Science, 3rd ed., pp. 287–342. Norwalk, CT, Appleton & Lange, 1991; reprinted by permission.)

E. Peripheral Nerve
   1. Morphology (Fig. 1–72)—The peripheral nerve is a highly organized structure comprised of nerve fibers, blood vessels, and connective tissues. Axons, coated with a fibrous tissue called **endoneurium,** are grouped into nerve bundles called **fascicles** that in turn are covered with connective tissue called **perineurium.** Peripheral nerves are composed of one (mono-), a few (oligo-), or several (poly-) fascicles and surrounding areolar connective tissue (**epineurium**) enclosed within an epineural sheath. The perineurium and endothelial cells of endoneurium make up the blood–nerve barrier.
   2. Nerve Fibers (Axons) (2–25 μm in diameter)—Three types of nerve fiber are shown in Table 1–26.
   3. Conduction—As has been previously discussed, myelinated axons conduct action potentials rapidly, facilitated by gaps between Schwann cells known as **nodes of Ranvier.**
   4. Blood Supply (Fig. 1–73)
      a. Extrinsic—Vessels run in loose connective tissue surrounding the nerve trunk.
      b. Intrinsic—Vascular plexuses in the epineurium, perineurium, and endoneurium (with interconnections between these three plexuses).
   5. Injury—Peripheral nerve injury leads to death of the distal axons and **Wallerian degeneration** (of myelin). Proximal axonal budding occurs (after a 1-month delay) and leads to regeneration at the rate of about 1 mm/day (possibly 3–5 mm/day in children). Pain is the first modality to return. Nerve injury is characterized as one of three types (Table 1–27). Nerve stretching also can affect function: 8% elongation diminishes microcirculation to the nerve, and 15% elongation disrupts axons. Nerve regeneration is influenced by contact guidance (attraction of regenerating nerve to basal lamina of the Schwann cell), neurotro-

TABLE 1–23. SUMMARY OF SPINAL REFLEXES

SEGMENTAL REFLEX	RECEPTOR ORGAN	AFFERENT FIBER
Phasic stretch reflex	Muscle spindle (primary endings)	Type Ia (large myelinated)
Tonic stretch reflex	Muscle spindle (secondary endings)	Type II (intermediate myelinated)
Clasp-knife response	Muscle spindle (secondary endings)	Type II (intermediate myelinated)
Flexion withdrawal reflex	Nociceptors (free nerve endings), touch and pressure receptors	Flexor-reflex afferents: small unmyelinated cutaneous afferents (A-delta, C and muscle afferents, group III)
Autogenic inhibition	Golgi tendon organ	Type Ib (large myelinated)

From Simon, S.R.: Orthopaedic Basic Science, 2nd ed., p. 350. Rosemont, IL, American Academy of Orthopaedic Surgeons, 1994, reprinted by permission.

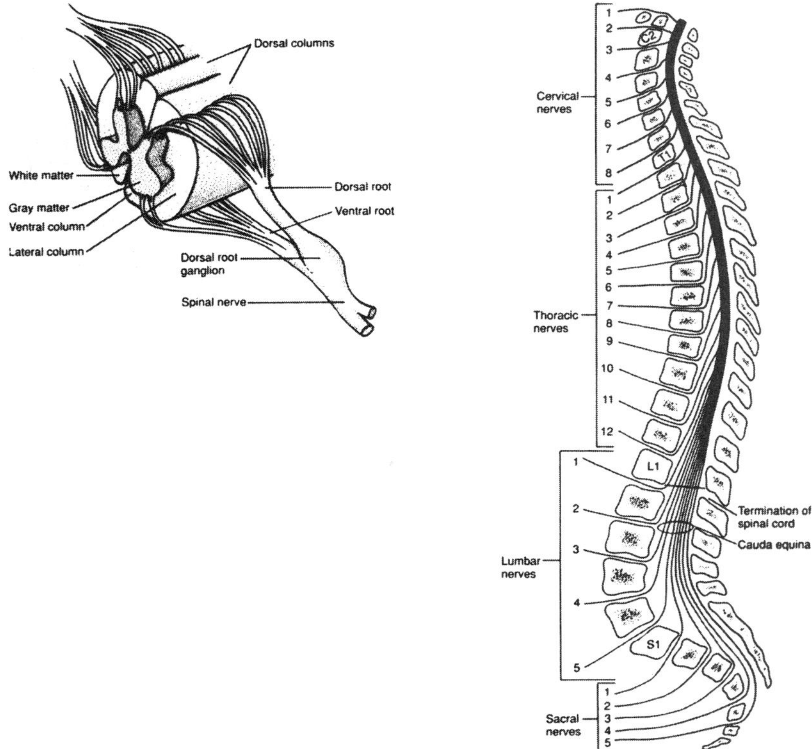

FIGURE 1–71. Spinal cord anatomy. *Left,* Each spinal nerve has a doral (sensory) and ventral (motor) root. Dorsal roots are branches from dorsal root ganglia cells; ventral roots are motor axons from cells in the ventral horn. *Right,* Note that the spinal cord terminates at the border of L1. The dorsal and ventral roots of the lumbar and sacral nerves are collectively called the cauda equina. (From Kandel, E.R., Schwartz, J.H., and Jessell, T.M.: Principles of Neural Science, 3rd ed., pp. 285–286. Norwalk, CT, Appleton & Lange, 1991; reprinted by permission.)

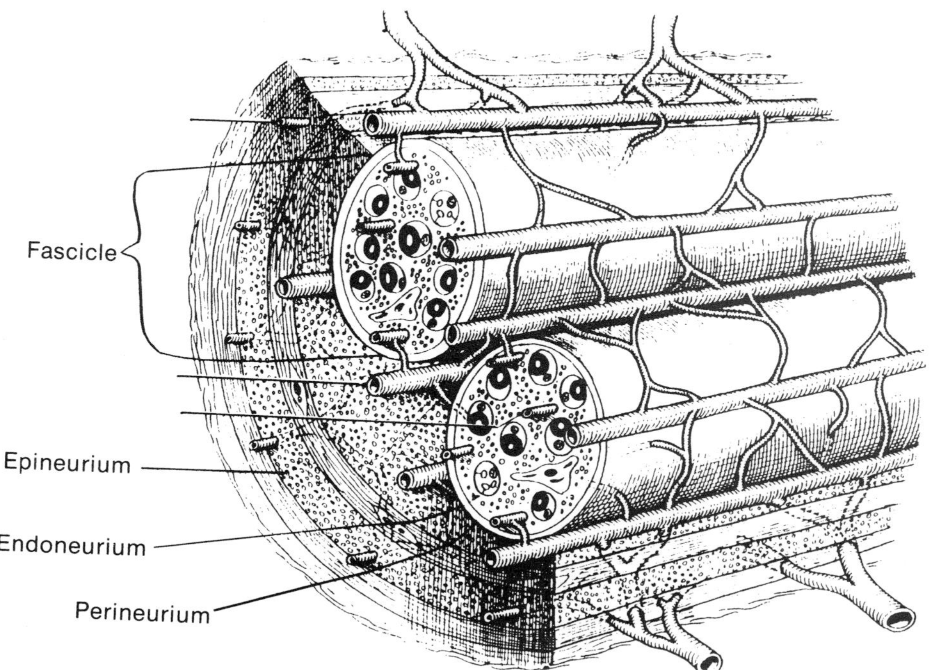

FIGURE 1–72. Peripheral nerve microstructure. (From Tubiana, R.: The Hand, p. 421. Philadelphia, WB Saunders, 1988; reprinted by permission.)

TABLE 1–24. GENERAL CHARACTERISTICS OF MOTOR UNIT TYPES

PARAMETER	Motor Unit Types		
	FF	FR	S
Muscle Unit Physiology[a]			
Contraction time	Fastest	Slightly slower	Slowest
Sag	Present	Present	Absent
Maximum tension	Largest	Smaller	Smallest
Fatigue index	<0.25	<0.75–1.00	0.7–1.0
Muscle Unit Anatomy[b]			
Innervation ratio	2.9	2.1	1.0
Fiber cross-sectional area	1.3	0.98	1.0
Specific tension	1.4	1.2	1.0
Muscle Unit Metabolism			
Fiber type	FG	FOG	SO
Myosin heavy chain	IIB	IIA	I
Glycogen	High	High	Low
Hexokinase	Low	Intermediate	High
Glycolytic enzymes	High	High	Low
Oxidative enzymes	Low	High	High
Cytochrome c	Low	High	High
Capillary supply	Sparse	Rich	Very rich
Motoneuron			
Cell body size	Largest	Slightly smaller	Smallest
Conduction velocity	Fastest	Slightly slower	Slowest
After-hyperpolarization duration	Shortest	Slightly shorter	Longest
Input Resistance	Lowest	Slightly higher	Highest

From Simon, S.R.: Orthopaedic Basic Science, 2nd ed., p. 344. Rosemont, IL, American Academy of Orthopaedic Surgeons, 1994; reprinted by permission.
FF, fast fatigable; FR, fast fatigue-resistant; S, fatigue-resistant; FG, fast glycolytic; FOG, fast oxidative glycolytic; SO, slow oxidative.
[a] Data relative to the FF unit.
[b] Data relative to the slow unit.

phism (factors enhancing growth), and neurotropism (preferential attraction toward nerves rather than other tissues). **"Stingers"** (or "burners") (**) refers to neuropraxia from a stretch injury to the brachial plexus; it is seen most commonly in football players.

6. Repair—Several methods are available.
   a. Direct Muscular Neurotization—Inserts the proximal stump of the nerve into the affected muscle belly. Results in less than normal function but is indicated in selected cases.
   b. Epineural Repair—Primary repair of the outer connective tissue layer of the nerve at the site of injury after resecting the proximal neuroma and distal glioma. Care is taken to ensure proper rotation and lack of tension on the repair.
   c. Grouped Fascicular Repair—Primary repair is also done after resection of the neuroma and glioma, but individual fascicles are reapproximated under microscopic control. Used for large nerves, but no significant improvement in results over epineural repair has been demonstrated.

TABLE 1–25. FINDINGS IN UPPER AND LOWER MOTONEURON LESIONS

FINDINGS	UPPER MOTONEURON LESIONS	LOWER MOTONEURON LESIONS
Strength	Decreased	Decreased
Tone	Increased	Decreased
Deep tendon reflexes	Increased	Decreased
Superficial tendon reflexes	Decreased	Decreased
Babinski's sign	Present	Absent
Clonus	Present	Absent
Fasciculations	Absent	Present
Atrophy	Absent	Present

From Simon, S.R.: Orthopaedic Basic Science, 2nd ed., p. 354. Rosemont, IL, American Academy of Orthopaedic Surgeons, 1994; reprinted by permission.

TABLE 1–26. TYPES OF NERVE FIBER

TYPE	DIAMETER (μm)	MYELINATION	SPEED	EXAMPLES
A	10–20	Heavy	Fast	Touch
B	<3	Intermediate	Medium	ANS
C	<1.3	None	Slow	Pain

ANS, autonomic nervous system.

TABLE 1–27. TYPES OF NERVE INJURY

INJURY	PATHOPHYSIOLOGY	PROGNOSIS
Neurapraxia	Reversible conduction block—local ischemia	Good
Axonotmesis	More severe injury but endoneurium intact	Fair
Neurotmesis	Complete nerve division	Poor

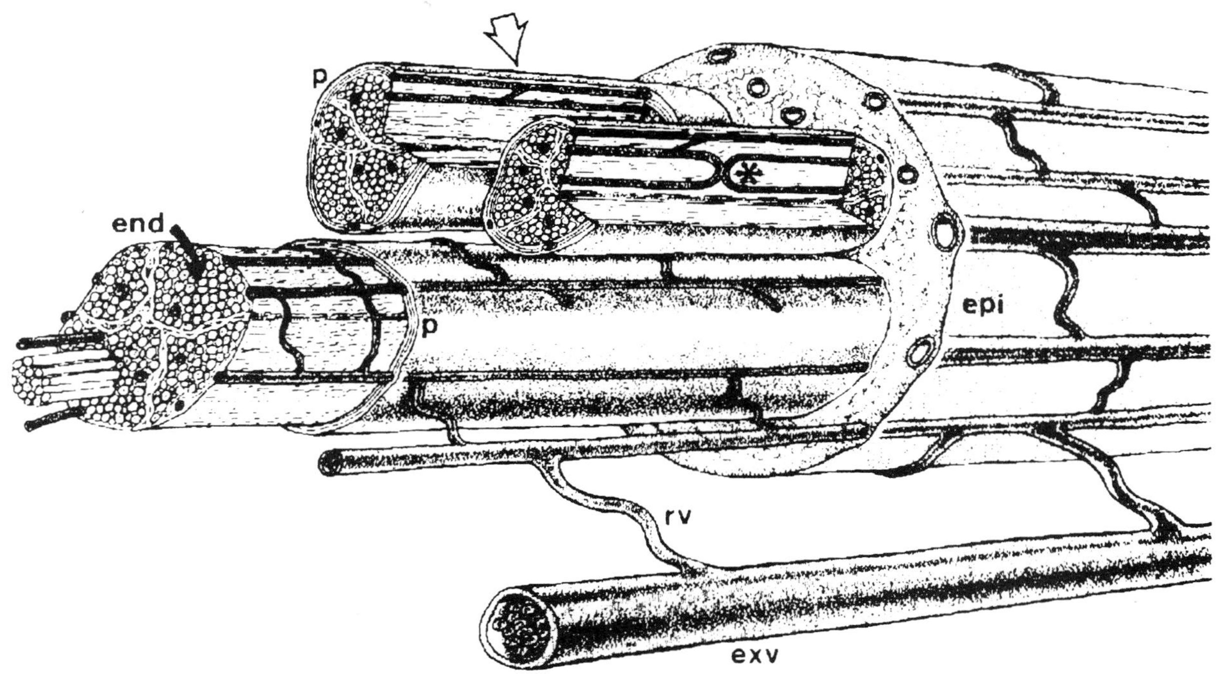

FIGURE 1–73. Interneural vascularization. exv, extrinsic vessels; rv, regional vessels; epi, epineurium; p, perineurium; end, endoneurium. Vessels penetrate the perineurium obliquely (arrows). * Intrafascicular "double loop formations." (From Lundgorg, G.: Nerve Injury and Repair, p. 43. New York, Churchill Livingstone, 1988; reprinted by permission.)

TEST QUESTIONS ON THE NERVOUS SYSTEM

TEST	QUESTION NUMBERS
1995 OSAE—Adult Reconstruction Hip/Knee	18, 99
1995 OSAE—Pediatric Orthopaedics	7, 17
1995 OSAE—Sports Medicine	85, 91
1994 OITE	
1994 OSAE—Adult Spine	80
1994 OSAE—Foot and Ankle	62, 82
1994 OSAE—M/S Trauma	
1993 OITE	158
1993 OSAE—M/S Tumors and Diseases	82
1993 OSAE—Shoulder and Elbow	
1992 OITE	
1992 OSAE—Adult Reconstruction Hip/Knee	
1992 OSAE—Pediatric Orthopaedics	
1992 OSAE—Sports Medicine	
1991 OITE	
1991 OSAE—Adult Spine	31
1991 OSAE—Anatomy and Imaging	
1991 OSAE—Foot and Ankle	54
1991 OSAE—M/S Trauma	

III. Connective Tissues

A. Tendons (Fig. 1–74)—Dense, regularly arranged tissues that attach muscle to bone. Composed of fascicles (groups of collagen bundles) separated by **endotenon,** surrounded by **epitenon,** and enclosed within a **paratenon (tendon sheath).** Tendons consist of fibroblasts (predominant cell type) arranged in parallel rows (Fig. 1–75) in fascicles (composed of fibrils) with surrounding loose areolar tissue (peritenon). Fibroblasts produce mostly type I collagen (85% dry weight of tendon). Insertion into bone is by way of transitional, **calcified fibrocartilage (Sharpey's fibers),** which helps dissipate stress. Although all tendons have some form of blood supply for nutrition, "vascular" tendons are surrounded by a vascular paratenon (Fig. 1–76), whereas "avascular" tendons are nourished by vincula within tendon sheaths (Fig. 1–77). Other sources of nutrition include synovial folds, periosteal attachments, and surrounding tissue. Tendinous structures tend to orient themselves along stress lines. Tendinous healing in response to injury is initiated by fibroblasts that originate in the epitenon and macrophages that initiate healing and remodeling. Treatment of injuries affects the repair process. Tendon healing occurs in large part through intrinsic capabilities. Tendon repairs are **weakest at 7–10 days;** they regain most of their original strength at 21–28 days and **achieve maximum strength in 6 months.** Early mobilization allows increased ROM but results in decreased strength. Immobilization leads to increased strength in the tendon substance, at the expense of ROM. However, immobilization tends to decrease the strength at the tendon–bone interface.

B. Ligaments—Composed of type I collagen (70% dry weight of ligament), these structures have a role in stability of joints. Their ultrastructure is similar to that of tendons, but the fibers are more variable and have a **higher elastin content.** Ligaments have a "uniform microvascularity," which receives its supply at the insertion site. They also possess mechanoreceptors and free nerve endings that may play a role in stabilizing joints. Ligament insertion into bone represents a transition from one material to another and can be classified into two types: **indirect insertion** (more common) and **direct insertion.** With an indirect insertion, the superficial fibers of the ligament insert at acute angles into the periosteum. Direct insertions display superficial and deep fibers; the deep fibers attach to bone at 90 degree angles, and the transition from ligament to bone occurs in four phases: ligament, fibrocartilage, mineralized fibrocartilage, and bone. The superficial fibers join the periosteum. Healing (in three phases, as in bone) is benefited from normal stress and strain across the joint. Early healing is with type III collagen that is later converted to type I collagen. **Avulsion of ligaments** typically occurs **between the unmineralized and mineralized fibrocartilage layers.** Immobilization adversely affects the strength of repair. Exercise causes a decrease in the number but an increase in the size of collagen fibrils and leads to decreased stiffness. The most common mechanism of ligament failure is **rupture of sequential series of collagen fiber bundles** (*). The most common site of failure

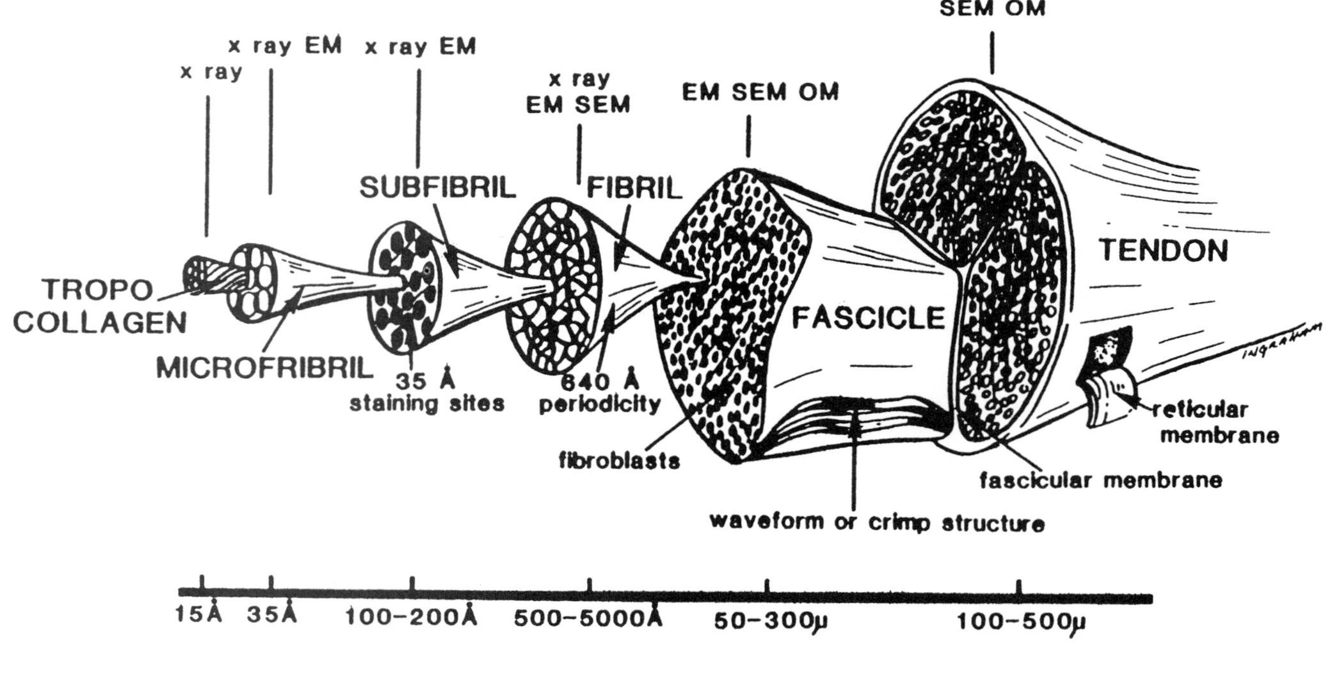

FIGURE 1–74. Tendon microstructure. (From Orthopaedic Science Syllabus, p. 35. Park Ridge, IL, American Academy of Orthopaedic Surgery, 1986; reprinted by permission.)

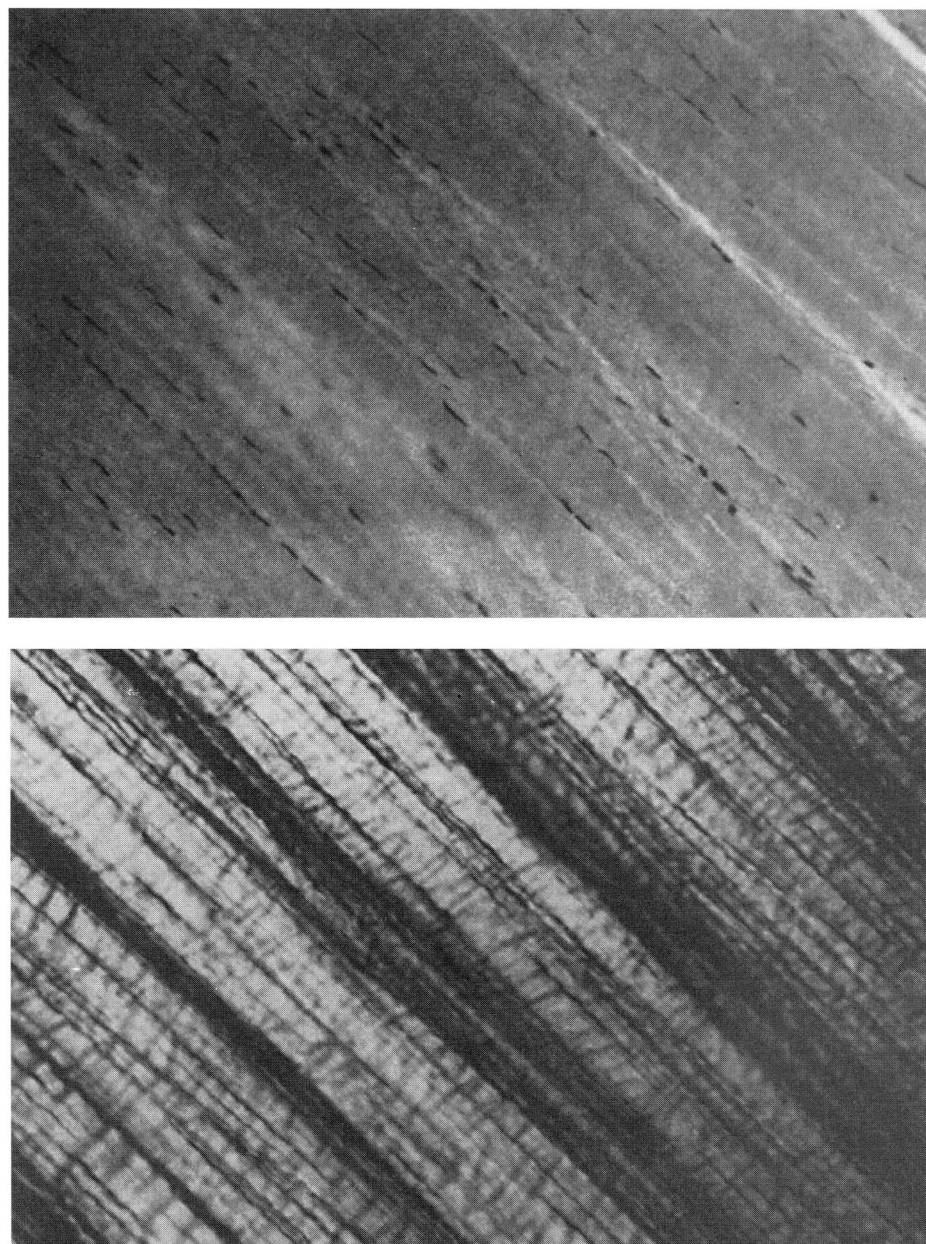

FIGURE 1–75. *Top,* Photomicrograph of flexor tendon with parallel rows of fibroblasts and collagen bundles. *Bottom,* Polarized light photograph of same section illustrating parallel, longitudinally arranged collagen bundles. (From Simon, S.R., ed.: Orthopaedic Basic Science, 2nd ed., p. 49. Rosemont, IL, American Academy of Orthopaedic Surgeons, 1994; reprinted by permission.)

during the immediate postoperative period of a bone–patellar tendon–bone anterior cruciate ligament (ACL) reconstruction is the fixation site (**). The major blood supply of the cruciate ligaments is the **middle genicular artery** (*).

C. Intervertebral Discs—Allow motion and stability of the spine. Composed of two components: the central nucleus pulposus (a hydrated gel with compressibility: high GAG/low collagen) and a surrounding annulus fibrosis (allows for extensibility and increased tensile strength: high collagen/low GAG). Composed of 85% water (decreases with age), proteoglycans (smaller and with more keratin sulfate than young cartilage), and **collagen types I and II** (type I in annulus; type II in nucleus pulposus). The aging disc shows decreased water content, decreased proteoglycan content, and increased collagen (*).

D. Soft Tissue Healing
   1. Four phases of soft tissue healing have been described.

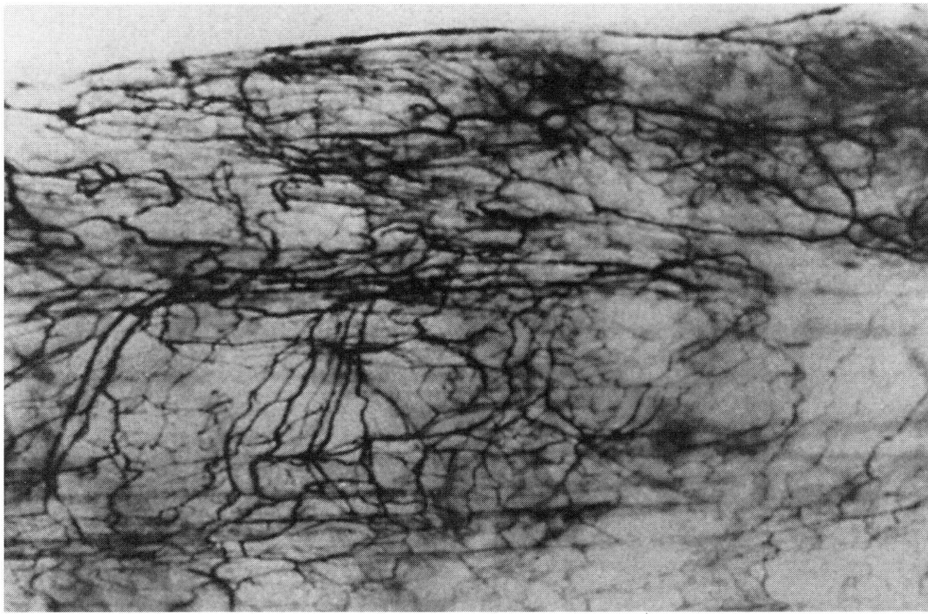

FIGURE 1–76. India ink injection of rabbit calcaneal tendon (Spalteholz technique) demonstrating the vasculature of the paratenon. (From Simon, S.R., ed.: Orthopaedic Basic Science, 2nd ed., p. 50. Rosemont, IL, American Academy of Orthopaedic Surgeons, 1994; reprinted by permission.)

a. Hemostasis—Primary platelet plug is formed within 5 minutes. Secondary clotting (via the coagulation cascade) uses fibrin and occurs within the first 10–15 minutes of injury. Fibronectin, a large glycoprotein, binds fibrin and cells and acts as a chemotactic factor. Platelets release factors that activate the next phase of healing.
b. Inflammation—Involves débridement of injured/necrotic tissue utilizing macrophages and occurs within the first week after injury. It has three stages: (1) activation (immediate); (2) amplification (48–72 hours); and (3) débridement (using bacteria, phagocytosis, and matrix [biochemical] means). Prostaglandins help to mediate the inflammatory response.
c. Organogenesis—Occurs at 7–21 days and consists of tissue modeling. Mesenchymal precursors differentiate into myofibroblasts. Angiogenesis occurs. Further differentiation leads to the final stage of healing.
d. Remodeling—Of individual tissue lines begins shortly after repair and continues for up to 18 months. Realignment and cross-linking of collagen fibers allows increased tensile strength.

2. Growth factors—Require activation, are redundant, and function with feedback loop mechanisms.
   a. Chemotactic Factors—Attract cells. The factors include prostaglandins (PMNs), prostanoids (PMNs), complement (PMNs and macrophages), PDGF (macrophages and fibroblasts), and angiokines (endothelial cells).
   b. Competence Factors—Activate dormant (G_0) cells. Include PDGF and prostaglandins.
   c. Progression Factors—Allow cell growth. Induce epidermal growth factor, IL-1, and somatomedins.
   d. Inductive Factors—Stimulate differentiation. Include angiokines, bone morphogenic protein, and specific tissue growth factors.
   e. Transforming Factors—Cause dedifferentiation and proliferation.
   f. Permissive Factors—Enhancing factors; include fibronectin and osteonectin.

E. Soft Tissue Implants
   1. Introduction—Usually used around the knee (ACL); implants can be allografts, autografts, and synthetics.
   2. Allografts—Have no donor site morbidity but incite an immune response and may transmit infection. The immunogenic response can be reduced with treatment (freeze-drying), but it decreases strength (deep freezing without drying does not significantly affect strength). If not harvested under sterile conditions, treatment with cold ethylene oxide gas may have adverse affects (**graft failure**) (*) particularly if >3 M rad irradiation is used in conjunction (2 M rad with ethylene oxide does not appear to significantly decrease the mechanical properties). Allograft ligaments exhibit slower, less predictable histologic recovery than autografts (*).
   3. Synthetic Ligaments—Unlike autografts or allografts, these structures have no initial period of weakness. However, they suffer from wear (debris) and are associated with **sterile joint effusions** (*) with increased levels of neutral proteinases (**collagenase** and gelatinase) and chondrocyte activation factor (IL-1) (*).

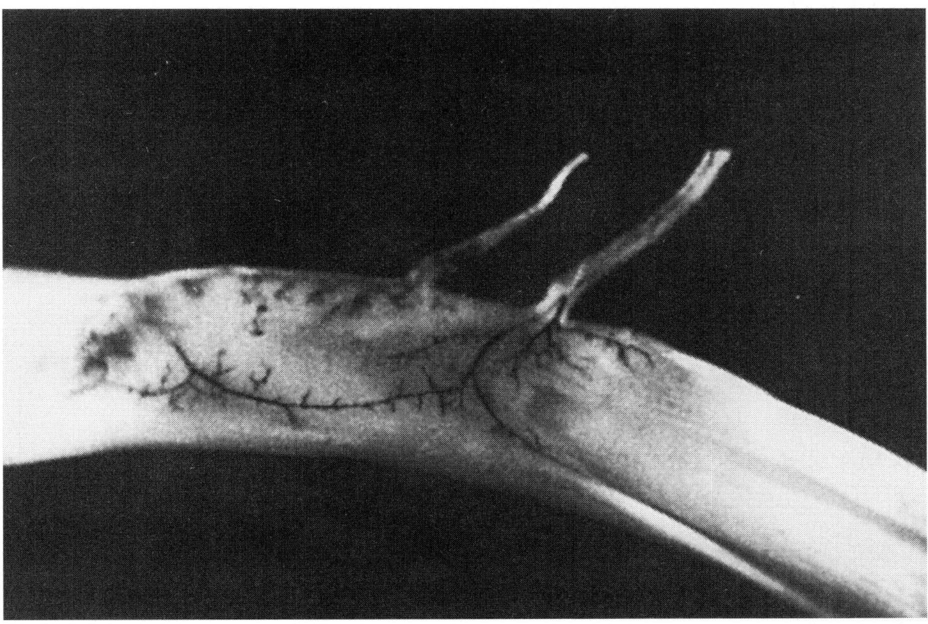

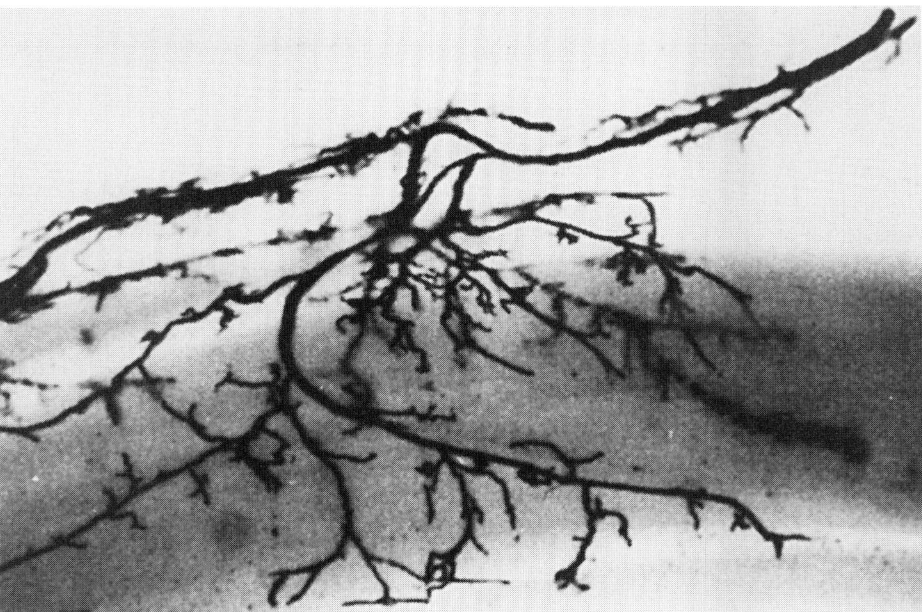

FIGURE 1–77. *Top*, India ink specimens demonstrating the vascular supply of the flexor tendons via vincula. *Bottom*, Closeup of specimen. (From Simon, S.R., ed.: Orthopaedic Basic Science, 2nd ed., p. 51. Rosemont, IL, American Academy of Orthopaedic Surgeons, 1994; reprinted by permission.)

TEST QUESTIONS ON CONNECTIVE TISSUES

TEST	QUESTION NUMBERS
1995 OSAE—Adult Reconstruction Hip/Knee	
1995 OSAE—Pediatric Orthopaedics	
1995 OSAE—Sports Medicine	89, 93
1994 OITE	
1994 OSAE—Adult Spine	
1994 OSAE—Foot and Ankle	
1994 OSAE—M/S Trauma	
1993 OITE	193
1993 OSAE—M/S Tumors and Diseases	
1993 OSAE—Shoulder and Elbow	
1992 OITE	
1992 OSAE—Adult Reconstruction Hip/Knee	
1992 OSAE—Pediatric Orthopaedics	
1992 OSAE—Sports Medicine	60, 71, 73, 79, 94, 102
1991 OITE	
1991 OSAE—Adult Spine	13
1991 OSAE—Anatomy and Imaging	28
1991 OSAE—Foot and Ankle	
1991 OSAE—M/S Trauma	

SECTION 4

Cellular and Molecular Biology, Immunology, and Genetics of Orthopaedics

The field of molecular biology is rapidly expanding. Recent advancements have been made in this area specifically in the field of musculoskeletal science. It is the intent of this section on Cellular and Molecular Biology, Immunology, and Genetics of Orthopaedics to serve as an introduction to the basic concepts of these fields.

I. Cellular and Molecular Biology

A. Chromosomes—Humans have 23 pairs (46) of chromosomes. Chromosomes are located in the nucleus of every cell in the body. Each chromosome contains at least 150,000 **genes.** Although every cell has 46 chromosomes, the genes located on these chromosomes are regulated so a relatively small number of genes are expressed for any given cell. In this way the regulation of **gene expression** determines the unique biologic qualities of each cell. Chromosomes contain both deoxyribonucleic acid (DNA) and ribonucleic acid (RNA).

B. DNA—Located within the chromosome (in the cell nucleus), DNA is responsible for regulating cellular functions via **protein synthesis.** DNA has been classically described as a double helix (double-stranded) that contains **two sugar molecules,** each of which has one of four nitrogenous bases (adenine, guanine, cytosine, thymine) (Fig. 1–78). The nitrogenous bases from one strand are linked to those of the other strand via hydrogen bonds. (In DNA, adenine is always linked to thymine, and guanine is always linked to cytosine.) DNA is important to three cellular processes: (1) DNA replication; (2) transcription of messenger RNA (mRNA); (3) regulation of cell di-

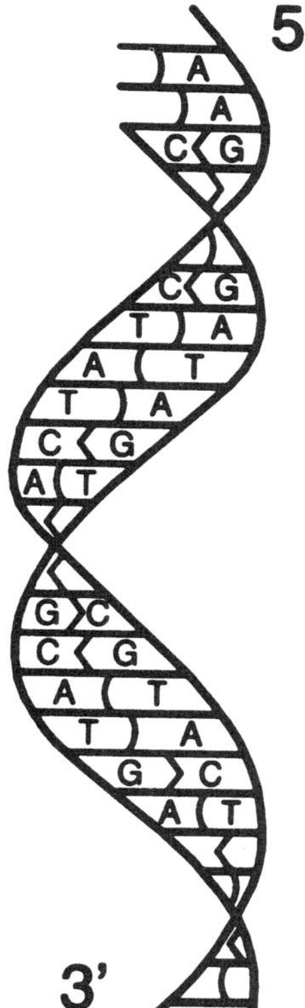

FIGURE 1–78. DNA structure. The two deoxyribose strands are connected by a pair of nucleotides (the rungs of the ladder) connected by hydrogen bonds. A, adenine; T, thymine; C, cytosine; G, guanine. (From Simon, S.R., ed.: Orthopaedic Basic Science, 2nd ed., p. 221. Rosemont, IL, American Academy of Orthopaedic Surgeons, 1994; reprinted by permission.)

vision and the production of mRNA. All nuclear DNA is housed in the 23 chromosome pairs.

C. Nucleotide—Made up of the sugar molecule plus its phosphate and nitrogen bases. Nucleotides code for specific amino acids. The nucleotide sequence in one strand of DNA determines the sequence in the other (adenine to thymine, guanine to cytosine).

D. Gene—Portion of DNA that codes for a specific protein.

E. Transcription (Fig. 1–79)—In order to produce a specific protein (to regulate cellular functions) the DNA of the gene that is coding for that specific protein must be transcribed to an mRNA (via RNA polymerase).

F. Translation (Fig. 1–79)—Process by which mRNA builds proteins from amino acids.

G. Protein Coding and Regulation—A **codon** is a sequence of three nucleotides in a strand of DNA or RNA that provides the genetic code information for a specific amino acid (Fig. 1–80). Between functional coding sequences are large noncoding sequences known as **regulating DNA.** The **gene promoter** is an important portion of the regulatory DNA and is required for the initiation of transcription. **Consensus sequences** (named for a specific nucleotide sequence) serve as binding sites for specific proteins involved in gene regulation. **Gene enhancers** are binding sites for proteins involved in the regulation of transcription. Protein coding and regulation are shown in Figure 1–81.

H. Techniques of Study—Used to study genetic (inherited) disorders.

1. Restriction Enzymes—Used to cut DNA at a precise, reproducible cleavage location. Fragments of DNA that have been cleaved using restriction enzymes are known as **restriction fragments.**
2. Agarose Gel Electrophoresis—When exposed to an electrical field, negatively charged DNA is attracted toward the positive pole of the field and moves through the agarose gel in which it has been placed. The gel acts as a "sieve" to the extent that small DNA fragments move more easily (migrate further from the original position) through the gel than large fragments. Agarose gel is commonly used following the use of (and in conjunction with) restriction enzymes.
3. DNA Ligation—Process of attaching genes removed from human DNA to pieces of nonhuman DNA known as **plasmids.** The purpose of this pro-

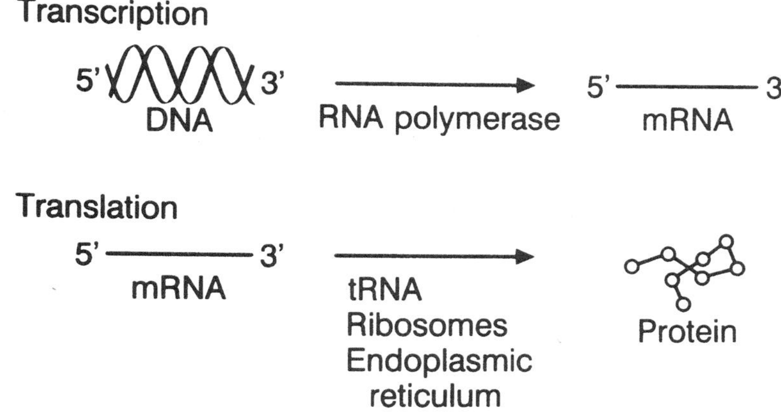

FIGURE 1–79. DNA information is transcribed into RNA in the nucleus. mRNA is then transported to the cytoplasm where translation into proteins occurs in the endoplasmic reticulum. DNA, deoxyribonucleic acid; RNA, ribonucleic acid; mRNA, messenger RNA; tRNA, transfer RNA. (From Simon, S.R., ed.: Orthopaedic Basic Science, 2nd ed., p. 222. Rosemont, IL, American Academy of Orthopaedic Surgeons, 1994; reprinted by permission.)

Codon	Amino acid	Codon	Amino acid	Codon	Amino acid	Codon	Amino acid
A A G	Lys	C A G	Gln	G A G	Glu	T A G	Stop
A A A		C A A		G A A		T A A	
A A C	Asn	C A C	His	G A C	Asp	T A C	Tyr
A A T		C A T		G A T		T A T	
A C G	Thr	C C G	Pro	G C G	Ala	T C G	Ser
A C A		C C A		G C A		T C A	
A C C		C C C		G C C		T C C	
A C T		C C T		G C T		T C T	
A G G	Arg	C G G	Arg	G G G	Gly	T G G	Trp
A G A		C G A		G G A		T G A	Stop
A G C	Ser	C G C		G G C		T G C	Cys
A G T		C G T		G G T		T G T	
A T G	Met	C T G	Leu	G T G	Val	T T G	Leu
A T A	Ile	C T A		G T A		T T A	
A T C		C T C		G T C		T T C	Phe
A T T		C T T		G T T		T T T	

FIGURE 1–80. Genetic dictionary for translation of mRNA into amino acid proteins. A, adenine; T, thymine; C, cytosine; G, guanine. (From Simon, S.R., ed.: Orthopaedic Basic Science, 2nd ed., p. 222. Rosemont, IL, American Academy of Orthopaedic Surgeons, 1994; reprinted by permission.)

cess is to facilitate the study of specific genes. Two DNA fragments linked together (via the ligation process) form **recombinant DNA.**

4. Plasmid Vectors—A gene to be studied is ligated into a plasmid (which is then known as a **recombinant plasmid**) and inserted into a bacterium using a process known as **transformation.** The recombinant plasmid then replicates and increases the amount of recombinant DNA inside the bacterium.
5. Genomic Library (Fig. 1–82)
6. Transgenic Animals (Fig. 1–83)—Used to investigate the function of cloned genes. A transgenic animal is produced by inserting a foreign gene (**transgene**) into a single-cell embryo, which then duplicates repeatedly and carries the transgene to every cell in the body.
7. Southern Hybridization—Technique used to identify a particular DNA sequence in an extract of mixed DNA.

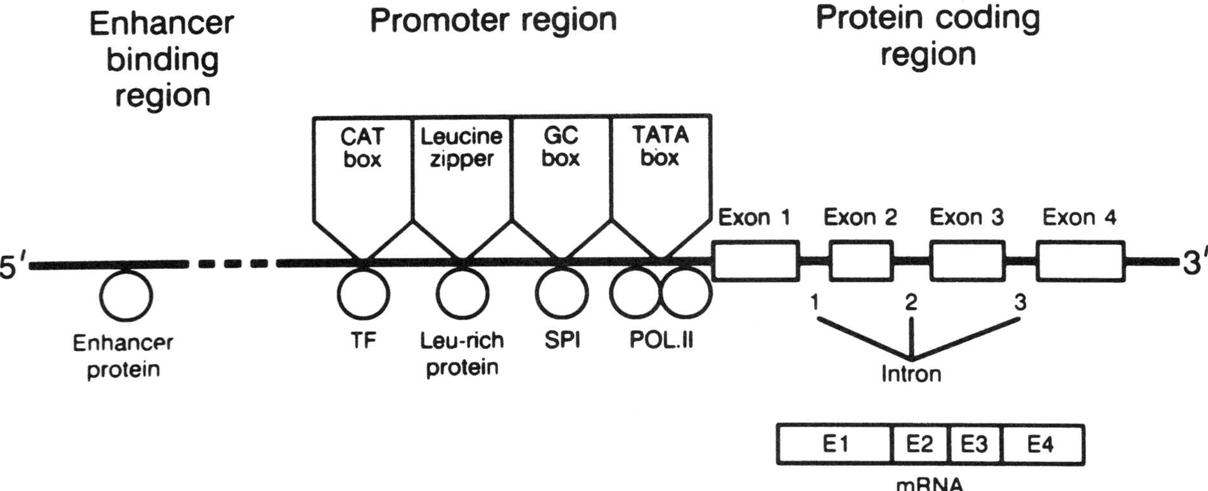

FIGURE 1–81. Protein coding and regulation. mRNA, messenger ribonucleic acid; TF, transcription factor; POL II, RNA polymerase II; SPI, serum promotor. (From Simon, S.R., ed.: Orthopaedic Basic Science, 2nd ed., p. 223. Rosemont, IL, American Academy of Orthopaedic Surgeons, 1994; reprinted by permission.)

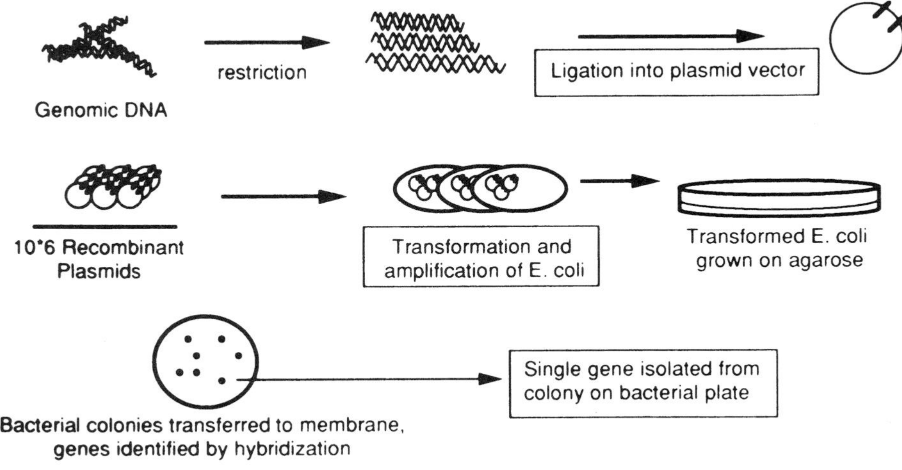

FIGURE 1–82. Genomic library of recombinant plasmids with fragments of all the DNA in the chromosome. The entire genome, restricted into small fragments, is ligated into plasmid vectors restricted by the same enzymes. These recombinant plasmids transform bacteria, which can be screened to isolate specific genes of interest. (From Simon, S.R., ed.: Orthopaedic Basic Science, 2nd ed., p. 227. Rosemont, IL, American Academy of Orthopaedic Surgeons, 1994; reprinted by permission.)

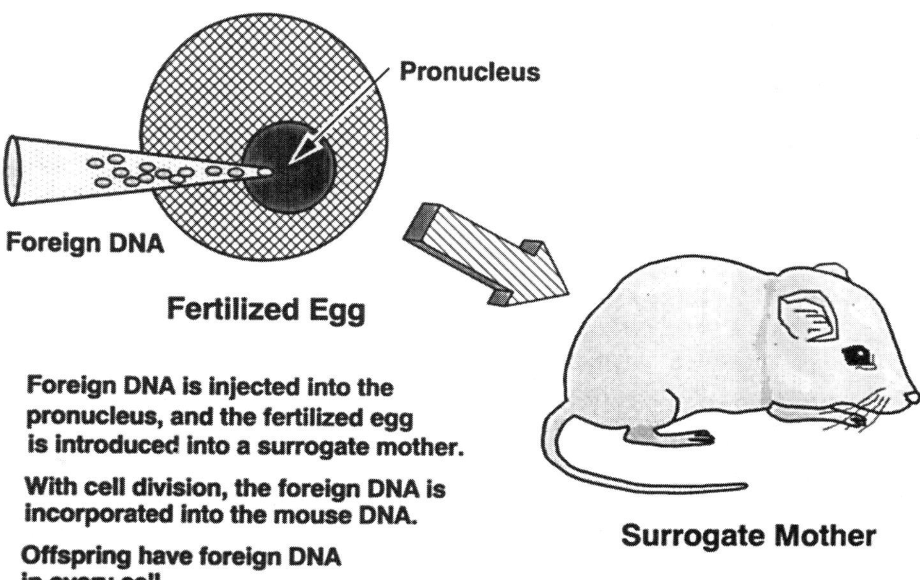

FIGURE 1–83. Transgenic mice. Recombinant DNA is injected into a fertilized mouse egg. The foreign DNA incorporates into the chromosome with cell division. As the egg develops into an embryo, every cell in the animal contains the foreign DNA. (From Simon, S.R., ed.: Orthopaedic Basic Science, 2nd ed., p. 228. Rosemont, IL, American Academy of Orthopaedic Surgeons, 1994; reprinted by permission.)

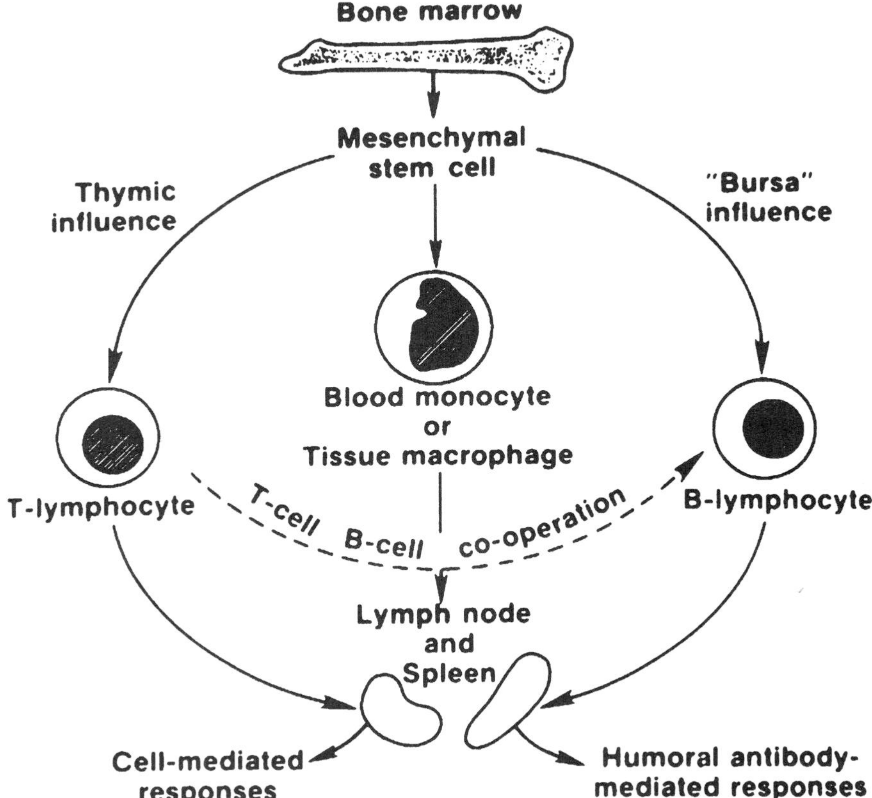

FIGURE 1–84. Bone marrow primitive mesenchymal cells differentiate into B and T lymphocytes and macrophages and cooperate in cell-mediated and humoral responses. (From Friedlander, G.E.: Immunology. In The Scientific Basis of Orthopaedics, 2nd ed., Albright, J.A., and Brand, R.A., eds., p. 484. Norwalk, CT, Appleton & Lange, 1987; reprinted by permission.)

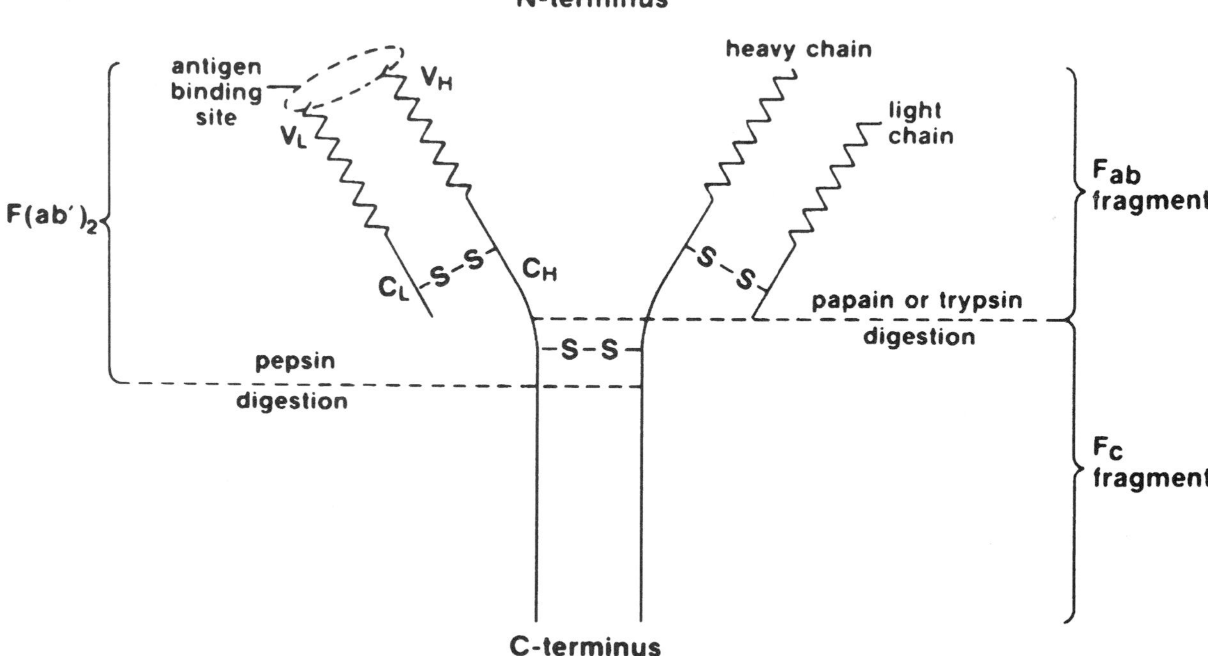

FIGURE 1–85. Basic subunit structure of the immunoglobulin molecule. (From Friedlander, G.E.: Immunology. In The Scientific Basis of Orthopaedics, 2nd ed., Albright J.A., and Brand, R.A., eds., p. 486. Norwalk, CT, Appleton & Lange, 1987; reprinted by permission.)

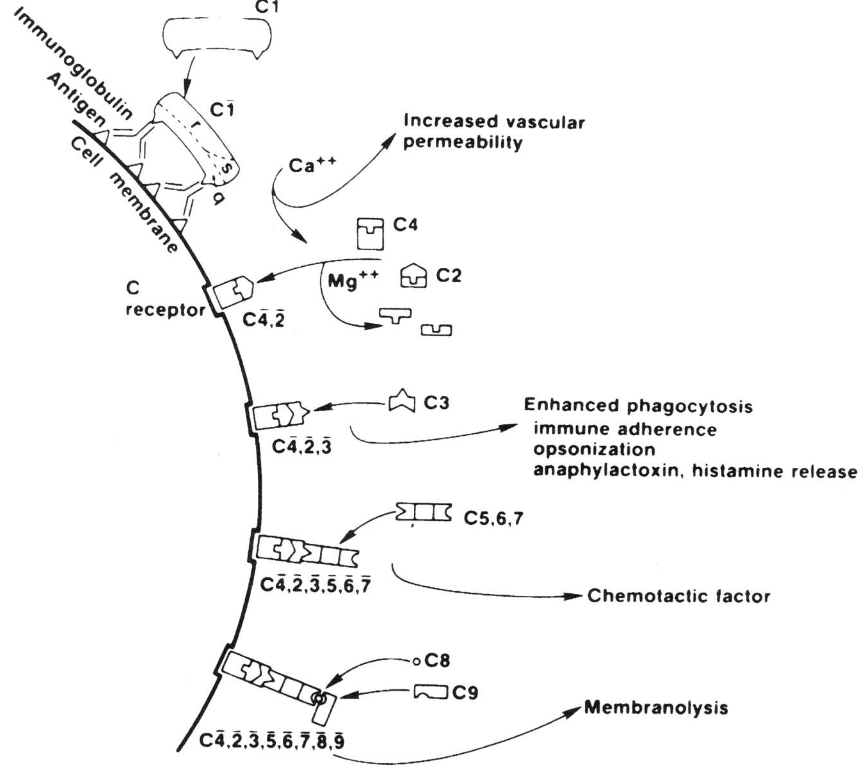

FIGURE 1–86. Complement cascade. (From Friedlander, G.E.: Immunology. In The Scientific Basis of Orthopaedics, 2nd ed., Albright, J.A., and Brand, R.A., eds., p. 491. Norwalk, CT, Appleton & Lange, 1987; reprinted by permission.)

8. Northern Hybridization—Technique used to identify a particular RNA in an extract of mixed RNA.
9. Polymerase Chain Reaction (PCR) Amplification—Method used to repetitively synthesize a specific DNA sequence in vivo such that the number of DNA copies doubles each cycle. PCR amplification has gained widespread use and has been employed for the prenatal diagnosis of sickle cell disease and screening DNA for gene mutations.

II. Immunology

A. Overview—Immunology is the study of the body's defense mechanisms. Areas of particular relevance to the musculoskeletal system are infection, transplantation, tumors, autoimmune disorders (e.g.,

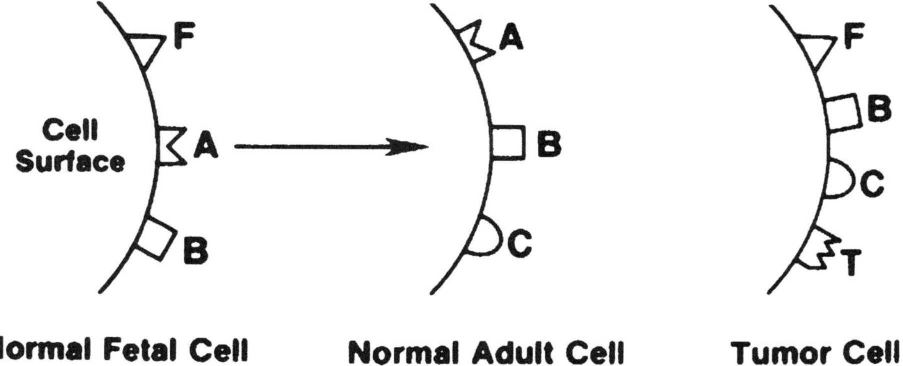

FIGURE 1–87. Tumor cells have cell-surface antigens common to other normal cells reflecting the tissue of origin (*B, C*). They may also demonstrate antigens normally present only on fetal cells (*F*) and loose antigens common to the cell type of origin (*A*). In addition, they acquire new tumor-associated antigens (*T*). (From Friedlander, G.E.: Immunology. In The Scientific Basis of Orthopaedics, 2nd ed., Albright, J.A., and Brand, R.A., eds., p. 502. Norwalk, CT, Appleton & Lange, 1987; reprinted by permission.)

rheumatoid arthritis), and bone remodeling. Two types of immune response have been described: nonspecific and specific.

B. Nonspecific Immune Response—**Inflammatory reaction** that begins when an antigen is recognized as foreign. This response may arise as a result of a fracture, soft tissue injury, or foreign body. Histamine is released and results in local vasodilation (exudate) with phagocytic cells that enzymatically digest "offending material." The inflammatory response may be enhanced by activation of the complement system or quieted by anti-inflammatory medication.

C. Specific Immune Response (Fig. 1–84)—Includes **cell-mediated** and **humoral** immune responses, which involve macrophages, B lymphocytes, and T lymphocytes.
   1. Antigens—Evoke an immune response.
   2. Macrophages—Responsible for processing antigen so it is able to stimulate lymphocytes.
   3. B Lymphocytes—Differentiate into **plasma cells** upon stimulation and produce immunoglobulins (Ig antibodies) against specific antigens. B lymphocytes are different from T lymphocytes because B lymphocytes are associated with immunoglobulins and the HLA system.
   4. Immunoglobulins—Produced by plasma cells in a "Y" configuration (Fig. 1–85). Five classes of immunoglobulin have been described.
      a. IgA—Mucosal surfaces.
      b. IgM—Produced earliest by fetus; largest.
      c. IgG—Most common; arises in response to infection.
      d. IgD—Acts as a receptor.
      e. IgE—Allergic responses.
   5. T Lymphocytes (T cells)—Originate in bone marrow and mature in the thymus. Produce cytokines. T cells include helper T cells, suppressor T cells, and "killer" T cells.

TABLE 1–28. AGE OF MANIFESTATION OF SOME GENETIC DISEASES

AGE	DISORDER
Conception	Chromosomal rearrangements (miscarriage)
Birth	Club feet
	Dislocated hip
	Skeletal dysplasias
Childhood	Morquio syndrome
	Multiple exostoses
	Vitamin D-resistant rickets
	Duchenne's muscular dystrophy
Adolescence	Scoliosis
	Ankylosing spondylitis
Middle age	Dupuytren's contracture

Adapted from Simon, S.R.: Orthopaedic Basic Science, 2nd ed., p. 211. Rosemont, IL, American Academy of Orthopaedic Surgeons, 1994, reprinted by permission.

TABLE 1–29. GENETIC MUTATIONS KNOWN TO CAUSE MUSCULOSKELETAL DISEASES

GENETIC DISEASE	ABNORMAL GENE
Osteogenesis imperfecta	Type I collagen
Marfan syndrome	Fibrillin gene
Selected chondrodystrophies	Type II collagen
Vitamin D-resistant rickets	Vitamin D receptor
Familial aortic aneurysm	Type III collagen

From Simon, S.R.: Orthopaedic Basic Science, 2nd ed., p. 230. Rosemont, IL, American Academy of Orthopaedic Surgeons, 1994, reprinted by permission.

   6. Cytokines—Proteins (or glycoproteins) that are cell products secreted in response to a foreign antigen. They regulate inflammatory and immune responses. Cytokines have been described in four broad categories.
      a. Interferons
      b. Growth Factors
      c. Colony-Stimulating Factors
      d. Interleukins
   7. Complement System (Fig. 1–86)—Group of 25 proteins that act in a "cascading sequence" to amplify an immune response.
   8. Immunogenetics—Human leukocyte antigens (HLA) contribute to the "specificity of immune recognition." The HLA gene is located on chromosome 6 (short arm); there are 6 class I loci and 14 class II loci. Table 1–19 shows gene variants for some of the rheumatoid conditions.
   9. Transplantation
      a. Allogenic Grafting—Transplantation between nonidentical members of the same species.
      b. Xenografting—Transplantation of tissues across species.
      c. Graft preparation
         1. Freezing—Cellular response diminished.
         2. Freeze-drying (Lyophilization)—Cellular response nearly undetectable.
   10. Oncology (Fig. 1–87)

III. Genetics of Orthopaedics—Although more than 3000 genetic disorders have been identified, the genes responsible for the disorders have been identified in but a small number of the musculoskeletal diseases (Tables 1–28, 1–29). Bone tumors arise as a result of a mutation in the genes responsible for regulating cell growth. It is believed that tumor cells (clones) arise as a result of inappropriately stimulated DNA transcription, translation, and replication along with inhibition of the mechanisms responsible for the suppression of growth. Our goal in understanding genetic disorders is to discover the specific gene responsible for the disorder and analyze the mutation.

Test Questions continued on opposite page

TEST QUESTIONS ON CELLULAR AND MOLECULAR BIOLOGY, IMMUNOLOGY, AND GENETICS OF ORTHOPAEDICS

TEST	QUESTION NUMBERS
1995 OSAE—Adult Reconstruction Hip/Knee	
1995 OSAE—Pediatric Orthopaedics	75, 76
1995 OSAE—Sports Medicine	
1994 OITE	
1994 OSAE—Adult Spine	
1994 OSAE—Foot and Ankle	
1994 OSAE—M/S Trauma	
1993 OITE	211
1993 OSAE—M/S Tumors and Diseases	
1993 OSAE—Shoulder and Elbow	
1992 OITE	
1992 OSAE—Adult Reconstruction Hip/Knee	
1992 OSAE—Pediatric Orthopaedics	
1992 OSAE—Sports Medicine	
1991 OITE	49, 193
1991 OSAE—Adult Spine	64
1991 OSAE—Anatomy and Imaging	
1991 OSAE—Foot and Ankle	23
1991 OSAE—M/S Trauma	

SECTION 5
Orthopaedic Infections and Microbiology

I. **Musculoskeletal Infections**—The following should serve as an overview of orthopaedic infections. Specific infections unique to particular orthopaedic areas are covered in detail in the appropriate chapters that follow.

A. Soft Tissue Infections

1. Cellulitis—Inflammatory infection of the subcutaneous tissues, usually due to staph or strep (and *Hemophilus* in children). Local erythema, tenderness, and occasionally lymphangitis/lymphadenopathy make up the clinical picture. Ordinarily, mild cases of cellulitis can be treated with an oral penicillinase-resistant synthetic penicillin (PRSP) or cephalosporin (cefazolin). Patients with high fever, systemic toxicity, poor host resistance, or underlying skin disease should be admitted for IV antibiotic therapy.

2. Significant Streptococcal Infections—Several serious diseases are related to specific streptococcal infections.

a. Erysipelas—**Group A (hemolytic) strep** causes this acute, progressively enlarging, red, raised, painful plaque seen predominantly in infants, diabetics, the elderly, and patients with predisposing skin ulcers. Severe toxicity, fever, leukocytosis, and bacteremia are common. Treatment is with high doses of PRSP or cefazolin.

b. Necrotizing Fasciitis—Aggressive, **life-threatening fascial infection** that is often associated with underlying vascular disease (especially diabetes). Usually follows insignificant trauma (can follow abdominal surgery in diabetics) and progresses rapidly. Can be associated with strep gangrene and may be polymicrobial with both aerobes and anaerobes. **Wide surgical I&D** and IV antibiotics are required **emergently.**

3. Gas Gangrene—Classically caused by ***Clostridium*** species (**gram-positive [G+] anaerobic rod**) but also can develop from gram-negative (G−) and sometimes G+ (strep) infections. Clinical presentation usually includes progressive pain; edema (distant from wound); foul-smelling, serosanguineous discharge. May be associated with bowel cancer. Radiographs typically show widespread **gas in tissues.** Treatment is with high dose penicillin G and clindamycin (or ceftriaxone, erythromycin), hyperbaric oxygen (inhibits toxins), and **surgical I&D.**
4. Tetanus—Potentially lethal neuroparalytic disease caused by an exotoxin of ***Clostridium tetani.*** Treatment is centered on prophylaxis with proper wound care and tetanus toxoid administration (and tetanus immunoglobulin [TIG] for patients with severe wounds and without known previous immunizations) (Table 1–30). Late management is largely symptomatic.
5. Toxic Shock Syndrome—Severe staph infection that usually develops postoperatively; **represents toxemia (from toxins produced), not septicemia. Fever, hypotension,** systemic symptoms, an **erythematous macular rash,** and a **serous exudate** (with G+ cocci) are present. Wounds may look benign but require immediate I&D and IV antibiotics; the patient may also require emergent fluid resuscitation (*).
6. Surgical Wound Infection—There has been a recent increase in the incidence of *Staph. epidermidis* wound infections. *Staph. aureus* is still the most common infection overall and is the most common in trauma patients. Methicillin-resistant *Staphylococcus* species infections are also increasing and are best treated with vancomycin.
7. Puncture Wounds of the Foot—Commonly are infected with *Pseudomonas* (classically from punctures through the sole of a tennis shoe) (***). *Pseudomonas* infections (**G− rod**) require aggressive débridement and appropriate antibiotics (aminoglycoside and piperacillin early). *Pseudomonas* infections require a two-antibiotic regimens ciprofloxacin may also be used in patients over 15 years of age. The prophylactic antibiotic treatment for a patient presenting with a recent (hours) puncture wound through the sole of a tennis shoe (without infection) remains controversial.
8. Diabetic Foot—Cultures of a recurrent, life-threatening diabetic foot show a **polymicrobial** picture (***) (including aerobic cocci, aerobic bacilli, and anaerobes). The antibiotic regimen includes ciprofloxacin (Cipro) and clindamycin; for septic patients, use imipenem/cilastatin, Timentin, or piperacillin-tazobactam. The most common organism in a limited number of cases of diabetic foot is aerobic G+ cocci, which should be treated with clindamycin or a first generation cephalosporin.
9. Paronychia—Most common organisms acquired from nail biting and manicuring are *Staph. aureus* and anaerobes (clindamycin or erythromycin). In **dentists** and anesthesiologists, consider **herpes simplex (whitlow)** and treat with acyclovir.
10. Bites—Bite injuries are summarized in Table 1–31.
11. Fungal Infections—Fungi are multicellular organisms with mycelia (branches) that induce a hypersensitivity reaction in tissues, causing chronic granuloma, abscess, and necrosis. Surgical treatment and **amphotericin B** administration are often required. Oral ketoconazole is effective for some limited infections.
12. Human Immunodeficiency Virus (HIV) Infection—Incidence is high in the homosexual male population and is becoming increasingly common in heterosexual patients. Additionally, more than half of the hemophiliac population is af-

TABLE 1–30. ANTITETANUS PROPHYLAXIS, WOUND CLASSIFICATION, IMMUNIZATION

Wound Classification[a]		
CLINICAL FEATURES	TETANUS PRONE	NONTETANUS PRONE
Age of wound	>6 Hours	≤6 Hours
Configuration	Stellate, avulsion	Linear
Depth	>1 cm	≤1 cm
Mechanism of injury	Missile, crush, burn, frostbite	Sharp surface (glass, knife)
Devitalized tissue	Present	Absent
Contaminants (e.g., dirt, saliva)	Present	Absent

Immunization Schedule[b]				
HISTORY OF TETANUS IMMUNIZATION	*Tetanus-Prone Wound* Td[c]	*Tetanus-Prone Wound* TIG	*Non-Tetanus-Prone Wound* Td	*Non-Tetanus-Prone Wound* TIG
Unknown or <3 doses	Yes	Yes	Yes	No
Three or more doses	No[d]	No	No[e]	No

Adapted from Sanford, J.P., Guide to Antimicrobial Therapy, p. 116. Dallas, Antimicrobial Therapy, Inc., 1994, reprinted by permission.
Td, tetanus and diphtheria toxoids (adults); TIG, tetanus immune globulin (human).
[a] Data from ACS Bulletin 69(10):22–23, 1984.
[b] Data from Morbidity and Mortality Weekly Report 39:37, 1990.
[c] Yes if wound >24 hours old. For children <7 years, DPT (DT if pertussis vaccine contraindicated); for persons ≥7 years, Td preferred to tetanus toxoid alone.
[d] Yes if >5 years since last booster.
[e] Yes if >10 years since last booster.

TABLE 1–31. BITE INJURIES

SOURCE OF BITE	ORGANISM(S)	PRIMARY ANTIMICROBIAL (OR DRUG) REGIMEN
Human	*Strep. viridans* (100%) *Bacteroides* *Staph. epidermidis* *Corynebacterium* *Staph. aureus* *Peptostreptococcus* *Eikenella*	Amoxicillin/clavulanate (Augmentin) [*Eikenella* → cefoxitan or ampicillin]
Dog	*Strep. viridans* *Pasteurella multocida* *Bacteroides* *Fusobacterium*	Penicillin V or ampicillin consider antirabies treatment
Cat	*Pasteurella multocida* *Staph. aureus* Possibly tularemia	Amoxicillin/clavulanate (Augmentin) *or* penicillin V
Rat	*Streptobacillus moniliformis*	Ampicillin antirabies treatment *not* indicated
Pig	Polymicrobic (aerobes and anerobes)	Amoxicillin/clavulanate (Augmentin)
Skunk, raccoon, bat	?	Ampicillin antirabies treatment indicated
Pit viper (snake)	*Pseudomonas* Enterobacteriaceae *Staph. epidermidis* *Clostridium*	Antivenom therapy ceftriaxone tetanus prophylaxis
Brown recluse spider	—	Dapsone
Catfish sting	Toxins (may become secondarily infected)	Amoxicillin/clavulanate (Augmentin)

Adapted from Sanford J.P.: Guide to Antimicrobial Therapy, pp. 30–31. Dallas, Antimicrobial Therapy, Inc., 1994, reprinted by permission.

fected. Fetal acquired immunodeficiency syndrome (AIDS) is transmitted across the placenta, and affected children typically have a box-like forehead, wide eyes, a small head, and growth failure. The virus primarily affects the lymphocyte and macrophage cell lines and **decreases the number of T helper cells (T4 lymphocytes).** This disease has increased the importance of blood and body fluid handling precautions during trauma management and surgery. Only advanced stages of HIV infection are classified as AIDS [class 6 of 6 in the Walter Reed classification scheme]. **HIV positivity is not a contraindication to performing required surgical procedures.** There is a 0.3% risk of HIV conversion following parenteral inoculation. HIV-positive patients (even those who are asymptomatic) with traumatic orthopaedic injuries (especially open fractures) or those undergoing certain orthopaedic surgical procedures appear to be at increased risk for developing wound infections as well as nonwound-related complications (e.g., urinary tract infection, pneumonia). Patients with HIV can develop secondary rheumatologic conditions such as Reiter's syndrome (*).

13. Hepatitis—Three types are commonly recognized.
    a. Hepatitis A—Common in areas with poor sanitation and public health concerns. Not a major problem of surgical transmission.
    b. Hepatitis B—Approximately 200,000 people are infected with the hepatitis B virus each year, and there are more than 1 million carriers. Screening and use of a vaccine has reduced the risk of transmission for health care workers. Immune globulin is administered after exposure in nonvaccinated individuals. Neither vaccine nor immune globulin administration has been documented as causing HIV transmission.
    c. Hepatitis Non-A, Non-B—The offending virus has been identified (hepatitis C virus). It is the **most common transfusion-associated hepatitis.**
14. Marine Injuries—To identify the pathogen, culture the specimen at 30°C (86°F) (*).

B. Bone and Joint Infections—A summary of common organisms found in osteomyelitis and septic arthritis are shown in Tables 1–32 and 1–33, respectively.
   1. Acute Hematogenous Osteomyelitis—Bone and bone marrow infection caused (most commonly) by blood-borne organisms. Commonly affects children (boys > girls). ***Staph. aureus* is the most common offender.** Anaerobic infections are also frequently seen, with *Peptococcus magnus* (G+) appearing more frequently than *Bacteroides* (G−). The infection is most common in the metaphyses or epiphyses of long bones (lower extremity > upper extremity). Radiographic changes include soft tissue swelling (early), demineralization (10 days to 2 weeks), and **sequestra** (dead bone with surrounding granulation tissue) and **involucrum** (periosteal new bone) later. Pain, loss of function, and sometimes a soft tissue abscess are present. Elevated WBC count and ESR and positive blood cultures are usually seen. Bone scan (delayed uptake in bone [pinhole views may be helpful]) ± gallium (for spinal infections) or indium (for extremity infections) scans may be helpful in equivocal cases. MRI shows the changes usually before plain films (nonspecific low signal intensity in marrow spaces on both T_1 and T_2 images). Aspiration is helpful for antibiotic choice. IV antibiotics followed by a course of oral antibiotics after the tem-

TABLE 1–32. ORGANISMS FOUND IN OSTEOMYELITIS

AGE AND CIRCUMSTANCES	ORGANISM	PRIMARY REGIMEN
Newborn	*Staph. aureus* Enterobacteriaceae Group A streptococcus Group B streptococcus	PRSP + third generation cephalosporin
Child ≤4 years	*H. influenzae* Streptococci *Staph. aureus*	Cefuroxime *or* third generation cephalosporin
Child >4 years	*Staph. aureus* Streptococci *H. influenzae*	PRSP *or* first generation cephalosporin
Adult	*Staph. aureus* Enterobacteriaceae Strep. species	PRSP *or* first generation cephalosporin
Puncture to foot through tennis shoe	*Pseudomonas* *Staph. aureus*	Cipro *or* Timentin *or* imipenem/cilastatin *or* third generation cephalosporin

Adapted from Sanford J.P.: Guide to Antimicrobial Therapy, p. 1. Dallas, Antimicrobial Therapy, Inc., 1994, reprinted by permission.
PRSP, penicillinase-resistant synthetic penicillin; Cipro, Ciprofloxacin.

perature has normalized (total of 6 weeks or until the ESR returns to normal), immobilization, and surgical drainage, when indicated, is the treatment regimen of choice. The indications for operative intervention include (1) drainage of an abscess; (2) débridement of infected tissues to save bone from further destruction; and (3) refractory cases that fail to show improvement after nonoperative treatment. Recurrence is high for metatarsal lesions (50%), around the knee (25%), and with late diagnosis (25%). Long-term morbidity is >25%. The treatment of acute osteomyelitis may be summarized as follows: (1) identification of organism; (2) selection of appropriate antibiotics; (3) delivery of antibiotics to the site of infection; and (4) halting tissue destruction.

TABLE 1–34. INFECTED HOST TYPES

TYPE	DESCRIPTION	RISK
A	Normal immune response; nonsmoker	Minimal
B	Local or mild systemic deficiency; smoker	Moderate
C	Major nutritional or systemic disorder	High

2. Subacute Osteomyelitis—Usually discovered radiologically in a patient with a painful limp and no systemic (and often no local) signs or symptoms. Subacute osteomyelitis may arise secondary to partially treated acute osteomyelitis or occasionally develops in a fracture hematoma. Unlike acute osteomyelitis, WBC count and blood cultures are frequently normal. ESR, bone cultures, and radiographs are often useful. It most commonly affects the femur and tibia; and unlike acute osteomyelitis, it can cross the physis even in older children. Radiographic changes include **Brodie's abscess** (a localized radiolucency usually seen in the metaphyses of long bones). It is sometimes difficult to differentiate from Ewing's sarcoma. When localized to the epiphysis only, other lesions (e.g., chondroblastoma) must be ruled out. **Epiphyseal osteomyelitis is caused almost exclusively by *Staph, aureus.*** Treatment of Brodie's abscess in the metaphysis includes surgical curettage. Epiphyseal osteomyelitis requires surgical drainage only if pus is present (48 hours of IV antibiotics followed by 6 weeks of oral antibiotics is curative otherwise).
3. Chronic Osteomyelitis—May arise as a result of inappropriately treated acute osteomyelitis, trauma, or soft tissue spread, especially in the Cierney type C elderly host, the immunosuppressed, diabetics, and IV drug abusers (*Pseudomonas*) (*) (Table 1–34). *Staph. aureus,* G– rods, and anaerobes are frequent offending organisms. It is often classified anatomically (Cierney) (Fig. 1–88). Skin and soft tissue are often involved, and **fistulous tracts** occasionally develop into **epidermoid carcinoma.** Periods of quiescence are often followed by **acute exacerbations.** Nuclear medicine studies are often helpful for

TABLE 1–33. ORGANISMS FOUND IN SEPTIC ARTHRITIS

AGE AND CIRCUMSTANCES	ORGANISM	PRIMARY REGIMEN
<3 Months	*Staph. aureus* Enterobacteriaceae Group B strep.	PRSP + third generation cephalosporin
3 Months to 6 years	*Staph. aureus* *H. influenzae* Streptococci Enterobacteriaceae	(PRSP or first generation cephalosporin) + third generation cephalosporin
Adult	*Staph. aureus* Group A streptococci Enterobacteriaceae	[(PRSP or first generation cephalosporin) + (APAG or Cipro)] *or* Timentin *or* piperacillin tazobactam *or* Unasyn
Adults with joint replacement	*Staph. epidermidis* *Staph. aureus* Enterobacteriaceae *Pseudomonas*	Vancomycin + Cipro *or* aztreonam *or* APAG

Adapted from Sanford J.P.: Guide to Antimicrobial Therapy, p. 17. Dallas, Antimicrobial Therapy, Inc., 1994, reprinted by permission.
PRSP, penicillinase-resistant synthetic penicillin; APAG, antipseudomonal aminoglycosidic antibiotic.

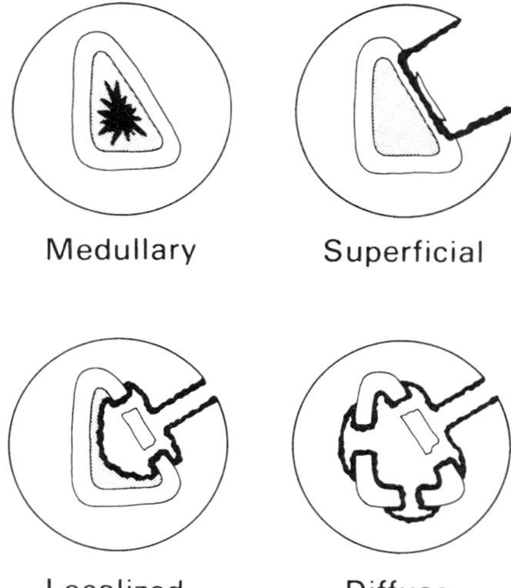

FIGURE 1–88. Cierney's anatomic classification of adult chronic osteomyelitis. (From Cierney, G., III: Chronic osteomyelitis: Results of treatment. Instr. Course Lect. 39:495, 1990; reprinted by permission.)

determining the activity of the disease. A combination of IV antibiotics (based on deep cultures), surgical débridement, bone grafting (open, vascularized, or bypass [proximal and distal to infected area]), stabilization (avoid IM devices following external fixator use with associated pin tract infections), and soft tissue coverage (flaps) are often required. Amputations are still frequently necessary.

4. Chronic Sclerosing Osteomyelitis—An unusual infection that involves primarily diaphyseal bones of adolescents. Typified by intense proliferation of the periosteum leading to bony deposition, it may be caused by anaerobic organisms. Insidious onset, dense progressive sclerosis on radiographs, and localized pain and tenderness are common. Malignancy must be ruled out. Surgical and antibiotic therapy are usually not curative.
5. Chronic Multifocal Osteomyelitis—Caused by an infectious agent, it appears in children without systemic symptoms. Normal laboratory values, except for an elevated ESR, are common. Radiographs demonstrate multiple metaphyseal lytic lesions, especially in the medial clavicle, distal tibia, and distal femur. Symptomatic treatment only is recommended because this condition usually resolves spontaneously.
6. Osteomyelitis with Unusual Organisms—Several unusual organisms occur in certain clinical settings (Table 1–35). Radiographs show characteristic features in syphilis (*Treponema pallidum*) (radiolucency in metaphysis from granulation tissue) and tuberculosis (joint destruction on both sides of a joint). Histology can also be helpful (e.g., tuberculosis with granulomas and Langerhan's giant cells).
7. Septic Arthritis (see Table 1–33)—Commonly follows hematogenous spread or extension of metaphyseal osteomyelitis in children. Can also arise as a complication of a diagnostic or therapeutic procedure. Most cases involve infants (hip) and children. **The metaphysis of the proximal femur, proximal humerus, radial neck, and distal fibula are within their respective joint capsules; metaphyseal osteomyelitis can rupture into the joint in these areas.** The most common site at which septic arthritis follows acute osteomyelitis is the proximal femur/hip (*). RA (tuberculosis most characteristic, *Staph. aureus* most common) and IV drug abuse (*Pseudomonas* most characteristic) predispose adults. Surgical drainage (often arthroscopically) or daily aspiration is the mainstay of treatment. Open drainage is required for septic hip joints. SI joint sepsis is unusual and is best diagnosed by physical examina-

TABLE 1–35. UNUSUAL ORGANISMS FOUND IN OSTEOMYELITIS

ORGANISM	RISK FACTOR(S)	SYMPTOMS/SIGNS/FINDINGS	TREATMENT
Serratia marcescens	IV drug abuse	Axial skeleton	Cotrimoxazole
Pseudomonas aeruginosa	IV drug abuse	Nonspecific	Aminoglycoside
Brucella (G−)	Meat handling	Flat bones	Tetracycline/Septra
Salmonella	Sickle cell disease	Asymptomatic	Ampicillin
Anaerobes	Skin contamination	Tissue culture	Clindamycin/cephalosporin
Fungi	Skin contamination	Special study	Amphotericin B
Treponema pallidum	Sexual contact	Nontender swelling	Penicillin
Mycobacteria	TB/leprosy/fishermen	PPD/granuloma/culture at 30°C	PAS, isoniazid

TB, tuberculosis, PPD, purified protein derivative; PAS, *p*-aminosalicylic acid.

TABLE 1–36. OVERVIEW OF ANTIMICROBIAL AGENTS

PENICILLINS

Natural

Penicillin G
Penicillin V (Pen·Vee K)

Penicillinase Resistant (PRSP)

Methicillin (Staphcillin, Celbenin)
Nafcillin (Unipen, Nafcil)
Oxacillin (Prostaphlin, Bactocill)
Cloxacillin (Tegopen)
Dicloxacillin (Dynapen, Pathocil)
Flucloxacillin

Aminopenicillins

Ampicillin (Omnipen, Polycillin)
Amoxacillin (Amoxil)
Bacampicillin (Spectrobid)
Amoxicillin clavulanate (Augmentin)
Ampicillin/sulbactam (Unasyn)

Antipseudomonal Agents

Indanyl carbenicillin (Geocillin)
Ticarcillin (Ticar)
Ticarcillin/clavulanate (Timentin)
Mezlocillin (Mezlin)
Piperacillin (Pracil)
Piperacillin tazobactam (Zosyn)

CEPHALOSPORINS

First Generation

Cephalothin (Keflin, Seffin)
Cefazolin (Ancef, Kefzol)
Cephapirin (Cefadyl)
Cephradine (Velosef)
Cephalexin (Keflex, Keftab)
Cefadroxil (Duricef, Ultracef)

Second Generation

Cefaclor (Ceclor)
Cefamandole (Mandol)
Cefoxitin (Mefoxin)
Cefuroxime (Zinacef, Kefurox)
Cefuroxime axetil (Ceftin)
Cefmetazole (Zefazone)
Cefotetan (Cefotan)
Cefprozil (Cefzil)
Cefonicid (Monocid)
Loracarbef (Lorabid)
Ceftibuten (Cedax)

Third Generation

Cefetamet pivoxil (R. 15-8075)
Cefoperazone (Cefobid)
Cefotaxime (Claforan)
Ceftizoxime (Cefizox)
Ceftriaxone (Rocephin, Nitrocephin)
Ceftazidime (Fortaz)
Cefixime (Suprax)
Cefpodoxime proxetil (Vantin)

Fourth Generation

Cefpirome
Cefepime

CARBAPENEMS

Imipenem [+ cilastatin (Primaxin)]

MONOBACTAMS

Aztreonam (Azactam)

AMINOGLYCOSIDES

Amikacin (Amikin)
Gentamicin (Garamycin)
Kanamycin (Kantrex)
Netilmicin (Netromycin)
Tobramycin (Nebcin)

FLUOROQUINOLONES

Norfloxacin (Noroxin)
Ciprofloxacin (Cipro)
Ofloxacin (Floxin)
Enoxacin (Penetrex)
Lomefloxacin (Maxaquin)
Pefloxacin

MACROLIDES

Azithromycin (Zithromax)
Clarithromycin (Biaxin)
Erythromycin

OTHER ANTIBACTERIAL AGENTS

Chloramphenicol (Chloromycetin)
Clindamycin (Cleocin)
Vancomycin (Vancocin, Vancoled)
Teicoplanin (Targocid)
Doxycycline (Vibramycin)
Minocycline (Minocin)
Tetracycline (Terramycin)
Polymixin B (Aerosporin)
Fusidic acid (Fucidin)
Fosfomycin
Sulfisoxazole (Gantrisin)
Trimethoprim/sulfamethoxazole (Bactrim, Septra)
Metronidazole (Flagyl)

ANTIFUNGAL AGENTS

Amphotericin B (Fungizone)
Fluconazole (Diflucan)
Flucytosine (Ancobon)
Ketoconazole (Nizoral)
Itraconazole (Sporanox)

ANTIMYCOBACTERIAL AGENTS

Isoniazid [INH (nydrazid)]
Rifampin (Rifadin)
Ethambutol (Myambutol)
Streptomycin
Pyrazinamide
Ethionamide
Cycloserine (Seromycin)
Amikacin (Amikin)
Capreomycin (Capastat)
Thioacetazone
Rifabutin (Mycobutin)

ANTIPARASITIC AGENTS

Albendazole (Zentel)
Atovaquone (Mepron)
Dapsone
Mefloquine (Lariam)
Pentamidine (Pentam 300)
Pyrimethamine (Daraprim)
Praziquantel (Biltricide)

ANTIVIRAL AGENTS

Acyclovir (Zovirax)
Amantadine (Symmetrel)
Didanosine (Videx)
Foscarnet (Foscavir)
Ganciclovir (Cytovene)
Zalcitabine (HIVID)
Zidovudine [AZT (Retrovir)]

Adapted from Sanford J.P.: Guide to Antimicrobial Therapy, pp. 45–60. Dallas, Antimicrobial Therapy, Inc., 1994, reprinted by permission.

tion (flexion abduction external rotation [FABER] most specific), ESR, bone scan, CT scan, and aspiration. A pannus (much as in inflammatory arthritis) can be seen in tuberculosis infections. Late sequelae of septic arthritis include soft tissue contractures that can sometimes be treated with soft tissue procedures such as quadricepsplasty.

8. Septic Bursitis—Most commonly caused by a *Staph. aureus* infection. Treated with PRSP.

C. Other Infections

1. Infected Total Joint Arthroplasty—Covered in Chapter 4, Adult Reconstruction, but bears some mention here. Perioperative IV antibiotics are the most effective method for decreasing its incidence, although good operative technique, laminar flow (avoiding obstruction between the air source and the operative wound), and special "space" suits also have a role. The ESR is the most sensitive indicator of infection, but it is nonspecific. Culture of the hip aspirate is sensitive and specific. C-reactive protein may be helpful also. Acute infections (within 2–3 weeks) can usually be treated with prosthesis salvage (provided the components are stable), but delayed or chronic infections require removal. ***Staph. epidermidis*** (and *Staph. aureus*) are the most common offenders. Polymicrobial organisms may form an overlying glycocalyx, making infection control difficult without removing the prosthesis and vigorous débridement. However, according to Cierney, the host is more important than the organism in terms of risk (see Table 1–34). Use of antibiotic-impregnated cement in revision arthroplasties and antibiotic spacers/beads in infected total joints may be helpful. Reimplantation after thorough débridement and use of polymethyl methacrylate (PMMA) with antibiotics has been successful at variable intervals. Some advocate frozen sections at the time of reimplantation to ensure that local tissues have fewer than 5–10 PMNs per high power field.
2. Allograft Infection—May involve up to 20% of allografts; requires aggressive measures to control.
3. Meningococcemia—Can develop in patients with multiple infarcts, such as those with **electrical burns.**
4. Marjolin's Ulcer—Squamous cell carcinoma that develops in patients with chronic drainage from sinus tracts. Seen in untreated chronic osteomyelitis.
5. Nutritional Status and Infection—Nutrition is critical to decreasing the incidence of postoperative infection. Malnutrition is common after multiple trauma.
6. Postsplenectomy Patients—Susceptible to streptococcal infections and respond poorly to them.

TABLE 1–37. ANTIBIOTICS, INDICATIONS, AND SIDE EFFECTS

ANTIBIOTIC	ORGANISMS	COMPLICATIONS/OTHER
CELL WALL SYNTHESIS INHIBITORS		
Penicillin	Strep, G+	Hypersensitivity/resistance, hemolytic
Methicillin/oxacillin/nafcillin	Penicillinase-resistant	Same as penicillin; nephritis (methicillin); subcut. skin slough (nafcillin)
Carbenicillin/ticarcillin/piperacillin	Better against G−	Bleeding diathesis (carbenicillin)
Cephalosporins		
First generation	Prophylaxis (surgical)	Cephazolin the drug of choice
Second generation	Some G+/G−	
Third generation	G−, fewer G+	Hemolytic anemia (bleeding diathesis [moxalactam])
INHIBITORS OF CELL MEMBRANE FUNCTION		
Polymyxin/nystatin	GU	Nephrotoxic
Amphotericin	Fungi	Nephrotoxic
INHIBITORS OF PROTEIN SYNTHESIS		
Aminoglycosides	G−, PM	Nephrotoxicity, ototoxicity (dose-related)
Clindamycin	G+, anaerobes	Pseudomembranous enterocolitis
Chloramphenicol	*H. influenzae*, anaerobes	Bone marrow aplasia
Erythromycin	G+ (PCN allergy)	Ototoxic
Tetracycline	G+ (PCN allergy)	Stains teeth/bone (up to age 8)
FLUOROQUINOLONES		
Ciprofloxacin	G−, methicillin-resistant *S. aureus*	Cartilage erosion (children); oral therapy increases theophylline levels; antacids reduce absorption
INHIBITORS OF NUCLEIC ACID SYNTHESIS		
Vancomycin	Methicillin-resistant *S. aureus, C. difficile*	Ototoxic, erythema with rapid IV delivery
Sulfonamides	GU	Hemolytic anemia
CARBAPENEMS		
Imipenem	G+, some G−	Resistance, seizure
Azactam	G−, no anaerobes	

G+, gram positive; G−, gram negative; GU, genitourinary; PM, polymicrobial; PCN, penicillin; subcut, subcutaneous.

II. Antibiotics

A. Indications—Used for prevention of postoperative sepsis, treatment of incipient infection, and treatment of established infections. Perioperative use of first-generation cephalosporins is efficacious in cases requiring insertion of hardware. Grade I and II open fractures require a first generation cephalosporin, Grade IIIA require a first generation cephalosporin and an aminoglycoside; penicillin is added for grossly contaminated (grade IIIB) open fractures. Prophylaxis against hematogenous seeding of a TJA in patients undergoing dental manipulation includes Pen·Vee K (2 g) 1 hour prior to dental manipulation and 1 g 6 hours after the first dose (*).

B. Overview—An overview of antimicrobial agents is shown in Table 1–36.

C. Specific Antibiotics—Selected antibiotics, their indications, and side effects (*) are listed in Table 1–37.

D. Other Forms of Antibiotic Delivery

1. Antibiotic Beads or Spacers—PMMA impregnated with antibiotics (usually an aminoglycoside); useful when treating infections with TJA or for osteomyelitis with bony defects. Antibiotic powder is mixed with cement powder; the type of antibiotic to be used is guided by the microorganism present, and dosage depends on the specific antibiotic selected and type of PMMA used. Antibiotics that have been used with PMMA for infection are tobramycin, gentamicin, cefazolin (Ancef) and other cephalosporins, oxacillin, cloxacillin, methicillin, lincomycin, clindamycin, colistin, fucidin, neomycin, kanamycin, and ampicillin. Chloramphenicol and tetracycline appear to be inactivated during polymerization. Antibiotics are eluted from PMMA beads with an exponential decline in elution over a 2-week period and then cease to be present in significant levels locally by 6–8 weeks (*). Local tissue concentrations of antibiotic are much higher than can be achieved with systemic administration and do not seem to cause problems in doses that are typically used. Increased surface area of PMMA (e.g., with oval beads) enhances elution of antibiotics. Beads are inserted only after thorough débridement. Because PMMA itself is associated with inducing infection (*), the beads should always be removed. Antibiotic powder in doses of 2 g per 40 g of powdered PMMA (simplex P) does not appreciably affect the compressive strength of PMMA. Much higher concentrations (4–5 g of antibiotic powder per 40 g of PMMA) significantly reduce the compressive strength (important in cemented joint arthroplasties).
2. Osmotic Pump—Method for delivering high concentrations of antibiotics locally. Used mainly for osteomyelitis.
3. Home IV Therapy—Cost-effective alternative for patients requiring long-term IV antibiotics. This treatment is facilitated by the use of a Hickman or Broviac indwelling catheter.
4. Immersion Solution—Contaminated bone from an open fracture may be sterilized (100% effective) by immersion in chlorhexidine gluconate scrub and an antibiotic solution (*).

TEST QUESTIONS ON MUSCULOSKELETAL INFECTIONS AND ANTIBIOTICS

TEST	QUESTION NUMBERS
1995 OSAE—Adult Reconstruction Hip/Knee	25, 40, 94
1995 OSAE—Pediatric Orthopaedics	18, 24, 73, 84
1995 OSAE—Sports Medicine	
1994 OITE	13, 32, 102, 110, 137, 148, 187
1994 OSAE—Adult Spine	1, 2, 68, 70, 73
1994 OSAE—Foot and Ankle	44, 85, 87, 121
1994 OSAE—M/S Trauma	12, 43, 71, 88, 90
1993 OITE	52, 118, 186, 225
1993 OSAE—M/S Tumors and Diseases	7, 64, 69, 75, 77
1993 OSAE—Shoulder and Elbow	
1992 OITE	26, 36, 133, 154, 198, 201, 204, 205, 236
1992 OSAE—Adult Reconstruction Hip/Knee	19, 30, 31, 32, 87
1992 OSAE—Pediatric Orthopaedics	14, 19, 22
1992 OSAE—Sports Medicine	92
1991 OITE	12, 24, 35, 36, 40, 63, 82, 177, 178, 224, 231, 232, 238, 250
1991 OSAE—Adult Spine	88
1991 OSAE—Anatomy and Imaging	
1991 OSAE—Foot and Ankle	47, 48, 60, 66, 67, 81, 82
1991 OSAE—M/S Trauma	11, 12, 13, 14, 15, 17, 18, 20, 29, 87, 99

SECTION 6

Perioperative Problems

I. Pulmonary Problems

A. General Considerations—Pulmonary function tests and blood gas measurements are often helpful for evaluating baseline status. Thoracic and abdominal surgery can significantly affect these values.

B. Blood Gas Evaluation—The following is a simple working formula and is useful for evaluating blood gases:

$$pO_2 = 7(FiO_2) - pCO_2$$

where pO_2 is the **anticipated or normal pO_2** for a given FiO_2 in a normal individual, FiO_2 is the percent inspired oxygen, and pCO_2 is the value obtained by the blood gas assay.

Example: A 63-year-old man has acute onset of shortness of breath 12 hours after a THA. When you arrive at his bed he has on a face mask with an inspired oxygen (FiO_2) of 60%. Using our working formula the anticipated, or normal, pO_2 for a normal individual would be:

$$pO_2 = 7(60) - pCO_2 = 420 - pCO_2$$

Now let us assume that a blood gas assay (blood obtained 15 minutes after placing the patient on 60% oxygen) reveals the following **observed values:**

$$pO_2 = 120$$

$$pCO_2 = 60$$

With a pCO_2 of 60 the anticipated, or normal, pO_2 would be

$$pCO_2 = 420 - 60 = \underline{\underline{360}}$$

Therefore for the patient on 60% oxygen with a pCO_2 of 60 we would anticipate a pO_2 of 360 if all were normal. Because the observed pO_2 is only 120, there is obviously a problem with this patient's pulmonary status. To quantify the extent of the patient's problem we must next calculate the **Aa gradient:**

$$\textbf{Aa gradient} = \textbf{(anticipated or normal } pO_2 \textbf{ [for a given } FiO_2\textbf{])} - \textbf{(observed } pO_2\textbf{)}$$

Continuing with the example:

$$\text{Aa gradient} = (360) - (120) = \underline{\underline{240}}$$

Finally, the **percent physiologic shunt** may be calculated as follows:

$$\textbf{Percent physiologic shunt} = \frac{\textbf{Aa gradient}}{\textbf{20}}$$

Continuing with the example:

$$\text{Percent physiologic shunt} = \frac{240}{20} = \underline{\underline{12\%}}$$

C. Thromboembolism—A common problem in orthopaedic patients, especially in those with procedures about the hip. Risk is increased with a history of thromboembolism, obesity, malignancy, aging, congestive heart failure (CHF), birth control pill use, varicose veins, smoking, use of **general anesthetics (in contrast to continuous epidural anesthesia,** which has a lower incidence of thromboemboli) (*), increased blood viscosity, immobilization, paralysis, and pregnancy.

1. Deep Venous Thrombosis (DVT)—Clinical suspicion is more helpful than the physical examination findings (pain, swelling, Homan's sign) for DVT. Useful studies include venography (the "gold standard"), which is 97% accurate (70% for iliac veins), ^{125}I-labeled fibrinogen (operative site artifact causes false positives), impedence plethysmography (poor sensitivity), duplex ultrasonography (B-mode)—90% accurate for DVT proximal to trifurcation, and Doppler imaging (immediate bedside tool, often best for the first study). Prophylaxis is the most important factor in decreasing morbidity and mortality, and the methods commonly used are listed in Table 1–38. The anticoagulation effects of **warfarin (Coumadin) can be reversed with vitamin K or more rapidly with fresh frozen plasma** (*). The diagnosis of DVT postoperatively requires initiation of heparin therapy (followed by later conversion to long-term [3 months] warfarin therapy) (*). Treatment is recommended for all thigh DVTs; however, treatment of DVTs occurring below the pop-

TABLE 1–38. THROMBOEMBOLISM PROPHYLAXIS

METHOD	EFFECT	ADVANTAGES	DISADVANTAGES
Heparin			
Intravenous	Coagulation cascade—antithrombin III	Reversible, effective	Control, embolization
Subcutaneous	Antithrombin III inhibitor	Reversible	No effect in extremity surgery
Coumadin	Coagulation cascade—vitamin K	Most effective, oral	3–5 Days to full effect, control
Aspirin	Inhibits platelet aggregation	Easy, no monitoring	Limited efficacy
Dextran	Dilutional	Effective	Fluid overload, bleeding
Pneumatic compression (and foot pumps)	Mechanical	Inexpensive, no bleeding	Bulky
Enoxaparin (Lovenox), a low-molecular-weight heparin	Inhibits clotting—forms complexes between antithrombin III and factors IIa and Xa	Fixed dose, no monitoring	Bleeding

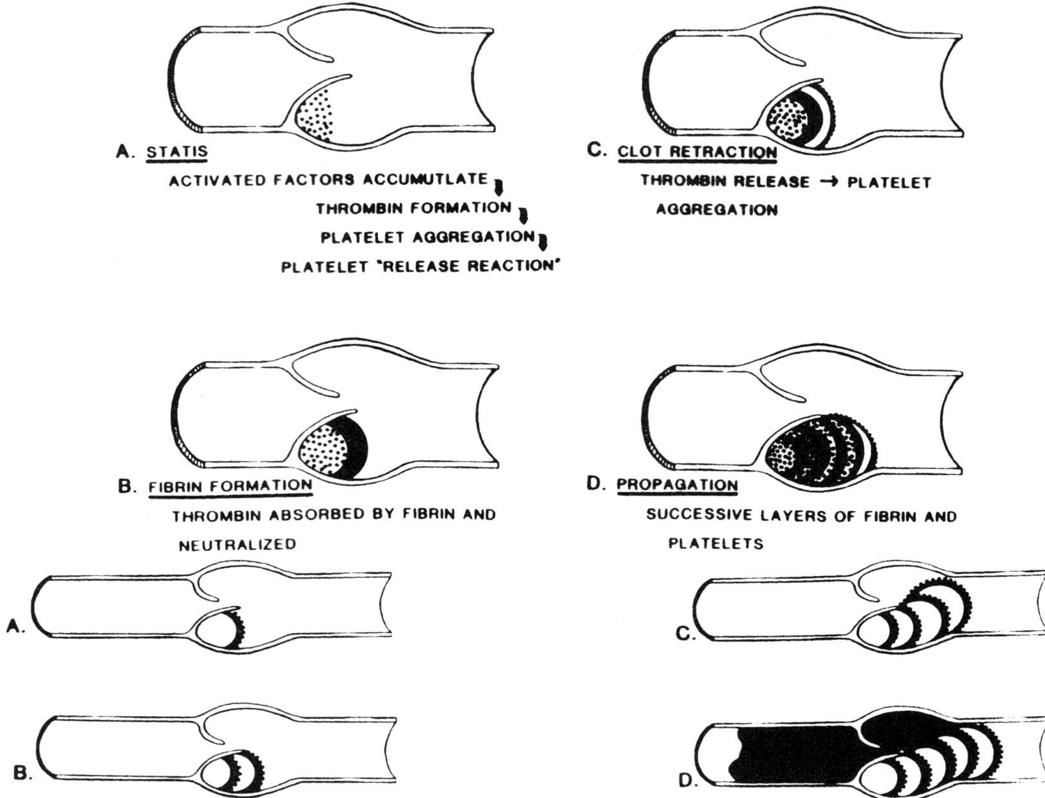

FIGURE 1–89. Venous thromboembolus formation. (From Simon, S.R., ed.: Orthopaedic Basic Science, 2nd ed., p. 492. Rosemont, IL, American Academy of Orthopaedic Surgeons, 1994; reprinted by permission.)

liteal fossa is controversial. Preoperative identification of a DVT in a patient with lower extremity trauma is an indication for placement of a **vena cava filter** (*). **Virchow's triad** of factors involved in venous thrombosis are stasis, hypercoagulability, and intimal injury (*). Thromboembolism formation is summarized in Figure 1–89.

2. Pulmonary Embolism—Pulmonary embolism (PE) should be suspected in postoperative patients with acute onset of pleuritic pain, tachypnea (90%), and tachycardia (60%). Initial workup includes EKG (right bundle branch block [RBBB], right axis deviation [RAD] in 25%; may also show ST depression or T wave inversion in lead III), chest radiograph (hyperlucency rare), and ABGs (normal PaO_2 does not exclude PE). Nuclear medicine ventilation–perfusion (V/Q) scan may be helpful, but pulmonary angiography (the "gold standard") is required to make the diagnosis if there is any question. Heparin therapy (continuous IV infusion) is initiated for the patient with a proved PE and is monitored by the partial thromboplastin time (PTT). More aggressive therapy (thrombolytic agents, vena cava interruption, and other surgical measures) is usually not required. Seven to ten days of heparin therapy is followed by 3 months of oral warfarin (monitored by the prothrombin time [PT]). Approximately 700,000 people in the United States have an asymptomatic PE each year, of which 200,000 are fatal. The most important factor for survival is early diagnosis with prompt therapy initiation. The incidence of DVT and fatal PE **in unprotected patients** is summarized in Table 1–39.
3. Coagulation (Fig. 1–90)—A cascading sequence of enzymatic reactions that begins with prothrombin-converting activity and concludes with the formation of a **fibrin** clot (as fibrinogen is converted to fibrin). Two interconnecting pathways have been described.

TABLE 1–39. FREQUENCY OF DEEP VEIN THROMBOSIS AND FATAL PULMONARY EMBOLISM (DIAGNOSED BY VENOGRAPHY)

	Frequency (%)	
UNPROTECTED PATIENTS	DVT	FATAL PE
Elective hip arthroplasty	70	2
Elective knee arthroplasty	80	1
Open meniscectomy	20	?
Hip fracture	60	3.5
Spinal fracture with paralysis	100	~1
Polytrauma patients	35	?
Pelvic/acetabular fracture	20	?

From Simon, S.R.: Orthopaedic Basic Science, 2nd ed., p. 489. Rosemont, IL, American Academy of Orthopaedic Surgeons, 1994, reprinted by permission.

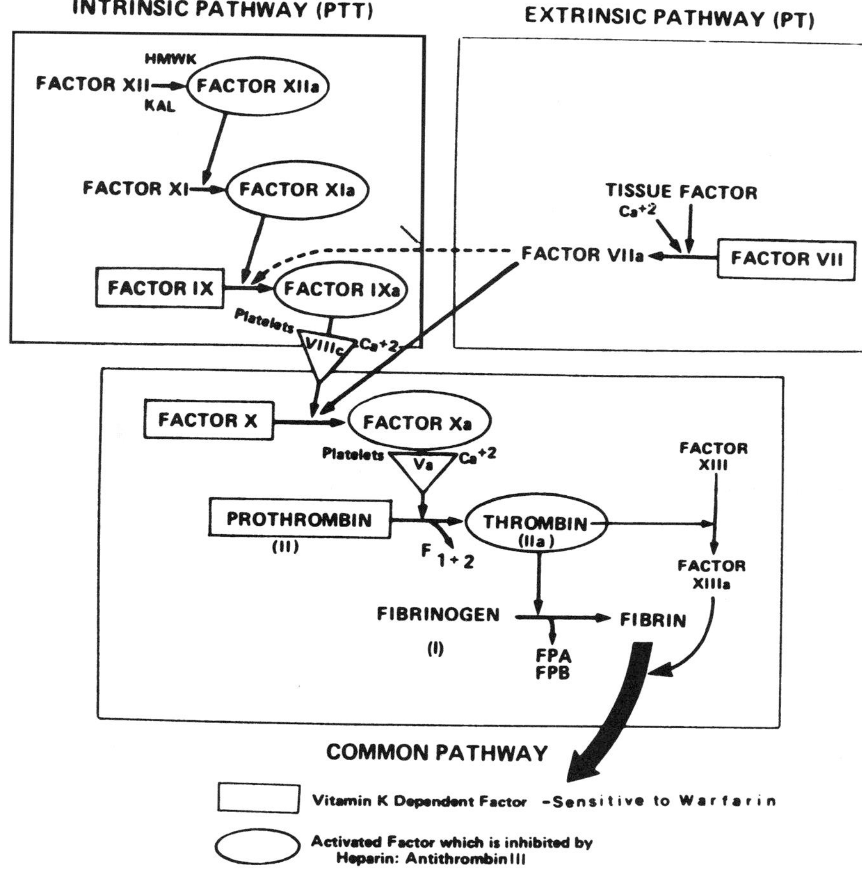

FIGURE 1–90. Coagulation cascade. (From Stead, R.B.: Regulation of hemostasis. In Pulmonary Embolism and Deep Venous Thromboembolism, Goldhaber, S.Z., ed., p. 32. Philadelphia, WB Saunders, 1985; reprinted by permission.)

a. Intrinsic Pathway—Monitored by **PTT.** Pathway is activated when factor XII makes contact with the collagen of damaged vessels.
b. Extrinsic Pathway—Monitored by **PT.** Pathway is activated by release of thromboplastin into the circulation secondary to cellular injury.
c. The **bleeding time test measures platelet function** (*). The **fibrinolytic system** is responsible for dissolving clots. Plasminogen is converted to plasmin (with the help of tissue activators, factor XIIa, and thrombin); plasmin dissolves fibrin clot.

D. Adult Respiratory Distress Syndrome (ARDS)—Acute respiratory failure secondary to pulmonary edema following trauma, shock, infection, and so on. Etiologies of ARDS include pulmonary infection, sepsis, fat embolism, microembolism, aspiration, fluid overload, atelectasis, oxygen toxicity, pulmonary contusion, and head injury. Tachypnea, dyspnea, hypoxemia, and decreased lung compliance are manifestations of ARDS. The clinical diagnosis of ARDS following a long-bone fracture is best made using ABGs (*). Normal supportive care is often unsuccessful, and a 50% mortality rate is not uncommon. Fluid overload, aspiration, and microscopic emboli may contribute to the development of ARDS. Activation of the complement system leads to further progression. Ventilation with PEEP is important; steroids have not been proven to be efficacious. Early stabilization of long-bone fractures (particularly the femur) decreases the risk of pulmonary complications (**).

E. Fat Embolism (Fig. 1–91)—Usually seen 24–72 hours after trauma (3–4% of patients with long-bone fractures). It is fatal in 10–15% of cases. Onset may be heralded by tachypnea, tachycardia, mental status changes, and upper extremity petechiae. May be caused by bone marrow fat (**mechanical theory**), chylomicron changes as a result of stress (**metabolic theory**), or both. Metabolism to free fatty acids, initiation of the clotting cascade, pulmonary capillary leakage, bronchoconstriction, and alveolar collapse result in a **ventillation–perfusion deficit** (hypoxemia) consistent with ARDS. Treatment includes mechanical ventilation with **high levels of PEEP.** Steroids do not appear to have a prophylactic role. Prevention with early fracture stabilization is key.

F. Pneumonia—Aspiration pneumonia can occur in patients with decreased mentation, supine positioning, and decreased GI motility. Simple preventive measures such as raising the head of the bed and the use of antacids and metoclopramide (Reglan) can

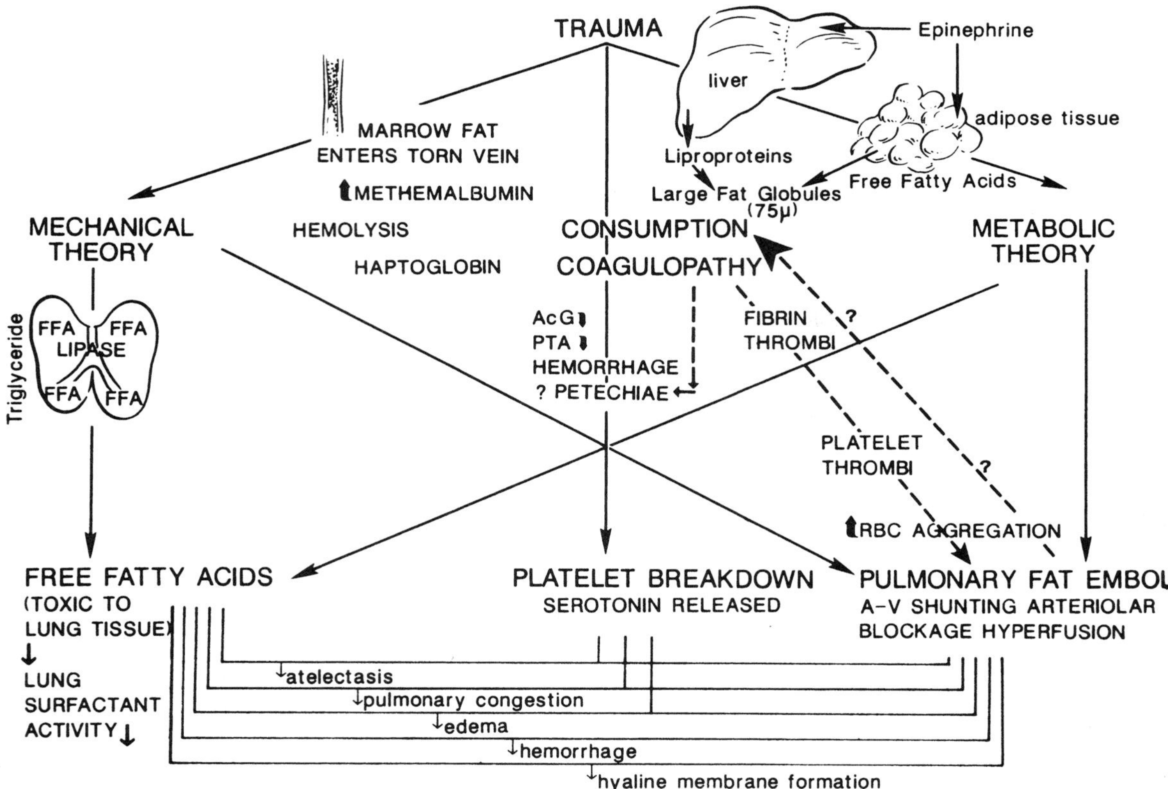

FIGURE 1–91. Pathological events of fat embolism syndrome. (From Simon, S.R., ed.: Orthopaedic Basic Science, 2nd ed., p. 502. Rosemont, IL, American Academy of Orthopaedic Surgeons, 1994; reprinted by permission.)

help to avoid problems. Appropriate IV antibiotics and pulmonary toilet are required.

G. Pulmonary Complications of Orthopaedic Disorders—Scoliosis of significant magnitude can cause pulmonary dysfunction. Spontaneous pneumothorax is common in patients with Marfan syndrome.

II. Other Medical Problems (Nonpulmonary)

A. Nutrition—Adequate nutrition should be ensured prior to elective surgery. Malnutrition may be present in 50% of patients on a surgical ward. Several indicators exist (e.g., anergy panels, albumin levels, transferrin level), but **arm muscle circumference measurement is the best indicator of nutritional status.** Wound dehiscence and infection, pneumonia, and sepsis can result from poor nutrition. Lack of enteral feeding can lead to **atrophy of the intestinal mucosae** (*), leading in turn to bacterial translocation. Nutritional requirements are significantly elevated as a result of stress. Full enteral or parenteral nutrition (nitrogen 200 mg/kg per day) should be provided for patients who cannot tolerate normal intake. Early elemental feeding through a jejunostomy tube can decrease complications in the multiple trauma patient. Enteral protein supplements have proved effective in patients at risk of developing multiple organ system failure (*). The metabolic changes of starvation and stress are compared in Table 1–40.

B. Myocardial Infarction (MI)—Acute chest pain, radiation, and EKG changes are classic and warrant monitoring in an appropriate critical care environment where cardiac enzymes and the EKG can be monitored on a continuing basis. Risk factors of MI include increased age, smoking, elevated cholesterol, hypertension, aortic stenosis, a history of coronary artery disease, and a variety of other factors.

C. GI Complications—Can range from ileus (treated with nasogastric suction [NG tube] and antacids) to upper GI bleeding. Postoperative ileus is common in diabetics with neuropathy. Upper GI bleeding is more likely in patients with a history of ulcers, NSAID use, and smoking. Treatment includes lavage, antacids, and H_2-blockers. Vasopressin (left gastric artery) may be required for more serious cases. Ogilvie syndrome, which includes cecal distention, can follow total joint replacement surgery. If the cecum is >10 cm on an abdominal flat plate radiograph, it must be decompressed (usually can be done colonoscopically).

D. Decubitus Ulcers—Associated with advanced age, critical illness, and neurologic impairment. Common sites include the sacrum, heels, and buttocks, which may be a source of infection and increased morbidity. Prevention with constant changing of position, special mattresses, and treatment of systemic illness and malnutrition is essential. Once established, débridement and sometimes soft tissue flaps are required for treatment.

TABLE 1–40. METABOLIC CHANGES OF STARVATION AND STRESS

METABOLIC ACTIVITY	STARVATION: EARLY	STARVATION: LATE	STRESS: HYPERMETABOLISM	STRESS: MULTISYSTEM
Energy expenditure	↓	↓↓	↑↑	Organ failure
Mediator activation	None	None	+ +	+ +
Metabolic responsiveness	Intact	Intact	Abnormal	Abnormal
Primary fuel	CHO	KB	"Mixed" (no KB)	"Mixed" (no KB)
Hepatic gluconeogenesis	↓	↓	↑	↑ or ↓
Hepatic protein synthesis	↓	↓	↑	↑ or ↓
Whole-body protein catabolism	Sl. ↑	Sl. ↑	↑↑	↑↑↑
Urinary nitrogen excretion	Sl. ↑	Sl. ↑	↑↑	↑↑↑
Malnutrition	Slow	Slow	Rapid	Rapid

Adapted from Simon, S.R.: Orthopaedic Basic Science, 2nd ed., p. 510. Rosemont, IL, American Academy of Orthopaedic Surgeons, 1994, reprinted by permission.
CHO, carbohydrate; Sl., slight; KB, ketone bodies.

E. Urinary Tract Infection (UTI)—Most common nosocomial infection (6–8%). Causes increased risk for joint sepsis following TJA (but may not be from direct seeding). Established UTIs should be adequately treated preoperatively. Perioperative catheterization (removed 24 hours postoperatively) may reduce the rate of postoperative UTI.

F. Prostatic Hypertrophy—Causes postoperative urinary retention. If the history, physical examination (prostate), and urine flow studies (<17 ml/sec peak flow rate) are suggestive, urologic referral should be accomplished preoperatively.

G. Acute Tubular Necrosis—Can cause renal failure in trauma patients. Alkalization of urine is important during the early treatment of this disorder.

H. Genitourinary (GU) Injury—NSAIDs can affect the kidney, and appropriate screening laboratories are required at regular intervals. Retrograde urethrogram best evaluates lower GU injuries with displaced anterior pelvic fractures (*).

I. Shock—Capillary blood flood is insufficient for the perfusion of vital tissues and organs. There are four types of shock.
   1. Hypovolemic Shock—"Volume loss": ↓ cardiac output (CO), ↑ peripheral vascular resistance (PVR), venous constriction.
   2. Cardiogenic Shock—"Ineffective pumping": ↓ CO, ↑ PVR, venous dilation.
   3. Vasogenic Shock (PE or pericardial tamponade)—Arteriolar constriction, venous dilation.
   4. Neurogenic Shock/Septic Shock—"Blood pooling": arteriolar, capillary, and venous dilation.

The preferred initial fluid for hypovolemic shock is Ringer's lactate (*). For patients in shock with a suboptimal response to Ringer's lactate, add blood transfusion (*); massive blood replacement requires concomitant fresh frozen plasma and platelets (**). The best indicator of adequate fluid resuscitation is urine output (**). Patients with inadequate fluid resuscitation show metabolic acidosis on ABGs (*).

J. Compartment Syndrome (****************)—Covered in detail in Chapter 10, Trauma. This subject matter is always tested heavily. Questions regarding compartment syndrome of the foot (*****) and thigh (**) seem to be "popular."

III. Intraoperative Considerations

A. Anesthesia—Regional anesthesia may allow quicker recovery, decreased blood loss, and fewer postoperative complications, including reduced blood loss and incidence of DVT/PE in THA patients. Controlled hypotension during surgery helps with blood loss and is a widely accepted technique, especially with THA and spinal arthrodesis (nitroprusside, nitroglycerine, and isoflurane are all effective). Transient decreases in BP with PMMA insertion are well known. The use of the fiberoptic bronchoscope has benefited surgery on RA patients and others with C-spine abnormalities. The use of local anesthetics for arthroscopy has also gained popularity. **Malignant hyperthermia** (******), an autosomal dominant (*), hypermetabolic disorder of skeletal muscle, can be triggered by the use of various anesthetics (especially halothane and succinylcholine) in susceptible patients (e.g., neuromuscular disorders). Patients with Duchenne's muscular dystrophy, arthrogryposis, and osteogenesis imperfecta are especially at risk. Cell membrane defects affect calcium transport, leading to muscle rigidity and hypermetabolism. Masseter muscle spasm, increased temperature, rigidity, and acidosis are the hallmarks of the disease. Early diagnosis and treatment [with **dantrolene** (***), balancing of electrolytes, increasing urinary output, respiratory support, cooling] are essential. The most accurate method for diagnosing malignant hyperthermia is **muscle biopsy** (in vitro muscle fiber testing) (*).

B. Spinal Cord Monitoring—Usually involves testing the posterior column, but monitoring of other areas is under investigation. Electrical monitoring includes the use of somatosensory cortical evoked potentials (SCEPs) to record summed input from stimulation of peripheral areas. Somatosensory spinal evoked potentials (SSEPs) are more invasive, but can be more sensitive. Preoperative recordings are compared to readings (especially latency and amplitude) at critical times during the procedure. The wake-up test is still the standard for monitoring and relies on the lightening of anesthesia and the patient moving selected extremities upon command.

C. Tourniquet—Injuries usually involve the area directly underneath the tourniquet and include nerve and muscle damage. Careful application, wide cuffs, lower pressures (200 mm Hg in upper extremity and 250 Hg mm in lower extremity [or 100–150 mm Hg above systolic BP for lower extremity]) (*), and double cuffs help avoid these problems. Equilibrium can be reestablished within 5 minutes following 90 minutes of tourniquet application but requires 15 minutes following the use of a tourniquet for 3 hours. EMG abnormalities have been reported in 70% of patients after routine surgery using a tourniquet.

IV. Other Problems

A. Pain Control—Acute pain implies the presence of potential tissue damage, whereas chronic pain (3–6 months) does not. Nociceptors transduce stimuli through substances, allowing transmission along peripheral nerves (types A and C fiber) to the dorsal column, spinothalamic tract, and thalamus. Modulation is via brain stem centers and endogenous opiates. Postoperative pain control can be targeted at any step. Local prostaglandin inhibitors and long-acting local anesthetics target transduction of pain. Perispinal opiates affect modulation, and systemic opiates affect perception and modulation of pain.

B. Transfusion—Because of the possibility of disease transmission, transfusion has become an important issue.

1. Transfusion Reactions—Include allergic, febrile, and hemolytic reactions.
   a. Allergic Reaction—Most common; occurs toward the end of transfusion. Symptoms include chills, pruritus, erythema, and urticaria. It usually subsides spontaneously. Pretreatment with diphenhydramine (Benadryl) and hydrocortisone may be appropriate in patients with a history of allergic reactions.
   b. Febrile Reaction—Also common; occurs after the initial 100–300 cc of packed RBCs have been transfused. Chills and fever are caused by antibodies to foreign WBCs. Treatment is similar to that for an allergic reaction.
   c. Hemolytic Reaction—Less common but most serious. It occurs early in the transfusion with symptoms that include chills, fever, tachycardia, chest tightness, and flank pain. Treatment comprises stopping the transfusion, administering IV fluids, having appropriate laboratory studies done, and monitoring in an intensive care setting.
2. Transfusion Risks—Include transmission of hepatitis (non-A, non-B [2–3%], B [<1%]), cytomegalovirus (CMV; highest incidence but not clinically important), HTLV-1, and HIV (<0.04%). Donor deferral for high-risk individuals and more effective screening methods are decreasing these risks.
3. Alternatives to Homologous Blood Transfusion
   a. Autologous Deposition—Requires a hemoglobin level of approximately 11 (and a hematocrit of 33%), and some lead time. Iron supplementation during donation is routine. Allows storage of several units prior to elective procedures with significant blood loss anticipated. Most donations significantly reduce the risk of developing non-A, non-B hepatitis (*).
   b. "Cell-Saver"—Intraoperative autotransfusion. Usually requires 400 ml of blood loss to recover 1 unit (250 ml). Can be used for only 4 hours at one time.
   c. Autotransfusion—Allows postoperative drain recuperation and use.
   d. Acute Preoperative Normovolemic Hemodilution—Allows storage of autologous blood (replace with crystalloid) immediately preoperatively for use intra/postoperatively.
   e. Pharmacologic Intervention—Alternatives including desmopressin (antidiuretic hormone [ADH] analogue that increases levels of plasma factor VIII), recombinant erythropoietin (stimulates erythrogenesis), and synthetic erythrocyte substitutes.
   f. Judicious Use of Blood Products—Platelet transfusion with massive bleeding or coagulopathies is performed based on clinical parameters rather than set platelet thresholds. Fresh frozen plasma is reserved for patients with massive bleeding and significantly abnormal coagulation tests. Cryoprecipitate is used for hemophilia (with less exposure than factor concentrates) and as a source of fibrinogen for consumptive coagulopathies.

C. Heterotopic Ossification—See Chapter 4, Adult Reconstruction. Seen most commonly following THA, in head-injured patients, and in those with elbow injuries. Indomethacin is effective for prophylaxis during THA. Diphosphonates do not prevent formation of osteoid matrix; after discontinuation of medication the matrix calcifies, and therefore diphosphonates are not good for prophylaxis. Etidronate sodium inhibits bone resorption at low doses and bone mineralization at high doses (*).

Test Questions continued on opposite page

TEST QUESTIONS ON PERIOPERATIVE PROBLEMS

TEST	QUESTION NUMBERS
1995 OSAE—Adult Reconstruction Hip/Knee	
1995 OSAE—Pediatric Orthopaedics	
1995 OSAE—Sports Medicine	
1994 OITE	74, 139, 144, 173, 219
1994 OSAE—Adult Spine	77
1994 OSAE—Foot and Ankle	77, 124
1994 OSAE—M/S Trauma	22, 24, 25, 35, 51, 54, 56, 58, 85, 95
1993 OITE	9, 47, 67, 96, 161, 162
1993 OSAE—M/S Tumors and Diseases	
1993 OSAE—Shoulder and Elbow	
1992 OITE	19, 52, 62
1992 OSAE—Adult Reconstruction Hip/Knee	
1992 OSAE—Pediatric Orthopaedics	
1992 OSAE—Sports Medicine	82
1991 OITE	15, 28, 33, 50, 70, 106, 112, 121, 134, 136, 164, 188, 193
1991 OSAE—Adult Spine	
1991 OSAE—Anatomy and Imaging	
1991 OSAE—Foot and Ankle	10, 51, 52
1991 OSAE—M/S Trauma	19, 21, 49, 54, 55, 56, 57, 58, 60, 61, 63, 64, 78, 79, 80, 82, 88, 90, 94, 100

SECTION 7
Imaging and Special Studies

I. Nuclear Medicine

A. Bone Scan—Technetium 99m–phosphate complexes reflect increased blood flow and metabolism and are absorbed onto the hydroxyapatite crystals of bone (*) in areas of infection, trauma, neoplasia, and so on. Whole-body views and more detailed (pinhole) views can be obtained. It is particularly useful for the diagnosis of subtle fractures; avascular necrosis (no focal uptake early, increased uptake during the reparative phase); osteomyelitis (especially when triple-phase study is done or in conjunction with gallium or indium scan); and THA and TKA loosening (especially femoral components; can be used with gallium scan to rule out concurrent infection). Three-stage or even four-stage studies may be helpful for evaluating diseases such as reflex sympathetic dystrophy and osteomyelitis. Delayed-phase scans may be negative in pediatric septic arthritis (*). Triple-phase bone scan is the most reliable test for assessing whether a nondisplaced scaphoid fracture exists (*).

B. Gallium Scan—Gallium 67 citrate localizes in site of inflammation and neoplasia probably because of exudation of labeled serum proteins. Delayed imaging (usually 24–48 hours or more) is required. Frequently used in conjunction with bone scan—a "double tracer" technique. Gallium is less dependent on vascular flow than technetium and may identify foci that would otherwise be missed. It is difficult to differentiate cellulitis from osteomyelitis.

C. Indium Scan—Indium 111-labeled WBCs accumulate in areas of inflammation and do not collect in areas of neoplasia. Useful for evaluation of acute osteomyelitis and possibly TJA infections. Unlike gallium, it is also useful in the presence of pseudarthrosis.

D. Technetium-Labeled WBC Scan—Similar to indium scan.

E. Radiolabeled Monoclonal Antibodies—May have a role in identifying primary malignancies and metastatic disease.

F. Other Studies

1. Bone Mineral Analysis—Single-photon absorptiometry (usually of the distal radius and cortical

bone; has limited utility), dual-photon absorptiometry (vertebral bodies and femoral neck), and quantitative CT (large radiation exposure and may be inaccurate but can pick up early changes in trabecular bone) can be used to measure bone mineral content for diagnosing osteoporosis and predicting fracture risk.

2. Deep Venous Thrombosis/Pulmonary Embolism (DVT/PE) Scan—Radioactive iodine-labeled fibrinogen accumulates in clot and shows up on scanning. Its limitations include inaccuracy in areas of surgical wounds. Radioisotope scanning of lungs may also help in evaluating regional pulmonary blood flow, but it too is limited at present.
3. Single-Photon Emission Computed Tomography (SPECT)—Uses scintigraphy and CT to evaluate overlapping structures. Femoral head ON, patellofemoral syndrome, and healing spondylolytic defects have been evaluated with this technique.

II. Arthrography

A. Shoulder—Can be used with single- or double-contrast technique (better detail). Used for the following studies.
   1. Rotator Cuff Tear Diagnosis—Extravasation of contrast through the tear into the subacromial bursa.
   2. Adhesive Capsulitis—Diagnosed by demonstrating diminished joint capsule size and loss of the normal axillary fold. May have a role in therapy also by distending the capsule.
   3. Recurrent Dislocations—Arthrography may demonstrate a distended capsule or disruption of the glenoid labrum. Can be used in conjunction with tomograms or CT (computed arthrotomography) to better demonstrate capsular or labral pathology.
   4. Other Uses—Include diagnosis of bicipital tendon abnormalities, articular pathology, and impingement syndrome.

B. Elbow—Especially when used with tomography, elbow arthrography can be helpful for diagnosing articular cartilage defects/loose bodies and osteochondral fractures.

C. Wrist—Most useful for evaluation of the posttraumatic wrist to demonstrate ligamentous disruption. Digital subtraction techniques are helpful in this area. Demonstration of communication between compartments is used to determine pathology; however, communication is common in asymptomatic patients in the over-40 age group. If a communication is observed at the radius-carpus and midcarpal joint, an S-L or L-T ligament tear should be suspected. Communication at the radius-carpus and distal radius-ulna suggests a TFCC tear.

D. Hip—Different indications in children and adults.
   1. Infants and Children—arthrography is useful for diagnosing the septic hip (obtain aspirate and assess joint damage), congenital dysplasia of the hip (degree of joint incongruity—interposed limbus), and Legg-Calvé-Perthes disease (severity of deformity).
   2. Adolescents and Adults—Used to evaluate arthritis (cartilage destruction and loose bodies), osteochondral fractures, chondrolysis, and THA loosening. Digital subtraction arthrography can be useful in patients with suspected loose THAs.

E. Knee—Can be a useful screening tool in patients with an equivocal history or findings. Accurate for diagnosing most meniscal tears (except in posterior horn of lateral meniscus) and demonstrates discoid lateral menisci well. Evaluation of cruciate ligaments is less accurate. Abnormalities of articular cartilage, evaluation of loose bodies (air contrast only is recommended), and pathologic synovial tissue (PVNS, popliteal cysts, synovial chondromatosis, plicas) can be demonstrated as well.

F. Ankle—Helpful for evaluating torn ligaments acutely and assessing chronic osseous and osteocartilaginous abnormalities.

G. Spine—May be useful in conjunction with therapeutic injections (of anesthetics and steroids) into facet joints.

III. Magnetic Resonance Imaging (MRI)

A. Introduction—Excellent study for soft tissue evaluation (*). Used frequently to evaluate ON, neoplasms, infection, and trauma. Allows both axial and sagittal representations. It is contraindicated in patients with pacemakers, cerebral aneurysm clips, or shrapnel or hardware in certain locations.

B. Basic Principles of MRI (Table 1–41)—Uses radiofrequency (Rf) pulses on tissues in a magnetic field and displays images in any plane desired without the use of ionizing radiation. MRI aligns nuclei with odd numbers of protons/neutrons (with a normally random spin) parallel to a magnetic field. Most magnets used have a strength of about 0.5–1.5 Telsa (1 Telsa is 10,000 Gauss). Rf pulses cause deflection of these particles' nuclear magnetic moments, resulting in an image. The use of surface coils decreases the signal-to-noise ratio. Body coils are used for large joints, smaller coils are available for other studies. Sequences have been developed that have either short (T_1) or long (T_2) relaxation times for atoms to return to their normal spin. **T_1 images are weighted toward fat; T_2 images are weighted toward water.** Typically, T_1-weighted images have TR values <1000, and T_2 images have TR values >1000. Some tissues appear differently on T_1- and T_2-weighted scans. Water, CSF, acute hemorrhage, and soft tissue tumors appear dark on T_1 studies and light on T_2 studies. Other

TABLE 1–41. PHYSICAL PROPERTIES OF MAGNETIC RESONANCE IMAGING

TISSUE	T1-WEIGHTED IMAGE[a]	T2-WEIGHTED IMAGE[b]
Cortical bone	Black	Black
Ligaments	Black	Black
Fibrocartilage	Black	Black
Hyaline cartilage	Gray	Gray
Bone marrow (fatty—appendicular)	Bright	Gray
Bone marrow (hematopoietic—axial)	Bright	Gray
Normal fluid	Dark	Bright
Abnormal fluid (pus)	Gray	Bright
Muscle	Gray	Gray
Intervertebral disc (central)	Gray	Bright
Intervertebral disc (peripheral)	Dark	Gray

From Simon, S.R.: Orthopaedic Basic Science, 2nd ed., p. 319. Rosemont, IL, American Academy of Orthopaedic Surgeons, 1994, reprinted by permission.
[a] Time to echo (TE), short <1000; time to repetition (TR), short <80.
[b] TE, long >1000; TR, long >80.

tissues remain basically the same color on both studies. Cortical bone, rapidly flowing blood, and fibrous tissue are all dark; muscle and hyaline cartilage are gray; and fatty tissue, nerves, slowly flowing (venous) blood, and bone marrow are light. T_1 images best demonstrate anatomic structure (high signal-to-noise ratio), whereas T_2 images are most useful for contrasting normal and abnormal tissues.

C. Specific Applications of MRI
   1. Osteonecrosis—MRI may be the **most sensitive method for early detection** of ON (detects early marrow necrosis and ingrowth of vascularized mesenchymal tissue); tomography is the best method for **staging** ON (of the hip) (*). It is highly specific (98%) and reliable for estimating age and extent of disease. T_1 images demonstrate diseased marrow as dark. MRI allows direct assessment of overlying cartilage.
   2. Infection and Trauma—MRI makes use of its excellent sensitivity to increases in free water to demonstrate areas of infection and fresh hemorrhage (dark on T_1 and light on T_2 studies).
   3. Neoplasms—MRI has many applications in the study of primary and metastatic bone tumors. Primary tumors, particularly soft tissue components (extraosseous and marrow), are well demonstrated on MRI. Although nuclear medicine studies remain the procedure of choice for seeking metastatic foci in bone, MRI has a role in evaluating skip lesions and spinal metastases. Benign tumors are typically bright on T_1 images and dark on T_2 images. Malignant bony lesions are often bright on T_2 images. Differential diagnosis, however, is best made based on plain films.
   4. Spine—Disc disease is well demonstrated on T_2 images. Degenerated discs lose their water content and become dark on T_2-weighted studies. Herniated discs and their extent are well shown. Recurrent disc herniation can be differentiated from scar based on the following characteristics: On T_1 image: scar ↓, free fragment ↑, extruded disc ↓. On T_2 image: scar ↑, free fragment ↑, extruded disc ↓. Gadolinium-DTPA can also be used to differentiate scar from disc; it enhances edematous structures in T_1 images. MRI is the best study for diagnosing early diskitis (*).
   5. Bone Marrow Changes—Best demonstrated by MRI (but nonspecific). Five groups of disorders have been described and are shown in Table 1–42.

TABLE 1–42. IMAGING BONE MARROW DISORDERS

DISORDER	PATHOLOGY	EXAMPLES	MRI CHANGES
Reconversion	Yellow → red	Anemia, metastasis	↓ T_1 image
Marrow infiltration		Tumor, infection	↓ T_1 image
Myeloid depletion		Anemia, chemotherapy	↑ T_1 image
Marrow edema		Trauma, RSD	↓ T_1, ↑ T_2 image
Marrow ischemia		Osteonecrosis	↓ T_1 image

RSD, reflex sympathetic dystrophy; ↑, increased; ↓, decreased.

TABLE 1–43. MRI CHANGES OF MENISCAL PATHOLOGY

GROUP	CHARACTERISTICS
I	Globular areas of hyperintense signal
II	Linear hyperintense signal
III	Linear hyperintense signal that communicates with the meniscal surface (tears)
IV	Vertical longitudinal tear/truncation

   6. Knee MRI—Arthrography with MRI can be accomplished with installation of saline, creating an iatrogenic effusion. This technique can improve joint definition. Knee derangements are well demonstrated on MRI. ACL rupture is correctly diagnosed in 95% of cases. Meniscal pathology has been classified into four groups of myxoid changes (Lotysch) (Table 1–43). MRI is the best **radiologic test** to demonstrate a posterior cruciate ligament (PCL) rupture (*).
   7. Shoulder MRI
      a. Rotator Cuff Tears—Results are improving with use (sensitivity and specificity are about 90%). Grade 0 tears show a normal signal, and grade 1, 2, and 3 tears show an increased signal. The morphology of grade 0 and 1 tears is normal; grade 2 tears show abnormal morphology; and Grade 3 tears show discontinuity.
      b. Capsular/Labral Tears—MRI is equal to CT arthrography in the presence of an effusion.
   8. MRI Spectroscopy—May help with the measurement of metabolic changes (especially ischemic changes).

IV. Other Imaging Studies

A. Computed Tomography (CT)—Continues to be important for evaluating many orthopaedic areas. Hounsfield units are used to identify tissue types (−100 = air, −100 to 0 = fat, 0 = water, 100 = soft tissue, 1000 = bone). **Demonstrates bony anatomy better than any other study.** Also shows herniated nucleus pulposis better than myelography alone and may be helpful in differentiating recurrent disc herniation from scar (like MRI). IV contrast material is administered and taken up in scar tissue but not disc material. Used frequently in conjunction with contrast (e.g., arthrogram CT, myelogram CT). Sagittal and three-dimensional reconstruction techniques may expand its indications. Cine-CT (and MRI) may be helpful for evaluating many joint disorders. CT digital radiography (CT scannogram) can be used for accurate demonstrations of leg-length discrepancy with minimal radiation exposure. Best demonstrates joint incongruity following closed reduction of a dislocated hip (*). CT is also important for evaluating injuries involving the subtalar joint (****) and for tarsal coalitions (*).

B. Ultrasonography—Has been used successfully in several areas of orthopaedics.
   1. Shoulder—May be useful for diagnosing rotator cuff tears.
   2. Hip—Has been shown to be effective in the diagnosis and follow-up of developmental hip dysplasia and to identify iliopsoas bursitis in adults.
   3. Knee—Used to assess articular cartilage thickness, identify intraarticular fluid, and so on.
   4. Other Areas—Helpful for evaluating soft tissue masses, hematoma, tendon rupture, abscesses,

TABLE 1–44. NERVE CONDUCTION STUDY RESULTS

CONDITION	LATENCY	CONDUCTION VELOCITY	EVOKED RESPONSE
Normal study	Normal	Upper extremities: >45 m/sec Lower extremities: >40 m/sec	Biphasic
Axonal neuropathy	Increased	Normal or slightly decreased	Prolonged, ↓ amplitude
Demyelinating neuropathy	Normal	Decreased (10–50%)	Normal or prolonged, with ↓ amplitude
Anterior horn cell disease	Normal	Normal (rarely decreased)	Normal or polyphasic with prolonged duration and ↓ amplitude
Myopathy	Normal	Normal	↓ Amplitude, may be normal
Neuropraxia			
Proximal to lesion	Absent	Absent	Absent
Distal to lesion	Normal	Normal	Normal
Axonotmesis			
Proximal to lesion	Absent	Absent	Absent
Distal to lesion	Absent	Absent	Normal
Neurotmesis			
Proximal to lesion	Absent	Absent	Absent
Distal to lesion	Absent	Absent	Absent

Modified from Jahss, M.H.: Disorders of the Foot. Philadelphia, WB Saunders, 1982; reprinted by permission.
↓, decreased.

foreign body location, and intraspinal disorders in infants.

C. Guided Biopsies—Aspiration and core biopsy (using a trephine Craig needle) is helpful in the work-up of musculoskeletal lesions; is commonly used in conjunction with CT.

D. Myelography—Still useful for evaluating cervical radiculopathy, subarachnoid cysts, and the failed back syndrome. It is the procedure of choice for extramedullary intradural pathology. Can be used in conjunction with other studies (CT).

E. Discography—Although its use is controversial, it is helpful for evaluating symptomatic disc degeneration. Reproduction of pain with injection and characteristic changes on discograms help identify pathologic discs. It is commonly used in conjunction with CT.

V. Electrodiagnostic Studies

A. Nerve Conduction Studies—Allow evaluation of peripheral nerves and their sensory and motor responses anywhere along their course. Nerve impulses are stimulated and recorded by electronic surface electrodes, allowing calculation of a conduction velocity. Latency (the time between the onset of the stimulus and the response) and the amplitude of the response are measured. Late responses (F and H) allow evaluation of proximal lesions (impulse travels to spinal cord and returns). Somatosensory evoked potentials (SEPs) can be used to study brachial plexus injuries and for spinal cord monitoring.

B. Electromyography (EMG)—Uses intramuscular needle electrodes to evaluate muscle units. Most studies are done to evaluate denervation, which demonstrates fibrillations (earliest sign usually at 4 weeks), sharp waves, and an abnormal recruitment pattern.

C. Interpretation—For peripheral nerve entrapment syndromes, distal motor and sensory latencies >3.5 m/s, nerve conduction velocities of <50 m/s, and changes over a distinct interval are considered abnormal (Tables 1–44, 1–45).

TABLE 1–45. ELECTROMYOGRAPHIC FINDINGS

CONDITION	INSERTIONAL ACTIVITY	ACTIVITY AT REST	MINIMAL CONTRACTION	INTERFERENCE
Normal study	Normal	Silent	Biphasic and triphasic potentials	Complete
Axonal neuropathy	Increased	Fibrillations and positive sharp waves	Biphasic and triphasic potentials	Incomplete
Demyelinating neuropathy	Normal	Silent (occasional activity)	Biphasic and triphasic potentials	Incomplete
Anterior horn cell disease	Increased	Fibrillations, positive sharp waves, fasciculations	Large polyphasic potentials	Incomplete
Myopathy	Increased	Silent or increased spontaneous activity	Small polyphasic potentials	Early
Neuropraxia	Normal	Silent	None	None
Axonotmesis	Increased	Fibrillations and positive sharp waves	None	None
Neurotmesis	Increased	Fibrillations and positive sharp waves	None	None

Modified from Jahss, M.H.: Disorders of the Foot. Philadelphia, WB Saunders, 1982; reprinted by permission.

TEST QUESTIONS ON IMAGING AND SPECIAL STUDIES

TEST	QUESTION NUMBERS
1995 OSAE—Adult Reconstruction Hip/Knee	5, 31, 85
1995 OSAE—Pediatric Orthopaedics	19
1995 OSAE—Sports Medicine	48, 73, 105
1994 OITE	
1994 OSAE—Adult Spine	22, 24, 27, 36, 39, 48, 54, 64, 83
1994 OSAE—Foot and Ankle	26, 46, 70, 92, 105, 118
1994 OSAE—M/S Trauma	
1993 OITE	21, 87
1993 OSAE—M/S Tumors and Diseases	28
1993 OSAE—Shoulder and Elbow	50
1992 OITE	38, 61, 67, 184, 189
1992 OSAE—Adult Reconstruction Hip/Knee	94, 95, 97, 99
1992 OSAE—Pediatric Orthopaedics	73
1992 OSAE—Sports Medicine	36, 66
1991 OITE	101
1991 OSAE—Adult Spine	14, 22, 34, 71
1991 OSAE—Anatomy and Imaging	
1991 OSAE—Foot and Ankle	31, 53, 87
1991 OSAE—M/S Trauma	46, 61, 65, 84, 85

SECTION 8
Biomaterials and Biomechanics

I. Basic Concepts

A. Definitions
1. Biomechanics—Science of the action of forces, internal or external, on the living body. (Know how to solve these problems!) (****)
2. Statics—Study of the action of forces on bodies at rest (in equilibrium).
3. Dynamics—Study of the motion of bodies and forces that produce the motion. There are three subtypes.
   a. Kinematics—Study of motion in terms of displacement, velocity, and acceleration without reference to the cause of the motion.
   b. Kinetics—Relates the action of forces on bodies to their resulting action.
   c. Kinesiology—Study of human movement/motion.

B. Principal Quantities
1. Basic Quantities—Described by the International System of units (SI) or the metric system.
   a. Length—Meter (m).
   b. Mass—Amount of matter (kilogram [kg]).
   c. Time—Second (s).
2. Derived Quantities (derived from basic quantities)
   a. Velocity—Time rate of change of displacement (m/s).
   b. Acceleration—Time rate of change of velocity (m/s^2).
   c. Force—Action of one body on another ($kg \cdot m/s^2$ [N])

C. Newton's Laws
1. First Law: Inertia—If a zero net external force acts on a body, the body will remain at rest or move uniformly. This law allows us to do static analysis with the equation $\Sigma F = 0$ (the sum of the external forces applied to a body equals zero).
2. Second Law: Acceleration—$F = ma$ (the acceleration a of an object of mass m is directly proportional to the force applied to the object). Helps in dynamic analysis.

3. Third Law: Reactions—For every action there is an equal and opposite reaction. Leads to free body analysis.

D. Scalar and Vector Quantities
   1. Scalar Quantities—Have magnitude but no direction. Examples include volume, time, mass, and speed (not velocity).
   2. Vector Quantities—Have magnitude and direction. Examples include force and velocity. Vectors have four characteristics: (1) magnitude (length of the vector); (2) direction (head of the vector); (3) point of application (tail of the vector); and (4) line of action (orientation of the vector). Vectors can be added, subtracted, and split into components (resolved) for analysis. The resultant of two vectors follows the principle of "parallelogram of forces."

E. Free Body Analysis (****)—Uses forces, moments, and free body diagrams to analyze the action of forces on bodies. Know how to do these problems!
   1. Forces—A push or a pull causing external (acceleration) and internal (strain) effects. Forces can be split into their **components** (usually in the *x* and *y* directions) for easier analysis. Some elementary knowledge of trigonometry is helpful ($F_x = F \cos \theta$, $F_y = F \sin \theta$). Also, remember the following simple approximations:

$$\sin 30° = \cos 60° \cong 0.5$$

$$\sin 45° = \cos 45° \cong 0.7$$

$$\sin 60° = \cos 30° \cong 0.9$$

   Representation of forces acting at a point is often an idealized situation and actually is an integration of a distributed load over its applied area. The **resultant force** is represented as a single force equivalent to a system of forces acting on a body. The **equilibrant force** is of equal magnitude and opposite to the resultant force.
   2. Moment—The rotational effect of a force on a body about a point (N·m). Any force acting at a distance from a point can produce a moment. The moment (or "torque") equals the force multiplied by the perpendicular distance from a specified point (moment arm): $M = F \times d$. **Mass moment of inertia** is resistance to rotation (*).
   3. Free Body Diagram (FBD)—Sketch of a body or portion thereof isolated from all other bodies and showing all forces acting on it. Weights of objects act through the center of gravity (CG). **The CG for the human body is just anterior to S2.**
   4. Free Body Analysis—Can proceed after all forces are represented on the FBD; using the concept of equilibrium ($\Sigma F = 0$ and $\Sigma M = 0$), solve for unknowns. Assumes no change in motion, deformation, or friction. The following steps are used in the analysis.
      a. Identify the system (objective, knowns, assumptions).
      b. Select a coordinate system.
      c. Isolate free bodies—FBD.
      d. Apply Newton's laws ($\Sigma F = 0$; $\Sigma M = 0$).
      e. Solve for unknowns.
   5. Example—Calculate the biceps force necessary to suspend the weight of the forearm (20 N) with the elbow flexed to 90 degrees; assume the biceps insertion is 5 cm distal to the elbow, and the CG of the forearm is 15 cm distal to the elbow (Fig. 1–92). (Answer: 60 N.) Also solve for the joint force (J) (Fig. 1–92). (Answer: 40 N.)

F. Other Important Basic Concepts
   1. Work—Force acts on the body to cause displacement. Work (W) = force (only components parallel to the displacement) × distance. Units: N·m [joules].

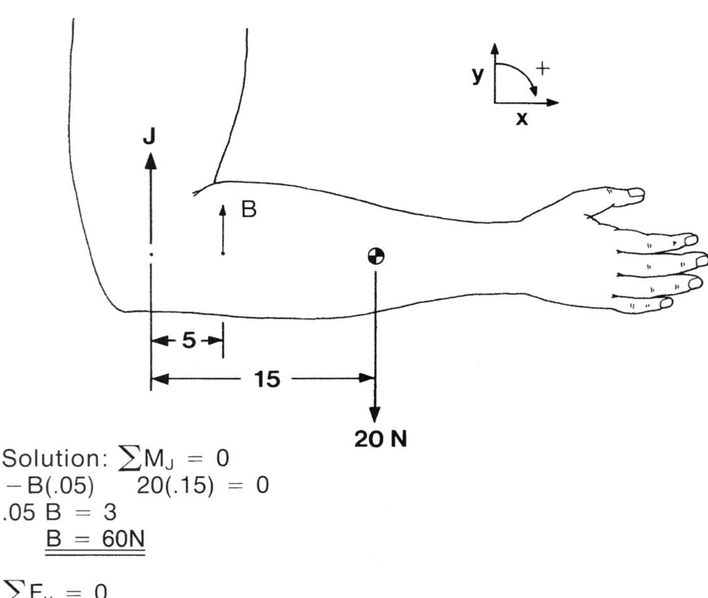

FIGURE 1–92. Biceps free body diagram (see text for explanation).

2. Energy—Ability to perform work (also joules). According to the law of conservation of energy, energy is neither created nor destroyed; it is transferred from one condition to another.
   a. Potential Energy—Stored energy; the ability of a body to do work as a result of its position or configuration (strain energy).
   b. Kinetic Energy—Energy of an object due to its motion (velocity): $KE = \frac{1}{2} mv^2$.
3. Friction (f)—Resistance between two bodies when one slides over the other. Oriented opposite to the applied force. When the applied force is > f, motion begins (*).
4. Piezoelectricity—Electrical charge from deformation of crystalline structures when forces are applied. Concave (compression) side = electronegative; convex (tension) side = electropositive.

TEST QUESTIONS ON BASIC CONCEPTS (BIOMATERIALS AND BIOMECHANICS)

TEST	QUESTION NUMBERS
1995 OSAE—Adult Reconstruction Hip/Knee	
1995 OSAE—Pediatric Orthopaedics	
1995 OSAE—Sports Medicine	
1994 OITE	195
1994 OSAE—Adult Spine	
1994 OSAE—Foot and Ankle	
1994 OSAE—M/S Trauma	
1993 OITE	145, 204
1993 OSAE—M/S Tumors and Diseases	
1993 OSAE—Shoulder and Elbow	
1992 OITE	147
1992 OSAE—Adult Reconstruction Hip/Knee	46
1992 OSAE—Pediatric Orthopaedics	
1992 OSAE—Sports Medicine	
1991 OITE	
1991 OSAE—Adult Spine	63
1991 OSAE—Anatomy and Imaging	
1991 OSAE—Foot and Ankle	
1991 OSAE—M/S Trauma	

II. Biomaterials

A. Strength of Materials
1. Definition—Branch of mechanics that deals with relations between externally applied loads and the resulting internal effects and deformations induced in the body subjected to these loads.
   a. Loads—Forces that act on a body (compression, tension, shear, torsion).
   b. Deformations—Temporary (elastic) or permanent (plastic) change in the shape of a body.

   Changes in load produce changes in deformation.
2. Stress—Intensity of internal force: **Stress = force/area.** Used to analyze the internal resistance of a body to a load. Helps in selection of materials. Normal stresses (compressive or tensile) are perpendicular to the surface on which they act. Shear stresses are parallel to the surface on which they act. Stress has the units N/m^2 (pascals [Pa]).
3. Strain—Relative measure of the deformation of a body as a result of loading. **Strain = change in length/original length of an object.** It can also be normal or shear. Strain is a proportion and therefore has no units.
4. Hooke's Law—Basically, stress is proportional to strain up to a limit (the proportional limit).
5. Young's Modules (of Elasticity, E)—Measure of the stiffness of a material or its ability to resist deformation: **E = stress/strain** (in the elastic range of the stress–strain curve it is the slope). Modulus of elasticity is the critical factor in load-sharing capacity (*).
6. Stress–Strain Curve—Derived by axially loading a body and plotting stress versus strain (Fig. 1–93).
   a. Proportional Limit (Yield Point)—Transition point from elastic to plastic range. Usually 0.2% strain in most metals.
   b. Ultimate Strength—Maximum strength obtained by material.
   c. Breaking Point—Point where the material fractures.
   d. Plastic Deformation—Change in length after removing load (before the breaking point) in the plastic range (*).

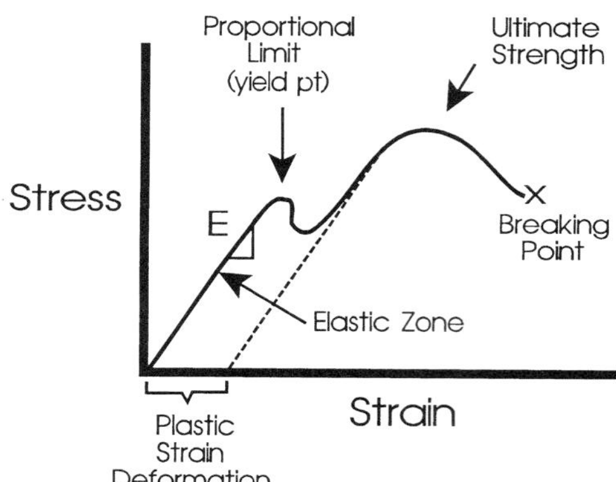

FIGURE 1–93. Stress–strain curve.

e. Strain Energy—Area under the curve (*). Total strain energy = recoverable strain energy (resilience) + dissipated strain energy. A measure of the toughness of a material.

B. Materials Versus Structures

1. Material—Related to a substance or element. Defined by mechanical properties (force, stress, strain) and rheologic properties (elasticity [ability to regain original shape], plasticity [permanent deformation], viscosity [resistance to flow or shear stress], strength).
   a. Brittle Materials (e.g., PMMA)—Exhibit a linear stress–strain curve up to the point of failure.
   b. Ductile Materials (e.g., Metal)—Undergo a large amount of plastic deformation prior to failure (*).
   c. Viscoelastic Materials (e.g., Bone and Ligaments)—Exhibit stress–strain behavior that is time-rate dependent and varies with the material. For example, at a bone–ligament interface, a slow rate of loading results in an avulsion fracture of bone, whereas a fast rate of loading causes ligament failure. During application of a constant load the material gradually deforms (*).
   d. Isotropic Materials—Possess the same mechanical properties in all directions.
   e. Anisotropic Materials—Have mechanical properties that vary with the orientation of loading (e.g., bone) (*).
   f. Homogeneous Materials—Have a uniform structure or composition throughout.
2. Structure—Related to both the material and shape of an object and its loading characteristics. A load deformation curve can be constructed similar to a stress–strain curve. The slope of the curve in the elastic range is referred to as the rigidity (versus stiffness) of the structure. Bending rigidity is proportional to the base multiplied by the height cubed for a rectangular structure ($bh^3/12$) and is proportional to the radius to the fourth power for a cylinder (torsional rigidity $\propto \pi r^4/L$). It is closely related to the moment of inertia (I, resistance to bending) (*), which is a function of the width and thickness of a structure, and the polar moment of inertia (J), which represents the resistance to torsion (twisting). The following equations use these concepts:

$$\sigma = my/I$$

$$\tau = Tr/J$$

C. Orthopaedic Materials

1. Metals—Demonstrate stress–strain curves as discussed above. Other important concepts follow.
   a. Fatigue Failure—Occurs with repetitive loading cycles at stress below the ultimate tensile strength. Fatigue failure depends on the magnitude of the stress and number of cycles. If the stress is less than a predetermined amount of stress, called the **endurance limit**, the material may be loaded cyclically an infinite number of times ($>10^6$·cycles) without breaking. Above the endurance limit, the fatigue life of a material is expressed by the stress (S) versus the number of loading cycles (n), or S–n, curve.
   b. Creep (a.k.a. Cold Flow)—Progressive deformation of metals over an extended period. If sudden stress followed by constant loading causes a material to continue to deform, it demonstrates creep (*). This process can produce a permanent deformity and may affect mechanical function (e.g., in a TJA).
   c. Corrosion—Chemical dissolving of metals as may occur in the high-saline environment of the body. Several types of corrosion may occur (Table 1–46). The risk of galvanic corrosion is high between stainless steel and cobalt–chromium (Co-Cr) (*). Corrosion can be decreased by using similar metals (e.g., with plates and screws), with proper design of implants, and with passivation (a thin layer that effectively separates the metal from the solution [e.g., stainless steel coated by chromium oxide]).
   d. Types of Metal—Implants used in orthopaedics are typically made of 316L (L = low carbon) stainless steel (iron, chromium, and nickel), "supermetal" alloys (e.g., cobalt–chromium–molybdenum [65% Co, 35% Cr, 5% Mo] made with a special forging process), and titanium alloy (Ti-6Al-4V). Each possesses a **different stiffness (E)** that is compared with other materials (Fig. 1–94) (***). Problems associated with certain metals include wear, stress shielding (increased with higher E metals), and ion release (Co-Cr causes macrophage proliferation and synovial degeneration). Titanium has poor resistance to wear (notch sensitivity) (*); particulates may incite a histiocytic response; and there is an uncertain association between titanium and neoplasms. One advantage of titanium is its relatively low E and high yield strength (***).

TABLE 1–46. TYPES OF CORROSION

CORROSION	DESCRIPTION
Galvanic	Dissimilar metals[a]; electrochemical destruction
Crevice	Occurs in fatigue cracks with low O_2 tension
Stress	Occurs in areas with high stress gradients
Fretting	From small movements abrading outside layer
Other	Includes inclusion, intergranular, and others

[a] Metals such as 316L stainless steel and Co-Cr-Mo produce galvanic corrosion.

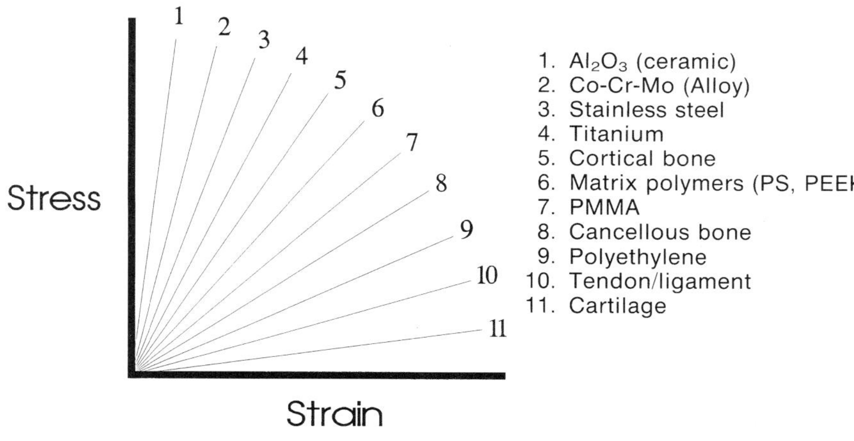

FIGURE 1–94. Comparison of Young's modulus (relative values, not to scale) for various orthopaedic materials.

2. Nonmetals—Include polyethylene, PMMA (bone cement), silicone, and ceramics.
   a. Polyethylene—Ultra-high-molecular-weight polyethylene (UHMWPE) polymer consists of long chains of carbons used in weight-bearing components of TJAs such as acetabular cups and tibial trays. These materials have wear characteristics superior to those of high-density polyethylene (HDP); they are tough, ductile, resilient, and resistant to wear, and they exhibit low friction. Polyethylenes are viscoelastic and susceptible to abrasion. They are also thermoplastic and may be altered by high dose radiation. They are weaker than bone in tension and have a low *E*. Wear debris is associated with a histiocytic osteolytic response. Wear is increased with thinner (<6 mm), flatter, carbon fiber-reinforced polyethylene. Metal backing may help minimize plastic deformation of HDP (and loosening) but decreases its effective thickness (wear). Catastrophic wear of polyethylene tibial inserts is associated with varus knee alignment, thin inserts (<6 mm), flat nonconforming inserts, and heat treatments of the insert (**). Polyethylene wear debris is the main factor affecting longevity of THAs (*).
   b. Polymethylmethacrylate (PMMA; Bone Cement)—Used for fixation (as a grout, not an adhesive) and load distribution for implants. It has poor tensile strength, is weaker than bone in compression, and has a low *E*. Reduction in the number of voids (porosity) with insertion (vacuum, centrifugation, good technique) increases its cement strength and decreases cracking (**). **PMMA functions by mechanically interlocking with bone. Insertion can lead to a precipitous drop in blood pressure.** Wear particles can incite a macrophage response that leads to loosening of a prosthesis. Cement failure is often caused by microfracture and fragmentation of cement (*).
   c. Silicones—Polymers used for replacement in non-weight-bearing joints. Their poor strength and wear capability are responsible for frequent synovitis with extended use.
   d. Ceramics—Broad class of materials that contain metallic and nonmetallic elements bonded ionically in a highly oxidized state. Include biostable (inert) materials such as Al_2O_3 and bioactive (degradable) substances such a bioglass. They typically have a "high *E*," high compressive strength, and **low tensile strength;** are brittle; have poor crack resistance characteristics; but have best wear characteristics with polyethylene (*). Their high conductiveness to tissue bonding is due to **high surface wetability and high surface tension,** which is also responsible for less friction and wear ("smooth surface") (*). Additionally, small grain size allows for an ultrasmooth finish and less friction. Calcium phosphates (e.g., hydroxyapatite) may have application as a coating (plasma sprayed) to allow increased strength of attachment and promote bone healing.
   e. Other Materials—Such as polylactic acid-coated carbon, which serves as a biodegradable scaffolding, and new polymer composites, some with carbon fiber reinforcement, are still investigational. Fabrication of these newer devices involves assembling "piles" of carbon fibers impregnated with matrix polymer (polysulfone or polyetheretherketone). Difficulties with abrasion and impact resistance, radiolucency, and manufacturing are still present.
3. Biomaterials—Possess certain unique characteristics including viscoelasticity (time-dependent stress–strain behavior), creep, and stress relaxation (internal stresses decrease with time). They also are capable of self-adaptation and repair; and characteristics change with aging and sampling.

4. Comparison of Common Orthopaedic Materials—Young's modules of elasticity (E) for various orthopaedic materials are compared in Figure 1–94.

D. Orthopaedic Structures

1. Bone
   a. Composite of Collagen and Hydroxyapatite—Collagen has a low E, good tensile strength, and poor compressive strength. Calcium apatite is a stiff, brittle material with good compressive strength. The combination is an anisotropic material that resists many forces; it is **strongest in compression,** weakest in shear, and intermediate in tension. Cancellous bone is 25% as dense, 10% as stiff, and 500% as ductile as cortical bone. Bone is a dynamic material because of its ability to self-repair, to change with aging (becomes stiffer and less ductile), and to change with prolonged immobilization (weaker). Stress concentration effects, which occur at points of defects within the bone or implant–bone interface (stress risers), reduce overall strength with loading. Stress shielding by implants results in osteoporosis of adjacent bone due to lack of normal physiologic stresses. This situation occurs commonly under plates and at the femoral calcar in high-riding total hip arthroplasties. A hole of 20–30% of the bone diameter, regardless of whether it is filled with a screw, reduces overall strength up to 50%, which does not return to normal until 9–12 months after screw removal. Cortical defects can reduce strength 70% or more (less with oval defects, as compared to rectangular, due to smaller stress riser). Bone is anisotropic and viscoelastic. Cortical bone is excellent versus torque; cancellous bone is good versus compressive and shear forces.
   b. Fracture—Type is based on mechanism.
      1. Tension—By muscle pull, typically transverse, perpendicular to load and bone axis.
      2. Compression—By axial loading of cancellous bone.
      3. Shear—Commonly around joints; load parallel to bone surface, and fracture parallel to load.
      4. Bending—By eccentric loading or direct blows. Fracture begins on tension side and continues transversely/obliquely.
      5. Torsion—Shear and tensile stresses result in spiral fractures (*).
   c. Comminution—Function of the amount of energy transmitted to bone (*).
2. Ligaments and Tendons—These structures can sustain 5–10% tensile strain before failure (versus bone, 1–4%). Tension rupture of fibers and shear failure between fibers occurs commonly. Most ligaments can undergo plastic strain to the point at which they cannot function effectively but are still in continuity. Soft tissue implants include stents, ligament augmentation devices, and scaffolding. **Tendons** are strong in tension only; E is only 10% that of bone but increases with slower loading. Fibers are oriented parallel. Demonstrates stress relaxation and creep. **Ligament** fibers can be oriented parallel if they are required to resist major joint stress or more randomly if they must resist forces from different directions. Stiffness = force/strain, as depicted on a force deformation graph (similar to E but does not consider the cross-sectional area). The bone–ligament complex is softer (less stiff—decreased E) and has a lower yield point and tensile strength with prolonged immobilization. Bone resorption at the tendon insertion site also occurs.
   a. Stents—Internal splint devices. These include the Proplast Tendon Transfer Stabilizer using synthetic polymers, Goretex Prosthetic ligaments, Xenotech (bovine tendon), and polyester implants. All are limited by not allowing adequate collagen ingrowth and so eventually fail. Synthetic ligaments produce wear particles that increase levels of proteinases, collagenase, gelatinase, and chondrocyte activation factor.
   b. Ligament Augmentation Devices (LADs)—Such as the Kennedy LAD (polypropylene yarn) and Dacron. LADs do allow some fibrous ingrowth, but their use is limited.
   c. Biodegradable Tissue Scaffolding—Allows immediate stability and long-term replacement with host tissue. Carbon fiber and polylactic acid (PLA)-coated carbon fiber devices have been used with limited success (slow ingrowth is improved with PLA coating).
3. Articular Cartilage—Contains 60% water, 25% collagen, and 15% proteoglycan. The ultimate tensile strength of cartilage is only 5% of bone, and E is 0.1% that of bone; nevertheless, because of its highly viscoelastic properties, it is well suited for compressive loading. Deformation and shift of water to and from cartilage are largely responsible.
4. Metal Implants
   a. Screws—Characterized by **pitch** (distance between threads), **lead** (distance advanced in one revolution), **root diameter** (minimal/inner diameter $\propto$ tensile strength), and **outer diameter** (determines holding power [pullout strength]). To maximize pullout strength a screw should have a large outer diameter, small root diameter, and fine pitch (*). Pullout strength of a pedicle screw is most affected by the degree of osteoporosis (*).
   b. Plates—Strength related to material and moment of inertia (thickness (t) is most important: rigidity $\propto t^3$). **Plates are most effective when placed on the tension side of a fracture.** Types of plates include static compression (best in upper extremity; can be stressed for compression), dynamic compression (e.g., tension band plate), neutralization (resists torsion), and buttress (protects bone graft). Stress concentration at open screw holes can lead to implant failure. Blade plates provide increased resistance to torsional deformation in subtrochanteric fractures.
   c. Intramedullary (IM) Nails—Require a high J to maximize torsional rigidity and strength.

Reaming allows increased torsional resistance owing to the increased contact area and allows use of a larger nail with increased rigidity and strength. IM nails are better at resisting bending than rotational forces. Unslotted nails allow stronger fixation and a smaller diameter (at the expense of flexibility). The greatest mechanical advantage of closed section IM nails over slotted nails is increased torsional stiffness (*). Posterior starting points for femoral nails decrease hoop stresses and comminution of fractures. Implant failure occurs more frequently with smaller-diameter, unreamed IM nails (*).

d. External Fixators—**Increased rigidity with larger-diameter pins** (most important), more pins, decreased bone–rod distance, and placement of central pins closer to the fracture site and peripheral pins further from fracture site (near-near, far-far), and pins in different planes. The rigidity of the frame itself is of secondary importance. The use of half-pins may provide more secure fixation and lower the incidence of pin loosening, particularly when separated >45 degrees. Addition of a second bar in the same plane provides increased resistance to bending moments in the sagittal plane.

e. Total Hip Arthroplasty (THA)—Design has evolved to help reduce biomechanical constraints. Femoral components are designed for use with and without cement. Stem length is directly related to rigidity. Minimum compressive and tensile stresses in adjacent structures result from a design with a broad medial surface, a broader lateral surface, and a large moment of inertia. Femoral component design must account for rotational forces. Placement of the femoral component should be in neutral or slight valgus to decrease the moment arm, cement stress, and abductor length. Femoral head size should be a compromise between small (22 mm) components with decreased friction and torque but decreased ROM/stability and large (36 mm) components with increased friction and torque but increased ROM/stability. A 26- or 28-mm head seems to be ideal in most instances. Metal backing of acetabular components decreases the stress in cement and cancellous bone. Use of different metal alloys and titanium (with *E* closer to cortical bone) is being investigated. **The use of titanium on weight-bearing surfaces (poor resistance to wear, notch sensitivity) may lead to fretting, wear debris, and blackening of soft tissues.** UHMWPE serves as a "shock absorber" and should be at least 6 mm thick to prevent creep. Wear rate of UHMWPE in the acetabulum is about 0.1 mm/year (*). Other new concepts include computer design of THA stems, modularity, custom designs, and more flexible stems. Forging of components appears to be superior to casting.

f. Total Knee Arthroplasty (TKA)—Design has evolved significantly after original design errors that did not take kinematics of the human knee into consideration (i.e., original hinge design). An appropriate compromise between total contact designs with excess stability (and less motion) but less wear and a low-contact design with less stability and increased wear is being approached. Metal alloys are typically used.

g. Compression Hip Screws—Demonstrate loading characteristics superior to blade plates. Higher-angled plates are subjected to lower bending loads but may be more difficult to insert. Sliding of the screw is proportional to the screw/side plate angle and the length of the screw in the barrel.

5. Implant Fixation—Three basic forms exist: interference fit, interlocking, and biologic.
   a. Interference Fit—Mechanical or press fit components rely on the formation of a fibrous tissue interface. Loosening can occur if stability is not maintained and high-*E* substances are used (leading to increased bone resorption/remodeling).
   b. Interlocking Fit—With PMMA as a grout and a low *E,* allows a gradual transfer of stresses to bone (microinterlocking of cement within cancellous bone). Microinterlock may not be achievable when doing a cemented revision of a previously cemented TKA (*). Aseptic loosening can occur over time. Careful technique with limiting of porosities and gaps and using a 3–5 mm cement thickness yields best results. Other improvements include low viscosity cement, better bone bed preparation, plugging and pressurization, and better (vacuum) cement mixing.
   c. Biologic Fit—Tissue ingrowth makes use of fiber–metal composites, void metal composites, or microbeads to create pore sizes of 50–400 μm (ideally 100–250 μm). Mechanical stability is required for ingrowth, which has been limited to 10–30% of the surface area. Problems include fiber/bead loosening, increased cost, proximal bone resorption (monocyte/macrophage-mediated), corrosion, and decreased implant fatigue strength. Bone ingrowth in the tibial component of an uncemented TKA occurs adjacent to fixation pegs and screws (*). Bone ingrowth of uncemented TJA components is dependent on the avoidance of micromotion (may be seen on follow-up radiographs as radiodense reactive lines about the prosthesis) at the bone–implant interface (**). Canal filling (maximal endosteal contact) of more fully coated femoral stems is an important factor for bone ingrowth (**).
6. Bone–Implant Unit—The integrated unit is a composite structure that has shared properties. The more accurately the bone cross section is reconstructed with metallic support, the better the loading characteristics. Plates should act as tension bands. Materials with increased *E* may result in bone resorption, whereas materials with decreased *E* may result in implant failure. **Placement of the implant initiates a race between bone healing and implant failure.**

TEST QUESTIONS ON BIOMATERIALS

TEST	QUESTION NUMBERS
1995 OSAE—Adult Reconstruction Hip/Knee	7, 8, 20, 23, 41, 57, 68, 83, 89, 98
1995 OSAE—Pediatric Orthopaedics	
1995 OSAE—Sports Medicine	
1994 OITE	45, 117, 183, 195, 207, 213, 244
1994 OSAE—Adult Spine	61, 64, 82
1994 OSAE—Foot and Ankle	33
1994 OSAE—M/S Trauma	11, 23, 40
1993 OITE	26, 30, 34, 35, 37, 42, 107, 154, 155, 197, 200, 227, 238
1993 OSAE—M/S Tumors and Diseases	
1993 OSAE—Shoulder and Elbow	
1992 OITE	15, 35, 50, 53, 101, 137, 167
1992 OSAE—Adult Reconstruction Hip/Knee	12, 13, 38, 40, 41, 42, 48, 49, 50, 71, 72, 84
1992 OSAE—Pediatric Orthopaedics	
1992 OSAE—Sports Medicine	1
1991 OITE	5, 38, 184, 214, 215, 216
1991 OSAE—Adult Spine	56, 69
1991 OSAE—Anatomy and Imaging	
1991 OSAE—Foot and Ankle	41
1991 OSAE—M/S Trauma	

III. Biomechanics

A. Joint Biomechanics: General

1. Degrees of Freedom—Joint motion is described based on rotation and translation in the *x, y,* and *z* directions. Therefore **six positions, or degrees of freedom,** are used to describe motion. Fortunately, translations are usually relatively insignificant and can be safely ignored for most joints.
2. Joint Reaction Force (R)—Force generated within a joint in response to external forces (both intrinsic and extrinsic). Muscle contractions about a joint are a major contributory factor to R (*). Values (of R) correlate to the predisposition to degenerative changes.
3. Coupled Forces—Certain joints move in such a way that rotation about one axis is accompanied by an obligatory rotation about another axis, and these movements are coupled. For example, lateral bending of the spine is accompanied by axial rotation, and these movements/forces are coupled.
4. Joint Congruence—Relates to the fit of two articular surfaces to each other and is a necessary condition for joint motion. It can be evaluated radiographically. Movement out of a position of congruity causes increased stress in cartilage by allowing less contact area for distribution of the joint reaction force, predisposing the joint to degeneration.
5. Instant Center—Point at which a joint rotates. In joints such as the knee, the location of the instant center changes during the arc of motion (due to joint translation) (*), following a curved path. The instant center normally lies on a line perpendicular to the tangent of the joint surface at all points of contact. If the instant center lies on the joint surface, a pure rolling motion occurs. Pure sliding motion occurs with no angular change in position and therefore has no instant center.
6. Friction and Lubrication—Resistance between two bodies when one slides over the other ($Ff = \mu N$). It is not a function of the contact area. Lubrication decreases the coefficient of friction between surfaces. Articular surfaces lubricated with synovial fluid have a coefficient of friction 10 times less than the best synthetic systems. **Boundary and hydrostatic lubrication are largely responsible.**

B. Hip Biomechanics

1. Kinematics
   a. Range of Motion (Table 1–47)
   b. Instant Center—Simultaneous motion in all three planes for this ball-and-socket joint makes analysis impossible.
2. Kinetics—The joint reaction force (R) in the hip is three to six times body weight (W) and is primarily due to contraction of muscles crossing the hip. This phenomenon can be demonstrated with the free body diagram (FBD) in Figure 1–95. If $A = 5$ and $B = 12.5$, using standard FBD analysis:

$$\sum MR = 0$$
$$-5\ M_y + 12.5\ W = 0$$
$$M_y = 2.5\ W$$
$$\sum F_y = 0$$
$$-M_y - W + R_y = 0$$
$$R_y = 3.5\ W$$
$$R = R_y/(\cos 30°)$$
$$R = \underline{\underline{\text{(approx) } 4\ W}}$$

TABLE 1–47. HIP BIOMECHANICS: RANGE OF MOTION

MOTION	AVERAGE RANGE (DEGREES)	FUNCTIONAL RANGE (DEGREES)
Flexion	115	90 (120 squat)
Extension	30	
Abduction	50	20
Adduction	30	
Internal rotation	45	0
External rotation	45	20

One can see that an increase in the ratio of *A/B* (e.g., with medialization of the acetabulum or long-neck prosthesis, or lateralization of the greater trochanter) decreases the joint reaction force. If $A = 7.5$ and $B = 10$, *R* would equal approximately 2.3 *W*. *R* can also be reduced with shifting body weight over the hip (Trendelenburg gait) and with a **cane in the contralateral hand (produces an additional moment—and can reduce *R* up to 60%!)** (*). Energy expenditure is 264% of normal with a resection arthroplasty of the hip (such as after a THA infection) (*).

3. Other Considerations
   a. Stability—Largely based on intrinsic stability of deep-seated "ball-and-socket" design.
   b. Sourcil—Condensation of subchondral bone under the superomedial acetabulum. At this point *R* is maximal (Pauwels).
   c. Gothic Arch—Remodeled bone supporting the acetabular roof with the sourcil at its base (Bombelli).
   d. Neck–Shaft Angle—Varus angle results in decreased *R* and increased shear across the neck. Valgus angle creates increased *R* and decreased shear. Neutral or valgus is better for THA because PMMA resists shear poorly.
   e. Arthrodesis—**Position for hip arthrodesis should be 25–30 degrees of flexion and 0 degrees of abduction and rotation (ER better than IR).** Increases oxygen consumption; gait efficiency is 53%; increases transpelvic rotation of contralateral hip (*).

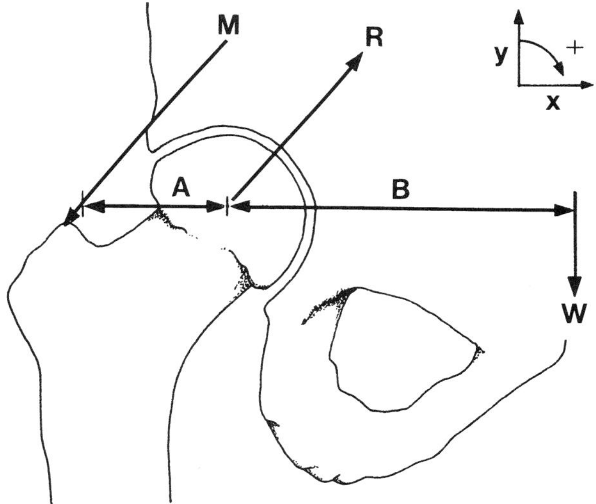

FIGURE 1–95. Pelvis free body diagram (see text for explanation).

C. Knee Biomechanics
1. Kinematics
   a. Range of Motion—ROM of the knee is from 10 degrees of extension (recurvatum) to about 130 degrees of flexion. Functional ROM is from near full extension to about 90 degrees of flexion (117 degrees is required for squatting and lifting). Flexion to approximately 110 degrees is required to arise from a chair following TKA (*). Rotation varies with flexion. At full extension there is minimal rotation. At 90 degrees flexion, 45 degrees of external and 30 degrees of internal rotation are possible. Abduction/adduction is essentially 0 degrees (a few degrees of passive motion is possible at 30 degrees of flexion normally). Motion about the knee is a complex series of movements about a changing instant center of rotation (i.e., polycentric rotation). There is 0.5 cm of excursion of the medial meniscus and 1.1 cm of excursion of the lateral meniscus during a 0- to 120-degree arc of knee motion (*).
   b. Joint Motion—The instant centers (*), when plotted, describe a J-shaped curve about the femoral condyle. Flexion and extension of the knee involve both rolling and gliding motions. The femur internally rotates (external tibial rotation) during the last 15 degrees of extension ("screw home" mechanism related to size and convexity of the medial femoral condyle [MFC] and musculature). **Posterior rollback of the femur on the tibia during knee flexion increases maximum knee flexion.** Normal femoral rollback is compromised when the PCL is sacrificed, as in some TKAs (*). The axis of rotation of the intact knee is in the MFC. The patellofemoral joint is a sliding articulation (patella slides 7 cm caudally with full flexion), with an instant center near the posterior cortex above the condyles.
2. Kinetics—Extension is via the quadriceps mechanism, through the patellar apparatus; the hamstring muscles are primarily responsible for flexion at the knee.
   a. Knee Stabilizers—Although bony contours have a role in knee stability, it is the ligaments and muscles of the knee that play the major role (Table 1–48). The ACL typically is subjected to peak loads of 170 N during walking and up to 500 N with running. The ultimate

TABLE 1–48. KNEE STABILIZERS

DIRECTION	STRUCTURES
Medial	Superficial MCL (1°), joint capsule, med. meniscus, ACL/PCL
Lateral	Joint capsule, IT band, LCL (mid), lat. meniscus, ACL/PCL (90°)
Anterior	ACL (1°), joint capsule
Posterior	PCL (1°), joint capsule; PCL tightens with IR
Rotatory	Combinations—MCL checks ER; ACL checks IR

IR, internal rotation; ER, external rotation; MCL, medial collateral ligament complex; LCL, lateral collateral ligament complex; IT, illiotibial; ACL, anterior cruciate ligament; PCL, posterior cruciate ligament.

strength of the ACL in young patients is about 1750 N. The ACL fails by serial tearing at 10–15% elongation.

b. Joint Forces
   1. Tibiofemoral Joint—Joint surfaces in the knee are subjected to a loading force equal to **three times the body weight during level walking** and up to **four times the body weight with walking steps.** Menisci help with load transmission (bear one-third to one-half of body weight), and removal of these structures increases contact stresses (up to four times load transfer to bone).
   2. Patellofemoral Joint—The patella aids in knee extension by increasing the lever arm and in stress distribution. This joint has the thickest cartilage in the body because it must bear the greatest load—ranging from 1/2 *W* with normal walking to seven times *W* with squatting and jogging. Loads are proportional to the quadriceps force/knee flexion ratio. The quadriceps provides an anterior subluxing force at 0–45 degrees ROM. During TKA the following enhance patella tracking: external rotation of the femoral component, lateral placement of the femoral and tibial components, medial placement of the patellar component, and avoidance of malrotation of the tibial component (avoid internal rotation) (**).

c. Axes (Fig. 1–96)
   1. Mechanical Axis—Femoral head to center of ankle.
   2. Vertical Axis—From center of gravity to ground.
   3. Anatomic Axis—Along shafts of femur and tibia.
   4. Relationships—Mechanical axis is 3 degrees valgus from vertical axis. Anatomic axis of femur is 6 degrees valgus from mechanical axis (9 degrees versus vertical axis). Anatomic axis of tibia is 2–3 degrees varus from mechanical axis.

d. Arthrodesis—**Position for knee arthrodesis should be 0–7 degrees of valgus and 10–15 degrees of flexion.**

D. Ankle and Foot Biomechanics
   1. Ankle
      a. Kinematics—Instant center is within the talus, and the lateral and posterior points are at the tips of the malleoli; they change slightly with movement. The talus is described as forming a cone with the body and trochlea wider anteriorly and laterally. Therefore the talus and fibula must externally rotate slightly with dorsiflexion. Ankle dorsiflexion and abduction are coupled movements in the ankle. Average ROM is 25 degrees dorsiflexion, 35 degrees plantar flexion, and 5 degrees rotation.
      b. Kinetics—The tibial/talar articulation is the major weight-bearing surface of the ankle, supporting compressive forces up to five times body weight on level surfaces and shear (backward-to-forward) forces up to body weight. A large weight-bearing surface area allows for decreased stress (force/area) at this joint. The fibula/talar joint transmits about one-sixth of the force.

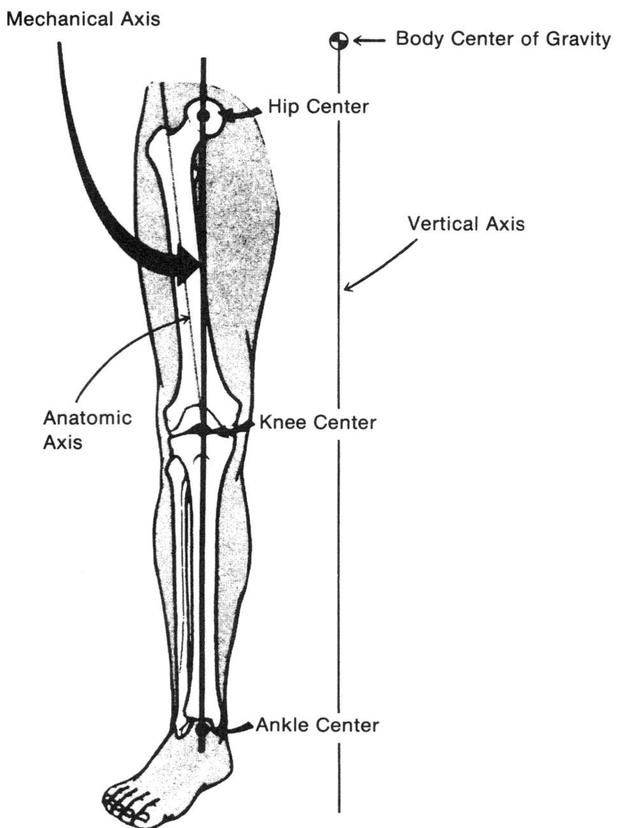

FIGURE 1–96. Knee axes. (Modified from Rohr, W.L.: Primary total knee arthroplasty. In Chapman's Operative Orthopaedics, p. 718. Philadelphia, JB Lippincott, 1988; reprinted by permission.)

      c. Other Considerations—Stability is based on the shape of the articulation (mortise that is maintained by talar shape) and ligamentous support. The best stability is in dorsiflexion. During weight-bearing (loaded), the tibial and talar articular surfaces contribute most to joint stability (*). A windlass action has been described in the ankle, where full dorsiflexion is limited by the plantar aponeurosis, and further tension on the aponeurosis (e.g., with toe dorsiflexion) causes the arch to rise. A syndesmosis screw limits primarily external rotation (*). **Arthrodesis should be performed in neutral or < 5 degrees equinus with 5–10 degrees external rotation** (anticipate loss of 70% of sagittal plane motion) (*).
   2. Subtalar Joint (Talus–Calcaneus–Navicular)—Axis of rotation is 42 degrees in the sagittal plane and 16 degrees in the transverse plane. Described as functioning like an oblique hinge; its motions are also coupled with dorsiflexion, abduction, and eversion in one direction (pronation) and plantar flexion, adduction, and inversion (supination) in the other. Average ROM of pronation is 5 degrees; supination is 20 degrees. Functional ROM is approximately 6 degrees.
   3. Transverse Tarsal Joint (Talus–Navicular, Calcaneal–Cuboid)—Motion is based on foot position with two axes of rotation (talonavicular and calca-

TABLE 1–49. ARCHES OF THE FOOT

ARCH	COMPONENTS	KEYSTONE	LIGAMENT SUPPORT	MUSCLE SUPPORT
Medial longitudinal	Calcaneus, talus, navicular, 3 cuneiforms, 1st–3rd metatarsals	Talus head	Spring (calcaneonavicular)	Tibialis post., flexor digitorum longus, flexor hallucis longus, adductor hallucis
Lateral longitudinal	Calcaneus, cuboid, 4th and 5th metatarsals		Plantar aponeurosis	Abductor digiti minimi, flexor digitorum brevis
Transverse	3 Cuneiforms, cuboid, metatarsal bases			Peroneus longus, tibialis post., adductor hallucis (oblique)

neocuboid). With eversion of the foot (as during the early stance phase), the two joints are parallel and ROM is permitted. With foot inversion (late stance), external rotation of the lower extremity causes the joints to no longer be parallel, and motion is limited.

4. Foot—Transmits about 1.2 times body weight with walking and three times body weight with running. It is composed of three arches (Table 1–49). The second MT Lisfranc joint is "key-like" and stabilizes the second MT, allowing it to carry the most load with gait (first MT bears the most load while standing).

E. Spine Biomechanics
1. Kinematics—ROM varies with anatomic segment (Table 1–50). Analysis is based on the functional unit (**motion segment = two vertebrae and their intervening soft tissues**). Six degrees of freedom exist about all three axes. Coupled motion is also demonstrated, especially with axial rotation and lateral bending. The instant center lies within the disc.
2. Supporting Structures—Anteriorly includes the anterior longitudinal ligament, posterior longitudinal ligament, and vertebral discs. Posteriorly includes the intertransverse ligaments, capsular ligaments and facets, and ligamentum flavum (yellow ligament).
   a. Apophyseal Joints—Resist torsion during axial loading, and the attached capsular ligaments resist flexion. They guide the motion of the motion segment. Direction of motion is determined by the orientation of the facets of the apophyseal joint, which varies with each level. **In the C-spine the facets are oriented 45 degrees to the transverse plane and parallel to the frontal plane. In the T-spine the facets are oriented 60 degrees to the transverse plane and 20 degrees to the frontal plane. In the L-spine the facets are oriented 90 degrees to the transverse plane and 45 degrees to the frontal plane** (i.e., they progressively tilt up [transverse plane] and in [frontal plane]).
3. Kinetics
   a. Disc—Behaves viscoelastically and demonstrates creep (deforms with time) and hysteresis (absorbs energy with repeated axial loads and later decreases in function). Compressive stresses are highest in the nucleus pulposus and tensile stresses in the annulus fibrosus. Stiffness of the disc increases with increasing compressive load. With higher loads increased deformation and faster creep can be expected. Repeated torsional loading may separate the nucleus pulposus from the annulus and end plate and may force nuclear material out through an annular tear (produced by shear forces). Loads are increased with bending and torsional stresses. Disc pressures are lowest in the lying supine position (**). When carrying loads, disc pressures are lowest when the load is carried close to the body (***).
   b. Vertebrae—Strength is related to the bone mineral content and size of the vertebrae (increased in the lumbar spine). Fatigue loading may lead to pars fractures. Compression fractures occur at the end plate. Decreased vertebral body stiffness in osteoporosis is caused by loss of horizontal trabeculae (*).

F. Shoulder Biomechanics
1. Kinematics—The scapular plane is 30 degrees anterior to the coronal plane and is the preferred reference for ROM. Abduction of the shoulder requires external rotation of the humerus to prevent greater tuberosity impingement. With internal rotation contractures, patients cannot abduct past 120 degrees. Abduction is a result of glenohumeral motion (120 degrees) and scapulothoracic motion (60 degrees) in a 2:1 ratio (*). Movement at the acromioclavicular (AC) joint is responsible for the early part of scapulothoracic motion, and sternoclavicular (SC) movement is responsible for the later portion, with clavicular rotation along the long axis. Surface joint motion in the glenohumeral joint is a combination of rotation, rolling, and translation.

TABLE 1–50. RANGE OF MOTION OF SPINAL SEGMENTS

LEVEL	FLEXION/EXTENSION (DEGREES)	LATERAL BENDING (DEGREES)	ROTATION (DEGREES)	INSTANT CENTER
Occiput–C1	13	8	0	Skull, 2–3 cm above dens
C1–C2	10	0	45	Waist of odontoid
C2–C7	10–15	8–10	10	Vertebral body below
T-spine	5	6	8	Vertebra below/disc centrum
L-spine	15–20	2–5	3–6	Disc annulus

TABLE 1–51. SHOULDER BIOMECHANICS: MUSCLE FORCES

MOTION	MUSCLE FORCES	COMMENTS
GLENOHUMERAL		
Abduction	Deltoid, supraspinatus	Cuff depresses head
Adduction	Latissimus dorsi, pectoralis major, teres major	
Forward flexion	Pectoralis major, deltoid (ant.), biceps	
Extension	Latissimus dorsi	
IR	Subscapularis, teres major	
ER	Infraspinatus, teres minor, deltoid (post.)	
SCAPULAR		
Rotation	Upper trapezius, levator scapula (ant.), serratus ant., lower trapezius	Works through a force couple
Adduction	Trapezius, rhomboid, latissimus dorsi	
Abduction	Serratus ant., pectoralis minor	

2. Kinetics (Table 1–51)—The zero position (Saha)—165 degrees of abduction in the scapular plane—minimizes deforming forces about the shoulder. This position is ideal for reducing shoulder dislocations (or "fractures with traction"). Free body analysis of the deltoid force (Fig. 1–97) reveals the following:

$$\Sigma M_0 = 0$$
$$3D - 0.05\ W(30) = 0$$
$$\underline{\underline{D = 0.5\ W}}$$

3. Stability—Limited about the glenohumeral joint. The humeral head has a surface area larger than the glenoid (48 × 45 versus 35 × 25). Bony stability is limited and relies only on inclination (125 degrees) and retroversion (25 degrees) of the humeral head and slight retrotilt of the glenoid. The ligaments (especially the middle and **inferior glenohumeral** [most important]) (*) and rotator cuff are largely responsible for stability about the shoulder. Stress on the posterior shoulder capsule is greatest during follow-through of throwing (*). **The position for arthrodesis is 30–50 degrees of true abduction, 20–30 degrees of forward flexion, and 25–30 degrees of internal rotation. Avoid excessive external rotation.**
4. Other Joints—The AC joint allows scapular rotation (through the conoid and trapezoid ligaments) and scapular motion (through the AC joint itself). The SC joint allows clavicular protraction/retraction in a transverse plane (through the coracoclavicular ligament), clavicular elevation and depression in the frontal plane (also through the coracoclavicular ligament), and clavicular rotation around the longitudinal axis.

G. Elbow Biomechanics

1. Introduction—The elbow serves three functions: (1) as a component joint of the lever arm when positioning the hand; (2) as a fulcrum for the forearm lever; and (3) as a weight-bearing joint in patients using crutches. During throwing, the elbow functions primarily as a positioner and a means of transferring energy from the shoulder and trunk (*).
2. Kinematics—Motion about the elbow includes flexion and extension (0–150 degrees with **functional ROM 30–130 degrees;** axis of rotation is the center of the trochlea) and pronation (P) and supination (S): P 80 degrees and S 85 degrees with **functional P and S of 50 degrees each;** the axis is a line from the capitellum through the radial head and to the distal ulna (defines a cone). The normal carrying angle (valgus angle at the elbow) is 7 degrees for males and 13 degrees for females. This angle decreases with flexion.
3. Kinetics—The forces that act about the elbow have short lever arms and are relatively inefficient, resulting in large joint reaction forces that subject the elbow to degenerative changes. Flexion is primarily by the brachialis and biceps, extension by the triceps, pronation by the pronators (teres and quadratus), and supination by the biceps and supinator. Static loads approach, and dynamic loads exceed, body weight. The FBD in Figure 1–98 demonstrates the inefficiency of elbow flexion.

$$\Sigma M_0 = 0$$
$$-5B + 15W = 0$$
$$\underline{\underline{B = 3W}}$$

Because the biceps inserts so close to the joint, it is relatively inefficient and must support three times the weight of the arm and any objects it holds.

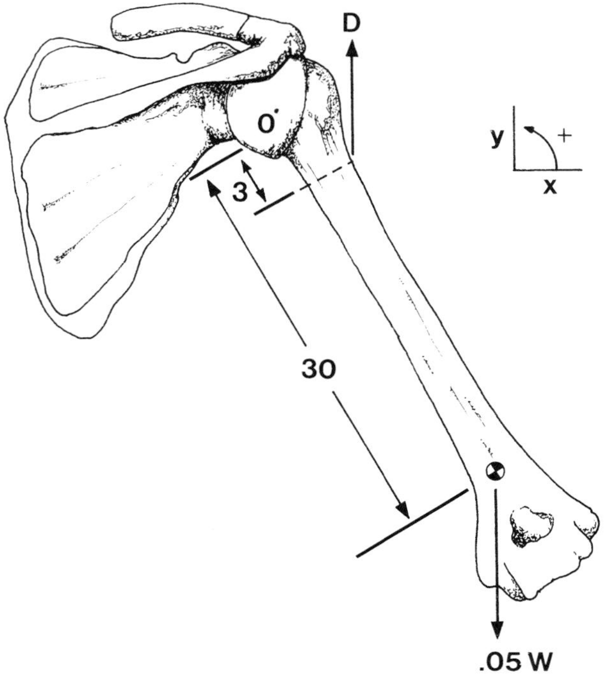

FIGURE 1–97. Shoulder free body diagram (see text for explanation).

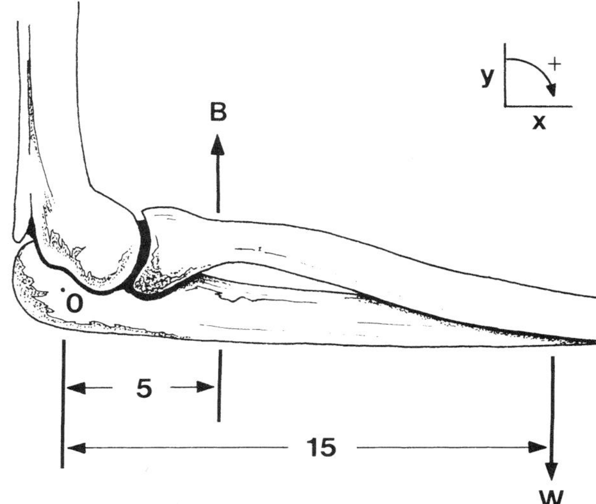

FIGURE 1–98. Elbow free body diagram (see text for explanation).

4. Stability—Provided partially by articular congruity. Radial head provides about 30% of valgus stability and is more important in 0–30 degrees of flexion and pronation. The greatest stability of the elbow comes from the medial side, where the **medial collateral ligament (MCL) is the most important stabilizer (especially the anterior oblique fibers)** (***). The MCL stabilizes the elbow to both valgus and distractional force with forearm flexion ≥90 degrees (*). Valgus extension overload of the elbow occurs during the late cocking and early acceleration phases of throwing (**). In extension, the capsule is the primary restraint to distractional forces. Laterally, stability is provided by the lateral collateral ligament (LCL), anconeus, and joint capsule. Position for unilateral arthrodesis is about 90 degrees of flexion; for bilateral arthrodesis one elbow is placed at 110 degrees of flexion (to reach the mouth) and the other at 65 degrees of flexion (for hygiene needs). Arthrodesis is difficult and fortunately is rarely required.
5. Forearm—About 17% of the axial load is transmitted by the ulna. The line of the center of rotation runs from the radial head to the distal ulna.

H. Wrist and Hand Biomechanics
 1. Wrist—Part of an intercalated link system.
  a. Kinematics—Motions about the wrist include flexion (65 degrees normal, 10 degrees functional), extension (55 degrees normal, 35 degrees functional), radial deviation (15 degrees normal, 10 degrees functional), and ulnar deviation (35 degrees normal, 15 degrees functional). Flexion and extension are primarily radiocarpal (two-thirds), but intercarpal movement is also important (one-third). Radial deviation is primarily due to intercarpal movement, whereas ulnar deviation relies on radiocarpal and intercarpal motion. The instant center for wrist motion is the head of the capitate but is variable.
  b. Columns—Three columns are described for the wrist (Taleisnik) (Table 1–52).

TABLE 1–52. COLUMNS OF THE WRIST

COLUMN	FUNCTION	COMMENTS
Central	Flexion-extension	Distal carpal row and lunate (link)
Medial	Rotation	Triquetrum
Lateral	Mobile	Scaphoid

  c. Link System—The carpus makes up a system of three links in a chain (Gilford): radius–lunate–capitate. This arrangement allows for less motion to be required at each link but adds to the instability of the "chain." Stability, however, is enhanced by strong volar ligaments and the scaphoid, which bridges both carpal rows.
  d. Relationships—Carpal collapse can be evaluated based on the ratio of carpal height/third MC height (normally 0.54). Ulnar translation can be determined using the ulna-to-capitate length/third MC height ratio (normal is 0.30). The distal radius normally bears about 80% of the distal radioulnar joint load and the distal ulna 20%. Ulnar load-bearing can be increased with ulnar lengthening (e.g., for treatment of Kienböck's disease) or decreased with ulnar shortening (e.g., for degenerative triangular fibrocartilage complex [TFCC] tears). Wrist arthrodesis is relatively common. A position of 10–20 degrees of dorsiflexion is good for unilateral fusion; and if bilateral fusion is necessary (avoid if possible), the other wrist should be fused in 0–10 degrees of palmar flexion.
 2. Hand
  a. Kinematics—ROM at the MCP joint (universal joint, 2 degrees of freedom) (*) includes 100 degrees of flexion and 60 degrees of abduction–adduction. PIP joints usually have about 110 degrees of flexion and DIP joints 80 degrees.
  b. Arches—The hand has two transverse arches (proximal ridge through the carpus and distal through the MC heads) and five longitudinal arches (through each of the rays).
  c. Stability—MCP stability is provided by the volar plate and the collateral ligaments. The PIPs and DIPs rely more on joint congruity. Also there is a large ligament/articular surface ratio in these joints.
  d. Other Concepts—The pulleys in the hand prevent bowstringing and decrease tendon excur-

TABLE 1–53. RECOMMENDED POSITIONS OF FLEXION FOR ARTHRODESIS OF THE JOINTS OF THE HAND

JOINT	DEGREES OF FLEXION	OTHER FACTORS
MCP	20–30	
PIP	40–50	Less radial than ulnar
DIP	15–20	
Thumb CMC		MC in opposition
Thumb MCP	25	
Thumb IP	20	

sion. Bowstringing increases the moment arm to the joint instant center. The sagittal bands allow extension at the MCP joint. With hyperextension at the MCPs, the intrinsics must function for PIP extension because the extensor tendon is lax. Normal grasp for males is 50 kg and for females 25 kg (only 4 kg is required for daily function). Normal pinch for males is 8 kg and for females 4 kg (1 kg is needed for day-to-day activities).

e. Kinetics—Joint loading with pinch is mostly in the MCP; but because the MCPs have a larger surface area, the contact pressures (joint load/contact area) at the MCPs are less. The DIPs have the most contact pressures and subsequently develop the most degenerative change with time (Heberden's nodes). Grasping contact pressures are less but focus on the MCPs; therefore patients with MCP arthritis frequently have had occupations that required grasping activities. Compressive loads at the thumb with pinching include 3 kg at the interphalangeal (IP), 5 kg at the MCP, and 12 kg at the thumb CMC joint (an unstable joint), which frequently leads to its degeneration.

f. Arthrodesis—Recommended positions of flexion for arthrodesis of joints in the hand are shown in Table 1–53.

TEST QUESTIONS ON BIOMECHANICS

TEST	QUESTION NUMBERS
1995 OSAE—Adult Reconstruction Hip/Knee	19, 44, 65, 99
1995 OSAE—Pediatric Orthopaedics	
1995 OSAE—Sports Medicine	10, 11, 19, 110
1994 OITE	5, 41, 83, 99, 103, 120, 155, 224, 239
1994 OSAE—Adult Spine	21
1994 OSAE—Foot and Ankle	74
1994 OSAE—M/S Trauma	
1993 OITE	18, 36, 110, 111, 232
1993 OSAE—M/S Tumors and Diseases	
1993 OSAE—Shoulder and Elbow	9, 41
1992 OITE	8, 9, 54, 116, 147, 174
1992 OSAE—Adult Reconstruction Hip/Knee	3, 4, 29, 34, 46, 47, 75
1992 OSAE—Pediatric Orthopaedics	
1992 OSAE—Sports Medicine	49, 75
1991 OITE	86, 89, 213
1991 OSAE—Adult Spine	7, 80, 95
1991 OSAE—Anatomy and Imaging	
1991 OSAE—Foot and Ankle	18
1991 OSAE—M/S Trauma	5, 6, 22, 25

Selected Bibliography

Histology of Bone

Azuma, H.: Intraosseous pressure as a measure of hemodynamic changes in bone marrow. Angiology 15:396–406, 1964.

Blair, W.F., Brown, T.D., and Greene, E.R.: Pulsed ultrasound doppler velocimetery in the assessment of microvascular hemodynamics. J. Orthop. Res. 6:300–309, 1988.

Branemark, P.: Experimental investigation of microcirculation in bone marrow. Angiology 12:293–306, 1961.

Bright, R.W., Burstein, A.H., and Elmore, S.M.: Epiphyseal-plate cartilage: A biomechanical and histological analysis of failure modes. J. Bone Joint Surg. 56A:688–703, 1974.

Brighton, C.T.: Clinical problems in epiphyseal plate growth and development. In American Academy of Orthopaedic Surgeons Instructional Course Lectures, XXIII, pp. 105–122. St. Louis, CV Mosby, 1974.

Brighton, C.T.: Structure and function of the growth plate. Clin. Orthop. 136:22–32, 1978.

Brinker, M.R., Lippton, H.L., Cook, S.D., et al.: Pharmacological regulation of the circulation of bone. J. Bone Joint Surg. [Am.] 72: 964–975, 1990.

Brookes, M.: The Blood Supply of Bone: An Approach to Bone Biology. London, Butterworth and Company, 1971.

Buckwalter, J. A.: Proteoglycan structure in calcifying cartilage. Clin. Orthop. 172:207–232, 1983.

Canalis, E.: Effect of growth factors on bone cell replication and differentiation. Clin. Orthop. 193:246–263, 1985.

Carter, D.R., Orr, T.E., Fyhrie, D.P., et al.: Influences of mechanical

stress on prenatal and postnatal skeletal development. Clin. Orthop. 219:237–250, 1987.
Cumming, J.D.: A study of blood flow through the bone marrow by a method of venous effluent collection. J. Physiol. (Lond.); 162: 13–20, 1962.
Driessens, M., and VanHoutte, P.M.: Vascular reactivity of the isolated tibia of the dog. Am. J. Physiol. 236:H904–H908, 1979.
Edholm, O.G., Howarth, S., and McMichael, J.: Heart failure and bone blood flow in osteitis deformans. Clin. Sci. 5:249–260, 1945.
Frymoyer, J.W., ed., Bone Metabolism and Metabolic Bone Disease. Orthopaedic Knowledge Update 4: Home Study Syllabus, p. 77. Rosemont, IL, American Academy of Orthopaedic Surgeons, 1993.
Guyton, A.C.: Local control of blood flow by tissues, and nervous and humoral regulation. In Textbook of Medical Physiology, 7th ed., pp. 230–243. Philadelphia, WB Saunders, 1986.
Heinegard, D., and Oldberg, A.: Structure and biology of cartilage and bone matrix noncollagenous macromolecules. FASEB J. 3: 2042–2051, 1989.
Houghton, G.R., and Rooker, G.D.: The role of the periosteum in the growth of long bones: An experimental study in the rabbit. J. Bone Joint Surg. 61B:218–220, 1979.
Iannotti, J.P.: Growth plate physiology and pathology. Orthop. Clin. North Am. 21:1–17, 1990.
Iannotti, J.P., Brighton, C.P., Iannotti, V., et al.: Mechanism of action of parathyroid hormone-induced proteoglycan synthesis in the growth plate chondrocyte. J. Orthop. Res. 8:136–145, 1990.
Iannotti, J.P., Goldstein, S., and Kuhn, J.: Growth plate and bone development. In Orthopaedic Basic Science, Simon, S.R., ed., pp. 185–217. Rosemont, IL, American Academy of Orthopaedic Surgeons, 1994.
Kaplan, F.S., Hayes, W.C., and Keaveny, T.M.: Form and function of bone. In Orthopaedic Basic Science, Simon, S.R., ed., pp. 127–184. Rosemont, IL, American Academy of Orthopaedic Surgeons, 1994.
Kelly, P.J., and Bronk, J.T.: Venous pressure and bone formation. Microvasc. Res. 39:364–375, 1990.
Kessler, S.B., Hallfeldt, K.K.J., Perren, S.M., et al.: The effects of reaming and intramedullary nailing on fracture healing. Clin. Orthop. 212:18–25, 1986.
Klein, M.P.M., Rahan, B.A., Frigg, R., et al.: Reaming versus non-reaming in medullary nailing: Interference with cortical circulation of the canine tibia. Arch. Orthop. Trauma Surg., 109:314–316, 1990.
Li, G., Bronk, J.T., and Kelly, P.J.: Canine bone blood flow estimated with microspheres. J. Orthop. Res. 7:61–67, 1989.
McPherson, A., Scales, J.T., and Gordon, L.H.: A method of estimating qualitative changes of blood-flow in bone. J. Bone Joint Surg. [Br.] 43:791–799, 1961.
Morris, M.A., Lopez-Curto, J.A., Hughes, S.P.F., et al.: Fluid spaces in canine bone and marrow. Microvasc. Res. 23:188–200, 1982.
Ogden, J.A.: Injury to the growth mechanisms of the immature skeleton. Skeleton Radiol. 6:237–253, 1981.
Ostrum, R.F., Chao, E.Y.S., Bassett, C.A.L., et al.: Bone injury, regeneration, and repair. In Simon SR (ed): Orthopaedic Basic Science, Simon, S.R., ed., pp. 277–323. Rosemont, IL, American Academy of Orthopaedic Surgeons, 1994.
Rhinelander, F.W.: Effects of medullary nailing on the normal blood supply of diaphyseal cortex. In American Academy of Orthopaedic Surgeons Instructional Course Lectures, XXII, pp. 161–187. St. Louis, CV Mosby, 1973.
Rhinelander, F.W.: Tibial blood supply in relation to fracture healing. Clin. Orthop. 105:34, 1974.
Rhinelander, F.W., Phillips, R.S., Steel, W.M., et al.: Microangiography in bone healing. II. Displaced closed fractures. J. Bone Joint Surg. [Am.] 50A:643–662, 1968.
Salter, R.B., and Harris, W.R.: Injuries involving the epiphyseal plate. J. Bone Joint Surg. 45A:587–622, 1968.
Shim, S.S.: Physiology of blood circulation. J. Bone Joint Surg. [Am.] 50A:812–824, 1968.
Shim, S.S., Copp, D.H., and Patterson, F.P.: An indirect method of bone blood-flow measurement based on the bone clearance of a circulating bone-seeking radioisotope. J. Bone Joint Surg. [Am.] 49:693–702, 1967.
Smith, S.R., Bronk, J.R., and Kelly, P.J.: Effect of fracture fixation on cortical bone blood flow. J. Orthop. Res. 8:471–478, 1990.
Stueker, R.D., Dunlap, J., Cook, S.D., et al.: Blood flow to the immature hip—the steal effect: A possible factor in the development of avascular necrosis in the treatment of congenital hip dislocation. Presented at the Annual Pediatric Orthopaedic Society of North America, Newport, RI, May 1992.
Swiontkowski, M.F.: Criteria for bone debridement in massive lower limb trauma. Clin. Orthop. 243:41–47, 1989.
Van Dyke, D., Anger, H.O., Yano, Y., et al.: Bone blood flow shown with F^{18} and the positron camera. Am. J. Physiol. 209:65–70, 1965.
White, N.B., Ter-Pogossian, M.M., and Stein, A.H.: A method to determine the rate of blood flow in long bone and selected soft tissues. Surg. Gynecol. Obstet. 119:535–540, 1964.
Whiteside, L.A., Lesker, P.A., and Simmons, D.J.: Measurement of regional bone and bone marrow blood flow in the rabbit using the hydrogen washout technique. Clin. Orthop. 122:340–346, 1977.
Wray, J.B.: Acute changes in femoral arterial blood flows after closed tibial fractures in dogs. J. Bone Joint Surg. [Am.] 46:1262–1268, 1964.

Bone Injury and Repair

Boskey, A.L.: Current concepts of the physiology and biochemistry of calcification. Clin. Orthop. 157:225–257, 1981.
Brighton, C.T.: Principles of fracture healing: Part I: The biology of fracture repair. In American Academy of Orthopaedic Surgeons Instructional Course Lectures XXXIII, Murray, J.A., ed., pp. 60–87. St. Louis, CV Mosby, 1984.
Canalis, E.: Effect of growth factors on bone cell replication and differentiation. Clin. Orthop. 193:246–263, 1985.
Chandler, H.P., and Pennenberg, B.L.: Bone Stock Deficiency in Total Hip Replacement. Thorofare, NJ, Slack, 1989.
Costantino, P.D., and Friedman, D.C.: Synthetic bone graft substitutes. Otolaryngol. Clin. North Am. 27:1037–1073, 1994.
Evans, F.G.: Mechanical Properties of Bone. Springfield, IL, Charles C Thomas, 1973.
Friedlaender, G.E.: Immune responses to osteochondral allografts: Current knowledge and future directions. Clin. Orthop. 174:58, 1983.
Friedlaender, G.E.: Bone grafts: The basic science rationale for clinical applications. J. Bone Joint Surg. [Am.] 69:786–790, 1987.
Friedlaender, G.E., ed.: Bone grafting. Orthop. Clin. North Am. (2), 1987.
Friedlaender, G.E., Mankin, H.J., and Sell, K.W., eds.: Osteochondral Allografts: Biology, Banking, and Clinical Applications. Boston, Little, Brown and Company, 1983.
Goldberg, V.M., and Stevenson, S.: Natural history of autografts and allografts. Clin. Orthop. 225:7–16, 1987.
Mankin, H.J., Doppelt, S.H., and Tomford, W.W.: Clinical experience with allograft implantation: The first ten years. Clin. Orthop. 174:69–86, 1983.
McKibbin, B.: The biology of fracture healing in long bones. J. Bone Joint Surg. [Br.] 60:150–162, 1978.
Ostrum, R.F., Chao, E.Y.S., Bassett, C.A.L., et al.: Bone injury, regeneration, and repair. In Orthopaedic Basic Science, Simon, S.R., ed., pp. 277–323. Rosemont, IL, American Academy of Orthopaedic Surgeons, 1994.
O'Sullivan, M.E., Chao, E.Y.S., and Kelly, P.J.: Current concepts review. The effects of fixation on fracture-healing. J. Bone Joint Surg. [Am.] 71:306, 1989.
Rhinelander, F.W.: Tibial blood supply in relation to fracture healing. Clin. Orthop. 105:34–81, 1974.
Springfield, D.S.: Massive autogenous bone grafts. Orthop. Clin. North Am. 18:249–256, 1987.
Stevenson, S., Dannucci, G.A., Sharkey, N.A., et al.: The fate of articular cartilage after transplantation of fresh and cryopreserved tissue-antigen-matched and mismatched osteochondral allografts in dogs. J. Bone Joint Surg. [Am.] 71:1297–1307, 1989.
Stevenson, S., Quing, L.X., and Martin, B.: The fate of cancellous and cortical bone after transplantation of fresh and frozen tissue-antigen-matched and mismatched osteochondral allografts in dogs. J. Bone Joint Surg. [Am.] 73:1143, 1991.

Conditions of Bone Mineralization, Bone Mineral Density, and Bone Viability

Aglietti, P., and Bullough, P.G.: Osteonecrosis. In Surgery of the Knee, Insall, J.N., ed., pp. 527–549. New York, Churchill Livingstone, 1984.

Aglietti, P., Insall, J.N., Buzzi, R., et al.: Idiopathic osteonecrosis of the knee: Aetiology, prognosis, and treatment. J. Bone Joint Surg. [Br.] 65:588–593, 1983.
Albright, J.A.: Management overview of osteogenesis imperfecta. Clin. Orthop. 159:80–87, 1981.
Alexander, A.H., and Lichtman, D.M.: Surgical treatment of transchondral talar dome fractures (osteochondritis dessicans). J. Bone Joint Surg. [Am.] 62A:646–652, 1980.
Arlet, J.: Non-traumatic avascular necrosis of the femoral head. In Recent Advances in Avascular Necrosis: Clinical Orthopaedics and Related Research, Ono, K., ed., pp. 12–21. Philadelphia, JB Lippincott, 1992.
Austin, L.A., and Heath, H., III: Calcitonin: Physiology and pathophysiology. N. Engl. J. Med. 304:269–278, 1981.
Barth, R.W., and Lane, J.M.: Osteoporosis. Orthop. Clin. North Am. 19:845–858, 1988.
Boden, S.D., and Kaplan, F.S.: Calcium homeostasis. Orthop. Clin. North Am., 21:31–42, 1990.
Boyer, D.W., Mickelson, M.R., and Ponseti, I.V.: Slipped capital femoral epiphysis: Long term follow-up and study of 121 patients. J. Bone Joint Surg. [Am.] 63:85, 1981.
Brinker, M.R., Rosenberg, A.G., Kull, L., et al.: Primary total hip arthroplasty using noncemented porous-coated femoral components in patients with osteonecrosis of the femoral head. J. Arthroplasty 9:457–468, 1994.
Buckwalter, J.A., and Cruess, R.L.: Healing of the musculoskeletal tissues. In Rockwood, C.A., Jr., and Green, D.P. Fractures in Adults. pp. 181–264. Philadelphia, JB Lippincott, 1991.
Bullough, P.G., Bansal, M., and DiCarlo, E.F.: The tissue diagnosis of metabolic bone disease: Role of histomorphometry. Orthop. Clin. North Am. 21:65–79, 1990.
Canale, S.T.: Fractures of the hip in children and adolescents. Orthop. Clin. North Am. 21:341–352, 1990.
Canale, S.T., and King, R.E.: Part II: Fractures of the hip. In Fractures in Children, vol. 3, Rockwood, C.A., Jr., Wilkins, K.E., and King, R.E., eds., pp. 1046–1120. Philadelphia, JB Lippincott, 1991.
Casey, R.H., Hamilton, H.W., and Bobechko, W.P.: Reduction of acutely slipped upper femoral epiphysis. J. Bone Joint Surg. [Br.] 54:607, 1972.
Chesney, R.W.: Current clinical applications of vitamin D metabolite research. Clin. Orthop. 161:285–314, 1981.
Cofield, R.H.: Degenerative and arthritic problems of the glenohumeral joint. In The Shoulder, vol. 2, Rockwood, C.A. Jr., and Matsen, F.A., III, eds, p. 697. Philadelphia, WB Saunders, 1990.
Davison, B.L., and Weinstein, S.L.: Hip fractures in children: A long-term follow-up study. J. Pediatr. Orthop. 12:355–358, 1992.
Ficat, R.P.: Idiopathic bone necrosis for the femoral head: Early diagnosis and treatment. J. Bone Joint Surg. [Br.] 67:3–9, 1985.
Ficat, R.P., and Arlet, J.: Ischemia and Necroses of Bone. Baltimore, Williams & Wilkins, 1980.
Fitzgerald, R.H., Jr., ed.: Ankle and foot: Trauma. In Orthopaedic Knowledge Update 2: Home Study Syllabus, pp. 447–454. Park Ridge, IL, American Academy of Orthopaedic Surgeons, 1987.
Frymoyer, J.W., ed.: Bone Metabolism and Metabolic Bone Disease. In Orthopaedic Knowledge Update 4: Home Study Syllabus, p. 77. Rosemont, IL, American Academy of Orthopaedic Surgeons, 1993.
Frymoyer JW (ed): Congenital abnormalities. In Orthopaedic Knowledge Update 4: Home Study Syllabus, pp. 127–128. Rosemont, IL, American Academy of Orthopaedic Surgeons, 1993.
Glimcher, M.J., and Kenzora, J.E.: The biology of osteonecrosis of the human femoral head and its clinical implications: I. Tissue biology. II. The pathological changes in the femoral head as an organ and in the hip joint. III. Discussion of the etiology and genesis of the pathological sequelae; Comments on treatment. Clin. Orthop. 138:284–309; 139:283–312; 140:273–312, 1979.
Greech, P., Martin, T.J., Barrington, N.A., and Ell, P.J.: Diagnosis of Metabolic Bone Disease. Philadelphia, WB Saunders, 1985.
Hagglund, G., Hanson, L.I., and Sandstrom, S.: Slipped capital femoral epiphysis in southern Sweden. Clin. Orthop. 217:190, 1987.
Hall, J.E.: The results of treatment of slipped femoral epiphysis. J. Bone Joint Surg. [Br.] 39:659, 1957.
Hansen, S.T., Jr.: Foot injuries. In Skeletal Trauma, vol. 2, Browner, B.D., Jupiter, J.B., Levine, A.M., et al., eds., pp. 1960–1965. Philadelphia, WB Saunders, 1992.
Heckman, J.D.: Fractures and dislocations of the foot. In Fractures in Adults, vol. 2, Rockwood, C.A., Green, D.P., and Bucholz, R.W., eds., p. 2100. Philadelphia, JB Lippincott, 1991.
Hungerford, D.S., ed.: Avascular necrosis of the femoral head. Hip 11:247–330, 1983.
Kanis, J.A.: Vitamin D metabolism and its clinical application. J. Bone Joint Surg. [Br.] 64:542–560, 1982.
Kaplan, F.S., Hayes, W.C., and Keaveny, T.M.: Form and function of bone. In Orthopaedic Basic Science, Simon, S.R., ed., pp 127–184. Rosemont, IL, American Academy of Orthopaedic Surgeons, 1994.
Kleerekoper, M.B., Tolia, K., and Parfitt, A.M.: Nutritional endocrine, and demographic aspects of osteoporosis. Orthop. Clin. North Am. 12:547–558, 1981.
Koshino, T.: The treatment of spontaneous osteonecrosis by high tibial osteotomy with and without bone grafting or drilling of the lesion. J. Bone Joint Surg. [Am.] 64:47–58, 1982.
Lane, J.M., Healey, J.H., Schwartz, E., et al.: Treatment of osteoporosis with sodium fluoride and calcium: Effects on vertebral fracture incidence and bone histomorphometry. Orthop. Clin. North Am. 15:729–745, 1984.
Lane, J.M., and Vigorita, V.J.: Osteoporosis. J. Bone Joint Surg. [Am.] 65:274–278, 1983.
Leventen, E.O.: The chevron procedure. Orthopaedics 13:973–976, 1990.
Lotke, P., Abend, J., and Ecker, M.: The treatment of osteonecrosis of the medial femoral condyle. Clin. Orthop. 171:109–116, 1982.
Lotke, P., and Ecker, M.: Current concepts review: osteonecrosis of the knee. J. Bone Joint Surg. [Am.] 70:470–473, 1988.
Mankin, H.J.: Rickets, osteomalacia, and renal osteodystrophy: An update. Orthop. Clin. North Am. 21:81–96, 1990.
Mann, R.A., and Coughlin, M.J.: Keratotic disorders of the plantar skin. In Surgery of the Foot and Ankle, 6th ed., vol. 1, Mann, R.A., and Coughlin, M.J., eds., p. 435. St. Louis, CV Mosby, 1993.
Mayo, K.A.: Fractures of the talus: Principles of management and techniques of treatment. Techniques Orthop 2:42–54, 1987.
Meier, P.J., and Kenzora, J.E.: The risks and benefits of distal foot metatarsal osteotomies. Foot Ankle 6:7–17, 1985.
Morrissy, R.T.: Slipped capital femoral epiphysis. In Lovell and Winter's Pediatric Orthopaedics, 3rd ed., vol. 2, Morrissy, R.T., ed., pp. 885–904. Philadelphia, JB Lippincott, 1990.
Morrissy, R.T., and Wilkins, K.E.: Deformity following distal humeral fracture in childhood. J. Bone Joint Surg. [Am.] 66:557–562, 1984.
Nordin, B.E.C., Horsman, A., Marshall, D.H., et al.: Calcium requirement and calcium therapy. Clin. Orthop. 140:216–239, 1979.
Ostrum, R.F., Chao, E.Y.S., Bassett, C.A.L., et al.: Bone injury, regeneration, and repair. In Orthopaedic Basic Science, Simon, S.R., ed., pp. 277–323. Rosemont, IL, American Academy of Orthopaedic Surgeons, 1994.
Prockop, D.J.: Mutations in collagen genes: Consequences for rare and common diseases. J. Clin. Invest. 75:783–787, 1985.
Sillence, D.: Osteogenesis imperfecta: An expanding panorama of variants. Clin. Orthop. 159:11–25, 1981.
Syszkowitz, R., Reschauer, R., and Seggl, W.: Eighty-five talus fractures treated by ORIF with five to eight years of follow-up study of 69 patients. Clin. Orthop. 199:97–107, 1985.
Tooke, S.M., Nugent, P.J., Bassett, L.W., et al.: Results of core decompression for femoral head osteonecrosis. Clin. Orthop. 228: 99–104, 1998.
Wallach, S.: Hormonal factors in osteoporosis. Clin. Orthop. 144: 284–292, 1979.
Wilkins, K.E.: Fractures and dislocations of the elbow region: Fractures of the distal humerus. In Fractures in Children, vol. 3, Rockwood, C.A., Wilkins, K.E., and King, R.E., eds., pp. 476–480. Philadelphia, JB Lippincott, 1984.

Articular Tissues

Anderson, P.A., Rivara, F.P., Maier, R.V., et al.: The epidemiology of seatbelt-associated injuries. J. Trauma 31:60–67, 1991.
Armstrong, C.P., Vander Spuy, J.: The fractured scapula: Importance and management based on a series of 62 patients. Injury 15: 324–329, 1984.
Arnoczky, S., Adams, M., DeHaven, K., et al.: Meniscus. In Injury and Repair of the Musculoskeletal Soft Tissues, Woo, S.L-Y., and

Buckwalter, J.A., eds., pp. 487–537. Park Ridge, IL, American Academy of Orthopaedic Surgeons, 1988.
Arnoczky, S.P., and Warren, R.F.: Miocrovasculature of the human meniscus. Am. J. Sports Med. 10:90–95, 1982.
Arnoczky, S.P., Warren, R.F., and McDevitt, C.A.: Meniscal replacement using a cryopreserved allograft: An experimental study in the dog. Clin. Orthop. 252:121–128, 1990.
Baker, J., Deitch, E., Berg, R., et al.: Hemorrhagic shock induces bacterial translocation from the gut. J. Trauma 28:896–905, 1988.
Barnes, R.W., Shankik, G.D., and Slaymaker, E.E.: An index of healing in below-knee amputation: Leg blood pressure by Doppler ultrasound. Surgery 79:13–20, 1976.
Bone, L., and Bucholz, R.: The management of fractures in the patient with multiple trauma. J. Bone Joint Surg. [Am.] 68:945–949, 1986.
Bone, L., Johnson, K., Weigelt, J., et al.: Prospective randomized study of femoral fractures: Early vs. delayed stabilization. J. Bone Joint Surg. [Am.] 70:3365–340, 1989.
Bone, L.B.: Emergency treatment of the injured patient. In Skeletal Trauma: Fractures, Dislocations and Ligamentous Injuries, Browner, B.D., Jupiter, J.B., Levine, A.M., et al., eds., p. 138. Philadelphia, WB Saunders, 1992.
Bostman, O., Hrykas, J., Hirvensalo, E., et al.: Blood loss, operating time and positioning of the patient in lumbar disc surgery. Spine 15:350, 1990.
Buckwalter, J.A., and Hunziker, E.B.: Articular cartilage biology and morphology. In Structure and Function of Articular Cartilage, Mow, V.C., and Ratcliffe, A., eds. Boca Raton, FL, CRC Press, 1993.
Buckwalter, J.A., Kuettner, K.E., and Thonar, E.J.: Age-related changes in articular cartilage proteoglycans: Electron microscopic studies. J. Orthop. Res. 3:251–257, 1985.
Cannon, W.D., and Morgan, C.D.: Meniscal repair. Part II. Arthroscopic repair techniques. J. Bone Joint Surg. [Am.] 76:294–311, 1994.
Colapinto, V.: Trauma to the pelvis: Urethral injury. Clin. Orthop. 151:46–55, 1980.
Collicott, P.: Initial assessment of the trauma patient. In Trauma Mattox, K., Moore, E., Feliciano, D., et al., eds., p. 115. Norwalk, CT, Appleton & Lange, 1988.
Cowley, R.A., and Dunham, C.M., eds.: Initial evaluation and management of the trauma patient. In Shock Trauma/Critical Care Manual: Initial Assessment and Management, p. 30. Baltimore, University Park Press, 1982.
DeHaven, K.E., and Arnoczky, S.P.: Meniscal repair. Part I. Basic science, indications for repair and open repair. J. Bone Joint Surg. [Am.] 76:140–152, 1995.
Duis, J.H., Nijsten, M.W.N., Kalausen, H.J., et al.: Fat embolism in patients with an isolated fracture of the femoral shaft. J. Trauma 28:383–390, 1988.
Eie, N., Solgaard, T., and Kleppe, H.: The knee-elbow position in lumbar disc surgery: A review of complications. Spine 8:897–900, 1983.
Fitzgerald, R.H., Jr., ed.: Trauma: Pelvis and acetabulum. In Orthopaedic Knowledge Update 2: Home Study Syllabus, p. 342. Park Ridge, IL, American Academy of Orthopaedic Surgeons, 1987.
Front, P., Aprile, F., Mitrovic, D.R., et al.: Age-related changes in the synthesis of matrix macromolecules by bovine articular cartilage. Connect. Tissue. Res. 19:121–133, 1989.
Frymoyer, J.W., ed.: Multiple trauma: Pathophysiology and management. In Orthopaedic Knowledge Update 4: Home Study Syllabus, pp. 141–153. Rosemont, IL, American Academy of Orthopaedic Surgeons, 1993.
Gleis, G.E., and Seligson, D.: Diagnosis and treatment of complications. In Skeletal Trauma: Fractures, Dislocations and Ligamentous Injuries, vol. 1., Browner, B.D., Jupiter, J.B.V., Levine, A.M., et al., eds., p. 444. Philadelphia, WB Saunders, 1992.
Grood, E.S.: Meniscal function. Adv. Orthop. Surg. 7:193–197, 1984.
Guthrie, D., ed.: Initial assessment and management. In Advanced Trauma Life Support Course, p. 5. Chicago, American College of Surgeons, 1989.
Guthrie, D., ed.: Shock. In Advanced Trauma Life Support Course, pp. 53–54, chap. 3. Chicago, American College of Surgeons, 1989.
Guthrie, D., ed.: Thoracic trauma. In Advanced Trauma Life Support Course, pp. 75, 79. Chicago, American College of Surgeons, 1989.
Guthrie, D., ed.: Upper airway management. In Advanced Trauma Life Support Course, p. 26. Chicago, American College of Surgeons, 1989.
Hardingham, T.E.: The role of link-protein in the structure of cartilage proteoglycan aggregates. Biochem. J. 177:237–247, 1979.
Hardingham, T.E., and Fosang, A.J.: Proteoglycans: Many forms and many functions. FASEB J. 6:861–870, 1992.
Heinegard, D., and Oldberg, A.: Structure and biology of cartilage and bone matrix noncollagenous macromolecules. FASEB J. 3: 2042–2051, 1989.
Iannotti, J.P., Goldstein, S., Kuhn, J.L., et al.: Growth plate and bone development. In Orthopaedic Basic Science, Simon, S.R., ed., pp. 185–217. Rosemont, IL, American Academy of Orthopaedic Surgeons, 1994.
Johnson, K.D., Cadambi, A., and Seibert, G.B.: Incidence of adult respiratory distress syndrome in patients with multiple musculoskeletal injuries: Effect of early operative stabilization of fractures. J. Trauma 24:375–384, 1985.
Mankin, H.J.: Current concepts review: The response of articular cartilage to mechanical injury. J. Bone Joint Surg. 64A:460–466, 1982.
Mankin, H.J., and Brandt, K.D.: Biochemistry and metabolism of articular cartilage in osteoarthritis. In Osteoarthritis: Diagnosis and Medical/Surgical Management, ed. 2, Moskowitz, R.W., Howell, D.S., Goldberg, V.M., et al., eds., pp. 109–154. Philadelphia, WB Saunders, 1992.
Mankin, H.J., Mow, V.C., Buckwalter, J.A., et al.: Form and function of articular cartilage. In Orthopaedic Basic Science, Simon, S.R., ed., pp. 1–44. Rosemont, IL, American Academy of Orthopaedic Surgeons, 1994.
Mankin, H.J., and Thrasher, A.Z.: Water content and binding in normal and osteoarthritic human cartilage. J. Bone Joint Surg. 57A: 76–80, 1975.
Mayne, R., and Irwin, M.H.: Collagen types in cartilage. In Articular Cartilage Biochemistry, Kuettner, K.E., Schleyerbach, R., and Hascall, V.C., eds., pp. 23–38. New York. Raven Press, 1986.
Mow, V.C., Flatow, E.L., and Foster, R.J.: Biomechanics. In Orthopaedic Basic Science, Simon, S.R., ed., pp. 397–446. Rosemont, IL, American Academy of Orthopaedic Surgeons, 1994.
Mow, V.C., Zhu, W., and Ratcliffe, A.: Structure and function of articular cartilage and meniscus. In Basic Orthopaedic Biomechanics, Mow, V.C., and Hayes, W.C., eds., pp. 143–198. New York, Raven Press, 1991.
Oreck, S.L., Burgess, A., and Levine, A.M.: Traumatic lateral displacement of the scapula: A radiographic sign of neurovascular disruption. J. Bone Joint Surg. [Am.] 66:758–763, 1984.
Osborn, K.D., Trippel, S.B., and Mankin, H.J.: Growth factor stimulation of adult articular cartilage. J. Orthop. Res. 7:35–42, 1989.
Peltier, L.F.: Fat embolism: A perspective. Clin. Orthop. 232: 263–270, 1988.
Poss, R., ed.: Polytrauma. In Orthopaedic Knowledge Update 3: Home Study Syllabus, pp. 81–91. Park Ridge, IL, American Academy of Orthopaedic Surgeons, 1990.
Rosenberg, L.C., and Buckwalter, J.A.: Cartilage proteoglycans. In Articular Cartilage Biochemistry, Kuettner, K.E., Schleyerbach, R., and Hascall, V.C., eds., pp. 39–58. New York, Raven Press, 1986.
Salter, R.B., Minster, R.R., Clements, N., et al.: Continuous passive motion and the repair of full thickness articular cartilage defects: A one-year follow-up. Orthop. Trans. 6:266–267, 1982.
Salter, R.B., Simmonds, D.F., Malcolm, B.W., et al.: The biological effect of continuous passive motion on the healing of full-thickness defects in articular cartilage: An experimental investigation in the rabbit. J. Bone Joint Surg. 62A:1232–1251, 1980.
Schenk, R.K., Eggli, P.S., and Hunziker, E.B.: Articular cartilage morphology. In Articular Cartilage Biochemistry, Kuettner, K.E., Schleyerbach, R., Hascall, V.C., eds., pp. 3–22. New York, Raven Press, 1986.
Skalak, R., and Chien, S.: Handbook of Bioengineering. New York, McGraw-Hill, 1987.
van der Rest, M., and Garrone, R.: Collagen family of proteins. FASEB J. 5:2814–2823, 1991.
Wagner, F.W., Jr.: The diabetic foot and amputations of the foot. In Surgery of the Foot, 5th ed., Mann, R.A., ed., pp. 421–455. St. Louis, CV Mosby, 1986.

Webber, R.J., York, L., Vander Schilden, J.L., et al.: An organ culture model for assaying wound repair of the fibrocartilaginous knee joint meniscus. Am. J. Sports Med. 17:393, 1989.

Weiss, C., and Parisien, J.S.: Basic Structure of Diarthrodial Joints in Arthroscopic Surgery, p. 3. New York, McGraw-Hill, 1988.

Weiss, C., Rosenberg, L., and Helfet, A.J.: An ultrastructural study of normal young adult human articular cartilage. J. Bone Joint Surg. [Am.] 50:663–674, 1968.

Woo, S.L., An, K., Arnoczky, S.P., et al.: Anatomy, biology, and biomechanics of tendon, ligament and meniscus. In Simon SR (ed): Orthopaedic Basic Science, Simon, S.R., ed., pp. 45–88. Rosemont, IL, American Academy of Orthopaedic Surgeons, 1994.

Woo, S.L.-Y., and Buckwalter, J.A., eds. Injury and Repair of the Musculoskeletal Soft Tissues. Park Ridge, IL. American Academy of Orthopaedic Surgeons, 1988.

Arthroses

Ahlberg, A.K.M.: On the natural history of hemophilic pseudotumor. J. Bone Joint Surg. [Am.] 57:1133–1136, 1975.

Ansell, B.M., and Swann, M.: The management of chronic arthritis of children. J. Bone Joint Surg. [Br.] 65:536–543, 1983.

Barry, P.E., and Stillman, J.S.: Characteristics of juvenile rheumatoid arthritis: Its medical and orthopaedic management. Orthop. Clin. North Am. 6:641–651, 1975.

Berquist, T.A.: Radiology of the Foot and Ankle, pp. 223–228. New York, Raven Press, 1989.

Brinker, M.R., Rosenberg, A.G., Kull, L., et al.: Primary noncemented total hip arthroplasty in patients with ankylosing spondylitis: A clinical and radiographic review at five years average follow-up. J. Arthroplasty, In press.

Buchanan, W.W.: Clinical features of rheumatoid arthritis. In Copeman's Textbook of the Rheumatoid Diseases, 5th ed., Scott, J.T., ed., pp. 318–364. Edinburgh, Churchill Livingstone, 1978.

Byers, P.D., Cotton, R.E., Decon, O.W., et al.: The diagnosis and treatment of pigmented villonodular synovitis. J. Bone Joint Surg. [Br.]; 50:290–305, 1968.

Calamia, K.T., and Hunder, G.G.: Clinical manifestations of giant cell arteritis. Clin. Rheum. Dis. 6:389–403, 1980.

Calin, A.: Ankylosing spondylitis. In Textbook of Rheumatology, Kelley, W.N., Harris, E.D., Ruddy, S., et al., eds., pp. 1021–1037. Philadelphia, WB Saunders, 1989.

Chand, Y., and Johnson, K.: Foot and ankle manifestations of Reiter's syndrome. Foot Ankle 1:167, 1980.

Chylack, L.T., Jr.: The ocular manifestations of juvenile rheumatoid arthritis. Arthritis Rheum. 20:217–223, 1977.

Clohisy, D.R., and Thompson, R.C.: Fractures associated with neuropathic arthroplasty in adults who have juvenile diabetes. J. Bone Joint Surg. [Am.] 70A:1192, 1988.

Cofield, R.H., Morrison, M.J., and Beabout, J.W.: Diabetic neuroarthropathy in the foot: Patient characteristics and patterns of radiographic change. Foot Ankle 4:15–22, 1983.

Culp, R.W., Eichenfield, A.H., Davidson, R.S., et al.: Lyme arthritis in children: An orthopaedic perspective. J. Bone Joint Surg. [Am.] 69:96–99, 1987.

Currey, H.L.F.: Aetiology and pathogenesis of rheumatoid arthritis. In Copeman's Textbook of the Rheumatoid Diseases, 5th ed., Scott, J.T., eds., pp. 261–272. Edinburgh, Churchill Livingstone, 1978.

De Lange, E.E., and Keats, T.E.: Localized chondrocalcinosis in traumatized joints. Skeletal Radiol. 14:249–256, 1985.

Firooznia, H., Seliger, G., Genieser, N.B., et al.: Hypertrophic pulmonary osteoarthropathy in pulmonary metastases. Radiology 115: 269–274, 1975.

Fisseler-Eckhoff, A., and Muller, K.M.: Arthroscopy and chondrocalcinosis. Arthroscopy 8:98–104, 1992.

Ford, D.: The clinical spectrum of Reiter's syndrome and similar postenteric arthropathies. Clin. Orthop. 143:59–65, 1979.

Fredrickson, B., and Yuan, H.: Nonoperative treatment of the spine: External immobilization. In Skeletal Trauma: Fractures, Dislocations and Ligamentous Injuries, Browner, B.D., Jupiter, J.B., Levine, A.M., et al., eds., p. 639. Philadelphia, WB Saunders, 1992.

Frymoyer, J.W., ed.: Arthritis. In Orthopaedic Knowledge Update 4: Home Study Syllabus, pp. 89–106. Rosemont, IL, American Academy of Orthopaedic Surgeons, 1993.

Gardner, D.L.: Pathology of rheumatoid arthritis. In Copeman's Textbook of the Rheumatoid Diseases, 5th ed., Scott, J.T., ed., pp. 273–317. Edinburgh, Churchill Livingstone, 1978.

Harrelson, J.: Tumors of the foot. In Disorders of the Foot and Ankle, Jahss, M.H., ed., p. 1674. Philadelphia, WB Saunders, 1991.

Heckman, J.D.: Fractures and dislocations of the foot. In Fractures in Adults, 3rd ed., vol. 1, Rockwood, C.A., Jr., Green, D.P., Bucholz, R.W., eds., pp. 2061–2064. Philadelphia, JB Lippincott, 1991.

Hockberg, M.C.: Epidemiology of rheumatoid disease. In Primer on the Rheumatic Disease, 9th ed., Schumacher, H.R., Jr., ed., pp. 48–51. Atlanta, Arthritis Foundation, 1988.

Jacobs, R.L.: Charcot foot. In Disorders of the Foot and Ankle, 2nd ed., vol. 3, Jahss, M.H., ed., p. 2164. Philadelphia, WB Saunders, 1991.

Jaffe, H.L.: Metabolic, Degenerative and Inflammatory Diseases of Bones and Joints, pp. 847–866. Philadelphia, Lea & Febiger, 1972.

Kelley, W.N., and Fox, I.H.: Gout and related disorders of purine metabolism. In Textbook of Rheumatology, 2nd ed., Kelley, W.N., Harris, E.D., Jr., Ruddy, S., et al., eds., p. 1382. Philadelphia, WB Saunders, 1985.

Leventen, E.O.: Charcot foot: A technique for treatment of chronic plantar ulcer by saucerization and primary closure. Foot Ankle 6:295–299, 1985.

Mankin, H.J., and Brandt, K.D.: Biochemistry and metabolism of articular cartilage in osteoarthritis. In Osteoarthritis: Diagnosis and Medical/Surgical Management, ed 2, Moskowitz, R.W., Howell, V.C., Goldberg, V.M., et al., eds., pp. 109–154. Philadelphia, WB Saunders, 1992.

Mankin, H.J., Dorfman, H., Lippiello, L., et al.: Biochemical and metabolic abnormalities in articular cartilage from osteo-arthritic human hips: II. Correlation of morphology with biochemical and metabolic data. J. Bone Joint Surg. 53A:523–537, 1971.

Mankin, H.J., Johnson, M.E., and Lippiello, L.: Biochemical and metabolic abnormalities in articular cartilage from osteoarthritic human hips: III. Distribution and metabolism of amino sugar-containing macromolecules. J. Bone Joint Surg. 63A:131–139, 1981.

Mankin, H.J., Mow, V.C., Buckwalter, J.A., et al.: Form and function of articular cartilage. In Orthopaedic Basic Science, Simm, S.R., ed., pp. 1–44. Rosemont, IL, American Academy of Orthopaedic Surgeons, 1994.

Mankin, H.J., and Thrasher, A.Z.: Water content and binding in normal and osteoarthritic human cartilage. J. Bone Joint Surg. 57A: 76–80, 1975.

Masuda, I., Ishikawa, K.: Clinical features of pseudogout attack, a survey of 50 cases. Clin. Orthop. 229:173–181, 1988.

Pearlman, S.G., and Barth, W.F.: Psoriatic arthritis: Diagnosis and management. Compr. Ther. 5:60–66, 1979.

Poss, R., ed.: Arthritis. In Orthopaedic Knowledge Update 3: Home Study Syllabus, p. 63. Park Ridge, IL, American Academy of Orthopaedic Surgeons, 1990.

Poss, R., Thornhill, T., Ewald, F., et al.: Factors influencing the incidence and outcome of infection following total joint arthroplasty. Clin. Orthop. 182:117–126, 1984.

Postel, M., and Kerboull, M.: Total prosthetic replacement in rapidly destructive arthrosis of the hip joint. Clin. Orthop. 72:138–144, 1970.

Rana, N.: Rheumatoid arthritis, other collagen diseases, and psoriasis of the foot. In Disorders of the Foot, ed 1, Jahss, M.H., ed., pp. 1057–1058. Philadelphia, WB Saunders, 1982.

Rana, N.A.: Rheumatoid arthritis, other collagen diseases, and psoriasis of the foot. In Disorders of the Foot and Ankle, 2nd ed., Jahss, M.H., ed., p. 1745. Philadelphia, WB Saunders, 1991.

Resnick, D.: Radiology of seronegative spondyloarthropathies. Clin. Orthop. 143:38–45, 1979.

Rhoades, C.E., Neff, J.R., Rengachary, S.S., et al.: Diagnosis of the post-traumatic syringohydromyelia presenting as neuropathic joints: Report of two cases and review of the literature. Clin. Orthop. 180:182–187, 1993.

Richards, R.R., and Delaney, J.: Syringomyelia presenting as shoulder instability. J. Shoulder Elbow Surg. 1:155–161, 1992.

Rodnan, G.P., and Schumacher, H.R., eds.: Primer on the Rheumatic Disease, 8th ed., pp. 128–131. Atlanta, Arthritis Foundation, 1983.

Romness, D.W., and Rand, J.A.: The role of continuous passive motion following total knee arthroplasty. Clin. Orthop. 226:34–37, 1988.

Rosenberg, Z.S., Shankman, S., Steiner, G.C., et al.: Rapid destructive osteoarthritis: Clinical, radiographic, and pathologic features. Radiology 182:213–216, 1993.

Roth, S.: Nonsteroidal anti-inflammatory drugs: Gastropathy, deaths, and medical practice. Ann. Intern. Med. 109:353–354, 1988.

Ryan, L.M., and McCarty, D.J.: Calcium pyrophosphate crystal deposition disease; pseudogout; articular chondrocalcinosis. In Arthritis and Allied Conditions, 12th ed., vol. 2, McCarty, D.J., and Koopmen, W.J., eds., pp. 1835–1855. Philadelphia, Lea & Febiger, 1993.

Salvati, E., Robinson, R., Zeno, S., et al.: Infection rates after 2,175 total hip and total knee replacements performed with and without a horizontal unidirectional filtered airflow system. J. Bone Joint Surg. [Am.] 64:525–535, 1982.

Sammarco, G.J.: Diabetic arthropathy. In The Foot in Diabetes, Sammarco, G.J., ed., pp. 153–172. Philadelphia, Lea & Febiger, 1991.

Schumacher, R.H., ed.: Primer of Rheumatic Disease, 9th ed., p. 149. Atlanta, Arthritis Foundation, 1988.

Schumacher, H.R., Jr.: Pathology of crystal deposition diseases. Rheum. Dis. Clin. North Am. 14:269–288, 1988.

Shaller, J.G.: Chronic arthritis in children: Juvenile rheumatoid arthritis. Clin. Orthop. 182:79–89, 1984.

Simmon, E.H.: The surgical correction of flexion deformity of the cervical spine in ankylosing spondylitis. Clin. Orthop. 86: 132–143, 1972.

Smith, J.H., and Pugh, D.G.: Roentgenographic aspects of articular pigmented villonodular synovitis. A.J.R. Am. J. Roentgenol. 87: 1146–1156, 1962.

Smukler, N.: Arthritic disorders of the spine. In The Spine, 2nd ed., Rothman, R.H., and Simeone, F.A., eds., pp. 906–941. Philadelphia, WB Saunders, 1982.

Springfield, D.S., Bolander, M.E., Friedlaender, G.E., et al.: Molecular and cellular biology of inflammation and neoplasia. In Orthopaedic Basic Science, Simon, S.R., ed., pp. 219–276. Rosemont, IL, American Academy of Orthopaedic Surgeons, 1994.

Thompson, F.M., and Mann, R.A.: Arthritides. In Surgery of the Foot, ed 5, Mann, R.A., ed., pp. 158–179. St. Louis, CV Mosby, 1986.

Thompson, F.M., and Mann, R.A.: Arthritides. In Surgery of the Foot and Ankle, 6th ed., vol. 1., Mann, R.A., and Coughlin, M.J., eds., p. 618. St. Louis, CV Mosby, 1993.

Wade, J.P., and Liang, M.H.: Avoiding common pitfalls in the diagnosis of gout. J. Musculoskel. Med. 6:16–24, 1988.

Wagner, F.W.: The diabetic foot and amputations of the foot. In Surgery of the Foot, ed 5, Mann, R.A., ed., pp. 421–455. St. Louis, CV Mosby, 1986.

Williams, B.: Orthopaedic features in the presentation of syringomyelia. J. Bone Joint Surg. [Br.] 61:314–323, 1979.

Wilson, M.G., Kelley, K., and Thornhill, T.S.: Infection as a complication of total knee replacement arthroplasty: Risk factors and treatment in sixty-seven cases. J. Bone Joint Surg. [Am.]; 72: 878–883, 1990.

Wood, G.W.: Other disorders of the spine. In Campbell's Operative Orthopaedics, 7th ed., vol. 4, Crenshaw, A.H., ed., p. 3363. St. Louis, CV Mosby, 1987.

Wright, V.: Psoriatic arthritis: A comparative radiographic study of rheumatoid arthritis and arthritis associated with psoriasis. Ann. Rheum. Dis. 20:123–132, 1961.

Yuh, W.T., and Corson, J.D.: Osteomyelitis of the foot in diabetic patients: Evaluation with plain film, ^{99m}Tc-MDP bone scintigraphy and MR imaging. A.J.R. Am. J. Roentgenol. 152:795–800, 1989.

Zvaifler, N.J.: Etiology and pathogenesis of rheumatoid arthritis. In Arthritis and Allied Conditions: A Textbook of Rheumatology, ed 10, McCarty, D.J., ed., pp. 557–570. Philadelphia, Lea & Febiger, 1985.

Skeletal Muscle and Athletics

AMA Council on Scientific Affairs. Drug abuse in athletes: Anabolic steroids and human growth hormone. J.A.M.A. 259:1703–1705, 1988.

American Academy of Orthopaedic Surgeons Position Statement: Anabolic Steroids to Enhance Athletic Performance. Park Ridge, IL, American Academy of Orthopaedic Surgeons, 1991.

American College of Sports Medicine position on the use of anabolic-androgenic steroids in sports. Med Sci Sports Exerc 19: 534–539, 1987.

American College of Sports Medicine position stand on weight loss in wrestlers. Med Sci Sports Exerc 8:xi–xiii, 1976.

American College of Sports Medicine position stand: The recommended quantity and quality of exercise for developing and maintaining cardiorespiratory and muscular fitness in healthy adults: The official position papers of the American College of Sports Medicine. Med Sci Sports Exerc 22:265–274, 1990.

Amsterdam, E.A., Laslett, L., and Holly, R.: Exercise and sudden death. Clin. Cardiol. 5:337–343, 1987.

Andersson, G.B.J.: Methods and applications of functional muscle testing. In Clinical Efficacy and Outcome in the Diagnosis and Treatment of Low Back Pain, Weinsten, J.N., ed., New York, Raven Press, 1992.

Asher, M.A., ed.: Health maintenance of the musculoskeletal system. In Orthopaedic Knowledge Update I: Home Study Syllabus, pp. 1–8. Park Ridge, IL, American Academy of Orthopaedic Surgeons, 1984.

Baldwin, K.M., Winder, W.W., and Holloszy, J.O.: Adaptation of actomyosin ATPase in different types of muscle to endurance exercise. Am. J. Physiol. 229:422–426, 1975.

Berquist, D.: Abdominal injury from sporting activities. Br. J. Sports Med. 16:76–79, 1982.

Best, T.M., and Garret, W.E.: Basic science of soft tissue: Muscle and tendon. In Orthopaedic Sports Medicine: Principles and Practice, vol. 1, DeLee, J., and Drez, D., eds., p. 17. Philadelphia, WB Saunders, 1994.

Bodine, S.C., and Lieber, R.L.: Peripheral nerve physiology, anatomy, and pathology. In Orthopaedic Basic Science, Simon, S.R., ed., pp. 325–396. Rosemont, IL, American Academy of Orthopaedic Surgeons, 1994.

Booth, F.W.: Physiologic and biochemical effects of immobilization on muscle. Clin. Orthop. 219:15–20, 1987.

Booth, F.W.: Physiologic and biochemical effects in immobilization of muscle. Clin. Orthop. 219:25–27, 1987.

Brower, K.J.: Anabolic steroids. Psychiatr. Clin. North Am. 16: 97–103, 1993.

DeLee, J.C.: Tissue remodeling and response to therapeutic exercise. In Sports-Induced Inflammation, Leadbetter, W.B., Buckwalter, J.A., and Gordon, S.L., eds., pp. 547–552. Park Ridge, IL, American Academy of Orthopaedic Surgeons, 1989.

DeLee, J.C.: Tissue remodeling in response to therapeutic exercise. In Sports-Induced Inflammation, Leadbetter, W.B., Buckwalter, J.A., and Gordon, S.L., eds., pp. 549–551. Park Ridge, IL, American Academy of Orthopaedic Surgeons, 1990.

Ellison, A.E., ed.: Special medical considerations: Environmental problems. In Athletic Training and Sports Medicine, 1st ed., p. 530. Park Ridge, IL, American Academy of Orthopaedic Surgeons, 1986.

Epstein, S.E., and Maron, B.J.: Sudden death and the competitive athlete: Retrospectives on preparticipation screening studies. J. Am. Coll. Cardiol. 7:220–230, 1986.

Faulkner, J.A.: New perspectives in training for maximum performance. J.A.M.A. 205:741–746, 1968.

Fitzgerald, R.H., Jr., ed.: Lumbar spine. In Orthopaedic Knowledge Update 2: Home Study Syllabus, p. 312. Park Ridge, IL, American Academy of Orthopaedic Surgeons, 1987.

Fromeli, J., Mubarak, S.J., Hargens, A.R., et al.: Management of chronic anterior compartment syndrome of the lower extremity. Clin. Orthop. 220:217–227, 1987.

Frymoyer, J.W., ed.: Bone metabolism and bone metabolic disease. In Orthopaedic Knowledge Update 4: Home Study Syllabus, p. 82. Rosemont, IL, American Academy of Orthopaedic Surgeons, 1993.

Frymoyer, J.W., and Gordon, S.L.: New Perspectives on Low Back Pain, pp. 304–307. Park Ridge, IL, American Academy of Orthopaedic Surgeons, 1988.

Ganong, W.F.: Review of Medical Physiology, 6th ed. New York, Lange Medical Publications, 1973.

Garrett, W.E., and Best, T.M.: Anatomy, physiology, and mechanics of skeletal muscle. In Orthopaedic Basic Science, Simon, S.R., ed., pp. 89–126. Rosemont, IL, American Academy of Orthopaedic Surgeons, 1994.

Garrett, W.E., Jr., Califf, J.C., Bassett, F.H., III: Histochemical correlates of hamstring injuries. Am. J. Sports Med. 12:98–103, 1984.

Garrett, W.E., Jr., Seaber, A.V., Boswick, J., et al.: Recovery of skeletal muscle after laceration and repair. J. Hand Surg. [Am.] 9:683–692, 1984.
Gollnick, P.D., Armstrong, R.B., Saltin, B., et al.: Effect of training on enzyme activity and fiber composition of human skeletal muscle. J. Appl. Physiol. 34:107–111, 1973.
Golub, L.J., Menduke, H., and Lang, W.R.: Exercise and dysmenorrhea in young teenagers: A three-year study. Obstet. Gynecol. 32: 508–511, 1968.
Grandjean, A.C.: Fluids and electrolytes. In Office Management of Sports Injuries and Athletic Problems, Mellion, M.B., ed., pp. 59–64. Philadelphia, Hanley & Belfus, 1988.
Grandjean, A.C.: Sports nutrition. In The Team Physician's Handbook, Mellion, M.B., Walsh, W.M., and Shelton, G.L., eds., pp. 78–91. Philadelphia, Hanley & Belfus, 1990.
Grood, E.S., Suntay, W.J., Noyes, F.R., et al.: Biomechanics of the knee-extension exercise: Effects of cutting the anterior cruciate ligament. J. Bone Joint Surg. [Am.] 66:725–734, 1984.
Haupt, H.A.: Current concepts: Anabolic steroids and growth hormone. Am. J. Sports Med., 21:468–474, 1993.
Holloszy, J.O.: Biochemical adaptations in muscle: Effects of exercise on mitochondrial oxygen uptake and respiratory enzyme activity in skeletal muscle. J. Biol. Chem. 242:2278–2282, 1967.
Huxley, A.F.: Muscular contraction. J. Physiol. (Lond.) 243:1–43, 1974.
Huxley, H.E.: Electron microscope studies on the structure of natural and synthetic protein filaments from striated muscle. J. Mol. Biol. 7:281–308, 1963.
Huxley, H.E.: The mechanism of muscular contraction. Science 164: 1356–1365, 1969.
Irrgang, J.: Modern trends in anterior ligament rehabilitation: Nonoperative and postoperative management. Clin. Sports Med. 12: 797–813, 1993.
Johnson, M.A., Polgar, J., Weightman, D., et al.: Data on the distribution of fibre types in thirty-six human muscles: An autopsy study. J. Neurol. Sci. 18:111–129, 1973.
Kibble, M.W., and Ross, M.B.: Adverse effects of anabolic steroids in athletes. Clin. Pharm. 6:686–692, 1987.
Kibler, W.B.: Physiology of exercising muscle. AAOS Instr. Course Lect. 43:3–4, 1994.
Kibler, W.B.: Racquet sports. In Sports Injuries: Mechanisms, Prevention and Treatment, Fu, F., and Stone, D., eds., pp. 531–551. Baltimore, Williams & Wilkins, 1994.
Kibler, W.B., Chandler, T.J., and Reuter, B.H.: Advances in conditioning. In Orthopaedic Knowledge Update: Sports Medicine, Griffin, L.Y., ed., pp. 65–73. Rosemont, IL, American Academy of Orthopaedic Surgeons, 1994.
Lebrun, C.: Effects of menstrual cycle and birth control pill on athletic performance. In Medical and Orthopaedic Issues of Active and Athletic Women, Agostini, R., ed., pp. 78–91. Philadelphia, Hanley & Belfus, 1994.
Lowey, S., and Risby, D.: Light chains from fast and slow muscle myosins. Nature 234:81–85, 1971.
Lutz, G.E., Palmitier, R.A., An, K.N., et al.: Comparison of tibiofemoral joint forces during open-kinetic-chain and closed-kinetic-chain exercises. J. Bone Joint Surg. [Am.] 75:732–739, 1993.
MacDougall, J.D., Elder, C.G., Sale, D.G., et al.: Effects of strength training and immobilization on human muscle fibres. Eur. J. Appl. Physiol. 43:25–34, 1980.
Maron, B.J., Epstein, S.E., and Roberts, W.C.: Causes of sudden death in competitive athletes. J. Am. Coll. Cardiol. 7:204–214, 1986.
Matthews, P.B.C.: Muscle spindles and their motor control. Physiol. Rev. 44:219–288, 1964.
McMaster, W.C., Stoddard, T., Duncan, W.: Enhancement of blood lactate clearance following maximal swimming: Effect of velocity of recovery swimming. Am. J. Sports Med. 17:472, 1989.
Murphy, C.P., and Drez, D.: Jejunal rupture in a football player. Am. J. Sports Med. 15:2, 1987.
Nattiv, A., and Lynch, L.: Female athlete triad. Phys. Sports. Med. 22:60–68, 1994.
Nelson, R.A.: Nutrition and physical performance. Phys. Sports Med. 10:55–63, 1982.
Noonan, T.J., and Garrett, W.E.: Injuries at the myotendinous junction. Clin. Sports Med. 11:783–806, 1992.
Nordin, M., and Frankel, V.H.: Biomechanics of collagenous tissues. In Basic Biomechanics of the Musculoskeletal System, 2nd ed., Frankel, V.H., and Nordein, M., eds., pp. 97–101. Philadelphia, Lea & Febiger, 1989.
Pedowitz, R.A., Hargens, A.R., Mubarak, S.J., et al.: Modified criteria for the objective diagnosis of chronic compartment syndrome of the leg. Am. J. Sports Med. 18:35–40, 1990.
Peterson, L., and Renstrom, P.: Sports Injuries: Their Prevention and Treatment, p. 465. Chicago, Year Book Medical Publishers, 1986.
Poss, R., ed.: Exercise and athletic conditioning. In Orthopaedic Knowledge Update 3: Home Study Syllabus, pp. 50–51. Park Ridge, IL, American Academy of Orthopaedic Surgeons, 1990.
Poss, R., ed.: Exercise and athletic conditioning: Drug use. In Orthopaedic Knowledge Update 3: Home Study Syllabus, p. 50. Park Ridge, IL, American Academy of Orthopaedic Surgeons, 1990.
Poss, R., ed.: General knowledge: Exercise and athletic conditioning; effect of warmup activities. In Orthopaedic Knowledge Update 3: Home Study Syllabus, p. 47. Park Ridge, IL, American Academy of Orthopaedic Surgeons, 1990.
Poss, R., ed.: Rehabilitation: Amputation, prosthetics, and orthotics, In Orthopaedic Knowledge Update 3: Home Study Syllabus, pp. 274–275. Park Ridge, IL, American Academy of Orthopaedic Surgeons, 1990.
Scott, M.J., III., and Scott, A.M.: Effects on anabolic androgenic steroids on the pilosebaceous unit. Cutis 50:113–116, 1992.
Simon, S.R., ed.: Anatomy: Muscle. In Orthopaedic Science: A Resource and Self-Study Guide for the Practitioner, p. 28. Park Ridge, IL, American Academy of Orthopaedic Surgeons, 1986.
Simon, R.A., ed.: Biomechanics: Biomechanics of materials; musculoskeletal tissues. In Orthopaedic Science: A Resource and Self-Study Guide for the Practitioner, p. 163. Park Ridge, IL, American Academy of Orthopaedic Surgeons, 1986.
Strauss, R.H.: Side effects of anabolic steroids in weight trained men. Phys. Sports Med. 11:87–88, 91–95, 1983.
Strauss, R.H.: Sports Medicine, p. 484. Philadelphia, WB Saunders, 1984.
Taylor, D.C., Dalton, J.D., Seaber, A.V., et al.: Viscoelastic properties of muscle-tendon units: The biomechanical effects of stretching. Am. J. Sports Med. 18:300–309, 1990.
Teitz, C.C.: Scientific Foundation of Sports Medicine, p. 247. Philadelphia, BC Decker, 1989.
Waddler, G.I., and Hainline, B.: Drugs in the Athlete, p. 65. Philadelphia, FA Davis, 1989.
Waters, R.L., Campbell, J.M., and Perry, J.: Energy cost of three-point crutch ambulation in fracture patients. J. Orthop. Trauma 1: 170–173, 1987.
Wiche, M.K.: Quenching the athlete's thirst. Phys. Sports Med. 14: 228–232, 1986.
Williams, C.: Diet and endurance fitness. Am. J. Clin. Nutr. 49: 1077–1083, 1989.
Yack, H.J., Collins, C.E., and Whieldon, T.J.: Comparison of closed and open kinetic chain exercises in the anterior cruciate ligament-deficient knee. Am. J. Sports Med. 21:49–54, 1993.

Nervous System

Aminoff, M.J., ed.: Electrodiagnosis in Clinical Neurology, ed 3. New York, Churchill Livingstone, 1992.
Battista, A., and Lusskin, R.: The anatomy and physiology of the peripheral nerve. Foot Ankle 7:69, 1986.
Bodine, S.C., and Lieber, R.L.: Peripheral nerve physiology, anatomy, and pathology. In Orthopaedic Basic Science, Simon, S.R., ed., pp. 325–396. Rosemont, IL, American Academy of Orthopaedic Surgeons, 1994.
Brown, A.G., ed. Organization in the Spinal Cord: The Anatomy and Physiology of Identified Neurones. Berlin, Springer-Verlag, 1981.
Burke, R.E.: Motor units: Anatomy, physiology and functional organization. In Handbook of Physiology, Section I, The Nervous System, Brooks, V.B., ed., pp. 345–422. Bethesda, MD, American Physiological Society, 1981.
Gelberman, R.H., ed. Operative Nerve Repair and Reconstruction. Philadelphia, JB Lippincott, 1991.
Guyton, A.C.: Basic Neuroscience: Anatomy and Physiology, ed 2. Philadelphia, WB Saunders, 1992.
Lusskin, R., and Battista, A.: Evaluation and therapy after injury to peripheral nerves. Foot Ankle 7:71–73, 1986.
Makely, J.T.: Prostaglandins: A mechanism for pain mediation in osteoid osteoma. Orthop. Trans. 6:72, 1982.

Omer, G.E., Jr.: The evaluation of clinical results following peripheral nerve suture. In Management of Peripheral Nerve Problems, Omer, G.E., Jr., and Spinner, M. eds., pp. 431–442. Philadelphia, WB Saunders, 1988.

Rall, W.: Core conductor theory and cable properties of neurons. In Kandel ER (ed): Handbook of Physiology, Section 1: The Nervous System, Kandel, E.R., ed., pp. 39–97. Bethesda, MD, American Physiological Society, 1977.

Seddon, H.J.: Surgical Disorders of the Peripheral Nerves, ed 2. Edinburgh, Churchill Livingstone, 1975.

Wold, L.E., Pritchard, D.J., Bergert, J., et al.: Prostaglandin synthesis by osteoid osteoma and osteoblastoma. Mod. Pathol. 1:129–131, 1988.

Connective Tissues

Arnoczky, S.P.: Anatomy of the anterior cruciate ligament. Clin. Orthop. 172:19–25, 1983.

Butler, D.L., Grood, E.S., Noyes, F.R., et al.: Biomechanics of ligaments and tendons. Exerc. Sports Sci. Rev. 6:125–181, 1976.

Frymoyer, J.W., ed.: Knee and leg: Soft-tissue trauma. In Orthopaedic Knowledge Update 4: Home Study Syllabus, pp. 593–602. Rosemont, IL, American Academy of Orthopaedic Surgeons, 1993.

Frymoyer, J.W., and Gordon, S.L., eds.: Intervertebral disk. In New Perspectives on Low Back Pain, pp. 131–214. Park Ridge, IL, American Academy of Orthopaedic Surgeons, 1989.

Holden, J.P., Grood, E.S., Butler, D.L., et al.: Biomechanics of fascia latae ligament replacements: Early postoperative changes in the goat. J. Orthop. Res. 6:639–647, 1988.

Indelicato, P.A., Pascale, M.S., and Huegel, M.O.: Early experience with the Gore-Tex polytetrafluoroethylene anterior cruciate ligament prosthesis. Am. Sports Med. 17:55–62, 1989.

Jackson, D.W., Windler, G.E., and Simon, T.M.: Intraarticular reaction associated with the use of freeze-dried, ethylene oxide-sterilized bone-patella tendon-bone allografts in the reconstruction of the anterior cruciate ligament. Am. J. Sports Med. 18:1, 1990.

Kurosaka, M., Yoshiya, S., and Andrish, J.T.: A biomechanical comparison of different surgical techniques of graft fixation in anterior cruciate ligament reconstruction. Am. J. Sports Med. 15:225–229, 1987.

Noyes, F.R., Butler, D.L., Grood, E.S., et al.: Biomechanical analysis of human ligament grafts used in knee ligament repairs and reconstructions. J. Bone Joint Surg. 66A:344–352, 1984.

Noyes, F.R., DeLucas, J.L., and Torvik, P.J.: Biomechanics of anterior cruciate ligament failure: An analysis of strain-rate sensitivity and mechanisms of failure in primates. J. Bone Joint Surg. [Am.] 56: 236–253, 1974.

Olson, E.J., Kang, J.D., Fu, F.H., et al.: The biomechanical and histological effects of artificial ligament wear particles: In vitro and in vivo studies. Am. J. Sports Med. 16:558–570, 1988.

Poss, R., ed.: Soft tissue implants. In Orthopaedic Knowledge Update 3: Home Study Syllabus, pp. 178–179. Park Ridge, IL, American Academy of Orthopaedic Surgeons, 1990.

Roberts, T.S., Drez, D., McCarthy, W., et al.: Anterior cruciate ligament reconstruction using freeze dried ethylene oxide sterilized bone-patella tendon-bone allografts: 2 years of results in 35 patients. Am. J. Sports Med. 19:35–41, 1991.

Robertson, D.B., Daniel, D.M., and Biden, E.: Soft tissue fixation to bone. Am. J. Sports Med. 14:398–403, 1986.

Sabiston, P., Frank, C., Lam, T., et al.: Allograft ligament transplantation: A morphological and biomechanical evaluation of a medial collateral ligament complex in a rabbit model. Am. J. Sports Med. 18:160, 1990.

Woo, S.L., An, K., Arnoczky, S.P., et al.: Anatomy, biology, and biomechanics of tendon, ligament and meniscus. In Orthopaedic Basic Science, Simon, S.R., ed., pp. 45–88. Rosemont, IL, American Academy of Orthopaedic Surgeons, 1994.

Woo, S.L-Y., and Buckwalter, J.A., eds.: Injury and Repair of the Musculoskeletal Soft Tissues. Park Ridge, IL, American Academy of Orthopaedic Surgeons, 1988.

Cellular and Molecular Biology, Immunology, and Genetics of Orthopaedics

Alberts, B., Bray, D., Lewis, J., et al., eds. Molecular Biology of the Cell, ed 2. New York, Garland Publishing, 1989.

Antonarakis, S.E.: Diagnosis of genetic disorders at the DNA level. N. Engl. J. Med. 320:151–163, 1989.

D'Astous, J., Drouin, M.A., and Rhine, E.: Intraoperative anaphylaxis secondary to allergy to latex in children who have spina bifida: Report of two cases. J. Bone Joint Surg. [Am.] 74:1084–1086, 1992.

Goldberg, V.M.: The immunology of articular cartilage. In Osteoarthritis Diagnosis and Management, Moskowitz, R.W., Howell, D.S., Goldberg, V.M., et al., eds., pp. 81–82. Philadelphia, WB Saunders, 1984.

Harrod, M.J., Friedman, J.M., Currarino, G., et al.: Genetic heterogeneity in spondyloepiphyseal dysplasia congenita. Am. J. Med. Genet. 18:311–320, 1984.

Leonard, M.A.: The inheritance of tarsal coalition and its relationship to spastic flat foot. J. Bone Joint Surg. [Br.] 56B:520, 1974.

McKusick, V.A.: Mapping and sequencing the human genome. N. Engl. J. Med. 320:910–915, 1989.

Schumacher, H.R., Jr.: Pathology of crystal deposition diseases. Rheum. Dis. Clin. North Am. 14:269–288, 1988.

Watson, J.D., Tooze, J., and Kurtz, D.T.: Recombinant DNA: A Short Course. New York, Scientific American Books, 1983.

Meehan, P.L., Galina, M.P., and Daftari, T.: Intraoperative anaphylaxis due to allergy to latex: Report of two cases. J. Bone Joint Surg. [Am.] 74:1087–1089, 1992.

Meeropol, E., Frost, J., Pugh, L., et al.: Latex allergy in children with myelodysplasia: A survey of Shriners hospitals. J. Pediatr. Orthop. 13:1–4, 1993.

Tolo, V.T.: Spinal deformity in short stature syndromes. AAOS Instr. Course Lact. 39:399–405, 1990.

White, R., and Lalouel, J.-M.: Chromosome mapping with DNA markers. Sci. Am. 258:40–48, 1988.

Zvaifler, N.J.: Etiology and pathogenesis of rheumatoid arthritis. In Arthritis and Allied Conditions: A Textbook of Rheumatology, ed 10, McCarty, D.J., ed., pp. 557–570. Philadelphia, Lea & Febiger, 1985.

Musculoskeletal Infections

Aalto, K., Osterman, K., Peltola, H., et al.: Changes in erythrocyte sedimentation rate and C-reactive protein after total hip arthroplasty. Clin. Orthop. 184:118–1209, 1984.

AAOS Task Force on AIDS and Orthopaedic Surgery: Recommendations for the Prevention of Human Immunodeficiency Virus (HIV) Transmission in the Practice of Orthopaedic Surgery. Park Ridge, IL, American Academy of Orthopaedic Surgeons, 1989.

Bansal, M.B., Chuah, S.K., and Thaldepalli, H.: In vitro activity and in vivo evaluation of ticarcillin; use of clavulanic acid against aerobic and anaerobic bacteria. Am. J. Med. 78:33–38, 1985.

Barnes, R.W., Shanik, G.D., and Slaymaker, E.E.: An index of healing in below-knee amputation: Leg blood pressure by Doppler ultrasound. Surgery 79:13, 1976.

Bartlett, P., Reingold, A.L., Graham, D.R., et al.: Toxic shock syndrome associated with surgical wound infections. J.A.M.A. 247: 1448–1451, 1982.

Birke, J.A., Sims, D.S., and Buford, W.L.: Walking casts: Effect on plantar foot pressures. J. Rehab. Res. Dev. 22:18–22, 1985.

Bordelon, R.L.: Surgical and Conservative Foot Care, pp. 139–140. Thorofare, NJ, Slack Inc, 1988.

Brand, R.A., and Black, H.: Pseudomonas osteomyelitis following puncture wounds in children. J. Bone Joint Surg. [Am.] 56: 1637–1642, 1974.

Brodsky, J.W., and Schneidler, C.: Diabetic foot infections. Orthop. Clin. North Am. 22:473–489, 1991.

Buchholz, H.W., Elson, R.A., Engelbrecht, E., et al.: Management of deep infection of total hip replacement. J. Bone Joint Surg. [Br.] 63:342–353, 1981.

Cabanela, M.E., Sim, F.H., Beabout, J.W., et al.: Osteomyelitis appearing as neoplasms: A diagnostic problem. Arch. Surg. 109: 68–72, 1974.

Calabrese, L.H.: The rheumatic manifestations of infections with the human immunodeficiency virus. Semin. Arthritis Rheum. 18: 255–239, 1989.

Centers for Disease Control: Recommendations for venting transmission of infection with human T-lymphotropic virus type III/lymphadenopathy-associated virus in the workplace. M.M.W.R. 34 (45):682–695, 1985.

Cierney, G., III: Chronic osteomyelitis: Results of treatment. Instr. Course Lect. 39:495–508, 1990.
Caudle, R.J., and Stern P.J.: Severe open fractures of the tibia. J. Bone Joint Surg. [Am.] 67:801–807, 1987.
Choi, I.H., Pizzutillo, P.D., Bowen, J.R., et al.: Sequelae and reconstruction after septic arthritis of the hip in infants. J. Bone Joint Surg. [Am.] 72:1150–1165, 1990.
Croall, J., and Chandhri, S.: Non-menstrual toxic shock syndrome complicating orthopaedic surgery [letter to editor]. J. Infect. 18: 195–196, 1989.
Dabezies, E.J., and D'Ambrosia, R.D.: Fracture treatment for the multiple injured patient. AAOS Instr. Course Lect. 35:13–21, 1986.
Dajani, A.S., Bisno, A.L., and Chung, K.J.: Prevention of bacterial endocarditis. J.A.M.A. 264:2919–2922, 1990.
Dalinka, M.K., Dinnenberg, S., Greendyk, W.H., et al.: Roentgenographic features of osseous coccidioidomycosis and differential diagnosis. J. Bone Joint Surg. [Am.] 53:1157–1164, 1971.
Del Curling, O., Jr., Gower, J.D., and McWhorter, J.M.: Changing concepts in spinal epidural abscess: A report of 29 cases. Neurosurgery 27:185–192, 1990.
Digby, J.M., and Kersley, J.B.: Pyogenic non-tuberculous spinal infection: An analysis of thirty cases. J. Bone Joint Surg. [Br.] 61: 47–55, 1979.
Dupont, J.A.: Significance of operative cultures in total hip arthroplasty. Clin. Orthop. 211:122–127, 1986.
Eismont, F.J., Bohlman, H.H., Soni, P.L., et al.: Pyogenic and fungal vertebral osteomyelitis with paralysis. J. Bone Joint Surg. [Am.] 65:19–29, 1983.
Emery, S.E., Chan, D.P., and Woodward, H.R.: Treatment of hematogenous pyogenic vertebral osteomyelitis with anterior debridement and primary bone grafting. Spine 14:284–291, 1989.
Fee, N.F., Dobranski, A., and Bisla, R.S.: Gas gangrene complicating open forearm fractures: Report of five cases. J. Bone Joint Surg. [Am.] 59:135–138, 1977.
Ferree, B.A., Stambough, J.L., and Greiner, A.L.: Spinal epidural abscess: A case report and literature review. Orthop. Rev. 18: 75–80, 1989.
Fitzgerald, R.H., Jr., ed.: Infection. In Orthopaedic Knowledge Update 2: Home Study Syllabus, pp. 71–82. Park Ridge, IL, American Academy of Orthopaedic Surgeons, 1987.
Fitzgerald, R.H., Jr., ed.: Knee and leg: Bone trauma. In Orthopaedic Knowledge Update 2: Home Study Syllabus, p. 429. Park Ridge, IL, American Academy of Orthopaedic Surgeons, 1987.
Fitzgerald, R.H., Jr.: Orthopaedic sepsis in osteomyelitis: Antimicrobial therapy for the musculoskeletal system. Instr. Course Lect. 31:1–9, 1982.
Fitzgerald, R.H., and Cowan, J.D.E.: Puncture wounds of the foot. Orthop. Clin. North Am. 6:965–972, 1975.
Frierson, J.G., and Pfeffinger, L.L.: Infections of the foot. In Surgery of the Foot and Ankle, 6th ed., Mann, R.A., and Coughlin, M.J., eds., p. 860. St. Louis, C.V., Mosby, 1993.
Frymoyer, J.W., ed.: Hip: Adult joint reconstruction. In Orthopaedic Knowledge Update 4: Home Study Syllabus, pp. 546–547. Rosemont, IL, American Academy of Orthopaedic Surgeons, 1993.
Frymoyer, J.W., ed.: Infection. In Orthopaedic Knowledge Update 4: Home Study Syllabus, p. 162. Rosemont, IL, American Academy of Orthopaedic Surgeons, 1993.
Frymoyer, J.W., ed.: Knee and leg: reconstruction. In Orthopaedic Knowledge Update 4: Home Study Syllabus, pp. 603–624. Rosemont, IL, American Academy of Orthopaedic Surgeons, 1993.
Garcia, A., and Grantham, S.A.: Hematogenous pyogenic vertebral osteomyelitis. J. Bone Joint Surg. [Am.] 42:429–436, 1960.
Garvin, K.L., Salvati, E.A., and Brause, B.D.: Role of gentamicin-impregnated cement in total joint arthroplasty. Orthop. Clin. North Am. 19:605–610, 1988.
Ghormley, R.K., Bickel, W.H., and Dickson, D.D.: A study of acute infectious lesions of the intervertebral discs. South. Med. J. 33: 347–353, 1940.
Gledhill, R.B.: Subacute osteomyelitis in children. Clin. Orthop. 96: 57–69, 1973.
Goulet, J.A., Pellicci, P.M., Brause, B.D., et al.: Prolonged suppression of infection in total hip arthroplasty. J. Arthroplasty 3: 109–116, 1988.
Grogan, T.J., Dorey, F., Rollins, J., et al.: Deep sepsis following total knee arthroplasty: Ten-year experience at the University of California at Los Angeles Medical Center. J. Bone Joint Surg. [Am.] 68:226–234, 1986.
Gustilo, R.B., Gruninger, R.P., and Davis, T.: Classification of type III (severe) open fractures relative to treatment and results. Orthopaedics 10:1781–1788, 1987.
Gustilo, R.B., Gruninger, R.P., and Tsukayama, D.T.: Orthopaedic Infection: Diagnosis and Treatment. Philadelphia, WB Saunders, 1989.
Gustilo, R.B., Merkow, R.L., and Templeman, D.: The management of open fractures: Current concepts. J. Bone Joint Surg. [Am.] 72: 299–304, 1990.
Harrelson, J.: Management of the diabetic foot. Orthop. Clin. North Am. 20:605, 1989.
Hawkins, L.G.: Pasteurella multocida infections. J. Bone Joint Surg. [Am.] 51:362–366, 1969.
Helm, P.A., and Walker, S.C.: Total contact casting in diabetic patients with neurotrophic foot ulcerations. Arch. Phys. Med. Rehab. 65:691–693, 1984.
Heydemann, J.S., and Morrissy, R.T.: Bone and joint sepsis in childhood: Problems in diagnosis. Orthop. Trans. 10:504, 1986.
Hill, C., Flamont, R., Mazas, F., et al.: Prophylactic cefazolin versus placebo in total hip replacement: Report of a multicentre double-blind randomized trial. Lancet 1:795–796, 1981.
Hlavin, M.L., Kaminiski, H.J., Ross, J.S., et al.: Spinal epidural abscess: A ten-year perspective. Neurosurgery 27:177–184, 1990.
Hollmann, M.W., and Horowitz, M.: Femoral fractures secondary to low velocity missiles: Treatment with delayed intramedullary fixation. J. Orthop. Trauma 4:64–69, 1990.
Insall, J., Thompson, F., and Brause, B.: Two-stage reimplantation for the salvage of infected total knee arthroplasty. J. Bone Joint Surg. [Am.] 65:1087–1098, 1983.
Jackson, M.A., and Nelson, J.D.: Etiology and medical management of acture suppurative bone and joint infections in pediatric patients. J. Pediatr. Orthop. 2:312, 1982.
Jacobs, R.F., Adelman, L., Sack, C.M., et al.: Management of Pseudomonas osteochondritis complicating puncture wounds of the foot. Pediatrics 69:432–435, 1982.
Kind, A.C., and Williams, D.N.: Antibiotics in open fractures. In Management of Open Fractures and Their Complications, Gustillo, R.B., ed., pp. 55–59, Philadelphia, WB Saunders, 1982.
Kuland, D.N.: The Injured Athlete, 1st ed., p. 43. Philadelphia, JB Lippincott, 1982.
Kuo, K.N., Lloyd-Robers, G.C., Orme, I.M., et al.: Immunodeficiency in infantile bone and joint infection. Arch. Dis. Child. 50:51, 1975.
Lange, R.H., Bach, A.W., Hansen, S.T., Jr., et al.: Open tibial fractures with associated vascular injuries: Prognosis for limb salvage. J. Trauma 25:203–208, 1985.
MacAusland, W.R., Jr.: The management of sepsis following intramedullary fixation for fractures of the femur. J. Bone Joint Surg. [Am.] 44:1643–1653, 1963.
Maggiore, P., and Echols, R.M.: Infections in the diabetic foot. In Disorders of the Foot and Ankle, 2nd ed., vol. 2, Jahss, M.H., ed., pp. 1951–1952. Philadelphia, WB Saunders, 1991.
McDonald, D.J., Fitzgerald, R.H., and Ilstrup, D.M.: Two-stage reconstruction of a total hip arthroplasty. J. Bone Joint Surg. [Am.] 71: 828–834, 1989.
Mallouh, A., and Talab, Y.: Bone and joint infection in patients with sickle cell disease. J. Pediatr. Orthop. 5:158–162, 1985.
Wagner, F.W., Jr.: The diabetic foot and amputations of the foot. In Surgery of the Foot, ed 5, Mann, R.A., ed., pp. 421–455. St Louis, CV Mosby, 1986.
Morrey, B.F., Bianco, A.J., and Rhodes, K.H.: Septic arthritis in children. Orthop. Clin. North Am. 6:923, 1975.
Morrissy, R.T.: Bone and joint infections. In Lovell and Winter's Pediatric Orthopaedics, 3rd ed., vol. 1., Morrissy, R.T., ed., pp. 539–561. Philadelphia, JB Lippincott, 1990.
Nelson, J.D.: Antibiotic concentrations in septic joint effusions. N. Engl. J. Med. 284:349, 1971.
Nelson, J.D., and Koontz, W.C.: Septic arthritis in infants and children: A review of 117 cases. Pediatrics 92:131, 1978.
Nelson, J.P., Fitzgerald, R.H., Jr., Jaspers, M.T., et al.: Prophylacctic antimicrobial coverage in arthroplasty patients [editorial]. J. Bone Joint Surg. [Am.] 72:1, 1990.
O'Connor, B.T., Steel, W.M., and Sanders, R.: Disseminated bone tuberculosis. J. Bone Joint Surg. [Am.] 52:537–542, 1970.

Ogden, J.A.: Pediatric osteomyelitis in septic arthritis: The pathology of neonatal disease. Yale J. Biol. Med. 52:423, 1979.
Paiement, G.D., Hymes, R.A., LaDouceur, M.S., et al.: Postoperative infections in asymptomatic HIV seropositive orthopaedic trauma patients. J. Trauma 37:545–551, 1994.
Pappas, A.M., Filler, R.M., Eraklis, A.J., et al.: Clostridial infections (gas gangrene): Diagnosis and early treatment. Clin. Orthop. 76: 177–184, 1971.
Patzakis, M.J., Harvey, J.P., Jr., and Ivler, D.: The role of antibiotics in the management of open fractures. J. Bone Joint Surg. [Am.] 56:532–541, 1974.
Patzakis, M.J., and Wilkins, J.: Factors influencing infection rate in open fracture wounds. Clin. Orthop. 343:36–40, 1989.
Patzakis, M.J., and Wilkins, J.: Surgical findings in clenched-fist injuries. Clin. Orthop. 220:237–240, 1987.
Patzakis, M.J., Wilkins, J., Brien, W.W., et al.: Wound site as a predictor of complications following deep nail punctures to the foot. West. J. Med. 150:545–547, 1989.
Patzakis, M.J., Wilkins, J., and Moore, T.M.: Considerations in reducing the infection rate in open tibial fractures. Clin. Orthop. 178: 36–41, 1983.
Patzakis, M.J., Wilkins, J., and Wiss, D.A.: Infection following intramedullary nailing of long bones. Clin. Orthop. 212:182–191, 1986.
Pinto, M.R., Racette, J.W., and Fitzgerald, R.H.: Staged hip reconstruction following cemented total hip arthroplasty. Orthop. Trans. 13:162, 1989.
Poss, R., ed.: Knee and leg: Reconstruction. In Orthopaedic Knowledge Update 3: Home Study Syllabus, pp. 583–601. Park Ridge, IL, American Academy of Orthopaedic Surgeons, 1990.
Riegler, H.F., and Rouston, G.W.: Complications of deep puncture wounds of the foot. J. Trauma 19:18–22, 1979.
Roberts, J.M., Drummond, D.S., Breed, A.L., et al.: Subacute hematogenous osteomyelitis in children: A retrospective study. J. Pediatr. Orthop. 2:249–254, 1982.
Rovner, R.A., Baird, R.A., and Malerick, M.M.: Fatal toxic shock syndrome as a complication of orthopaedic surgery: A case report. J. Bone Joint Surg. [Am.] 66:952–954, 1984.
Salvati, E.A., Callaghan, J.J., Brause, B.D., et al.: Reimplantation in infection: Elution of gentamicin from cement and beads. Clin. Orthop. 207:83–93, 1986.
Sanford, J.P., Gilbert, D.N., and Gerberding, J.L.: Guide to Antimicrobial Therapy. Dallas, Antimicrobial Therapy, Inc., 1994.
Sapico, F.L., Canawati, H.N., Witte, J.L., et al.: Quantitative aerobic and anaerobic bacteriology of infected diabetic feet. J. Clin. Microbiol. 12:413–420, 1980.
Sapico, F.L., Witte, J.L., and Canawati, H.N.: The infected foot of the diabetic patient: Quantitative microbiology and analysis of clinical features. Rev. Infect. Dis. 6:S171–S176, 1984.
Silverman, J.F., and Marrow, H.G.: Fine needle aspiration of granulomatous disease of the lung including nontuberculous mycobacterium infection. Acta Cytol. 29:535–541, 1985.
Stone, J.L., Cybulski, G.R., Rodriguez, J., et al.: Anterior cervical debridement and strut grafting for osteomyelitis of the cervical spine. J. Neurosurg. 70:879–883, 1989.
Sullivan, P.M., Johnston, R.C., and Kelky, S.S.: Late infection after total hip replacement, caused by an oral organism after dental manipulation. J. Bone Joint Surg. [Am.] 72:121–123, 1990.
Swiontkowski, M.F.: Criteria for bone debridement in massive lower limb trauma. Clin. Orthop. 243:41–47, 1989.
Tachdjian, M.O.: Pediatric Orthopaedics, 2nd ed., vol. 2, pp. 1415–1441. Philadelphia, WB Saunders, 1990.
Thelander, U., and Larsson, S.: Quantitation of C-reactive protein levels and erythrocyte sedimentation rate after spinal surgery. Spine 17:400–404, 1992.
Torholm, C., Lidgren, L., Lindberg, L., et al.: Total hip joint arthroplasty with gentamycin-impregnated cement: A clinical study of gentamycin excretion kinetics. Clin. Orthop. 181:99–106, 1983.
Turker, R., Lubicky, J.P., and Vogel, L.C.: Toxic shock syndrome in patients with external fixators. J. Pediatr. Orthop. 12:658–662, 1992.
Van Winkle, B.A., and Neustein, J.: Management of open fractures with sterilization of large, contaminated extruded cortical fragments. Clin. Orthop. 223:275–281, 1987.
Veitch, J.M., and Omer, G.E.: Case report: Treatment of catbite injuries of the hand. J. Trauma 19:201–202, 1989.
Wahlig, H., Dingeldein, E., Bergmann, R., et al.: The release of gentamycin from polymethylmethacrylate beads: An experimental and pharmacokinetic study. J. Bone Joint Surg. [Br.] 60:270, 1978.
Waldvogel, F.A., and Papageorgiou, P.S.: Osteomyelitis: The past decade. N. Engl. J. Med. 303:360–370, 1980.
Weissberg, E.D., Smith, A.L., and Smith, D.H.: Clinical features of neonatal osteomyelitis. Pediatrics 53:505, 1974.
Wheat, L.J., Allen, S.D., Henry, M., et al.: Diabetic foot infections: Bacteriologic analysis. Arch. Intern. Med. 146:1935–1940, 1986.
Wilde, A., and Ruth, J.: Two-stage reimplantation in infected total knee arthroplasty. Clin. Orthop. 236:23–35, 1988.
Windsor, R.E., Insall, J.N., Urs, W.K., et al.: Two-stage reimplantation for the salvage of total knee arthroplasty complicated by infection: Further follow-up and refinement of indications. J. Bone Joint Surg. [Am.] 72:272–278, 1990.
Wiss, D.A., Brien, W.W., and Becker, V., Jr.: Interlocking nailing for the treatment of femoral fractures due to gunshot wounds. J. Bone Joint Surg. [Am.] 73:598–606, 1991.
Wopperer, J.M., White, J.J., Gillespie, R., et al.: Long term follow-up of infantile hip sepsis. J. Pediatr. Orthop. 8:322–325, 1988.
Wroblewski, B.M.: One-stage revision of infected cemented total hip arthroplasty. Clin. Orthop. 211:103–107, 1986.

Perioperative Problems

Aiach, M., Michaud, A., Balian, J.L., et al.: A new low molecular weight heparin derivative: In vitro and in vivo studies. Thromb. Res. 31:611–621, 1983.
Amato, J.J., Rheinlander, H.F., and Cleveland, R.J.: Post-traumatic adult respiratory distress syndrome. Orthop. Clin. North Am. 9: 693–713, 1978.
Awbrey, B.J., Sienkiewicz, P.S., and Mankin, H.J.: Chronic exercise-induced compartment pressure elevation measured with a miniaturized fluid pressure monitor. A laboratory and clinical study. Am. J. Sports Med. 16:610–615, 1988.
Cerra, F.B.: Hypermetabolism, organ failure, and metabolic support. Surgery 101:1–14, 1987.
Colwell, C.W., Spiro, T.E., Trowbridge, A.A., et al.: Use of enoxaparin, a low-molecular-weight heparin, and unfractionated heparin for the prevention of deep venous thrombosis after elective hip replacemnt: A clinical trial comparing efficacy and safety. J. Bone Joint Surg. [Am.] 76:3–14, 1995.
Culver, D., Crawford, J.S., Gardiner, J.H., et al.: Venous thrombosis after fractures of the upper end of the femur: A study of incidence and site. J. Bone Joint Surg. [Br.] 52:61–69, 1970.
Davey, J.R., Rorabeck, C.H., and Fowler, P.J.: The tibialis posterior muscle compartment. An unrecognized cause of exertional compartment syndrome. Am. J. Sports Med. 12:391–397, 1984.
DeLee, J.C., and Rockwood, C.A., Jr.: Current concepts review. The use of aspirin in thromboembolic disease. J. Bone Joint Surg. [Am.] 62:149–152, 1980.
Einhorn, T.A., Bonnarens, F., and Burstein, A.H.: The contributions of dietary protein and mineral to the healing of experimental fractures: A biomechanical study. J. Bone Joint Surg. 68A:1389–1395, 1986.
Gossling, H.R., and Pellegrini, V.D., Jr.: Fat embolism syndrome: A review of the pathophysiology and physiological basis of treatment. Clin. Orthop. 165:68–82, 1982.
Jardon, O.M., Wingard, D.W., Barak, A.J., and Connolly, J.F.: Malignant hyperthermia. A potentially fatal syndrome in orthopaedic patients. J. Bone Joint Surg. [Am.] 61:1064–1070, 1979.
Kakkar, V.V., Hose, C.T., Flanc, C., et al.: Natural history of postoperative deep vein thrombosis. Lancet 2:230–232, 1969.
Karlestrom, G., Lonnerholm, T., and Olerud, S.: Cavus deformity of the foot after fracture of the tibial shaft. J. Bone Joint Surg. [Am.] 57A:893–900, 1975.
Kudsk, K.A., Fabian, T.C., Baum, S., et al.: Silent deep vein thrombosis in immobilized multiple trauma patients. Am. J. Surg. 158: 515–519, 1989.
Leach, R.E.: Fractures of the tibia and fibula. In Fractures in Adults, ed 2, Rockwood, C.A., Jr., and Green, D.P., eds., p. 1647. Philadelphia, JB Lippincott, 1984.
Levy, D.: The fat embolism syndrome: A review. Clin. Orthop. 261: 281–2886, 1990.
Lotke, P.A., and Elia, E.A.: Thromboembolic disease after total knee surgery: A critical review. In American Academy of Orthopaedic

Surgeons Instructional Course Lectures XXXIX, Green, W.B., ed., pp. 409–412. Park Ridge, IL, American Academy of Orthopaedic Surgeons, 1990.
MacLean, L.D.: Shock: Causes and management of circulatory collapse. In Davis-Christopher Textbook of Surgery, ed 12, Sabiston, D.C., Jr., ed., pp. 58–90. Philadelphia, WB Saunders, 1981.
Martens, M.A., Backaert, M., Vermaut, G., et al.: Chronic leg pain in athletes due to a recurrent compartment syndrome. Am. J. Sports Med. 12:148–151, 1984.
Matsen, F.A., and Clawson, D.K.: The deep posterior compartmental syndrome of the leg. J. Bone Joint Surg. [Am.] 57A:34–39, 1975.
Messmer, K.F.: Mechanisms of traumatic shock and their consequences. In Blunt Multiple Trauma, Border, J.R., Allgöwer, M., and Hansen, S.T., Jr., eds. pp. 39–49. New York, Marcel Dekker, 1990.
Mubarak, S.J.: Compartment syndromes in operative technique. In Operative Orthopaedics, vol. 1, Chapman, M.W., ed., pp. 179–202. Philadelphia, JB Lippincott, 1988.
Mubarak, S.J., Hargens, A.R., and Akeson, W.H.: Compartment Syndromes and Volkmann's Contracture, pp. 214–217. Philadelphia, WB Saunders, 1981.
Mull, J.R., Reuben, J.D., Parker, J.R., et al.: Comparison of General Epidural and Spinal Anesthesia in Patients Undergoing Total Hip Replacement. Presented at the 62nd Annual Academy of Orthopaedic Surgeons Meeting (Paper 89, p. 99), Orlando, FL, 1995.
Myerson, M.S.: Experimental basis for fasciotomy of the foot and decompression in acute compartment syndromes. Foot Ankle 8: 308–314, 1988.
Myerson, M.: Compartment syndromes of the foot. Bull. Hosp. Jt. Dis. Orthop. Inst. 47:251–261, 1987.
Peltier, L.F.: Fat embolism: A perspective. Clin. Orthop. 232: 263–270, 1988.
Poss, R., ed.: Polytrauma. In Orthopaedic Knowledge Update 3: Home Study Syllabus, p. 88. Park Ridge, IL, American Academy of Orthopaedic Surgeons, 1990.
Reid, H.S., Camp, R.A., and Jacob, W.H.: Tourniquet hemostasis: A clinical study. Clin. Orthop. 177:230, 1983.
Vinazzer, H., and Woler, M.: A new low molecular weight heparin fragment (PK 10169): In vitro and in vivo studies. Haemostatus 16:106–115, 1986.
Webb, L.X., Rush, P.T., Fuller, S.B., et al.: Greenfiled filter prophylaxis of pulmonary embolism in undergoing surgery for acetabular fractures. J. Orthop. Trauma 6:139–145, 1992.

Imaging and Special Studies

Aminoff, M.J., ed. Electrodiagnosis in Clinical Neurology, ed 3. New York, Churchill Livingstone, 1992.
Bernier, D.R., Christian, P.E., Langan, J.K., et al. eds.: Nuclear Medicine Technology and Techniques, ed 2. St Louis, CV Mosby, 1989.
Gilmer, P.W., Herzenberg, J., Frank, J.L., et al.: Computerized tomographic analysis of acute calcaneal fractures. Foot Ankle 6: 184–193, 1986.
Grogan, D., Gasser, S., and Ogden, J.: The painful accessory navicular: A clinical and histopathological study. Foot Ankle 10: 164–169, 1989.
Guyer, B.H., Levinsohn, E.M., Fredericksohn, B.E., et al.: Computer tomography of calcaneal fractures: Anatomy, pathology, and clinical relevance. Am. J. Radiol. 145:911–919, 1985.
Harcke, H.T., Grissom, L.E., and Finkelstein, M.S.: Evaluation of the musculoskeletal system with sonography. AJR 150:1253–1261, 1988.
Hauzeur, J.P., Pasteels, J.L., Schoutens, A., et al.: The diagnostic value of magnetic resonance imaging in nontraumatic osteonecrosis of the femoral head. J. Bone Joint Surg. [Am.] 71:641, 1989.
Kneeland, J.B., Middleton, W.D., Carrera, G.F., et al.: MR imaging of the shoulder: Diagnosis of rotator cuff tears. AJR 149:333–337, 1987.
Marchisello, P.J.: The use of computerized axial tomography for the evaluation of talocalcaneal coalition. J. Bone Joint Surg. [Am.] 69A:609–611, 1987.
Mitchell, M.D., Kundel, H.L., Steinberg, M.E., et al.: Avascular necrosis of the hip: Comparison of MR, CT, and scintigraphy. AJR 147:67–71, 1986.
Pykett, I.L., Newhouse, J.H., Buonanno, F.S., et al.: Principles of nuclear magnetic resonance imaging. Radiology 143:157–168, 1982.
Robinson, H.J., Jr., Hartleben, P.D., Lund, G., et al.: Evaluation of magnetic resonance imaging in the diagnosis of osteonecrosis of the femoral head. Accuracy compared with radiographs, core biopsy, and intra-osseous pressure measurements. J. Bone Joint Surg. [Am.] 71:650, 1989.
Watanabe, A.T., Carter, B.C., Tettelbaum, G.P., et al.: Common pitfalls in magnetic resonance imaging of the knee. J. Bone Joint Surg. [Am.] 71:857, 1989.

Biomaterials and Biomechanics: Basic Concepts

Frankel, V.H., and Burstein, A.H.: Orthopaedic Biomechanics. Philadelphia, Lea & Febiger, 1970.
Fung, Y.C.: Biomechanics: Mechanical Properties of Living Tissues. New York, Springer-Verlag, 1981.
Fung, Y.C.: Biomechanics: Motion, Flow, Stress and Growth. New York, Springer-Verlag, 1990.
Mow, V.C., and Hayes, W.C., eds.: Basic Orthopaedic Biomechanics. New York, Raven Press, 1991.
Pauwels, F.: Biomechanics in the Normal and Diseased Hip, p. 26. Berlin, Springer-Verlag, 1976.
Stillwell, W.T.: The Art of Total Hip Arthroplasty, p. 26. Orlando, FL, Grune & Stratton, 1987.
White, A.A., and Panjabi, M.M.: Clinical Biomechanics of the Spine. Philadelphia, JB Lippincott, 1978.

Biomaterials

Black, J.: Orthopaedic Biomaterials in Research and Practice. New York, Churchill Livingstone, 1988.
Bobyn, J.D., Pilliar, R.M., Cameron, H.U., and Weatherly, G.C.: The optimum pore size for the fixation of porous-surfaced metal implants by bone ingrowth. Clin. Orthop. 150:263–270, 1980.
Bordelon, L.: Surgical and Conservative Foot Care, p. 37. Thorofare, NJ, Slack Inc, 1988.
Carter, D.R., and Spengler, D.M.: Mechanical properties and composition of cortical bone. Clin. Orthop. 135:192–217, 1978.
Charnley, J.: Acrylic Cement in Orthopaedic Surgery. Baltimore, Williams & Wilkins, 1970.
Claes, L.: Biomechanical properties of human ligaments. Aktuel Probl. Chir. Orthop. 26:10–17, 1983.
Glass, M.K., and Karno, M.L.: An office based orthotic system in the treatment of the arthritic foot. Foot Ankle 3:37, 1982.
Kourosh, S., Stills, M., and Mooney, J.: Objective evaluation of insert material for diabetic and athletic footwear. Foot Ankle 3:11–116, 1988.
Park, J.B.: Biomaterials Science and Engineering. New York, Plenum Press, 1984.

Biomechanics

Fung, Y.C.: Biomechanics: Mechanical Properties of Living Tissues. New York, Springer-Verlag, 1981.
Frankel, V.H., and Burnstein, A.H.: Orthopaedic Biomechanics. Philadelphia, Lea & Febiger, 1970.
Mann, R.A.: Surgical implications of biomechanics of the foot and ankle. Clin. Orthop. Rel. Res. 146:111–118, 1980.
Morrey, B.F., and Wiedeman, G.P.: Complications and long-term results of ankle arthrodeses following trauma. J. Bone Joint Surg. [Am.] 62A:777–784, 1980.
Mow, V.C., and Hayes, W.C., eds.: Basic Orthopaedic Biomechanics. New York, Raven Press, 1991.
Palmer, A.K., Werner, F.W., Murphy, D., and Glisson, R.: Functional wrist motion: A biomechanical study. J. Hand Surg. [Am.] 10: 39–46, 1985.
Perry, J.: Anatomy and biomechanics of the hindfoot. Clin. Orthop. 177:9–15, 1983.
Samuelson, K.M., Harrison, R., and Freeman, M.A.R.: A roentgenographic technique to evaluate and document hindfoot position. Foot Ankle 1:286–289, 1981.

2

PEDIATRIC ORTHOPAEDICS

RAYMOND M. STEFKO AND DENNIS R. WENGER

I. **Embryology**—Beginning at day 12 after conception, the **primitive streak** appears, and beginning caudally ectodermal cells migrate between endoderm and ectoderm to form the **mesoderm. Mesenchyme** comes from mesoderm and gives rise to connective tissues, muscles, vessels, blood cells, and the GU system. Between days 5 and 21, the **notochord** is formed at the cranial end of the primitive streak as ectoderm forms a primitive knot that becomes a blastopore and eventually differentiates into the notochord (Fig. 2–1). **Neural crest** cells also differentiate at this time and later form the peripheral nervous system (**PNS**), automatic nervous system (**ANS**), and Schwann cells. **Somites** are formed from mesoderm, line both sides of the notochord, and eventually total 42–44 pairs. Each somite develops into a lateral dermatome, a medial myotome, and a ventral sclerotome, forming skin, muscle, and skeletal elements, respectively (Fig. 2–2). **Limb buds** develop between 4 and 6 weeks (Fig. 2–3) and quickly form the upper extremity, with pronated forearms that then rotate externally. A few days later the lower extremity forms and eventually rotates internally. Although finger rays are present at 7 weeks, the hand continues to differentiate until week 13 (Fig. 2–4). The median artery, which intially supplies the hand, evolves at about 6 weeks. **Bone** is formed through mesenchymal aggregation into a cartilage model that is systematically replaced by bone (except for a few bones that are formed without a cartilage model through intramembranous ossification: skull and scapula. **Primary centers of ossification** appear in the diaphyses of bones between 7 and 12 weeks. Most secondary centers for ossification (except the distal femur) are not present until after birth.

II. **Bone Dysplasias (Dwarfs)**

A. Introduction—According to Rubin, **dysplasia** refers to deformities caused by intrinsic bone disturbance (e.g., achondroplasia); **dystrophy** alludes to deformities caused by metabolic or nutritional deficiencies (e.g., mucopolysaccharidoses); and **dysostosis** is the term used when there are underlying mesodermal or ectodermal abnormalities (e.g., diastrophic dysplasia). Histologic changes common to all dysplasias include horizontal orientation of primary trabeculae adjacent to the physis. **Proportionate** dwarfism displays symmetric decrease in both truncal and limb length (e.g., mucopolysaccharidoses, metaphyseal chon-

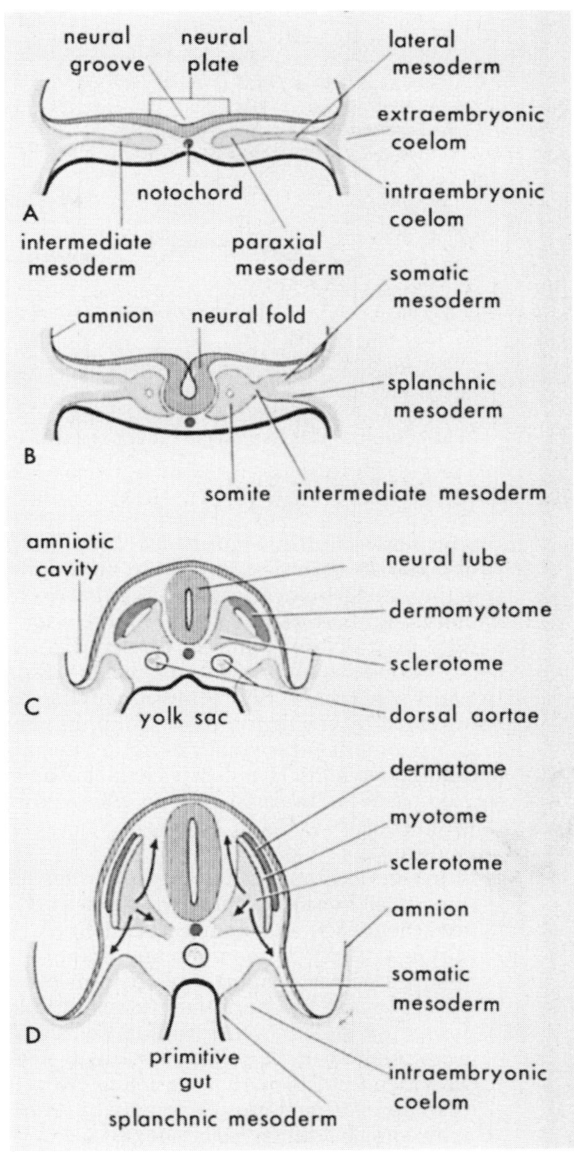

FIGURE 2–1. Formation of the neural tube (*A–D*, 18, 22, 26, and 28 days' gestation, respectively). (From Moore, K.L.: The Developing Human. Philadelphia, WB Saunders, 1982; reprinted by permission.)

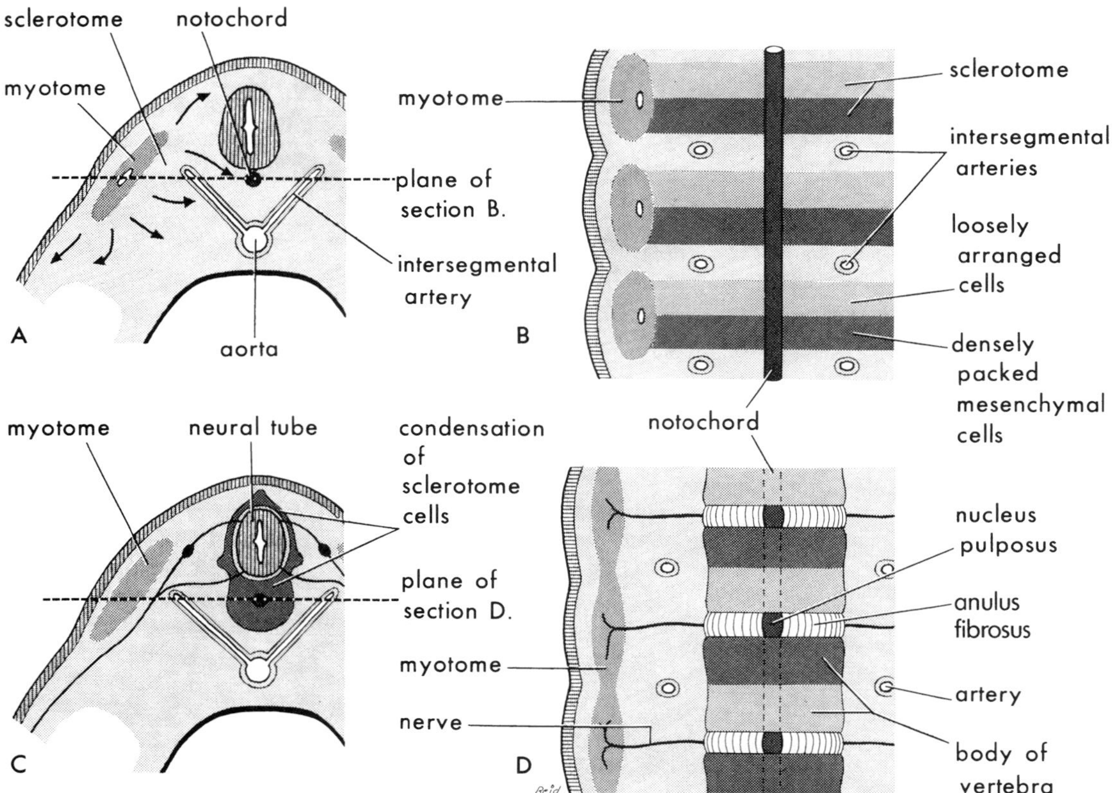

FIGURE 2–2. Further development of the axial skeleton. *A, B,* Transverse and frontal sections, respectively, of 4-week embryo. *C, D,* Similar sections of 5-week embryo. Note that the vertebral body forms from the cranial and caudal halves of two successive sclerotome masses. (From Moore, K.L.: The Developing Human. Philadelphia, WB Saunders, 1982; reprinted by permission.)

drodysplasia, multiple epiphyseal dysplasia). **Disproportionate** dwarfing conditions are subdivided into the short-trunk variety (e.g., Kneist syndrome, spondyloepiphyseal dysplasia) or the short-limb variety (e.g., achondroplasia, diastrophic dysplasia, chondroectodermal dysplasia—Ellis-van Creveld syndrome). Short-limb dwarfism can be subdivided by the region of the limb that is short (e.g., rhizomelic—proximal, mesomelic—middle, acromelic—distal). Dysplasias can also be characterized based on the area of bone where growth is affected (Fig. 2–5; Table 2–1).

B. Achondroplasia

1. Introduction and Etiology—Achondroplasia, the most common form of disproportionate dwarfism, is an autosomal dominant (AD) condition with 80% spontaneous mutation. This disproportionate, short-limbed form of dwarfism is caused by abnormal endochondral bone formation (defect in the proliferative zone). It is a quantitative, not a qualitative, cartilage defect. Endochondral growth is much more affected than appositional growth. It may be associated with late childbirth (after age 36).
2. Signs and Symptoms—Clinical features include a normal trunk and short limbs (rhizomelic). Typically, these patients have prominent foreheads, button noses, small nasal bridges, trident hands (inability to approximate extended middle and ring fingers), thoracolumbar kyphosis (the most common spinal deformity), lumbar stenosis and excessive lordosis (short pedicles with decreased interpedicular distances), radial head subluxation, and hypotonia during the first year of life.

   Involved children have normal intelligence but delayed walking and other motor milestones. Although sitting height may be normal, standing height is in the lower 3%. Radiographs show narrowed interpedicular distance L1–S1, T12/L1 wedging, generalized posterior vertebral scalloping, delayed appearance of growth plates, and broad, short iliac wings ("champagne glass" pelvic outlet). Achondroplasia may also be associated with radial or tibial bowing (ulna and fibula less affected), coxa valga, genu varum (with disproportionately long fibula), and metaphyseal flaring with an "inverted **V**"-shaped distal femoral physis. Neurologic symptoms are usually related to nerve root or spinal cord compression, which can occur at any level, including the foramen magnum (which may cause periods of apnea). The growth of the foramen magnum is severely impaired, especially during the first year of life, predominantly in the transverse diameter. The mean size of an adult achondroplastic foramen magnum is the same as that of a nonachondro-

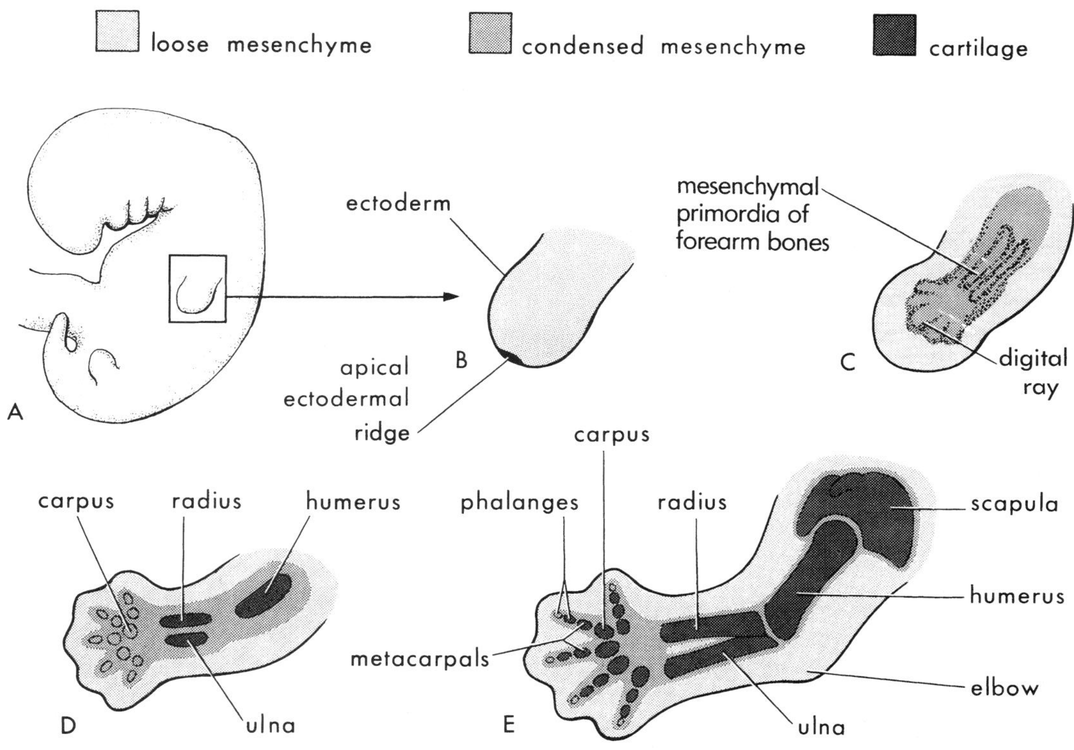

FIGURE 2–3. Development of the limb bud. *A, B,* Appearance of limb bud at 28 days. *C,* Mesenchymal primordium at 33 days. *D, E,* Further development at 6 weeks. (From Moore, K.L.: The Developing Human. Philadelphia, WB Saunders, 1982; reprinted by permission.)

plastic individual at birth in its transverse dimension.

3. Treatment—Nonoperative treatment includes weight loss (typically a problem), bracing, and exercises (unpredictable). Surgical options include decompression of the spine plus bone grafting for a developing neurologic deficit. In rare cases, young children have progressive kyphosis without neurologic problems. In such cases, anterior fusion with strut grafting and posterior fusion are indicated for kyphosis >60 degrees. Preoperative pulmonary evaluation is indicated for associated pulmonary problems. Fibular epiphysiodesis, osteotomies, or both are indicated for genu varum. Limb-lengthening procedures including chondrodiatasis (lengthening through the growth plate) or callodiatasis (lengthening through a metaphyseal corticotomy) have been well described and generally are well tolerated with a low rate of complications. The patients are still left with the other underlying problems, however, and limb-

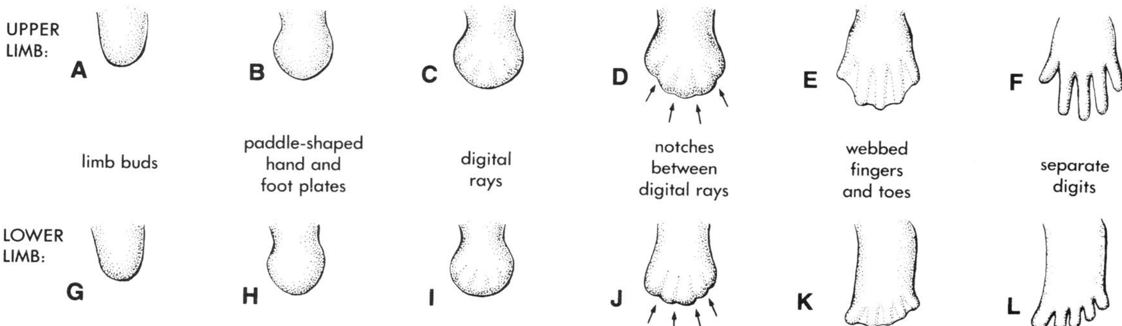

FIGURE 2–4. Development of the hands and feet. *A–F,* Development of the hand (4–8 weeks). *G–L,* Development of the foot ($4\frac{1}{2}$–$8\frac{1}{2}$). (From Moore, K.L.: The Developing Human. Philadelphia, WB Saunders, 1982; reprinted by permission.)

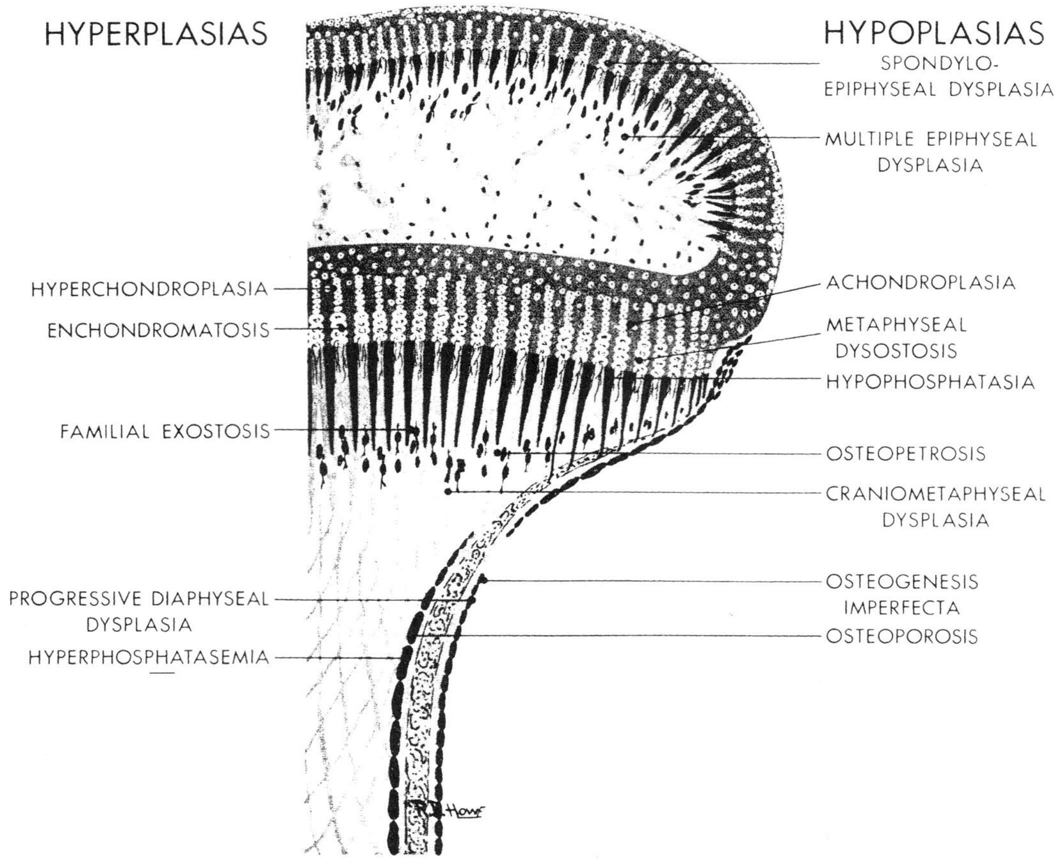

FIGURE 2–5. Location of abnormalities leading to dysplasias. (From Rubin, P.: Dynamic Classification of Bone Dysplasias. Chicago, Year Book Medical Publishers, 1964; reprinted by permission.)

lengthening procedures remain controversial in achondroplastic patients.

C. Spondyloepiphyseal Dysplasia—Three forms are generally recognized.

1. Congenita Form—Short-trunked dwarfism associated with primary involvement of the vertebra (beaking) and epiphyseal centers (affects the proliferative zone), clinical heterogenicity, and AD inheritance. The clinical and radiographic differences are frequently age-related and not distinguishable at birth. Delayed appearance of the epiphysis, flattened facies, platyspondyly, scoliosis, odontoid hypoplasia, coxa vara, and genu valgum are common. Patients should also be screened for associated retinal detachment and myopia.
2. Tarda Form—These patients typically have a variable inheritance pattern and late (age 8–10) manifestations of the disorder, which affects primarily the spine and large joints. Hips may be dislocated, and affected children often are susceptible to premature osteoarthritis (osteotomies may be helpful) and scoliosis (treated like idiopathic scoliosis).
3. Pseudoachondroplastic Dysplasia—Although considered separately in some classifications, this disorder, which has an AD inheritance pattern, is clinically similar to achondroplasia, although affected children have normal facies. Radiographs demonstrate metaphyseal flaring and delayed epiphyseal ossification. Orthopaedic manifestations of the disorder include cervical instability, scoliosis with increased lumbar lordosis, significant lower extremity bowing, and hip, knee, and elbow flexion contractures with precocious osteoarthritis.

D. Chondrodysplasia Punctata—Characterized by multiple punctate calcifications seen on radiographs during infancy. The AD (Conradi-Hünermann) form has a wide variation of clinical expression. The severe autosomal recessive (AR) rhizomelic form is usually fatal during the first year of life. Cataracts, asymmetric limb shortening that may require surgical correction, and spinal deformities are common.

E. Kneist Syndrome—AD, short-limbed, short-trunked, disproportionate dwarfism with joint stiffness/contractures, scoliosis, kyphosis, dumbbell-shaped femora, and hypoplastic pelvis and spine. May be related to an abnormality of cartilage proteoglycan metabolism, and physes may have a characteristic "Swiss cheese" appearance histologically. Radiographs show osteoporosis and platyspondyly or hypoplasia. Respiratory problems and cleft palate are common; associated retinal detachment and myopia require an oph-

TABLE 2–1. RUBIN'S CLASSIFICATION OF BONE DYSPLASIAS

I. Epiphyseal dysplasias
  A. Epiphyseal hypoplasias
    1. Failure of articular cartilage: spondyloepiphyseal dysplasia
    2. Failure of ossification of center: multiple epiphyseal dysplasia
  B. Epiphyseal hyperplasia
    1. Excess of articular cartilage: dysplasia epiphysealis hemimelica
II. Physeal dysplasia
  A. Cartilage hypoplasia
    1. Failure of proliferating cartilage: achondroplasia
    2. Failure of hypertrophic cartilage: metaphyseal dysostosis; cartilage–hair hypoplasia
  B. Cartilage hyperplasias
    1. Excess of proliferating cartilage: hyperchondroplasia (Marfan syndrome)
    2. Excess of hypertrophic cartilage: enchondromatosis
III. Metaphyseal dysplasias
  A. Metaphyseal hypoplasias
    1. Failure to form primary spongiosa: hypophosphatasia
    2. Failure to absorb primary spongiosa: osteopetrosis
    3. Failure to absorb secondary spongiosa: craniometaphyseal dysplasia
  B. Metaphyseal hyperplasia
    1. Excessive spongiosa: multiple exostoses
IV. Diaphyseal dysplasias
  A. Diaphyseal hypoplasias
    1. Failure of periosteal bone formation: osteogenesis imperfecta
    2. Failure of endosteal bone formation: idiopathic osteoporosis, congenita and tarda
  B. Diaphyseal hyperplasias
    1. Excessive periosteal bone formation: progressive diaphyseal dysplasia (Engelmann's disease)
    2. Excessive endosteal bone formation: hyperphosphatasemia (including juvenile Paget's disease and van Buchem's disease)

Adapted from Rubin, P.: Dynamic Classification of Bone Dysplasias. Chicago, Year Book Medical Publishers, 1964.

thalmology consult. Early therapy for joint contractures is required. Reconstructive procedures may be required for early hip degenerative arthritis. Otitis media and hearing loss are frequent.

F. Metaphyseal Chondrodysplasia—Heterogeneous group of disorders characterized by metaphyseal changes of tubular bones with normal epiphyses. The physis (proliferative and hypertrophic zones) appears histologically to be more affected than the metaphysis; hence the term metaphyseal dysostoses has fallen out of favor. Several types are recognized, including the following.
  1. Jansen (Rare)—AD, retarded, short-limbed dwarf with wide eyes, monkey-like stance, and hypercalcemia.
  2. Schmid—AD, short-limbed dwarf not diagnosed until older, with stunting of growth and bowing of legs due to coxa vara and genu varum. Metaphyseal lesions heal with bed rest but recur with weight-bearing. Often confused with rickets, but laboratory tests are normal.
  3. McKusick—AR, cartilage–hair dysplasia (hypoplasia of cartilage and small diameter of hair) seen most commonly among the Amish population and in Finland. Atlantoaxial instability is common and requires flexion-extension lateral radiographs for proper evaluation. Ankle deformity develops owing to fibular overgrowth distally. These patients may have abnormal immunologic competence (susceptible to chickenpox).

G. Multiple Epiphyseal Dysplasia—Short-limbed disproportionate dwarfism that often does not manifest until age 5–14. A mild form (Ribbing) and a more severe form (Fairbank) exist. The disorder is characterized by irregular or delayed (or both) ossification at multiple epiphyses. Short, stunted metacarpals/metatarsals, irregular femora (mimics Legg-Calvé-Perthes disease but is bilateral and symmetric, not associated with metaphyseal cysts, and often has early acetabular changes), abnormal ossification (tibial "slant sign" and flattened femoral condyles), T12/L1 notching and deformed ring apophysis, valgus knees (consider early osteotomy), waddling gait, and early hip arthritis are common.

H. Dysplasia Epiphysealis Hemimelica (Trevor's Disease)—Essentially an osteochondroma that causes half of the epiphysis (usually the medial half) to enlarge (with an irregular mass). Most common at the knee. Partial excision of the prominent overgrowth (if symptomatic) and later osteotomies may be required.

I. Progressive Diaphyseal Dysplasia (Camurati-Engelmann Disease)—AD; affected children are often "late walkers" (because of associated muscle weakness), with symmetric cortical thickening of long bones. Radiographs demonstrate widened, fusiform diaphyses with increased bone formation and sclerosis. The tibia, femur, and humerus are most often affected (in that order), affecting only the diaphyseal portion of bone. Symptomatic treatment includes salicylates, nonsteroidal anti-inflammatory drugs (NSAIDs), and steroids for refractory cases. Watch for leg-length inequality.

J. Mucopolysaccharidosis—In contrast to the above conditions, these forms of dwarfism are easily differentiated based on the presence of complex sugars found in the urine. They produce a proportionate dwarfism caused by accumulation of mucopolysaccharides (MPSs) due to a hydrolase enzyme deficiency. MPSs consist of glycosaminoglycans attached to a link protein with a hyaluronic acid core (see Chapter 1, Basic Sciences). Four main types include Hurler, Hunter, Sanfilippo, and Morquio syndromes (Table 2–2). Morquio syndrome is the most common form and presents by age 18 months to 2 years with waddling gait, knock knees, thoracic kyphosis, cloudy corneas, and normal intelligence. Bony changes include a thickening skull, wide ribs, anterior beaking of vertebrae, wide flat pelvis, coxa vara with unossified femoral heads, and bullet-shaped metacarpals. C1–C2 instability (due to odontoid hypoplasia) can be seen with Morquio syndrome presenting with myelopathy and requires decompression and cervical fusion.

K. Diastrophic Dysplasia—AR; severe, short-limbed dwarfism associated with a disorder of type II collagen in the physis. This "twisted" dwarf classically has a cleft palate, severe joint contractures (especially hip and knees), cauliflower ears, hitchhiker thumb, rigid club feet, midthoracic kyphoscoliosis, cervical kyphosis (requires immediate

TABLE 2–2. MAIN TYPES OF MUCOPOLYSACCHARIDOSIS

SYNDROME	INHERITANCE	INTELLIGENCE	CORNEA	URINARY EXCRETION	OTHER
I Hurler	AR	MR	Cloudy	Dermatan/heparan sulfate	Worst prognosis
II Hunter	XR	MR	Clear	Dermatan/heparan sulfate	
III Sanfilippo	AR	MR	Clear	Heparan sulfate	Normal until 2 years old
IV Morquio	AR	Normal	Cloudy	Keratan sulfate	Most common

AR, autosomal recessive; XR, sex-linked recessive; MR, mental retardation.

treatment with neurologic sequela), thoracolumbar kyphoscoliosis, spina bifida occulta, and atlantoaxial instability due to odontoid hypoplasia. Surgical release of club feet, osteotomies for contractures, and spinal fusion are often required.

L. Cleidocranial Dysplasia (Dysostosis)—AD; proportionate dwarfism that affects bones formed intramembranously. Patients present with dwarfism (or stunted growth), with aplasia of part or all of the clavicle. Usually unilateral, often the lateral part of the clavicle is missing, and there is delayed skull suture closure, frontal bossing, coxa vara (consider intertrochanteric osteotomy if varus is <100 degrees), delayed ossification of the pubis, and wormian-type bone.

M. Dysplasias Associated with Benign Bone Growths—Includes multiple hereditary exostosis (osteochondromatosis), fibrous dysplasia, Ollier's disease (enchondromatosis), and Maffucci syndrome (enchondromatosis plus hemangiomas). These entities are discussed in Chapter 8, Orthopaedic pathology.

N. Dysplasia Summary—The various types of dysplasia are summarized in Table 2–3.

III. Chromosomal and Teratologic Disorders

A. Down Syndrome (Trisomy 21)—Most common chromosomal abnormality; its incidence increases with maternal age. Usually associated with increased growth, ligament laxity, hypotonia, mental impairment, heart disease (50%), endocrine disorders (hypothyroidism and diabetes), and premature aging. Orthopaedic problems include metatarsus primus varus, pes planus, spinal abnormalities (atlantoaxial instability, scoliosis, spondylolisthesis), hip instability (open reduction ± osteotomy usually required), slipped capital femoral epiphysis, patellar dislocation, and symptomatic planovalgus feet. Atlantoaxial instability is evaluated with flexion-extension radiographs of the C-spine. Asymptomatic children with instability should avoid contact sports, diving, and gymnastics. Atlantoaxial fusion has a high complication rate and is usually reserved for patients with progressive instability, instability >10 mm, or neurologic symptoms. Preoperative cardiac evaluation is essential.

B. Turner Syndrome—45,XO females with short stature, sexual infantilism, web neck, and cubitus valgus. Hormonal therapy can exacerbate scoliosis by increasing preexisting osteopenia. Renal anomalies (usually minor) in two-thirds and cardiac anomalies in one-third. Genu valgum and shortening of the fourth and fifth metacarpals usually require no treatment. Malignant hyperthermia is common with anesthetic use.

C. Noonan Syndrome—Short stature, web neck, and cubitus valgus deformities in boys with normal sexual genotypes. Increased risk for malignant hyperthermia with anesthetics.

D. Prader-Willi Syndrome—Chromosome 15 abnormality, causing a floppy, hypotonic infant who becomes an intellectually impaired, obese adult with an insatiable appetite. Growth retardation, hip dysplasia, hypoplastic genitalia, and scoliosis are common.

E. Menkes' Syndrome—X-linked recessive disorder of copper transport that affects bone growth and

TABLE 2–3. TYPES OF DYSPLASIA

DYSPLASIA	TYPE	INHERITANCE	ZONE	CLINICAL FINDINGS	RADIOGRAPHIC FEATURES
Achondroplasia	Dis	AD/SM	Epi	Facies, spine abnormalities	Stenosis, leg bowing
SED (congenita)	Dis	AD	Epi	Cleft palate, lordosis	Platyspondyly
SED (pseudoachondroplastic)	Dis	AD/AR	Epi	Normal facies	Fragmented epiphysis
SED (tarda)	Dis	XR	Epi	Kyphosis, hip pain	Hip dysplasia, thick vertebrae
Chondrodysplasia punctata	Dis	AD	Phy	Flat facies	Stippled epiphyses
Kneist syndrome	Dis	AD	Phy	Retinal detachment, scoliosis	Dumbbell femora
Metaphyseal chondrodysplasia	Dis	AD/AR	Met	Wide eyes, leg bowing	Bowed legs
Multiple epiphyseal	Dis	AD	Epi	Late—waddling gait	Irregular epiphyseal ossification
Dysplasia epiphysealis hemimelica	Dis	—	Met	Bowed legs	Hemi-enlarged epiphysis
Diaphyseal	Dis	AD	Dia	Delayed walking	Symmetric cortical thickening
Mucopolysaccharidosis	Pro	AD/XR	Hyp	Cornea, urinary sugars, AAI	Thick bone, bullet metacarpals
Diastrophic	Pro	AR	Phy	Palate, ear, thumb	Kyphoscoliosis
Cleidocranial dysostosis	Pro	AR	Met	Absent clavicles	Delayed physeal closure

Dis, disproportionate; Pro, proportionate; AD, autosomal dominant; AR, autosomal recessive; SM, spontaneous mutation; XR, sex-linked recessive; Epi, epiphyseal; Phy, physical; Met, metaphyseal; Dia, diaphyseal; Hyp, hypophyseal; SED, spondyloepiphyseal dysplasia; AAI, atlantoaxial instability.

causes characteristic "kinky" hair. May be differentiated from occipital horn syndrome (which also affects copper transport) by the characteristic bony projections from the occiput of the skull in that disorder.

F. Rett Syndrome—Progressive impairment and stereotaxic abnormal hand movements characterize this disorder. It is seen in girls at 6–18 months of age who present with developmental delay much like that seen with cerebral palsy. Affected children typically have scoliosis with a C-shaped curve unresponsive to bracing. Anterior diskectomy and interbody fusion combined with posterior fusion and instrumentation are indicated for curves >40 degrees. Spasticity results in joint contractures, which are treated as in cerebral palsy patients.

G. Teratogens
1. Fetal Alcohol Syndrome—Maternal alcoholism can cause growth disturbances, CNS dysfunction, dysmorphic facies, hip dislocation, C-spine vertebral and upper extremity fusions, congenital scoliosis, and myelodysplasia.
2. Maternal Diabetes—May lead to heart defects, sacral agenesis, and anencephaly. Careful management of pregnant diabetics is essential.
3. Other Teratogens—Includes drugs (e.g., aminopterin, phenytoin, thalidomide), trace metals, maternal conditions, infections, and intrauterine factors; may also lead to orthopaedic manifestations in affected children.

IV. Hematopoietic Disorders

A. Gaucher's Disease—Aberrant AR lysosomal storage disease (also known as familial splenic anemia) characterized by accumulation of cerebroside in cells of the reticuloendothelial system (RES). Commonly seen in children of Jewish descent, it is associated with osteopenia, metaphyseal enlargement (failure of remodeling), femoral head necrosis (head-within-head deformity) moth-eaten trabeculae, patchy sclerosis, and "Erlenmeyer flask" distal femora. Affected patients may complain of bone pain and occasionally experience a "bone crisis" (similar to sickle cell anemia). Bleeding abnormalities are also common. Histologic examination demonstrates characteristic lipid-laden histiocytes. Treatment is basically supportive; new enzyme therapy is available but is extremely expensive.

B. Niemann-Pick Disease—Caused by accumulation of phospholipid in RES cells. Seen commonly in Eastern European Jews. Marrow expansion and cortical thinning are common in long bones; coxa valga is also seen.

C. Sickle Cell Anemia—Sickle cell disease (affects 1% of African-Americans) is more severe but less common than sickle cell trait (8% prevalence). Crises usually begin at age 2–3 and may lead to characteristic bone infarctions. Growth retardation/skeletal immaturity; osteonecrosis of femoral and humeral heads; osteomyelitis (often in diaphysis); septic arthritis (probably best treated with a third generation cephalosporin). *Salmonella* is more commonly seen in children with sickle cell disease than in those without it. Despite this tendency, *Staphylococcus aureus* is still the most common cause of osteomyelitis in sickle cell patients. Dactylitis (acute hand/foot swelling) is also common. Aspiration and culture are necessary to differentiate infarction from osteomyelitis. Radiographs commonly show osteoporosis and cortical thinning. Preoperative oxygenation and exchange transfusion are helpful for affected patients requiring surgery. Hydroxyurea, a cancer chemotherapeutic agent, has produced dramatic relief of pain when utilized for bone crises.

D. Thalassemia—Similar to sickle cell anemia in presentation. Most common in people of Mediterranean descent. Common symptoms include bone pain and leg ulceration. Radiographs show osteoporosis and distorted trabeculae.

E. Hemophilia—Sex-linked recessive (XR) disorder with decreased factor VIII (hemophilia A), abnormal factor VIII with platelet dysfunction (von Willebrand's disease), or factor IX (hemophilia B—Christmas disease); associated with bleeding episodes and skeletal/joint sequelae. Can be mild (5–25% of factor present), moderate (1–5% available), or marked (<1% of factor present).

Hemarthrosis presents with painful swelling and decreased range of motion of affected joints. Deep intramuscular bleeding is also common and can lead to the formation of a pseudotumor (blood cyst), which may occur in soft tissue or bone. Ultrasonography can help diagnose bleeding into muscles (most commonly in the lower extremity). Intramuscular hematomas can lead to compression of adjacent nerves (e.g., an iliacus hematoma may cause femoral nerve paralysis and may mimic a bleed into the hip joint). Factor levels should be elevated to at least 25% after major bleeding episodes. Radiographic findings in hemophilia include squaring of the patellas and condyles, epiphyseal overgrowth with leg-length discrepancy, and generalized osteoporosis with resulting fractures, commonly around the knee. Fractures heal in normal time with proper clotting. Cartilage atrophy due to enzymatic matrix degeneration is frequent. Therapy includes fracture management, contacture release, osteotomies, open synovectomy, arthroscopic synovectomy (better motion, shorter hospitalization), radiation synovectomy (useful in patients with antibody inhibitors and poor medical management), and total joint arthroplasty (TJA). Treatment of hemophilia has become more complex owing to the risk of HIV transmission in factor VIII replacement. Mild to moderate hemophilia A can be treated with desmopressin (DDAVP). Factor VIII levels should be increased for prophylaxis in the following situations: vigorous physical therapy (20%), treatment of hematoma (30%), acute hemarthrosis or soft tissue surgery (>50%), skeletal surgery (approach 100% preoperatively and maintain >50% for 10 days postoperatively). Tourniquets can be used, vessels should be ligated rather than cauterized, and rigid fixation of fractures decrease postoperative bleeding. **Antibody inhibitors** are present in 4–20% of hemophiliacs and **are a relative contraindication to surgery.** Large levels of factor VIII, or Autoplex (activated prothrombin), are required to offset these inhibitors. Inhibitor levels of <10 Bethesda units are treatable with high dose factor VIII. If levels are >10 Bethesda units, more sophisticated treatment (factor IX, VII) is required. Because of the amount of blood component therapy required to treat this disorder, a large percentage of hemophiliacs are HIV-positive. The incidence of HIV positivity in the older hemophiliac population (before donor screening and the more recent component treatment) approaches 100%.

F. Leukemia—Most common malignancy of childhood. Causes demineralization of bones and septic arthritic and occasionally lytic lesions. One-fourth to one-third of children present with musculoskeletal complaints (back, pelvic, leg pains). Radiolucent "leukemia" lines may be seen in the metaphyses of affected bones in older children. Management of leukemia includes chemotherapy.

G. Acquired Immunodeficiency Syndrome (AIDS)—Caused by HIV. Children born with AIDS are becoming more common in neonatal units, and supportive care is indicated. Protection for surgeons with patients at risk (e.g., IV drug abusers, homosexuals, hemophiliacs) is essential (see Chapter 1, Basic Sciences, part 5: Orthopaedic Infections and Microbiology).

V. Metabolic Disease/Arthritides (see also Chapter 1, Basic Sciences)

A. Rickets (Referred to as Osteomalacia in Adults)—Decrease in calcium (and sometimes phosphorus), affecting mineralization at the epiphyses of long bones. Classically, brittle bones with **physeal cupping/widening,** bowing of long bones, transverse radiolucent (Looser's) lines, ligamentous laxity, flattening of the skull, enlargement of costal cartilages (rachitic rosary), and dorsal kyphosis (cat back) characterize this disorder. There are several varieties of rickets based on the underlying abnormality (e.g., GI, kidney, diet, end-organ), which is discussed in detail in Chapter 1, Basic Sciences. Histologically, **widened osteoid seams** and "Swiss cheese" trabeculae are characteristic in bone; at the growth plate there is gross distortion of the maturation zone (enlarged and distorted) and a poorly defined zone of provisional calcification.

B. Osteogenesis Imperfecta (OI)—Defect in collagen (procollagen to type 1 collagen sequence and abnormal cross-linking) that leads to decreased collagen secretion, bone fragility (brittle "wormian" bone), short stature, scoliosis, tooth defects, hearing defects, and ligamentous laxity. Four types have been identified (Sillence), although the disorder is probably best considered as a continuum with different inheritance patterns and severity.

TYPE	INHERITANCE	SCLERAE	FEATURES
I	AD	Blue	Preschool age (tarda), hearing loss (IA = teeth involved; IB = teeth not affected)
II	AR	Blue	Lethal; concertina femur, beaded ribs
III	AR	Normal	Fractures at birth; progressive, short stature
IV	AD	Normal	Milder form, normal hearing (IVA = teeth involved; IVB = teeth not affected)

Radiographs demonstrate thin cortices. Histologically, increased diameters of haversian canals and osteocyte lacunae, increased numbers of cells, and replicated cement lines are noted, which result in the thin cortices seen on radiographs. Fractures are common; the initial healing is normal, but bone typically does not remodel. Fractures occur less frequently with advancing age (usually cease at puberty). Spinal deformities, including scoliosis (50%, bracing ineffective, fuse at 50 degrees), and compression fractures (codfish vertebrae) occur. The goal of treatment is fracture management and long-term rehabilitation. Bracing is indicated early to prevent deformity and minimize fractures. Sofield osteotomies ("shish kebab" bone with either fixed-length Rush rods or telescoping [Bailey-Dubow] intramedullary [IM] rods) are sometimes required for progressive bowing of long bones. Fractures in children under age 2 are treated similarly to those in children without OI. After age 2 years, telescoping IM rods (Bailey-DuBow) can be considered. Although synthetic salmon calcitonin and calcium supplements have been suggested to decrease the number of fractures in some OI patients, no medical therapy has been unequivocally proved effective.

C. Idiopathic Juvenile Osteoporosis—Rare, self-limited disorder that appears at ages 8–14 with osteopenia, growth arrest, and bone and joint pain. Serum calcium and phosphorus levels are normal. Typically, there is spontaneous resolution 2–4 years after onset of puberty. One must differentiate this disorder from other causes of osteopenia (e.g., osteogenesis imperfecta, malignancy, Cushing's disease).

D. Osteopetrosis—Failure of osteoclastic and chondroclastic resorption, probably secondary to a defect in the thymus leading to dense bone, "rugger jersey" spine, marble bone, and an "Erlenmeyer flask" proximal humerus/distal femur. Mild form is AD; "malignant" form is AR. Bone marrow transplant may be helpful for treating the malignant form (see Chapter 1, Basic Sciences).

E. Infantile Cortical Hyperostosis (Caffey's Disease)—Soft tissue swelling and bony cortical thickening (especially the jaw and ulna) that follows a febrile illness in infants 0–9 months old. Radiographs show characteristic periosteal reaction. This disorder may be differentiated from trauma (and child abuse) based on single bone development in the latter. A similar presentation may occur in older children (>6 months) with hypervitaminosis A. Caffey's disease, however, does not produce bleeding gums, fissures at the corners of the mouth, or the liver enzyme abnormalities associated with hypervitaminosis A. Infection, scurvy, and progressive diaphyseal dysplasia may also be items in the differential diagnosis for all-age children. Condition is benign and self-limiting.

F. Connective Tissue Syndrome—Heterogeneous group of disorders with a broad spectrum of features.

1. Marfan Syndrome—AD disorder of collagen synthesis (possibly the α_1 subunit) associated with arachnodactyly, long slender "sedia" finders, pectus deformities, scoliosis, cardiac (valvular) abnormalities, and ocular findings (superior lens dislocation). Other abnormalities may

include dural ectasia and meningocele. Joint laxity is treated conservatively; scoliosis and spondylolisthesis are treated aggressively. Bracing is ineffective. The presence of kyphosis with scoliosis requires anterior diskectomy and fusion with posterior fusion and instrumentation. Protrusio acetabuli can be treated with early triradiate cartilage fusion.

2. Ehlers-Danlos Syndrome—AD disorder with hyperextensibility of "cigarette paper" skin, joint hypermobility and dislocation, soft tissue/bone fragility, and soft tissue calcification. Failure of other supporting connective tissues can lead to vascular and visceral tears as well. Types II and III (of XI) are the most common and least disabling. Treatment consists of physical therapy, orthotics, and arthrodesis (soft tissue procedures fail).
3. Homocystinuria—AR inborn error of methionine metabolism (decreased enzyme cystathionine β-synthase). Accumulation of the intermediate metabolite homocysteine in the production of the amino acid cysteine can lead to osteoporosis, a marfanoid-like habitus (but with stiffening joints), and inferior lens dislocation. Diagnosis is made by demonstrating increased homocysteine in urine (cyanide-nitroprusside test). This disorder is differentiated from Marfan syndrome based on the direction of lens dislocation and the presence of osteoporosis in homocystinuria. Spontaneous thrombotic episodes can be intiated by minor procedures, anesthesia, and surgery. CNS effects, including mental retardation, are common in this disorder. Early treatment with vitamin B_6 and a decreased methionine diet is often successful.

G. Juvenile Rheumatoid Arthritis (JRA; Juvenile Chronic Arthritis)—Persistent noninfectious arthritis lasting more than 6 weeks to 3 months after other possible etiologies have been ruled out. The term juvenile chronic arthritis is gradually being adopted. To confirm the diagnosis, one of the following is required: rash, presence of rheumatoid factor, iridocyclitis, C-spine involvement, pericarditis, tenosynovitis, intermittent fever, or morning stiffness. JRA affects girls more than boys and commonly involves the wrist (flexed and ulnar-deviated) and hand (fingers extended, swollen, radially deviated). C-spine involvement can lead to kyphosis, facet ankylosis, and atlantoaxial subluxation. Lower extremity problems include flexion contractures (hip and knee flexed, ankle dorsiflexed), subluxation, and other deformities (hip protrusio, valgus knees, equinovarus feet). Five types of JRA are usually identified (Schaller) (Table 2–4). Synovial proliferation leads to joint destruction (chondrolysis) and soft tissue destruction. Radiographs can show rarefaction of juxta-articular bone. In 50% of patients symptoms resolve with sequelae, 25% are slightly disabled, and 20–25% have crippling arthritis/blindness. Therapy includes night splinting, salicylates, and rarely synovectomy (for chronic swelling refractory to medical management). Arthrodesis and arthroplasty may be required for severe JRA. Slit-lamp examination is required twice yearly, as progressive iridocyclitis can lead to rapid loss of vision if left untreated.

H. Ankylosing Spondylitis (AS)—Typically affects adolescent boys with asymmetric lower extremity large joint arthritis, heel pain, and sometimes eye symptoms; hip and back pain (cardinal symptom) may develop later. HLA-B27 test is positive in 90–95% of patients with AS or Reiter syndrome but also is positive in 4–8% of all white Americans. Therefore HLA-B27 is not a good screening test for AS. Radiographs show bilateral, symmetric sacroiliac erosion, followed by joint space narrowing, later ankylosis, and late vertebral spasms. NSAIDs and physical therapy are the mainstays of treatment.

I. Acute Rheumatic Fever—Autoimmune process that affects children 5–15 years old; it follows an untreated streptococcal infection by 2–4 weeks. Can present with migratory arthritis, fever, carditis, subcutaneous nodules, and **erythema marginatum** (pink rash on trunk and extremities but not the face ± history of strep infection). The Jones criteria are used for diagnosis (see Chapter 1, Basic Sciences). Treatment includes salicylates and appropriate antibiotics.

VI. Birth Injuries

A. Brachial Plexus Palsy—Decreasing in severity as a result of better obstetric management but still 2 per 1000 births have an injury associated with stretching or contusion of the brachial plexus. Occurs most commonly with large babies; shoulder dystocia, forceps delivery, breech position, and prolonged labor. Three types are commonly recognized.

TYPE	ROOTS	DEFICIT	PROGNOSIS
Erb-Duchenne	C5,6	Deltoid, cuff, elbow flexors, wrist and hand dorsiflexors; "waiter's tip" deformity	Best
Total plexus	C5–T1	Sensory and motor; flaccid arm	Worst
Klumpke	C8–T1	Wrist flexors, intrinsics; Horner	Poor

TABLE 2–4. TYPES OF JUVENILE RHEUMATOID ARTHRITIS

TYPE	%	JOINTS	ANA	RF	SYSTEMIC SYMPTOMS AND SIGNS	PROGRESS (%)
Systemic—Still's	25	Many	–	–	Fever, rash, organomegaly	25
Polyarticular/RF –	15	Many	1/3	–	Mild fever	30
Polyarticular/RF +	15	Many	1/3	+	Mild	25
Pauciarticular I (F)	30	Large	+	–	Iridocyclitis[a]	15
Pauciarticular II (M)	15	Large	–	–	HLA-B27 +, spondylitis	15

ANA, antinuclear antibodies; RF, rheumatoid factor; F, female; M, male.
[a] Slit-lamp examination is important to identify iridocyclitis, which is seen early in the pauciarticular form.

The key to therapy is maintaining passive range of motion and awaiting return of motor function (up to 18 months). As many as 90% or more cases eventually resolve without intervention. However, **lack of biceps function 3 months after injury** carries a poor prognosis and **may be an indication for surgery** (nerve grafting). Late musculoskeletal surgery can improve functional motion. Options include releasing contractures (Fairbanks), latissimus and teres major transfer to the shoulder external rotators (L'Episcopo), tendon transfers for elbow flexion (Clarke's pectoral transfer and Steindler's flexorplasty), proximal humerus rotational osteotomy (Wickstrom), and microsurgical nerve grafting. Reports have shown that release of the subscapularis tendon for internal rotation contacture, if performed by age 2 years, may result in improved active external rotation of the shoulder with muscle transfer to assist in active external rotation.

B. Torticollis—Congenital deformity resulting from contracture of the sternocleidomastoid muscle and associated with other "molding disorders," such as hip dysplasia and metatarsus adductus (up to 20% association with hip dysplasia). The differential diagnosis includes C-spine anomalies, ophthalmologic disorders that may require the child to tilt the head to see normally, and posterior fossa brain tumors. The etiology of congenital muscular torticollis remains uncertain, although most cases follow a difficult labor and delivery. Studies suggest that the muscle abnormality may be the result of an intrauterine compartment syndrome involving the sternocleidomastoid muscle compartment. Fibrosis of the muscle and a palpable mass are noted within the first 4 weeks of life. Most patients (90%) respond to passive stretching within the first year. Surgery (release of the muscle distally or proximally and distally) may be required if torticollis persists beyond the first year in order to prevent development of permanent plagiocephaly. Torticollis may also be associated with congenital atlanto-occipital abnormalities.

C. Congenital Pseudarthrosis of the Clavicle—May be confused with a fracture but involves the middle third of the clavicle; it does not have associated fracture callus and is not painful at birth. It almost always occurs on the right side. Surgical repair should be considered for pain and sometimes cosmesis.

VII. Cerebral Palsy (CP)

A. Introduction—Nonprogressive neuromusclular disorder with onset before age 2 years resulting from injury to the immature brain. Etiology includes prenatal intrauterine factors, perinatal infections (TORCH), prematurity (most common), anoxic injuries, head injuries, and meningitis. This upper motor neuron disease results in a mixture of muscle weakness and spasticity. Initially, the abnormal muscle forces cause a dynamic deformity at joints. Persistent spasticity leads to short muscles, contractures, bony deformity, and ultimately joint subluxation/dislocation.

B. Classification—CP can be classified based on physiology (according to the movement disorder) or topography (according to geographic distribution).

1. Physiologic Classification
   a. Spasticity—Characterized by increased muscle tone and hyperreflexia, with slow, restricted movements (because of co-contraction of agonist and antagonists). This form of CP is the most common and is most amenable to improvement of musculoskeletal function by operative intervention.
   b. Athetosis—Characterized by a constant succession of slow, writhing, involuntary movements, this form of CP is less common and more difficult to treat.
   c. Ataxia—Characterized by an inability to coordinate muscles for voluntary movement, resulting in an unbalanced, wide-based gait. Also less amenable to orthopaedic treatment.
   d. Mixed—Typically involves a combination of spasticity and athetosis with total body involvement.
2. Topographic Classification
   a. Hemiplegia—Involves the upper and lower extremities on the same side, usually with spasticity. These children often develop early "handedness." All children with hemiplegia are eventually able to walk regardless of treatment.
   b. Diplegia—Patients have more extensive involvement of the lower extremity than the upper extremity. Most diplegics eventually walk. IQ may be normal; strabismus is common.
   c. Total Involvement—These children have extensive involvement, low IQ, and high mortality; they usually are unable to walk.

C. Orthopaedic Assessment—Based on thorough birth and developmental history taking, and examination. A patient's locomotor profile is based on the persistence of primitive reflexes; the presence of two or more usually means the child will be a nonambulator. Commonly tested reflexes include the Moro startle reflex (disappears by age 6 months) and the parachute reflex (normally appears by 12 months of age). Surgery to improve function is considered for the child over 3 years old with spastic CP and voluntary motor control. Muscle imbalance yields later bony changes; therefore the general surgical plan is to perform soft tissue procedures early and, if necessary, bony procedures later. Surgery is commonly performed on patients who have no potential for walking or independence, particularly to keep the hips located (to avoid painful arthritis) and to maintain spinal stability (scoliosis surgery) to maintain sitting posture. Use of intramuscular botulinum A toxin to temporarily decrease dynamic spasticity is being investigated at several centers in the United States and Europe. The reduction of dynamic tone with use of botulinum toxin may promote normal muscle growth and avoid development of soft tissue contractures. Selective dorsal root rhizotomy is a neurosurgical procedure designed to decrease lower extremity spasticity. This treatment, indicated only for spastic CP, includes resection of dorsal rootlets not exhibiting a myographic or clinical response upon stimulation. It may help reduce spasticity and complement orthopaedic management in spastic diplegic patients. It requires multilevel laminectomy, which may include posterior stabilization to prevent development of late instability and deformity. Laminoplasty is now recommended rather than laminectomy. Discussion of specific disorders follows. Discussion of hand disorders is included in Chapter 6, Hand.

D. Gait Disorders—Probably the most common problem seen by the orthopaedist. Hemiplegics usually present with toe walking only. The use of three-dimensional computerized gait analysis with dynamic EMG and force plate studies have allowed a more scientific approach to preoperative decision making and postoperative analysis of the results of cerebral palsy surgery. Specific abnormal gait patterns have been identified (Table 2–5) and surgical procedures devised to treat them. The use of gait analysis has allowed a more individualized treatment plan for patients with CP. Lengthening of continuously active muscles and transfer of muscles out of phase is often helpful. Timing and indications for surgery require experience and skill because surgeries often should be done in tandem to best correct the problem (e.g., often heel cord lengthening alone exacerbates a crouched gait). In general, surgery is typically performed in the 4- to 5-year age group. A few generalized guidelines are given in Table 2–6.

E. Spinal Disorders—Most commonly involve scoliosis, which can be severe, making proper wheelchair sitting difficult. Surgical indications include curves >45–50 degrees, documented progression of >10 degrees, or deterioration of function. Two types of curves occur. Group I curves are double curves with thoracic and lumbar components and little pelvic obliquity. Group II curves are larger

TABLE 2–6. SURGICAL OPTIONS FOR GAIT DISORDERS

PROBLEM	DIAGNOSIS	SURGICAL OPTIONS
Hip flexion	Contraction (Thomas)	Psoas tenotomy or recession
Spastic hip	Decreased abduction/ uncovered head	Adductor release, osteotomy (late)
Hip adduction	Scissoring gait	Adductor release
Femoral anteversion	Prone internal rotation decreased	Osteotomy, VDRO, hamstring lengthening
Knee flexion	Contraction, increased popliteal angle	Hamstring lengthening
Knee hypertension	Recurvatum	Rectus femoris lengthening
Stiff leg gait	EMG—hamstring, quadriceps continuous, passive knee flexion decreased with hip extension	Distal rectus transfer to hamstrings
Talipes equinus	Toe walking	Achilles lengthening, Achilles transfer
Talipes varus	Standing position	Split ant. or post. tibialis transfer (based on EMG findings)
Talipes valgus	Standing position	Peroneal lengthening, Grice subtalar fusion
Hallux valgus	Exam/ radiographs	Osteotomy, MTP fusion

VDRO, varus derotation osteostomy.

TABLE 2–5. COMMON GAIT ABNORMALITIES OF THE KNEE IN CEREBRAL PALSY

	Phase					
	STANCE			SWING		
ABNORMALITY	IDS	SLS	SDS	I	M	T
Jump knee	↑F	V	V	V	V	↑F
Crouch knee	↑F	↑F	↑F	V	V	↑F
Stiff knee	V	V	V	↓F	↓F	V
Recurvatum knee	V	↑E	↑E	V	V	V

From Sutherland, D.H., and Davids, J.R.: Common gait abnormalities of the knee in cerebral palsy. Clin. Orthop. 288:139–147, 1993; reprinted by permission.
IDS, initial double stance; SLS, single limb stance; SDS, second double stance; I, initial swing; M, mid swing; T, terminal swing; F, flexion; V, variable; E, extension.

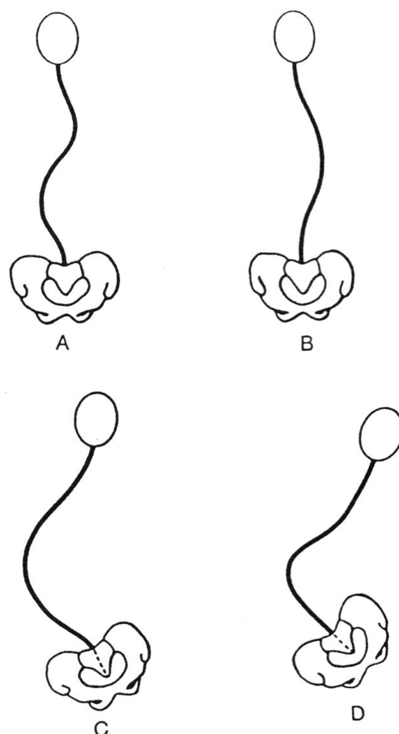

FIGURE 2–6. Curve patterns of cerebral palsy scoliosis. Group I curves are double curves with thoracic and lumbar components. There is little pelvic obliquity; the curve may be well balanced (*A*); or if the thoracic curve is more significant, there may be some imbalance (*B*). Group II curves are large lumbar or thoracolumbar curves with marked pelvic obliquity. There may be a short fractional curve between the end of the curve and the sacrum (*C*); or the curve may continue into the sacrum, with the sacral vertebrae forming part of the curve (*D*) (From Weinstein, S.L.: The Pediatric Spine: Principles and Practice. New York, Raven Press, 1994; reprinted by permission.)

lumbar or thoracolumbar curves with marked pelvic obliquity (Fig. 2–6). Treatment is tailored to the needs of the patient. Custom-molded seat inserts allow better positioning but do not prevent curve progression. Small curves with no loss of function or large curves in severely involved patients may require observation alone. Group I curves in ambulators are treated as idiopathic scoliosis with posterior fusion alone. Group I curves in sitters, or group II curves, require anterior and posterior fusion with Luque rods and sublaminar wires, as well as pelvic fixation with the Galveston technique and unit rod variation. The decision about one-stage versus two-stage interior and posterior fusion is based on the surgeon's skill and speed, blood loss, and the presence of other factors. Kyphosis is also common and may require fusion and instrumentation. It is important to assess nutritional status preoperatively and consider Nissen fundoplication/gastrostomy tube placement prior to spinal surgery if indicated.

F. Hip Subluxation/Dislocation—Treated initially with a soft tissue release (adductor/psoas) plus abduction bracing. Later it may require femoral or acetabular osteotomies (Dega) (or both) to maintain hip stability. The goal is to keep the hip reduced. Spastic dislocation often leads to painful arthritis, which is difficult to treat. This entity is characterized by four stages.
   1. Hip at risk—This situation is the only exception to the general rule of avoiding surgery in CP patients during the first 3 years of life. Characterized by abduction of <45 degrees with partial uncovering of the normal head on radiographs. May benefit from adductor and psoas release. Neurectomy of the anterior branch of the obturator nerve is now rarely performed because by converting an upper motor neuron lesion to a lower motor neuron lesion the muscle is made stiff and fibrotic.
   2. Hip Subluxation—Best treated with adductor tenotomy in children with abduction of <20 degrees, sometimes with psoas release/recession. Femoral or pelvic osteotomies may be considered with femoral coxa valga and acetabular dysplasia.
   3. Spastic Dislocation—May benefit from open reduction, femoral shortening, varus derotation osteotomy, and Salter, Dega (Fig. 2–7), triple or Chiari osteotomy. The type of pelvic osteotomy indicated is best determined by three dimensional CT scan, which will demonstrate the area of acetabular deficiency (anterior, lateral or posterior) and the congruency of the joint surfaces. Late dislocations may best be left out or treated with a Shanz abduction osteotomy. In extremely severe cases, a Girdlestone resection arthroplasty is performed.
   4. Windswept Hips—Characterized by abduction of one hip and adduction of the contralateral hip. Treatment is best directed at attempting to abduct the adducted hip with bracing or tenotomies and releasing the abduction contracture of the contralateral hip.

G. Knee Abnormalities—Usually includes flexion contractures and decreased range of motion. Hamstring lengthening is often helpful (sometimes increases lumbar lordosis). Distal transfer of an out-of-phase rectus femoris muscle to semitendinosis or gracilis has demonstrated superior results over proximal or distal rectus release in improving knee flexion and foot clearance during the early swing phase of gait.

H. Foot and Ankle Abnormalities—Common in CP gait, and dynamic EMG evaluation is often helpful.
   1. Equinovalgus Foot—More common in spastic diplegia. Caused by spastic peroneals, contracted heel cords, and ligamentous laxity. Peroneus brevis lengthening is often helpful to correct moderate valgus. Medial sliding calcaneal osteotomy is gradually replacing the Grice-Green bone block procedure for correcting hindfoot valgus because it maintains subtalar motion.
   2. Equinovarus Foot—More common in spastic hemiplegia; caused by overpull of the posterior or anterior tibialis tendons (or both). Lengthening of the posterior tibialis is rarely indicated because of recurrence and development of a calcaneovalgus foot. Likewise, transfer of an entire muscle (posterior or anterior tibialis) is rarely recommended. **Split muscle transfers are helpful** in certain circumstances, especially **when the affected muscle is spastic during both**

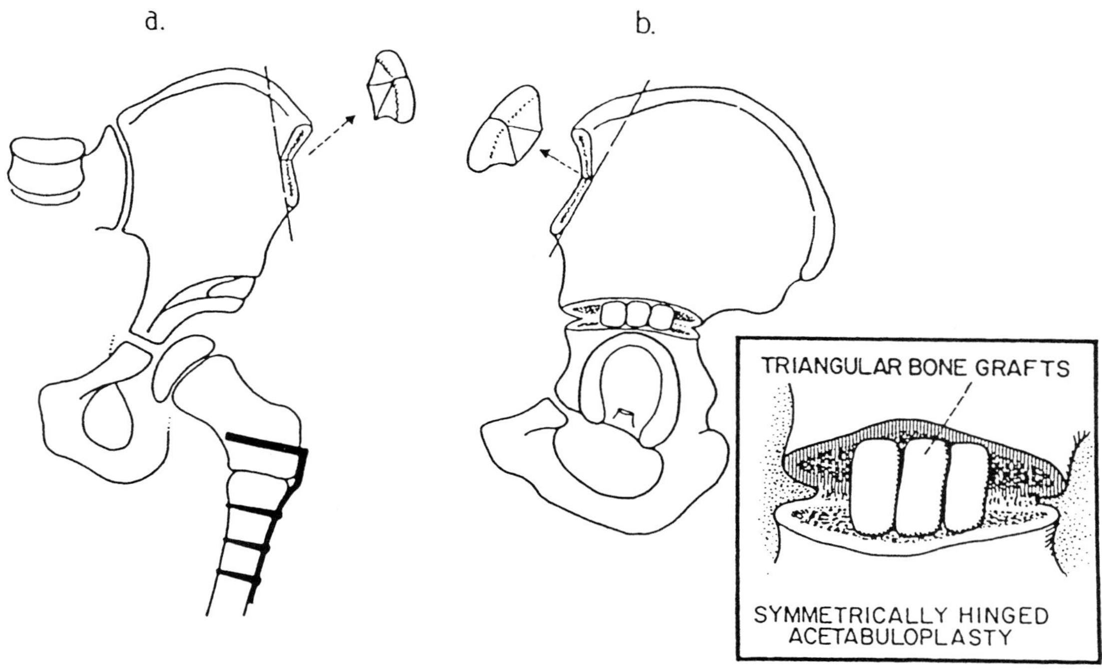

FIGURE 2–7. Placement of graft for Dega acetabuloplasty. A bone graft is obtained from the anterosuperior iliac crest and converted to three small triangles, with the base measuring 1 cm (*a*). The grafts are placed in the osteotomy site with the largest placed in the area where maximum improvement of coverage is desired (*b*). The triangular wedges are packed close to each other to prevent collapse, turning, or dislodgement; and the result is a symmetric hinging on the triradiate cartilage (*inset*). With the medial wall of the pelvis maintained, the elasticity of the osteotomy keeps the wedges in place. No pins are necessary to maintain the osteotomy. (Adapted from Mubarak, S.J., Valencia, F.G., and Wenger, D.R.: One stage reconstruction of the spastic hip. J. Bone Joint Surg. [Am.] 74:1352, 1992; reprinted by permission.)

stance and swing phases of gait. The split posterior tibialis transfer (rerouting half of the tendon dorsally to the peroneus brevis) is used in cases with spasticity of the muscle, flexible varus foot, and weak peroneals. Complications include decreased foot dorsiflexion. Split anterior tibialis transfer (rerouting half of its tendon lateral to the cuboid) is used in patients with spasticity of the muscle and a flexible varus deformity. Complications of this procedure include overcorrection. Most recently, combined split anterior tibial tendon transfer and intramuscular lengthening of the posterior tibial tendon has been recommended for dynamic varus of the hindfoot and adduction of the forefoot during both stance and swing phases of the gait.

VIII. Neuromuscular Disorders

A. Arthrogrypotic Syndromes

1. Arthrogryposis Multiplex Congenita (Amyoplasia)—Nonprogressive disorder of multiple etiologies with multiple congenitally rigid joints; believed to be caused by oliogohydramnios or any condition limiting fetal movement. This disorder, which can be myopathic, neuropathic, or mixed, is associated with loss of anterior horn cells and other neural elements of the spinal cord, possibly secondary to an in utero viral infection. In some ways, arthrogryposis resembles polio, as sensory function is maintained and motor function is lost. Evaluation should include neurologic studies, enzyme tests, and muscle biopsy (at 3–4 months). Affected patients typically have normal facies, normal intelligence, multiple joint contractures, and no visceral abnormalities. Upper extremity involvement usually includes adduction and internal rotation of the humerus, elbow extension and wrist flexion, and ulnar deviation. Treatment consists in passive stretching, serial casts for elbow contractures, and possibly osteotomies after 4 years of age to allow independent eating. One upper extremity should be left in extension at the elbow for positioning and perineal care and one elbow allowed flexion for feeding. In the lower extremity, rigid club feet, hip dislocation, and knee contractures are common. The spine may be involved with characteristic "C-shaped" (neuromuscular) scoliosis. Fractures are also common (25%). Treatment includes soft tissue releases (especially hamstrings), open reduction of hip dislocation, aggressive surgical treatment of club feet with an initial attempt at posteromedial release (followed by bony procedures if the deformity recurs) and attempts at achieving ambulation. The goal is a stiff, plantigrade foot that enables shoe wear and possibly ambulation. Knee contractures should be corrected before hip reduction in order to maintain the reduction.
2. Larsen Syndrome—Similar to arthrogryposis in

clinical appearance, but joints are less rigid. The disorder primarily is associated with multiple joint dislocations (including bilateral congenital knee dislocations), abnormal (flattened) facies, scoliosis, and cervical kyphosis.

3. Distal Arthrogryposis Syndrome—AD disorder that predominantly affects the hands and feet. Ulnarly deviated fingers (at MCP joints), MCP and PIP flexion contractures, and adducted thumbs with web space thickening are common. Club feet and vertical talus are common in the feet.
4. Multiple Pterygium Syndrome—AR disorder characterized by cutaneous flexor surface webs, congenital vertical talus, and scoliosis.

B. Myelodysplasia (Spina Bifida)

1. Introduction—Disorder of spinal cord development/closure or secondary rupture of the developing cord secondary to hydrocephalus (two theories are proposed for the etiology). Includes spina bifida occulta (defect in the vertebral arch with confined cord and meninges); meningocele (sac with neural elements protruding through the defect); myelomeningocele (spina bifida; with protrusion of the sac with neural elements); and rachischisis (neural elements exposed with no covering). Can be diagnosed in utero (increased α-fetoprotein) in a high risk infant (usually with a positive family history). Muscle imbalance and intrauterine positioning frequently lead to hip dislocations, knee hyperextension, and club feet. Function is primarily related to the level of the defect and the associated congenital abnormalities. **Sudden changes in function (rapid increase of scoliotic curvature, spasticity, and new neurologic deficit) can be associated with tethered cord, hydrocephalus (most common), or hydromyelia** (increased fluid in the central canal of the cord), among other defects. Head CT (70% of myelodysplastics have hydrocephalus) and a myelogram or spinal MRI are required. **Fractures are also common in myelodysplasia,** most often about the knee and hip in 3- to 7-year-olds and frequently can be diagnosed only by noting **redness, warmth,** and **swelling.** Treatment is conservative (avoid disuse). Fractures usually heal with abundant callus. The myelodysplasia level is based on the lowest functional level (Table 2–7). L4 is a key level because quadriceps can function and allow community ambulation.
2. Treatment Principles—Careful observation of patients with myelodysplasia is important. Several myelodysplasia "milestones" have been developed to assess progress.

AGE (mo)	FUNCTION	TREATMENT
4–6	Head control	Positioning
6–10	Sitting	Supports/orthotics
10–12	Prone mobility	Prone board
12–15	Upright stance	Standing orthosis
15–18	Upright mobility	Trunk/extremity orthosis

Treatment utilizes a team approach to allow maximum function consistent with the patient's level and other abnormalities and as normal development as possible. Proper use of orthotics is essential in myelodysplasia. Determination of ambulation potential is based on the level of the deficit. Surgery for myelodysplasia focuses on balancing of muscles and correction of deformities. Increased attention has been focused on latex sensitivity in myelodysplastic patients. Allergic reactions are now well described in the literature. Consideration should be given to providing a latex-free environment whenever surgical procedures are performed in spina bifida patients.

3. Hip Problems—Flexion contractures occur commonly in patients with thoracic/high lumbar myelomeningocele owing to unopposed hip flexors or in patients who are sitters. Treatment for these patients consists of anterior hip release with tenotomy of the iliopsoas, sartorius, rectus femoris, and tensor fascia lata. For low lumbar level patients the psoas should be preserved for independent ambulation. Hip abduction contracture can cause pelvic obliquity and scoliosis; it is treated with proximal division of the fascia lata and distal iliotibial band release (Ober-Yount procedure). Adduction contractures are treated with adductor myotomy. Hip dislocation occurs frequently in myelodysplastic patients because of paralysis of the hip abductors and extensors with unopposed hip flexors and adductors. **Hip dislocation is most common at the L3/L4 level.** Treatment of hip dislocation is controversial, but in general containment is considered essential only in patients with a functioning quadriceps. The aim of hip surgery is to maintain range of motion and achieve full hip extension. Containment is a secondary concern. Treatment of hip dislocation is based on the level of the defect: If L2 or higher, leave both hips symmetric; if L4 or lower (and neurologically stable) the dislocation should be reduced. The latter usually requires (1) correction of muscle imbalance by transfer of the external oblique to augment the

TABLE 2–7. CHARACTERISTICS OF MYELODYSPLASIA LEVELS

LEVEL	HIP	KNEE	FEET	ORTHOSIS	AMBULATION
L1	External rotation/flexed	—	Equinovarus	HKAFO	Nonfunctional
L2	Adduction/flexed	Flexed	Equinovarus	HKAFO	Nonfunctional
L3	Adduction/flexed	Recurvatum	Equinovarus	KAFO	Household
L4	Adduction/flexed	Extended	Cavovarus	AFO	Household plus
L5	Flexed	Limited flexion	Calcaneal valgus	AFO	Community
S1			Foot deformities	Shoes	Near normal

HKAFO, hip–knee–ankle–foot orthosis; KAFO, knee–ankle foot orthosis; AFO, ankle foot orthosis.

hip external rotators; (2) release of soft tissue contractures; (3) correction of coxa valga with varus derotational osteotomy (VDRO) and acetabular dysplasia with a Pemberton or Shelf acetabuloplasty; (4) correction of capsular laxity with capsular plication. Stiffness is rarely a problem if all procedures are carried out at one time but may occur after multiple operations. Redislocation may occur no matter what treatment is used to maintain the reduction. Late dislocation at the low lumbar level may be a sign of neurologic decompensation due to a tethered cord, which must be released prior to reducing the hip.

4. Knee Problems—Usually includes quadriceps weakness (usually treated with knee-ankle-foot orthoses [KAFOs]). Flexion deformities (associated with hip flexion deformities, calcaneovalgus feet, and tethered cord) are not important in wheelchair-bound patients but can be treated with hamstring release and posterior capsular release. Recurvatum (associated with club feet and hip dislocation) is rarely a problem and can be treated early with serial casting and KAFOs. Tenotomies (quadriceps lengthening) are sometimes required. Valgus deformities are usually not a problem. Sometimes iliotibial band release or late osteotomies are needed.
5. Ankle and Foot Deformities—Objectives are to obtain braceable, plantigrade feet and muscle balance. Affected patients may present with a valgus foot. Total contact AFOs often are helpful, but clubfoot release, tendon release (anterior tibialis, Achilles), posterior tibialis lengthening, and other procedures may be required. Triple arthrodesis should be avoided in most myelodysplastic patients and is used only for severe deformities with sensate feet. Ankle valgus (resulting from a disparity in fibular versus tibial growth) is addressed by tibial osteotomy or hemiepiphysiodesis (older patients) if the fibula is shortened or Achilles tendon tenodesis to the fibula (patients <8 years old).

   Rigid clubfoot, secondary to retained activity or contracture of tibialis posterior and tibialis anterior, is common in L4 level patients. Treatment consists of complete subtalar release via a transverse (Cincinnati) incision, lengthening of tibialis posterior and Achilles tendons, and transfer of tibialis anterior tendon to the dorsal midfoot.

   Secondary hindfoot valgus due to overlengthening of posterior tibial tendon can be treated with a medial displacement calcaneal sliding osteotomy. For severe rotational deformities distal tibial osteotomy may be required. Subtalar procedures, in general, should be avoided and AP radiographs of the ankle should be carefully reviewed to rule out more common involvement of this joint.
6. Spine Problems—Deformity can result from the spine disorder itself, resulting in an upper lumbar kyphosis, or other congenital malformation (hemivertebrae, diastomatomyelia, unsegmented bars) of the spine due to a lack of segmentation or formation. Scoliosis can also occur with severe lordosis as a result of muscular imbalance due to thoracic level paraplegia. Spinal deformities are often severe and progressive. Nearly all patients with thoracic level paraplegia develop scoliosis. Attempts at bracing (TLSO) may fail and require subcutaneous rodding for very young children with fusion later. **Rapid curve progression** can be associated with hydrocephalus or a **tethered cord,** which may manifest as lower extremity spasticity (MRI helpful for evaluation). Segmental Luque sublaminar wiring with fixation to the pelvis (Galveston technique) or to the front of the sacrum (Dunn technique) (Fig. 2–8), usually preceded by anterior release and fusion, is often required for curves >60 degrees. Kyphosis in myelodysplasia is a difficult problem. Resection of the kyphosis with local fusion (Lindseth procedure (Figs. 2–9, 2–10) or fusion to the pelvis is required in severe cases. Infection rates are high owing to frequent septicemia and poor skin quality over the lumbar spine.

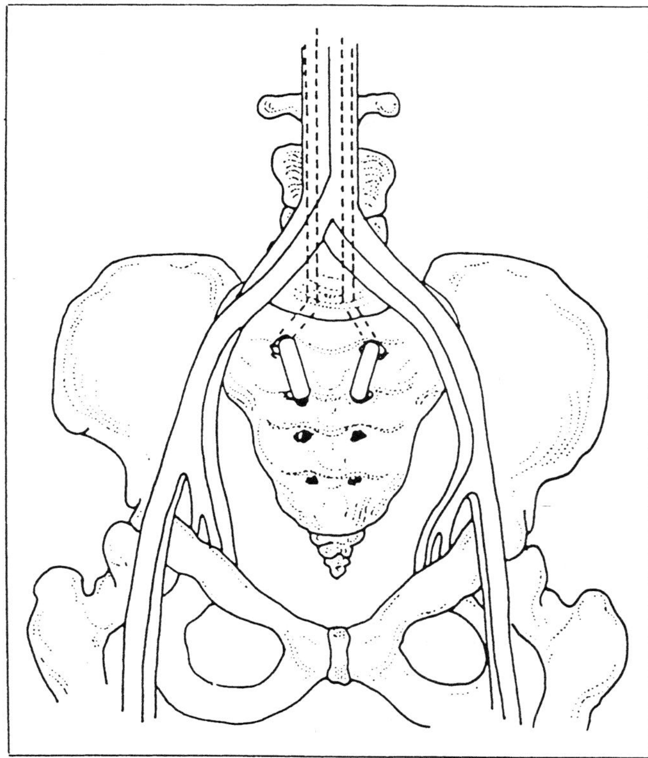

FIGURE 2–8. Anterior placement of Luque rods through the first sacral foramina. The first sacral foramina are medial to the internal iliac vessels. (From Warner, W.C., and Fackler, C.D.: Comparison of two instrumentation techniques in treatment of lumbar kyphosis in myelodysplasia. J. Pediatr. Orthop. 13:704–708, 1993; reprinted by permission.)

7. Pelvic Obliquity—Can occur in myelodysplasia as a result of prolonged unilateral hip contractures or scoliosis. Custom seat cushions, thoracolumbosacral orthosis (TLSO), spinal fusion, and ultimately pelvis osteotomies may be required for treatment.

C. Myopathies (Muscular Dystrophies)—Noninflammatory inherited disorders with progressive mus-

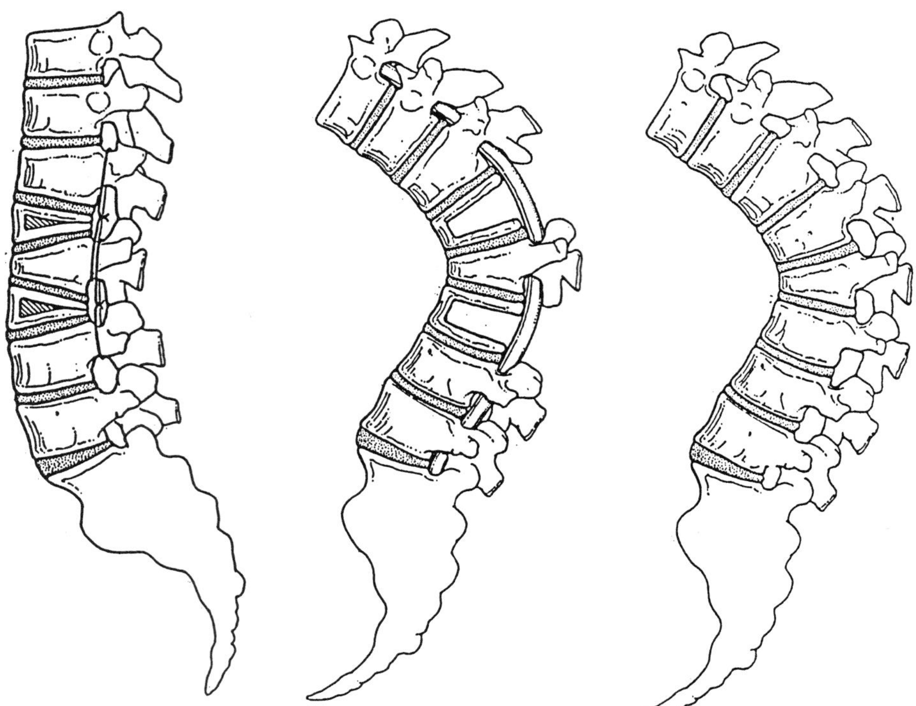

FIGURE 2–9. *L → R,* C-Shaped kyphosis before removal of the ossific nucleus from its vertebrae. *Center,* Spinous process, lamina pedicle, and ossific nucleus have been removed from the vertebrae above and below the apical vertebrae. Growth plate, disc, and anterior cortex are left intact. *Right,* Deformity is reduced by pushing the apical vertebrae forward and placing tension-band wiring around the pedicles. (From Lindseth, R.E.: Spine deformity in myelomeningocele. Instr. Course Lect. 40:276, 1991; reprinted by permission.)

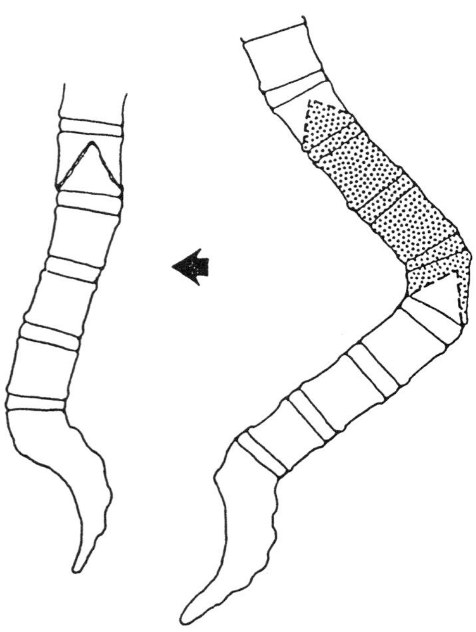

FIGURE 2–10. Rigid S-shaped kyphosis is corrected by excising the vertebrae between the apex of the kyphosis and the lordosis and fusing the apical vertebrae. (From Lindseth, R.E.: Myelomeningocele. In Lovell and Winters' Pediatric Orthopaedics, 3rd ed., Morrisy, R.T., ed., p. 522. Philadelphia, JB Lippincott, 1990; reprinted by permission.)

cle weakness. Treatment focuses on physical therapy, orthotics, genetic counseling, and surgery for severe problems (includes tibialis posterior transfers, release of flexion contractures, and early fusion for neuromusculasr scoliosis). Fusion (often T2 to sacrum) should be done earlier than in idiopathic scoliosis (often at 25 degrees of curvature) before pulmonary status deteriorates. Several types of muscular dystrophy are classified based on their inheritance pattern.

1. Duchenne—Sex-linked recessive abnormality of young boys, manifested as clumsy walking, decreased motor skills, lumbar lordosis, calf pseudohypertrophy, positive Gowers sign (rises by walking the hands up the legs to compensate for gluteus maximus and quadriceps weakness), **markedly elevated CPK,** and absent dystrophin protein on muscle biopsy DNA testing. Hip extensors are typically the first muscle group affected. Muscle biopsy shows foci of necrosis and connective tissue infiltration. Treatment is based on keeping the patient ambulatory as long as possible. They lose independent ambulation by age 10, although use of KAFOs and release of contractures can extend walking ability for 2–4 years. Patients are usually wheelchair-bound by age 15 years. With no muscle support scoliosis progresses rapidly between age 13 and 14 years. They become bedridden by age 16 owing to spinal deformity and are unable to sit for more than 8 hours (see neuromuscular section of spine deformity for treatment of

scoliosis). These children usually die of cardiorespiratory complications before age 20. Differential diagnosis includes **Becker's** dystrophy (also sex-linked recessive), which is often seen in 7-year-old, red/green color-blind boys with a similar, but less severe, picture. This diagnosis applies for all who live beyond age 22 years without respiratory support. Abnormal dystrophin protein is present on muscle biopsy DNA testing.

2. Fascioscapulohumeral—AD disorder typically seen in patients 6–20 years old with facial muscle abnormalities, normal CPK, and winging of the scapula (stabilizes with scapulothoracic fusion).
3. Limb–Girdle—AR disorder; seen in those 10–30 years old with pelvic or shoulder girdle involvement and decreased CPK values.
4. Others—**Gowers** (distal involvement, high incidence in Sweden); **ocular, oculopharyngeal** (high incidence in French-Canadians).

D. Myotonic Myopathies—AD disorders with inability of muscles to relax after contractures. There are three basic types.

1. Myotonia Congenita (Thomsen's)—Defect localized to chromosome 7 region of human skeletal muscle chloride channel. Widespread involvement, no weakness, increased hypertrophy. Improves with exercise.
2. Dystrophic Myotonia (Steinert's)—Defect in chromosome 19. Small gonads, heart disease, low IQ distal/lower extremity involvement, "dive bomber" EMG.
3. Paramyotonia Congenita (Eulenburg's)—Defect in chromosome 17 skeletal sodium channel. Myotonic symptoms develop with exposure to cold, especially in the hands (symptoms often respond to quinine or mexiletine).

E. Congenital Myopathies—Nonprogressive AD disorders that present as a "floppy baby." Hypotonia is predominant in the pelvic and shoulder girdles. Muscle biopsy histochemical analysis is required for differentiation of the four types.

F. Polymyositis, Dermatomyositis—Characterized by a febrile illness that may be acute or insidious. Females predominate and typically exhibit photosensitivity and increased CPK and ESR values. Muscles are tender, brawny, and indurated. Biopsy demonstrates the pathognomonic inflammatory response.

G. Hereditary Neuropathies—Disorders associated with multiple CNS lesions, including the following.

1. Friedreich's Ataxia—Spinocerebellar degenerative disease with onset before age 10 years. Present with staggering, wide-based gait, nystagmus, cardiomyopathy, cavus foot (treated with plantar release ± metatarsal and calcaneal osteotomies early, and triple arthrodesis later), and scoliosis (treated much like Duchenne muscular dystrophy scoliosis). **Involves motor and sensory defects.** Ataxia limits ambulation by age 30, and death occurs by age 40–50.
2. Charcot-Marie-Tooth Disease (Peroneal Muscular Atrophy)—Autosomal dominant motor sensory demyelinating neuropathy. Two forms are described: a hypertrophic form (CMT-1) with onset during the second decade of life, and a neuronal form (CMT-2) with onset during the third or fourth decade but with more extensive foot involvement. Orthopaedic manifestations include pes cavus, hammer toes with frequent corns/calluses, peroneal weakness, and "stork legs." Low nerve conduction velocities with prolonged distal latencies are noted in peroneal, ulnar, and median nerves. Intrinsic wasting is noted in hands. Treatment includes plantar release, posterior tibial tendon transfer (if flexible), triple arthrodesis versus calcaneal and metatarsal osteotomies (if bony deformity not fixed and foot not too short), Jones procedure for hammer toes, and intrinsic minus procedures for hand deformity. **Involves motor defects much more than sensory defects.**
3. Dejerine-Sottas Disease—AR hypertrophic neuropathy of infancy (CMT-3). Delayed ambulation, pes cavus foot, footdrop, stocking–glove dysesthesia, and spinal deformities are common. Confined to wheelchair by third or fourth decade.
4. Riley-Day Syndrome (Dysautonomia)—One of five inherited (AR) sensory and autonomic neuropathies. This disease is found only in patients of Ashkenazic Jewish ancestry. Clinical presentation includes dysphagia, alacrima, pneumonia, excessive sweating, postural hypotension, and sensory loss.

H. Myasthenia Gravis—Chronic disease with insidious development of easy muscle fatigability after exercise. Caused by competitive inhibition of acetylcholine receptors at the motor end plate by antibodies produced in the thymus gland. Treatment consists of cyclosporin, anti-acetylcholinesterase agents or thymectomy.

I. Anterior Horn Cell Disorders

1. Poliomyelitis—Viral destruction of anterior horn cells in the spinal cord and brain stem motor nuclei; all but disappeared in the United States after vaccine was developed. Many surgical procedures still used were developed for treatment of polio. The hallmark of polio is muscle weakness with normal sensation.
2. Spinal Muscle Atrophy—AR; loss of horn cells from the spinal cord. Most common diagnosis in girls with progressive weakness. **Werdnig-Hoffman** form—present at birth, short life-span. **Kugelberg-Wellander** form—later onset, long life-span. Often associated with progressive scoliosis that is best treated surgically like Duchenne muscular dystrophy curves, except that fusion may be required while patients are still ambulatory (may result in loss of ambulation ability). Patients have symmetric paresis with more involvement of the lower extremity and proximal muscles. Four types of spinal muscle atrophy (Table 2–8) are commonly recognized (Evans and Drennan), but they probably represent the spectrum of a single disease.

J. Acute Idiopathic Postinfectious Polyneuropathy (**Guillain-Barré Syndrome**)—Symmetric ascending motor paresis caused by demyelination following viral infection. **CSF protein is typically elevated.** Usually self-limited; better prognosis with the acute form.

TABLE 2–8. TYPES OF SPINAL MUSCLE ATROPHY

TYPE	ONSET	AMBULATION	SCOLIOSIS FIRST DECADE (DEGREES)	SURVIVAL AGE (YEARS)	COMMENTS
I[a]	Birth	None	60+	0–10	Severe respiratory involvement
II	6 Months	None	50	>35	Has head control
III	1 Year	Orthotics	20	>45	Fusion for scoliosis
IV[b]	Child	Can run	Variable	>55	Lose ambulation by mid-30s

[a] Werdnig-Hoffman disease.
[b] Kugelberg-Welander disease.

K. Overgrowth Syndromes

1. Proteus Syndrome—Overgrowth of hands and feet with bizarre facial disfigurement, scoliosis, genu valum, hemangiomas, lipomas, and nevi.
2. Klippel-Trenaunay Syndrome—Overgrowth caused by underlying AV malformations. Associated with cutaneous hemangiomas and varicosities. Severely hypertrophied extremities often require amputation.
3. Hemihypertrophy—Can be caused by various syndromes, but most are idiopathic. Most commonly known cause is neurofibromatosis. This disorder is often associated with renal abnormalities (especially Wilms' tumor). Management of associated leg-length discrepancy is discussed below.

IX. Pediatric Spine

A. Idiopathic Scoliosis

1. Introduction—Lateral deviation and rotation of the spine without an identifiable cause but may be related to a hormonal, brain stem, or proprioception disorder. Most patients have a positive family history, but there is variable expressivity. The curve description is characterized by its apex. Right thoracic curves, with apex T7 or T8, are the most common, followed by double major (right thoracic and left lumbar), left lumbar, and right lumbar curves, in that order. In adolescents **left thoracic curves** are rare, and **evaluation of the spinal cord by MRI** is suggested to rule out cord abnormalities. The adolescent form of idiopathic scoliosis is the most common, but one also sees the infantile form (left thoracic curves are seen in England that may be related to supine positioning of neonates) and juvenile form (right thoracic with earlier onset than adolescent form). Curve progression is more likely with greater curve magnitudes (>20 degrees), younger age (<12 years), and lesser Risser stage (0–1) at presentation (Table 2–9). About 75% of immature patients with curves of 20–30 degrees will progress at least 5 degrees. Severe curves (>90 degrees) may be associated with cardiopulmonary dysfunction, early death, pain, and a decreased self-image.
2. Diagnosis—Patients are often referred via school screening-based truncal rotation with forward bending as measured by scoliometer. A threshold level of 7 degrees is thought to be an acceptable compromise between overreferral and a high false-negative rate. Physical findings include shoulder or pelvic asymmetry, trunk shift, limb-length inequality, asymmetric umbilical reflex, spinal curvature, and asymmetric rib hump (seen with forward bending). Careful neurologic examination of spinal cord pathology is important (especially with left thoracic curves). Standing posteroanterior radiographs (and lateral view if abnormalities are suspected) are obtained, and curves are measured based on the Cobb method (measured perpendicular to end plate of most tilted [end] vertebra) (Fig. 2–11). Typically there is hypokyphosis of the apical vertebrae. Inclusion of the iliac crest on radiographs allows determination of skeletal maturity (based on ossification of the iliac crest apophysis and graded 0–5 [Risser stage]). A lateral radiograph to assess for spondylolisthesis is often recommended. An MRI scan is obtained for skeletal cases with structural abnormalities on plain films, excessive kyphosis, early-onset scoliosis (age <11 years), rapid curve progression, neurologic signs/symptoms, associated syndromes, and left thoracic/thoracolumbar curves.
3. Treatment—Based on the maturity of the patient (Risser stage and presence of menarche), degree of curve, and curve progression. Treatment options include observation, bracing, and surgery. Exercise and electrical stimulation have not been shown to affect the normal history of curve progression. Bracing only helps to halt curve progression and does not improve cosmetic appearance. The Milwaukee brace or Boston underarm brace with Milwaukee superstructure are used for curves with the apex at or above T7. The Boston-type underarm TLSO brace is used for curves with the apex at T8 or below. Patients with thoracic lordosis or hypo-

TABLE 2–9. INCIDENCE OF PROGRESSION AS RELATED TO THE MAGNITUDE OF THE CURVE AND THE RISSER SIGN

RISSER SIGN	PERCENT OF CURVES THAT PROGRESSED 5–19° CURVES	20–29° CURVES
0, 1	22	68
2, 3, 4	1.6	23

From Lonstein, J.E., and Carlson, J.M.: The prediction of curve progression in untreated idiopathic scoliosis during growth. J. Bone Joint Surg. [Am.] 66: 1067, 1984; reprinted by permission.

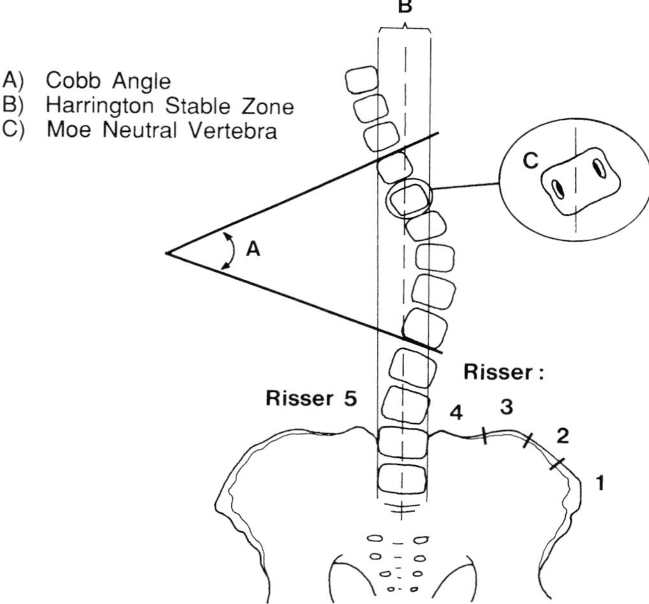

FIGURE 2–11. Measurements for idiopathic scoliosis. Note the Cobb angle (*A*), Harrington's stable zone (*B*), Moe's neutral vertebra (*C*), and Risser staging.

kyphosis are poor candidates for bracing. **The effectiveness of bracing patients with idiopathic scoliosis is dose-related** (the more the brace is worn each day, the more effective it is). Although the efficacy of full-time wear has been well demonstrated, long-term prospective studies on part-time brace wear are still lacking. Use of the Charleston nighttime brace is still under investigation. Surgical options include instrumentation without fusion for infantile and juvenile forms of scoliosis and a variety of methods for adolescent idiopathic scoliosis. Posterior fusion and instrumentation with Harrington distraction rods has been the traditional standard. Sublaminar wiring (Luque) offers excellent fixation, but because of its slightly greater risk for neurologic injury it is now used only for neuromuscular scoliosis. The Drummond technique of spinous process wiring provides improved fixation with less risk of neurologic sequelae. Cotrel-Dobousset and TSRH implants allow for segmental fixation and some rotational correction while maintaining sagittal plane contours; they generally do not require long-term immobilization. They are more expensive, however, and concern has been raised about the increasing incidence of late reaction to metal wear debris leading to low grade infections with these modular systems. As a result of these late problems the new modular systems are more likely to require late instrumentation removal. Dwyer or Zielke anterior instrumentation is useful for selected lumbar or thoracolumbar curves. Anterior instrumentation may result in more correction and save lower fusion levels; but it may be associated with higher pseudarthrosis rates, development of lumbar kyphosis, and an uncosmetic scar. The following general treatment guidelines apply.

CURVE (degrees)	PROGRESSION (degrees)	RISSER	THERAPY
0–25	—	Immature	Serial observation
25–30	5–10	Immature	Brace
30–40	—	Immature	Brace
>40	—	Immature	Surgery
>50	—	Mature	Surgery (young adults)

4. Fusion Levels—Successful surgery is based on picking appropriate fusion levels, among other considerations. Several methods have been developed to select the correct levels. Harrington recommended fusion one level above and two levels below the end vertebrae if these levels fell within the **stable zone** (within parallel lines drawn vertically up from the lumbosacral facet joints). Moe recommended fusion to the **neutral vertebrae** (without rotation—pedicles symmetric) (Fig. 2–11). It is almost never necessary to fuse to the pelvis in adolescent idiopathic scoliosis. Cochran identified a markedly **increased incidence of late low back pain with fusion to L5** and some increase with fusion to L4; every attempt therefore should be made to stop the fusion at L3 or above. King and Moe identified five patterns and treatment options (Table 2–10; Fig. 2–12). Bridwell noted thoracic decompensation after use of CD instrumentation for right thoracic idiopathic scoliosis. He reviewed his results with five different hook patterns for the King–Moe II, III, and IV curves and recommended stopping the fusion one segment short of the stable vertebra with all hooks in a distraction mode, or reversal of rod bend and hook on the left side between the neutral

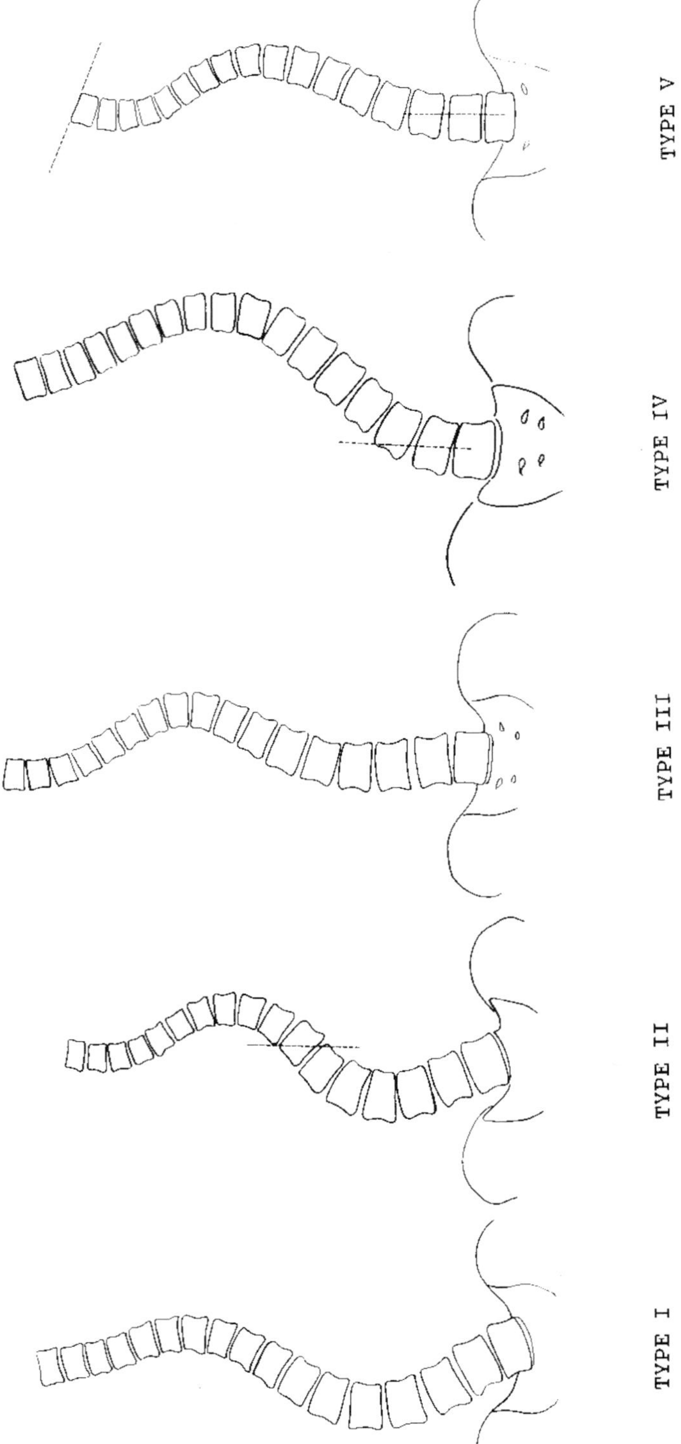

FIGURE 2–12. Five types of scoliotic curves (I–V). See text for description. (From King, H.A., Moe, J.H., Bradford, D.S., and Winter, R.B.: The selection of fusion levels in thoracic idiopathic scoliosis. J. Bone Joint Surg. [Am.] 65:1302–1313, 1983; reprinted by permission.)

TABLE 2–10. PATTERNS OF IDIOPATHIC SCOLIOSIS AND TREATMENT OPTIONS (AFTER KING)

TYPE	DEFINITION	FLEXIBILITY (FLEXION-EXTENSION)	TREATMENT
I	S-Shaped thoracolumbar curve; crosses midline	Lumbar < thoracic (or lumbar curve larger)	Fuse lumbar and thoracic vertebrae
II	S-Shaped thoracolumbar curve; crosses midline	Lumbar > thoracic (and thoracic curve larger)	Fuse thoracic vertebrae[a]
III	Thoracic curve; lumbar vertebrae do not cross midline	Lumbar vertebrae highly flexible	Fuse thoracic vertebrae
IV	Long thoracic curve	L4 tilts to thoracic curve	Fuse through L4
V	Double thoracic curve	T1 tilts to upper curve	Fuse through T2

[a] Experience with lumbar curves >50 degrees suggests that large lumbar curves should be included in the fusion for rotational correction.

and stable vertebra to decrease the incidence of decompensation (Table 2–11; Fig. 2–13). King–Moe type V curves require careful preoperative analysis. If the left shoulder is elevated on presentation, the upper curve must be included in the fusion or the left shoulder will be even more elevated postoperatively. If the shoulders are level and the upper curve is flexible, the upper thoracic curve alone may be fused. If the shoulders are level and the upper thoracic curve is rigid, both the upper and lower curves must be incorporated into the fusion.

5. Complications—The most disastrous complication of spinal surgery is a neurologic deficit that was not present preoperatively. Successful surgical intrevention is based on careful technique (intraoperative monitoring [SSEP] is helpful ± Stagnara wake-up test and clonus tests). Apel described the use of SSEP with temporary occlusion of segmental spinal arteries to avoid ischemic neurologic injury during thoracic anterior spinal fusion. It is especially useful in patients with congenital kyphoscoliosis. Attempting excessive correction or placement of sublaminar wires is associated with an increased risk of neurologic damage. Minimizing blood loss and the use of autologous blood is important to avoid transfusion-associated problems. Surgical complications include pseudarthrosis (1–2%), wound infection (1–2%), and implant failure (early hook cutout and late rod breakage). Late rod breakage frequently signifies failure of fusion. Only an asymptomatic pseudarthrosis (no pain or loss of curve correction) should be observed because the results of the late repair do not differ from those performed earlier. Use of a compression implant facilitates pseudoarthrosis repair. Creation of a "flat back syndrome," or early fatigability and pain due to loss of lumbar lordosis, can be minimized with rod contouring and effective use of compression and distraction devices. Treatment of this condition requires posterior closing wedge osteotomies; and the results appear to be improved, with maintenance of correction, if anterior release and fusion precede the posterior osteotomies. The Crankshaft phenomenom occurs in the setting of continued ante-

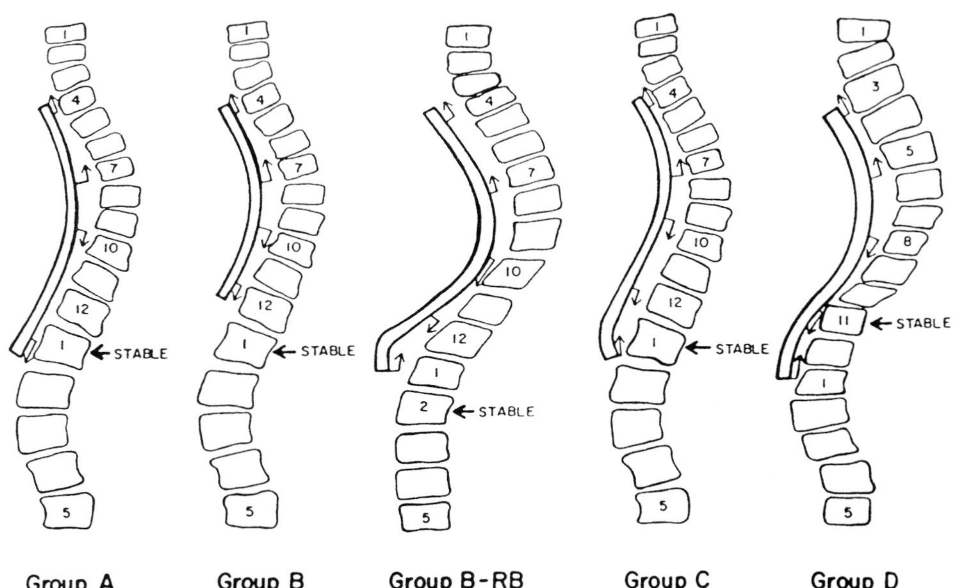

FIGURE 2–13. Groups A, B, B-RB, C, and D, as described in Table 2–11. See text for further description. (From Bridwell, K.H., McAllister, J.W., Betz, R.R., et al.: Coronal decompensation produced by Cotrel-Dubousset "derotation' maneuver for idiopathic right thoracic scoliosis. Spine 16:769–777, 1991; reprinted by permission.)

TABLE 2–11. SEGMENTAL INSTRUMENTATION PATTERNS FOR PREVENTION OF CORONAL DECOMPENSATION FOR TREATMENT OF THORACIC SCOLIOSIS

GROUP	CRITERIA FOR HOOK SELECTION
A	Fused to stable vertebra: one mode of hook orientation on left-sided rod, one rod contour (four hook sites)
B	Fused to one above stable: one mode of hooks, one rod contour (four hook sites)
B-RB	Fused to one above stable: terminal reverse bend and reversal of last two hooks (five hook sites)
C	Fused to stable, with terminal reverse bend between neutral and stable and reverse rod bend (contour) (five hook sites)
D	Fused beyond stable: reverse bend and reversal of hook direction between the stable or neutral vertebra and the distally fused segment (five hook sites)

From Bridwell, K.H., McAllister, J.W., and Betz, R.R.: Coronal decompensation produced by Cotrel-Dubousset "derotation" maneuver for idiopathic right thoracic scoliosis. Spine 16:769–777, 1991; reprinted by permission.

rior spinal growth after posterior fusion in skeletally immature patients. It results in increased rotation of the spine, as an anterior growth causes a spin around the posterior tether. This situation is best avoided by anterior diskectomy and fusion in immature patients with curves of >50 degrees (Risser 0–1; girls <11 years, boys 13 years).

6. Infantile Idiopathic Scoliosis—Presents at age 2 months to 3 years with left-sided thoracic scoliosis, male predominance, plagiocephaly (skull flattening), and other congenital defects. Most cases have been reported from Great Britain. The rib–vertebra angle difference (RVAD) (Mehta) of the apical vertebra (>20 degrees) and overlap of the apical vertebral body and rib (phase II) are associated with increased likelihood of progression. Treatment is as follows.

CURVE (degrees)	PROGRESSION (degrees)	RVAD (degrees)	TREATMENT
<25	—	<20	Serial observation
25–35	10	20–25	Cast/brace
>35	>10		Neuro/MRI work-up, instrumentation without fusion or combined ant. and post. fusion

7. Juvenile Idiopathic Scoliosis—Scoliosis in 3- to 10-year-olds is similar to adolescent scoliosis in terms of presentation and treatment. A high risk of curve progression is seen; 70% require treatment, with 50% needing bracing (generally Milwaukee type) and 50% requiring surgery (poor prognosis for bracing with a curve >45 degrees or RVAD >20 degrees). Fusion should be delayed until the onset of the adolescent growth spurt if possible (unless curve magnitude is >60 degrees). The use of spinal instrumentation without fusion (as for infantile scoliosis) may facilitate this delay.

B. Neuromuscular Scoliosis—Many children with neuromuscular disorders develop scoliosis or other spinal deformities. In general, neuromuscular curves are longer, involve more vertebrae, and are less likely to have compensatory curves than idiopathic scoliosis. Additionally, neuromuscular curves progress more rapidly and may progress after maturity. These curves may be associated with pelvic obliquity, bony deformities, and cervical involvement—again distinguishing them from idiopathic curves. Pulmonary complications are also more frequent, including decreased pulmonary function, pneumonia, and atelectasis. For patients who are already wheelchair-bound curve progression may make them bedridden. Orthotic use is advised until age 10–12 years, at which time corrective fusion is usually performed to provide permanent stability. Underarm (Boston type) braces are most often used, with Milwaukee braces contraindicated (pressure sores). Fusion often involves more levels than for idiopathic curves. Fusion to the pelvis may be required for fixed pelvic obliquity, with the Galveston technique of pelvic fixation most commonly used (bending the caudal end of the rods from the lamina of S1 to pass into the posterosuperior iliac spine and between the tables of the ilium just anterior to the sciatic notch). The goal of treatment is stability and balance. Patients with upper motor neuron disease (CP) are initially treated with a body jacket or seat orthotics but require fusion for curve progression of >50 degrees. Children with severe involvement require fusion to the sacrum and may require both anterior and posterior procedures. Posterior fusion alone is associated with higher pseudarthrosis rates and development of the "crankshaft" phenomenon (fusions at an early age and delayed bone age in neuromuscular patients). Lower motor neuron disease (polio and spinal muscular atrophy) is treated with orthotics initially. If this treatment fails, instrumentation without fusion is carried out in young children (<10 years old) with fusion reserved for older children (girls >12 years, boys >14 years). Severe curves require early correction, usually with Luque instrumentation. Myopathic disease (muscular dystrophy) often results in rapidly progressive, severe scoliosis and markedly decreased pulmonary function soon after the child is wheelchair-bound. Bracing is not recommended, and fusion (with Luque instrumentation) is usually done for >20 degree curves in patients with pulmonary function adequate to allow sitting, prolonging their life-span.

C. Congenital Spinal Disorders—Due to a developmental defect in the formation of the mesenchymal anlage during the 4th to 6th weeks of development. Three basic types of defect are noted: **failure of segmentation** (typically results in a vertebral bar), **failure of formation** (due to lack of material, may result in hemivertebrae), and **mixed.** Three-dimensional CT is helpful for defining the type (Fig. 2–14) of vertebral anomaly. Spinal MRI scans should be obtained prior to any surgery to assess for intraspinal anomalies. Associated anomalies include GU (25%), cardiac (10%), and dysraphism (25%, usually diastomatomyelia—cleft in the spine). Renal ultrasonography is used to rule out associated kidney abnormalities.

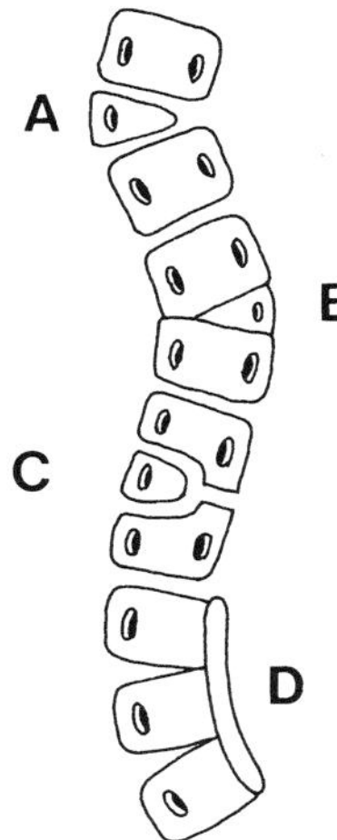

FIGURE 2–14. Vertebral anomalies leading to congenital scoliosis. *A*, Fully segmented hemivertebra. *B*, Unsegmented hemivertebra. *C*, Incarcerated hemivertebra. *D*, Unilateral unsegmented bar.

1. Congenital Scoliosis—Most common congenital spinal disorder. The worst prognosis (most likely to progress) is seen with a unilateral unsegmented bar with a contralateral fully segmented hemivertebra. Best prognosis is with a block vertebra (bilateral failure of segmentation). A **unilateral unsegmented bar is a common disorder and is likely to progress.** An incarcerated hemivertebra (within the lateral margins of the vertebrae above and below) has a better prognosis than an unincarcerated (laterally positioned) hemivertebra. A fully segmented hemivertebra is free with normal disc spaces on both sides (higher risk of progression), whereas an unsegmented hemivertebra is fused above and below (lower risk) (see Fig. 1–14). **Unilateral unsegmented bars should be treated operatively when diagnosed;** other deformities should demonstrate progression before surgical options are considered. Bracing may be effective for compensatory curves or for smaller, supple curves above a vertebral anomaly; but it is ineffective for controlling congenital curves. Anterior and posterior hemivertebral excision may be indicated for lumbosacral hemivertebrae associated with progressive curves and imbalance. Isolated hemivertebral excision can destabilize the spine on the convex side and should be accompanied by anterior/posterior arthrodesis (possibly with use of internal fixation (instrumentation) to bring the adjacent vertebrae together). Anterior and posterior convex hemiepiphysiodesis/arthrodesis is safer, but correction of imbalance is less predictable.

   Posterior fusion, with or without instrumentation, is the mainstay of treatment for most progressive curves. In young patients (girls <10 years, boys <12 years) the "crankshaft" phenomenon may occur because of continued anterior spinal growth; in these cases anterior/posterior fusion may be required. A summary of treatment recommendations for congenital scoliosis follows.

RISK OF PROGRESSION (HIGHEST TO LOWEST)	CHARACTER OF CURVE PROGRESSION	TREATMENT OPTIONS
Unilateral unsegmented bar with contralateral hemivertebra	Rapid and relentless	Posterior spinal fusion (add anterior fusion for girls <10, boys <12)
Unilateral unsegmented bar	Rapid	Same
Fully segmented hemivertebra	Steady	Anterior spinal fusion Ant/post convex hemiepiphysiodesis (age <5, curve <70°, no kyphosis Hemivertebra excision
Partially segmented hemivertebra	Less rapid; curve usually <40° at maturity	Observation Hemivertebra excision
Incarcerated hemivertebra	May slowly progress	Observation
Nonsegmented hemivertebra	Little progression	Observation

2. Congenital Kyphosis—May be secondary to failure of formation (type I), failure of segmentation (type II), or mixed abnormalities (type III), with **failure of formation (type I, most common) having the worst prognosis** for progression (95% progress) and neurologic involvement of all spinal deformities. Type I congenital kyphosis is also the most likely to result in paraplegia (neurofibromatosis is second). The presence of significant congenital kyphosis secondary to failure of formation (type I) is an indication for surgery. Posterior fusion is favored in young children (<5 years) with curves less than 50 degrees. Combined anterior/posterior fusion is reserved for older children or more severe curves. Anterior vertebrectomy, spinal cord decompression, and anterior fusion followed by posterior fusion are indicated for curves associated with neurologic deficits. A type II congenital kyphosis can be observed to document progression, but progressive curves should be fused posteriorly.

D. Neurofibromatosis—AD disorder of neural crest origin, often associated with neoplasia and skeletal abnormalities. Two of the following seven findings are necessary to establish the diagnosis.

DIAGNOSTIC CRITERIA	REQUIREMENTS
At least six café-au-lait spots	>5 mm (prepubital); >15 mm (mature)
Neurofibromas	Two or more (or one plexiform type)
Axillary/inguinal freckles	Multiple
Osseous lesion	Sphenoid dysplasia, cortical thinning
Optic glioma	Present
Lish nodules	Two or more iris lesions by slit-lamp examination
Family history	First-degree relative with neurofibromatosis

The spine is the most common site of skeletal involvement. Careful screening of scoliosis radiographs for vertebral scalloping, **enlarged foramina,** pencilling of transverse processes or ribs, severe apical rotation, short, tight curves, or a paraspinal mass may differentiate this condition from idiopathic scoliosis. Spinal deformity secondary to neurofibromatosis is characteristically kyphoscoliosis in the thoracic region with dystrophic changes, but nondystrophic scoliosis or cervical involvement may also be noted. Nondystrophic scoliosis is treated as appropriate for idiopathic scoliosis; but with dystrophic deformities nonoperative treatment of curves >20 degrees is futile. Surgical treatment consists in posterior fusion with instrumentation for patients without significant kyphosis (<50 degrees) and combined anterior fusion with strut grafting and posterior fusion with instrumentation for patients with more severe kyphosis. If fusion is required in the juvenile age group, anterior and posterior fusion are routinely performed to avoid the "crankshaft" phenomenon. Neurologic involvement is common in neurofibromatosis and may be caused by the deformity itself, an intraspinal tumor, a soft tissue mass, or dural ectasia. Anterior decompression with strut grafting followed by posterior fusion is required in these cases. Because of a high pseudarthrosis rate, some authors recommend routine augmentation of the posterior fusion mass at 6 months postoperatively with repeat iliac crest bone graft. C-spine involvement includes kyphosis or atlantoaxial instability. Posterior fusion with autologous grafting and halo immobilization is recommended for severe C-spine deformity with instability. Isolated kyphosis of the T-spine is treated with anterior decompression of the kyphotic angular cord compression, followed by anterior and posterior fusion.

E. Other Spinal Abnormalities
   1. Diastomatomyelia—Fibrous, cartilaginous, or osseous bar creating a longitudinal cleft in the spinal cord. Usually occurs in the lumbar spine and can lead to tethering of the cord with associated neurologic deficits. Intrapedicular widening on plain radiographs is suggestive, and myelo-CT or MRI is necessary to fully define the pathology. A diastomatomyelia must be resected prior to correction of a spinal deformity; but if otherwise asymptomatic and without neurologic sequelae, it may be simply observed.
   2. Sacral Agenesis—Partial or complete absence of the sacrum and lower lumbar spine. Highly associated with maternal diabetes, it is often accompanied by GI, GU, and cardiovascular abnormalities. Clinically, children have a prominent lower lumbar spine and atrophic lower extremities; and they may sit in a "Buddha" position. Motor impairment is at the level of the agenesis, but sensory innervation is largely spared. Management may include amputation or spinal–pelvic fusion.

F. Low Back Pain—In children, complaints of low back pain and especially painful scoliosis should be taken seriously. Acute back pain can be associated with diskitis (presents as refusal to sit or walk, increased ESR, and later disc space narrowing—takes 3 weeks to appear on plain films) or osteomyelitis (systemic illness, leukocytosis). Ring and Wenger discussed the difficulty of differentiating between diskitis and osteomyelitis, and they recommended use of the term infectious spondylitis to describe disc-space infections in children. Occasionally herniated nucleus pulposis (HNP), presenting as sciatica and back pain in older children, occurs and may require operative intervention. Spondylolysis is common after athletic injuries, and conservative treatment is usually adequate. Painful scoliosis often signifies a tumor (e.g., osteoid osteoma) or spinal cord anomaly and should be investigated aggressively. A bone scan is an excellent screening method for the child or adolescent with back pain. The use of single emission positron computed tomography (SPECT scanning) has improved detection of occult spondylolysis and osteoid osteoma, and it should be undertaken if plain radiographs are negative and pain continues more than 1 month. Further specificity in a still unclear clinical setting may be garnered from CT scanning (spondylolysis, HNP), or MRI (infection, HNP).

G. Kyphosis
   1. Congenital Kyphosis—Discussed above: see Congenital Spinal Disorders.
   2. Scheuermann's Disease—Classic definition is increased thoracic kyphosis (>45 degrees) **with 5 degrees or more anterior wedging at three sequential vertebrae.** Other radiographic findings include disc narrowing, end plate irregularities, spondylolysis (30–50%), scoliosis (33%), and Schmorl's nodes (Sorenson). Scheuermann's disease is more common in males and typically presents in adolescents with poor posture and occasionally aching pain. Physical examination characteristically shows hyperkyphosis that does not reverse on attempts at hyperextension and tight hamstrings. Neurologic sequelae secondary to disc herniation or extradural spinal cysts are rare but have been reported. Treatment consists in bracing (modified Milwaukee brace) for a progressive curve in a patient with 1 year or more of skeletal growth remaining (Risser 3 or below). Bracing may effect 5–10 degrees of permanent curve correction but is less effective for kyphosis of >75 degrees. In the skeletally mature patient with severe kyphosis (>65 degrees) surgical correction may be indicated. Posterior fusion with dual rod segmentally attached compression instrumentation is the treatment of choice, preceded by anterior release and interbody fusion for curves of >75 degrees or those not correcting to <55 degrees on hyperextension. Thorascopic anterior diskectomy and interbody fusion have been utilized to decrease the morbidity associated with thoracotomy for anterior release and fusion. Lumbar Scheuermann's disease is less common than the thoracic variety but may cause back pain on a mechanical basis (more common in athletes and manual laborers). The pain is usually self-limited. Lumbar Scheuermann's disease also demonstrates irregular vertebral end plates with Schmorl's nodes and decreased disc height, but it is not associated with vertebral wedging.
   3. Postural Round Back—Also associated with kyphosis but does not demonstrate vertebral body

changes. Forward bending demonstrates kyphosis, but there is no sharp angulation as in Scheuermann's disease. Correction with backward bending and prone hyperextension is typical. Treatment includes a hyperextension exercise program. Occasionally bracing is required, but surgery is rarely indicated.

4. Other Causes of Kyphosis—Include trauma, infections, spondylitis, bone dysplasias (mucopolysaccharidoses, Kneist syndrome, diastrophic dysplasia), and neoplasms. Additionally, postlamimectomy kyphosis can be severe and requires anterior and posterior fusion early. Performance of total laminectomy in immature patients without stabilization is contraindicated.

H. Cervical Spine Disorders—Many disorders.

1. Klippel-Feil Syndrome—Multiple fused cervical segments due to failure of normal segmentation of cervical somites at 3–8 weeks' gestation. Often associated with congenital scoliosis, renal disease (aplasia 33%), synkinesis (mirror motions), Sprengel's deformity, congenital heart disease, brain stem abnormalities, or congenital cervical stenosis. The classic triad of low posterior hairline, short "web" neck, and limited cervical ROM is seen in fewer than 50% of cases. Most therapy is conservative, but chronic pain with myelopathy associated with instability may require surgery. Three high risk fusion patterns are more apt to cause neurologic problems: (1) C2/C3 fusion with occipitalization of the atlas; (2) long fusion with abnormal occipital–cervical junction; and (3) single open cervical interspace. Affected children should avoid collision sports.

2. Atlantoaxial Instability

   a. Anteroposterior Instability—Associated with Down syndrome (trisomy 21), JRA, various osteochondrodystrophies, os odontoidium, and other abnormalities. In patients with Down syndrome and a normal neurologic examination, simple avoidance of contact sports is appropriate, but with >10 mm of subluxation on flexion-extension films, spinal fusion is indicated (high complication rate). An atlanto-dens interval (ADI) of >5 mm should be treated with activity restriction in the absence of myelopathy.

   b. Rotatory Atlantoaxial Subluxation—May present with torticollis; can be caused by retropharyngeal inflammation (Grisel's disease). It is probably caused by secondary ligamentous laxity and is best treated with traction and bracing early. Current diagnosis is by CT scans at the C1–C2 level with the head straightforward, in maximal rotation to the right, and then in maximum rotation to the left (Fig. 2–15). Late diagnosis may require C1–C2 fusion. Traumatic atlantoaxial subluxation may present as torticollis, which can be treated initially with a soft collar for up to 1 week. If symptoms persist past this point, cervical traction should be initiated. If discovered late (>1 month), fusion may be required for fixed rotary subluxation. Rotary subluxation can also be caused by rheumatoid arthritis, ankylosing spondylitis, Down syndrome, congenital anomalies, and cervical tumors.

3. Os Odontoideum—Previously thought to be due to failure of fusion of the base of the odontoid, it appears like a type II odontoid fracture. Evidence suggests that it may represent the residuals of an old traumatic process. Usually seen in place of the normal odontoid process (orthotopic type), but it may fuse to the clivus (dystopic type—more often seen with neurologic compromise). Therapy is conservative unless instability (>3 mm translation on flexion-extension radiographs) or neurologic symptoms are present, which require posterior C1–C2 fusion.

4. Pseudosubluxation of the Cervical Spine—Subluxation of C2 on C3 (and occasionally of C3 on C4) of up to 40% or 4 mm can be normal in children <8 years old because of the orientation of the facets. Rapid resolution of pain, relatively minor trauma, lack of anterior swelling, continued alignment of the posterior interspinous distances and the posterior spinolaminar line (Schwischuk's line) on radiographs, and reduction of the subluxation with neck extension help differentiate this entity from more serious disorders.

5. Intervertebral Disc Calcification Syndrome—Pain, decreased ROM, low grade fevers, increased ESR, and radiographic disc calcification (within the annulus) without erosion characterize this disorder, which usually involves the C-spine. Conservative treatment is indicated for this self-limited condition.

6. Basilar Impression/Invagination—Bony deformity at the base of the skull causes cephalad migration of the odontoid into the foramen magnum (see Fig. 7–2). Sagittal MRI scan best demonstrates impingement of the dens on the brain stem. Weakness, parasthesias, and hydrocephalus may result. Treatment is often operative and may include transoral resection of the dens, occipital laminectomy, and occipitocervical fusion and wiring.

X. Upper Extremity Problems (see also Chapter 6, Hand)

A. Sprengel's Deformity—Undescended scapula often associated with winging, hypoplasia, and omovertebral connections (30%). It is the most common congenital anomaly of the shoulder in children. Affected scapulae are usually small, relatively wide, and medially rotated. Increased association with Klippel-Feil syndrome, kidney disease, scoliosis, and diastematomyelia. Surgery for cosmetic or functional deformities (decreased abduction) includes distal advancement of the associated muscles (and scapula) (Woodward) or detachment and movement of the scapula. (Schrock, Green). Surgery is best done in the 3- to 8-year-old.

B. Congenital Pseudarthrosis of the Clavicle—Failure of union of the medial and lateral ossification centers of the right clavicle. Etiology may be related to pulsations of the underlying subclavian artery. Presents as an enlarging, painless, nontender mass. Radiographs show rounded sclerotic bone at the pseudarthrosis site. Surgery (open reduction/internal fixation with bone grafting) is indicated for unacceptable cosmetic deformities or with significant

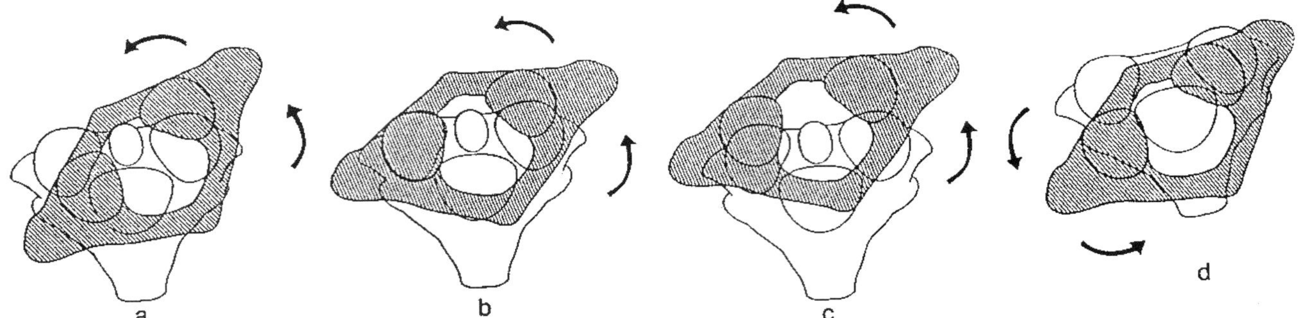

FIGURE 2–15. Four types of rotary fixation. *a*, Type I—rotary fixation with no anterior displacement and the odontoid acting as the pivot. *b*, Type II—rotary fixation with anterior displacement of 3–5 mm, one lateral process acting as the pivot. *c*, Type III—rotary fixation with anterior displacement of more than 5 mm. *d*, Type IV—rotary fixation with posterior displacement. (From Fielding, J.W., and Hawkins, R.J.: Atlanto-axial rotatory fixation. J. Bone Joint Surg. [Am.] 59:42, 1977; reprinted by permission.)

functional symptoms (mobility of the fragments and winging of the scapula). Successful union is predictable (in contrast to congenital pseudoarthrosis of the tibia).

C. Deltoid Fibrotic Problems—Short fibrous bands replace the deltoid muscle and cause abduction contractures at the shoulder, with elevation and winging of the scapula when the arms are adducted. Surgical resection of these bands is often required.

XI. Lower Extremity Problems

A. Introduction—Lower extremity problems that are best considered as a whole are presented in this section to provide a basis for understanding and comparison.

B. Rotational Problems of the Lower Extremities—Include femoral anteversion, tibial torsion, and metatarsus adductus. All of these problems may be a result of intrauterine positioning and commonly present with an intoeing gait. These deformities are usually bilateral, and the clinician should be wary of asymmetric findings. Evaluation should include the measurements noted in Table 2–12 and illustrated in Fig. 2–16.

1. Metatarsus Adductus—Forefoot is adducted at the tarsal-metatarsal joint. **Usually seen during the first year of life.** May be associated with hip dyplasia (10–15%). Approximately 85% resolve spontaneously; feet that can be actively corrected to neutral require no treatment. Stretching exercises are used on feet that can be passively corrected to neutral (heel bisector line lines up with the second MT). Feet that cannot be passively corrected usually require serial casting. MT osteotomies and limited medial release are indicated in resistant cases in children >1 year. The Heyman-Herndon procedure (complete tarsometatarsal capsulotomy) has fallen into disfavor because of a high incidence of failures at long-term follow-up. Rigidity and heel valgus should be identified and treated with early casting.
2. Tibial Torsion—Most common cause of intoeing. Usually **seen during the second year** of life and can be associated with metatarsus adductus. It is often bilateral (left > right) and may be secondary to excessive medial ligamentous tightness. Medial rotation of the tibia at the knee causes the intoeing gait. Usually improves with growth. Denis Browne night splinting can be used if symptoms persist, but its efficacy is questionable. Operative correction is seldom necessary except in severe cases, which are addressed with a supramalleolar osteotomy.
3. Femoral Anteversion—Internal rotation of the femur, **seen in 3- to 6-year-olds.** Increased medial rotation and decreased lateral rotation noted on examination of a child with an intoeing gait and whose patellas are medially rotated. Children with this problem classically sit in a W position. If associated with tibial torsion, femoral anteversion may lead to patellofemoral problems. This disorder usually corrects spontaneously by age 10, but in the older child with <10 degrees of medial rotation femoral derotational osteotomy (intertrochanteric is best) may be considered for cosmesis.

XII. Hip and Femur

A. Developmental Dysplasia of the Hip (DDH)

1. Introduction—Previously called congenital

TABLE 2–12. EVALUATION OF ROTATIONAL PROBLEMS OF THE LOWER EXTREMITIES

MEASUREMENT	TECHNIQUE	NORMAL VALUES (DEGREES)	SIGNIFICANCE
Foot-progression angle	Foot vs. straight line	−5 to +20	Nonspecific rotation
Medial rotation	Prone hip ROM	20–60	>70°, femoral anteversion
Lateral rotation	Prone hip ROM	30–60	<20°, femoral anteversion
Thigh-foot angle	Knee bent—foot up	0–20	<−10°, tibial torsion
Foot lateral border	Convex, medial crease	Straight, flexible	Metatarsus adductus

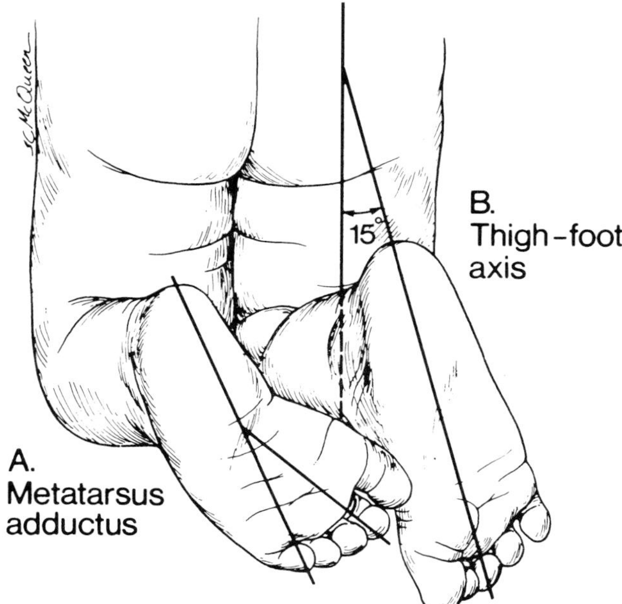

FIGURE 2–16. *A*, Deviation of the forefoot in metatarsus adductus. *B*, Note also the normal thigh–foot angle (15 degrees); negative thigh–foot angles (<10 degrees) are seen in tibial torsion. (From Fitch, R.D.: Introduction to pediatric orthopedics. In Sabiston's Essentials of Surgery, Sabiston, D.C., Jr., ed. Philadelphia, WB Saunders, 1987; reprinted by permission.)

dysplasia of the hip (CDH), this disorder represents abnormal development or dislocation of the hip secondary to capsular laxity and mechanical factors (e.g., intrauterine positioning). Breech positioning and female sex are risk factors. Decreased intrauterine space explains the increased incidence of DDH in the first-born child. Commonly associated with other "packaging problems," such as torticollis (20%) and metatarsus adductus (10%), it is partially characterized by increased amounts of type III collagen. DDH is seen most commonly in the left hip (67%) in females (85%) with a positive family history (20+%), increased maternal estrogens, and breech births (30–50%). This disorder includes the spectrum of complete dislocation, subluxation, instability, and acetabular dysplasia. The teratologic form is most severe and usually requires early surgery. If left untreated, muscles about the hip contract, and the acetabulum becomes flatter (dysplastic) and filled with fibrofatty debris (pulvinar). The capsule and labrum become redundant, and the head may be trapped by the iliopsoas tendon (causing an "hourglass" constriction) or may block reduction (inverted limbus), and an abnormal femoral head and "false acetabulum" may develop.

2. Diagnosis—Early diagnosis is possible with the Ortolani test (elevation and abduction of femur relocates a dislocated hip) and Barlow test (adduction and depression of femur dislocates a dislocatable hip). Three phases are commonly recognized: (1) **dislocated** (Ortolani-positive, early; Ortolani-negative, late when femoral head cannot be reduced); (2) **dislocatable** (Barlow-positive); and (3) **subluxatable** (Barlow-suggestive). Later diagnosis is made with asymmetry of hip abduction as the laxity resolves and stiffness becomes more clinically evident. (*Caution:* Abduction may be decreased symmetrically with bilateral dislocations.) Other signs of dislocation include a positive Galeazzi sign demonstrated by a short knee on the affected side with the feet held together and knees flexed (a congenitally short femur can also cause a positive Galeazzi sign), asymmetric gluteal folds (less reliable), or positive Trendelenburg stance. Repeat examination, especially in the infant, is important because a child's irritability can prevent proper evaluation. Radiographs may be helpful in the older child (>3 months); and measurement of the acetabular index (normal <25 degrees), Perkins line (normally the ossific nucleus of femoral head is medial to this line), and evaluation of Shenton's line are useful (Fig. 2–17). Later, delayed ossification of the femoral head on the affected side may be seen. Dynamic ultrasonography is also useful for making the diagnosis, especially in young children prior to ossification of the femoral head (which occurs at age 4–6 months). It is also useful for assessing reduction in a Pavlik harness and diagnosing acetabular dysplasia or capsular laxity; however, it is operator-dependent. Arthography is helpful after closed reduction to determine concentric reduction (<6 mm widening).

3. Treatment—Based on achieving and maintaining early "concentric reduction" in order to prevent future degenerative joint disease. Specific therapy is based on the child's age and includes the Pavlik harness, which is designed to maintain infants (<6 months) reduced in about 100 degrees of flexion and mild abduction (the "human position" [Salter]). Reduction should be confirmed by radiographs or ultrasound scans after placement in the harness and the

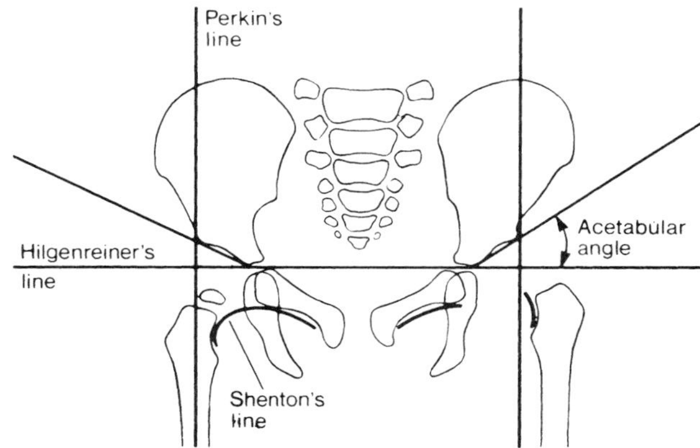

FIGURE 2–17. Common measurements used to evaluate developmental dysplasia of the hip. Note the delayed ossification, disruption of Shenton's line, and increased acetabular index on the left dislocated hip. (From Fitch, R.D.: Introduction to pediatric orthopaedics. In Sabiston's Essentials of Surgery, Sabiston, D.C., Jr., ed. Philadelphia, WB Saunders, 1987, reprinted by permission.)

brace adjusted accordingly. The position of the hip should be within the "safe zone" of Ramsey (between maximum adduction before redislocation and excessive abduction causing a high risk of avascular necrosis [impingement of the posterosuperior retinacular branch of the medial femoral circumflex artery]). Patients with a narrow safe zone should be considered for an adductor tenotomy. The child is placed in the harness, and radiographs or ultrasound scans are obtained to assess reduction. If unsatisfactory, the harness is adjusted (usually by increasing the amount of flexion [excessive flexion may result in transient femoral nerve palsy], and the study is repeated. A stable reduction must be demonstrated in the harness early (within 2–4 weeks). Treatment continues until the hip is reduced and stable. Weaning from the harness is generally done over a period twice as long as the treatment duration. Use of abduction bracing may be considered for residual acetabular dysplasia in a child who is ambulating. Children between 6 and 18 months, and younger infants in whom the Pavlik treatment fails, require closed reduction. Prereduction traction is controversial. One study has shown that home traction is as safe and efficacious as inpatient traction. Several studies have demonstrated similar rates of osteonecrosis of the femoral head with closed or open reduction with or without preliminary traction. An arthrogram is usually obtained at the time of closed reduction to check for a medial dye pool, which should be ≤5 mm with an acceptable reduction. The arthrogram may show an inverted limbus or an hourglass constriction of the capsule indicating an incomplete reduction. Alternatively, ultrasonography can be used in the operating room to assess the results of closed reduction. Casting after reduction should be done for at least 4 months, followed by nighttime bracing. Open reduction is reserved for 12- to 18-month-olds who fail closed reduction, have an obstructed limbus, or have an unstable safe zone and for 18-month-old to 6-year-old children initially. It is usually done through an anterior approach (less risk to the medial femoral circumflex artery) and may include capsulorrhaphy, adductor tenotomy, or perhaps femoral shortening. The major risk associated with both open and closed reductions is osteonecrosis (due to direct vascular injury or impingement versus disruption of the circulation from osteotomies). Failure of open reduction is difficult to treat surgically owing to the high complication rate of revision surgery (50% osteonecrosis, 33% pain and stiffness in a recent study). The following treatment guidelines are appropriate.

SITUATION	FINDINGS	TREATMENT
Newborn		
Dislocated	+Ortolani test	Pavlik harness
Dislocatable	+Barlow test	Pavlik harness
Subluxatable	Barlow test rides up edge	Supportive/Pavlik
<6 Months Old		
Dislocatable/ reducible	+Ortolani test	Pavlik harness
Unreducible	−Ortolani test	Pavlik harness → traction, closed reduction
>6 Months Old		
Unreducible	−Ortolani test	Traction and closed reduction
Failed closed reduction	Medial dye pool >5 mm	Open reduction, psoas tenotomy, capsulorrhaphy, ± femoral shortening osteotomy, ± pelvic osteotomy
>3 Years Old		
Dislocated	Trendelenburg gait, leg asymmetry (Allis test)	Open reduction, psoas tenotomy, capsulorrhaphy, femoral shortening osteotomy, ± pelvic osteotomy

4. Osteotomies—May be required in toddlers and school-age children. Osteotomies are required for instability, failure of acetabular development, or progressive femoral head subluxation after reduction. Osteotomies should be done only after congruent reduction, with satisfactory ROM, and after reasonable femoral sphericity is achieved by closed or open methods. Diagnosis after age 8 years (younger in patients with bilateral DDH) may contraindicate reduction because the acetabulum has little chance to remodel, although reduction may be indicated in conjunction with salvage procedures. The choice of femoral versus pelvic osteotomy (Fig. 2–18) is sometimes a matter of the surgeon's choice. Some surgeons prefer to perform pelvic osteotomies after age 4 and femoral osteotomies prior to this age. In general, pelvic osteotomies should be done when severe dysplasia is accompanied by significant radiographic changes on the acetabular side (i.e., increased acetabular index, failure of lateral acetabular ossification), whereas changes on the femoral side (e.g., marked anteversion, coxa valga) are best treated by femoral osteotomies. Femoral osteotomies rarely correct hip dysplasia successfully after age 5 years. The following are common reconstructive osteotomies.

OSTEOTOMY	PROCEDURE	REQUIREMENT
Femoral	Intertrochanteric osteotomy (VDRO)	Concentric reduction
Salter	Innominate osteotomy, open wedge	Concentric reduction
Sutherland (double)	Salter + pubic osteotomy	Concentric reduction
Steel (triple)	Salter + osteotomy of both rami	Concentric reduction

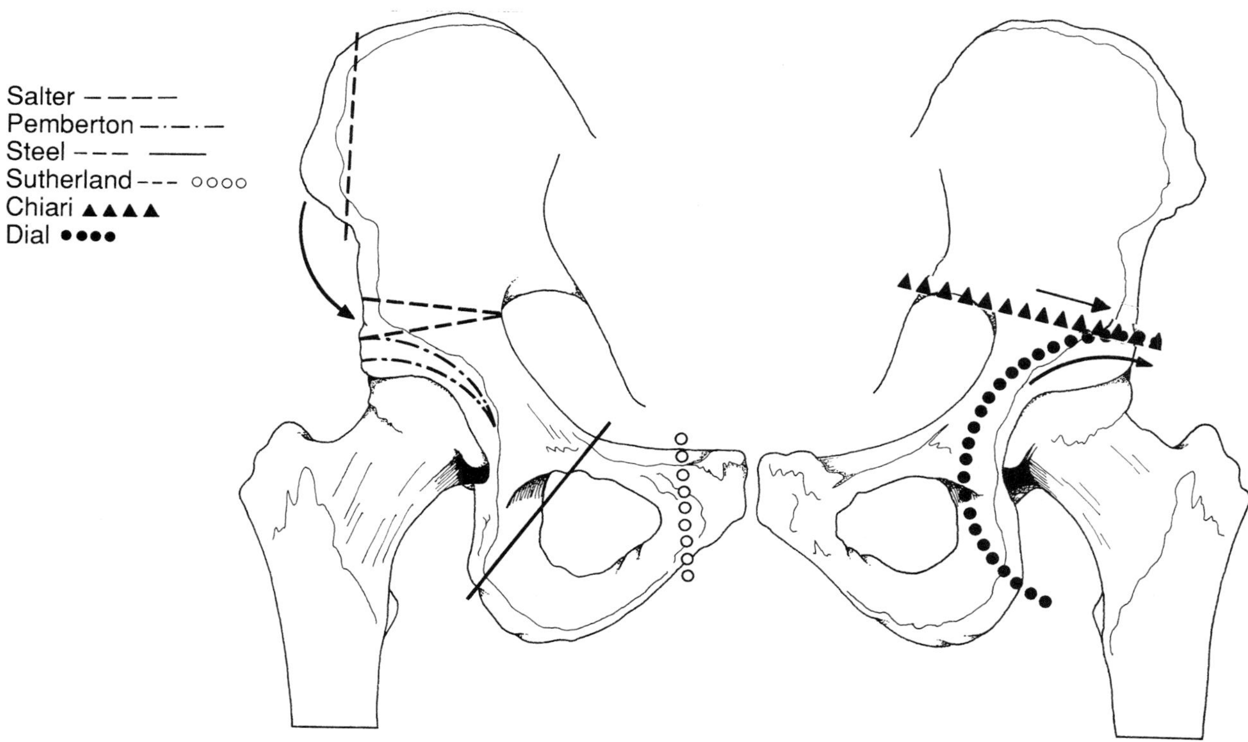

FIGURE 2–18. Common pelvic osteotomies for treatment of developmental dysplasia of the hip.

OSTEOTOMY	PROCEDURE	REQUIREMENT
Dial	Periacetabular osteotomy	Surgeon's experience
Pemberton	Through acetabular roof to triradiate cartilage	Concentric reduction
Chiari	Through ilium above acetabulum (makes new roof)	Salvage procedure for asymmetric incongruity
Shelf	Slotted lateral acetabular augmentaion	Salvage procedure for asymmetric incongruity

The **Salter osteotomy may lengthen the affected leg** up to 1 cm. The Pemberton acetabuloplasty is a good choice for residual dysplasia because it reduces acetabular volume (bends on triradiate cartilage). The Steel (triple) innominate osteotomy is favored in older children because their symphysis pubis does not rotate as well. Dega type osteotomies are often favored for paralytic dislocations and patients with posterior acetabular deficiency. This osteotomy is more versatile and is sometimes used for DDH. The Dial osteotomy is technically difficult and rarely used. The Chiari osteotomy is recommended for patients with inadequate femoral head coverage and an incongruous joint but is considered a salvage procedure. The **Chiari osteotomy shortens the affected leg** and requires periarticular soft tissue metaplasia for success. Other procedures include the Shelf lateral acetabular augmentation procedure for patients with inadequate lateral coverage or increased trochanteric advancement in a patient >8 years old with increased trochanteric overgrowth (improves hip abductor biomechanics).

B. Congenital Coxa Vara—Decreased neck–shaft angle due to a defect in ossification of the femoral neck. It is bilateral in one-third to one-half of cases. Coxa vara can be congenital (noted at birth and differentiated from DDH by MRI), developmental (AD, progressive), or acquired (e.g., trauma, LCP, slipped capital femoral epiphysis). May present with a waddling gait (bilateral) or a painless limp (unilateral). Radiographs classically demonstrate a triangular ossification defect in the inferomedial femoral neck in developmental coxa vara. Evaluation of Hilgenreiner's epiphyseal angle (the angle between Hilgenreiner's line and a line through the proximal femoral physis) is the key to treatment. An angle of <45 degrees spontaneously corrects, whereas an angle of >60 degrees (and a neck–shaft angle of <110 degrees) usually requires surgery (corrective valgus osteotomy of the proximal femur). Proximal femoral (valgus) ± derotation osteotomy (Pauwel) is indicated for a neck–shaft angle <90 degrees, a vertically oriented physeal plate, progressive deformities, or significant gait abnormalities. Concomitant distal/lateral transfer of the greater trochanter may also be indicated to restore more normal hip abductor mechanics.

C. Legg-Calvé-Perthes Disease (Coxa Plana)—Noninflammatory, self-limited deformity of the weight-bearing surface of the femur probably secondary to a vascular insult leading to osteonecrosis of the proximal femoral epiphysis. Usually seen in a 4- to 8-year-old boy with delayed skeletal maturation. There is an increase incidence with a positive family history, low birth weight, and abnormal birth presentation. Symptoms include pain (**often knee pain!**), effusion (from synovitis), and limp. Decreased hip ROM (especially abduction and internal rotation) and a Trendelenburg stance are also common. **Age is the key to prognosis; presentation after age 8 years is associated with a poor prognosis.** Up to 12% of cases are bilateral but are at different stages and are asymmetric (versus multiple epiphyseal dysplasia). Differential diagnosis includes septic arthritis, blood dyscrasias, hypothyroidism, and epiphyseal dysplasia. Bony necrosis is followed by revascularization and resorption via creeping substitution that eventually allows remodeling and fragmentation. Radiographic findings vary with the stage of disease but include cessation of growth of the ossific nucleus, medial joint space widening, and development of a "crescent sign" representing subchondral fracture. Four radiographic stages (Waldenström) are usually described based on the appearance of the capital femoral epiphysis.

STAGE	CHARACTERISTICS
Initial	Physeal irregularity, metaphyseal blurring, radiolucencies
Fragmentation	Radiolucencies and radiodensities
Reossification	Normal density returns
Healed	Residual deformity

Catterall has defined four stages based on the amount of femoral involvement (seen as the crescent sign). This grouping has been simplified by Salter and Thompson based on whether the lateral margin of the capital femoral epiphysis (CFE) is involved (Fig. 2–19).

CATERALL	SALTER AND THOMPSON	LOCATION	PROGNOSIS
I	A	Anterior (seen on lateral view)	Good
II	A	Anterior and partial lateral	Good
III	B	Anterior and lateral margin	Poor
IV	B	Throughout CFE dome	Poor

The crescent sign represents a pathologic fracture of the resorbing femoral head and is best seen on a frog-leg view of the pelvis. Bone scans and MRI may help identify early involvement but do not correlate with the extent of involvement. Newer, magnified bone scans may help identify the revascularization pattern. These sophisticated studies (bone scan, MRI) are not required for routine cases. Herring et al. described the lateral pillar classification of femoral head involvement in the fragmentation stage of Perthes disease (Fig. 2–20). This radiographic classification is based on the degree of involvement at the lateral pillar of the femoral head. **Group A** has no involvement of the lateral pillar and a uniformly good outcome. **Group B** has >50% lateral pillar height maintained and a good outcome in patients <9 years old but a less fortunate outcome in older patients. **Group C** has <50% of lateral pillar height maintained, and most CFEs in all age groups become aspherical and show a longer duration of fragmentation and reossification stages. This classification has a high correlation for predicting the amount of femoral head flattening at skeletal maturity and is a strong predictor of final outcome at the onset. Maintaining the sphericity of the femoral head is the most important factor in achieving a good result. Use of circular templates (Mose) is helpful for evaluating this parameter. Early hip degenerative joint disease (DJD) results from aspherical femoral heads. Poor prognosis is associated with older children (>8 years), female sex, advanced stages (with lateral margin of the CFE involved), loss of containment, and decreased hip ROM (decreased abduction). Radiographic findings associated with poor prognosis (Catterall's "head at risk" signs) include (1) lateral calcification; (2) Gage's sign (V-shaped defect at lateral physis); (3) lateral subluxation; (4) metaphyseal cyst formation; and (5) horizontal growth plate. In general, the goals of treatment are relief of symptoms, restoration of ROM, and containment of CFE. Use of outpatient or inpatient traction, anti-inflammatory medications, and partial weight-bearing with crutches for periods of 1–2 days to several weeks is helpful for relieving symptoms. ROM is maintained with traction, muscle releases, exercise, and/or use of a Petrie cast. Containment of CFE by use of traction, muscle releases, abduction bracing, or varus femoral versus pelvic osteotomy is helpful for maintaining CFE sphericity. Herring has described a treatment plan based on age and the lateral pillar classification of disease involvement.

AGE	LATERAL PILLAR CLASSIFICATION	GOALS OF TREATMENT	TREATMENT RECOMMENDATION
<6 Years	Any	Relief of symptoms	NSAIDs, home traction, avoid weight-bearing
6–8 Years	A	Relief of symptoms	Same as above
	B	Containment	Traction, muscle releases, abdominal brace, VDRO vs. Salter osteotomy
	C	Containment	Same as type B, but bracing ineffective due to difficulty centering CFE
>9 Years	A	Relief of symptoms	NSAIDs, home traction, avoid weight-bearing
	B	Containment	Bracing difficult due to loss of motion and poor compliance, VDRO, Salter, muscle release, Petrie cast (B and C)
	C	Containment	

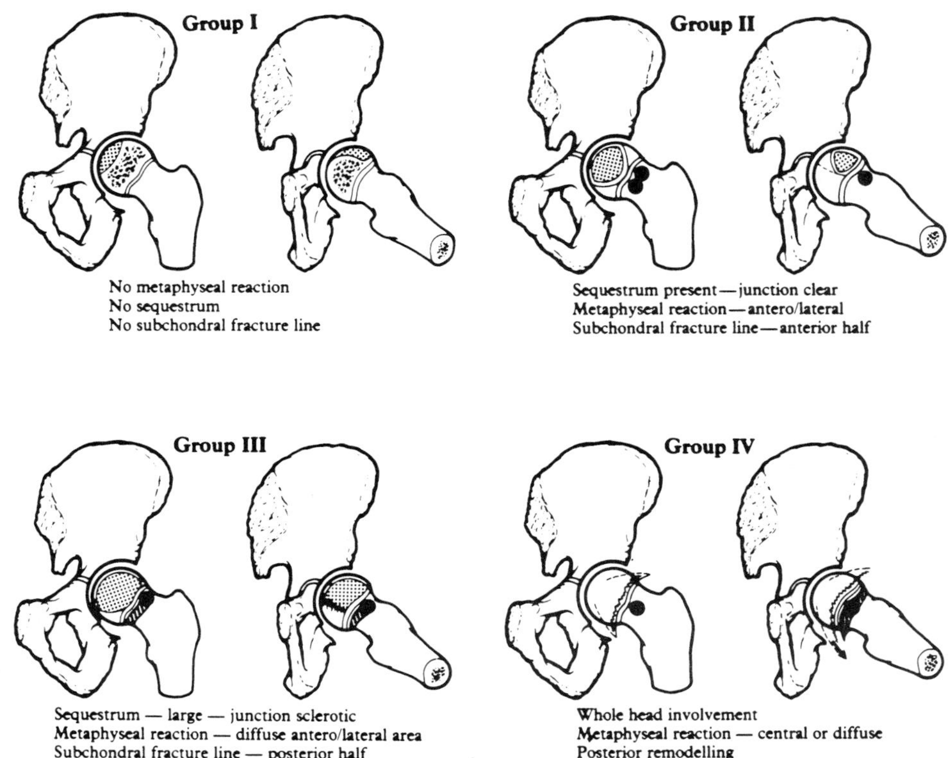

FIGURE 2–19. Catterall classification of Legg-Calvé-Perthes disease. Note the significant involvement of the lateral margin of the capital femoral epiphysis in groups III and IV (Salter and Thompson "B"). (From Fitch, R.D.: Introduction to pediatric orthopedics. In Sabiston's Essentials of Surgery, Sabiston, D.C., Jr., ed. Philadelphia, WB Saunders, 1987; reprinted by permission.)

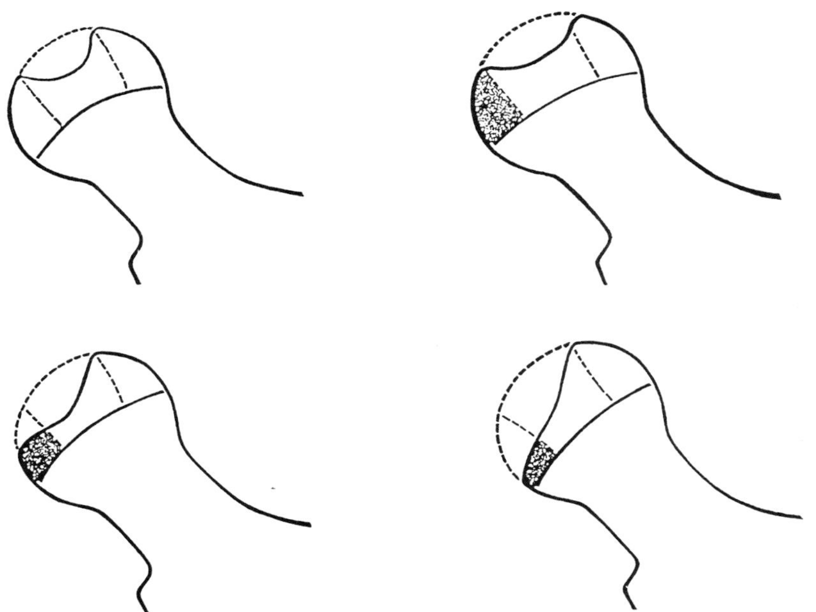

FIGURE 2–20. Lateral pillar classification of Legg-Calvé-Perthes disease. *Normal Pillars,* The pillars were derived by noting the lines of demarcation between the central sequestrum and the remainder of the epiphysis on the anteroposterior radiograph. *Group A,* Normal height of the lateral pillar is maintained. *Group B,* More than 50% height of lateral pillar is maintained. *Group C,* Less than 50% height of lateral pillar is maintained. (Adapted from Herring, J.A., Neustadt, J.B., Williams, J.J., Early, J.S., and Brown, R.H.: The lateral pillar classification of Legg-Calvé-Perthes disease. J. Pediatr. Orthop. 12:143–150, 1992; reprinted by permission.)

Bracing should continue until the increased density on radiographs disappears, representing the end of the fragmentation stage (usually 1 year after onset of symptoms). Some recommend continuing bracing until new bone is seen on the anterolateral portion of the femoral head. Advanced flattening of the femoral head can make it "noncontainable." Because abduction results in hinging and subluxation, bracing at this stage is not effective. Treatment options include Chiari osteotomy, cheilectomy (of the femoral head prominence), and valgus osteotomy (a technique with some promise). Distal transfer of the greater trochanter is occasionally required to offset overgrowth of the greater trochanter (which is not affected and continues to grow).

D. Slipped Capital Femoral Epiphysis (SCFE)—Disorder of the proximal femoral epiphysis of the femur seen during puberty caused by weakness of the perichondral ring and slip through the hypertrophic zone of the growth plate. The femoral head remains in the acetabulum, and the neck displaces anteriorly and externally rotates. SCFE is seen commonly in African-American, obese, adolescent boys with a positive family history. Up to 25% of cases are bilateral. May be associated with hormonal changes in young children, hypothyroidism, or advanced renal disease. May present with coxalgic, externally rotated gait, decreased internal rotation, thigh atrophy, and hip or knee pain. Symptoms vary with acuteness of the slip.

SLIP	DURATION OF SYMPTOMS (WEEKS)	SYMPTOMS
Acute	<3	Prodrome of knee pain
Chronic	>3	Insidious onset
Acute on chronic		Acute pain with old slipped CFE

Loder et al. described a new classification of SCFE based on the ability to bear weight. **Stable slips** are those with which weight-bearing with or without crutches is possible. **Unstable slips** are those with which weight-bearing is not possible because of severe pain. No patients with stable slips developed osteonecrosis, whereas 50% of the unstable slips developed osteonecrosis in this study of 55 patients (all treated with single pin fixation). Satisfactory results were obtained in 47% of unstable hips and 96% of stable hips. Radiographs show the slip, which is classified based on the percent of slip: grade I, 0–33%; grade II, 33–50%; and grade III, >50%. In mild cases loss of the lateral overhang of the femoral ossific nucleus (Klein's line) and blurring of the proximal femoral metaphysis may be all that is seen on the AP film. If seen acutely (within 3 weeks), limited closed reduction and pinning are indicated. Later, recommended therapy is pinning in situ or epiphysiodesis if deformity is severe in a heavy patient. **Forceful reduction** before pinning **is never indicated.** Pin placement can be percutaneous with one pin. The pin should be placed anteriorly on the femoral neck, ending in the central portion of the femoral head. Prophylactic pinning of the opposite hip is no longer recommended. Intertrochanteric (Kramer) or subtrochanteric (Southwick) osteotomies may be required with severe slips to increase ROM in patients who do not have adequate remodeling and have limited flexion (<90 degrees). Cuneiform osteotomy at the femoral neck has the potential to correct a higher degree of deformity but remains controversial owing to the high reported rates of osteonecrosis (37%) and future osteoarthritis (37%). Complications from the disorder itself or therapy include chondrolysis (narrowed joint space and decreased motion seen; treatment includes traction, NSAIDs, and physical therapy); osteonecrosis (can result from traction and manipulation, especially with acute slips; also can be the result of of superior screw placement; treatment is partial weight-bearing and observation); and perhaps DJD (pistol grip deformity of the proximal femur).

E. Proximal Femoral Focal Deficiency (PFFD)—Developmental defect of the proximal femur recognizable at birth. Clinically, patients with PFFD have a short, bulky thigh that is flexed, abducted, and externally rotated. PFFD can be associated with coxa vera or fibular hemimelia (50%). Congenital knee ligamentous laxity and contracture are also common. Treatment must be individualized based on leg-length discrepancy, adequacy of proximal musculature, femoral rotation, and proximal joint stability. The percentage of shortening is constant during growth, allowing assessment of the final outcome. Four groups exist (Fig. 2–21) that can be subdivided into two categories based on the requirement for amputation: Aitken classes A and B have a femoral head present (and may be treated with limb-lengthening procedures), whereas classes C and D do not (usually require amputation or ankle disarticulation with knee fusion (or Van Ness rotationplasty—with a stable ankle and patient and parent acceptance).

F. Leg-Length Discrepancy (LLD)—There are many causes of leg-length discrepancy, including congenital disorders (e.g., hemihypertrophy dysplasias, PFFD, DDH), paralytic disorders (e.g., spasticity, polio), infection (pyogenic disruption of the growth plate), tumors, and trauma. Long-term problems associated with LLD include inefficient gait, equinus contractures of the ankle, postural scoliosis, and low back pain. The discrepancy must be measured accurately (e.g., with blocks of set height under the affected side, scanogram) and can be tracked with the Green Anderson or Mosely graph (with serial leg-length films or CT scanograms and bone age determinations). In general, projected discrepancies at maturity of <2 cm are ignored or treated with shoe lifts; 2- to 5-cm differences can be treated with epiphysiodesis of the unaffected side (usually done percutaneously with the aid of a C-arm [or shortening at maturity]). Discrepancies of >5 cm are treated with lengthening. Using standard techniques, distraction of 1 mm/day is typical. The Ilizarov principles are followed, including metaphyseal corticotomy (preserving the medullary canal and blood supply) followed by gradual lengthening. Rarely one can consider physeal distraction. This procedure must be done near skeletal maturity because the physis almost always fuses after limb lengthening. Gross estimate

TYPE		FEMORAL HEAD	ACETABULUM	FEMORAL SEGMENT	RELATIONSHIP AMONG COMPONENTS OF FEMUR AND ACETABULUM AT SKELETAL MATURITY
A	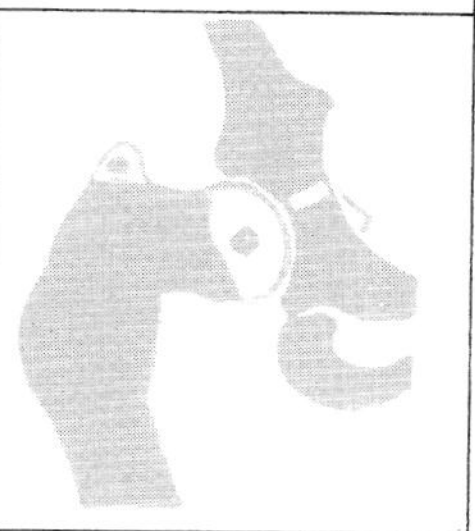	Present	Normal	Short	Bony connection between components of femur Femoral head in acetabulum Subtrochanteric varus angulation, often with pseudarthrosis
B	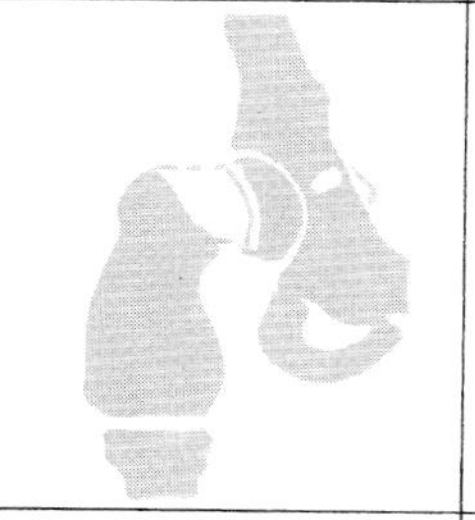	Present	Adequate or moderately dysplastic	Short, usually proximal bony tuft	No osseous connection between head and shaft Femoral head in acetabulum
C	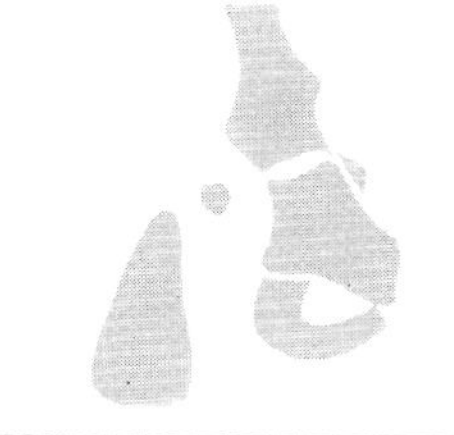	Absent or represented by ossicle	Severely dysplastic	Short, usually proximally tapered	May be osseous connection between shaft and proximal ossicle No articular relation between femur and acetabulum
D		Absent	Absent Obturator foramen enlarged Pelvis squared in bilateral cases	Short, deformed	(none)

FIGURE 2–21. Aiken classification of proximal femoral focal deficiency. Note lack of femoral head in types C and D. (From Tachdjian, M.O.: Pediatric Orthopaedics, 2nd ed. Philadelphia, WB Saunders, 1990; reprinted by permission.)

of LLD can be made using the following assumption of growth per year up to age 16 in boys and age 14 in girls: distal femur, 3/8 inch/year; proximal tibia, 1/4 inch/year; and proximal femur 1/8 inch/year. Use of the Mosely data gives more accurate data.

G. Lower Extremity Inflammation and Infection (see also Chapter 1, Basic Sciences, Part 5: Orthopaedic Infections and Microbiology)

1. Transient Synovitis—Most common cause of painful hips during childhood, but it is a diagnosis of exclusion. Can be related to viral infection, allergic reaction, or trauma; however, etiology is unknown. Onset can be acute or insidious. Symptoms, which are self-limited, include voluntary limitation of motion and muscle spasm. With transient synovitis, the ESR is usually <20 mm/hr. Rule out septic hip with aspiration (especially in children with fever, leukocytosis, or elevated ESR); then observe in Buck's traction for 24–48 hours.
2. Osteomyelitis—More common in children because of their rich metaphyseal blood supply and thick periosteum. Most common organism is *Staph. aureus* (except in neonates in whom **group B strep is more common**). *Hemophilus influenzae* is also common in children 6 months to 4 years of age. A history of trauma is common and may predispose children to osteomyelitis. Osteomyelitis in children usually begins through hematogenous seeding of a bony metaphysis in the small arterioles that bend just beyond the physis, where blood flow is sluggish and there is poor phagocytosis, creating a bone abscess (Fig. 2–22). Pus lifts the thick periosteum and puts pressure on the cortex, causing coagulation. Cortical bone may die and become a sequestrum. Finally, subperiosteal new bone

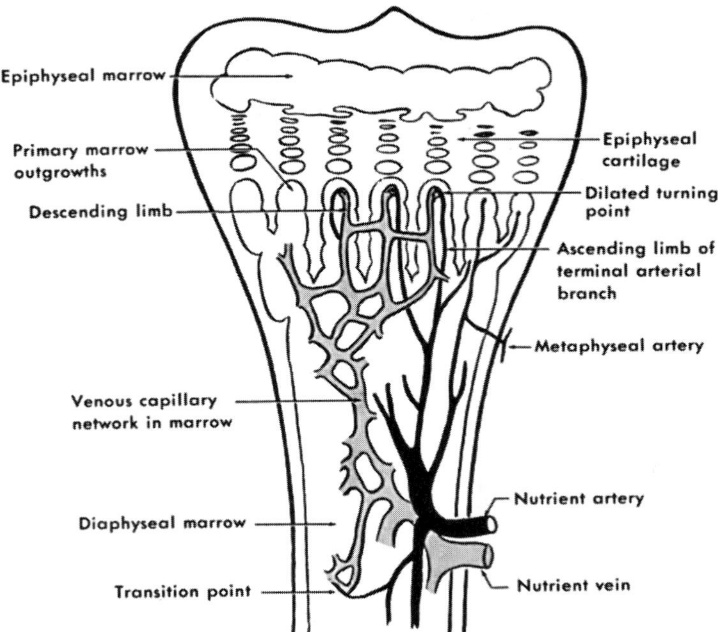

FIGURE 2–22. Metaphyseal sinusoids where sluggish blood flow increases susceptibility to osteomyelitis. (From Tachdjian, M.O.: Pediatric Orthopaedics, 2nd ed. Philadelphia, WB Saunders, 1990; reprinted by permission.)

forms around the dead sequestrum, creating an involucrum. Chronic bone abscesses may become surrounded by thick, fibrous tissue and sclerotic bone (Brodie's abscess). Clinically, the child presents with a tender, warm, sometimes swollen area over a long bone metaphysis. Fever may or may not be present. Laboratory tests may be helpful (blood cultures, WBC, ESR, C-reactive protein [CRP]), and radiologic studies are also useful (radiographs with only soft tissue edema early, metaphyseal rarefaction late, and bone scans). Definitive diagnosis is made with aspiration (50% positive cultures). IV antibiotics (usually a third generation cephalosporin [e.g., cefataxime {Claforan}] in neonates and a first generation cephalosporin [e.g., cefazolin {Ancef}] in older children; followed by antibiotics specific for organisms cultured) are the best initial treatment if osteomyelitis is caught early with no radiographic changes and rapid response to treatment. Failure to respond to antibiotics, frank pus on aspiration, or the presence of a sequestered abscess (not accessible to antibiotics), requires operative drainage and débridement are required. Specimens should be sent for histology and culture. Some tumors (with necrosis) look like infections. The wound can be closed over a drain. IV antibiotics can be changed to appropriate PO antibiotics after a good response to treatment (usually at 7–10 days) and with sensitive oral antibiotics. Antibiotics should be continued until the ESR (or CRP) returns to normal.

3. Septic Arthritis—Can develop from osteomyelitis (especially in neonates, in whom transphyseal vessels allow proximal spread into the joint) in joints with an intra-articular metaphysis (hip, elbow, shoulder); or it can be from hematogenous spread of infection. Because pus is chondrolytic, septic arthritis in children is an acute surgical emergency. Organisms vary with age.

AGE	COMMON ORGANISMS	EMPIRIC ANTIBIOTICS
<12 mo	Staph, group B strep	First generation cephalosporin
6 mo–5 yr	Staph, *H. influenzae*	Second or third generation cephalosporin
5–12 yr	*S. aureus*	First generation cephalosporin
12–18 yr	*S. aureus, N. gonorrhoeae*	Oxacillin/ cephalosporin

Decreased ROM and severe pain with passive motion may be accompanied by systemic symptoms of infection. Radiographs may show widened joint space or even dislocation. Joint fluid aspirate shows a high WBC count, glucose level 50 mg/dl less than serum levels, and in patients with gram-positive cocci or gram-negative rods a high lactic acid level. Ultrasonography can be helpful for identifying the presence of an effusion. Aspiration should be followed by I&D in major joints (especially in the hip, culture of synovium is also recommended). Lumbar punture (LP) should be considered in a septic joint caused by *Hemophilus influenzae* because of increased incidence of meningitis. LP may not be necessary if an antibiotic is selected that is known to cross the blood–brain barrier. IV antibiotics are changed to specific oral antibiotics after a good response to treatment is seen and only for reliable patients/ parents and for those with good drug tolerance. Prognosis is usually good except in young patients, those with associated osteomyelitis, and those with infection in the hip joint. Patients with *N. gonorrhoea* septic arthritis usually have a preceding migratory polyarthralgia, small red papules, and multiple joint involvement. This organism typically elicits less WBC response (50,000 versus >100,000 WBCs/mm^3 in other septic arthritides) and usually does not require surgical drainage. Large doses of penicillin are required to eliminate this organism.

XIII. Knee and Leg

A. Genu Valgum—Normally genu varum (bowed legs) evolves naturally to genu valgum (knocked knees) by age 21/2 years, with a gradual transition to physiologic valgus by age 4 years. Observation of gait is important when evaluating patients to determine if there is a thrust at the onset of weight-bearing. This sign indicates weak restraints and connotes an increased likelihood of progression.

1. Genu Varum (Bowed Legs)—Normal in children <2 years old. Radiographs in physiologic bowing typically show flaring of the tibia and femur in a symmetric fashion. Pathologic conditions that can cause genu varum include osteogenesis imperfecta, osteochondromas, trauma, various dysplasias, and most commonly Blount's disease. **Blount's disease** (tibia varum) differs from physiologic genu varum because it is caused by a disorder of the posterior medial tibial physis. Affected children are most commonly African-American, obese males. Radiographs may show a metaphyseal–diaphyseal angle abnormality. Drennan's angle of >11 degrees is considered abnormal. This angle is formed between the metaphyseal beaks and is perpendicular to the long axis of the tibia (Fig. 2–23). The epiphyseal–metaphyseal angle is also useful (Fig. 2–24). The infantile form of Blount's disease (most common) is usually bilateral and is associated with internal tibial torsion. Adolescent Blount's is less severe and predominantly unilateral. Treatment is based on age and the stage of disease (Langinskiold I–VI with VI characterized by a metaphyseal–epiphyseal bony bridge).

AGE	STAGE	TREATMENT
<18 mo	I–II	None
18–24 mo	I–II	A-frame/Blount brace (night)
2–3 yr	I–II	Modified locked KAFO
3–8 yr	III–V	Valgus rotational osteotomy
3–8 yr	VI	Resection of bony bridge

2. Genu Valgum (Knock-Knees)—Up to 15 degrees at the knee is common in 2- to 6-year-old children. Pathologic genu valgum may be associated, for example, with renal osteodystrophy (most common cause if bilateral), tumors (e.g., osteochondromas), infections (may stimulate proximal asymmetric tibial growth), or

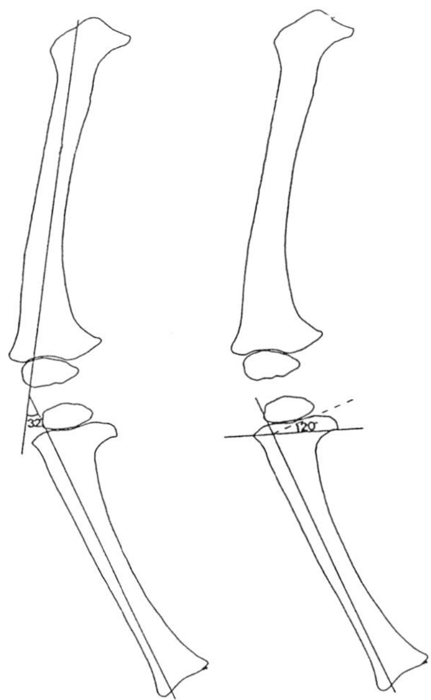

FIGURE 2–23. Comparison of tibiofemoral angle with Levine and Drennan's metaphyseal–diaphyseal angle in tibia vara. *Tibiofemoral Angle,* Method used to determine the tibiofemoral angle. A line is drawn along the longitudinal axis of the tibia and the femur, the angle between the lines is the tibiofemoral angle (32 degrees). *Metaphyseal–Diaphyseal Angle,* Method used to determine the metaphyseal-diaphyseal angle in the same extremity. A line is drawn perpendicular to the longitudinal axis of the tibia, and another is drawn through the two beaks of the metaphysis to determine the transverse axis of the tibial metaphysis. The metaphyseal-diaphyseal angle is the angle bisected by the two lines. (Adapted from Levine, A.M., and Drennan, J.C.: Physiological bowing and tibia vara. J. Bone Joint Surg. [Am.] 64:1159, 1982; reprinted by permission.)

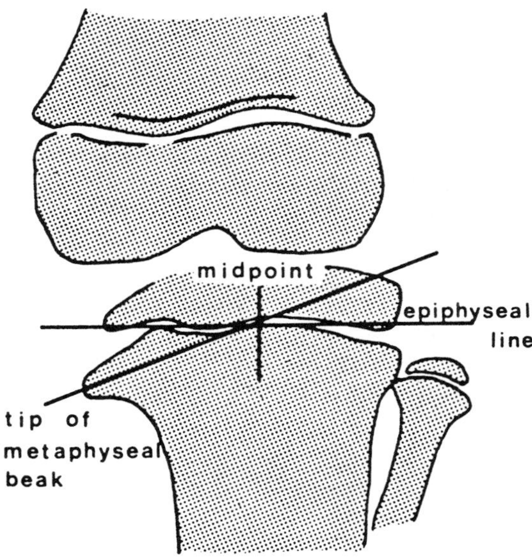

FIGURE 2–24. Blount's disease and measurement of the epiphyseal-metaphyseal angle. (From Tachdjian, M.O.: Pediatric Orthopaedics, 2nd ed. Philadelphia, WB Saunders, 1990; reprinted by permission.)

trauma. Conservative treatment is ineffective. Consider surgery (at the site of the deformity) only in children >10 years old with >10 cm between the medial malleoli or >15–20 degrees of valgus. Hemiepiphysiodesis or physeal stapling of the medial side is effective prior to the end of growth for severe deformities.

B. Tibial Bowing—Three types based on the apex of the curve.
   1. Posteromedial—Physiologic bowing usually of the middle and distal thirds of the tibia may be the result of abnormal intrauterine positioning. It is commonly associated with calcaneovalgus feet and tight anterior structures. Spontaneous correction is the rule, but follow the patient to evaluate late leg-length discrepancy (LLD). Late contralateral epiphysiodesis may be required for an average LLD of 3–4 cm. Tibial osteotomies are not indicated.
   2. Anteromedial Tibial Bowing—Typically caused by fibular hemimelia. A congenital longitudinal deficiency of the fibula is the most common long-bone deficiency and the **most common skeletal deformity in the leg.** It is usually associated with anteromedial bowing and is often accompanied by ankle instability, equinovarus foot (± absent lateral rays), tarsal coalition, and femoral shortening. Classically, skin dimpling is seen over the tibia. Significant LLD often results from this disorder. Hemimelia can be intercalary, which involves the whole bone (absent fibula), or terminal. Fibular hemimelia is frequently associated with femoral abnormalities such as coxa vara and PFFD. Treatment varies from a simple shoe lift or bracing to Syme amputation. Amputation is usually done at about 10 months of age. For less severe cases, lengthening and reconstruction of the mortise (Gruca) may be an alternative. This procedure should include resection of the fibular anlage to avoid future foot problems.
   3. Anterolateral Tibial Bowing—Congenital pseudarthrosis of the tibia is the most common cause of anterolateral bowing. It is often accompanied by neurofibromatosis (50%—but only 10% of patients with neurofibromatosis have this disorder). Classification (Boyd) is based on bowing and the presence of cystic changes, sclerosis, or dysplasia; dysplasia and cystic changes are most common. Early treatment includes a total contact brace to protect from fractures, intramedullary fixation with excision of hamartomatous tissue, and autogenous bone grafting (osteosynthesis) for nonhealing fractures. Vascularized fibular graft or Ilizarov methods should be considered if bracing fails. Osteotomies and electrical stimulation alone are contraindicated. Amputation (Symes) and prosthetic fitting are indicated after two or three failed surgical attempts.
   4. Other Lower Limb Deficiencies—Include tibial hemimelia, an AD disorder that is a congenital longitudinal deficiency of the tibia. It is much less common than fibular hemimelia and is often associated with other bony abnormalities (especially lobster-claw hand). Clinically, the extremity is shortened and anterolaterally bowed with a prominent fibular head and equinovarus foot, with the sole of the foot facing the perineum. Treatment may include Symes or a below-knee amputation. Severe deformities with an absent tibia require knee disarticulation. Fibular transposition (Brown) has been unsuccessful, especially with absent quadriceps function and absent proximal tibias.

C. Osteochondritis Dissecans—Intra-articular lesion, usually of the knee, with disorderly enchondral ossification of epiphyseal growth. Common in 10- to 15-year-olds and can affect many joints, especially the knee and elbow (capitellum). The lesion is thought to be secondary to trauma, ischemia, or abnormal epiphyseal ossification. The lateral intercondylar portion of the medial femoral condyle is most frequently involved (seen best on notch view). Classified into three categories based on age at appearance (Pappas).

CATEGORY	AGE GROUP	PROGNOSIS	TREATMENT
I	Birth to adolescence	Excellent	Rest, immobilize
II	Teenage children	Intermediate	Rest, arthroscopic fixation of large defects
III	Adult (20+); closed physis	Poor; fragments/ defects	Operative

Symptoms include activity-related pain, localized tenderness, stiffness, and swelling ± mechanical symptoms. Radiographs should include the tunnel (notch) view to evaluate the condyles. Differential diagnosis includes anomalous ossification centers. Surgical therapy includes drilling with multiple holes, fixation of large fragments, and bone grafting of large lesions in patients with closed physes. Commonly treated arthroscopically. Poor prognosis is associated with lesions in the lateral femoral condyle and patella. The arthroscopic classification and treatment of osteochondritis dissecans (after Guhl) is as follows.

CLASSIFICATION	TREATMENT
Intact lesion	K wire drilling
Early-sepated lesion	In situ pinning
Partially detached lesion Salvageable loose body	Débridement of base and reduction and pinning
Unsalvageable loose body	Removal and débridement of base

D. Osgood-Schlatter Disease—Osteochondritis or fatigue failure of the tibia tubercle apophysis due to stress from the extensor mechanism in a growing child. Radiographs may show irregularity and fragmentation of the tibial tubercle. Usually self-limited; late excision of separate ossicles is occasionally required.

E. Discoid Meniscus—Abnormal development of the lateral meniscus leads to the formation of a disc-shaped (or hypertrophic), rather than the normal crescent-shaped, meniscus. Typically, radiographs demonstrate widening of the cartilage space on the affected side (up to 11 mm). If symp-

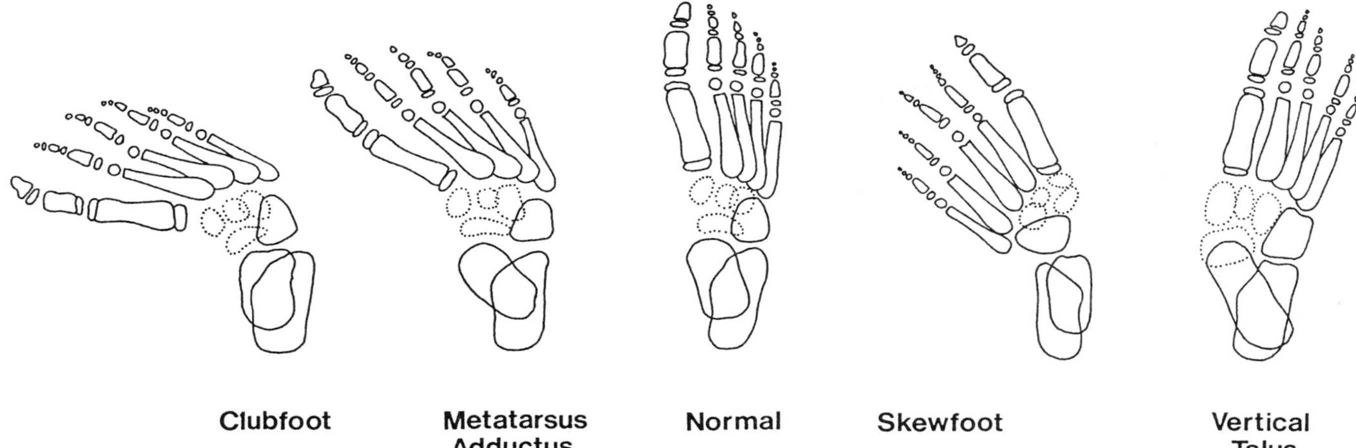

FIGURE 2–25. Anteroposterior view of common childhood foot disorders. *A,* Varus position of hindfoot and adducted forefoot in clubfoot. *B,* Normal hindfoot and adducted forefoot in MTA. *C,* Normal foot. *D,* Valgus hindfoot (with increased talocalcaneal angle) and adducted forefoot in skewfoot. *E,* Increased talocalcaneal angle and lateral deviation of the calcaneus in congenital vertical talus.

tomatic and torn, it can be arthroscopically débrided.

XIV. Feet (Fig. 2–25)

A. Clubfoot (Congenital Talipes Equinovarus)—Forefoot adduction and hindfoot varus with the calcaneus inverted under the equinus talus. Talar neck deformity (medial and plantar deviation) with medial rotation of the calcaneus and medial displacement of the navicular and cuboid occurs. Clubfoot is more common in males, and half are bilateral. It is associated with shortened/contracted muscles (intrinsics, plantar flexors, invertors), joint capsules, ligaments, and fascia that lead to the associated deformities. Can be associated with hand anomalies (Streeter's dysplasia), diastrophic dwarfism, arthrogryposis, and myelomeningocele. Radiographs should include the **dorsiflexed lateral** view (Turco) in which a talocalcaneal angle of >35 degrees is normal; a smaller angle with a flat talar head is seen with clubfoot. On the AP view a talocalcaneal (Kite) angle of 20–40 degrees is normal (<20 degrees is seen with clubfoot). The talus–first metatarsal angle is normally 0–20 degrees (a negative talus-first metatarsal angle is seen with clubfoot.) (Fig. 2–26). "Parallelism" of the calcaneus and talus is seen on both views. Only 10–15% of those with true (rigid, structural) club-

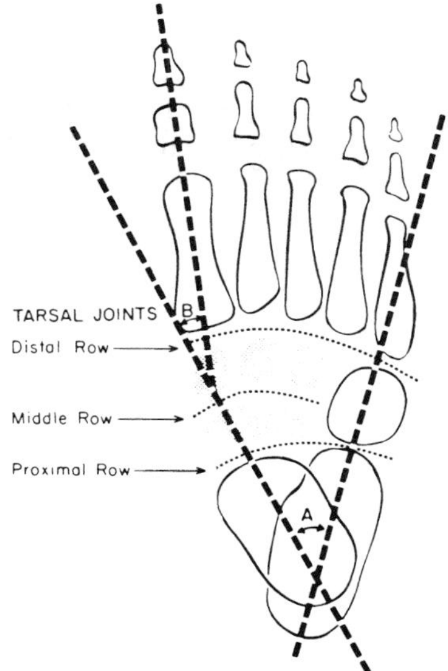

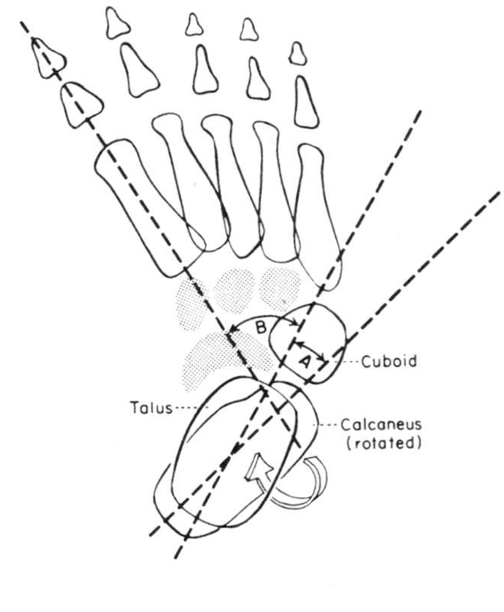

FIGURE 2–26. Radiographic evaluation of club feet. Note the "parallelism" of the talus and calcaneus with a talocalcaneal angle (*A*) of <20 degrees and negative talus–first metatarsal angle (*B*) on the clubfoot side. (From Simmons, G.W.: Analytical radiography of clubfeet. J. Bone Joint Surg. [Br.] 59:485–489, 1974; reprinted by permission.)

foot (refractory to casting with midfoot crease and small heel) respond to serial manipulation and casting. Nevertheless, 3 months of casting is the recommended therapy for children initially. Some cases can be fully corrected with serial casts, although many require corrective surgery. Surgical subtalar and posterior capsular release with tendon lengthening (Turco, posteromedial release with attention also to the posterolateral corner) is favored usually at 3–9 months. The following structures are addressed.

STRUCTURE	PROCEDURE
Achilles tendon	Z-lengthening
Calcaneal fibular ligament	Release
Post. talofibular ligament	Release
Post. tibialis tendon	Z-lengthening
Subtalar capsule	Release
Superficial deltoid	Release
Fibulocalcaneal ligament	Partial release
Tibiotalar, subtalar capsule	Complete release
Talonavicular tibionavicular (pseudo)	Release

The posterior tibial artery must be carefully protected. Often the dorsalis pedis artery is insufficient. Casting for several months is usually required postoperatively. In older patients (3–10 years old), medial opening or lateral column shortening osteotomies or cuboidal decancellization is recommended. For children who present with refractory clubfoot late (8–10 years old), triple arthrodesis is the only procedure possible to eliminate associated pain. Triple arthrodesis is contraindicated in patients with insensate feet because it causes a rigid foot that may lead to ulceration. Talectomy may be a better procedure in these patients.

B. Forefoot Adduction (see Fig. 2–19)
  1. Metatarsus Adductus (MTA) (see Section XI: Lower Extremity Problems, B: Rotational Problems of the Lower Extremities, above)—Adduction of the forefoot is commonly associated with DDH. A simple clinical grading system has been described by Bleck based on the heel bisector line (Fig. 2–27); normally the heel bisector should line up with the second/third toe interspace). Four subtypes have been identified (Berg).

TYPE	FEATURES
Simple MTA	MTA
Complex MTA	MTA + lateral shift of midfoot
Skew foot	MTA + valgus hindfoot
Complex skew foot	MTA, lateral shift, valgus hindfoot

If peroneal stimulation corrects MTA, usually it responds to stretching. Otherwise, manipulation and special off-the-shelf orthotics or serial casting may be required. Surgery in refractory cases (usually those with a medial skin crease) includes abductor hallucis longus recession (for an atavistic first toe), medial capsular release with Evans calcaneal osteotomy (lateral column shortening), or medial opening cuneiform and lateral closing cuboid osteotomies, ± metatarsal osteotomies based on the severity of deformity.
  2. Medial Deviation of the Talar Neck—Benign disorder of the foot that generally corrects spontaneously.
  3. Serpentine ("Z") Foot (Complex Skew Foot)—Associated with residual tarsometatarsal adductus, talonavicular lateral subluxation, and hindfoot valgus. No good nonoperative therapy. Surgical treatment of this difficult problem is demanding and may include medial calcaneal sliding osteotomy (for hindfoot valgus), opening wedge cuboid osteotomy and closing wedge cuneiform osteotomy (to correct midfoot lateral subluxation), and metatarsal osteotomies (to correct forefoot adductus).

C. Pes Cavus—Cavus deformity of the foot (elevated longitudinal arch) due to fixed plantar flexion of the forefoot. There are four basic types of pes cavus.

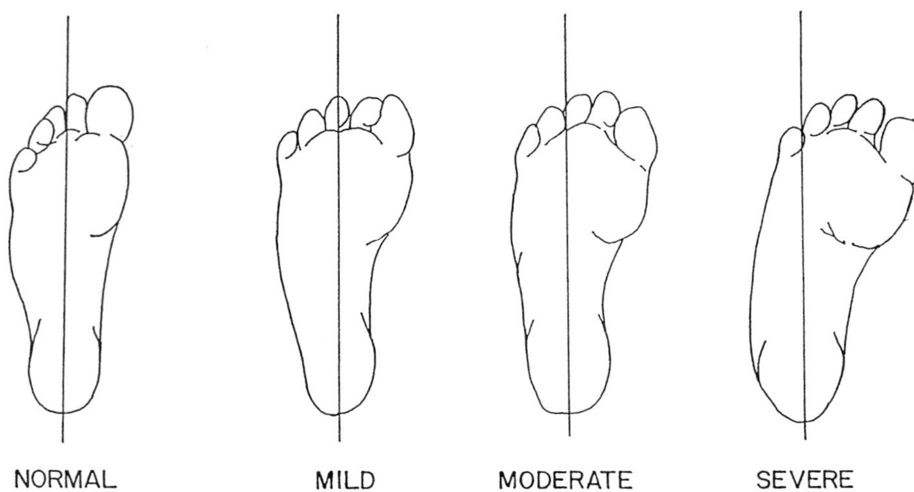

FIGURE 2–27. Classification of metatarsus adductus. (From Bleck, E.E.: Metatarsus adductus: Classification and relationship to all kinds of treatment. J. Pediatr. Orthop. 3:2–9, 1983, reprinted by permission.)

TYPE	FOREFOOT	HINDFOOT	RADIOGRAPHS
Simple	Balanced	Neutral	Decreased talus–calcaneus angle
Cavorvarus	Plantar flexed	Varus	
Calcaneus	Fixed equinus	Calcaneus	
Equinocavus	Equinus	Equinus	

Pes cavus is commonly associated with neurologic disorders including polio, CP, Friedreich's ataxia, and Charcot-Marie-Tooth disease. Full neurologic work-up is mandatory. Lateral block test (Coleman) assesses hindfoot flexibility of the cavovarus foot (flexible feet correct to normal with a lift placed under lateral aspect of foot). Nonoperative management is rarely successful. Surgery includes plantar release, metatarsal osteotomies, tendon transfers (if a supple deformity); and if the lateral block test is abnormal (rigid deformity), a calcaneal osteotomy is done. In the past, triple arthrodesis has been used for rigid deformity in mature patients; the use of calcaneal sliding osteotomy, with multiple metatarsal extension osteotomies, may offer an alternative to subtalar fusion procedures.

D. Pes Calcaneovalgus

1. Congenital Vertical Talus (Rocker-Bottom Foot)—Irreducible dorsal dislocation of the navicular on the talus with a fixed talocalcaneal complex. Clinically, the talar head is prominent medially, the sole is convex, the forefoot is abducted and dorsiflexed, and the hindfoot is in equinovalgus (Persian slipper foot). Patients may demonstrate a "peg-leg" gait (awkward gait with limited forefoot pushoff). It is a common cause of a rigid flatfoot, which can be isolated or can occur with chromosomal abnormalities, myeloarthropathies, or neurologic disorders. **Plantar-flexed lateral radiographs** show that a line along the long axis of the talus passes below the metatarsal–cuneiform axis (Meary, tarsal–first metatarsal angle <60 degrees [normal 0–20 degrees dorsal tilt]) (Fig. 2–28). AP radiographs show a talocalcaneal angle of >40 degrees (normal 20–40 degrees). Differential diagnosis includes oblique talus (corrects with plantar flexion), tarsal coalition, and paralytic pes valgus. Three months of corrective casting (foot plantar flexed/inverted) or manipulative stretching is tried initially. Surgery at 6–12 months old includes soft tissue release/lengthening. Late treatment includes subtalar arthrodesis (21/2–6 years old) and triple arthrodesis (>6 years old).

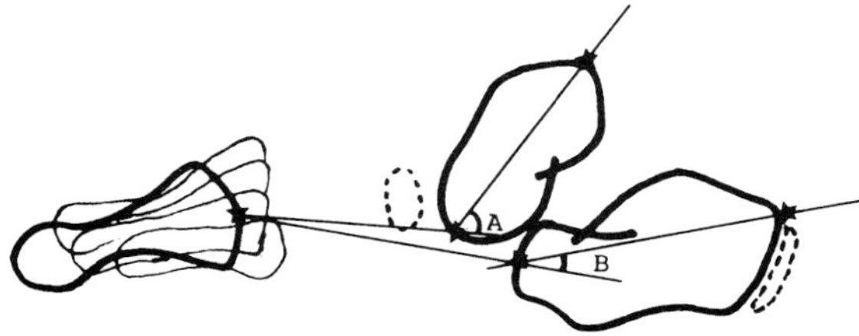

FIGURE 2–28. Plantar-flexed lateral radiographic features in congenital vertical talus. *A*, Talar axis–metatarsal base angle (normally 3 ± 6 degrees). *B*, Calcaneal axis–metatarsal base angle (normally −9 ± 5 degrees). Both angles are increased in congenital vertical talus. (From Hamanishi, C.: Congenital vertical talus. J. Pediatr. Orthop. 4:319, 1984; reprinted by permission.)

2. Oblique Talus—Talonavicular subluxation that reduces with plantar flexion of foot. Treatment is observation and sometimes a UCBL shoe insert. Some patients require pinning of the talonavicular joint in the reduced position and tendoachilles lengthening.

E. Tarsal Coalitions—AD disorder of mesenchymal segmentation leading to fusion of tarsal bones and rigid flatfoot. Most commonly involves talocalcaneal or calcaneonavicular joints and is the leading cause of peroneal spastic flatfoot. Symptoms, which appear by age 10–12 years, include calf pain due to peroneal spasticity, flatfoot, and limited subtalar motion. Coalitions may be fibrous, cartilagenous, or osseous. **Calcaneonavicular coalition is the most common in children** and is **seen on oblique radiographs of the foot (Sloman).** Lateral radiographs may demonstrate an elongated anterior process of the calcaneus (**"anteater" sign**). Talocalcaneal coalitions may demonstrate talar beaking on the lateral view (does not denote degenerative joint disease) or an irregular middle facet on Harris axial view. **The best study for identifying and measuring the cross-sectional area of a talocalcaneal coalition is a CT scan.** Early surgery is recommended to resect a symptomatic bar in cases involving <50% of the middle facet in talocalcaneal coalitions in order to avoid a triple arthrodesis later. Observation is reasonable for asymptomatic bars in young children. Older patients with calcaneonavicular bars may do well with fusion of talonavicular and calcaneocuboid joints only. Advanced cases require triple arthrodesis.

F. Calcaneovalgus Foot—Newborn condition associated with intrauterine positioning. Common in firstborn children. Presents with a dorsiflexed hindfoot with eversion and abduction of the hindfoot that is passively correctable to neutral. Treatment is passive stretching and observation. Also seen with myelomeningocele at the L5 level due to muscular imbalance between foot dorsiflexors/everters (L4 and L5 roots) and plantar flexors/inverters (S1 and S2 roots).

G. Juvenile Bunions—Often are bilateral and familial. This disorder is less common and usually less severe than the adult form. May be associated with ligamentous laxity and a hypermobile first ray. Usually found in adolescent girls. Wide shoes and arch supports help early. Surgery is indicated with an intermetatarsal angle (IMA) of >10 degrees (metatarsus primus varus) and a hallux valgus angle (HVA) of >20 degrees. Distal metatarsal procedures are more often successful than proximal ones. Metatarsus primus varus may require metatarsal osteotomy and distal capsular reefing. Complications include overcorrection and hallux varus. Recurrence is frequent (>50%), especially when only soft tissue procedures are performed. It is best to wait until maturity to reoperate.

H. Köhler's Disease—Osteonecrosis of the tarsal navicular; usually presents at about 5 years old. Pain is caused by recurring trauma to the maturing epiphysis. Radiographs show sclerosis of the navicular. Symptoms usually resolve spontaneously with decreased activity ± immobilization.

I. Flexible Pes Planus—Foot is flat only when standing and not with toe walking or foot hanging. Frequently familial and almost always bilateral. Commonly associated with minor lower extremity rotational problems and ligamentous laxity. Symptoms, including aching midfoot or pretibial pain, can occur. Lateral radiographic findings mimic those of vertical talus, but a plantar-flexed lateral view demonstrates that a line along the long axis of the talus passes above the metatarsal–cuneiform axis. Treatment is observation only, with no special shoes. Sometimes soft arch supports are helpful but not corrective. Thorough evaluation should be completed to rule out tight heel cords and decreased subtalar motion. UCBL heel cups are sometimes indicated for advanced cases with pain (symptomatic treatment only). Calcaneal osteotomy or select fusions may provide pain relief at the expense of inversion/eversion in adolescents with disabling pain refractory to every means of conservative treatment. The following radiographic views may be helpful.

VIEW	ASSESSMENT
Standing AP	Talar head coverage, talocalcaneal angle
Standing lateral	Calcaneal/talar equinus, talocalcaneal angle
Oblique	To rule out coalition

J. Habitual Toe Walker—Contracture of Achilles tendon. Usually responds to serial casting; sometimes requires tendoachilles lengthening.

K. Accessory Navicular—Normal variant seen in up to 12% of the population. Commonly associated with flat feet. Symptoms usually include medial arch pain with overuse. Symptoms usually abate with activity restriction and/or immobilization. External oblique radiographic views are often helpful for the diagnosis. Most cases respond spontaneously; occasionally excision of the accessory bone is done, which can correct symptoms (but not flatfoot) in most patients.

L. Ball and Socket Ankle—Abnormal formation with a spherical talus (ball) and a cup-shaped tibiofibular articulation (socket). It usually requires no treatment but should be recognized because of its high association with tarsal coalition (50%), absent lateral rays (50%), and leg-length discrepancies.

M. Congenital Toe Disorders
1. Syndactyly—Fusion of the soft tissues (simple) and sometimes bone (complex) of the toes. Simple syndactyly usually does not require treatment; complex syndactyly is treated as it is in the hand.
2. Polydactyly (Extra Digits)—May be AD and usually involves the lateral ray in patients with a positive family history. Treatment includes ablation of the supranumerary digit and any bony protrusion of the common metatarsal (typically the border digit is excised, not the best formed). The procedure is usually done at age 9–12 months, but some rudimentary digits can be ligated in the newborn nursery.
3. Oligodactyly—Congenital absence of the toes. May be associated with more proximal agenesis (i.e., fibular hemimelia) and tarsal coalition. The disorder usually requires no treatment.
4. Atavistic Great Toe (Congenital Hallux Varus)—Great toe adduction deformity that is often associated with supranumerary toes. Must be differentiated from metatarsus adductus. Usually the deformity occurs at the MTP joint and includes a short, thick first metatarsal and a firm band (abductor hallucis longus muscle) that may be responsible for the disorder. Surgery is sometimes required and includes release of the abductor hallucis longus muscle.
5. Overlapping Toe—The fifth toe overlaps the fourth (usually bilaterally) and may cause problems with footwear. Initial treatment includes passive stretching and buddy taping. Surgical options include tenotomy, dorsal capsulotomy, and syndactylization to the fourth toe (McFarland).
6. Underlapping Toe (Congenital Curly Toe)—Usually occurs at lateral three toes and is rarely symptomatic. Surgery (flexor tenotomies) is occasionally indicated.

Selected Bibliography

Embryology

Moore, K.L.: The Developing Human. Philadelphia, WB Saunders, 1982.

Bone Dysplasias

Bassett, G.S.: Lower extremity abnormalities in dwarfing conditions. Instr. Course Lect. 39:389–397, 1991.

Bassett, G.S.: Orthopedic aspects of skeletal dysplasias. Instr. Course Lect. 39:381–387, 1991.

Beals, R.K., and Rolfe, B.: Current concepts review: Vater association; a unifying concept of multiple anomalies. J. Bone Joint Surg. [Am.] 71:948–950, 1989.

Bethem, D., Winter, R.B., Lutter, L., et al.: Spinal disorders of dwarfism. J. Bone Joint Surg. [Am] 63:1412–1425, 1981.

Dawe, C., Wynne-Davies, R., and Fulford, G.E.: Clinical variation in dyschondrosteosis: A report on 13 individuals in 8 families. J. Bone Joint Surg. [Br.] 64:377–381, 1982.

Goldberg, M.J.: The Dysmorphic Child: An Orthopedic Perspective. New York, Raven Press, 1987.

Hecht, J.T., Horton, W.A., Reid, C.S., Pyeritz, R.E., and Chakraborty, R.: Growth of the foramen magnum in achondroplasia. Am. J. Med. Genet. 32:528–535, 1989.

Jones, K.L., and Robinson, L.K.: An approach to the child with structural defects. J. Pediatr. Orthop. 3:238–244, 1983.

Kopits, S.E.: Orthopedic complications of dwarfism. Clin. Orthop. 114:153–179, 1976.

McKusick, V.A.: Heritable Disorders of Connective Tissue, 4th ed. St. Louis, CV Mosby, 1972.

Rubin, P.: Dynamic Classification of Bone Dysplasias. Chicago, Year Book Medical Publishers, 1964.

Stanscur, V., Stanscur, R., and Maroteaux, P.: Pathogenic mechanisms in osteochondrodysplasias. J. Bone Joint Surg. [Am.] 66: 817–836, 1984.

Swanson, A.B.: A classification for congenital limb malformation. J. Hand Surg. 1:8–22, 1976.

Chromosomal and Teratologic Disorders

Elliot, S., Morton, R.E., and Whitelaw, R.A.J.: Atlantoaxial instability and abnormalities of the odontoid in Down syndrome. Arch. Dis. Child 63:1484–1489, 1988.

Huang, T.J., Lubricky, J.P., and Hammerberg, K.W.: Scoliosis in Rhett syndrome. Orthop. Rev. 23:931–937, 1994.
Loder, R., Lee, C., and Richards, B.: Orthopedic aspects of Rhett syndrome: A multicenter review. J. Pediatr. Orthop. 9:557–562, 1989.
Pueschel, S.M., Herndon, J.H., Gelch, M.M., et al.: Symptomatic atlantoaxial subluxation in persons with Down syndrome. J. Pediatr. Orthop. 4:682–688, 1984.
Rees, D., Jones, M.W., Owen, R., et al.: Scoliosis surgery in the Prader-Willi syndrome. J. Bone Joint Surg. [Br.] 71:685–688, 1989.
Segal, L.S., Drummond, D.S., Zanott, R.M., Ecker, M.L., and Mubarak, S.J.: Complications of posterior arthrodesis of the cervical spine in patients who have Down syndrome. J. Bone Joint Surg. [Am.] 73:1547–1554, 1991.
Smith, D.W.: Recognizable Pattern of Human Malformation, 2nd ed. Philadelphia, WB Saunders, 1983.

Hematopoietic Disorders

Diggs, L.W.: Bone and joint lesions in sickle-cell disease. Clin. Orthop. 52:119–143, 1967.
Gill, J.C., Thometz, J.C., and Scott, J.P., Montgomery: Musculoskeletal Problems in Hemophilia in the Child and Adult. New York, Raven Press, 1989.
Triantafylluo, S., Hanks, G., Handal, J.A., and Greer, R.B., III: Open and arthroscopic synovectomy in hemophilic arthropathy of the knee. Clin. Orthop. 283:196–204, 1992.

Metabolic Disease/Arthritides

Albright, J.A., and Miller, E.A.: Osteogenesis imperfecta [editorial comment]. Clin. Orthop. 159:2, 1981.
Birch, J.G., and Herring, J.A.: Spinal deformity in Marfan syndrome. J. Pediatr. Orthop. 7:546–552, 1987.
Certner, J.M., and Root, L.: Osteogenesis imperfecta. Orthop. Clin. North Am. 21:151–162, 1990.
Gamble, J.G., Strudwick, W.J., Rinsky, L.A., and Bleck, E.E.: Complications of intramedullary rods in osteogenesis imperfecta: Bailey-Dubow rods versus nonelongating rods. J. Pediatr. Orthop. 8: 645–649, 1989.
Hensinger, R.N., DeVito, P.D., and Ragsdale, C.G.: Changes in the cervical spine in juvenile rheumatoid arthritis. J. Bone Joint Surg. [Am.] 68:189–199, 1986.
Mankin, H.J.: Rickets, osteomalacia and renal osteodystrophy: An update. Orthop. Clin. North Am. 21:81–96, 1990.
Robelo, I., Peredra, D.A., Silva, L., et al.: Effects of synthetic salmon calcitonin therapy in children with osteogenesis imperfecta. J. Int. Med. Res. 17:401–405, 1989.
Schaller, J.G.: Chronic arthritis in children: Juvenile rheumatoid arthritis. Clin. Orthop. 182:79–89, 1984.
Shapiro, F.: Consequences of an osteogenesis imperfecta diagnosis for survival and ambulation. J. Pediatr. Orthop. 5:456–462, 1985.
Sillence, D.O.: Osteogenesis imperfecta: An expanding panorama of variance. Clin. Orthop. 159:11, 1981.
Sofield, H.A., Miller, E.A.: Fragmentation realignment, and intramedullary rod fixation of deformities of the long bones in children. J. Bone Joint Surg. [Am.] 41:1371, 1959.

Birth Injuries

Canale, S.T., Griffin, T.W., and Hubbard, C.N.: Congenital muscular torticollis: A long term follow-up. J. Bone Joint Surg. [Am.] 64: 810–816, 1982.
Davids, J.R., Wenger, D.R., and Mubarak, S.J.: Congenital muscular torticollis: Sequelae of intrauterine or perinatal compartment syndrome. J. Pediatr. Orthop. 13:141–147, 1993.
Gilbert, A., Brockman, R., and Carlioz, H.: Surgical treatment of brachial plexus birth palsy. Clin. Orthop. 264:39–47, 1991.
Hentze, V.R., and Meyer, R.D.: Brachial plexus microsurgery in children. Microsurgery 12:175–185, 1991.
Jahnke, A.H., Bovill, D.F., McCarroll, H.R., and Ashley, J.P.: Persistent brachial plexus birth palsies. J. Pediatr. Orthop. 11:533–537, 1991.
Quinlan, W.R., Brady, P.G., and Regan, B.F.: Congenital pseudarthrosis of the clavical. Acta Orthop. Scand. 51:489–492, 1980.

Cerebral Palsy

Albright, A.L., Barron, W.B., Fasick, M.P., et al.: Continuous intrathecal baclofen infusion for spasticity of cerebral origin. J.A.M.A. 270:2475–2477, 1993.
Barnes, M.J., and Herring, J.A.: Combined-split anterior tibial-tendon transfer and intramuscular lengthening of the posterior tibial tendon. J. Bone Joint Surg. [Am.] 73:734–738, 1991.
Bleck, E.E.: Current concepts review: Management of the lower extremities in children who have cerebral palsy. J. Bone Joint Surg. [Am.] 72:140, 1990.
Bleck, E.E.: Orthopedic Management of Cerebral Palsy. Philadelphia, JB Lippincott, 1987.
Coleman, S.S., and Chestnut, W.J.: A simple test for hindfoot flexibility in the cavovarus foot. Clin. Orthop. 123:60–62, 1977.
Cosgrove, A.P., and Graham, H.K.: Botulinum toxin-A prevents the development of contractures in the hereditary spastic mouse. Dev. Med. Child Neurol. 36:379–385, 1994.
Elmer, E.B., Wenger, D.R., Mubarak, S.J., and Sutherland, D.H.: Proximal hamstring lengthening in the sitting cerebral palsy patient. J. Pediatr. Orthop. 12:329–336, 1992.
Ferguson, R.L., and Allen, B.L.: Considerations in the treatment of cerebral palsy patients with spinal deformities. Orthop. Clin. North Am. 19:419–425, 1988.
Gage, J.R.: Gait analysis: An essential tool in the treatment of cerebral palsy. Clin. Orthop. 288:126–134, 1993.
Gage, J.R.: The clinical use of kinetics for evaluation of pathologic gait in cerebral palsy. J. Bone Joint Surg. [Am.] 76:622–631, 1994.
Koman, L.A., Mooney, J.F., and et al.: Management of valgus hindfoot deformity in pediatric cerebral palsy patients by medial displacement osteotomy. J. Pediatr. Orthop. 13:180–183, 1993.
Koman, L.A., Mooney, J.F., Smith, B.P., et al.: Management of spasticity in cerebral palsy with botulinum-A toxin: Report of preliminary, randomized, double-blind trial. J. Pediatr. Orthop. 14: 299–303, 1994.
Mubarak, S.J., Valencia, F.G., and Wenger, D.R.: One stage correction of the spastic dislocated hip. J. Bone Joint Surg. [Am.] 74: 1347–1357, 1994.
Ounpuu, S., Muik, E., Davis, R.B., et al.: Rectus femoris surgery in children with cerebral palsy. Part II. A comparison between the effect of transfer and release of the distal rectus femoris on knee motion. J. Pediatr. Orthop. 13:331–335, 1993.
Rang, M., Silver, R., de la Garza, Jr., et al.: Cerebral palsy. In Lovell and Winter, eds. Pediatric Orthopedics, 2nd ed. Philadelphia, JB Lippincott, 1986.
Rang, M., and Wright, J.: What have 30 years of medical progress done for cerebral palsy? Clin. Orthop. 247:55–60, 1989.
Sutherland, D.H., and Davids, J.R.: Common gait abnormalities of the knee in cerebral palsy. Clin. Orthop. 288:139–147, 1993.

Neuromuscular Disorders

Allen, B.L., Jr., and Ferguson, R.L.: The Galveston technique of pelvic fixation with Luque-rod instrumentation of the spine. Spine 9:388–394, 1984.
Beaty, J.H., and Canale, S.T.: Current concepts review: Orthopedic aspects of myelomeningocele. J. Bone Joint Surg. [Am.] 72: 626–630, 1990.
Carlson, W.O., Speck, G.J., Vicari, V., and Wenger, D.R.: Arthrogryposis multiplex congenita: A long term follow-up study. Clin. Orthop. 194:115–123, 1985.
Carroll, N.J.: Assessment and management of the lower extremity in myelodysplasia. Orthop. Clin. North Am. 18:709–724, 1987.
Diaz, L.S.: Hip deformities in myelomeningocele. Instr. Course Lect. 40:281–286, 1991.
Drennan, J.C.: Foot deformities in myelomeningocele. Instr. Course Lect. 40:287–291, 1991.
Drummond, D.S., Moreau, M., and Cruess, R.L.: The results and complications of surgery for the paralytic hip and spine in myelomeningocele. J. Bone Joint Surg. [Br.] 62:49–53, 1980.
Emans, J.B.: Current concepts review: Allergy to latex in patients who have myelodysplasia. J. Bone Joint Surg. [Am.] 74: 1103–1109, 1992.
Evans, G.A., Drennan, J.C., and Russman, B.S.: Functional classification and orthopedic management of spinal muscular atrophy. J. Bone Joint Surg. [Br.] 63:516–522, 1981.
Hoffer, M.M., Feiwell, E., Perry, R., et al.: Functional ambulation in patients with myelomeningocele. J. Bone Joint Surg. [Am.] 55: 137–148, 1973.
Lindseth, R.E.: Spine deformity in myelomeningocele. Inst. Course Lect. 40:273–279, 1991.

Mazur, J.M., Shurtleff, D., Menelaus, M., et al.: Orthopedic management of high-level spina bifida: Early walking compared with early use of a wheelchair. J. Bone Joint Surg. [Am.] 71:56, 1989.
Mendell, J.R., and Sahenk, Z.: Recent advances in diagnosis and classification of Charcot-Marie-Tooth disease. Curr. Opin. Orthop. 4:39–45, 1993.
Shapiro, F., and Bresnan, M.J.: Orthopedic management of childhood neuromuscular disease. Part II. Peripheral neuropathies, Friedrich's ataxia, and arthrogryposis multiplex congenita. J. Bone Joint Surg. [Am.] 64:949–953, 1982.
Shapiro, F., and Specht, L.: Current concepts review: The diagnosis and orthopedic management of inherited muscular disorders of childhood. J. Bone Joint Surg. [Am] 75:439–454, 1993.
Sodergard, J., and Ryoppy, S.: Foot deformities in arthrogryposis multiplex congenita. J. Pediatr. Orthop. 14:768–772, 1994.
Thompson, G.H.: Arthrogryposis multiplex congenita [editorial]. Clin. Orthop. 194:2–3, 1985.

Pediatric Spine

Ali, M.S., and Hooper, G.: Congenital pseudarthrosis of the ulna due to neurofibromatosis. J. Bone Joint Surg. [Br.] 64:600–602, 1982.
Apel, D.M., Marrero, G., King, J., et al.: Avoiding paraplegia during anterior spinal surgery: The role of somatosensory evoked potentials monitoring with temporary occlusion of segmental spinal arteries. Spine 16:S365–S370, 1991.
Bellah, R.D., Summerville, D.A., Treves, S.T., and Micheli, L.J.: Low-back pain in adolescent athletes: Detection of stress injury to the pars intrarticularis with SPECT. Radiology 180:509–512, 1991.
Bollini, G., Bergion, M., Labriet, C., et al.: Hemivertebrae excision and fusion in children aged less than 5 years. J. Pediatr. Orthop. 1(part B):95–101, 1993.
Bradford, D.S., Ahmed, K.B., Moe, J.H., et al.: The surgical management of patients with Scheuerman's disease: A review of twenty-four cases managed by combined anterior and posterior spine fusion. J. Bone Joint Surg. [Am.] 62:705–712, 1980.
Bradford, D.S., and Hensinger, R.M., eds.: The Pediatric Spine. New York, Thieme-Stratton, 1985.
Bradford, D.S., Lonstein, J.E., Ogilvie, J.B., and Winter, R.B., eds: Moe's Textbook of Scoliosis and Other Spinal Deformities, 2nd ed. Philadelphia, WB Saunders, 1987.
Bridwell, K.H., McAllister, J.W., Betz, R.R., et al.: Coronal decompensation produced by Cotrel-Dubousset "derotation" maneuver for idiopathic right thoracic scoliosis. Spine 16:769–777, 1991.
Carr, W.A., Moe, J.H., Winter, R.B., and Lonstein, J.E.: Treatment of idiopathic scoliosis in the Milwaukee brace. J. Bone Joint Surg. [Am.] 62:599–612, 1980.
Crawford, A.H., Jr., and Bagamery, M.: Osseous manifestations of neurofibromatosis in childhood. J. Pediatr. Orthop. 6:72–88, 1986.
Denis, F.: Cotrel-Duboussetinstrumentation in the treatment of idiopathic scoliosis. Orthop. Clin. North Am. 19:291–311, 1988.
Dickson, J.H., Erwin, W.D., and Rossi, D.: Harrington instrumentation and arthrodesis for idiopathic scoliosis. A twenty-one year follow-up. J. Bone Joint Surg. [Am.] 72:678–683, 1990.
Dimeglio, A.: Growth of the spine before age 5 years. J. Pediatr. Orthop. 1(part B):102–107, 1993.
Engler, G.L.: Preoperative and intraoperative considerations in adolescent idiopathic scoliosis. Inst. Course Lect. 38:137–141, 1989.
Fielding, J.W., and Hawkins, R.J.: Atlantoaxial rotatory fixation. J. Bone Joint Surg. [Am.] 59:37–44, 1977.
Fielding, J.W., Hensinger, R.N., and Hawkins, R.J.: Os odontoidium. J. Bone Joint Surg. [Am.] 62:376–383, 1980.
Fitch, R.D., Turi, M., Bowman, B.E., and Hardaker, W.T.: Comparison of Cotrel-Dubousset and Harrington rod instrumentation in idiopathic scoliosis. J. Pediatr. Orthop. 10:44–47, 1990.
Keller, R.B.: Nonoperative treatment of adolescent idiopathic scoliosis. Inst. Course Lect. 38:129–135, 1989.
King, H.A., Moe, J.H., Bradford, D.S., and Winter, R.B.: The selection of fusion levels in thoracic idiopathic scoliosis. J. Bone Joint Surg. [Am.] 65:1302–1313, 1983.
Koop, S.E., Winter, R.B., and Lonstein, J.E.: The surgical treatment of instability of the upper part of the cervical spine in children and adolescents. J. Bone Joint Surg. [Am.] 66:403–411, 1984.
Kostuik, J.P.: Current concepts review: Operative treatment of idiopathic scoliosis. J. Bone Joint Surg. [Am.] 72:1108–1112, 1990.
Lenke, L.G., Bridwell, K.H., Baldus, C., et al.: Cotrel-Dubousset instrumentation for idiopathic scoliosis. J. Bone Joint Surg. [Am.] 74:1056–1068, 1992.
Lonstein, J.E.: Adolescent idiopathic scoliosis: Screening and diagnosis. Inst. Course Lect. 38:105–113, 1989.
Lonstein, J.E., Bjorklunk, S., Wanninger, M.H., and Nelson, R.P.: Voluntary school screening for scoliosis in Minnesota. J. Bone Joint Surg. [Am.] 64:481–488, 1982.
Lonstein, J.E., and Carlson, J.M.: Prognostication in idiopathic scoliosis. Orthop. Trans. 5:22, 1981.
Lonstein, J.E., and Carlson, J.M.: The prediction of curve progression in untreated idiopathic scoliosis during growth. J. Bone Joint Surg. [Am.] 66:1061–1071, 1984.
Lowe, T.G.: Current concepts review: Scheuerman's disease. J. Bone Joint Surg. [Am.] 72:940–945, 1990.
Luque, E.R.: Segmental spinal instrumentation for correction of scoliosis. Clin. Orthop. 163:192–198, 1982.
McFarland, B.: Congenital deformity of the spine and limbs. In Modern Trends in Orthopedics, Platt, H., ed. New York, PB Hoeber, 1950.
McMaster, M.J., and Ohtsuka, K.: The natural history of congenital scoliosis: a study of two hundred and fifty-one patients. J. Bone Joint Surg. [Am.] 64:1128–1137, 1982.
Mehta, M.H.: The rib-vertebra angle in the early diagnosis between resolving and progressive infantile scoliosis. J. Bone Joint Surg. [Br.] 54:230–243, 1972.
Mielke, C.H., Lonstein, J.E., Denis, F., et al.: Surgical treatment of adolescent idiopathic scoliosis: A comparative analysis. J. Bone Joint Surg. [Am.] 71:1170–1177, 1989.
Miller, J.A.A., Nachemson, A.L., and Schultz, A.B.: Effectiveness of braces in mild idiopathic scoliosis. Spine 9:632–635, 1984.
Montgomery, S., and Hall, J.: Congenital kyphosis: Surgical treatment at Boston Children's Hospital. Orthop. Trans. 5:25, 1981.
Pang, D., and Wilberger, J.E., Jr.: Spinal cord injury without radiographic abnormalities in children. J. Neurosurg. 57:114–129, 1982.
Ring, D., and Wenger, D.R.: Magnetic resonance imaging scans in discitis: Sequential studies in a child who needed operative drainage; a case report. J. Bone Joint Surg. [Am.] 76:596–601, 1994.
Schrock, R.D.: Congenital abnormalities at the cervicothoracic level. Inst. Course Lect. 6:1949.
Scoles, P.V., and Quinn, T.P.: Intervertebral discitis in children and adolescents. Clin. Orthop. 162:31–36, 1982.
Smith, A.D., Koreska, J., and Moseley, C.F.: Progressive scoliosis in Duchenne muscular dystrophy. J. Bone Joint Surg. [Am.] 71: 1066–1074, 1989.
Sorenson, K.H.: Scheuermann's Juvenile Kyphosis. Copenhagen, Munksgaard, 1964.
Tolo, V.T.: Surgical treatment of adolescent idiopathic scoliosis. Inst. Course Lect. 38:143–156, 1989.
Tredwell, S.J., Newman, D.E., and Lockitch, G.: Instability of the upper cervical spine in Down syndrome. J. Pediatr. Orthop. 10: 602–606, 1990.
Weinstein, S.L.: Adolescent idiopathic scoliosis: Prevalence and natural history. Inst. Course Lect. 38:115–128, 1989.
Weinstein, S.L.: Idiopathic scoliosis: Natural history. Spine 11: 780–783, 1986.
Weinstein, S.L., and Ponseti, I.V.: Curve progression in idiopathic scoliosis. J. Bone Joint Surg. [Am.] 65:447–455, 1983.
Winter, R.B.: Congenital spine deformity: "What's the latest and what's the best?" Spine 14:1406–1409, 1989.
Winter, R.B., and Lonstein, J.E.: Adult idiopathic scoliosis treated with Luque or Harrington rods and sublaminar wiring. J. Bone Joint Surg. [Am.] 71:1308–1313, 1989.
Winter, R.B., Lonstein, J.E., Drogt, J., et al.: The effectiveness of bracing in the nonoperative treatment of idiopathic scoliosis. Spine 11:790–791, 1986.
Winter, R.B., Moe, J.H., Bradford, D.S., et al.: Spine deformity in neurofibromatosis: A review of 102 cases. J. Bone Joint Surg. [Am.] 61:677–694, 1979.
Winter, R.B., Moe, J.H., and Lonstein, J.E.: Posterior spinal arthrodesis for congenital scoliosis: An analysis of the cases of two hundred and ninty patients, five to nineteen years old. J. Bone Joint Surg. [Am.] 66:1188–1197, 1984.
Winter, R.B., Moe, J.H., and Lonstein, J.E.: The incidence of Klippel-

Feil syndrome in patients with congenital scoliosis and kyphosis. Spine 9:363–366, 1984.

Winter, R.B., Moe, J.H., and Lonstein, J.E.: The surgical treatment of congenital kyphosis: A review of 94 patients age 5 years or older, with 2 years or more follow-up in 77 patients. Spine 10: 224–231, 1985.

Upper Extremity Problems

Carson, W.G., Lovell, W.W., and Whitesides, T.E., Jr.: Congenital elevation of the scapula: Surgical correction by the Woodward procedure. J. Bone Joint Surg. [Am.] 62:1199–1207, 1981.

Fitch, R.D.: Introduction to pediatric orthopedics. In Sabiston's Essentials of Surgery, Sabiston, D.C., Jr., ed. Philadelphia, WB Saunders, 1987.

Green, W.T.: The surgical correction of congenital elevation of the scapula (Sprengel's deformity). J. Bone Joint Surg. [Am.] 149, 1957.

Liebovic, S.J., Erlich, M.G., and Zaleske, D.J.: Sprengel deformity. J. Bone Joint Surg. [Am.] 72:192–197, 1990.

Woodward, J.W.: Congenital elevation of the scapula, correction by release and transplantation of muscle origins. J. Bone Joint Surg. [Am.] 43:219–228, 1961.

Lower Extremity Problems

Berg, E.F.: A reappraisal of metatarsus adductus and skewfoot. J. Bone Joint Surg. [Am.] 68:1185–1196, 1986.

Bleck, E.E.: Metatarsus adductus: Classification and relationship to outcomes of treatment. J. Pediatr. Orthop. 3:2–9, 1983.

Crawford, A.H., and Gabriel, K.R.: Foot and ankle problems. Orthop. Clin. North Am. 18:649–666, 1987.

Green, W.B.: Metatarsus adductus and skewfoot. Inst. Course Lect. 43:161–178, 1994.

Kling, T.F., and Hensinger, R.N.: Angular and torsional deformities of the lower limbs in children. Clin. Orthop. 176:136–147, 1983.

Staheli, L.T., Clawson, D.K., and Hubbard, D.D.: Medial femoral torsion: Experience with operative treatment. Clin. Orthop. 146: 222–225, 1980.

Staheli, L.T., Corbett, M., Wyss, C., et al.: Lower extremity rotational problems in children: Normal values to guide management. J. Bone Joint Surg. [Am.] 67:39–47, 1985.

Hip and Femur

Abraham, E., Garst, J., and Barmada, R.: Treatment of moderate to severe slipped capital femoral epiphysis with extracapsular base-of-neck osteotomy. J. Pediatr. Orthop. 13:924–302, 1993.

Beaty, J.H.: Legg-Calvé-Perthes disease: Diagnostic and prognostic techniques. Instr. Course Lect. 38:291–296, 1989.

Berkeley, M.E., Dickson, J.H., Cain, T.E., and Donovan, M.M.: Surgical therapy for congenital dislocation of the hip in patients who are 12 to 36 months old. J. Bone Joint Surg. [Am.] 66:412–420, 1984.

Bialik, V., Fishman, J., Katzir, J., et al.: Clinical assessment of hip instability in the newborn by an orthopedic surgeon and a pediatrician. J. Pediatr. Orthop. 6:703–705, 1986.

Bialik, V., Reuvèni, A., Pery, M., et al.: Ultrasonography in developmental displacement of the hip: A critical analysis of our results. J. Pediatr. Orthop. 9:154–156, 1989.

Blanco, J.S., Taylor, B., and Johnston, C.E., II: Comparison of single pin vs multiple pin fixation in treatment of slipped capital femoral epiphysis. J. Pediatr. Orthop. 12:384–389, 1992.

Boal, D.K., and Schwennkter, E.P.: The infant hip: Assessment with real-time ultrasound. Radiology 157:667–672, 1985.

Boyer, D.W., Mickelson, M.R., and Ponseti, I.V.: Slipped capital femoral epiphysis: Long term follow-up study of 121 patients. J. Bone Joint Surg. [Am.] 63:85–95, 1981.

Canale, S.T.: Problems and complications of slipped capital femoral epiphysis. Inst. Course Lect. 38:281–290, 1989.

Canale, S.T., Harkness, R.M., Thomas, P.A., et al.: Does aspiration of bones and joints affect results of later bone scanning? J. Pediatr. Orthop. 5:23–26, 1985.

Castelein, R.M., and Sauter, A.J.M.: Ultrasound screening for congenital dysplasia of the hip in newborns: Its value. J. Pediatr. Orthop. 8:666–670, 1988.

Catterall, A.: Legg-Calvé-Perthes disease. Instr. Course Lect. 38: 297–303, 1989.

Catterall, A.: Legg-Calvé-Perthes syndrome. Clin. Orthop. 158: 41–52, 1981.

Chiari, K.: Medial displacement osteotomy of the pelvis. Clin. Orthop. 98:55–71, 1974.

Christensen, F., Soballe, K., Ejsted, R., et al.: The Catterall classification of Perthes disease: An assessment of reliability. J. Bone Joint Surg. [Br.] 68:614–615, 1986.

Clarke, N.M.P., Clegg, J., and Al-Chalabi, A.N.: Ultrasound screening of hips at risk for CDH: Failure to reduce the incidence of late cases. J. Bone Joint Surg. [Br.] 71:9–12, 1989.

Crawford, A.H.: The role of osteotomy in the treatment of slipped capital femoral epiphysis. Inst. Course Lect. 38:273–280, 1989.

Daoud, A., and Saighi-Bouaouina, A.: Treatment of sequestra, pseudarthroses and defects in the long bones of children who have chronic hematogenous osteomyelitis. J. Bone Joint Surg. [Am.] 71: 1448–1468, 1989.

Epps, C.H., Jr.: Current concepts review: Proximal femoral focal deficiency. J. Bone Joint Surg. [Am.] 65:867–870, 1983.

Fabry, F., and Meire, E.: Septic arthritis of the hip in children: Poor results after late and inadequate treatment. J. Pediatr. Orthop. 3: 461–466, 1983.

Faciszewski, T., Coleman, S.S., and Biddolpf, G.: Triple innominate osteotomy for acetabular dysplasia. J. Pediatr. Orthop. 13: 426–430, 1993.

Faciszewski, T., Keifer, G., and Coleman, S.S.: Pemberton osteotomy for residual acetabular dysplasia in children who have congenital dislocation of the hip. J. Bone Joint Surg. [Am.] 5:643–649, 1993.

Fackler, C.D.: Nonsurgical treatment of Legg-Calvé-Perthes disease. Instr. Course Lect. 38:305–308, 1989.

Gage, J.R., and Winter, R.B.: Avascular necrosis of the capital femoral epiphysis as a complication of closed reduction of congenital dislocation of the hip: A critical review of twenty years experience at Gillette Children's Hospital. J. Bone Joint Surg. [Am.] 54:373–388, 1972.

Galpin, R.D., Roach, J.W., Wenger, D.R., et al.: One stage treatment of congenital dislocation of the hip in older children including femoral shortening. J. Bone Joint Surg. [Am.] 71:734–741, 1989.

Green, N.E., and Edwards, K.: Bone and joint infections in children. Orthop. Clin. North Am. 18:555–576, 1987.

Harke, H.T., and Grissom, L.E.: Performing dynamic ultrasonography of the infant hip. A.J.R. Am. J. Roentgenol. 155:837–844, 1990.

Harris, I.E., Dickens, R., and Menelaus, M.B.: Use of the Pavlik harness for hip displacements: When to abandon treatment. Clin. Orthop. 281:29–33, 1992.

Herndon, W.A., Knaur, S., Sullivan, J.A., et al.: Management of septic arthritis in children. J. Pediatr. Orthop. 6:576–578, 1986.

Herring, J.A.: Current concepts review: The treatment of Legg-Calvé-Perthes disease. J. Bone Joint Surg. [Am.] 76:448–457, 1994.

Herring, J.A., Neustadt, J.B., Williams, J.J., Early, J.S., and Brown, R.H.: The lateral pillar classification of Legg-Calvé-Perthes disease. J. Pediatr. Orthop. 12:143–150, 1992.

Iwasaki, K.: Treatment of congenital dislocation of the hip by the Pavlik harness: Mechanisms of reduction and usage. J. Bone Joint Surg. [Am.] 65:760–767, 1983.

Jackson, M.A., and Nelson, J.D.: Etiology and medical management of acute suppurative bone and joint infections in pediatric patients. J. Pediatr. Orthop. 2:313–323, 1982.

Kalamchi, A., McFarland, R., III: The Pavlik harness: Results in patients over three months of age. J. Pediatr. Orthop. 2:3–8, 1982.

Kershaw, C.J., Ware, H.E., Pattinson, R., and Fixsen, J.A.: Revision of failed open reduction of congenital dislocated hip. J. Bone Joint Surg. [Br.] 75:744–749, 1993.

Koval, K.J., Lehman, W.B., Rose, D., et al.: Treatment of slipped capital femoral epiphysis with a cannulated screw technique. J. Bone Joint Surg. [Am.] 71:1370–1377, 1989.

Lewin, J.S., Rosenfield, N.H., Hoffer, P.B., et al.: Acute osteomyelitis in children: Combined Tc-99 and gallium-67 imaging. Radiology 158:795–804, 1986.

Loder, R.T., Arbor, A., and Richards, B.S.: Acute slipped capital femoral epiphysis: The importance of physeal stability. J. Bone Joint Surg. [Am.] 75:1134–1140, 1993.

Mausen, J.P.G.M., Rozing, P.M., and Obermann, W.R.: Intertrochanteric corrective osteotomy in slipped capital femoral epiphysis: A long term follow-up study of 26 patients. Clin. Orthop. 259: 100–109, 1990.

McAndrew, M.P., and Weinstein, S.L.: A long term follow-up of Legg-Calvé-Perthes disease. J. Bone Joint Surg. [Am.] 66:860–869, 1984.
Morrissey, R.T.: Principles of in situ fixation in chronic slipped capital epiphysis. Instr. Course Lect. 38:257–262, 1989.
Morrissey, R.T., ed.: Lovell and Winter's Pediatric Orthopedics, 3rd ed. Philadelphia, JB Lippincott, 1990.
Moseley, C.F.: Assessment and prediction in leg length discrepancy. Inst. Course Lect. 38:325–330, 1989.
Mubarak, S.J., Beck, L.R., and Sutherland, D.H.: Home traction in the management of congenital dislocation of the hips. J. Pediatr. Orthop. 6:721–723, 1986.
Mubarak, S.J., Garfin, S., Vance, R., et al.: Pitfalls in the use of the Pavlik harness for treatment of congenital dysplasia, subluxation, and dislocation of the hip. J. Bone Joint Surg. [Am.] 63:1239–1248, 1981.
Norlin, R., Hammerby, S., and Tkaczuk, H.: The natural history of Perthes disease. Int. Orthop. 15:13–16, 1991.
Paley, D.: Current techniques of limb lengthening. J. Pediatr. Orthop. 8:73–92, 1988.
Pizzutillo; P.D.: Developmental dysplasia of the hip. Instr. Course Lect. 43:179–184, 1994.
Price, C.T.: Metaphyseal and physeal lengthening. Instr. Course Lect. 38:331–336, 1989.
Ramsey, P.L., Lasser, S., and MacEwen, G.D.: Congenital dislocation of the hip: Use of the Pavlik harness in the child during the first 6 months of life. J. Bone Joint Surg. [Am.] 58:1000–1004, 1976.
Rennie, A.M.: The inheritance of slipped upper femoral epiphysis. J. Bone Joint Surg. [Br.] 64:180–184, 1982.
Richardson, E.G., and Rambach, B.E.: Proximal femoral focal deficiency: A clinical appraisal. South. Med. J. 72:166–173, 1979.
Ring, D., Wenger, D.R.: Magnetic resonance imaging scans in discitis. J. Bone Joint Surg. [Am.] 76:596–601, 1994.
Ritterbusch, J.F., Shantharam, S.S., and Gelinas, C.: Comparison of lateral pillar classification and Catterall classification of Legg-Calvé-Perthes disease. J. Pediatr. Orthop 13:200–202, 1993.
Salter, R.B., Hansson, G., and Thompson, G.H.: Innominate osteotomy in the management of residual congenital subluxation of the hip in young adults. Clin. Orthop. 182:53–68, 1984.
Simons, G.W.: A comparative evaluation of the current methods for open reduction of the congenitally displaced hip. Orthop. Clin. North Am. 11:161–181, 1980.
Southwick, W.O.: Compression fixation after biplane intertrochanteric osteotomy for slipped capital femoral epiphysis. J. Bone Joint Surg. [Am.] 55:1218–1224, 1973.
Staheli, L.T., and Chew, D.E.: Slotted acetabular augmentation in childhood and adolescence. J. Pediatr. Orthop. 12:569–580, 1992.
Staheli, L.T., Coleman, S.S., Hensinger, R.N., et al.: Congenital hip dysplasia. Instr. Course Lect. 33:350–363, 1984.
Steele, H.H.: Triple osteotomy of the innominate bone. J. Bone Joint Surg. [Am.] 55:343–350, 1973.
Stromqvist, B., and Sunden, G.: CDH diagnosed at 2 to 12 months of age. J. Pediatr. Orthop. 9:208–212, 1989.
Sutherland, D.H., and Greenfield, R.: Double innominate osteotomy. J. Bone Joint Surg. [Am.] 59:1082–1091, 1977.
Suzuki, S., and Yamamuro, T.: Avascular necrosis in patients treated with Pavlik harness for congenital dislocation of the hip. J. Bone Joint Surg. [Am.] 72:1048–1055, 1990.
Tachdjian, M.O.: Pediatric Orthopedics, 2nd ed. Philadelphia, WB Saunders, 1990.
Tetzlaff, T.R., McCracken, G.H., Jr., and Nelson, J.D.: Oral antibiotic therapy for skeletal infections in children. II. Therapy of osteomyelitis and arthritis. J. Pediatr. 92:485–490, 1978.
Tonnis, D., Storch, K., and Ulbrich, H.: Results of newborn screening for CDH with and without sonography and correlation of risk factors. J. Pediatr. Orthop. 10:145–152, 1990.
Tredwell, S.J., and Davis, L.A.: Prospective study of congenital dislocation of the hip. J. Pediatr. Orthop. 9:386–390, 1989.
Viere, R.G., Birch, J.F., Herring, J.A., et al.: Use of the Pavlik harness in congenital dislocation of the hip: An analysis of failures of treatment. J. Bone Joint Surg. [Am.] 72:238–244, 1990.
Weiner, D.S.: Bone graft epiphysiodesis in the treatment of slipped capital femoral epiphysis. Instr. Course Lect. 38:263–272, 1989.
Wenger, D.R.: Congenital hip disclocation. Instr. Course Lect. 38: 343–354, 1989.
Zionts, L.E., and MacEwen, G.D.: Treatment of congenital dislocation of the hip in children between the ages of one and three years. J. Bone Joint Surg. [Am.] 68:829–846, 1986.

Knee and Leg

Brown, F.W., and Pohnert, W.H.: Construction of a knee joint in meromelia tibia (congenital absence of the tibia): A 15 year follow-up study. J. Bone Joint Surg. [Am.] 54:1333, 1972.
Dickhaut, S.C., and DeLee, J.C.: The discoid lateral-meniscus syndrome. J. Bone Joint Surg. [Am.] 64:1068–1073, 1982.
Guhl, J.: Osteochondritis dissecans. In O'Conners Textbook of Arthroscopic Surgery, Shahriaree, H., ed. Philadelphia, JB Lippincott, 1984.
Hayashi, L.K., Yamaga, H., Ida, K., and Miura, T.: Arthroscopic meniscectomy for discoid lateral meniscus in children. J. Bone Joint Surg. [Am.] 70:1495–1499, 1988.
Insall, J.: Current concept review: Patellar pain. J. Bone Joint Surg. [Am.] 64:147–152, 1982.
Jacobsen, S.T., Crawford, A.H., Miller, E.A., and Steel, H.H.: The Syme amputation in patients with congenital pseudarthrosis of the tibia. J. Bone Joint Surg. [Am.] 65:533–537, 1983.
Langenskiold, A.: Tibia vara: osteochondrosis deformans tibiae: Blount's disease. Clin. Orthop. 158:77–82, 1981.
Letts, M., and Vincent, N.: Congenital longitudinal deficiency of the fibula (fibular hemimelia): Parental refusal of amputation. Clin. Orthop. 287:160–166, 1993.
Morrissey, R.T.: A symposium: Congenital pseudarthrosis. Clin. Orthop. 166:1–61, 1982.
Paterson, D.: Congenital pseudarthrosis of the tibia. Clin. Orthop. 247:44–54, 1989.
Poppas, A.M.: Osteochondrosis dissecans. Clin. Orthop. 158: 59–669, 1981.
Roach, J.W., Shindell, R., and Green, N.E.: Late onset pseudarthrosis of the dysplastic tibia. J. Bone Joint Surg. [Am.] 75:1593–1601, 1993.
Schoenecker, P.L., Capelli, A.M., Miller, E.A., et al.: Congenital longitudinal deficiency of the tibia. J. Bone Joint Surg. [Am.] 71: 278–287, 1989.
Schoenecker, P.L., Meade, W.C., Pierron, R.L., et al.: Blount's disease: A retrospective review and recommendations for treatment. J. Pediatr. Orthop. 5:181–186, 1985.

Feet

Adelar, R.S., Williams, R.M., and Gould, J.S.: Congenital convex pes valgus: Results of an early comprehensive release and a review of congenital vertical talus at Richmond Crippled Childrens Hospital and the University of Alabama at Birmingham. Foot Ankle 1: 62–73, 1980.
Chambers, R.B., Cook, T.M., and Cowell, H.R.: Surgical reconstruction for calcaneonavicular coalition: Evaluation of function and gait. J. Bone Joint Surg. [Am.] 64:829–836, 1982.
Coleman, S.S.: Complex Foot Deformities in Children. Philadelphia, Lea & Febiger, 1983.
Cowell, H.R.: The management of clubfoot [editorial]. J. Bone Joint Surg. [Am.] 67:991–992, 1985.
Crawford, A.H., Marxen, J.L., and Osterfeld, D.L.: The Cincinnati incision: A comprehensive approach for surgical procedures of the foot and ankle in childhood. J. Bone Joint Surg. [Am.] 64: 1355–1358, 1982.
Cummings, R.J., and Lovell, W.W.: Current concepts review: Operative treatment of congenital idiopathic clubfoot. J. Bone Joint Surg. [Am.] 70:1108–1112, 1988.
Hamanishi, C.: Congenital vertical talus: Classification with 69 cases and new measurement system. J. Pediatr. Orthop. 4:318–326, 1984.
Jacobs, R.F., Adelman, L., Sack, C.M., et al.: Management of Pseudomonas osteochondritis complicating puncture wounds of the foot. Pediatrics 69:432–435, 1982.
Jahss, M.H.: Evaluation of the cavus foot for orthopedic treatment. Clin. Orthop. 181:52–63, 1983.
McHale, K.A., and Lenhart, M.K.: Treatment of residual clubfoot deformity, the "bean-shaped" foot, by opening wedge medial cuneiform osteotomy and closing wedge cuboid osteotomy: Clinical review and cadaver correlations. J. Pediatr. Orthop. 11:374–381, 1991.
McKay, D.W.: New concept of and approach to clubfoot treatment:

Section I. Principles and morbid anatomy. J. Pediatr. Orthop. 2: 347–356, 1982.
Onley, B.W., and Asher, M.A.: Excision of symptomatic coalition of the middle facet of the talocalcaneal joint. J. Bone Joint Surg. [Am.] 69:539–544, 1987.
Oppenheim, W., Smith, C., and Christe, W.: Congenital vertical talus. Foot Ankle 5:198–204, 1985.
Pentz, A.S., and Weiner, D.S.: Management of metatarsus adductovarus. Foot Ankle 14:241–246, 1993.
Peterson, H.A.: Skewfoot (forefoot adduction with heel valgus). J. Pediatr. Orthop. 6:24–30, 1986.
Simons, G.W.: Analytical radiography of club feet. J. Bone Joint Surg. [Br.] 59:485–489, 1974.
Simons, G.W.: Complete subtalar release in club feet. Part I. A preliminary report. Part II. Comparison with less extensive procedures. J. Bone Joint Surg. [Am.] 67:1044–1065, 1985.
Thometz, J.G., and Simons, G.W.: Deformity of the calcaneocuboid joint in patients who have talipes equinovarus. J. Bone Joint Surg. [Am.] 75:190–195, 1993.
Turco, V.J.: Resistant congenital clubfoot—one-stage posteromedial release with internal fixation: A follow-up report of a 15 year experience. J. Bone Joint Surg. [Am.] 61:805–814, 1979.
Victoria-Diaz, A., and Victoria-Diaz, J.: Pathogenesis of idiopathic clubfoot. Clin. Orthop. 185:14–24, 1984.
Zinman, C., Wolfson, N., and Reis, N.D.: Osteochondritis dissecans of the dome of the talus: computed tomography scanning in diagnosis and follow-up. J. Bone Joint Surg. [Am.] 70:1017–1019, 1988.

3

SPORTS MEDICINE

MARK D. MILLER

I. Knee

A. Anatomy and Biomechanics—Although a thorough discussion of anatomy is included in Chapter 11, a brief review of knee anatomy is relevant.

1. Ligaments—Four major ligaments and several other supporting ligaments and structures provide stability to the knee joint.
   a. Anterior Cruciate Ligament (ACL) originates in a broad, irregular, diamond-shaped area just in front of the intercondylar eminence of the tibia and inserts in a semicircular area on the posteromedial aspect of the lateral femoral condyle. It is approximately 33 mm long and 11 mm in diameter. The ACL is often said to be composed of two "bundles"—an anteromedial bundle that is tight in flexion and a posterolateral bundle that is tight in extension. The blood supply to both cruciate ligaments is via branches of the middle geniculate artery. Mechanoreceptor nerve fibers within the ligament may have a proprioceptive role.
   b. Posterior Cruciate Ligament (PCL) originates from a broad, crescent-shaped area on the medial femoral condlye and inserts on the tibia in a sulcus that is below the articular surface. It also is composed of two "bundles"—an anterolateral portion that is tight in flexion and a posteromedial portion that is tight in extension. Variable meniscofemoral ligaments (Humphry—anterior; Wrisberg—posterior) originate from the lateral meniscus and insert into the substance of the PCL.
   c. Medial Collateral Ligament (MCL) is composed of superficial (tibial collateral ligament) and deep (medial capsular ligament) fibers. The ligament originates from the medial femoral epicondyle and inserts on the proximal tibia. The deep portion of the ligament is intimately associated with the medial meniscus (coronary ligaments).
   d. Lateral Collateral Ligament (LCL), or fibular collateral ligament, originates on the lateral femoral epicondyle and inserts on the lateral aspect of the fibular head.
   e. Medial and lateral supporting structures are best considered in layers (Fig. 3–1).

Medial Structures		Lateral Structures	
LAYER	**COMPONENTS**	**LAYER**	**COMPONENTS**
I	Sartorius and fascia	I	Iliotibial tract, biceps, fascia
II	Superfical MCL, posterior oblique ligament, semimembranosus	II	Patellar retinaculum, patellofemoral ligament
III	Deep MCL, capsule	III	LCL, arcuate ligament, fabellofibular ligament, capsule

2. Menisci are cresent-shaped fibrocartilagenous structures that are triangular in cross section. Only the peripheral 20–30% of the menisci are vascularized (medial and lateral genicular arteries). The medial meniscus is more C-shaped, and the lateral meniscus is more circular in shape (Fig. 3–1). These structures, which deepen the articular surfaces of the tibial plateau and have a role in stability, lubrication, and nutrition, are connected anteriorly by the transverse ligament.
3. Joint Relationships—The height of the lateral femoral condyle is greater than that of the medial condyle. The alignment of the condyles are also different; the lateral condyle is relatively straight, but the medial condyle is curved (allowing the medial tibial plateau to externally rotate in full extension—the "screw home mechanism"). The lateral condyle can also be identified by its terminal sulcus and groove of the popliteus insertion (Fig. 3–2). The patellofemoral joint is composed of the patella (with variably sized medial and lateral facets) and the femoral trochlea. The patella is restrained in the trochlea by valgus axis of the quadriceps mechanism (*Q angle*), oblique fibers of the vastus medialis and lateralis muscles (and their extensions—the patella retinacula), and the patellofemoral ligaments (Fig. 3–3).
4. Biomechanics
   a. Knee ligaments serve primarily as passive restraints to knee motion.

LIGAMENT	RESTRAINT
ACL	Anterior translation of the tibia
PCL	Posterior tibial displacement
MCL	Valgus angulation
LCL	Varus angulation

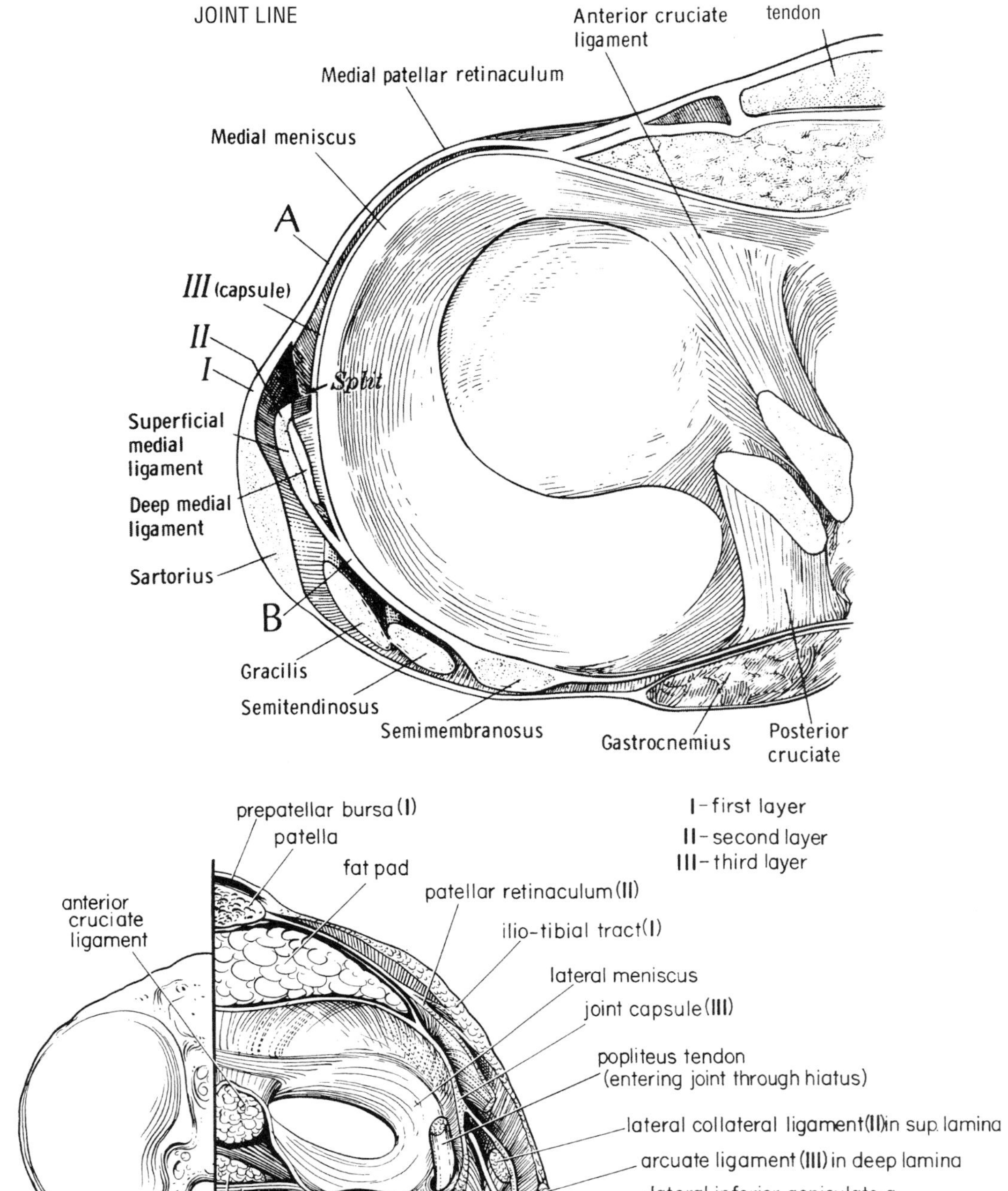

FIGURE 3–1. Medial and lateral supporting structures of the knee. *A,* Medial structures of the knee include the saritorius and its fascia and the patellar retinaculum (layer I); the hamstring tendons and superficial MCL (layer II); and the deep MCL (layer III). (From Warren, L.F., and Marshal, J.L.: The supporting structures and layers of the medial side of the knee. J. Bone Joint Surg. [Am.] 61:56–62, 1979; reprinted by permission.) *B,* Lateral structures of the knee include the IT tract and biceps (layer I), patellar retinaculum (layer II), and capsule and LCL (layer III). (From Seebacher, J.R., Ingilis, A.E., Marshall, J.L., and Warren, R.F.: The structure of the posterolateral aspect of the knee. J. Bone Joint Surg. [Am.] 64:536–541, 1982; reprinted by permission.)

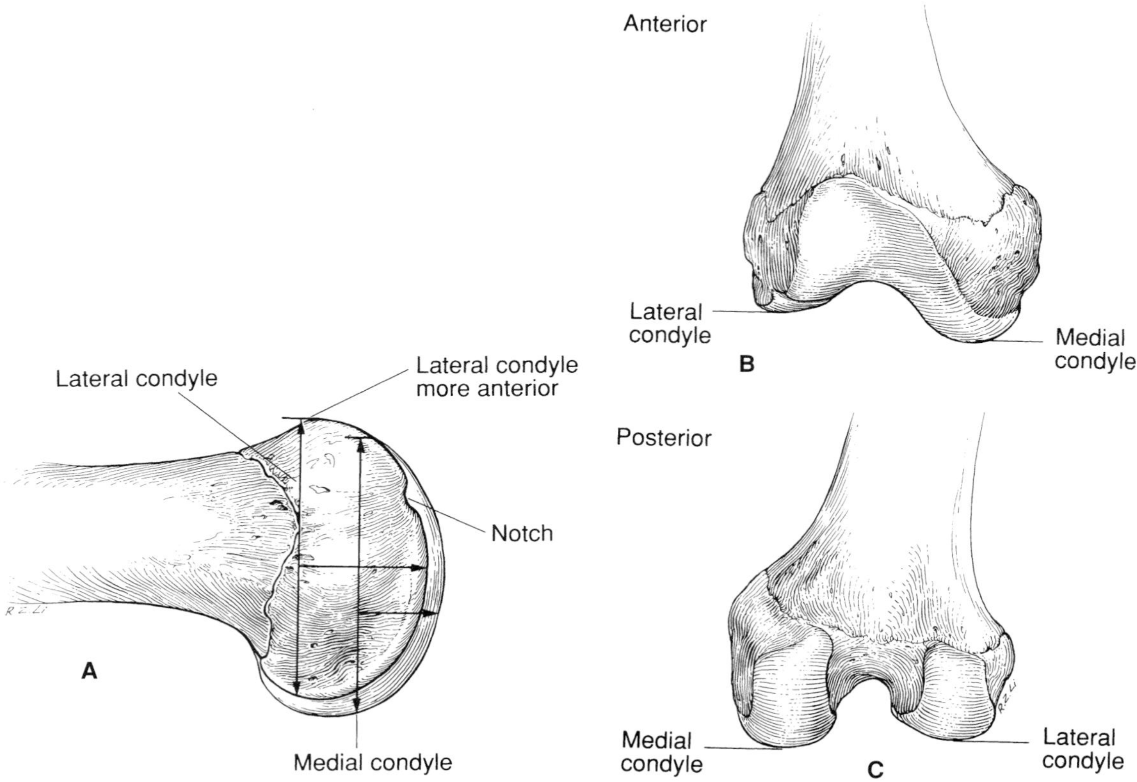

FIGURE 3–2. Relationships of the femoral condyles. *A*, On the lateral projection, the lateral condyle projects more anteriorly and is notched. AP (B) and PA (C) view demonstrating the difference in size and curvature of the medial femoral condyle. (From Tria, A.J., and Klein, K.S.: An Illustrated Guide to the Knee, p. 5. New York, Churchill Livingstone, 1992; reprinted by permission.)

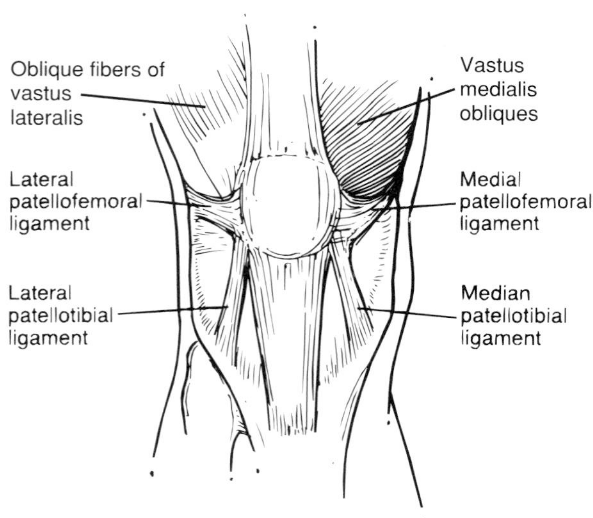

FIGURE 3–3. Patellar restraints include the patellofemoral and patellotibial ligaments as well as the oblique fibers of the vastus medialis and lateralis. (From Walsh, W.M.: Patellofemoral joint. In Orthopaedic Sports Medicine Principles and Practice, DeLee, J.C., and Drez, D., Jr., eds. Philadelphia: WB Saunders, 1994; reprinted by permission.)

The tensile strength of the ACL is approximately 2200 N. The tensile strength of a 10 mm patellar tendon graft (young specimens) is more than 2900 N and is about 30% stronger when rotated 90 degrees. However, this strength quickly diminishes in vivo. The concept of ligament "isometry" remains controversial. Reconstructed ligament should reapproximate normal anatomy and lie within the flexion axis in all positions of knee motion. Other considerations such as graft impingement and avoiding flexion contractures are equally important.

b. Menisci are composed of collagen fibers that are arranged radially and longitudinally (Fig. 3–4). The longitudinal fibers help dissipate the hoop stresses in the menisci, and the combination of fibers allows the meniscus to expand under compressive forces and increase the contact area of the joint. The lateral meniscus has twice the excursion of the medial meniscus during knee range of motion and rotation.

B. History and Physical Examination
   1. History—Several key historical points should be sought.

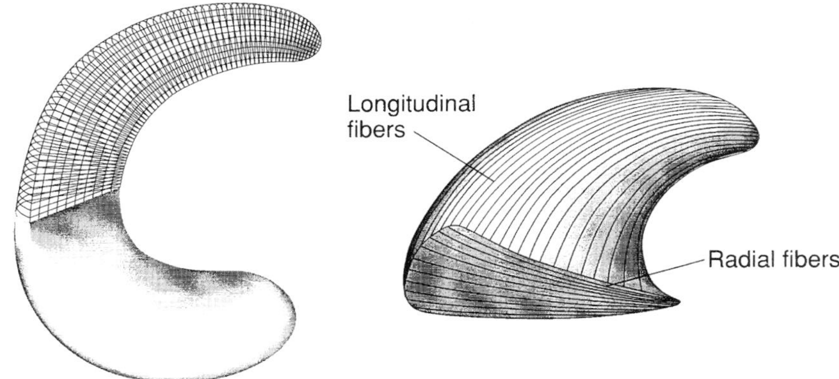

FIGURE 3–4. Longitudinal and radial fibers of the menisci. (From Tria, A.J., and Klein, K.S.: An Illustrated Guide to the Knee, p. 37. New York, Churchill Livingstone, 1992; reprinted by permission.)

HISTORY	SIGNIFICANCE
Pain after sitting/stair climbing	Patellofemoral etiology
Dashboard injury	PCL tear/dislocation
Locking/pain with squatting	Meniscal tear
Noncontact injury with "pop"	ACL tear
Contact injury with "pop"	Colateral ligament, meniscus, patellar dislocation
Acute swelling	ACL, peripheral meniscus tear, osteochondral fx, ± capsule tear
Knee "gives way"	Ligamentous laxity, patella subluxation/dislocation, meniscal tear, chondromalacia of patella
Anterior force—dorsiflexed foot	Patellar injury
Anterior force—plantar-flexed foot	PCL injury

2. Physical Examination—The following are key examination points and may be best elicited with an examination under anesthesia.

EXAMINATION	METHOD	SIGNIFICANCE
Standing/gait	Observe gait	Based on pathology
Deformity	Observe patient standing	Based on pathology
Effusion	Patella: ballot/milk	Ligament/meniscus injury (acute), arthritis (chronic)
PMT	Palpate for tenderness	Based on location (joint line tenderness = meniscus)
ROM	Active and passive	Block = meniscus injury (bucket handle), loose body, ACL tear impinging
Patella crepitus	With passive ROM	Patellofemoral pathology
Patella grind	Push patella with quadriceps contraction	Patellofemoral pathology
Patella apprehension	Push patella lat. at 20–30° flexion	Patella subluxation/dislocation
Q angle	ASIS-patella-tibial tubercle	Incr. with patella malalignment
J sign	Lateral deviation of the patella in extension	
Ext rotation recurvatum	Pick up great toes; **knee-varus and hyperextension**	
Patella tilt	Tilt up laterally	>15° = Lax <0° = tight lateral constraint
Patella glide	Like apprehension	>50° = Incr. medial const laxity
Active glide	Lat. excursion with quad. contraction	Lat. > prox. excursion = incr. functional Q angle quadriceps
Quadriceps circumference	10 cm (VMO), 15 cm (quad.)	Atrophy from inactivity
Symmetric extension	Heel from ground	Contracture, displaced meniscal tear, or other mechanical block
McMurray	Ext./int. rotation varus/valgus stress-extension	Meniscal pathology or chondromalacia of articular surface
Varus/valgus stress	30°	MCL/LCL laxity (grade I–IV)
Varus/valgus stress	0°	MCL/LCL and PCL/post. capsule
Apley's	Prone-flexion compression	DJD, meniscal path
Lachman	Tibia forward at 30° flexion	ACL (most sensitive)
Finacetto	Lachman with tibia subluxing beyond post. horns of menisci	ACL (severe)
Ant. drawer	Tibia forward at 90° flexion	ACL
Int. rotation drawer	Foot int. rotated with drawer	Tighter = (normal), looser = ALRI
Ext. rotation drawer	Foot ext. rotation with drawer	Loose (normal), looser = AMRI
Pivot shift	Flexion with int. rotation and valgus	ALRI
Flexion-rotation drawer	Shift with axial load, less valgus	ALRI
Slocum	On back/side flexion and pivot	ALRI

EXAMINATION	METHOD	SIGNIFICANCE
Pivot jerk	Extension with int. rotation and valgus	ALRI
Post. drawer	Tibia backward at 90° flexion	PCL
Tibia sag.	Flex 90°, observe	PCL
90° quad. act	Extend flexed knee	PCL
Ext. rotation recurvatum	Pick up great toes	PLRI
Reverse pivot	Extension with ext. rotation and valgus	PLRI
Ext. rotation at 30° + 90° flexion	Incr. and ext. rotation associated with PLRI	PLRI
Posterolateral drawer	Post. drawer, lat. > med.	PLRI

3. Instrumented Knee Laxity Measurement—KT-1000 (MED-metric, San Diego, CA) is the most commonly accepted device for standardized laxity measurement. The 30-pound and manual maximum anterior displacements are the most commonly reported values and are based on side-to-side comparison (>3 mm significant). PCL laxity can also be measured with this device, although it is less accurate.

C. Imaging the Knee—In addition to standard radiographs, certain other findings and views can be helpful.

VIEW/SIGN	FINDING	SIGNIFICANCE
Lateral—hip and knee flexed	Sag	PCL disruption
Varus/valgus stress view	Opening	Collateral ligament injury; Salter-Harris fracture
Lateral capsule (Segund) sign	Small tibial avulsion	ACL tear
Pellegrini-Stieda lesion	Med. femoral condyle avulsion	Chronic MCL injury
Lateral-high patella	Patella alta	Patellofemoral path
Congruence angle	$\mu = -6°$ $SD = 11°$	Patellofemoral path
Tooth sign	Irregular ant. patella	Patellofemoral chondrosis
Arthrogram	Dye outline	Meniscal tear
MRI	Intra-articular path	Specific for lesion
Square lateral condyle	Thick joint space	Discoid meniscus
Fairbank's changes	Square condyle, peak eminences, ridging, narrowing	Early DJD (post. meniscectomy)
PA flexion weight-bearing		Early DJD, OCD, notch evaluation
Bone scan		Stress fractures, early DJD, RSD
CT		Tibial plateau fractures, patellar tilt

Evaluation of patella height is accomplished by one of three commonly used methods (Fig. 3–5).

D. Knee Arthroscopy

1. Portals—Standard portals include a superomedial or superolateral inflow portal (made with the knee in extension) and inferomedial and inferolateral portals (made with the knee in flexion) for

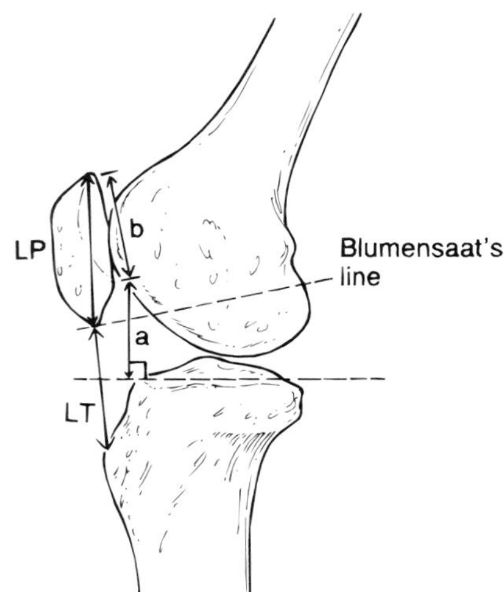

FIGURE 3–5. Three popular methods for evaluating patella alta and baja. (1) **Blumensaat's line**: With the knee flexed 30 degrees, the lower border of the patella should lie on a line extended brom the intercondylar notch. (2) **Insall-Salvati index**: Patella tendon length (LT) to patella length (LP) ratio, or index, should be 1.0. An index of >1.2 is alta and <0.8 is baja. (3) **Blackburne and Peel index**: Ratio of the distance from the tibial plateau to the inferior articular surface of the patella (a) to the length of the patella articular surface (b) should be 0.8. An index of >1.0 is alta. (From Harner, C.D., Miller, M.D. and Irrgang, J.J.: Management of the stiff knee after trauma and ligament reconstruction. In Traumatic Disorders of the Knee, Siliski, J.M., ed., p. 364. New York, Springer-Verlag, 1994; reprinted by permission.)

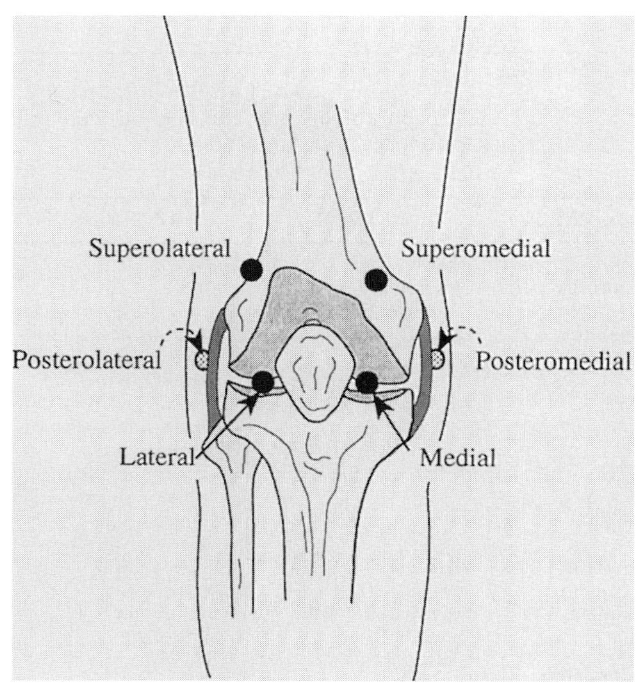

FIGURE 3–6. Commonly used arthroscopic portals. (From Reiman, P.R., and Gardner, W.G.: Septic arthritis. In Knee Surgery, Fu, F.H., Harner, C.D., and Vince, K.G., eds., p. 452. Baltimore, Williams & Wilkins, 1994; reprinted by permission.)

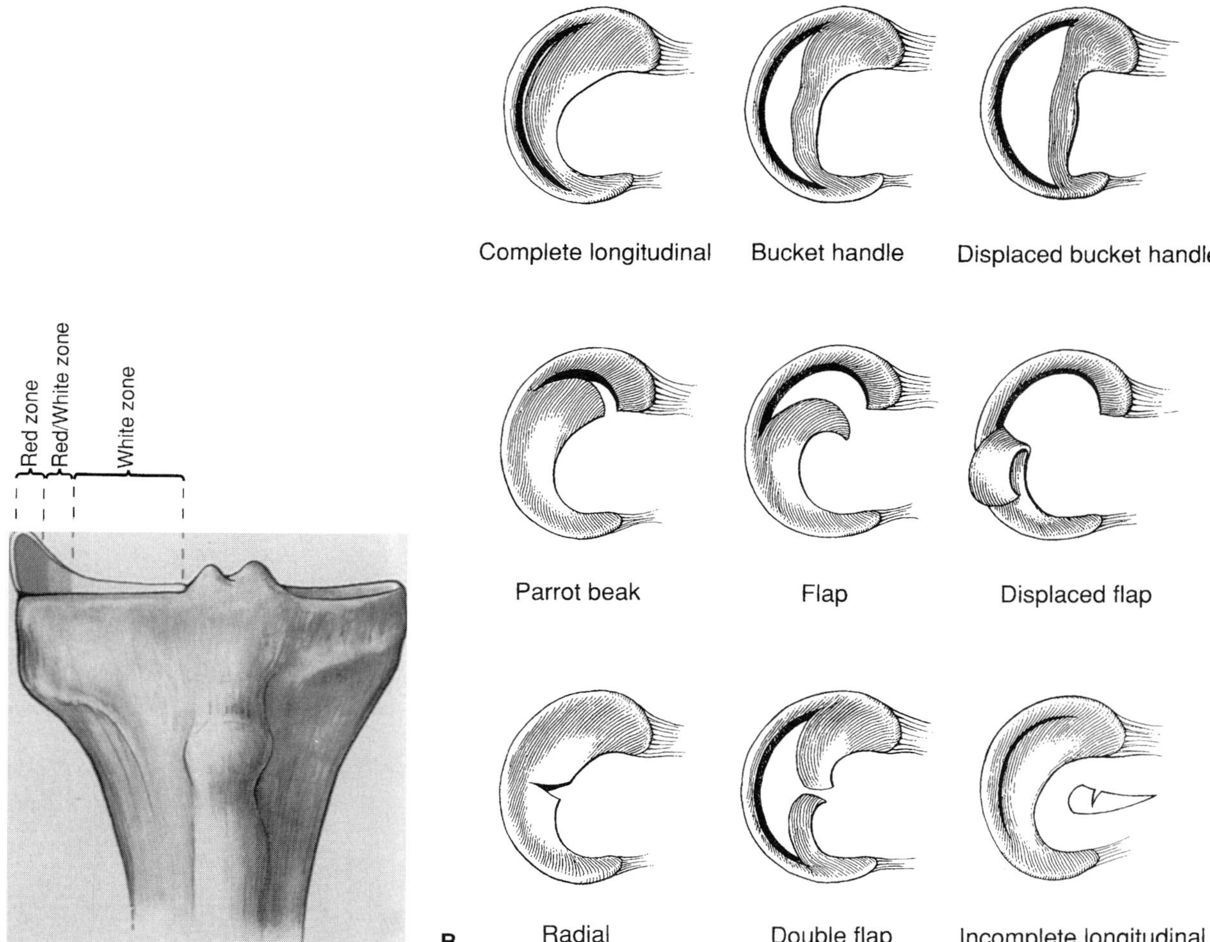

FIGURE 3–7. Classification of meniscal tears. *A,* Vascular zones. The red–red zone has the highest potential for meniscal healing and the white–white zone has essentially no healing potential for healing without enhancement. (Modified from Miller, M.D., Warner, J.J.P., and Harner, C.D.: Meniscal repair. In Knee Surgery, p. 616. Baltimore, Williams & Wilkins, 1994; reprinted by permission.) *B,* Common meniscal tear appearance and orientation. (From Tria, A.J., and Klein, K.S., An Illustrated Guide to the Knee. New York, Churchill Livingstone, 1992; reprinted by permission.)

instruments and the arthroscope, respectively (Fig. 3–6). Accessory portals, sometimes helpful for visualizing the posterior horns of the menisci and PCL, include the posteromedial portal (1 cm above the joint line behind the MCL [avoid saphenous nerve branches]) and the posterolateral portal (1 cm above the joint line between the LCL and biceps tendon [avoiding the common peroneal nerve]). The transpatellar portal (1 cm distal to the patella, splitting the patellar tendon fibers) can be used for central viewing or grabbing but should be avoided in patients requiring subsequent autogoneous patellar tendon harvesting. Other less commonly used portals include the medial and lateral mid-patellar portals and the proximal superomedial portal (4 cm proximal to the patella) used for anterior compartment visualization and the far medial and far lateral portals for accessory instrument placement (loose body removal).

2. Technique—A systematic examination of the knee should include evaluation of the patellofemoral joint, medial and lateral gutters, medial and lateral compartments, and the notch. The posteromedial corner can best be visualized with a 70 degree arthroscope placed through the notch (modified Gillquist view).

E. Menisci

1. Meniscal tear is the most common injury to the knee that requires surgery. The medial meniscus is torn approximately three times more frequently than the lateral meniscus. Traumatic meniscal tears are common in young patients with sports-related injuries. Degenerative tears usually occur in older patients and can have an insidious onset. Meniscal tears can be classified based on their location in relation to the vascular supply (and healing potential), their position (anterior, middle, or posterior third), and their appearance and orientation (Fig. 3–7).
   a. Partial Meniscectomy—Tears that are not amenable to repair (e.g., peripheral, longitudinal tears) excluding tears that do not require any treatment (e.g., partial thickness tears, tears <5

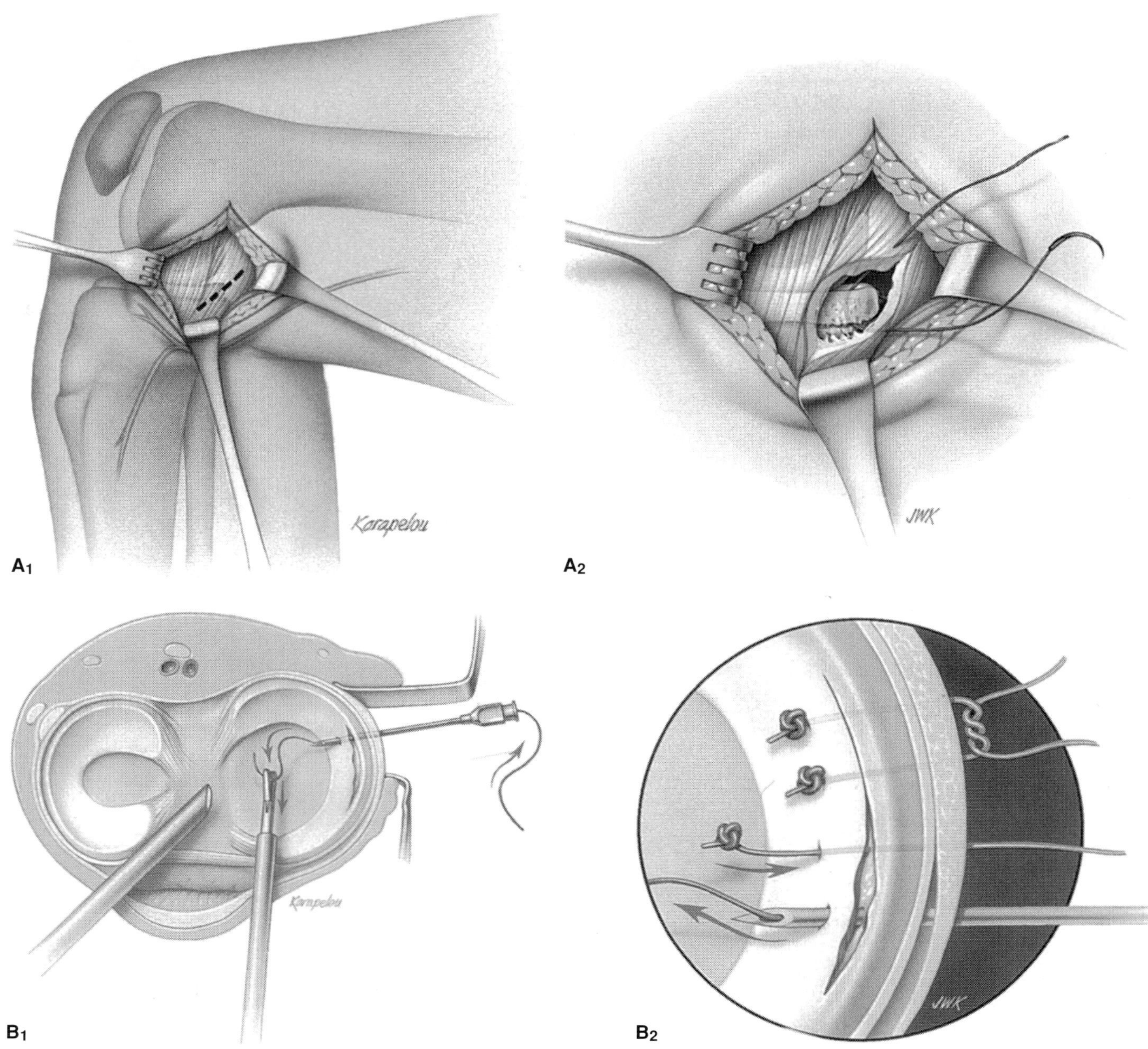

FIGURE 3–8. Meniscal repair techniques. *A,* Open repair of the medial meniscus (right knee). *B,* "Outside-in medial meniscal repair (right knee). *C,* "Inside-out" lateral meniscal repair (right knee). *D,* "All inside" lateral meniscal repair (right knee). (From Miller, M.D.: Atlas of meniscal repair. Op. Tech. Orthop. 5(1):70–71, 1995. *Illustration continued on opposite page*

mm in length, and tears that cannot be displaced >1–2 mm) are best treated by partial meniscectomy. In general, complex, degenerative, and central/radial tears are resected with minimal normal meniscus being resected. A motorized shaver is helpful for creating a smooth transition zone. The role of lasers for this purpose is still investigational.

b. Meniscal Repair—Should be accomplished for all peripheral longitudinal tears, especially in young patients. Augmentation techniques (fibrin clot, vascular access channels, synovial rasping) may extend the indications for repair. Four techniques are commonly used: open, "outside-in," "inside-out," and "all-inside" (Fig. 3–8). Regardless of the technique used, it is essential to protect the saphenous nerve branches during medial repairs and the peroneal nerve during lateral repairs (Fig. 3–9) Results of meniscal repair are good, especially with acute, peripheral tears in young patients undergoing concurrent ACL reconstruction.

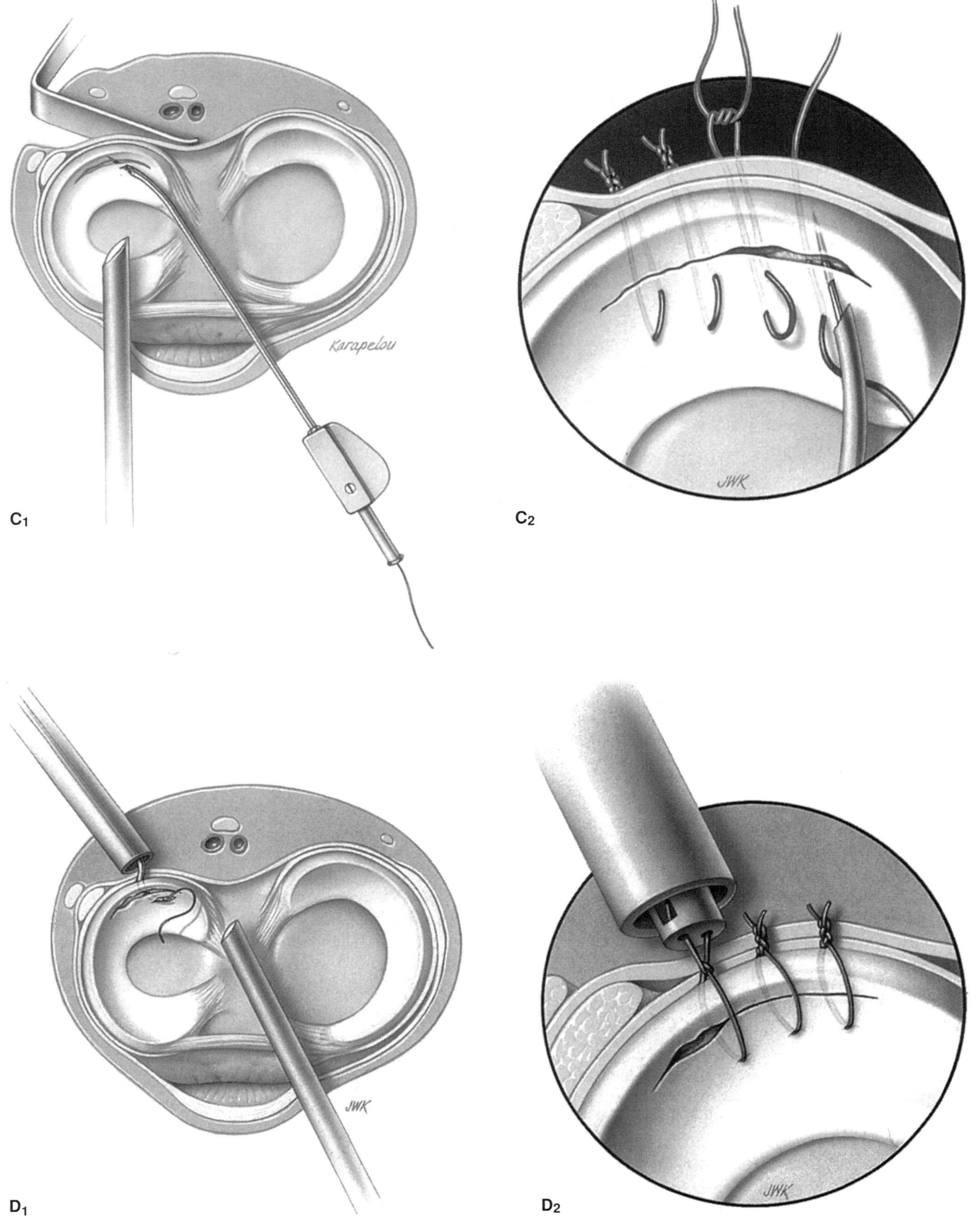

FIGURE 3–8. *Continued*

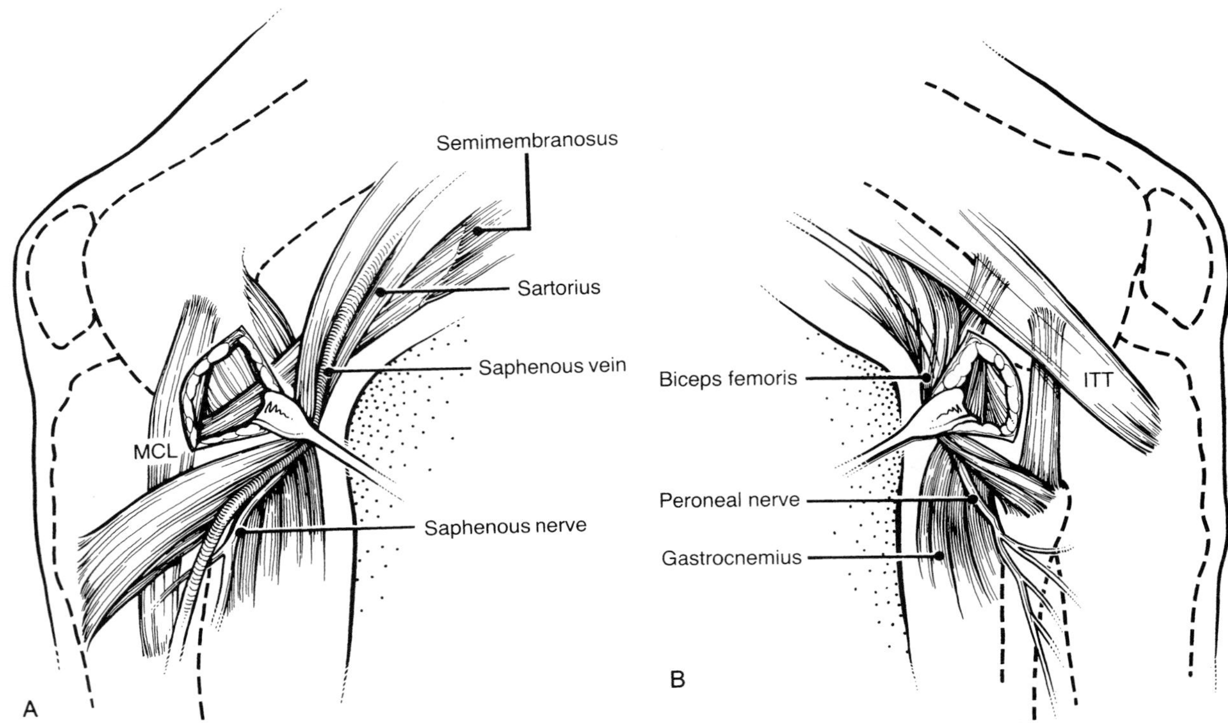

FIGURE 3–9. Incisions for meniscal repair must be planned to allow for retraction and protection of the saphenous nerve branches during medial meniscal repairs *(A)* and the Peroneal nerve during lateral meniscal repairs *(B)*. (From Scot, W.N., ed.: Arthroscopy of the Knee. Philadelphia, WB Saunders, 1990; reprinted by permission.)

2. Meniscal Cysts—Most commonly occur in conjunction with horizontal cleavage tears of the lateral meniscus (Fig. 3–10). Operative treatment consisting of arthroscopic partial meniscectomy and decompression through the tear (sometimes including "needling" of the cyst, has been shown to be efficacious. En bloc excision is no longer favored for most meniscal cysts. Popliteral (Baker's) cysts are also related to meniscal pathology and will usually resolve with treatment of meniscal pathology. They are classically located between the SM and Med Head of the semimembranosus and medial head of the gastrocnemius.
3. Discoid Menisci ("Popping Knee Syndrome")—can be classified as (1) incomplete, (2) complete, or (3) Wrisberg variant (Fig. 3–11). Patients may develop mechanical symptoms, or "popping," with the knee in extension. Plain radiographs may demonstrate a widened joint space, squaring of the lateral condyle, cupping of the lateral tibial plateau, and a hypoplastic lateral intercondylar spine. MRI can be helpful and can also show associated tears. Treatment includes partial meniscectomy (saucerization) for tears, meniscal repair for peripheral detachments (Wrisberg variant), and observation for discoid menisci unsuspected prior to arthroscopy.
4. Meniscal Transplantation—Remains controversial but may be indicated for young patients who have had near-total meniscectomy (especially lateral meniscectomy) and with early chondrosis. Indications and techniques are evolving.

F. Osteochondral Lesions
   1. Osteochondritis Dissecans (OCD)—Involves subchondral bone and overlying cartilage separation, most likely as a result of occult trauma. The lesion most often involves the lateral aspect of the me-

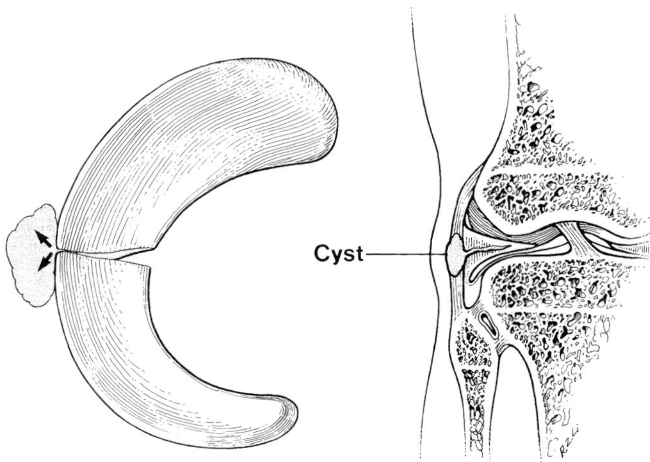

FIGURE 3–10. Meniscal cysts most commonly involve the lateral meniscus. (From Tria, A.J., and Klein, K.S.: An Illustrated Guide to the Knee, p. 101. New York, Churchill Livingstone, 1992; reprinted by permission.)

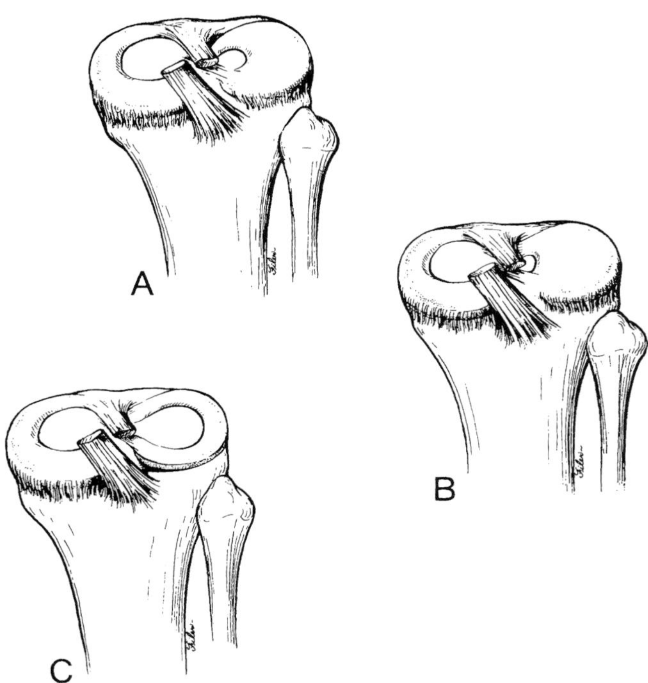

FIGURE 3–11. Classification of lateral discoid menisci. *A,* Incomplete. *B,* Complete. *C,* Wrisberg ligament varient. (From Neuschwander, D.C.: Discoid lateral meniscus. In Knee Surgery, p. 394. Baltimore, Williams & Wilkins, 1994; reprinted by permission.)

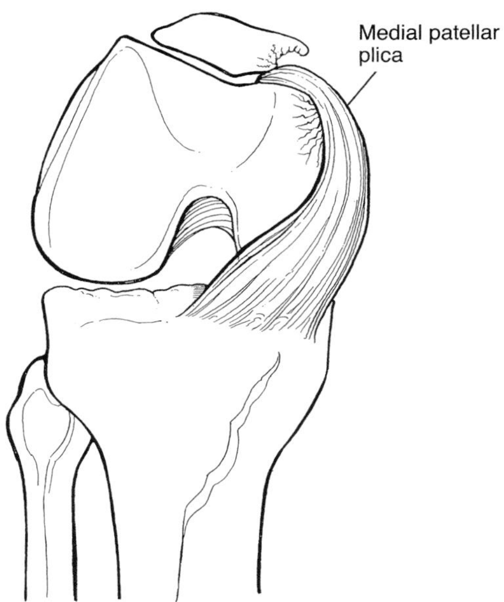

FIGURE 3–12. Medial patellar plica (shelf) with associated chondromalacia of the patella and medial femoral condyle. (From Miller, M.D., Cooper, D.E., and Warner, J.J.P.: Review of Sports Medicine and Arthroscopy, p. 36. Philadelphia, WB Saunders, 1995; reprinted by permission.)

dial femoral condyle. Children with open growth plates have the best prognosis, and often these lesions can be simply observed. In situ lesions can be treated with retrograde drilling. Detached lesions may require abrasion chondroplasty or allograft replacement.

2. Cartilage Injury—Usually occurs on the medial femoral condyle, often from shearing injuries. Débridement and chondroplasty are currently recommended for symptomatic lesions. Osteochondral injuries can sometimes be replaced and secured with small recessed screws or absorbable pins.

G. Synovial Lesions

1. Pigmented Villonodular Synovitis (PVNS)—Patients may present with pain and swelling and may have a palpable mass. Synovectomy is efficacious, but there is a high recurrence rate.
2. Other synovial lesions that respont to synovectomy include (osteo)chondromatosis, pauciarticular juvenile rheumatoid arthritis, and hemophilia. Additional arthroscopic portals are required for complete synovectomy.
3. Plicae—Synovial folds that are embryologic remnants. Occasionally, they are pathologic, particularly the medial patellar plica. This plica can cause abrasion of the medial femoral condyle (Fig. 3–12) and sometimes respond to arthroscopic excision.

H. Ligamentous Injuries

1. Anterior Cruciate Ligament Injury—Controversy continues regarding the development of late arthritis in ACL deficient versus reconstructed knees. Nevertheless, chronic ACL deficiency is associated with a higher incidence of complex meniscal tears not amenable to repair. Treatment decisions should be individualized based on age, activity level, instability, associated injuries, and other factors (Fig. 3–13). ACL injuries are often the result of noncontact pivoting injuries and are commonly associated with an audible "pop" with immediate swelling. The Lachman test is the most sensitive examination for acute ACL injuries. Intra-articular reconstruction (usually with bone–patella, tendon–bone, or hamstring autograft) is currently favored for patients with meet the criteria indicated in Fig. 3–13. Rehabilitation has evolved, and early motion and weight-bearing are encouraged in most protocols. Complications most commonly are a result of aberrant tunnel placement (often the femoral tunnel is place too far anteriorly) and early surgery (resulting in knee stiffness). The existence and treatment of "partial" ACL tears is also controversial, although clinical examination and functional stability remain the most important factors.
2. Posterior Cruciate Ligament Injury—Treatment is controversial, although reports suggest that nonoperative management may result in late patellar and medial femoral condyle chondrosis. Injuries occur most commonly as a result of a direct blow to the anterior tibia with the knee flexed (the "dashboard injury") or hyperflexion without a blow; hyperextension injuries can also result in PCL rupture. The key examination is the posterior drawer test with an absent or posteriorly directed tibial "step-off." Nonoperative treatment is favored for most isolated PCL injuries. Bony avulsion fractures can be repaired primarily with good results, although primary repair of mid-substance

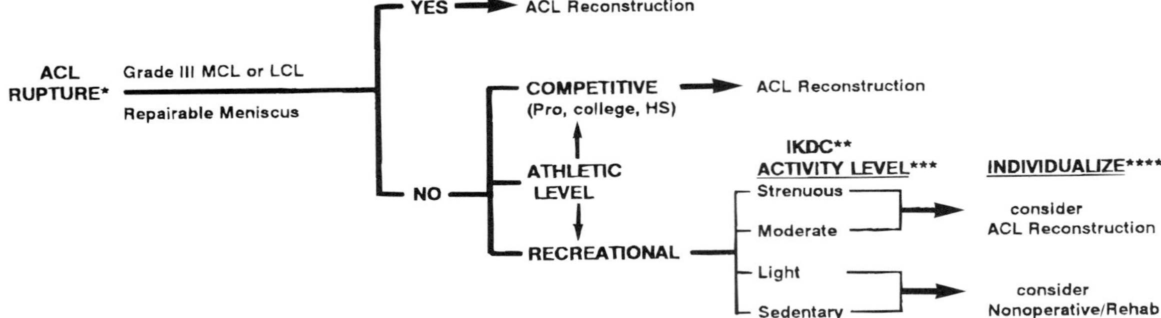

FIGURE 3–13. Algorithm for the treatment of ACL ruptures. *midsubstance tears; **IKKC (International Knee Documentation Committee Committee); ***activity level; strenuous, jumping/pivoting sports; moderate, heavy manual work, skiing; light, light manual work, running; sedentary, activities of daily living; ****individualize based on age, arthritis, occupation, activity modification, other medial conditions. (From Spindler, K.P., and Walker, R.N.: General approach to ligament surgery. In Knee Surgery, p. 652. Baltimore, Williams & Wilkins, 1994; reprinted by permission.)

PCL (and ACL) injuries has not been successful. PCL reconstruction is recommended for functionally unstable or combined injuries (Fig. 3–14).

3. Collateral Ligament Injury
   a. Medial Collateral Ligament (MCL)—Occur as a result of valgus stress to the knee. Pain and instability with valgus stress testing at 30 degrees of flexion (and not in full extension) is diagnostic. Injuries most commonly occur at the femoral insertion of the ligament. Nonoperative treatment (hinged knee brace) is highly successful for isolated MCL injuries. Prophylactic bracing may be helpful for football players. Rarely, advancement and reinforcement of the ligament is necessary for chronic injuries that do not respond to conservative treatment.
   b. Lateral Collateral Ligament (LCL)—Injury to this ligament is uncommon. Varus instability in 30 degrees of flexion is diagnostic. Isolated LCL injuries should be managed nonoperatively.
4. Posterolateral Corner Injuries—These injuries occur rarely as isolated injuries but more commonly are associated with other ligamentous injuries (especially the PCL). Because of poor results with chronic reconstructions, acute repair is advocated. Examination for increased external rotation, external rotation recurvatum test, posterolateral drawer test, and reverse pivot shift test is important. Early anatomic repair is often successful. Procedures recommended for chronic injuries include posterolateral corner advancement, popliteus bypass, biceps tenodesis, and more recently "split" grafts, which are used to reconstruct both the LCL and the popliteus/posterolateral corner (Fig. 3–15).
5. Multiple Ligament Injuries—Combined ligamentous injuries (especially ACL-PCL injuries) can be a result of a knee dislocation, and neurovascular injury must be suspected. Liberal use of vascular studies is recommended early (Fig. 3–16). Dislocations are classified based on the direction of tibial displacement (Fig. 3–17). Treatment is usually operative. Emergent surgical indications include popliteal artery injury, open dislocations and irreducible dislocations. Most surgeons recommend delaying surgery 5–7 days to ensure that there is no vascular injury. Avulsion injuries can be repaired primarily; however, interstitial injuries must be reconstructed.

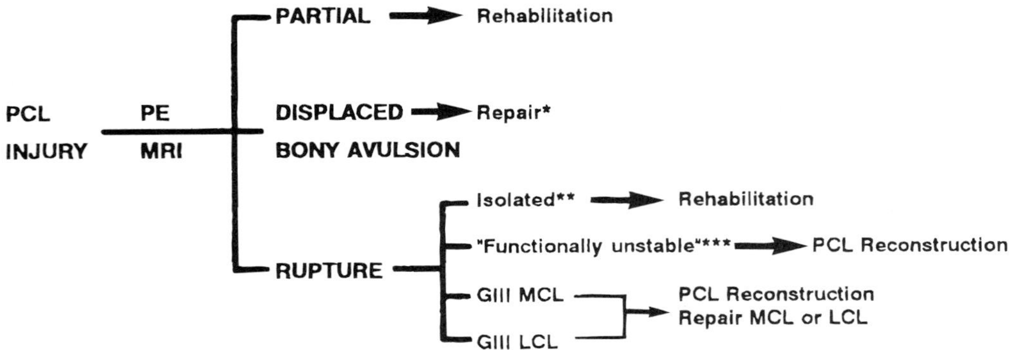

FIGURE 3–14. Algorithm for treatment of PCL injuries. *With an intact ligament; **without posterolateral injury or combined ligamentous injury; ***failed rehabilitation or unstable/symptomatic with activities of daily living. (From Spindler, K.P., and Walker, R.N.: General approach to ligament surgery. In Knee Surgery, p. 655. Baltimore, Williams & Wilkins, 1994; reprinted by permission.)

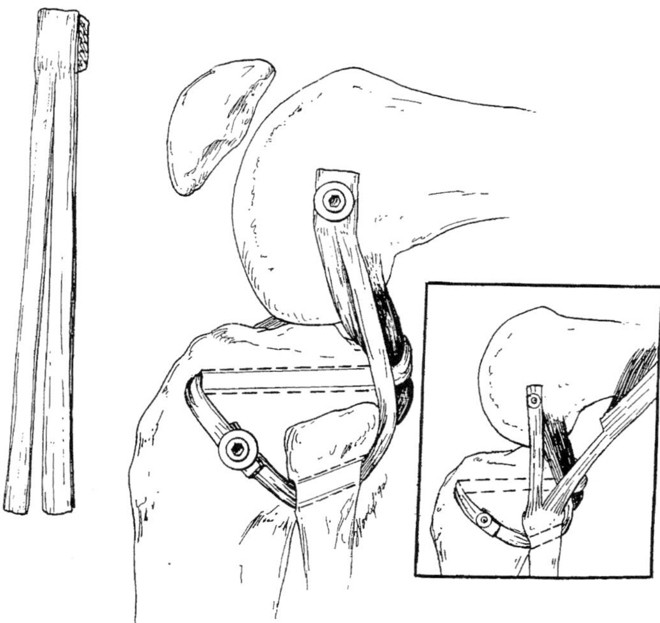

FIGURE 3–15. Split posterolateral corner graft. (From McKernan, D.J., and Paulos, L.E.: Graft selection. In Knee Surgery, p. 669. Baltimore, Williams & Wilkins, 1994; reprinted by permission.)

I. Anterior Knee Pain
   1. Introduction—Anterior knee pain is classified based on etiology (Table 3–1). The term "chondromalacia" should be replaced with a specific diagnosis based on this classification.
   2. Trauma—Includes fractures of the patella (discussed in Chapter 10) and tendon injuries.
      a. Tendon Ruptures—Quadriceps tendon ruptures are more common than patellar tendon ruptures and occur most commonly in patients over 40 years old with indirect trauma. Patellar tendon ruptures occur in young patients with direct trauma. Both types of tendon rupture are more common in patients with underlying disorders of the tendon. A palpable defect and inability to extend the knee is diagnostic. Primary repair with temporary stabilization is indicated.
      b. Overuse Injuries
         1. Patellar Tendinitis (Jumper's Knee)—This condition, most common in athletes who participate in sports such as basketball and volleyball, is associated with pain and tenderness near the inferior border of the patella (worse in extension than flexion). Treatment includes NSAIDs, physical therapy (strengthening and ultrasound), orthotics, and rarely surgery (excision of necrotic tendon fibers).
         2. Quadriceps Tendinitis—Less common but just as painful. Patients may note painful clicking and localized pain. Operative treatment is occasionally necessary.
         3. Prepatellar Bursitis (Housemaid's Knee)—It is the most common form of bursitis of the knee and is associated with a history of prolonged kneeling. Supportive treatment (knee pads, occasional steroid injections) and rarely bursal excision are recommended.
         4. Iliotibial Band Friction Syndrome—It can occur in runners and cyclist and is a result of abrasion between the iliotibial band and the lateral femoral condyle. Localized tenderness, worse with the knee flexed 30 degrees, is common. Rehabilitation is usually successful. Surgical excision of an ellipse of the iliotibial band is occasionally necessary.
         5. Semimembranosus Tendinitis—Most common in male athletes in their early thirties, this condition can be diagnosed with nuclear imaging and responds to stretching and strengthening.
      c. Late Effects of Trauma
         1. Patellofemoral Arthritis—Injury and malalignment can contribute to patellar DJD. Lateral release may be beneficial early; however, other procedures may be required for advanced patellar arthritis. Options include anterior or anteromedial transfer of the tibial tubercle, or patellectomy for severe cases.
         2. Anterior Fat Pad Syndrome (Hoffa Disease)—Trauma to the anterior fat pad can lead to fibrous changes and pinching of the fat pad, especially in patients with genu recurvatum. Activity modification, ice, and knee padding can be helpful. Occasionally arthroscopic excision is beneficial.

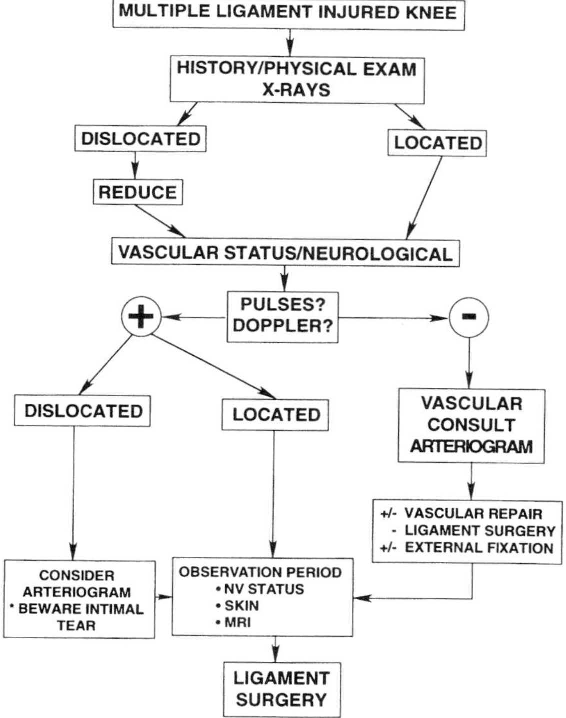

FIGURE 3–16. Algorithm for the treatment of multiple knee ligament injuries. (From Marks, P.H., and Harner, C.D.: The anterior cruciate ligament in the multiple ligament-injured knee. Clin. Sports Med. 12:825–838, 1993; reprinted by permission.)

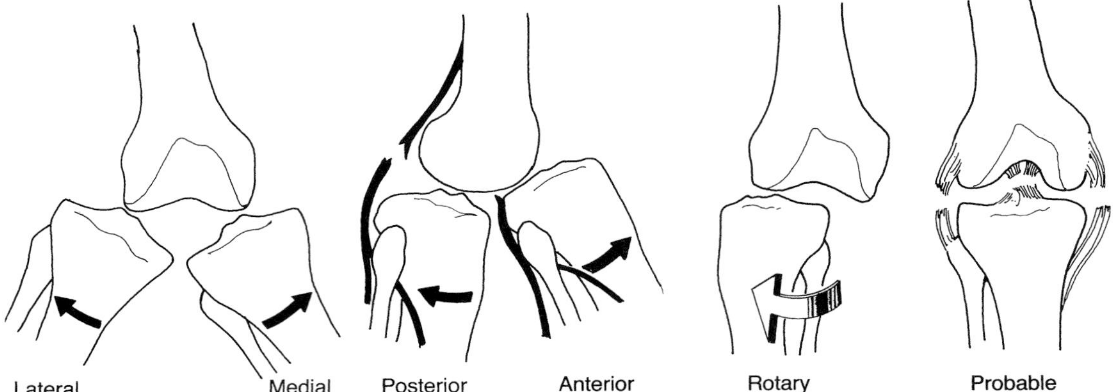

FIGURE 3–17. Classification of knee dislocations. (From Miller, M.D., Cooper, D.E., and Warner, J.J.P.: Review of Sports Medicine and Arthroscopy, p. 51. Philadelphia, WB Saunders, 1995; reprinted by permission.)

3. Reflex Sympathetic Dystrophy (RSD)—Characterized by pain out of proportion to physical findings, RSD is an exaggerated response to injury. Three stages, progressing from swelling, warmth, and hyperhidrosis to brawny edema and trophic changes and finally to glossy, cool, dry skin and stiffness, are typical. Patellar osteopenia, a "flamingo gait" are also common. Treatment includes nerve stimulation, NSAIDs, and sympathetic or epidural blocks.

d. Patellofemoral Dysplasia

1. Lateral Patellar Compression Syndrome—This problem is associated with a tight lateral retinaculum and excessive lateral tilt. Treatment includes activity modification, NSAIDs, and vastus medialis obiquus (VMO) strengthening. Arthroscopy and lateral release are occasionally required. Arthroscopic visualization through a superior portal demonstrates that the patella does not articulate medially by 40 degrees of knee flexion. Lateral release requires care to ensure that adequate hemostasis is achieved postoperatively and that the patella can be passively tilted 80 degrees.
2. Patellar Instability—Recurrent subluxation/dislocation of the patella can be characterized by lateral displacement of the patella, a shallow intercondylar sulcus, or patellar incongruence. When associated with femoral anteversion, genu valgum, and pronated feet, the symptoms can be exacerbated, especially in adolescents ("miserable malalignment syndrome"). Extensive rehabilitation is often currative. Surgical procedures include proximal and/or distal realignment procedures.

e. Chondromalacia—Although this term has fallen into disfavor, articular damage and changes to the patella are common. Treatment is usually symptomatic. Débridement procedures are of questionable benefit.

f. Abnormalities of Patellar Height—Patella alta (high-riding patella) and baja (low-riding patella) is determined based on various measurements made on lateral radiographs of the knee (Fig. 3–5). Patella alta can be associated with patellar instability because the patella may not articulate with the sulcus, which normally constrains the patella. Patella baja is often the result of fat pad and tendon fibrosis, and may require proximal transfer of the tubercle for refractory cases.

J. Pediatric Knee Disorders

1. Physeal Injuries—Most commonly involve Salter-Harris II fractures of the distal femoral physis. Pain, swelling, and an inability to ambulate are common. Stress radiographs may be necessary to make the diagnosis. Open reduction and internal fixation are indicated for Salter-Harris III and IV fractures, and Salter-Harris I and II fractures that cannot be adequately reduced.
2. Ligament Injuries—Most ligament injuries are treated similar to those in adults. Mid-substance ACL injuries in skeletally immature individuals remains a subject of considerable debate. Procedures that do not violate the growth plate are usually recommended for patients who fail nonoperative management. Avulsion fractures of the intercondylar eminence of the tibia are treated with closed treatment; if this treatment fails arthroscopic reduction and fixation of the fragment are undertaken.
3. Traction Apophysitis—Including Osgood-Schlatter disease and Sinding-Larsen-Johansson disease is usually treated symptomatically. Occasionally, procedures such as ossicle excision are indicated for refractory cases.

II. Other Lower Extremity Sports Medicine Problems

A. Nerve Entrapment Syndromes

1. Ilioinguinal Nerve Entrapment—This nerve can be constricted by hypertrophied abdominal muscles as a result of intensive training. Hyperextension of the hip may exacerbate the pain that patients experience, and hyperesthesia symptoms are common. Surgical release is occasionally necessary.
2. Obturator Nerve Entrapment—Can lead to chronic medial thigh pain, especially in athletes with well developed hip adductor muscles (e.g., skaters). Nerve conduction studies are helpful for establishing the diagnosis. Treatment is usually supportive.

TABLE 3–1. CLASSIFICATION OF PATELLOFEMORAL DISORDERS

I. Trauma (conditions caused by trauma in the otherwise normal knee)
  A. Acute trauma
    1. Contusion (924.11)
    2. Fracture
      a. Patella (822)
      b. Femoral trochlea (821.2)
      c. Proximal tibial epiphysis (tubercle) (823.0)
    3. Dislocation (rare in the normal knee) (836.3)
    4. Rupture
      a. Quadriceps tendon (843.8)
      b. Patellar tendon (844.8)
  B. Repetitive trauma (overuse syndromes)
    1. Patellar tendinitis ("jumper's knee") (726.64)
    2. Quadriceps tendinitis (726.69)
    3. Peripatellar tendinitis (e.g., anterior knee pain of the adolescent due to hamstring contracture) (726.699)
    4. Prepatellar bursitis ("housemaid's knee") (726.65)
    5. Apophysitis
      a. Osgood-Schlatter disease (732.43)
      b. Sinding-Larsen-Johansson disease (732.42)
  C. Late effects of trauma (905)
    1. Posttraumatic chondromalacia patellae
    2. Posttraumatic patellofemoral arthritis
    3. Anterior fat pad syndrome (posttraumatic fibrosis)
    4. Reflex sympathetic dystrophy of the patella
    5. Patellar osseous dystrophy
    6. Acquired patella infera (719.366)
    7. Acquired quadriceps fibrosis
II. Patellofemoral dysplasia
  A. Lateral patellar compression syndrome (LPCS) (718.365)
    1. Secondary chondromalacia patellae (717.7)
    2. Secondary patellofemoral arthritis (715.289)
  B. Chronic subluxation of the patella (CSP) (718.364)
    1. Secondary chondromalacia patellae (717.7)
    2. Secondary patellofemoral arthritis (715.289)
  C. Recurrent dislocation of the patella (RDP) (718.361)
    1. Associated fractures (822)
      a. Osteochondral (intra-articular)
      b. Avulsion (extra-articular)
    2. Secondary chondromalacia patellae (717.7)
    3. Secondary patellofemoral arthritis (715.289)
  D. Chronic dislocation of the patella (718.362)
    1. Congenital
    2. Acquired
III. Idiopathic chondromalacia patellae (717.7)
IV. Osteochondritis dissecans
  A. Patella (732.704)
  B. Femoral trochlea (732.703)
V. Synovial plicae (727.8916) (anatomic variant made symptomatic by acute or repetitive trauma)
  A. Medial patellar ("shelf") (727.89161)
  B. Suprapatellar (727.89163)
  C. Lateral patellar (727.89165)

Orthopaedic ICD-9-CM Expanded Diagnostic Codes in parentheses.
From Merchant AC: Classification of patellofemoral disorders. Arthroscopy 4:235, 1988, with permission.

3. Lateral Femoral Cutaneous Nerve Entrapment—Can lead to a painful condition termed **meralgia paresthetica.** Tight belts and prolonged hip flexion may exacerbate symptoms. Release of compressive devices, postural exercises, and anti-inflammatory medications are usually curative.
4. Saphenous Nerve Entrapment—Compressed at Hunter's canal or in the proximal leg, this nerve can cause painful symptoms inferior and medial to the knee.
5. Peroneal Nerve Entrapment—The common peroneal nerve can be compressed behind the fibula or injured by a direct blow to this area. The superficial peroneal nerve can be entrapped about 12 cm proximal to the tip of the lateral malleolus, where it exits the fascia of the anterolateral leg, as a result of inversion injuries. Fascial defects can be present as well, contributing to the problem. Compartment release is sometimes indicated. The deep peroneal nerve can be compressed by the inferior extensor retinaculum, leading to **anterior tarsal tunnel syndrome,** sometimes necessitating release of this structure.
6. Tibial Nerve Entrapment—When compressed behind the medial malleolus under the flexor retinaculum, it can lead to **tarsal tunnel syndrome.** EMG/NCS evaluation is helpful, and surgical release is sometimes indicated. Distal entrapment of the first branch of the lateral plantar nerve (to the adductor digiti quinti) has also been described.
7. Medial Plantar Nerve Entrapment—It occurs at the point where the flexor digitorum longus and flexor hallicus longus cross (knot of Henry) and is caused most commonly by external compression by orthotics. Commonly called **jogger's foot,** this condition usually responds to conservative measures.

B. Contusions
1. Iliac Crest Contusions—Direct trauma to this area can occur in contact sports; known commonly as a **hip pointer.** An avulsion of the iliac apophysis should be ruled out in adolescent athletes. Treatment consists in ice, compression, pain control, and placing the affected leg on maximum stretch. Additional padding is indicated after the acute phase.
2. Groin Contusions—An avulsion fracture of the lesser trochanter must be ruled out prior to supportive treatment.
3. Quadriceps Contusions—Can result in hemorrhage and late myositis ossificans. Acute management includes cold compression and **immobilization in flexion.** Close monitoring for compartment syndrome should be accomplished acutely.

C. Muscle Injuries
1. Hamstring Strain—This common injury is often the result of sudden stretch on the musculotendinous junction during sprinting. These injuries can occur anywhere in the posterior thigh. Treatment is supportive followed by stretching and strengthening. To prevent recurrence, return to play should be delayed until strength is approximately 90% of the opposite side.
2. Adductor Strain—Common in sports such as soccer, these injuries must be differentiated from subtle hernias.
3. Rectus Femoris Strain—Acute injuries are usually located more distally on the thigh, but chronic injuries are more commonly near the muscle origin. Tratment includes ice and stretching/strengthening.
4. Gastrocnemius–Soleus Strain—Nicknamed **tennis leg** because of its common association with that sport, this injury is probably much more common than rupture of the plantaris tendon. Supportive treatment is indicated.

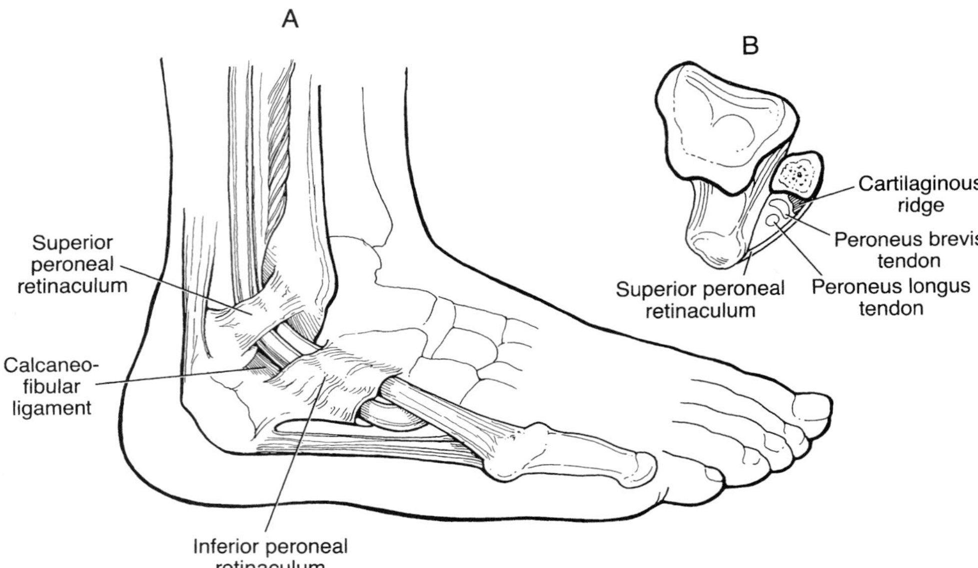

FIGURE 3–18. Normal relationship of the peroneal tendons. Note the superior and inferior retinacula and the cartilaginous rigege on the posterolateral fibula. A, Lateral view. B, Superior view. (From Miller, M.D., Cooper, D.E., and Warner, J.J.P.: Review of Sports Medicine and Arthroscopy, p. 82. Philadelphia, WB Saunders, 1995; reprinted by permission.)

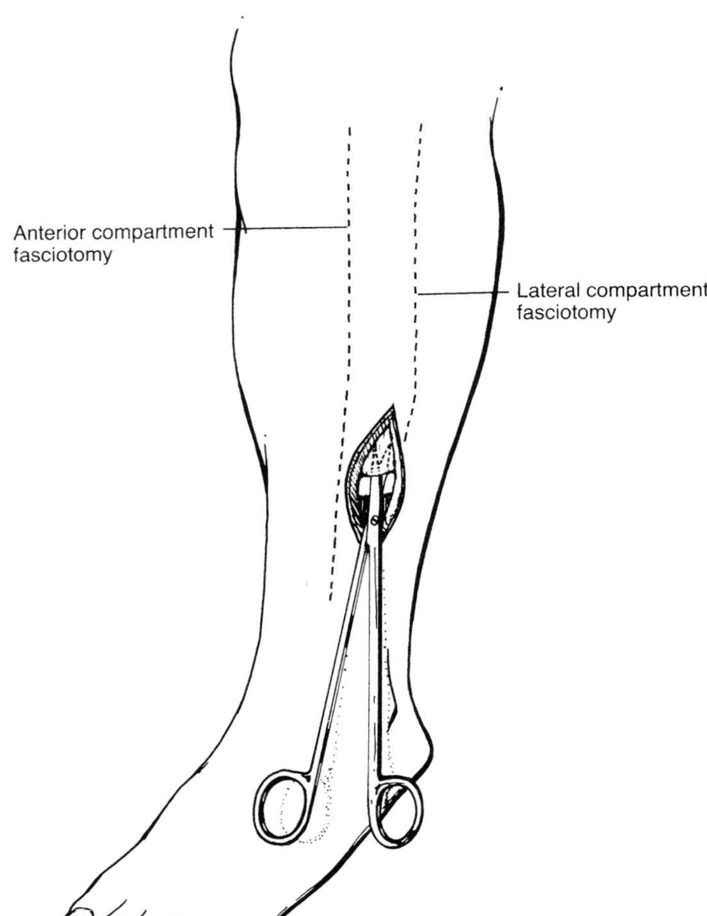

FIGURE 3–19. Anterior and lateral compartment release. (From DeLee, J.C., and Drez, D.: Orthopaedic Sports Medicine: Principles and Practice, p. 1618. Philadelphia, WB Saunders, 1994; reprinted by permission.)

D. Tendon Injuries
   1. Peroneal Tendon Injuries
      a. Subluxation/Dislocation—Violent dorsiflexion of the everted foot can result in injury of the fibro-osseous peroneal tendon sheath. Diagnosis is confirmed by observing the subluxation or dislocation with eversion and dorsiflexion of the foot. Plain radiographs may demonstrate a rim fracture of the lateral aspect of the distal fibula. Treatment of acute injuries includes restoration of the normal anatomy (Fig. 3–18). Chronic reconstruction involves groove-deepening procedures, tissue transfers, or bone block techniques.
      b. Longitudinal Tears of the Peroneal Tendons (Especially Brevis Tendon)—Recognized with increasing frequency. Repair and decompression are generally recommended.
   2. Posterior Tibialis Tendon Injury—This injury can occur in older athletes. Débridement of partial ruptures and flexor digitorum longus transfer for chronic injuries are recommended.
   3. Achilles Tendon Injuries
      a. Tendinitis—Overuse injury to the Achilles tendon usually responds to rest and physical therapy modalities. Progression to partial rupture may necessitate surgical excision of scar and granulation tissue.
      b. Rupture—Complete rupture of the tendon is caused by maximal plantar flexion with the foot planted. Patients may relate that they felt as if they were "shot." The Thompson test (squeezing the calf results in plantar flexion of the foot normally) is helpful for confirming the diagnosis. Treatment remains controversial; however, recurrence rates can be reduced with primary repair.

E. Chronic/Exertional Compartment Syndrome—Although more commonly encountered with trauma, sports-related compartment syndrome is becoming more frequently diagnosed. Athletes (especially runners and cyclists) may note pain that has a gradual onset during exercise, ultimately restricting their performance. Compartment pressures taken before, during, and after exercise (resting pressure >15 mm Hg or a delay in return to baseline after 5–10 minutes after exertion) can help establish the diagnosis. The anterior and deep posterior compartments of the leg are most often involved. Fasciotomy is sometimes indicated for refractory cases (Fig. 3–19).

F. Stress Fractures
   1. Common Characteristics—A history of overuse with an insidious onset of pain and localized tenderness and swelling are typical. Bone scan can be diagnostic, even with normal plain radiographs. Treatment includes protected weight-bearing, rest, cross-training, analgesic, and therapeutic modalities.
   2. Femoral Neck Stress Fractures—Tension, or transverse, fractures are more serious than compression fractures and may require operative stabilization.
   3. Femoral Shaft Fractures—Usually respond to protected weight-bearing but can progress to complete fractures if unrecognized.
   4. Tibial Shaft Fractures—Can be difficult. Persistence of the "dreaded black line" (Fig. 3–20) for more than 6 months, especially with a positive bone scan, can be an indication for bone grafting.
   5. Tarsal Navicular Fractures—Can be challenging. Immobilization and **non-weight-bearing** is important during the early management of these stress fractures.

G. Other Hip Disorders
   1. Snapping Iliotibial Band Syndrome—Condition in which the iliotibial band abruptly catches on the greater trochanter. The condition, more common in females with wide pelves and prominent trochanters, can be exacerbated by running on banked surfaces. The snapping may be reproduced with passive hip flexion from an adducted position. Stretching/strengthening modalities, such as ultrasound and occasionally surgical release may relieve the snapping. This condition must be differentiated from the less common snapping iliospoas tendon.
   2. Traumatic Avascular Necrosis—Traumatic hip subluxation can disrupt the arterial blood supply to the hip and result in avascular necrosis. Early recognition of these injuries, seen recently in football players, is essential.
   3. Proximal Femoral Fractures—Can occur in athletes, especially cross-country skiers (**skier's hip**). Release bindings may reduce the incidence of these injuries.

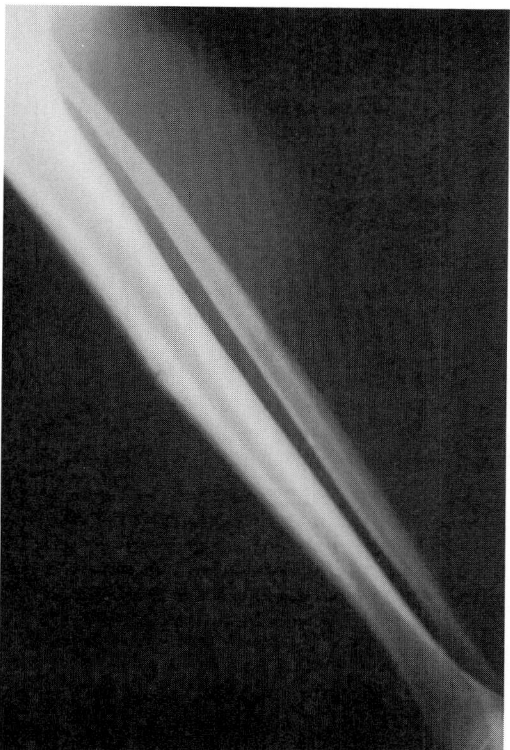

FIGURE 3–20. Radiograph demonstrating the "dreaded black line" associated with an impending complete fracture of the tibial shaft. (From Miller, M.D., Cooper, D.E., and Warner, J.J.P.: Review of Sports Medicine and Arthroscopy, p. 81. Philadelphia, WB Saunders, 1995; reprinted by permission.)

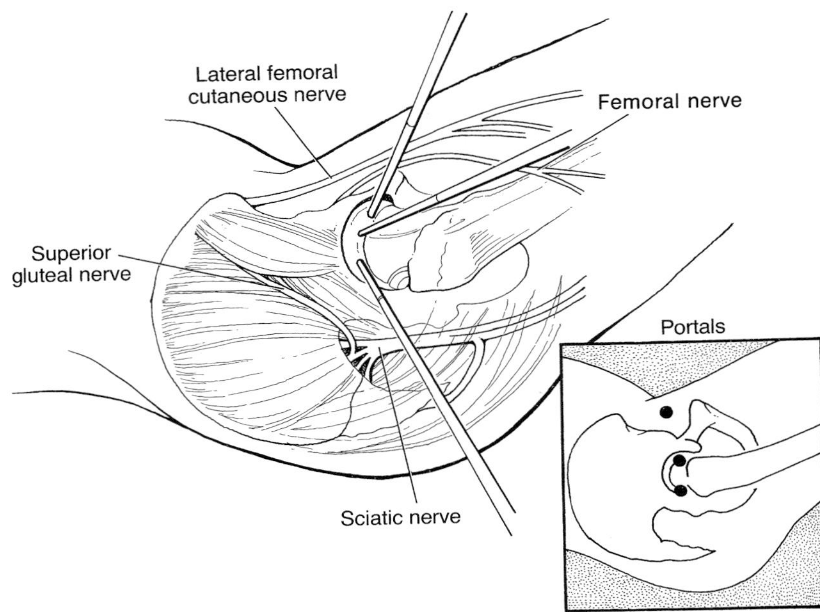

FIGURE 3–21. Portals for hip arthroscopy include the anterior portal and two portals adjacent to the greater trochanter. (From Miller, M.D., Cooper, D.E., and Warner, J.J.P.: Review of Sports Medicine and Arthroscopy, p. 107. Philadelphia, WB Saunders, reprinted by permission.)

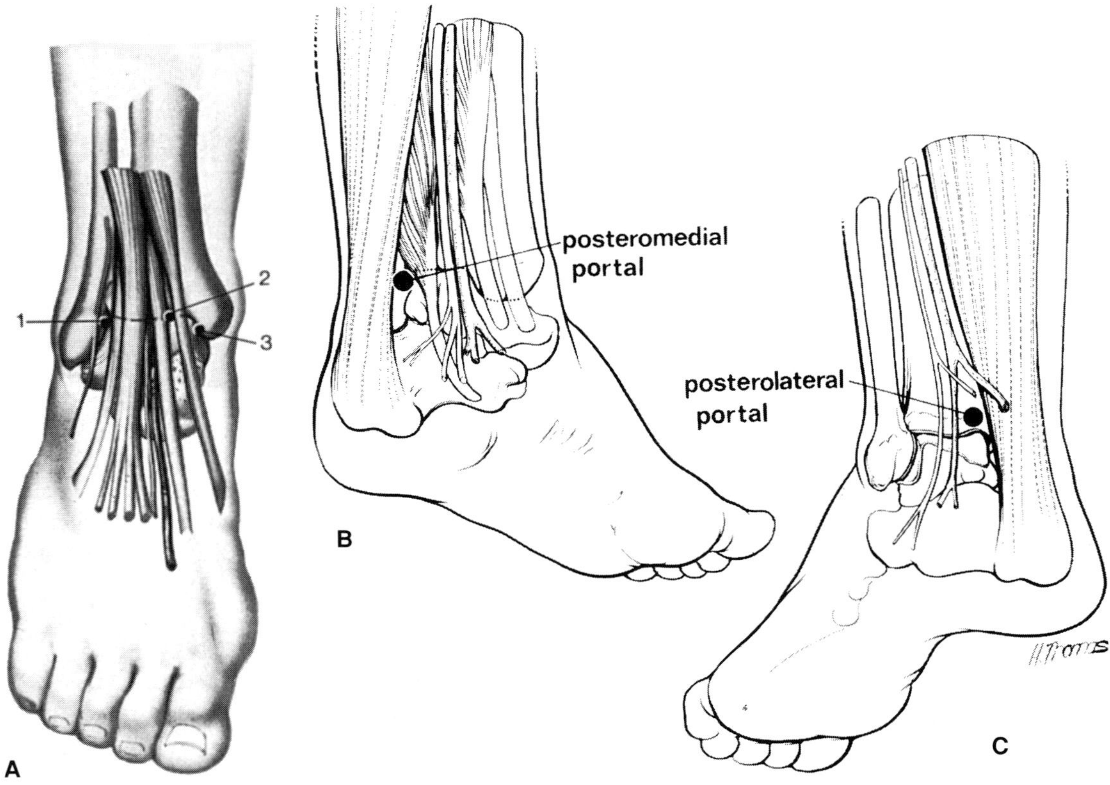

FIGURE 3–22. Arthroscopic portals for ankle arthroscopy. A, Anterior portals. 1, anterolateral portal, placed lateral to the peroneus tertius and extensor tendons; 2, anterocentral portal medial or lateral to the extensor hallicus tendon; 3, anteromedial portal, just medial the the tibialis anterior tendon. Posteromedial (B) and posterolateral (C) portals immediately adjacent to the Achilles tendon. (From Jahss, M.H.: Disorders of the Foot and Ankle, 2nd ed., p. 206. Philadelphia, WB Saunders, 1991; reprinted by permission.)

H. Other Foot and Ankle Disorders
   1. Plantar Fasciitis—Inflammation of the plantar fascia, usually in central to medial subcalcaneal region, is common in runners. Rest, orthotics, stretching, and anti-inflammatory medications are helpful. Occasionally, plantar fasciotomy is necessary, but recovery can be protracted.
   2. Os Trigonum—An unfused fractured os trigonum can cause impingement with dorsiflexion of the foot, especially in ballet dancers. Treatment may include local anesthetic injection and other supportive measures. Surgical excision of the offending bone is occasionally necessary.
   3. Recurrent Ankle Sprains—These injuries are common in athletes and most often involve the anterior talofibular ligament (ATFL). Surgical treatment is reserved for recurrent, symptomatic ankle instability with excessive tilt and drawer on examination/stress radiographs that has not responded to orthotics and peroneal strengthening over an extended period. Anatomic procedures (Brostrom) are usually successful. Involvement of the subtalar joint requires tendon rerouting procedures that include this joint. Patients with "high" ankle sprains involving the syndesmosis require recovery periods almost twice those for common ankle sprains.
   4. Turf Toe—Severe dorsiflexion of the MTP joint of the great toe can result in a tender, stiff, swollen toe. Treatment includes motion, ice, and taping. If symptoms persist, a stress fracture of the proximal phalanx should be ruled out with a bone scan.

I. Arthroscopy
   1. Hip Arthroscopy—A relatively new procedure; advocates suggest that loose body removal, synovectomy, and labral débridement are indications. Lateral decubitus or, more recently, supine positioning with approximatly 50 pounds of traction with a well padded peroneal post is recommended. Three portals are commonly used—one on each side of the greater trochanter and an additional anterior portal for instrumentation (Fig. 3–21).
   2. Ankle Arthroscopy—Indications include treatment of osteochondral injuries of the talus, débridement of posttraumatic synovitis, removal of anterior tibiotalar spurring, and cartilage débridement in conjunction with ankle fusions. Supine positioning with the leg over a well padded bolster and an external traction device is currently popular. Five portals have been suggested (Fig. 3–22), but most surgeons avoid the posteromedial portal because of risk to the posterial tibial artery and tibial nerve. Treatment of osteochondral injuries of the talus, including drilling of the base of these lesions and fixation of replaceable lesions, has been advocated. The Loomer et al. modification to the Berndt and Harty classification scheme (Fig. 3–23) is helpful in the management of these injuries.

III. Shoulder

A. Anatomy and Biomechanics—A more detailed description of shoulder anatomy appears in Chapter 11, but a brief review of important concepts is in order.

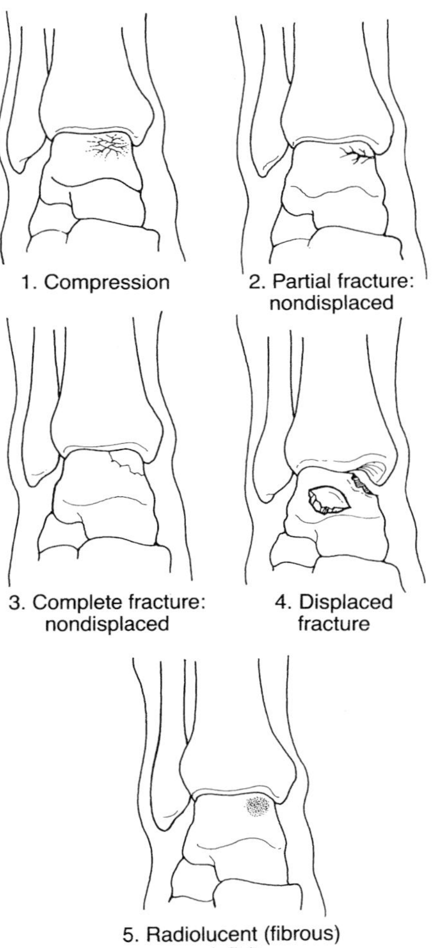

FIGURE 3–23. Loomer and coworkers' modification to the Berndt and Harty classification of osteochondral lesions of the talus. (From Miller, M.D., Cooper, D.E., and Warner, J.J.P.: Review of Sports Medicine and Arthroscopy, p. 95. Philadelphia, WB Saunders, 1995; reprinted by permission.)

   1. Joint—The shoulder is composed of the glenohumeral, sternoclavicular, acromioclavicular, and scapulothoracic joints, each with its own unique ligaments.
      a. Glenohumeral Joint—The glenohumeral joint, a spheroidal (ball and socket) joint is the principal articulation of the shoulder and is supported by the glenohumeral ligaments and labrum (Fig. 3–24). The glenohumeral ligaments are discrete capsular thickenings that limit excessive rotation and translation of the humeral head. These ligaments are named based on their relationship to the glenoid as inferior, middle, and superior. The **inferior glenohumeral ligament** is composed of an anterior and posterior band with an interposed axillary pouch. This "complex" is a major anterior stabilizer of the glenohumeral joint, especially with the arm abducted. The **middle glenohumeral ligament,** which runs obliquely over the

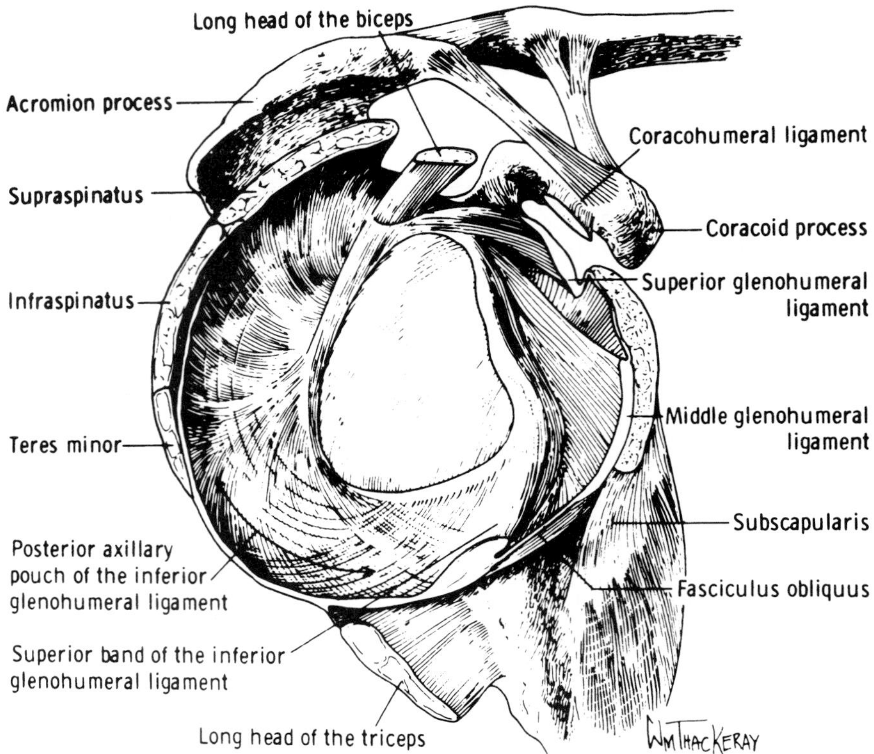

FIGURE 3–24. Important ligaments of the shoulder. (From Turkel, S.J., Panio, M.W., Marshall, J.L., and Girgis, F.G.: Stabilizing mechanisms preventing anterior dislocation of the gleno-humeral joint. J. Bone Joint Surg. [Am.] 63:1209, 1981; reprinted by permission.)

subscapularis, is highly variable in size and appearance. It functions principally to prevent anterior instability when the shoulder is externally rotated and abducted 45 degrees. The **superior glenohumeral ligament** works with the coracohumeral ligament to prevent inferior instability in the adducted arm. The **posterior capsule** is often thin and is not described as having any ligaments. The **labrum** is a fibrocartilaginous thickening surrounding the glenoid that deepens the glenoid cavity and serves as a "chock block," preventing abnormal motion. It also serves to anchor the inferior glenohumeral ligament complex.

b. Sternoclavicular Joint—A gliding joint with a disc, this joint serves to anchor the shoulder girdle to the chest wall.
c. Acromioclavicular Joint—Similar to the sternoclavicular joint but with a incomplete disc. This joint serves as an attachment for the acromion and clavicle. It is supported by the acromioclavicular ligament and the coracoclavicular ligaments (conoid and trapezoid) (Fig. 3–25).
d. Scapulothoracic Joint—The medial border of the scapula articulates with the posterior aspect of ribs 2–7. The ratio of glenohumeral to scapulothoracic motion during shoulder abduction is approximately 2:1.

2. Supporting Structures—Much like the knee, it is helpful to consider the shoulder in layers (Fig. 3–26).

LAYER	COMPONENTS
I	Deltoid, pectoralis major
II	Clavicopectoral fascia, conjoined tendon, pectoralis minor
III	Subdeltoid bursa, rotator cuff muscles
IV	Glenohumeral capsule, coracohumeral ligament

3. Biomechanics—The shoulder is stabilized by both static and dynamic restraints. Static restraints include the articular anatomy (humeral head diameter/glenoid diameter = 0.60–0.75); labrum (deepens the socket/"chock block"); negative intra-articular pressure; and the glenohumeral ligaments (may be "stretched" in addition to tearing with dislocations). Dynamic restraints include joint compression, barrier effect, and steering effect of the rotator cuff muscles.
4. Throwing—Significant forces are generated when throwing and can result in shoulder injury. The

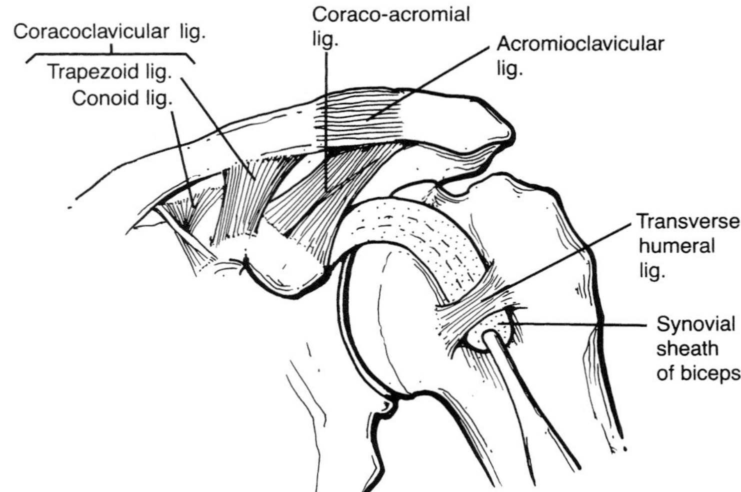

FIGURE 3–25. Acromioclavicular joint anatomy. (From Tibone, J., Patek, R., Jobe, F.W., Perry, J., and Pink, M.: Functional anatomy, biomechanics, and kinesiology; the shoulder. In Orthopaedic Sports Medicine Principles and Practice, DeLee, J.C., Drez, D., Jr., eds., p.465. Philadelphia, WB Saunders, 1994; reprinted by permission.)

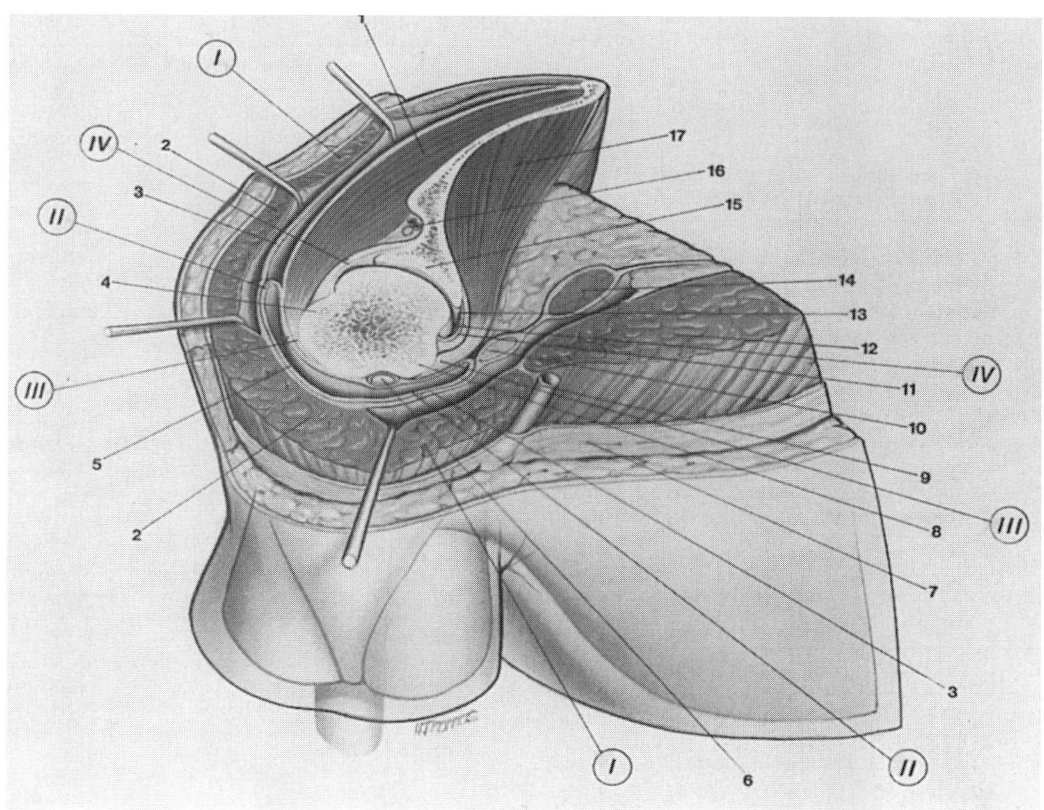

FIGURE 3–26. Cross-sectional view of the right shoulder at the level of the lesser tuberosity. Note the four layers of the shoulder and their components: I—deltoid (2), pectoralis major (12), cephalic vein (9); II—conjoined tendon (10), pectoralis minor (14), claviopectoral fascia (7); III—subdeltoid bursa (5), rotator cuff muscles (1, 17); glenohumeral capsule (11), greater tuberosity (4), long head of biceps (6), lesser tuberosity (8), fascia (3), synovium (13), glenoid (15). (From Cooper, D.E., O'Brien, S.J., and Warren, R.F.: Supporting layers of the glenohumeral joint: an anatomic study. Clin. Orthop. 289:144–155, 1993; reprinted by permission.)

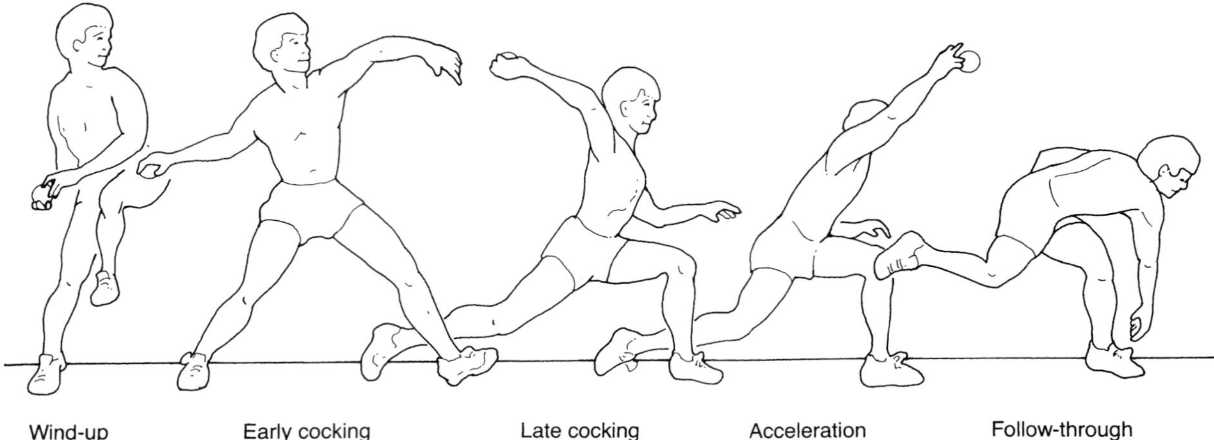

FIGURE 3–27. The five phases of throwing. (From Miller, M.D., Cooper, D.E., and Warner, J.J.P.: Review of Sports Medicine and Arthroscopy, p. 123. Philadelphia, WB Saunders, 1995; reprinted by permission.)

five phases of throwing include the following (Fig. 3–27).

PHASE	MAXIMUM STRESSES	COMMENTS
Wind-up	—	Upper extremity flexion
Early cocking	Rotator cuff, deltoid	Abduction, external rotation
Late cocking	Rotator cuff, deltoid, inferior capsule	Begins with foot contact
Acceleration	All structures	Minimum activity
Follow-through	Posterior capsule	Maximum activity

B. History and Physical Examination
   1. History—Age and chief complaint are two important considerations. Instability, acromioclavicular injuries, and distal clavicle osteolysis are more common in young patients. Rotator cuff tears, arthritis, and proximal humeral fractures are more common in older patients. Direct blows are usually responsible for acromioclavicular separations. Instability is related to injury to the abducted, externally rotated arm. Chronic overhead pain and night pain are associated with rotator cuff tears.
   2. Physical Examination—Observation and palpation can lead to important diagnostic clues.

FINDING	SIGNIFICANCE
Muscle wasting	Chronic rotator cuff tear, nerve injury
"Popeye" muscle	Proximal rupture of the biceps long head
Scapular winging	Serratus anterior (long thoracic nerve) injury
Superior prominence	Acromioclavicular separation/clavicle fracture
Anterior prominence	Glenohumeral dislocation, sternoclavicular injury
Systemic hyperlaxity	Multidirectional instability

Evaluation of range of motion (normally 160 degrees forward flexion, 30–60 degrees external rotation, and internal rotation T6) and strength testing are also important. Special testing includes the following examinations.

EXAMINATION	TECHNIQUE	SIGNIFICANCE
Impingement sign	Passive FF >90°	Pain = impingement syndrome
Impingement test	Same after subacromial lidocaine	Relief of pain = impingement syndrome
Hawkins test	Passive FF 90° and int. rotation	Pain = impingement syndrome
Apprehension test	Abd. 90° and ext. rotation	Apprehension = ant. shoulder instability
Relocation test (Fig. 3–28)	Supine apprehension with posterior force	Relief of apprehension = ant. shoulder instability
Posterior apprehension	Forward flexion 90°, internal rotation, posterior force	Apprehension = posterior instability
Sulcus sign	Downward traction on arm	Presence of sulcus below acromion = inferior laxity
Crossed chest adduction test	Passive FF 90° and adduction	Pain = acromioclavicular pathology
AC injection	Same after AC lidocaine injection	Relief of symptoms = acromioclavicular pathology
Bicipital tenderness	Localized tenderness	Bicipital tendinitis
Yergason test	Resisted supination	Pain = bicipital tendinitis
Speed test	Resisted forward elevation of arm	Pain = bicipital tendinitis
Lift-off sign	Arm behind back lifted posteriorly	Inability to accomplish = subscapularis rupture
Wright's test	Ext-Abd-ER arm, neck rotated away	Loss of pulse and reproduction of Sx = thoracic outlet syndrome
Spurling test (Fig. 3–29)	Lat. flexion, rotation and compression of neck	Cervical spine pathology

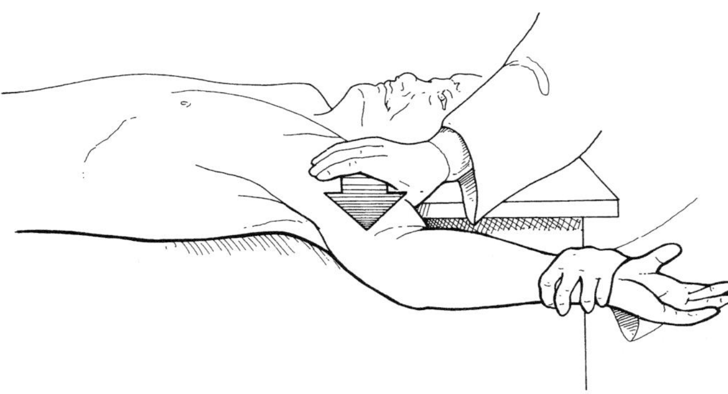

FIGURE 3–28. Relocation test. Anterior pressure on the proximal arm relocates the humerus and causes relief of apprehension. (From Miller, M.D., Cooper, D.E., and Warner, J.J.P.: Review of Sports Medicine and Arthroscopy. Philadelphia, WB Saunders, 1995; reprinted by permission.)

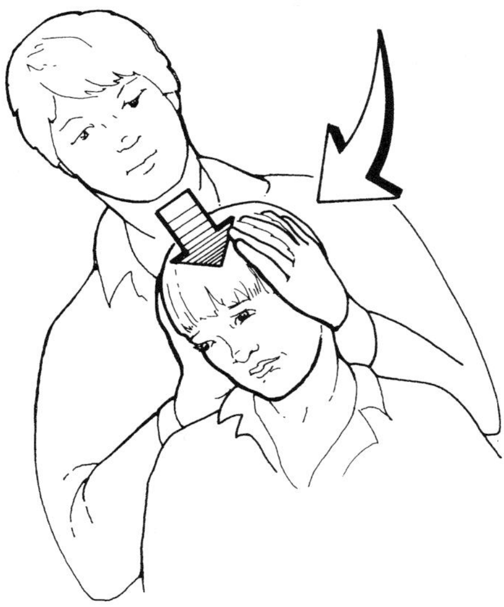

FIGURE 3–29. Spurling test. Lateral flexion and rotation with some compression may cause nerve root encroachment and pain on the ipsilateral side in patients with cervical nerve root impingement. (From Miller, M.D., Cooper, D.E., and Warner, J.J.P.: Review of Sports Medicine and Arthroscopy. Philadelphia, WB Saunders, 1995; reprinted by permission.)

C. Imaging the Shoulder—The trauma series of radiographs includes a "true" AP view (plate is placed parallel to the scapula, about 45 degrees from the plane of the thorax) and an axillary lateral view. Other views that are sometimes helpful include a scapular Y or transscapular view and AP radiographs in internal and external rotation. Special radiographic views have also been developed for certain other abnormalities.

D. Shoulder Arthroscopy
   1. Portals—Standard portals include the posterior portal (2 cm distal and medial to posterolateral border of acromion, used for the scope), anterior portals (lateral to the coracoid and below the biceps, used for instrumentation), lateral portal (for acromioplasty), and supraspinatus (Nevaiser) portal for anterior glenoid visualization (rarely used), as demonstrated in Fig. 3–31.

VIEW/SIGN	FINDINGS	SIGNIFICANCE
Supraspinatus outlet view (Fig. 3–30)	Acromial morphology (types I–III)	Type III (hooked) acromion associated with impingement
30° Caudal tilt view	Subacromial spurring	Area below level of clavicle = impingement area
Zanca 10° cephalic tilt	AC joint pathology	AC DJD, distal clavicle osteolysis
West Point	Anteroinferior glenoid evaluation	Bony Bankart lesion seen with instability
Garth view	Anteroinferior glenoid evaluation	Bony Bankart
Stryker notch	Humeral head evaluation	Hill-Sachs impression fracture with recurrent dislocation episodes
AP int. rot.	Humeral head evaluation	Hill-Sachs defect
Hobbs view	Sternoclavicular injury	Anteroposterior dislocations
Serendipity view	Sternoclavicular injury	Ant.-post. dislocation
45° Abduction true AP	Glenohumeral space	Subtle DJD
Arthrography	Rotator cuff injuries	Dye above cuff = tear
CT	Fractures	Classification easier
MRI ± arthro-MRI	Soft tissue evaluation	Labral, cuff, muscle tears

   2. Technique—Orderly evaluation of the biceps tendon, articular surfaces, rotator cuff, labrum, and glenohumeral ligaments should be accomplished. Subacromial bursoscopy can allow coracoacromial ligament resection, acromioplasty, and distal clavicle resection.

E. Shoulder Instability
   1. Diagnosis—The shoulder is the most commonly dislocated joint in the body. Anterior dislocations, by far the most common, are often classified based on the mechanism of injury. Diagnosis of instability is based upon history, physical examination, and imaging. *T*raumatic *U*nilateral dislocations with a *B*ankart lesion often require *S*urgery (*TUBS*) because they typically occur in young patients and have recurrence rates of up to 70–80% with nonoperative management. *A*traumatic *m*ultidirectional *b*ilateral shoulder dislocation/subluxation often responds to *r*ehabilitation, and sometimes an *i*nferior capsular shift is required (*AMBRI*).
   2. Treatment—Nonoperative management of anterior shoulder instability includes immobilization for 2–4 weeks based on the age of the patient (longer for young patients) followed by an aggressive rotator cuff strengthening program. Many procedures have been developed for recurrent instability, including the following.

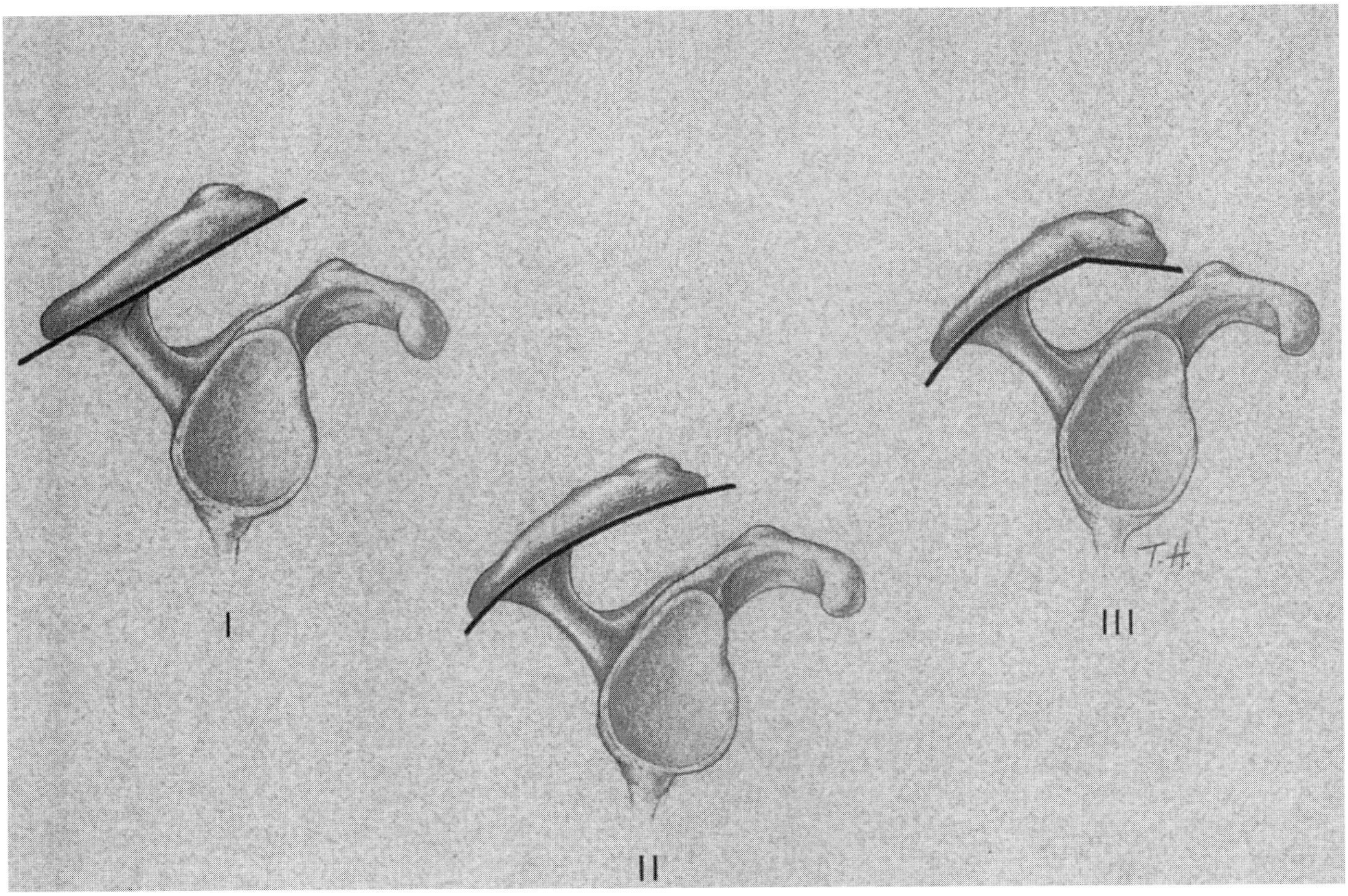

FIGURE 3–30. Acromion morphology is classified on the basis of the supraspinatus outlet view, as originally described by Bigliani. (From Esch, J.C.: Shoulder arthroscopy in the older age group. Op. Tech. Orthop. 1:200, 1991; reprinted by permission.)

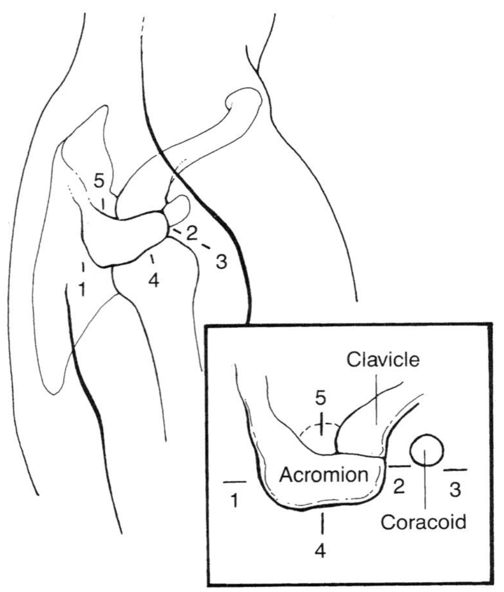

FIGURE 3–31. Arthroscopic portals of the shoulder. 1, posterior; 2, anterosuperior; 3, anteroinferior; 4, lateral; 5, supraspinatus (Neviaser) portal. (From Miller, M.D., Cooper, D.E., and Warner, J.J.P.: Review of Sports Medicine and Arthroscopy. Philadelphia, WB Saunders, 1995; reprinted by permission.)

PROCEDURE	ESSENTIAL FEATURES	COMPLICATIONS
Bankart	Reattachment of labrum (and IGHLC) to glenoid	"Gold standard"
Staple capsulorraphy	Capsular reattachment and tightening	Staple migration/ articular injury
Putti-Platt	Subscapularis advancement capsular coverage	Decreased external rotation
Magnuson-Stack	Subscapularis transfer to greater tuberosity	Decreased external rotation
Boyd-Sisk	Transfer of biceps laterally and posteriorly	Nonanatomic, recurrence
Bristow	Coracoid transfer to inferior glenoid	Nonunion, migration, recurrence
Bone block osteotomy	Anterior bone block	Nonunion, migration, articular injury
Capsular shift	Inferior capsule shifted superiorly—"pants over vest"	Overtightening, "gold standard" for multidirectional instability

In addition to these "open" procedures, several techniques for arthroscopic treatment of anterior instability have been developed. These procedures specifically address the Bankart lesion and not the capsule, and they are therefore not indicated for patients with multidirectional instability or multiple recurrences (with capsular stretching). The two most popular of these methods are transglenoid suture techniques (Caspari, Morgan, Maki) and staple (Johnson) or absorbable tack (Warren) fixation. Although the role for arthroscopic treatment of shoulder instability is still unclear, it is perhaps most efficacious for young patients who do not participate in contact sports with first (or second) time traumatic dislocations, without systemic laxity.

3. Posterior Shoulder Instability—Much less common and less amenable to surgical correction. Nonoperative treatment should emphasize external rotator and posterior deltoid strengthening. Surgical management is difficult because the posterior capsule is often very thin; however, posterior capsular shift procedures can be helpful in refractory cases.

F. Impingement Syndrome/Rotator Cuff Disease

1. Diagnosis—Although traditionally considered a disease of the older population, rotator cuff impingement and tears are becoming increasingly common in throwing athletes because of repetitive overuse. Neer identified three stages of subacromial impingement (Table 3–2). Patients typically present with pain during overhead activities and have characteristic physical examination findings and radiographs (see above).
2. Treatment—Nonoperative treatment includes activity modification, modalities such as ultrasound and ionophoresis, subacromial corticosteroid injection, and rotator cuff strengthening. Surgical treatment includes subacromial decompression (removal of the coracoacromial ligament and subacromial spur) and rotator cuff repair (into a bony trough at the greater tuberosity) if necessary. Arthroscopic subacromial decompression can be as successful as open decompression when correctly performed. Arthroscopically assisted rotator cuff repair can also be successful for small, easily mobilized tears.
3. Rotator Cuff Arthropathy—This condition is associated with glenohumeral joint degeneration in conjunction with a massive chronic tear of the cuff. Hemiarthroplasty with a large head may be helpful if the anterior deltoid is preserved.
4. Subcoracoid Impingement—This unusual condition is associated with a laterally placed coracoid that can impinge on the proximal humerus with forward flexion and internal rotation. CT with the arm in the provocative position and relief with local anesthetic injection in the area can reveal the diagnosis. Treatment may include resection of the lateral aspect of the coracoid process.

G. Biceps Tendon Injuries

1. Biceps Tendinitis—Often associated with impingement syndrome, it can also exist as an isolated entity. Tenderness along the bicipital groove, the Speed and Yergason sign (see above), can help confirm the diagnosis. Treatment of associated impingement syndrome often relieves symptoms. Rarely, tenodesis of the biceps tendon into the proximal humerus using a "keyhole" technique can be helpful in chronic injuries or tears.
2. Biceps Tendon Subluxation—Often associated with a subscapularis tear, this condition is associated with instability and medial displacement of the tendon out of its groove. Occasionally the tendon must be relocated into a deepened groove and stabilized operatively.
3. Superior Labral Lesions—*S*uperior *l*abral *a*ntero*p*osterior (SLAP) lesions have been classified into four varieties (Fig. 3–32).

TYPE	DESCRIPTION	TREATMENT
I	Biceps fraying, intact anchor on superior labrum	Arthroscopic débridement
II	Detachment of biceps anchor	Reattachment/stabilization

TABLE 3–2. STAGES OF SUBACROMIAL IMPINGEMENT SYNDROME

STAGE	AGE (years)	PATHOLOGY	CLINICAL COURSE	TREATMENT
I	<25	Edema and hemorrhage	Reversible	Conservative
II	25–40	Fibrosis and tendinitis	Activity-related pain	Therapy/operative
III	>40	AC spur and cuff tear	Progressive disability	Acromioplasty/repair

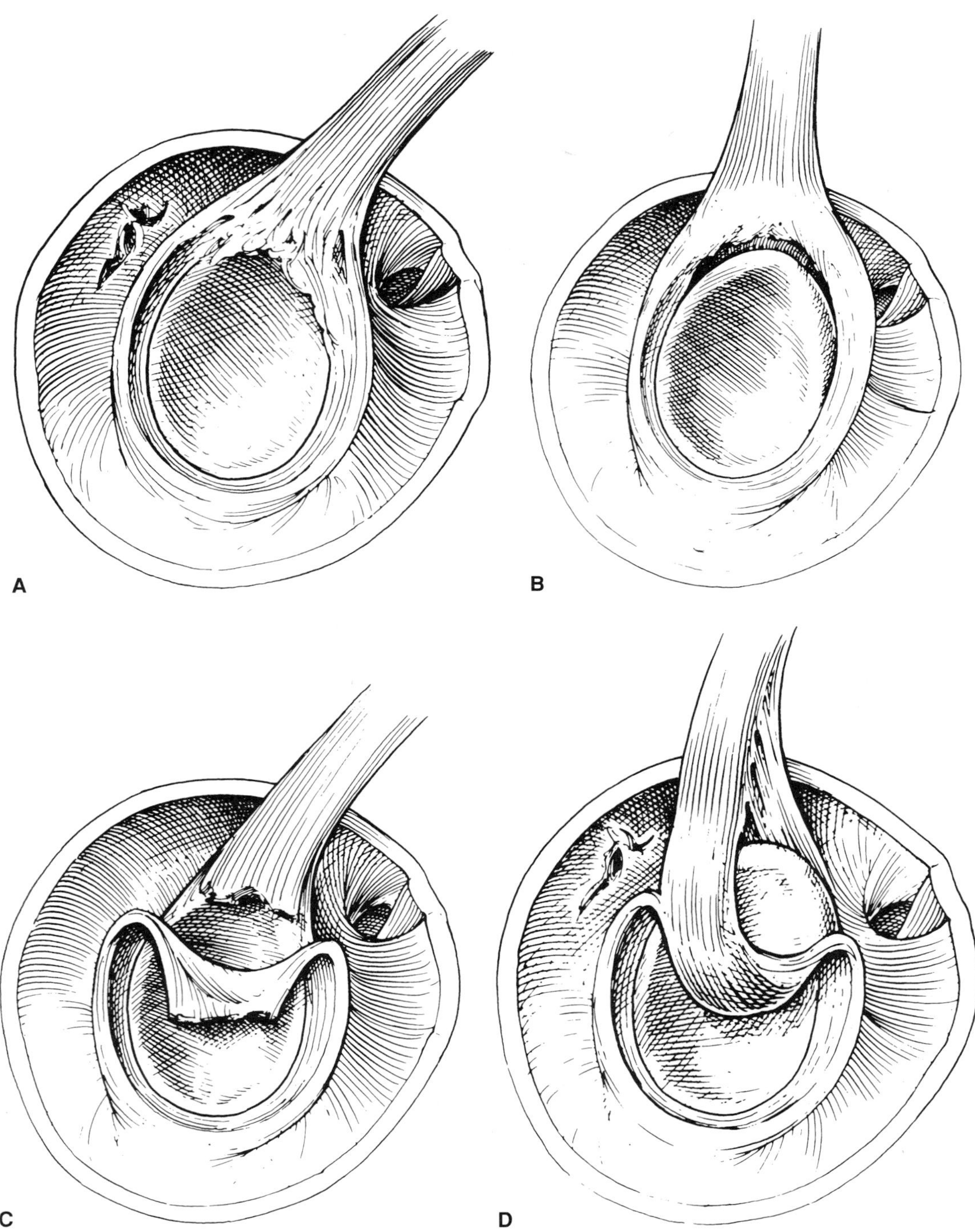

FIGURE 3–32. Superior labral anterior to posterior (SLAP) classification. *A,* Type I—superior labral fraying. *B,* Type II—detachment of the biceps anchor. *C,* Type III—superior lateral bucket-handle tear, biceps anchor intact. *D,* Type IV—superior labral bucket handle-tear involving biceps tendon. (From Snyder, S.J., and Wuh, H.C.K.: Arthroscopic evaluation and treatment of the rotator cuff superior labrum anterior posterior lesion. Op. Tech. Orthop. 1:218–219, 1991; reprinted by permission.)

TYPE	DESCRIPTION	TREATMENT
III	Bucket-Handle superior labral tear; biceps intact	Arthroscopic débridement
IV	Bucket-Handle tear of superior labrum into biceps	Repair or tenodesis of tendon based on symptoms and condition of remaining tendon

Complex tears (type V) represent some combination of tears described above and are treated on an individual basis.

H. Acromioclavicular and Sternoclavicular Injuries

1. Acromioclavicular Separation—This common athletic injury results from a direct fall onto the shoulder. Acromioclavicular separations are classified as shown in Fig. 3–33. Treatment of type III injuries is controversial, but most surgeons currently favor nonoperative management. Types IV–VI injuries should be reduced and stabilized

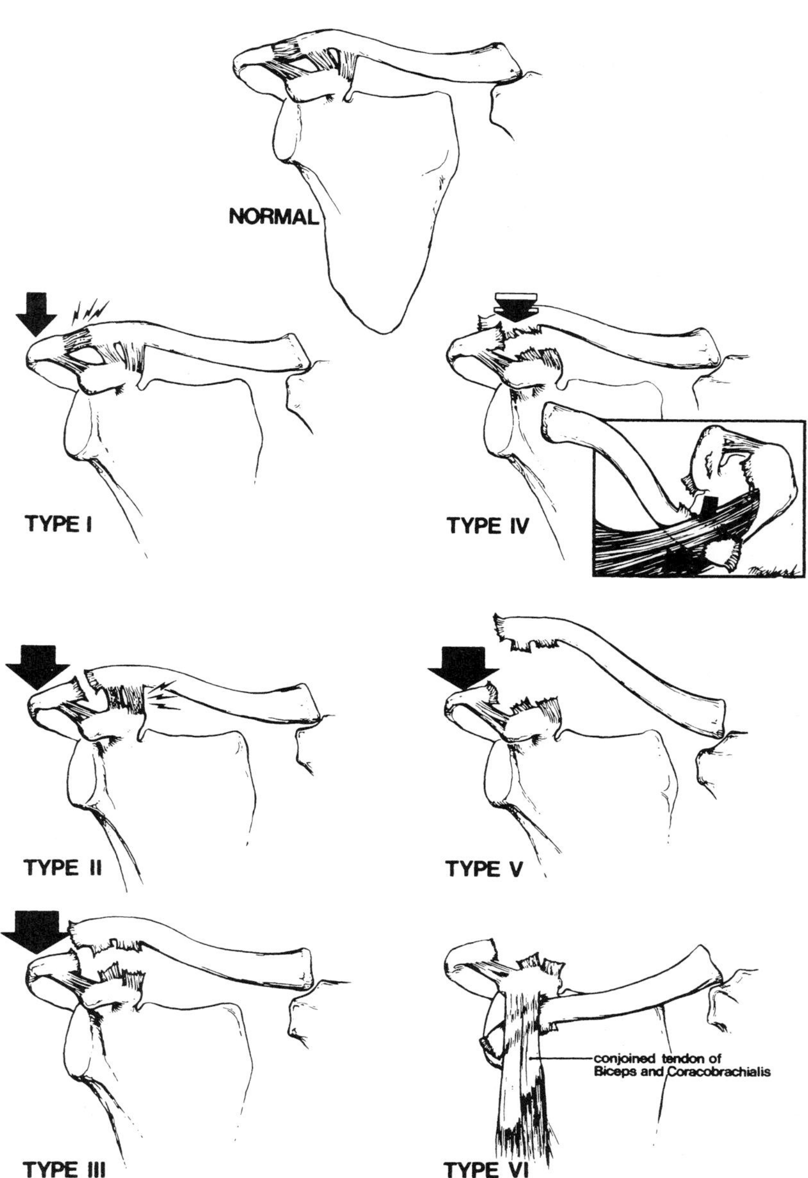

FIGURE 3–33. Classification of acromioclavicular. Type I injuries involve only an acromioclavicular (AC) sprain. Type II injuries are characterized by complete AC tear but intact coracoclavicular (CC) ligaments. Type II injuries involve both the AC and CC ligaments with a coracoclavicular distance of 125–200% of the opposite shoulder. Type IV injuries are associated with posterior displacement of the clavicle into the trapezius muscle. Type V injuries involve superior displacement with a coracoclaviclar distance of more than twice the opposite side. This injury is usually associated with rupture of the deltotrapezial fascia, leaving the distal end of the clavicle subcutaneous. Type VI injuries are rare and are defined based on inferior displacement of the clavicle below the coracoid. (From Rockwood, C.A., Jr., and Young, D.C.: Disorders of the acromioclavicular joint. In The Shoulder, p. 423. Rockwood, C.A., Jr., and Matsen, F.A., III, eds. Philadelphia, WB Saunders, 1990; reprinted by permission.)

with some form of temporary coracoclavicular fixation. Chronic injuries may require transfer of the coracoacromial ligament into the resected end of the distal clavicle (modified Weaver-Dunn procedure).

2. Distal Clavicle Osteolysis—Common in weightlifters, this condition is associated with osteopenia and cystic changes to the distal clavicle. It often responds to activity modification but occasionally requires distal clavicle resection.
3. Acromioclavicular Degenerative Joint Disease —May be present in conjunction with impingement syndrome. Localized tenderness, pain with crossed chest adduction, and joint narrowing and osteophytes on radiographs lead to the diagnosis. Treatment may include open or arthroscopic distal clavicle resection (Mumford procedure).
4. Sternoclavicular (SC) Subluxation/Dislocation —Often caused by motor vehicle accidents or direct trauma, SC injuries can be best diagnosed by CT. Closed reduction is often successful. Hardware should be avoided.

I. Muscle Ruptures

1. Pectoralis Major—Injury to this muscle is caused by excessive tension on a maximally eccentrically contracted muscle, often in weight lifters. Localized swelling and ecchymosis, a palpable defect, and weakness with adduction and internal rotation are characteristic. Surgical repair to bone is usually necessary.
2. Deltoid—Complete rupture of this muscle is unusual, and injuries are most often strains or partial tears. Repair to bone is required for complete injury.
3. Triceps—Most often associated with systemic illness or steroid use. Primary repair of avulsions is indicated.
4. Subscapularis—Can occur with anterior dislocations or following anterior shoulder surgery. Increased external rotation and a "lift-off sign" may be present. Surgical reattachment is indicated.

J. Calcifying Tendinitis and Adhesive Capsulitis

1. Calcifying Tendinitis—Usually involves the supraspinatus tendon and may be associated with tendon degeneration. Radiographs demonstrate characteristic calcification within the tendon. Physical therapy, modalities such as ultrasound and ionophoresis, and aspiration are usually successful. Operative treatment (removal of the deposit) is occasionally necessary.
2. Adhesive Capsulitis—Also known (inaccurately) as "frozen shoulder," this disorder is characterized by pain and restricted glenohumeral motion. Arthrography may demonstrate a loss of the normal axillary recess. Three clinical stages and four arthroscopic stages have been defined.

STAGE	CHARACTERISTICS
Clinical:	
Painful	Gradual onset of diffuse pain
Stiff	Decreased ROM; affects activities of daily living
Thawing	Gradual return of motion
Arthroscopic:	
1	Patchy fibrinous synovitis
2	Capsular contraction, fibrinous adhesions, synovitis
3	Increased contraction, resolving synovitis
4	Severe contraction

Treatment includes nonsteroidal antiinflammatory drugs (NSAIDs), passive motion, and occasionally manipulation under anesthesia. The role of arthroscopy in the treatment of adhesive capsulits is not yet established.

K. Nerve Disorders

1. Brachial Plexus Injury—Minor traction or compression injuries, commonly known by football players as "burners" or "stingers," can be serious if they are recurrent or persist for more than a short time. More significant injuries, such as root avulsions, can be devastating.
2. Thoracic Outlet Syndrome—Compression of the nerves and vessels that pass through the scalene muscles and first rib can result in this disorder. Patients may note pain and ulnar paresthesias. The Wright test, described previously, and neurological evaluation can be diagnostic. First-rib resection is occasionally required.
3. Long Thoracic Nerve Palsy—Injury to this nerve can result in scapular winging secondary to serratus anterior dysfunction. Bracing and rarely pectoralis major transfer are required.
4. Suprascapular Nerve Compression—Ganglia and other lesions can compress the suprascapular nerve resulting in weakness and atrophy of the supraspinatus and infraspinatus muscles. Neurologic studies and MRI can demonstrate nerve impingement, which usually responds to surgical release.

L. Other Shoulder Disorders

1. Glenohumeral Degenerative Joint Disease—Overuse injuries, aberrant hardware, and other conditions can result in arthritis of this joint. Arthroscopic débridement may have a role in the early stages of this disease, but occasionally arthroplasty is required. Progressive pain, decreased ROM, and inability to perform activities of daily living are reasonable indications for considering prosthetic replacement. Hemiarthroplasty is preferred to total shoulder arthroplasty unless the glenoid is significantly affected because of the problems with glenoid component loosening. The humeral component should be placed in 30–40 degrees of retroversion in most cases. Less retroversion is recommended for prosthetic replacement in fractures. Neutral rotation is favored in patients with posterior fracture-dislocations. Fusion is rarely indicated, but the position should be 20–30 degrees flexion, 40 degrees abduction, and 25–45 degrees internal rotation.
2. Snapping Scapula—This unusual disorder can be caused by irregularities of the medial scapula or the scapulothoracic bursa. Physical therapy, local injections, and other nonoperative treatment options are usually successful. Occasionally, resection of the medial border of the scapula is necessary.
3. Reflex Sympathetic Dystrophy—Much as in the knee, this disorder can be a difficult problem. Stellate ganglion blocks may be helpful in the management of this condition.

IV. Other Upper Extremity Sports Medicine Problems

A. Tendon Injuries

1. Lateral Epicondylitis (Tennis Elbow)—Degeneration at the extensor muscle group origin, principally in the extensor carpi radialis brevis, can be

a result of overuse injuries or poor technique in racket sports. Localized tenderness, exacerbated by resisted wrist extension is common. Therapy that includes stretching, strengthening, ultrasound, and electrical stimulation can be helpful for this condition. Orthotics that are designed to decentralize the area of stress (tennis elbow strap) are also useful. Equipment modifications (more flexible racket, larger head, larger grip) may also be efficacious. Surgical options include release of the common extensor origin and/or débridement of the pathologic tissue (Fig. 3–34).

2. Medial Epicondylitis (Golfer's Elbow)—This condition is less common and more difficult to treat than lateral epicondylitis. The affected area is at the pronator teres–flexor carpi radialis interface. Treatment is similar to that for lateral epicondylitis.
3. Distal Biceps Tendon Avulsion—Acute onset of pain in the antecubital fossa following a sudden force overload with the elbow partially flexed is common. Reattachment of the tendon with a two-incision (Boyd-Anderson) technique is favored.
4. Distal Triceps Tendon Avulsion—Sudden loss of elbow extension and a palpable defect is the classic history. Early repair is favored for this rare injury.
5. De Quervain Disease—Stenosing tenosynovitis of the first dorsal compartment of the wrist can occur with racket sports and in golfers. This site of tendinitis is only one of many in the wrist (Fig. 3–35). The Finkelstein test (ulnar deviation of the wrist with the thumb in the palm) is diagnostic. Treatment includes activity modification, local injection, and occasionally surgical release.
6. Flexor Carpi Radialis/Ulnaris Tendinitis—Associated with overuse, this condition usually responds to anti-inflammatory agents, rest, and rarely tenolysis.
7. Extensor Carpi Ulnaris—Tendinitis and even subluxation of this tendon can be treated with immobilization with the wrist in pronation. Occasionally, it is necessary to débride or stabilize the tendon in the sixth dorsal compartment.
8. Intersection Syndrome—Irritation and inflammation at the crossing point of the tendons of the first dorsal compartment (APL and EPB) and the second dorsal compartment (ECRL and ECRB) can cause pain and crepitus ("squeakers"). Splinting, local injections, and decompression may be indicated.
9. Other Extensor Tendon Tendinitis—Includes the EPL, EDQ, and EIP. Usually responds to local measures and rarely surgical release.
10. FDP Avulsion Injuries—Commonly known by the appropriate term "Jersey finger," these injuries require operative repair.
11. Mallet/Baseball Finger—Avulsion of the terminal extensor tendon in the finger usually can be treated with extension splinting of the DIP joint for 6+ weeks.

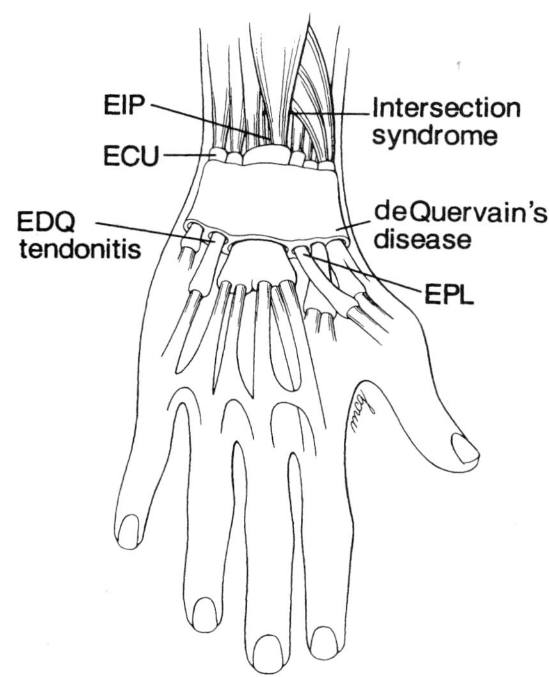

FIGURE 3–35. Location of common sites of tendinitis about the wrist. EIP, extensor indicis proprius; ECU, extensor carpi ulnaris; EDQ, extensor digiti quinti; EPL, extensor pollicus longus. (From Kiefhaber, T.R., and Stern, P.J.: Upper extremity tendinitis and overuse syndromes in the athlete. Clin. Sports Med. 11:43, 1992; reprinted by permission.)

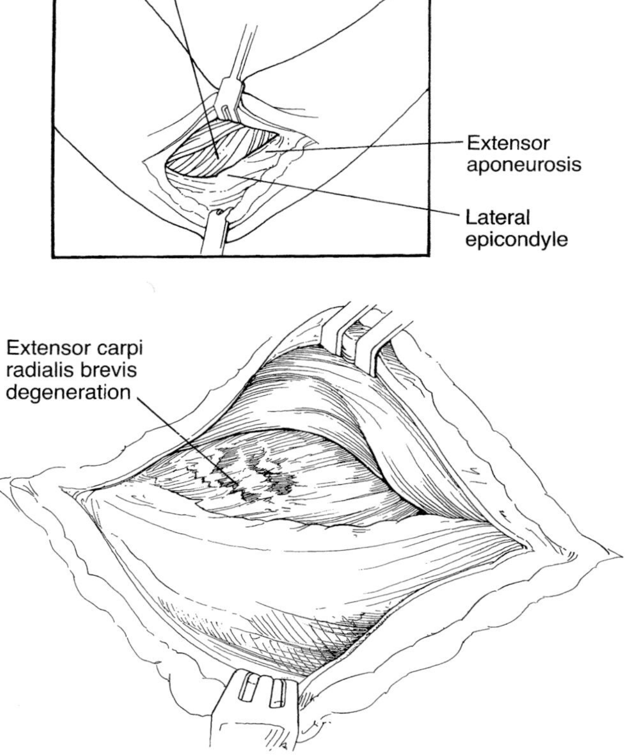

FIGURE 3–34. Operative exposure for lateral epicondylitis. (From Miller, M.D., Cooper, D.E., and Warner, J.J.P.: Review of Sports Medicine and Arthroscopy. p. 178. Philadelphia, WB Saunders, 1995; reprinted by permission.)

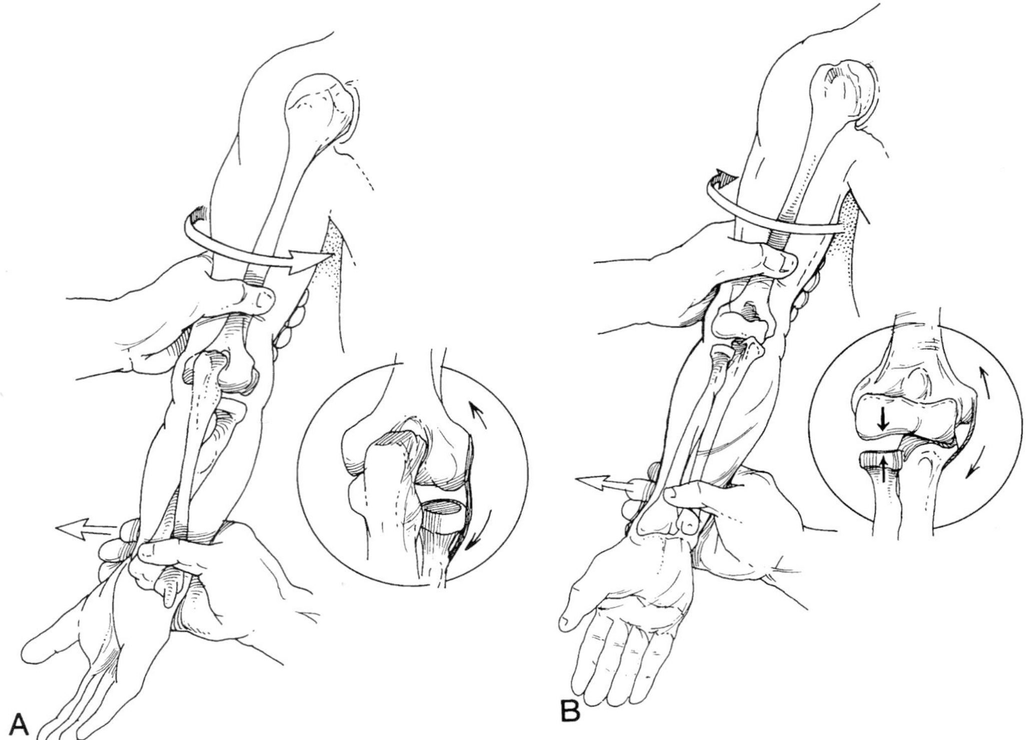

FIGURE 3–36. Varus *(A)* and valgus *(B)* instability testing of the elbow. Note the position and rotation of the arm. (From Morrey, B.F.: The Elbow and Its Disorders, 2nd ed., p. 83. Philadelphia, WB Saunders, 1994; reprinted by permission.)

B. Ligamentous Injuries
  1. Ulnar (Medial) Collateral Ligament of the Elbow—Injury to this ligament is usually the result of a valgus stress. The all-important anterior band of this ligament is commonly involved, especially in baseball pitchers. The diagnosis is based on clinical examination findings (Fig. 3–36) and sometimes MRI. Reconstruction using a palmaris longus tendon graft (Fig. 3–37) is occasionally required for chronic injuries. Repair of acute injuries is usually less successful.
  2. Lateral Collateral Ligament Injuries of the Elbow—This injury has only recently been characterized. Patients may complain of recurrent clicking or locking while extending the elbow. Clinically, posterolateral rotatory subluxation can be demonstrated by the lateral pivot shift test of the elbow (Fig. 3–38). The test is considered positive if the patient experiences apprehension. Reconstruction of the lateral ulnar collateral ligament is sometimes necessary for recurrent subluxation.
  3. Wrist Ligament Instabilities—Include scapholunate instability (DISI deformity), triquetrohamate instability (DISI or VISI deformity), and triquetrolunate instability (VISI deformity). (Fig. 3–39). The Watson test (radial deviation of the hand with volar pressure on the scaphoid) may reproduce pain or a clunk in patients with scapholunate instability. Radiographs may demonstrate an increased scapholunate interval as well. The ballotment test (palmar and dorsal displacement of the triquetrum with lunate stabilization using the opposite hand) can produce pain in patients with triquetrolunate instability. Limited arthrodesis is often required for treatment of chronic wrist instabilities.
  4. Ligament Injuries in the Hand—Includes collateral ligament injuries (treated with buddy taping) and volar plate injuries (associated with dorsal dislocations), among others. Injury to the ulnar collateral ligament of the thumb is commonly referred to as gamekeeper's, or skier's, thumb. Treatment of the incomplete injury is immobilization. Complete injuries (>15 degrees side–side difference or opening >45 degrees) require operative intervention because of interposition of the adductor aponeurosis between the two torn ends of the ulnar collateral ligament (Fig. 3–40).

C. Articular Injuries
  1. Medial Epicondyle Injuries—Stress fractures of the medial epicondyle are common in adolescents with repetitive valgus forces in throwing, **Little Leaguer's elbow.** Rest and activity modification can help reduce the incidence of a complete fracture.
  2. Osteochondritis Dissecans—Related to vascular insufficiency and repetitive microtrauma, this condition usually affects the capitellum but can also involve the radial head. If the fragment is stable, this condition can be treated with activity modification and supportive methods. Arthroscopy may be indicated for separated fragments. Osteochondrosis of the capitellum (Panner's disease) is seen in young children and is associated with a more benign course.

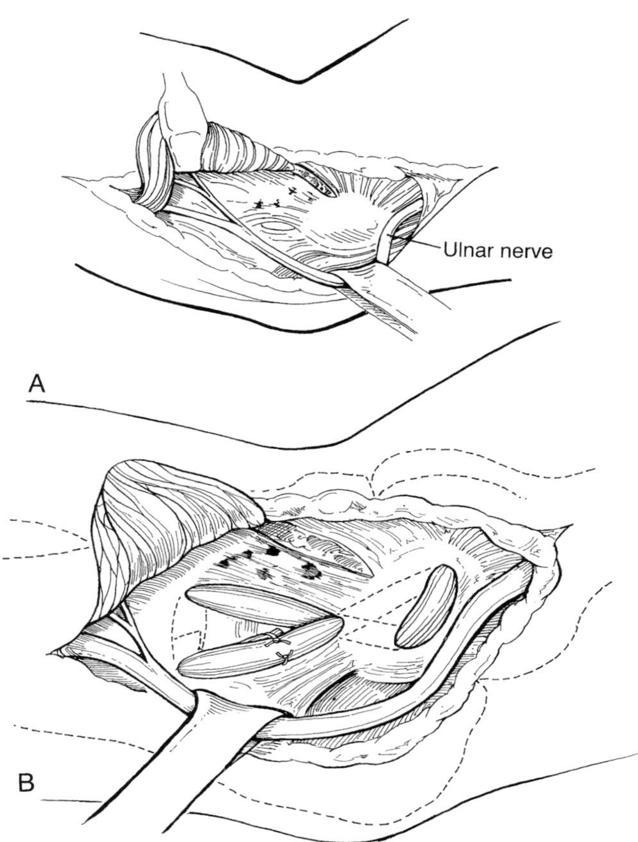

FIGURE 3–37. Reconstruction of the (medial) ulnar collateral ligament. (From Miller, M.D., Cooper, D.E., and Warner, J.J.P.: Review of Sports Medicine and Arthroscopy, p. 179. Philadelphia, WB Saunders, 1995; reprinted by permission.)

3. Osteoarthritis of the Elbow—This condition, common in football lineman, throwers, and athletes who participate in racket sports, is associated with pain at the endpoint of forced extension or flexion. Arthroscopic débridement, open decompression, distraction arthroplasty, and other procedures may be indicated for advanced cases. The ulnohumeral (Outerbridge-Kashiwagi) arthroplasty may allow decompression with minimal morbidity (Fig. 3–41).
4. Wrist Triangular Fibrocartilage Complex (TFCC) Injuries—Common cause of ulnar wrist pain; tears in this complex can be diagnosed based on arthrography or MRI. Treatment includes débridement or suture repair (Table 3–3).
5. Posttraumatic Problems of the Wrist—Kienböck's disease is avascular necrosis and collapse of the lunate, probably related to overuse and ulnar negative wrist variance. Ulnar lengthening or radial

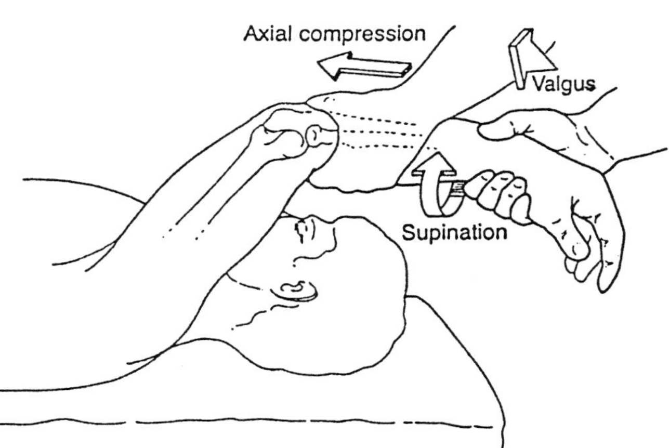

FIGURE 3–38. Lateral pivot shift test of the elbow for posterolateral rotatory instability. (Redrawn from O'Driscoll, S.W., Bell, D.F., and Morrey, B.F.: Posterolateral instability of the elbow. J. Bone Joint Surg. [Am.] 73:440–446, 1991.)

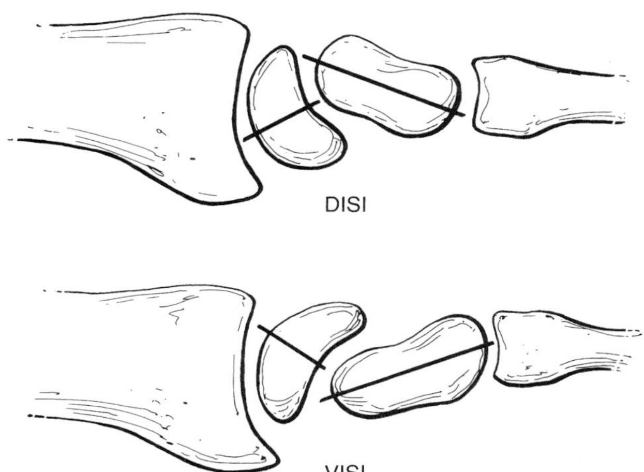

FIGURE 3–39. Scapholunate instability is associated with a dorsal intercalated instability (DISI) pattern. Triquetrolunate instability may have a volar intercalated instability (VISI) pattern. Note the increased scapholunate angle (>60 degrees) with the DISI pattern (normal 30 degrees) (From McCue, F.C., and Bruce, J.F.: The wrist. In Orthopaedic Sports Medicine, DeLee, J.C., and Drez, D., Jr., eds., p. 918. Philadelphia, WB Saunders, 1994; reprinted by permission.)

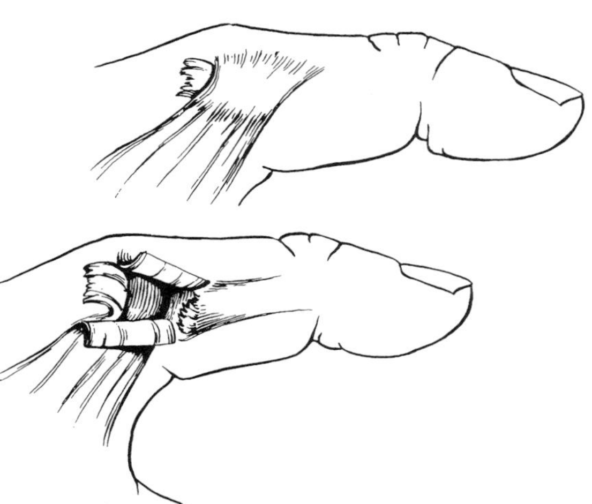

FIGURE 3–40. Stener lesion. The adductor aponeurosis separates the two ends of the ulnar collateral ligament, and it must be incised to repair the ligament. (From Green, D.P., and Strickland, J.W.: The hand. In Orthopaedic Sports Medicine, DeLee, J.C., and Drez, D., Jr., eds., p. 976. Philadelphia, WB Saunders, 1994; reprinted by permission.)

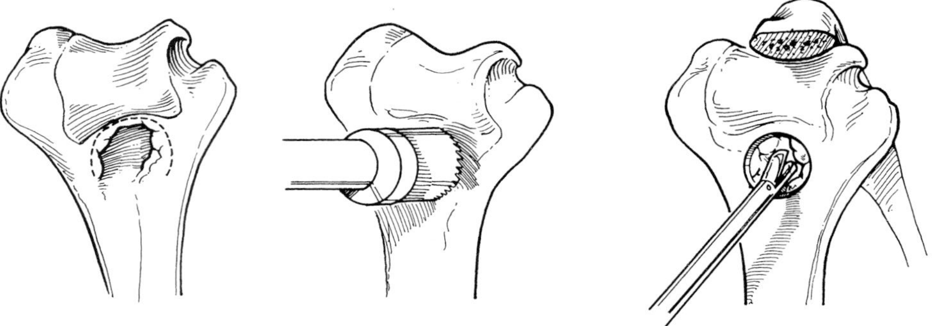

FIGURE 3–41. Outerbridge-Kashiwagi arthroplasty, performed through a triceps-splitting approach. The coranoid is approached through a Cloward drill hole in the olecranon fossa. The olecranon can also be débrided through this approach. (From Miller, M.D., Cooper, D.E., and Warner, J.J.P.: Review of Sports Medicine and Arthroscopy, p. 180. Philadelphia, WB Saunders, 1995; reprinted by permission.)

shortening is helpful early, but limited wrist fusions may be necessary for later stages. Osteochondrosis of the capitate can occur in gymnasts and may respond to débridement or limited fusions. Scaphoid avascular necrosis is relatively common owing to its tenuous blood supply. Bone grafting with internal fixation is usually curative. Unrecognized scapholunate injuries can lead to the development of collapse (SLAC wrist), which may require limited, or even total, wrist fusions.

D. Arthroscopy

1. Elbow Arthroscopy—Especially helpful for removing loose bodies, débridement, and synovectomy. Most surgeons prefer supine positioning with a wrist-holder and traction. Common portals include the anterolateral portal (1 cm distal and 1 cm anterior to the lateral epicondyle), the anteromedial portal (2 cm distal and 2 cm distal to the medial epicondyle), and the posterolateral portal (2 cm proximal to the olecranon, just lateral to the triceps) (Fig. 3–42). The "nick and spread" method is helpful for minimizing neurovascular risks.
2. Wrist Arthroscopy—Indications now include TFCC débridement, treatment of certain ligamentous injuries, management of ulnar abutment syndrome, and assessing reduction of certain intra-articular fractures. A 2.5- or 3.0-mm arthroscope is commonly used, and the patient is supine with a traction apparatus. Three radiocarpal portals and three midcarpal portals are commonly used. Portals are named in relation to the dorsal compartments of the wrist (Fig. 3–43). The 3–4 radiocarpal portal (located between the EPL and EDC tendons) is usually established first. The 4–5 radiocarpal portal (positioned between the EDC and

TABLE 3–3. CLASSIFICATION OF INJURIES OF THE TFCC

	CLASS DESCRIPTION	TREATMENT
	TRAUMATIC LESIONS (TYPE I)	
1A	Horizontal tear adjacent to sigmoid notch*	Débridement
1B	Avulsion from ulna +/− ulnar styloid fracture	Suture repair
1C	Avulsion from carpus; exposes pisiform	Débridement
1D	Avulsion from sigmoid notch	Débridement
	DEGENERATIVE LESIONS (TYPE 2)	
2A	Thinning of TFCC without perforation†	
2B	Thinning of disc with chondromalacia	
2C	Perforation of disc with chondromalacia	
2D	Perforation of disc, chondromalacia, partial tear of lunotriquetral ligament	
2E	Perforation of disc, chondromalacia, complete tear of lunotriquetral ligament, ulnocarpal degenerative joint disease	

* Most common.
† Treatment for degenerative lesions includes débridement of loose degenerated discs, intra-articular resection of the ulnar head, and débridement of lunotriquetral ligament tears with percutaneous pinning of the lunotriquetral joint based on the pathology present. From Miller M.D., Cooper D.E., and Warner J.J.P. et al.; Review of Sports Medicine and Arthroscopy, p. 188. Philadelphia, WB Saunders, 1995; reprinted by permission.

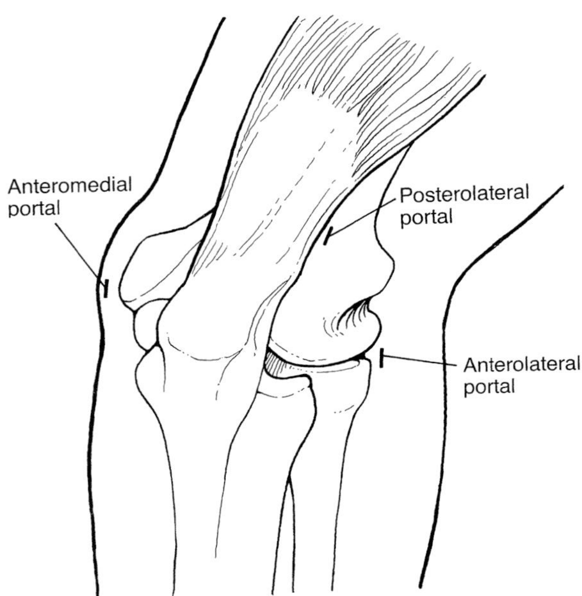

FIGURE 3–42. Portals for elbow arthroscopy. (From Miller, M.D., Cooper, D.E., and Warner, J.J.P.: Review of Sports Medicine and Arthroscopy, p. 174. Philadelphia, WB Saunders, 1995; reprinted by permission.)

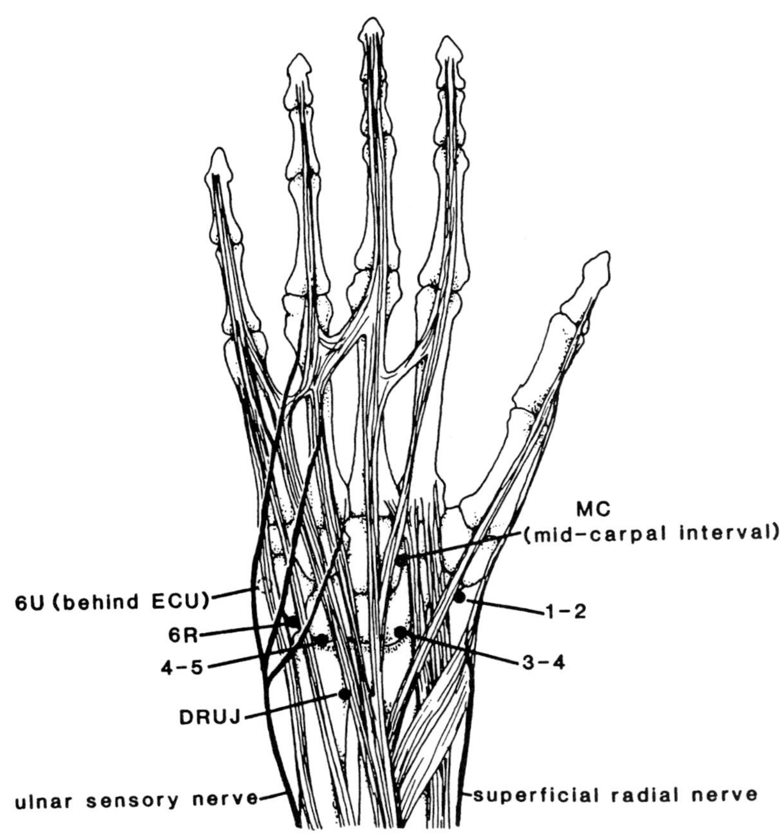

FIGURE 3–43. Portals for wrist arthroscopy. U, ulnar; R, radial; ECU, extensor carpi ulnaris; DRUJ, distal radioulnar joint; MC, midcarpal. (From Miller, M.D., Cooper, D.E., and Warner, J.J.P.: Review of Sports Medicine and Arthroscopy, p. 186. Philadelphia, WB Saunders, 1995; reprinted by permission.)

EDM tendons) is commonly used for instrumentation. The 6R portal (placed just radial to the ECU tendon) can be used for visualization or instrumentation. The midcarpal portals include the midcarpal radial (MCR) portal, the midcarpal ulnar (MCU) portal, and the scaphotrapezial–trapezoid portal. These portals are used only for pathology involving the midcarpal joints.

V. Head and Spine Injuries

A. Head Injuries

1. Diffuse Brain Injuries—Includes mild and "classic" cerebral concussion and diffuse axonal injury. Mild concussions occur without loss of consciousness and can be subdivided into three grades as follows (where RTP represents "return to play").

GRADE	SYMPTOMS	DURATION	RECOMMENDED RTP
1	Confusion, no amnesia	Minutes	When symptoms resolve
2	Retrograde amnesia	Hours to days	1 Week
3	Amnesia after impact	Days	1 Month

Postconcussion syndrome, characterized by persistent headaches, irritability, confusion, and difficulty concentrating, can occur with grade 2 and 3 mild concussions. "Classic" concussion includes a period of loss of consciousness. If it lasts >5 minutes, head CT should be obtained. Delay in return to play should be 1 week to 1 month after the first episode and for the entire season for a second episode. Diffuse axonal injury occurs with loss of consciousness lasting >6 hours, and athletes who suffer this injury should consider total avoidance of future contact sports.

2. Focal Brain Syndromes—Include contusions, intracranial hematomas, epidural hematomas, and subdural hematomas. CT scanning is helpful for distinguishing these entities (Fig. 3–44). Although epidural hematomas classically are said to be characterized by a period of lucidity followed by loss of consciousness, this sequence may not occur. Surgical treatment of intracranial hematomas may be indicated.

B. Cervical Spine Injuries—Catastrophic injury to the cervical spine is unfortunately an all too common event in contact sports. Underlying cervical stenosis, or narrowing of the AP diameter of the spine, can make these injuries worse (Fig. 3–45). Recommendations for return to play for athletes with cervical stenosis with transient symptoms are controversial. Football players who repeatedly use poor tackling techniques can develop a condition known as **spear tackler's spine,** which includes cervical stenosis, loss of lordosis, and other radiographic abnormalities. Return to contact sports should be avoided.

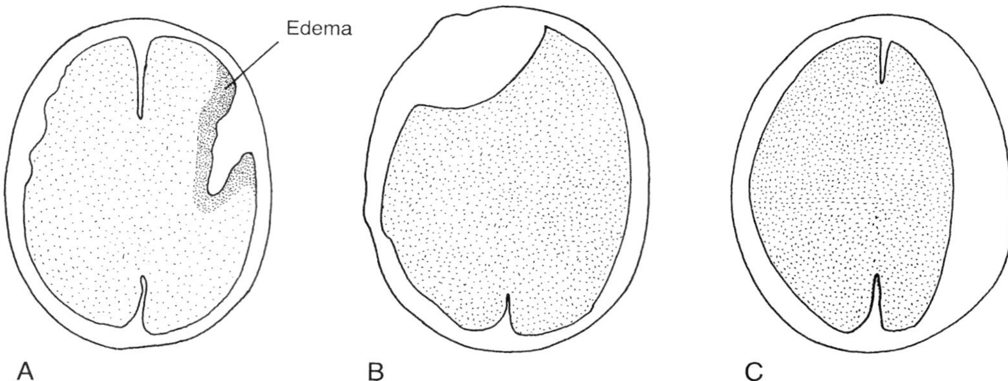

FIGURE 3–44. CT findings. *A*, Contusion includes a hemorrhagic area and surroundings edema. *B*, Epidural hematomas typically have a biconvex appearance. *C*, Subdural hematomas have a concave or crescentric appearance. (From Miller, M.D., Cooper, D.E., and Warner, J.J.P.: Review of Sports Medicine and Arthroscopy, p. 204. Philadelphia, WB Saunders, 1995; reprinted by permission.)

C. Thoracic and Lumbar Spine Injuries—Injuries commonly associated with sports include muscle injury, fractures, disc disease, and spondylolysis/spondylolisthesis. The latter condition is common in football interior lineman and gymnasts. Oblique radiographs, bone scan, and CT are all helpful for establishing the diagnosis. Treatment includes activity modification, bracing, and fusion for high grade slips.

VI. Medical Aspects of Sports Medicine

A. Ergogenic Drugs

1. Anabolic Steroids—Derivatives of testosterone are abused by athletes attempting to increase muscle mass and strength. Adverse effects include liver dysfunction, hypercholesterolemia, cardiomyopathy, testicular atrophy, gynecomastia, and alopecia.
2. Human Growth Hormone—Made from recombinant DNA; illegal use of this drug is common. Athletes attempting to increase muscle size and weight abuse this drug, which has similar side effects similar to those of steroids, as well as hypertension and gigantism.
3. Other commonly abused drugs include amphetamines, blood doping, diuretics, and laxatives.

B. Sudden Cardiac Death—Usually related to an underlying heart condition, especially hypertrophic cardiomyopathy in young athletes. Screening including EKG can identify this problem early.

C. Exercise—Done on a regular basis, exercise can decrease heart rate and blood pressure, decrease insulin requirements in diabetics, decrease cardiovascular risk, and increase lean body mass. The aerobic

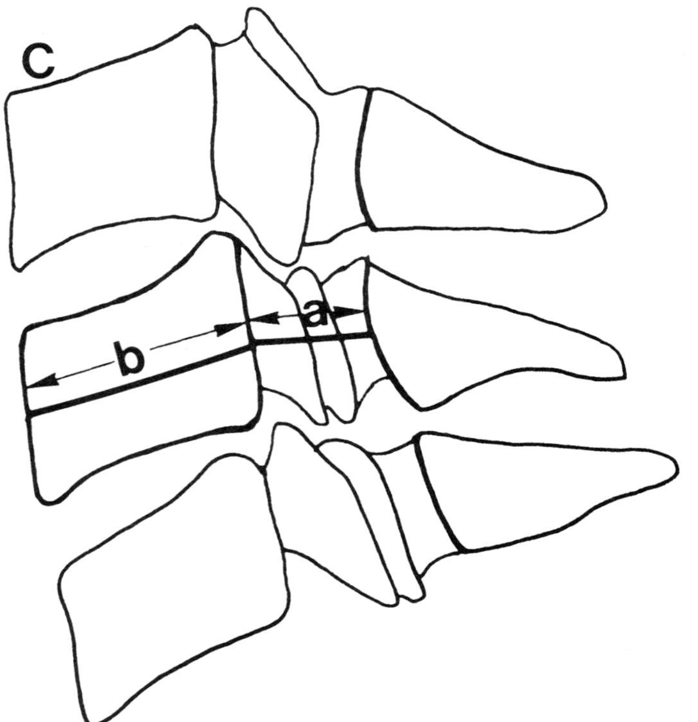

FIGURE 3–45. Pavlov ratio (a/b) of <0.8 is consistent with cervical stenosis. (From Pavlov, H., and Porter, I.S.: Criteria for cervical instability and stenosis. Op. Tech. Sports Med. 1:170, 1993; reprinted by permission.)

EXERCISE	DESCRIPTION	BENEFIT
Isometric	Muscle tension without change in unit length	Muscle hypertrophy; not endurance
Isotonic	Weight training with a constant resistance through arc of motion	Improved motor
Isokinetic	Weight training with a constant velocity, variable resistance	Increase strength; less time-consuming but more expensive
Functional	Aerobic fitness	Easily performed

threshold can be determined by measuring oxygen consumption and is useful for evaluating endurance athletes. Several exercise categories have been described. Stretching has also been shown to have a beneficial effect.

D. Female Athlete
   1. Physiologic Differences—Women are typically smaller, lighter, and have greater body fat. Lower MVO_2, cardiac output, hemoglobin, and muscular mass/strength are also important considerations. Other differences contribute to the increased incidence of patellofemoral disorders, stress fractures, and knee ligament injuries in females.
   2. Amenorrhea—This problem may be related to a low body fat percentage and/or stress. Dietary management and birth control pills are helpful for treating this problem.

Selected Bibliography

Knee

Anatomy and Biomechanics

Arnoczky, S.P.: Anatomy of the anterior cruciate ligament. Clin. Orthop. 172:19–25, 1983.

Arnoczky, S.P., and Warren, R.F.: Microvasculature of the human meniscus. Am. J. Sports Med. 10:90–95, 1982.

Cooper, D.E., Deng, X.H., Burnstein, A.L., and Warren, R.F.: The strength of the central third patellar tendon graft: A biomechanical study. Am. J. Sports Med. 21:818–824, 1993.

Daniel, D.M., Akeson, W.H., and O'Connor, J.J., eds.: Knee Ligaments: Structure, Function, Injury, and Repair. New York, Raven Press, 1990.

Fu, F.H., Harner, C.D., Johnson, D.L., et al.: Biomechanics of knee ligaments: Basic concepts and clinical application. J. Bone Joint Surg. [Am.] 75:1716–1725, 1993.

Girgis, F.G., Marshall, J.L., and Al Monajem, A.R.S.: The cruciate ligaments of the knee joint: Anatomical, functional and experimental analysis. Clin. Orthop. 106:216–231, 1975.

Noyes, F.R., Butler, D.L., Grood, E.S., et al.: Biomechanical analysis of human ligament grafts used in knee-ligament repairs and reconstructions. J. Bone Joint Surg. [Am.] 66:344–352, 1984.

Seebacher, J.R., Inglis, A.E., Marshall, J.L., and Warren, R.F.: The structure of the posterolateral aspect of the knee. J. Bone Joint Surg. [Am.] 64:536–541, 1982.

Thompson, W.O., Theate, F.L., Fu, F.H., and Dye, S.F. Tibial meniscal dynamics using three-dimensional reconstruction of magnetic resonance images. Am. J. Sports Med. 19:210–216, 1991.

Warren, L.F., and Marshall, J.L.: The supporting structures and layers of the medial side of the knee. J. Bone Joint Surg. [Am.] 61: 56–62, 1979.

Warren, R., Arnoczky, S.P., and Wickiewicz, T.L.: Anatomy of the knee. In The Lower Extremity and Spine in Sports Medicine, Nicholas, J.A., and Hershman, E.B., eds., pp. 657–694. St. Louis: CV Mosby, 1986.

History and Physical Examination

Fetto, J.F., and Marshall, J.L.: Injury to the anterior cruciate ligament producing the pivot shift sign. J. Bone Joint Surg. [Am.] 61: 710–714, 1979.

Fulkerson, J.P., Kalenak, A., Rosenberg, T.D., and Cox, J.S.: Patellofemoral pain. Instr. Course Lect. 41:57–71, 1992.

Galway, R.D., Beaupre, A., and MacIntosh, D.L.: Pivot shift. J. Bone Joint Surg. [Br.] 54:763, 1972.

Hosea, T.M., and Tria, A.J.: Physical examination of the knee: clinical. In Ligament and Extensor Mechanism Injuries of the Knee: Diagnosis and Treatment, Scott, W.N., ed. St. Louis, CV Mosby, 1991.

Ritchie, J.R., Miller, M.D., and Harner, C.D.: History and physical examination of the knee. In Knee Surgery, Fu, F.H., Harner, C.D., and Vince, K.G., eds. Baltimore, Williams & Wilkins, 1994.

Slocum, D.B., and Larson, R.L.: Rotatory instability of the knee. J. Bone Joint Surg. [Am.] 50:211, 1968.

Imaging

Blackburne, J.S., and Peel, T.E.: A new method of measuring patellar height. J. Bone Joint Surg. [Br.] 59:241–242, 1977.

Blumensaat, C.: Die lageabweichunger and verrenkungen der kniescheibe. Ergeb. Chir. Orthop. 31:149–223, 1938.

Insall, J., and Salvati, E.: Patella position in the normal knee joint. Radiology 101:101–104, 1971.

Jackson, D.W., Jennings, L.D., Maywood, R.M., and Bergere, P.E.: Magnetic resonance imaging of the knee Am. J. Sports Med. 16: 29–38, 1988.

Merchant, A.C., Mercer, R.L., Jacobsen, R.H., and Cool, C.R.: Roentgenographic analysis of patellofemoral congruence. J. Bone Joint Surg. [Am.] 56:1391–1396, 1974.

Newhouse, K.E., and Rosenberg, T.D.: Basic radiographic examination of the knee. In Knee Surgery, Fu, F.H., Harner, C.D., and Vince, K.G., eds, pp. 313–324. Baltimore, Williams & Wilkins, 1994.

Rosenberg, T.D., Paulos, L.E., Parker, R.D., Coward, D.B., et al.: The forty-five-degree posteroanterior flexion weight-bearing radiograph of the knee. J. Bone Joint Surg. [Am.] 70:1479–1483, 1988.

Thaete, F.L., and Britton, C.A.: Magnetic resonance imaging. In Knee Surgery, Fu, F.H., Harner, C.D., and Vince, K.G., eds. Baltimore, Williams & Wilkins, 1994.

Knee Arthroscopy

DeLee, J.C.: Complications of arthroscopy and arthroscopic surgery: Results of a national survey. Arthroscopy 4:214–220, 1988.

DiGiovine, N.M., and Bradley, J.P.: Arthroscopic equipment and setup. In Knee Surgery, Fu, F.H., Harner, C.D., and Vince, K.G., eds. Baltimore, Williams & Wilkins, 1994.

Gillquist, J.: Arthroscopy of the posterior compartments of the knee. Contemp. Orthop. 10:39–45, 1985.

Johnson, L.L.: Arthroscopic Surgery: Principles and Practice, 3rd ed. St. Louis, CV Mosby, 1986.

O'Connor, R.L.: Arthroscopy in the diagnosis and treatment of acute ligament injuries of the knee. J. Bone Joint Surg. [Am.] 56:333–337, 1974.

Rosenberg, T.D., Paulos, L.E., Parker, R.D., and Abbott, P.J.: Arthroscopic surgery of the knee. In Operative Orthopaedics, Chapman, M.W., ed., pp. 1585–1604. Philadelphia, JB Lippincott, 1988.

Small, N.C.: Complications in arthroscopy: The knee and other joints. Arthroscopy 2:253–258, 1986.

Wantanabe, M., and Takeda, S.: The number 21 arthroscope. J. Jpn. Orthop. Assoc. 34:1041, 1960.

Meniscus

Aichroth, P.M., Patel, D.V., and Marx, C.L.: Congenital discoid lateral meniscus in children: A follow-up study and evolution of management. J. Bone Joint Surg. [Br.] 73:932–936, 1991.

Arnoczky, S.P., Warren, R.F., and Spivak, J.M.: Meniscal repair using an exogenous fibrin clot—an experimental study in dogs. J. Bone Joint Surg. [Am.] 70:1209–1220, 1988.

Baratz, M.E., Fu, F.H., and Mengato, R.: Meniscal tears: The effect of meniscectomy and of repair on intra-articular contact areas and stresses in the human knee. Am. J. Sports Med. 14:270–275, 1986.

Cannon, W.D., Jr.: Arthroscopic meniscal repair. In Operative Arthroscopy, McGinty, J.B., ed., pp. 237–251. New York, Raven Press, 1991.

Cannon, W.D., and Vittori, J.M.: The incidence of healing in arthroscopic meniscal repairs in anterior cruciate ligament reconstructed knees versus stable knees. Am. J. Sports Med. 20: 176–181, 1992.

Cooper, D.E., Arnoczky, S.P., and Warren, R.F.: Arthroscopic meniscal repair. Clin. Sports Med. 9:589–607, 1990.

DeHaven, K.E.: Peripheral meniscal repair: An alternative to meniscectomy. J. Bone Joint Surg. [Br.] 63:463, 1981.

DeHaven, K.E., Black, K.P., and Griffiths, H.J.: Open meniscus repair: Technique and two to nine year results. Am. J. Sports Med. 17:788–795, 1989.

Dickhaut, S.C., and DeLee, J.C.: The discoid lateral meniscus syndrome. J. Bone Joint Surg. [Am.] 64:1068–1073, 1982.

Fairbank, T.J.: Knee joint changes after meniscectomy. J. Bone Joint Surg. [Br.] 30:664–670, 1948.

Glasgow, M.M.S., Allen, P.W., and Blakeway, C.: Arthroscopic treatment of cysts of the lateral meniscus. J. Bone Joint Surg. [Br.] 75: 299–302, 1993.

Henning, C.E., Lynch, M.A., Yearout, K.M., et al.: Arthroscopic meniscal repair using an exogenous fibrin clot. Clin. Orthop. 252: 64, 1990.

Miller, M.D., Ritchie, J.R., Royster, R.M., et al.: Meniscal repair: An experimental study in the goat. Am. J. Sports Med. 23(1):124–128, 1995.

Miller, M.D., Warner, J.J.P., and Harner, C.D.: Mensical repair. In Knee Surgery, Fu, F.H., Harner, C.D., and Vince, K.G., eds. Baltimore, Williams & Wilkins, 1994.

Morgan, C.D.: The "all-inside" meniscus repair: Technical note. Arthroscopy 7:120–125, 1991.

Neuschwander, D.C., Drez, D., and Finney, T.P.: Lateral meniscal variant with absence of the posterior coronary ligament. J. Bone Joint Surg. [Am.] 74:1186–1190, 1992.

Parisien, J.S.: Arthroscopic treatment of cysts of the menisci: A preliminary report. Clin. Orthop. 257:154–158, 1990.

Warren, R.F.: Meniscectomy and repair in the anterior cruciate ligament-deficient patient. Clin. Orthop. 252:55–63, 1990.

Osteochondral Lesions

Aichroth, P.M.: Osteochondral fracture and osteochondritis dissecans in sportsmen's knee injuries. J. Bone Joint Surg. [Br.] 59:108, 1977.

Bauer, M., and Jackson, R.W.: Chondral lesions of the femoral condyles: A system of arthroscopic classification. Arthroscopy 4: 97–102, 1988.

Garrett, J.C.: Osteochondritis dissecans. Clin. Sports Med. 10:569, 1991.

Guhl, J.: Arthroscopic treatment of osteochondritis dissecans. Clin. Orthop. 167:65–74, 1982.

Rand, J.A.: Arthroscopic diagnosis and management of articular cartilagee pathology. In Arthroscopy of the Knee, Scott, W.N., ed., pp. 113–128. Philadelphia, WB Saunders, 1990.

Vince, K.G.: Osteochondritis dissecans of the knee. In Arthroscopy of the Knee, Scott, W.N., ed. Philadelphia, WB Saunders, 1990.

Synovial Lesions

Collican, M.R., and Dandy, D.J.: Arthroscopic management of synovial chondromatosis of the knee: Findings and results in 18 cases. J. Bone Joint Surg. [Br.] 71:498, 1989.

Flandry, F., and Hughston, J.C.: Current concepts review: pigmented villonodular synovitis. J. Bone Joint Surg. [Am.] 69:942, 1987.

Johnson, D.P., Eastwood, D.M., and Witherow, P.J.: Symptomatic synovial plicae of the knee. J. Bone Joint Surg. [Am.] 75: 1485–1496, 1993.

Sims, F.H.: Synovial proliferative disorders: Role of synovectomy. Arthroscopy 1:198, 1985.

Wilson, W.J., and Parr, T.J.: Synovial chondromatosis. Orthopedics 11:1179, 1988.

Knee Ligament Injuries

Almeekinders, L.C., and Logan, T.C.: Results following treatment of traumatic dislocations of the knee joint. Clin. Orthop. 284: 203–207, 1992.

Clancy, W.G., Ray, J.M., and Zoltan, D.J.: Acute tears of the anterior cruciate ligament: Surgical versus conservative treatment. J. Bone Joint Surg. [Am.] 70:1483–1488, 1988.

Cooper, D.E., Speer, K.P., Wickiewicz, T.L., and Warren, R.F.: Complete knee dislocation without posterior cruciate disruption: A report of four cases and review of the literature. Clin. Orthop. 284: 228–244, 1992.

Cooper, D.E., Warren, R.F., and Warner, J.J.P.: The posterior cruciate ligament and posterolateral structures of the knee: Anatomy, function, and patterns of injury. Instr. Course Lect. 40:249–270, 1991.

Daniel, D.M., Akeson, W.H., and O'Connor, J.J., eds.: Knee Ligaments: Structure, Function, Injury and Repair. New York, Raven Press, 1990.

Feagin, J.A., ed.: The Crucial Ligaments: Diagnosis and Treatment of Ligamentous Injuries About the Knee. New York, Churchill Livingstone, 1988.

Fowler, P.J., and Messieh, S.S.: Isolated posterior cruciate ligament injuries in athletes. Am. J. Sports Med. 15:553–557, 1987.

Frassica, F.J., Sim, F.H., Staeheli, J.W., and Pairolero, P.C.: Dislocation of the kneee. Clin. Orthop. 263:200–205, 1991.

Harner, C.D., Irrgang, J.J., Paul, J., Dearwater, S., and Fu, F.H.: Loss of motion following anterior cruciate ligament reconstruction. Am. J. Sports Med. 20:507–515, 1992.

Howell, S.M., and Taylor, M.A.: Failure of reconstruction of the anterior cruciate ligament due to impingement by the intercondylar roof. J. Bone Joint Surg. [Am.] 75:1044–1055, 1993.

Indelicato, P.A., Hermansdorfer, J., and Huegel, M.: Nonoperative management of complete tears of the medial collateral ligament of the knee in intercollegiate football players. Clin. Orthop. 256: 174–177, 1990.

Johnson, R.J., Beynnon, B.D., Nichols, C.E., and Renstrom, P.A.F.H.: Current concepts review: The treatment of injuries of the anterior cruciate ligament. J. Bone Joint Surg. [Am.] 74:140–151, 1992.

Myers, M.H., and Harvey, J.P.: Traumatic dislocation of the knee joint: A study of eighteen cases. J. Bone Joint Surg. [Am.] 53:16–29, 1971.

Muller, W.: The Knee: Form, Function, and Ligament Reconstruction. New York, Springer-Verlag, 1983.

O'Brien, S.J., Warren, R.F., Pavlov, H., et al.: Reconstruction of the chronically insufficient anterior cruciate ligament with the central third of the patellar ligament. J. Bone Joint Surg. [Am.] 73: 278–286, 1991.

Paulos, L.E., Rosenberg, T.D., Drawbert, J., Manning, J., et al.: Infrapatellar contracture syndrome: An unrecognized cause of knee stiffness with patellar entrapment and patella infera. Am. J. Sports Med. 15:331–341, 1987.

Scott, W.N., ed.: Ligament and Extensor Mechanism of the Knee: Diagnosis and Treatment. St. Louis: CV Mosby, 1991.

Shelbourne, K.D., and Nitz, P.: Accelerated rehabilitation after anterior cruciate ligament reconstruction. Am. J. Sports Med. 18: 292–299, 1990.

Shelbourne, K.D., and Nitz, P.A.: The O'Donoghue triad revisited: Combined injuries involving the anterior cruciate and medial collateral ligament tears. Am. J. Sports Med. 19:474–477, 1991.

Sisto, D.J., and Warren, R.F.: Complete knee dislocation: A follow-up study of operative treatment. Clin. Orthop. 198:94–101, 1985.

Sitler, M., Ryan, J., Hopkinson, W., et al.: The efficacy of a prophylactic knee brace to reduce knee injuries in football: A prospective, randomized study at West Point. Am. J. Sports Med. 18:310–315, 1990.

Sommerlath, K., Lysholm, J., and Gillquist, J.: The long-term course after treatment of acute ACL ruptures. Am. J. Sports Med. 19: 156–162, 1991.

Warner, J.J.P., Warren, R.F., and Cooper, D.E.: Management of acute anterior cruciate ligament injury. Instr. Course Lect. 40:219–232, 1991.

Anterior Knee Pain

Cooper, D.E., and DeLee, J.C.: Reflex sympathetic dystrophy. In Knee Surgery, Fu, F.H., Harner, C.D., and Vince, K.G., eds. Baltimore, Williams & Wilkins, 1994.

Fulkerson, J.P.: Anteromedialization of the tibial tuberosity for patellofemoral malalignment. Clin. Orthop. 177:176–181, 1983.

Fulkerson, J.P., and Hungerford, D.S.: Disorders of the Patellofemoral Joint, 2nd ed. Baltimore, Williams & Wilkins, 1990.

Fulkerson, J.P., and Shea, K.P.: Disorders of patellofemoral alignment: Current concepts review. J. Bone Joint Surg. [Am.] 72: 1424–1429, 1990.

Hughston, J.C., and Walsh, W.M.: Proximal and distal reconstruction of the extensor mechanism for patellar subluxation. Clin. Orthop. 144:36–42, 1979.

Insall, J.: Patellar pain: Current concepts review. J. Bone Joint Surg. [Am.] 64:147, 1982.

Jacobsen, K.E., and Flandry, F.C.: Diagnosis of anterior knee pain. Clin. Sports Med. 8:179–196, 1989.

Kilowich, P., Paulos, L., Rosenberg, T., and Farnsworth, S.: Lateral release of the patella: Indications and contraindications. Am. J. Sports Med. 18:361, 1990.

Larson, R.L., Cabaud, H.E., Slocum, D.B., et al.: The patellar compression syndrome: Surgical treatment by lateral retinacular release. Clin. Orthop. 134:158–167, 1978.

Merchant, A.: Classification of patellofemoral disorders. Arthroscopy 4:235–240, 1988.

Merchant, A.C., Mercer, R.L., Jacobsen, R.J., and Cool, C.R.: Roentgenographic analysis of patello-femoral congruence. J. Bone Joint Surg. [Am.] 56:1391–1396, 1974.

Ray, J.M., Clancy, W.G., and Lemon, R.A.: Semimembranosus tendinitis: An overlooked cause of medial knee pain. Am. J. Sports Med. 16:347–351, 1988.

Childhood and Adolescent Knee Disorders

Angel, K.R., and Hall, D.J.: Anterior cruciate ligament injury in children and adolescents. Arthroscopy 4:197–201, 1989.

Baxter, M.P., and Wiley, J.J.: Fractures of the tibial spine in children: An evaluation of knee stability. J. Bone Joint Surg. [Br.] 70: 228–230, 1988.

Clanton, T.O., DeLee, J.C., Sanders, B., et al.: Knee ligament injuries in children. J. Bone Joint Surg. [Am.] 61:1195–1201, 1979.

McCarroll, J.R., Rettig, A.C., and Shelbourne, K.D.: Anterior cruciate ligament injuries in the young athlete with open physes. Am. J. Sports Med. 16:44–47, 1988.

Medlar, R.C., and Lyne, E.D.: Sinding-Larsen-Johansson disease: Its etiology and natural history. J. Bone Joint Surg. [Am.] 60: 1113–1116, 1978.

Meyers, M.H., and McKeever, F.M.: Fractures of the intercondylar eminence of the tibia. J. Bone Joint Surg. [Am.] 41:209–222, 1959.

Micheli, L.J., and Foster, T.E.: Acute knee injuries in the immature athlete. Inst. Course Lect. 42:473–481, 1993.

Ogden, J.A., Tross, R.B., and Murphy, M.J.: Fractures of the tibial tubereosity in adolescents. J. Bone Joint Surg. [Am.] 62:205–215, 1980.

Parker, A.W., Drez, D., and Cooper, J.L.: Anterior cruciate ligament injuries in patients with open physes. Am. J. Sports Med. 22: 44–47, 1994.

Riseborough, E.J., Barrett, I.R., and Shapiro, F.: Growth disturbances following distal femoral physeal fracture-separations. J. Bone Joint Surg. [Am.] 65:885–893, 1983.

Stanitski, C.L.: Knee overuse disorders in the pediatric and adolescent athlete. Instr. Course Lect. 42:483–495, 1993.

Other Lower Extremity Sports Medicine Problems

Nerve Entrapment Syndromes

Baxter, D.E.: Functional nerve disorders in the athlete's foot, ankle, and leg. Instr. Course Lect. 42:185–194, 1993.

Baxter, D.E., Pfeffer, G.B., and Thigpen, M.: Chronic heel pain treatment rationale. Orthop. Clin. North Am. 20:563–570, 1989.

Jordan, B.D., Tsairis, P., and Warren, R.F.: Sports Neurology. Rockville, MD, Aspen Press, 1989.

Styf, J.: Entrapment of the superficial peroneal nerve: Diagnosis and results of decompression. J. Bone Joint Surg. [Br.] 71:131–135, 1989.

Contusions

Campbell, J.D.: Injuries of the pelvis, hip and thigh. Clin. Sports Med., 1991.

Jackson, D.W., and Feagin, J.A.: Quadriceps contusions in young athletes. J. Bone Joint Surg. [Am.] 55:95–105, 1973.

Renstrom, P.A.H.F.: Tendon and muscle injuries in the groin area. Clin. Sports Med. 11:815–831, 1992.

Rooser, B., Bengston, S., and Hagglund, G.: Acute compartment syndrome from anterior thigh muscle contusion: A report of eight cases. J. Orthop. Trauma 5:57–59, 1991.

Ryan, J.B., Wheeler, J.H., Hopkinson, W.J., et al.: Quadriceps contusions: West Point update. Am. J. Sports Med. 19:299–304, 1991.

Muscle Injury

Burkett, L.N.: Investigation into hamstring strains: The case of the hybrid muscle. J. Sports Med. 3:228, 1975.

Clanton, T.O., and Schon, L.C.: Athletic injuries to the soft tissues of the foot and ankle. In Surgery of the Foot and Ankle, Mann, R.A., and Coughlin, M.J., eds. St. Louis, CV Mosby, 1993.

Renstrom, P.A.H.F.: Tendon and muscle injuries in the groin area. Clin. Sports Med. 11:815–831, 1992.

Zarins, B., and Ciullo, J.V.: Acute muscle and tendon injuries in athletes. Clin. Sports Med. 2:167, 1983.

Tendon Injuries

Arrowsmith, S.R., Flemming, L.L., and Allman, F.L.: Traumatic dislocations of the peroneal tendons. Am. J. Sports Med. 11:142, 1983.

Bassett, F.H., and Speer, K.P.: Longitudinal rupture of the peroneal tendons. Am. J. Sports Med. 21:354–357, 1993.

Biedert, R.: Dislocation of the tibialis posterior tendon. Am. J. Sports Med. 20:775–776, 1992.

Bradley, J.P., and Tibone, J.E.: Percutaneous and open surgical repairs of Achilles tendon ruptures: A comparative study. Am. J. Sports Med. 18:188–195, 1990.

Brage, M.E., and Hansen, S.T.: Traumatic subluxation/dislocation of the peroneal tendons. Foot Ankle 13:423–430, 1992.

Lutter, L.D.: Hindfoot problems. Instr. Course Lect. 42:195–200, 1993.

Millar, A.P.: Strains of the posterior calf musculature ("tennis leg"). Am. J. Sports Med. 7:172–174, 1979.

Ouzounian, T.J., and Myerson, M.S.: Dislocation of the posterior tibial tendon. Foot Ankle 13:215–219, 1992.

Renstrom, P.A.F.H.: Mechanism, diagnosis, and treatment of running injuries. Instr. Course Lect. 42:225–234, 1993.

Sobel, M., Geppert, M.J., Olson, E.J., et al.: The dynamics of peroneus brevis tendon splits: A proposed mechanism, technique of diagnosis, and classification of injury. Foot Ankle 13:413–421, 1992.

Thompson, F.M., and Patterson, A.H.: Rupture of the peroneus longus tendon: Report of three cases. J. Bone Joint Surg. [Am.] 71: 293–295, 1989.

Williams, J.G.P.: Achilles tendon lesions in sport. Sports Med. 3: 114–135, 1986.

Woods, L., and Leach, R.E.: Posterior tibial tendon rupture in athletic people. Am. J. Sports Med. 19:495–498, 1991.

Compartment Syndrome

Beckham, S.G., Grana, W.A., Buckley, P., et al.: A comparison of anterior compartment pressures in competitive runners and cyclists. Am. J. Sports Med. 21:36–40, 1993.

Bourne, R.B., and Rorabeck, C.H.: Compartment syndromes of the lower leg. Clin. Orthop. 240:97–104, 1989.

Clanton, T.O., and Schon, L.C.: Athletic injuries to the soft tissues of foot and ankle. In Surgery of the Foot and Ankle, 2nd ed., Mann,

R.A., and Coughlin, M.J., eds, pp. 1095–1224. St. Louis, CV Mosby, 1993.
Colosimo, A.J., and Ireland, M.L.: Thigh compartment syndrome in a football athlete: A case report an review of the literature. Med. Sci. Sports Exerc. 24:958–963, 1992.
Eisele, S.A., and Sammarco, G.J.: Chronic exertional compartment syndrome. Instr. Course Lect. 42:213–217, 1993.
James, S.L., Bates, B.T., and Osternig, L.R.: Injuries to runners. Am. J. Sports Med. 6:40–50, 1978.
Martens, M.A., and Moeyersoons, J.P.: Acute and recurrent effort-related compartment syndrome in sports. Sports Med. 9:62–68, 1990.
Pedowitz, R.A., Horgens, A.R., Mubarak, S.J., et al.: Modified criteria for the objective diagnosis of compartment syndrome of the leg. Am. J. Sports Med. 18:35–40, 1990.
Rorabeck, C.H., Bourne, R.B., and Fowler, P.J.: The surgical treatment of exertional compartment syndromes in athletes. J. Bone Joint Surg. [Am.] 65:1245, 1983.
Rorabeck, C.H., Fowler, P.J., and Nitt, L.: The results of fasciotomy in the management of chronic exertional compartment syndrome. Am. J. Sports Med. 16:224–227, 1986.

Stress Fractures

Anderson, E.G.: Fatigue fractures of the foot. Injury 274–279, 1990.
Blickenstaff, L.D., and Morris, J.M.: Fatigue fracture of the femoral neck. J. Bone Joint Surg. [Am.] 48:1031, 1966.
Eisele, S.A., and Sammarco, G.J.: Fatigue fractures of the foot and ankle in the athlete. Instr. Course Lect. 42:175–183, 1993.
Green, N.E., Rogers, R.A., and Lipscomb, A.B.: Nonunions of stress fractures of the tibia. Am. J. Sports Med. 13:171–176, 1985.
Hajek, M.R., and Noble, H.B.: Stress fractures of the femoral neck in joggers: Case reports and review of the literature. Am. J. Sports Med. 10:112, 1982.
Kadel, N.J., Teitz, C.C., and Kronmal, R.A.: Stress fractures in ballet dancers. Am. J. Sports Med. 20:445–449, 1992.
Khan, K.M., Fuller, P.J., Brukner, P.D., et al.: Outcome of conservative and surgical management of navicular stress fracture in athletes: Eighty-six cases proven with computerized tomography. Am. J. Sports Med. 20:657–661, 1992.
Lombardo, S.J., and Benson, D.W.: Stress fractures of the femur in runners. Am. J. Sports Med. 10:219, 1982.
McBryde, A.M.: Stress fractures in athletes. J. Sports Med. 3:212, 1973.
McBryde, A.M.: Stress fractures in runners. Clin. Sports Med. 4: 737–752, 1985.
Rettig, A.C., Shelbourne, K.D., McCarroll, J.R., et al.: The natural history and treatment of delayed union stress fractures of the anterior cortex of the tibia. Am. J. Sports Med. 16:250–255, 1988.
Shiraishi, M., Mizuta, H., Kubota, K., et al.: Stress fracture of the proximal phalanx of the great toe. Foot Ankle 14:28–34, 1993.
Stanitski, C.L., McMaster, J.H., and Scranton, P.E.: On the nature of stress fractures. Am. J. Sports Med. 6:391, 1978.

Other Hip Disorders

Cooper, D.E., Warren, R.F., and Barnes, R.: Traumatic subluxation of the hip resulting in aseptic necrosis and chondrolysis in a professional football player. Am. J. Sports Med. 19:322–324, 1991.
Frost, A., and Bauer, M.: Skier's hip: A new clinical entity? Proximal femur fractures sustained in cross-country skiing. J. Orthop. Trauma 5:57–50, 1991.
Holmes, J.C., Pruitt, A.L., and Whalen, N.J.: Iliotibial band syndrome in cyclists. Am. J. Sports Med. 21:419–424, 1993.
Jacobs, M., and Young, B.: Snapping hip phenomenon among dancers. Am. Correct. Ther. J. 32:92, 1973.
Martens, M., Libbrecht, P., and Burssens, A.: Surgical treatment of the iliotibial band friction syndrome. Am. J. Sports Med. 17: 651–654, 1989.
Stenger, A.: Bo's hip dislocates stellar athletic career. Phys. Sports Med. 19:17–18, 1991.
Stewart, W.J.: Aseptic necrosis of the head of the femur following traumatic dislocation of the hip joint: Case report and experimental studies. J. Bone Joint Surg. 15:413–438, 1933.

Other Foot and Ankle Disorders

Baxter, D.E.: The foot in running. In Surgery of the Foot and Ankle, Mann, R.A., and Coughlin, M.J., ed. St. Louis: CV Mosby, 1993.
Daly, P.J., Kitaoka, H.B., and Chao, E.Y.S.: Plantar fasciotomy for intractable plantar fascitis: Clinical results and biomechanical evaluation. Foot Ankle 13:188–196, 1992.
Garrick, J.G., and Requa, R.K.: The epidemiology of foot and ankle injuries in sports. Clin. Sports Med. 7:29–36, 1988.
Hamilton, W.G., Thompson, F.M., and Snow, S.W.: The modified Brostrom procedure for lateral ankle instability. Foot Ankle 14: 1–7, 1993.
Hopkinson, W.J., St. Pierre, P., Ryan, J.B., and Wheeler, J.H.: Syndesmosis sprains of the ankle. Foot Ankle 10:325–330, 1990.
Kwong, P.K., Kay, D., Voner, R.T., and White, M.W.: Plantar fasciitis: Mechanics and pathomechanics of treatment. Clin. Sports Med. 7:119–126, 1988.
Marotta, J.J., and Micheli, L.J.: Os trigonum impingement in dancers. Am. J. Sports Med. 20:533–536, 1992.
Raatikainen, T., Putkonen, M., and Puranen, J.: Arthrography, clinical examination, and stress radiograph in the diagnosis of acute injury to the lateral ligaments of the ankle. Am. J. Sports Med. 20: 2–6, 1992.
Rodeo, S.A., O'Brien, S., Warren, R.F., et al.: Turf toe: An analysis of metatarsal phalangeal joint pain in professional football players. Am. J. Sports Med. 18:280–285, 1990.
Sammarco, G.J.: Turf toe. Instr. Course Lect. 42:207–212, 1993.
Wilkerson, L.A.: Ankle injuries in athletes. Prim. Care 19:377–392, 1992.

Hip and Ankle Arthroscopy

Angermann, P., and Jensen, P.: Osteochondritis dissecans of the talus: Long term results of surgical treatment. Foot Ankle 10: 161–163, 1989.
Basset, F.H., Billy, J.B., and Gates, H.S.: A simple surgical approach to the posteromedial ankle. Am. J. Sports Med. 21:144–146, 1993.
Bassett, F.H., Gates, H.S., Billys, J.B., Morris, H.B., and Nikolaou, P.K.: Talar impingement by the anteroinferior tibiofibular ligament. J. Bone Joint Surg. [Am.] 72:55–59, 1990.
Dorfmann, H., Boyer, T., Henry, P., and DeBie, B.: A simple approach to hip arthroscopy. Arthroscopy 4:141–142, 1988.
Feder, K.S., Schonholtz, G.J.: Ankle arthroscopy: Review and long-term results. Foot Ankle 13:382–385, 1992.
Ferkel, R.D., and Scranton, P.E.: Current concepts review: Arthroscopy of the ankle and foot. J. Bone Joint Surg. [Am.] 75:1233–1243, 1993.
Glick, J.M.: Hip arthroscopy using the lateral approach. Instr. Course Lect. 37:223–231, 1988.
Glick, J.M., Sampson, T.G., Gordon, R.B., et al.: Hip arthroscopy by the lateral approach. Arthroscopy 3:4–12, 1987.
Guhl, J.: Ankle Arthroscopy. Pathology and Surgical Techniques, pp. 49–117. Thorofare, NJ, Slack, 1988.
Loomer, R., Fisher, C., Lloyd-Smith, R., et al.: Osteochondral lesions of the talus. Am. J. Sports Med. 21:13–19, 1993.
McCarroll, J.R., Schrader, J.W., Shelbourne, K.D., et al.: Meniscoid lesions of the ankle in soccer players. Am. J. Sports Med. 15:257, 1987.
Meislin, R.J., Rose, D.J., Parisien, S., and Springer, S.: Arthroscopic treatment of synovial impingement of the ankle. Am. J. Sports Med. 21:186–189, 1993.
Ogilvie-Harris, D.J., Lieverman, I., and Fitsalos, D.: Arthroscopically assisted arthrodesis for osteoarthritic ankles. J. Bone Joint Surg. [Am.] 75:1167–1174, 1993.
Okada, Y., Awaya, G., Ikeda, T., et al.: Arthroscopic surgery for synovial chondromatosis of the hip. J. Bone Joint Surg. [Br.] 71: 198–199, 1989.
Scranton, P.E., and McDermott, J.E.: Anterior tibiotalar spurs: A comparison of open versus arthroscopic débridement. Foot Ankle 13:125–129, 1992.
Taga, I., Shino, K., Inoue, M., et al.: Articular cartilage lesions in ankles with lateral ligament injury: An arthroscopic study. Am. J. Sports Med. 21:120–124, 1993.
Thein, R., and Eichenblat, M.: Arthroscopic treatment of sports-related synovitis of the ankle. Am. J. Sports Med. 20:496–499, 1992.

Shoulder

Anatomy and Biomechanics

Blasier, R.B., Guldberg, R.E., and Rothman, E.D.: Anterior shoulder stability: Contributions of rotator cuff forces and the capsular ligaments in a cadaver model. J. Shoulder Elbow Surg. 1:140–150, 1992.

Clark, J.M., and Harryman, D.T., II: Tendons, ligaments, and capsule of the rotator cuff: Gross and microscopic anatomy. J. Bone Joint Surg. [Am.] 74:713–725, 1992.

Cooper, D.E., Arnoczsky, S.P., O'Brien, S.J., et al.: Anatomy, histology, and vascularity of the glenoid labrum. J. Bone Joint Surg. [Am.] 74:46–52, 1992.

Cooper, D.E., O'Brien, S.J., and Warren, R.F.: Supporting layers of the glenohumeral joint: An anatomic study. Clin. Orthop. 289: 144–155, 1993.

Ferrari, D.A.: Capsular ligaments of the shoulder: Anatomical and functional study of the anterior superior capsule. Am. J. Sports Med. 18:20–24, 1990.

Flatow, E.L.: The biomechanics of the acromioclavicular, sternoclavicular, and scapulothoracic joints. Instr. Course Lect. 42: 237–245, 1993.

Harryman, D.T., II: Common surgical approaches to the shoulder. Inst. Course Lect. 41:3–11, 1992.

Howell, S.M., and Galinat, B.J.: The glonoid-labral socket: A constrained articular surface. Clin. Orthop. 243:122, 1989.

Iannotti, J.P., Gabriel, J.P., Schneck, S.L., et al.: The normal glenohumeral relationships: An anatomical study of one hundred and forty shoulders. J. Bone Joint Surg. [Am.] 74:491–500, 1992.

Jobe, C.M.: Gross anatomy of the shoulder. In The Shoulder, Rockwood, C.A., Jr., and Matsen, F.A., III, eds., pp. 34–97. Philadelphia, WB Saunders, 1990.

Morrey, B.F., and An, K-N.: Biomechanics of the shoulder. In The Shoulder, Rockwood, C.A., Jr., and Matsen, F.A., III, eds., pp. 209–245. Philadelphia, WB Saunders, 1990.

O'Brien, S.J., Neves, M.C., Rozbruck, S.R., et al.: The anatomy and histology of the inferior glenohumeral ligament complex of the shoulder. Am. J. Sports Med. 18:449, 1990.

O'Connell, P.W., Nuber, G.W., Mileski, R.A., and Lautenschlager, E.: The contribution of the glenohumeral ligaments to anterior stability of the shoulder joint. Am. J. Sports Med. 18:579–584, 1990.

Sarrafian, S.K.: Gross and functional anatomy of the shoulder. Clin. Orthop. 173:11, 1983.

Warner, J.J.P.: The gross anatomy of the joint surfaces, ligaments labrum, and capsule. In The Shoulder: A Balance of Mobility and Stability, Matsen, F.A., III, Fu, F.H., and Hawking, R.J., eds., pp. 7–28. Rosemont, IL, American Academy of Orthopaedic Surgeons, 1993.

Warner, J.J.P., and Caborn, D.N.: Overview of shoulder instability. Crit. Rev. Phys. Rehabil. Med. 4:145–198, 1992.

Warner, J.J.P., Deng, X.H., Warren, R.F., and Torzilli, P.A.: Static capsuloligamentous restraints to superior-inferior translation of the glenohumeral joint. Am. J. Sports Med. 20:675–685, 1992.

Warner, J.J.P., Deng, X., Warren, R.F., and Torzilli, P.A.: Superior-inferior translation in the intact and vented glenohumeral joint. J. Shoulder Elbow Surg. 2:99–105, 1993.

History and Physical Examination

Gerber, C., and Ganz, R.: Clinical assessment of instability of the shoulder with special reference to anterior an posterior drawer tests. J. Bone Joint Surg. [Br.] 66:551–556, 1984.

Hawkins, R.J., and Hobeika, P.: Physical examination of the shoulder. Orthopedics 6:1270–1278, 1983.

Hawkins, R.J., and Mohtadi, N.G.H.: Clinical evaluation of shoulder instability. Clin. J. Sports Med. 1:59–64, 1991.

Hawkins, R.J., and Bokor, D.J.: Clinical evaluation of shoulder problems. In The Shoulder, Rockwood, C.A., Jr., and Matsen, F.A., III, eds., pp. 149–177. Philadelphia, WB Saunders, 1990.

Hoppenfeld, S.: Physical Examination of the Spine and Extremities. Norwalk, CT, Appleton-Century-Crofts, 1976.

Neer, C.S., and Welsh, R.P.: The shoulder in sports. Orthop. Clin. North Am. 8:583–591, 1977.

Imaging of the Shoulder

Beltran, J.: The use of magnetic resonance imaging about the shoulder. J. Shoulder Elbow Surg. 1:287–295, 1992.

Bigliani, L.U., Morrison, D., and April, E.W.: The morphology of the acromion and its relationship to rotator cuff tears. Orthop. Trans. 10:228, 1986.

Garth, W.P., Jr., Slappey, C.E., and Ochs, C.W.: Roentgenographic demonstration of instability of the shoulder: The apical oblique projection—a technical note. J. Bone Joint Surg. [Am.] 66: 1450–1453, 1984.

Hill, H.A., Sachs, M.D.: The grooved defect of the humeral head: A frequently unrecognized complication of dislocations of the shoulder joint. Radiology 35:690–700, 1940.

Hobbs, D.W.: Sternoclavicular joint: A new axial radiographic view. Radiology 90:801–802, 1968.

Jahnke, A.H., Petersen, S.A., Neumann, C., et al.: A prospective comparison of computerized arthrotomography and magnetic resonance imaging of the glenohumeral joint. Am. J. Sports Med. 20: 695–701, 1992.

Kozo, O., Yamamuro, T., and Rockwood, C.A.: Use of a thirty-degree caudal tilt radiograph in the shoulder impingement syndrome. J. Shoulder Elbow Surg. 1:246–252, 1992.

Recht, M.P., and Resnick, D.: Instructional Course Lectures: Magnetic resonance imaging studies of the shoulder: Diagnosis of lesions of the rotator cuff. J. Bone Joint Surg. [Am.] 75:1244–1253, 1993.

Rockwood, C.A., Jr., Green, D.P., and Bucholz, R.W.: Rockwood and Green's Fractures in Adults, 3rd ed. Philadelphia, JB Lippincott, 1991.

Rockwood, C.A., Jr., Szalay, E.A., Curtis, R.J., et al.: X-ray evaluation of shoulder problems. In The Shoulder, Rockwood, C.A., Jr., and Matsen, F.A., III, eds., pp. 178–207. Philadelphia, WB Saunders, 1990.

Rokous, J.R., Feagin, J.A., and Abbott, H.G.: Modified axillary roentgenogram. Clin. Orthop. 82:84–86, 1972.

Zanca, P.: Shoulder pain: Involvement of the acromioclavicular joint; analysis of 1000 cases. AJR Am. J. Roentgenol. 112:493–506, 1971.

Arthroscopy of the Shoulder

Altchek, D.W., Warren, R.F., and Skyhar, M.J.: Shoulder arthroscopy. In The Shoulder, Rockwood, C.A., Jr., and Matsen, F.A., III, eds., pp. 258–277. Philadelphia, WB Saunders, 1990.

Caborn, D.M., and Fu, F.H.: Arthroscopic approach and anatomy of the shoulder. Op. Tech. Orthop. 1(2):126–133, 1991.

Nisbet, J.K., and Paulos, L.E.: Subacromial bursoscopy. Op. Tech. Orthop. 1(3):221–228, 1991.

Skyhar, M.J., Altchek, D.W., Warren, R.F., et al.: Shoulder arthroscopy with the patient in the beach chair position. Arthroscopy 4: 256–259, 1988.

Souryal, T.O., and Baker, C.L.: Anatomy of the supraclavicular portal in shoulder arthroscopy. Arthroscopy 6:297–300, 1990.

Warner, J.J.P.: Shoulder arthroscopy in the beach-chair position: Basic setup. Op. Tech. Orthop. 1(2):147–154, 1991.

Wolf, E.M.: Anterior portals in shoulder arthroscopy. Arthroscopy 5:201–208, 1989.

Shoulder Instability

Altchek, D.W., Warren, R.F., and Skyhar, M.J.: Shoulder arthroscopy. In The Shoulder, Rockwood, C.A., Jr., and Matsen, F.A., III, eds., pp. 258–277. Philadelphia, WB Saunders, 1990.

Altchek, D.W., Warren, R.F., Skyhar, M.J., and Ortiz, G.: T-Plasty modification of the Bankhart procedure for multidirectional instability of the anterior an inferior types. J. Bone Joint Surg. [Am.] 73:105–112, 1991.

Arciero, R.A., Wheeler, J.H. III, Ryan, J.B., and McBride, J.T.: Arthroscopic Bankart repair for acute, initial anterior shoulder dislocations. Am. J. Sports Med. 22:589–594, 1994.

Caspari, R.B.: Arthroscopic stabilization for shoulder instability. In Operative Techniques in Shoulder Surgery, pp. 57–63. Gaithersburg, MD, Aspen, 1991.

Cooper, R.A., and Brems, J.J.: The inferior capsular shift procedure for multi-directional instability of the shoulder. J. Bone Joint Surg. [Am.] 74:1516–1521, 1992.

Detrisac, D.A.: Arthroscopic shoulder staple capsulorrhaphy for traumatic anterior instability. In Operative Arthroscopy, McGinty, J.B., ed. New York, Raven Press. 1991.

Grana, W.A., Buckley, P.D., and Yates, C.K.: Arthroscopic Bankart suture repair. Am. J. Sports Med. 21:348–353, 1993.

Harryman, D.T., II, Sidles, J.A., Harris, S.L., and Matsen, F.A., III: Laxity of the normal glenohumeral joint: A quantitative in-vivo assessment. J. Shoulder Elbow Surg. 1:66–76, 1992.

Hawkins, R.B.: Arthroscopic stapling repair for shoulder instability; a retrospective study of 50 cases. Arthroscopy 5:122–128, 1989.

Hovelius, L., Thorling, J., and Fredin, H.: Recurrent anterior dislocation of the shoulder: Results after the Bankart and Putti-Platt operations. J. Bone Joint Surg. [Am.] 61:566–569, 1979.

Hurley, J.A., Anderson, T.E., Dear, W., et al.: Posterior shoulder instability: Surgical versus conservative results with evaluation of glenoid version. Am. J. Sports Med. 20:396–400, 1992.

Lippit, S., and Matsen, F.A., III: Mechanisms of glenohumeral joint stability. Clin. Orthop. 291:20–28, 1993.

Maki, N.J.: Arthroscoic stabilization: Suture technique. Op. Tech. Orthop. 1(2):180–183, 1991.

Mallon, W.J.: Shoulder instability. In Orthopaedic Knowledge Update 4 Home Study Syllabus, Frymoyer, J.W., ed., Rosemont, IL, American Academy of Orthopaedic Surgeons, pp. 297–302, 1993.

Morgan, C.D., and Bodenstab, A.B.: Arthroscopic Bankart suture repair; techniques and early results. Arthroscopy 3:111–112, 1982.

Neer, C.S., II, and Foster, C.R.: Inferior capsular shift for involuntary inferior and multidirectional instability of the shoulder: A preliminary report. J. Bone Joint Surg. [Am.] 62:897–908, 1980.

Rowe, C.R., and Sakellarides, H.T.: Factors related to recurrences of anterior dislocation of the shoulder. Clin. Orthop. 20:40–47, 1961.

Rowe, C.R., Patel, D., and Southmayd, W.W.: The Bankart procedure—a long-term end-result study. J. Bone Joint Surg. [Am.] 55: 445–460, 1973.

Turkel, S.J., Panio, M.W., Marshall, J.L., et al.: Stabilizing mechanisms preventing anterior dislocation of the glenohumeral joint. J. Bone Joint Surg. [Am.] 63:1208–1217, 1981.

Warner, J.J.P., and Warren, R.F.: Arthroscopic Bankart repair using a cannulated, absorbable fixation device. Op. Tech. Orthop. 1: 192–198, 1991.

Zuckerman, J.D., Matsen, F.A., III: Complications about the glenohumeral joint related to the use of screws and staples. J. Bone Joint Surg. [Am.] 66:175–180, 1984.

Impingement Syndrome/Rotator Cuff

Bigliani, L.U., Cordasco, F.A., McIlveen, S.J., and Musso, E.S.: Operative treatment of failed repairs of the rotator cuff. J. Bone Joint Surg. [Am.] 74:1505–1515, 1992.

Caspari, R.B., and Thal, R.: A technique for arthroscopic subacromial decompression. Arthroscopy 8:23–20, 1992.

Ellman, H., Kay, S.P., and Worth, M.: Arthroscopic treatment of full thickness rotator cuff tears: Two to seven year follow-up study. Arthroscopy 9:301–314, 1993.

Gerber, C., Terrier, F., and Ganz, R.: The role of the coracoid process in the chronic impingement syndrome. J. Bone Joint Surg. [Br.] 67:703–708, 1985.

Hawkins, R.J., and Kennedy, J.C.: Impingement syndrome in athletes. Am. J. Sports Med. 8:151–158, 1980.

Holsbeeck, E.: Subacromial impingement: Open versus arthroscopic decompression. Arthroscopy 8:173–178, 1992.

Kimio, N., Ozaki, J., Tomito, Y., and Tamai, S.: Magnetic resonance imaging of rotator cuff tearing and degenerative changes: Correlation with histologic pathology. J. Shoulder Elbow Surg. 2: 156–164, 1993.

Lazarus, M.D., Chansky, H.A., Misra, S., Williams, et al., Comparison of open and arthroscopic subacromial decompression. J. Shoulder Elbow Surg. 3:1–11, 1994.

Matsen, F.A., III, and Arntz, C.T.: Subacromial impingement. In The Shoulder, Rockwood, C.A., Jr., and Matsen, F.A., III, eds., pp. 623–646. Philadelphia, WB Saunders, 1990.

Neer, C.S., II: Anterior acromioplasty for the chronic impingement syndrome in the shoulder. J. Bone Joint Surg. [Am.] 54:41–50, 1972.

Rockwood, C.A., Jr., and Lyons, F.R.: Shoulder impingement syndrome: Diagnosis, radiographic evaluation, and treatment with a modified Neer acromioplasty. J. Bone Joint Surg. [Am.] 75: 409–424, 1993.

Ryu, R.K.N.: Arthroscopic subacromial decompression: A clinical review. Arthroscopy 8:141–147, 1992.

Speer, K.P., Lohnes, J., and Garrett, W.C.: Arthroscopic subacromial decompression: Results in advanced impingement syndrome. Arthroscopy 7:291–296, 1991.

Warner, J.J.P., Altchek, D.W., and Warren, R.F.: Arthroscopic management of rotator cuff tears with emphasis on the throwing athlete. Op. Tech. Orthop. 1(3):235–239, 1991.

Zuckerman, J.D., Kummer, F.J., Cuomo, F., et al.: The influence of coracoacromial arch anatomy on rotator cuff tears. J. Shoulder Elbow Surg. 1:4–14, 1992.

Biceps Injuries

Andrews, J., Carson, W., and McLeod, W.: Glenoid labrum tears related to the long head of the biceps. Am. J. Sports Med. 13: 337–341, 1985.

Burkhead, W.Z., Jr.: The biceps tendon. In The Shoulder, Rockwood, C.A., Jr., and Matsen, F.A., III, eds., pp. 791–836. Philadelphia, WB Saunders, 1990.

Froimson, A.I., and Oh, I.: Keyhole tenodesis of biceps origin at the shoulder. Clin. Orthop. 112:245–249, 1974.

Resch, H., Golser, K., Thoeni, H., and Sperner, G.: Arthroscopic repair of superior glenoid labral detachment (the SLAP lesion). J. Shoulder Elbow Surg. 2:147–155, 1993.

Snyder, S.J., and Wuh, H.C.K.: Arthroscopic evaluation and treatment of the rotator cuff and superior labrum anterior posterior lesion. Op. Tech. Orthop. 1(3):207–220.

Warren, R.F.: Lesions of the long head of the biceps tendon. Instr. Course Lect. 34:204–209, 1985.

Acromioclavicular and Sternoclavicular Injuries

Cahill, B.R.: Osteolysis of the distal part of the clavicle in male athletes. J. Bone Joint Surg. [Am.] 64:1053–1058, 1982.

Gartsman, G.M.: Arthroscopic resection of the acromioclavicular joint. Am. J. Sports Med. 21:71–77, 1993.

Richards, R.R.: Acromioclavicular joint injuries. Instr. Course Lect. 42:259–269, 1993.

Rockwood, C.A., Jr.: Disorders of the sternoclavicular joint. In The Shoulder, Rockwood, C.A., Jr., and Matsen, F.A., III, eds., pp. 477–525. Philadelphia, WB Saunders, 1990.

Rockwood, C.A., Jr.: Injuries to the acromioclavicular joint. In Fractures in Adults, 2nd ed., vol. 1, pp. 860–910. Philadelphia, JB Lippincott, 1984.

Rockwood, C.A., Jr., and Young, D.C.: Disorders of the acromioclavicular joint. In The Shoulder, Rockwood, C.A., Jr., and Matsen, F.A., III, eds., pp. 413–476. Philadelphia, WB Saunders, 1990.

Scavenius, M., and Iverson, B.F.: Nontraumatic clavicular osteolysis in weight lifters. Am. J. Sports Med. 20:463–467, 1992.

Muscle Ruptures

Berson, B.L.: Surgical repair of the pectoralis major rupture in an athlete. Am. J. Sports Med. 7:348–351, 1979.

Caughey, M.A., and Welsh, P.: Muscle ruptures affecting the shoulder girdle. In The Shoulder, Rockwood, C.A., Jr., and Matsen, F.A., III, eds., pp. 863–873. Philadelphia, WB Saunders, 1991.

Gerber, C., and Krushell, R.J.: Isolated rupture of the tendon of the subscapularis muscle. J. Bone Joint Surg. [Br.] 73:389–394, 1991.

Kretzler, H.H., Jr., and Richardson, A.B.: Rupture of the pectoralis major muscle. Am. J. Sports Med. 17:453–458, 1989.

Miller, M.D., Johnson, D.L., Fu, F.H., et al.: Rupture of the pectoralis major muscle in a collegiate football player. Am. J. Sports Med. 21:475–477, 1993.

Wolfe, S.W., Wickiewics, T.L., and Cananaugh, J.T.: Ruptures of the pectoralis major muscle: An anatomic and clinical analysis. Am. J. Sports Med. 20:587–593, 1992.

Calcific Tendinitis and Adhesive Capsulitis

Ark, J.W., Flock, T.J., Flatow, E.L., and Bigliani, L.U.: Arthroscopic treatment of calcific tendinitis of the shoulder. Arthroscopy 8: 183–188, 1992.

Coventry, M.B.: Problem of the painful shoulder. J.A.M.A. 151: 177–185, 1953.

Faure, G., and Daculsi, G.: Calcified tendinitis: A review. Ann. Rheum. Dis. 42(suppl):49–53, 1983.
Grey, R.G.: The natural history of "idiopathic" frozen shoulder. J. Bone Joint Surg. [Am.] 60:564, 1978.
Harmon, H.P.: Methods and results in the treatment of 2580 painful shoulders: With special reference to calcific tendinitis and the frozen shoulder. Am. J. Surg. 95:527–544, 1958.
Harryman, D.T., II: Shoulders: Frozen and stiff. Instr. Course Lect. 42:247–257, 1993.
Leffert, R.E.: The frozen shoulder. Instr. Course Lect. 34:199–203, 1985.
Miller, M.D., Wirth, M.A., and Rockwood, C.A., Jr.: Thawing the frozen shoulder: The "patient" patient. Orthopedics (in press).
Murnaghan, J.P.: Adhesive capsulitis of the shoulder: Current concepts and treatment. Orthopaedics 2:153–158, 1988.
Murnaghan, J.P.: Frozen shoulder. In The Shoulder, Rockwood, C.A., Jr., and Matsen, F.A., III, eds. Philadelphia, WB Saunders, 1990.
Neviaser, J.S.: Adhesive capsulitis and the stiff and painful shoulder. Orthop. Clin. North Am. 2:327–331, 1980.
Neviaser, T.J.: Adhesive capsulitis. In Operative Arthroscopy, McGinty, J.B., ed., pp. 561–566. New York, Raven Press, 1991.
Neviaser, R.J., and Neviaser, T.J.: The frozen shoulder: Diagnosis and management. Clin. Orthop. 223:59–64, 1987.
Shaffer, B., Tibone, J.E., and Kerlan, R.K.: Frozen shoulder: A long term follow-up. J. Bone Joint Surg. [Am.] 74:738–746, 1992.

Nerve Disorders

Black, K.P., and Lombardo, J.A.: Suprascapular nerve injuries with isolated paralysis of the infraspinatus. Am. J. Sports Med. 18:225, 1990.
Burkhead, W.Z., Scheinberg, R.R., and Box, G.: Surgical anatomy of the axillary nerve. J. Shoulder Elbow Surg. 1:31–36, 1992.
Drez, D.: Suprascapular neuropathy in the differential diagnosis of rotator cuff injuries. Am. J. Sports Med. 4:443, 1976.
Fechter, J.D., and Kuschner, S.H.: The thoracic outlet syndrome. Orthopedics 16:1243–1254, 1993.
Kauppila, L.I.: The long thoracic nerve: Possible mechanisms of injury based on autopsy study. J. Shoulder Elbow Surg. 2:244–248, 1993.
Leffert, R.D.: Neurological problems. In The Shoulder, Rockwood, C.A., Jr., and Matsen, F.A., III, eds., pp. 750–773. Philadelphia, WB Saunders, 1990.
Markey, K.L., DiBeneditto, M., and Curl, W.W. Upper trunk brachial plexopathy: The stinger syndrome. Am. J. Sports Med. 23: 650–655, 1993.
Marmor, L., and Bechtal, C.O.: Paralysis of the serratus anterior due to electric shock relieved by transplantation of the pectoralis major muscle. J. Bone Joint Surg. [Am.] 45:156–160, 1983.
Post, M., and Grinblat, E.: Suprascapular nerve entrapment: Diagnosis and results of treatment. J. Shoulder Elbow Surg. 2:190–197, 1993.
Vastamaki, M., and Kauppila, L.I.: Etiologic factors in isolated paralysis of the serratus anterior muscle: A report of 197 cases. J. Shoulder Elbow Surg. 2:244–248, 1993.
Warner, J.J.P., Krushell, R.J., Masquelet, A., and Gerber, C.: Anatomy and relationships of the suprascapular nerve: Anatomical constraints to mobilization of the supraspinatus and infraspinatus muscles in the management of massive rotator cuff tears. J. Bone Joint Surg. [Am.] 74A:36–45, 1992.

Other Shoulder Disorders

Matthews, L.S., Wolock, B.S., and Martin, D.F.: Arthroscopic management of degenerative arthritis of the shoulder. In Operative Arthroscopy, McGinty, J.B., ed., pp. 567–572. New York, Raven Press, 1991.
Miller, M.D., and Warner, J.J.P.: The abduction (weight bearing) radiograph of the shoulder. Poster American Academy of Orthopaedic Surgeons 61st Annual Meeting, New Orleans, 1994.

Other Upper Extremity Sports Medicine Problems

Tendon Injuries

Boyd, H.B., and Anderson, L.D.: A method for reinsertion of the distal biceps brachii tendon. J. Bone Joint Surg. [Am.] 43: 1041–1043, 1961.
Boyd, H.B., and McLeod, A.C.: Tennis elbow. J. Bone Joint Surg. [Am.] 55:1183, 1973.
Burhkhart, S.S., Wood, M.B., and Linscheid, R.L.: Posttraumatic recurrent subluxation of the extensor carpi ulnaris tendon. J. Hand Surg. 7:1, 1982.
Coonrad, R.W.: Tennis elbow. Instr. Course Lect. 35:94–101, 1986.
D'Alessandro, D.F., Shields, C.L., Tibone, J.E., and Chandler, R.W.: Repair of distal biceps tendon ruptures in athletes. Am. J. Sports Med. 21:114, 1993.
Dobyns, J.H., Sim, F.H., and Linscheid, R.L.: Sports stress syndromes of the hand and wrist. Am. J. Sports Med. 6:236, 1978.
Farrar, E.L., III, and Lippert, F.G., III: Avulsion of the triceps tendon. Clin. Orthop. 161:242–246, 1981.
Finkelstein, H.: Stenosing tendovaginitis at the radial styloid process. J. Bone Joint Surg. [Am.] 12:509, 1930.
Froimson, A.I.: Treatment of tennis elbow with forearm support band. J. Bone Joint Surg. [Am.] 53:183, 1971.
Green, D.P., and Strickland, J.W.: The hand. In Orthopaedic Sports Medicine, DeLee, J.C., and Drez, D., Jr., eds., pp. 945–1017. Philadelphia, WB Saunders, 1993.
Ilfeld, F.W.: Can stroke modification relieve tennis elbow? Clin. Orthop. 276:182–185, 1992.
Kiefhaber, T.R., and Stern, P.J.: Upper extremity tendinitis and overuse syndromes in the athlete. Clin. Sports Med. 11:39–55, 1992.
Leddy, J.P., and Packer, J.W.: Avulsion of the profundus tendon insertion in athletes. J. Hand Surg. 2:66–69, 1977.
Morrey, B.F.: Reoperation of failed surgical treatment of refractory lateral epicondylitis. J. Shoulder Elbow Surg. 1:47–55, 1992.
Moss, J.G., and Steingold, R.F.: The long term results of mallet finger injury: A retrospective study of one hundred cases. Hand 15: 151–154, 1983.
Nirschl, R.P.: Sports—and overuse injuries to the elbow. In The Elbow and Its Disorders, 2nd ed., Morrey, B.F., ed., pp. 537–552. Philadelphia, WB Saunders, 1993.
Nirschl, R.P., and Pettrone, F.: Tennis elbow: The surgical treatment of lateral epicondylitis. J. Bone Joint Surg. [Am.] 61:832, 1979.
Regan, W., Wold, L.E., Coonrad, R., and Morrey, B.F.: Microscopic histopathology of chronic refractory lateral epicondylitis. Am. J. Sports Med. 20:746–749, 1992.
Rettig, A.C.: Closed tendon injuries of the hand and wrist in the athlete. Clin. Sports Med. 11:77–99, 1992.
Strickland, J.W.: Management of acute flexor tendon injuries. Orthop. Clin. North Am. 14:827–849, 1983.
Tarsney, F.F.: Rupture and avulsion of the triceps. Clin. Orthop. 83: 177–183, 1972.
Wood, M.B., and Dobyns, J.H.: Sports-related extraarticular wrist syndromes. Clin. Orthop. 202:93–102, 1986.

Ligamentous Injuries

Alexander, C.E., and Lichtman, D.M.: Ulnar carpal instabilities. Orthop. Clin. North Am. 15:307–320, 1984.
Bennett, J.B., Green, M.S., and Tullos, H.S.: Surgical management of chronic medial elbow instability. Clin. Orthop. 278:62–68, 1992.
Betz, R.R., Browne, E.Z., Perry, G.B., and Resnick, E.J.: The complex volar metacarpophalangeal-joint dislocation. J. Bone Joint Surg. [Am.] 64:1374–1375, 1982.
Campbell, C.S.: Gamekeepers thumb. J. Bone Joint Surg. [Br.] 37: 148–149, 1955.
Conway, J.E., Jobe, F.W., Glousman, R.E., and Pink, M.: Medial instability of the elbow in throwing athletes: Surgical treatment by ulnar collateral ligament repair or reconstruction. J. Bone Joint Surg. [Am.] 74:67, 1992.
Cooney, W.P., III, Linscheid, R.L., and Dobyns, J.H.: Carpal instability: Treatment of ligament injuries of the wrist. Instr. Course Lect. 41:33–44, 1992.
Eaton, R.G., and Malerich, M.M.: Volar plate arthroplasty of the proximal interphalangeal joint: A review of ten years' experience. J. Hand Surg. 5:260–268, 1980.
Green, D.P., and Strickland, J.W.: The hand. In Orthopaedic Sports Medicine, DeLee, J.C., and Drez, D., Jr, eds., pp. 945–1017. Philadelphia, WB Saunders, 1993.
Habernek, H., and Ortner, F.: The influence of anatomic factors in elbow joint dislocation. Clin. Orthop. 274:226–230, 1992.
Hinterman, B., Holzach, P.J., Schultz, M., and Matter, P.: Skier's thumb: The significance of bony injuries. Am. J. Sports Med. 21: 800–804, 1993.

Hubbard, L.F.: Metacarpophalangeal dislocations. Hand Clin. 4: 39–44, 1988.

Isani, A., and Melone, C.P., Jr.: Ligamentous injuries of the hand in athletes. Clin. Sports Med. 5:757–772, 1986.

Jobe, F.W., and Kvitne, R.S.: Elbow instability in the athlete. Inst. Course Lect. 40:17, 1991.

Kaplan, E.B.: Dorsal dislocation of the metacarpophalangeal joint of the index finger. J. Bone Joint Surg. [Am.] 39:1081–1086, 1957.

Light, T.R.: Buttress pinning techniques. Orthop. Rev. 10:49–55, 1981.

McCue, F.C., and Bruce, J.F.: The wrist. In Orthopaedic Sports Medicine, DeLee, J.C., and Drez, D., Jr., eds., pp. 913–944. Philadelphia, WB Saunders, 1993.

McElfresh, E.C., Dobyns, J.H., and O'Brien, E.T.: Management of fracture-dislocation of the proximal interphalangeal joints by extension-block splinting. J. Bone Joint Surg. [Am.] 54:1705–1711, 1972.

McLaughlin, H.L.: Complex "locked" dislocation of the metacarpalphalangeal joints. J. Trauma 5:683–688, 1965.

Nestor, B.H., O'Driscoll, S.W., and Morrey, B.F.: Ligamentous reconstruction for posterolateral rotatory instability of the elbow. J. Bone Joint Surg. [Am.] 74:1235–1241, 1992.

O'Driscoll, S.W., and Morrey, B.F.: Arthroscopy of the elbow: Diagnostic and therapeutic benefits and hazards. J. Bone Joint Surg. [Am.] 74:84–94, 1992.

O'Driscoll, S.W., Morrey, B.F., Korinek, S., et al.: Elbow subluxation and dislocation: A spectrum of instability. Clin. Orthop. 280: 17–28, 1992.

Palmer, A.K., and Louis, D.S.: Assessing ulnar instability of the metacarpophalangeal joint of the thumb. J. Hand Surg. 3:542–546, 1978.

Redler, I., and Williams, J.T.: Rupture of a collateral ligament of the proximal interphalangeal joint of the fingers: Analysis of eighteen cases. J. Bone Joint Surg. [Am.] 49:322–326, 1967.

Stener, B.: Displacement of the ruptured collateral ligament of the metacarpophalangeal joint of the thumb: A clinical and anatomical study. J. Bone Joint Surg. [Br.] 44:869–879, 1962.

Watson, H.K., and Ballet, F.L.: The SLAC wrist: Scapholunate advanced collapse pattern of degenerative arthritis. J. Hand Surg. 9A:358–365, 1984.

Watson, H.K., and Hempton, R.F.: Limited wrist arthrodesis. I. The triscaphoid joint. J. Hand Surg. 5:320–327, 1980.

Wilson, F.D., Andrews, J.R., Blackburn, T.A., and McCluskey, G.: Valgus extension overload in the pitching elbow. Am. J. Sports Med. 11:83, 1983.

Articular Injuries

Almquist, E.E., and Burns, J.F.: Radial shortening for the treatment of Kienbock's disease—a 5 to 10 year follow-up. J. Hand Surg. 7: 348–352, 1982.

Armstead, R.B., Linscheid, R.L., Dobyns, J.H., et al.: Ulnar lengthening in the treatment of Kienbock's disease. J. Bone Joint Surg. [Am.] 64:170–178, 1982.

Aulicino, P.L., and Siegel, L.: Acute injuries of the distal radioulnar joint. Hand Clin. 7:283–293, 1991.

Bauer, M., Jonsson, K., Josefsson, P.O., and Linden, B.: Osteochondritis dissecans of the elbow: A long-term follow-up study. Clin. Orthop. 284:156–160, 1992.

Bennett, J.B.: Articular injuries in the athlete. In The Elbow and Its Disorders, 2nd ed., Morrey, B.F., ed., pp. 581–595. Philadelphia, WB Saunders, 1993.

Bowers, W.H.: The distal radioulnar joint. In Operative Hand Surgery, 3rd ed., Green, D.P., ed., pp. 973–1019. New York, Churchill Livingstone 1993.

DeHaven, K.E., and Evarts, C.M.: Throwing injuries of the elbow in athletes. Orthop. Clin. North Am. 1:801, 1973.

Dell, P.C.: Traumatic disorders of the distal radioulnar joint. Clin. Sports Med. 11:141–159, 1991.

Feldon, P., Belsky, M.R., and Terrono, A.L.: Partial ("wafer") distal ulna resection for triangular fibrocartilage tears and/or ulnar impaction syndrome. J. Hand Surg. 15A:826–827, 1990.

Gelberman, R.H., Salamon, P.B., Jurist, J.M., and Posch, J.L.: Ulnar variance in Kienbock's disease. J. Bone Joint Surg. [Am.] 57: 674–676, 1975.

Morrey, B.F.: Primary arthritis of the elbow treated by ulno-humeral arthroplasty. J. Bone Joint Surg. [Br.] 74:409, 1992.

Murakami, S., and Nakajima, H.: Aseptic necrosis of the capitate bone. Am. J. Sports Med. 12:170–173, 1984.

Nalebuff, E.A., Poehling, G.G., Siegel, D.B., and Koman, L.A.: Wrist and hand: Reconstruction. In Orthopaedic Knowledge Update 4 Home Study Syllabus, Frymoyer, J.W., ed., pp. 389–402. Rosemont, IL, American Academy of Orthopaedic Surgeons, 1993.

Osterman, A.L.: Arthroscopic debridement of triangular fibrocartilage complex tears. Arthroscopy 6:120–124, 1990.

Palmer, A.K.: Triangular fibrocartilage disorders: Injury patterns and treatment. Arthroscopy 6:125–132, 1990.

Pappas, A.M.: Elbow problems associated with baseball during childhood and adolescence. Clin. Orthop. 164:30, 1982.

Singer, K.M., and Roy, S.P.: Osteochondrosis of the humeral capitellum. Am. J. Sports Med. 12:351–360, 1984.

Watson, H.K., Ryu, J., and DiBella, W.S.: An approach to Kienbock's disease: Triscaphe arthrodesis. J. Hand Surg. 10A:179–187, 1985.

Woodward, A.H., and Bianco, A.J.: Osteochondritis dissecans of the elbow. Clin. Orthop. 110:35, 1975.

Arthroscopy

Andrews, J.R., and Carson, W.G.: Arthroscopy of the elbow. Arthroscopy 1:97, 1985.

Boe, S.: Arthroscopy of the elbow: Diagnosis and extraction of loose bodies. Acta Orthop. Scand. 57:52, 1986.

Carson, W.: Arthroscopy of the elbow. Instr. Course Lect. 37:195, 1988.

Cooney, W.P., Dobyns, J.H., and Linscheid, R.L.: Arthroscopy of the wrist: Anatomy and classification of carpal instability. Arthroscopy 6:133–140, 1990.

Guhl, J.: Arthroscopy and arthroscopic surgery of the elbow. Orthopedics 8:1290, 1985.

Lindenfeld, T.N.: Medial approach in elbow arthroscopy. Am. J. Sports Med. 18:413–417, 1990.

Lynch, G., Meyers, J., Whipple, T., and Caspari, R.: Neurovascular anatomy and elbow arthroscopy: Inherent risks. Arthroscopy 2: 191, 1986.

North, E.R., and Meyer, S.: Wrist injuries: Correlation of clinical and arthroscopic findings. J. Hand Surg. 15A:915–920, 1990.

Osterman, A.L.: Arthroscopic debridement of triangular fibrocartilage complex tears. Arthroscopy 6:120–124, 1990.

Poehling, G.G., Siegel, D.B., Koman, L.A., and Chabon, S.J.: Arthroscopy of the wrist and elbow. In Orthopaedic Sports Medicine, DeLee, J.C., and Drez, D., Jr., eds., pp. 189–214. Philadelphia, WB Saunders, 1993.

Roth, J.H., Poehling, G.G., and Whipple, T.L.: Arthroscopic surgery of the wrist. Instr. Course Lect. 37:183–194, 1988.

Whipple, T.L.: Diagnostic and surgical arthroscopy of the wrist. In The Upper Extremity in Sports Medicine, Nichols, J.A., and Hershman, E.B., eds., pp. 399–418. St. Louis, CV Mosby, 1990.

Head and Spine Injuries

Head Injuries

Bruno, L.A.: Focal intracranial hematoma. In Athletic Injuries to the Head, Neck and Face, 2nd ed., Torg, J.S., ed. St. Louis, Mosby-Year Book, 1991.

Cantu, R.C.: Criteria for return to competition after a closed head injury. In Athletic Injuries to the Head, Neck and Face, 2nd ed., Torg, J.S., ed. St. Louis, Mosby-Year Book, 1991.

Cantu, R.C.: Guidelines to return to sports after cerebral concussion. Phys. Sports Med. 14:76, 1986.

Gennarelli, T.A.: Head injury mechanisms, and cerebral concussion and diffuse brain injuries. In Athletic Injuries to the Head, Neck and Face, 2nd ed., Torg, J.S., ed. St. Louis: Mosby-Year Book, 1991.

Jordan, B.D., Tsairis, P., and Warren, R.F.: Sports Neurology. Rockville, MD, Aspen Press, 1989.

Lindsay, K.W., McLatchie, G., Jennett, B.: Serious head injuries in sports. B.M.J. 281:789–791, 1980.

Cervical Spine Injuries

Albright, J.P., Moses, J.M., Feldich, H.G., et al.: Non-fatal cervical spine injuries in interscholastic football. J.A.M.A. 236:1243–1245, 1976.

Bracken, M.D., Shepard, M.J., Collins, W.F., et al.: A randomized, controlled trial of methylprednisolone or naloxone in the treatment of acute spinal cord injury. N. Engl. J. Med. 322:1405, 1990.

Pavlov, H., Torg, J.S., Robie, B., and Jahre, C.: Cervical spinal stenosis: Determination with vertebral body radio method. Radiology 164:771–775, 1987.

Schneider, R.C. The syndrome of acute anterior spinal cord injury. J. Neurosurg. 12:95–123, 1955.

Thompson, R.C.: Current concepts in management of cervical spine fractures and dislocations. Am. J. Sports Med. 3:159, 1975.

Torg, J.S., and Gennarelli, T.A.: Head and cervical spine injuries. In Orthopaedic Sports Medicine: Principles and Practice, DeLee, J.C., and Drez, D., Jr., eds., pp. 417–462. Philadelphia, WB Saunders, 1994.

Torg, J.S., Pavolv, H., Genuario, S.E., et al.: Neuropraxia of the cervical spinal cord with transient quadriplegia. J. Bone Joint Surg. [Am.] 68:1354–1370, 1986.

Torg, J.S., Sennett, B., Pavlov, H., Leventhal, M.R., and Glasgow, S.G.: Spear tackler's spine: An entity precluding participation in tackle football and collision activities that expose the cervical spine to axial energy inputs. Am. J. Sports Med. 21:640–649, 1993.

Torg, J.S., Sennett, B., Vegso, J.J., and Pavlov, H.: Axial loading injuries to the middle cervical spine segment: An analysis and classification of twenty-five cases. Am. J. Sports Med. 19:6–20, 1991.

Torg, J.S., Vegso, J.J., O'Neill, J., and Sennett, B.: The epidemiologic, pathologic, biomechanical and cinematographic analysis of football-induced cervical spine trauma. Am. J. Sports Med. 18:50–57, 1990.

White, A.A., Johnson, R.M., and Panjabi, M.M.: Biomechanical analysis of clinical stability in the cervical spine. Clin. Orthop. 109: 85–93, 1975.

Thoracic and Lumbar Spine Injuries

Bradford, D.S., and Boachie-Adjei, O.: Treatment of severe spondylolisthesis by anterior and posterior reduction and stabilization: a long-term follow-up study. J. Bone Joint Surg. [Am.] 72:1060, 1990.

Eismont, F.J., and Currier, B.: Surgical management of lumbar intervertebral disc disease. J. Bone Joint Surg. [Am.] 71:1266, 1989.

Eismont, F.J., and Kitchel, S.H.: Thoracolumbar spine. In Orthopaedic Sports Medicine, DeLee, J.C., and Drez, D., Jr., eds., pp. 1018–1062. Philadelphia, WB Saunders, 1994.

Jackson, D., Wiltse, L., Dingeman, R., and Hayes, M.: Stress reactions involving the pars interarticularis in young athletes. Am. J. Sports Med. 9:305, 1981.

Jacobs, R.R., Asher, M.A., and Snider, R.K.: Thoracolumbar spine injuries. Spine 5:463, 1986.

Keene, J.S., Albert, M.J., Springer, S.L., Drummond, D.S., and Clancy, W.G.: Back injuries in college athletes. J. Spinal Disord. 2:190–195, 1989.

Mundt, D.J., Kelsey, J.L., Golden, A.L., et al.: An epidemiological study of sports and weightlifting as possible risk factors for herniated lumbar and cervical discs. Am. J. Sports Med. 21:854–860, 1993.

Medical Aspects

Ergogenic Drugs

Aronson, V.: Protein and miscellaneous ergogenic aids. Physician Sports Med. 14:209–212, 1986.

Bahrke, M.S., Wright, J.E., Strauss, R.H., and Catlin, D.H.: Psychological moods and subjectively perceived behavioral and somatic changes accompanying anabolic-androgenic steroid use. Am. J. Sports Med. 20:717–724.

Brien, A.J., and Simon, T.L.: The effects of red blood cell infusion on 10-km race time. J.A.M.A. 257:2761, 1987.

Cowart, V.S.: Human growth hormone: The latest ergogenic aid? Physician Sports Med. 16:175, 1988.

Coyle, E.F.: Ergogenic aids. Clin. Sports Med. 3:731–742, 1984.

Haupt, H.A.: Anabolic steroids and growth hormone: Current concepts. Am. J. Sports Med. 21:468–474, 1993.

Perlmutter, G., and Lowenthal, D.T. Use of anabolic steroids by athletes. Am. Fam. Physician 32:208, 1985.

Pope, H.G., Katz, D.L., and Champoux, R.: Anabolic-androgenic steroid use among 1,010 college men. Physician Sports Med. 16:75, 1988.

Robinson, J.B.: Ergogenic drugs in sports. In Orthopaedic Sports Medicine, DeLee, J.C., and Drez, D., Jr., eds., pp. 294–306. Philadelphia, WB Saunders, 1994.

Sawka, M.N.: Erythrocyte reinfusion and maximal aerobic power: An examination of modifying factors. J.A.M.A. 257:1496, 1987.

Sudden Cardiac Death

Alpert, S.A., et al.: Athletic heart syndrome. Physician Sports Med. 12:103–107, 1989.

Braden, D.S., and Strong, W.B.: Preparticipation screening for sudden cardiac death in high school and college athletes. Physician Sports Med. 16:128–140, 1988.

Epstein, S.E., and Maron, B.J.: Sudden death and the competitive athlete: Perspectives on preparticipation screening studies. J. Am. Coll. Cardiol. 7:220–230, 1986.

Finney, T.P., and D'Ambrosia, R.D.: Sudden cardiac death in an athlete. In Orthopaedic Sports Medicine, DeLee, J.C., and Drez, D., Jr., eds., pp. 404–416. Philadelphia, WB Saunders 1994.

James, T.N., Froggatt, P., and Marshall, T.K.: Sudden death in young athletes. Ann. Intern. Med. 67:1013–1021, 1967.

Maron, B.J., Epstein, S.E., and Roberts, W.C.: Causes of sudden death in competitive athletes. J. Am. Coll. Cardiol. 7:204–214, 1986.

Maron, B.J., Roberts, W.C., McAllister, H.A., Rosing, D.R., and Epstein, S.E.: Sudden death in young athletes. Circulation 62: 218–229, 1980.

Van Camp, S.P.: Exercise-related sudden deaths: Risks and causes. Physician Sports Med. 16:97–112, 1988.

Exercise Physiology

Fleck, S.J., and Schutt, R.C.: Types of strength training. Clin. Sports Med. 4(1):159–168, 1985.

Katch, F.I., and Drumm, S.S.: Effects of different modes of strength training on body composition and arthropometry. Clin. Sports Med. 5(3):413–459, 1986.

Paulos, L.E., Grauer, J.D.: Exercise. In Orthopaedic Sports Medicine: Principles and Practice, Delee, J.C., and Drez, D., Jr., eds., pp. 228–243. Philadelphia, WB Saunders, 1994.

Pipes, T.V.: Isokinetic vs isotonic strength training an adult men. Med. Sci. Sports 7:262–274, 1975.

Taylor, D.C., Dalton, J.D., Seaber, A.V., et al.: Viscoelastic properties of muscle-tendon units: The biomechanical effects of stretching. Am. J. Sports Med. 18:300–309, 1990.

Yamamoto, S.K., Hartman, C.W., Feagin, J.A., and Kimball, G.: Functional rehabilitation of the knee: A preliminary study. J. Sports Med. 3(6):228–291, 1976.

Female Athletes

Barrow, G., and Saha, S.: Menstrual irregularity and stress fractures in collegiate female distance runners. Am. J. Sports Med. 16: 209–215, 1988.

Clarke, K., and Buckley, W.: Women's injuries in collegiate sports. Am. J. Sports Med. 8:187–191, 1980.

Cox, J., and Lenz, H.: Women in sports: The Naval Academy experience. Am. J. Sports Med. 7:355–357, 1979.

Eisenberg, T., and Allen, W.: Injuries in a women's varsity athletic program. Physician Sports Med. 6:112–116, 1978.

Hunter, L., Andrews, J., Clancy, W., and Funk, F.: Common orthopaedic problems of the female athlete. Instr. Course Lect. 31: 126–152, 1982.

Powers, J.: Characteristic features of injuries in the knee in women. Clin. Orthop. 143:120–124, 1979.

Protzman, R.: Physiologic performance of women compared to men: Observations of cadets at the United States Military Academy. Am. J. Sports Med. 7:191–194, 1979.

Whiteside, P.: Men's and women's injuries in comparable sports. Physician Sports Med. 8:130–140, 1980.

4

ADULT RECONSTRUCTION

NICHOLAS SOTEREANOS, JOHN FERNANDEZ, and CHARLES A. ENGH

I. Hip Reconstruction

A. Arthrodesis—Favored in **young** patients with **unilateral** hip disease (usually posttraumatic) with a **good back and ipsilateral knee.** A return to normal activity, including manual labor, can be expected with excellent pain relief. Indications include arthritis, failed osteotomies, and failed cup arthroplasty in young patients. Preoperative immobilization (hip spica) is commonly used to acquaint the patient with postoperative expectations. Fusion in neutral adduction and rotation with **30 degrees of flexion** is recommended; **avoid abduction** and internal rotation. Fixation is with Barr bolts or the AO Cobra plate (more stable but disrupts abductors). Complications include nonunion, malposition (most common), degenerative joint disease (DJD), and/or instability of the ipsilateral knee, back, and contralateral hip. Arthrodesis should not be done bilaterally but can be done with a contralateral total hip arthroplasty (THA).

1. Conversion to total hip arthroplasty—Revising an ankylosed hip to a total hip arthroplasty is fraught with complications and should be reserved for those with strict indications such as painful malunions or non-union, and difficulties of the lumbar spine or knees refractory to conservative measures. Complications include component failure, dislocation and infection. Forty-eight percent of those patients with surgical ankylosis will have a complicated course after conversion to THA versus those patients with spontaneous ankylosis with a documented 5% complication rate. (This is probably related to preservation of hip abductors.) Also, an age of 50 or less does not correlate with a higher failure rate. The risk of failure does not correlate with length of time from ankylosis.

B. Resection Arthroplasty—Indicated for incurable infection (especially after failed THA), post-radiation osteonecrosis, or in patients with minimal or no ambulation potential with poor mental status and high medical risk. A shortening of 2–5 cm and severe Trendelenburg gait can be expected, and most patients require support to ambulate. When done bilaterally, there are significant increases in oxygen consumption.

C. Femoral Osteotomy—Although used commonly in Europe for advanced DJD, its use in the United States is usually restricted to localized structural defects that can be redirected to a nonweight bearing area. Intertrochanteric osteotomies are commonly done after examining radiographs in abduction, adduction, internal rotation are studied to plan for the best correction. Congruence achieved in *ad*duction is a major criterion for selecting a **valgus** osteotomy (also referred to as an *ab*duction osteotomy). An increased neck-to-shaft angle, superolateral joint space narrowing, sphericity of the femoral head, and congruence achieved in *ab*duction are all criteria for selecting a **varus** osteotomy (also referred to as an *ad*duction osteotomy). A varus osteotomy is the most common. The best results are in young, nonobese patients with good range of motion (ROM) and radiographs with focal defects. In summary, if the femoral head fits better with the head in *ab*duction, a varus or *ad*duction osteotomy is performed. In contrast, when the femoral head is more congruent with the hip in *ad*duction, a valgus or *ab*duction osteotomy is performed (Fig. 4–1).

D. Pelvic Osteotomies (see Chapter 2, Pediatric Orthopaedics)—Can allow redirection of acetabular cartilage (Steel, Sutherland, Salter, Dome/Dial) or augment the acetabulum with extra-articular bone (Chiari, shelf). Redirection osteotomies require a congruent joint space (relatively early arthritis with >50% joint space and >60% ROM remaining); the Chiari and shelf procedures are salvage procedures (articular cartilage reduced by >50%). Table 4–1 summarizes the salient features of each.

E. Resurfacing Arthroplasty—Femoral resurfacing implants became popular during the late 1970s; however, because of frequent failure (20–50% at 5 years) they are not currently indicated. Failure occurred frequently at the femoral neck due to disruption of the vascular supply and femoral neck osteolysis. Revision was difficult when loosening occurred due to large acetabular bone loss. Long-term follow-up reveals significant rates of osteolysis possibly secondary to a large femoral head articulation and thin polyethylene.

F. Hemiarthroplasty—Requires a normal acetabulum and therefore is rarely used for arthritis. This procedure may be indicated with osteonecrosis or hip fracture and can be converted later to a THA. No significant difference has been reported when comparing unipolar to bipolar implants (other than cost). There is a higher rate of acetabular protrusio when performed on patients with inflammatory arthritis and, therefore, is contraindicated in these patients.

G. Total Hip Arthroplasty

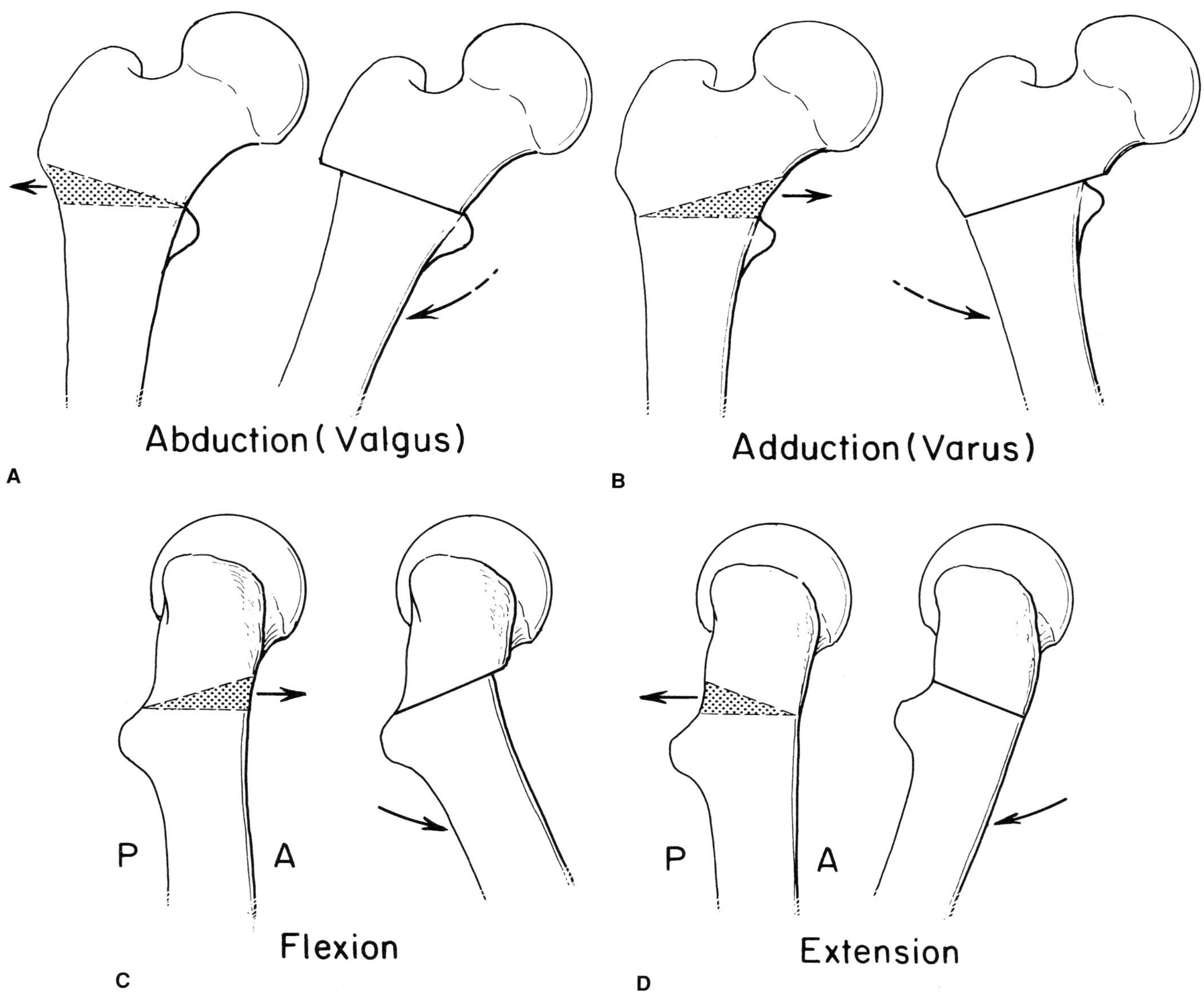

FIGURE 4–1. Femoral osteotomies.

1. Indications—Expanded from the original primary indication of incapacitating pain in >65 year-old patients refractory to all medical and surgical therapy (short of resection arthroplasty); now includes rheumatoid arthritis (RA), osteonecrosis, developmental dysplasia of the hip (DDH), fractures, failed reconstruction, and tumors. It should also be considered in young patients with significant back or ipsilateral knee DJD (who are not candidates for fusion). Conservative therapy, including weight loss, anti-inflammatory medications, limitation of activity, and use of a cane (in **contralateral** hand)

TABLE 4–1. FEATURES OF VARIOUS PELVIC OSTEOTOMIES

PROCEDURE	OSTEOTOMIES	INDICATION	OTHER
Salter	Innominate (open wedge)	Youth/anterior deficiency	Poor lateral coverage/length
Steel	Innominate and both rami	Increased dislocation	Increased instability, complex
Sutherland	Innominate and pubis	Can medially displace	Less rotation
Dome/Dial	Acetabulum subchondral	Good cartilage	Osteonecrosis and penetration
Chiari	Innominate (displaces roof)	Salvage	Loses cartilage and cartilage continuity (fibrocartilage metaplasia)

should be exhausted prior to considering THA. Persistent symptoms of pain with limited ambulation, night pain, and severe quality of life limitations despite conservative therapy are now recognized as the principal indications for THA. Contraindications include pre-existing medical problems that have not been optimized (e.g., cardiac, pulmonary, GI), physiologic age >80, nonambulators, and the skeletally immature. Specific contraindications include active infection, rapid destruction of bone, neurotrophic joint, abductor mass loss, and progressive neurologic disease.

2. Preoperative Assessment—Careful preoperative evaluation that includes medical and dental evaluation, laboratory studies, and surgical planning (e.g., approach, templating) is necessary. Pre- and postoperative antibiotics have been recommended (most important variable in controlling sepsis), and careful preparation of the patient and the room is indicated to decrease the incidence of infection. The use of laminar flow, special surgical exhaust systems, and special drapes may reduce rates of infection. Deep vein thrombosis (DVT) prophylaxis usually includes the use of Coumadin (Warfarin) perioperatively.
   a. Radiographic Evaluations—Minimum necessary views include an AP pelvis film, a cross-table lateral view centered at the hip and an AP view centered at the hip (preferably with a magnification marker) and leg internally rotated 15 degrees.
      When the femur is **internally rotated** 15 degrees, the **lesser trochanter** is less discernible and the anteversion is taken out of the femoral neck. This gives a "true" anterior/posterior view of the greater trochanter which facilitates templating.
      The quality of the bone is judged on both views and typed A, B, and C, per Goodman et al.
      Type A: Good cortical bone on both AP and lateral views
      Type B: Cortical thinning posteriorly on lateral view
      Type C: Cortical thinning on AP and lateral views
3. Surgical Approach—Many favor the anterolateral approach (with or without a greater trochanteric osteotomy); however, the posterior approach is also commonly used (possibly increased incidence of posterior dislocation but component positioning is the most critical factor).
4. Components
   a. Femoral Component—Designed for either cemented or noncemented (press fit and/or porous ingrowth) use. Other differences are based on metal type and design properties. Stainless steel or "supermetal" alloys (Co-Cr-Mo) have been used most frequently, but newer implants using titanium may allow increased implant load transmission to the cement and bone in the calcar region. Poor wear characteristics of titanium has lead to use of Co-Cr heads on titanium stems. Mechanical loosening is also a problem (loosening in torsion most common). Press-fit prostheses rely on bone formation about the stem to allow a tight fit. Porous-coated implants have surface openings of 150–400 μm to allow bone ingrowth. Initial stability is best achieved by maximum interference fit with less than 150 microns of motion. Stems are often not coated distally to allow later removal for revision. Proximally (as opposed to fully) porous coated implants, may (theoretically) decrease the amount of stress shielding to the proximal femur. This is related to where stress transfer occurs (proximal with proximally porous coated stems). Complications are still not fully understood but may include metal ion release and loosening. Additionally, **postoperative thigh pain** is common and may last up to a year or more. Newer materials, coatings, and designs may allow better results in the future. Hydroxyapatite coatings and fibermesh (as opposed to beaded design) allow better ingrowth in animal models. Cemented stems are best for older patients (>65 years physiologic age) with poor bone quality (e.g., type "C" bone with thin cortices and no fluting). Uncemented stems are best for young patients and for revision surgery. Collared designs appear to have decreased subsidence rates and higher load-to-failure ratios. Mechanical effect of collar decreases cement stress.
   b. Femoral Head—Available in different diameters. The smallest diameter heads (22 mm) allow less stress/torque but may result in increased central acetabular wear. Larger head sizes (up to 32 mm) allow increased ROM and may reduce dislocation but have less net wall thickness and increased volumetric wear. Heads of 26–28 mm appear to be the ideal compromise and are most commonly used. Controversy exits over corrosion between the morse taper and femoral head. Increased corrosion (fretting and galvanic) may occur between titanium stems and cobalt chrome heads.
   c. Acetabular component—Like the femoral component, it is designed either for cemented of non-cemented use. Noncemented prostheses which rely on a macrolock screw in design have increased incidence of loosening. Porous coated designs usually rely on temporary fixation with screws. Placement of these screws anteriorly has been demonstrated to be dangerous **(iliac vein is at risk with anterosuperior screws; obturator artery is at risk with anteroinferior screws).** Currently, under reaming and press fitting porous coated implants (without screws) is becoming popular.
   d. Acetabular Cup—Typically ultrahigh-molecular-weight polyethylene (UHMWPE). Thickness is based on femoral head size and can include a lip of 10–20 degrees ("dial-a-prayer") that may reduce the incidence of postoperative dislocation.
5. Component Position—The femoral component should be placed in slight valgus with the neck in 5–10 degrees of anteversion (Fig. 4–2). The acetabulum should be placed in 10–15 degrees of anteversion and 45 degrees of vertical inclination. Deviations increase the incidence of dislocation. Acetabulums placed in a more vertical orientation also are associated with increased polyethylene wear and osteolysis most likely related to edge loading of the polyethylene.

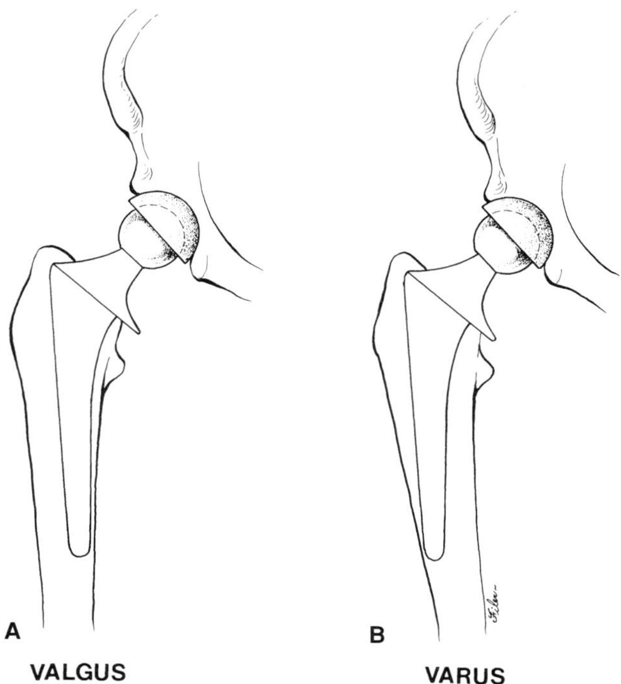

FIGURE 4–2. Femoral stem positioning. *A*, Valgus. *B*, Varus.

6. Complications
   a. Osteolysis—Significant cause for failure under intense investigation. Wear of biomaterials generates particulate debris to which the immune system responds. Macrophages and giant cells generate PGE_2, collagenase, and other humoral factors leading to resorption of bone at the bone–cement interface. Polyethylene particles are classically implicated but others include particulates of polymethylmethacralate and titanium. There is some experimental evidence which shows titanium particles to be more inflammatory than particles of cobalt chrome. Factors influencing wear include component conformity, contact stresses, material "tougheners," and metal fretting. Future directions are aimed at decreasing wear by improving characteristics of materials (i.e., ceramic heads and toughening polyethylene and possible metal on metal articulations).
   b. Loosening—The most common long-term complication of a cemented femoral prosthesis. It can be based on radiographic or clinical grounds. Radiographic grounds for loosening have been developed by Harris et al, into three groups: **Definitely** loose includes those with component migration, cement cracks, or component fracture. **Probably** loose includes those with radiolucent zones circumferentially including the entire prosthesis. **Possibly** loose are those with radiolucency of more than 50% but not the entire prosthesis. There is a 10–40% incidence of radiographic loosening at 10 years. Early loosening (first 5 years) is usually from the **femoral** component at the **prosthesis–cement interface;** late loosening is usually from the acetabular component. Loosening is more frequent with young patients, RA patients, heavy patients, and patients with prior hip surgery. The diagnosis and treatment of loosening are largely based on the patient's symptoms. Bone scans may be beneficial but are not specific. Arthrograms are not usually helpful but can sometimes be helpful, particularly if the patient is allowed to ambulate after injection. Aspiration and culture are often included with an arthrogram, but may be done separately to rule out septic loosening. False negative rates range from 15–30%. The injection of an anesthetic into the joint is also helpful in establishing the diagnosis of symptomatic loosening. The ultimate treatment for patients with increased symptoms, progressive radiographic loosening (subsidence), and failure to respond to conservative therapy may be surgical intervention, if necessary. Specific points regarding stem and cup loosening follow.
      1. Stem Loosening—Four modes of femoral stem loosening have been described for cemented hip replacement (Gruen) (Table 4–2; Fig. 4–3). **Cracks most commonly begin in the cement mantle on the anterolateral surface** of the femoral prosthesis. Uncemented stems with a porous surface fail if bone does not grow into the porous surface. This is usually an early post-operative event. Late loosening of a well fixed porous coated stem is rare.
      2. Cup Loosening—Description based on three zones (DeLee); I, superior; II, middle; III, inferior (Fig. 4–3). The acetabular cup is considered loose if there is a radiolucency >2 mm in all three zones, **progressive loosening** in one or two zones, or change in position of cup. Loosening between the cement and cup is unusual (versus femoral stem). The popular use of non-cemented press-fit components in the acetabulum, even with cemented stems (hybrid design), has reduced cup loosening problems. Loosening of cemented acetabular components may be related to osteolysis and not frank mechanical failure of the cement mantle.
      3. Cement technique—Centrifugation or vacuum mixing can decrease the porosity of cement (centrifugation is more effective), thus giving a theoretical advantage in terms of developing cement column stress fractures. Preparation of the canal, pulse lavage, and pressurization of the cement column also give theoretical advantages. The combination of canal plugging, reduced cement porosity, canal preparation, and cement column pressurization are referred to as third generation cementing technique.
   c. Implant Failure
      1. Stem Failure—Increased incidence with heavy, active patients; varus position of the stem; stems with decreased cross-sectional area and long necks; stainless steel components; and poor support in the proximal

TABLE 4–2. MODES OF CEMENTED FEMORAL STEM LOOSENING

MODE	MECHANISM	CAUSE	FINDINGS/RESULTS
I	Pistoning	Subsidence	Stem in cement or cement mantle
II	Medial stem pivot	Medial migration	Proximal medial, distal lateral shift
III	Calcar pivot	Distal toggle	Windshield wiper effect
IV	Cantilever bending[a]	Proximal resorption	Medial migration, defect, or *fracture of proximal stem*

[a] Most common

third (**bending cantilever fatigue**). A fracture usually begins in the middle third of the anterolateral aspect of the stem and progresses medially.

2. Acetabular Wear—Although initially a big concern, wear rates of **less than 0.1 mm/year** can be expected, partly due to UHMWPE. Wear rates can be increased with loose prostheses or acrylic debris. Metal backing on prostheses has reduced stresses in cement and trabecular bone but has not decreased polyethylene wear. Proximal femoral osteolysis is associated with polyethylene wear and can lead to loosening of cemented and uncemented stems (late loosening).

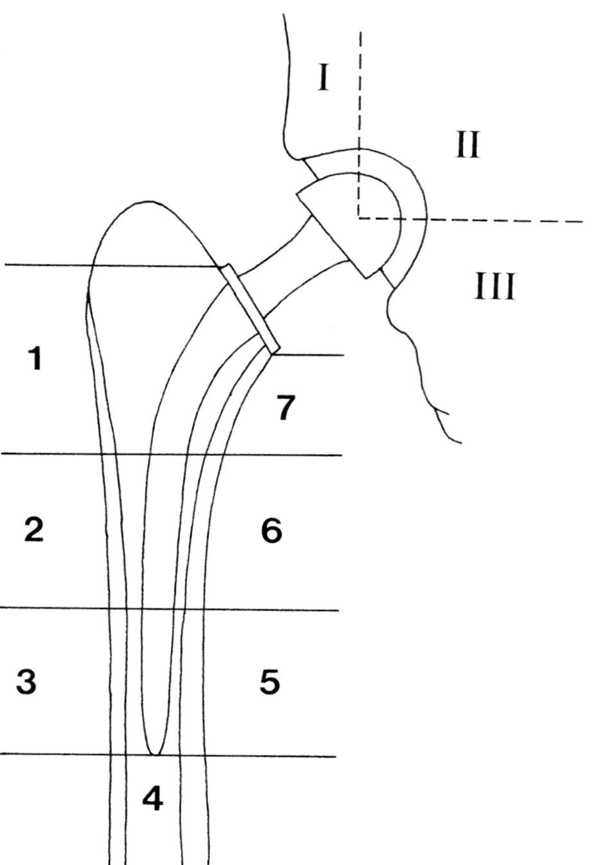

FIGURE 4–3. Zones of loosening in THA. (Modified from Gruen, T.A., McNeice, G.M., and Amstutz, H.C.: Modes of failure of cemented stem-type femoral components. Clin. Orthop. 141:17–27, 1979; and DeLee, J.C., and Charnley, J.: Radiologic demarcation of cemented sockets in total hip replacement. Clin. Orthop. 121:20–32, 1976; reprinted by permission.)

d. Dislocation—Occurs in 1–4% of primary THAs. Most commonly caused by "looseness" of the hip (improper neck length with subsequent "pistoning" and poor abductor tension) and component malposition (anteversion/anterior dislocation; retroversion/posterior dislocation). Dislocations are most common with revision THAs (revisions for dislocations especially). Careful testing with trial components for correction of neck length, impingement, and repair of the greater trochanter may avoid this complication. Late dislocation may be related to gradual stretching of the pseudocapsule. Patient education is also a critical factor. After reduction, treatment with 3–6 weeks of immobilization in abduction with a brace or hip spica may be indicated. Recurrent dislocation should be managed with aspiration (to rule out sepsis) and revision if indicated. Posterior dislocations are more common than anterior dislocations. Dislocation may be more common in radiation therapy osteonecrosis; acetabular components should be placed more horizontally in these patients.

e. Heterotopic Bone—Increased incidence in males those with ankylosing spondylitis, diffuse idiopathic skeletal hyperostosis (DISH), posttraumatic arthritis, heterotopic osteoarthritis, and patients who previously formed heterotopic bone. Treatment with low-dose radiation therapy (800–1000) cGy (rads) immediately postoperatively has been most effective for prophylactic treatment of patients at risk. Indomethacin (1 month preop to 3 months postop) has also been shown to be a useful prophylaxis. These agents may affect porous ingrowth and therefore are generally indicated for cemented components. Radiation can be used if the ingrowth areas of the components are shielded with lead.

f. Thromboembolic (TE) Disease—Most common serious complication of THA and a significant cause of postop mortality. An increased incidence can be expected with older patients, osteoarthritis (versus RA), history of TE disease, obesity, and long operations with large blood loss. Other factors include congestive heart failure (CHF), malignancy, and prolonged immobility. Adjusted dose warfarin appears to be the best prophylaxis. Other schemes include minidose heparin, enteric-coated aspirin, dextran, and pneumatic devices. B-mode ultrasonography can be helpful for diagnosing deep vein thrombosis (DVT), but venography is still best. Ventilation-perfusion (V/Q) scan and pulmonary angiography may be required to establish the diagnosis of pulmonary embolism (PE) prior to starting a heparin drip, which is followed by 3–6 months of warfarin therapy. Venous filters are reserved for high-risk patients. Low molecular weight heparin has also been effective in clinical trials (can be reversed with Protamine).

g. Intraoperative Complications—Can include fracture (especially medial calcar), which is treated with cerclage wiring and in some cases longer femoral stems; neurovascular injury (common peroneal branch of the sciatic is more common and results in footdrop); significant vascular injury from acetabular screws placed anteriorly [superiorly and inferiorly]); shaft penetrations (especially laterally during revision THA when the medial cement is not removed early); and various other catastrophes. Hypotension during cement insertion may be associated with complement activation; it is usually transient; however, at times it may be fatal. Prior to pressurizing the cement mantle, care must be taken to ensure the patient is hemodynamically stable with adequate volume resuscitation (inform anesthesiologist prior to pressurization) and that the cement is viscous. Postoperative "cement venograms" can occur, and are associated with hypotension and death.

h. Greater Trochanteric Problems—Nonunions of the trochanter after osteotomy may do well after wire removal or may require reapproximation. Fortunately, greater trochanteric osteotomy is used less commonly, although cable fixation devices may create a resurgence of its use. Greater trochanteric bursitis is common but usually responds to hip abductor strengthening and steroid injection.

i. Infection—Perhaps the most devastating and dreaded complication. It often results in removal of components, increased morbidity, and often mortality. The incidence of infection is increased with obesity, diabetes, sickle cell disease, osteonecrosis, alcoholism, RA, patients on immunosuppressive drugs (including steroids), and postoperative urinary catheterization. The chance of infection is increased with longer procedures and revisions. The use of IV antibiotics, ultraclean air, ultraviolet lights and decreased traffic and conversation in the operating room during surgery may help decrease infection. Prophylactic regimens of antibiotics for dental, oral, GI, GU, and respiratory procedures should be followed and patients counseled regarding their use (see Table 4–3). The most common organisms include *Staph. aureus* (penicillin, cefazolin), *streptococcus* (penicillin), *E. coli* (amphotericin ± gentamicin) and *Pseudomonas* (gentamicin, ticarcillin). The presentation of infection usually involves pain (especially at rest). Laboratory studies are often not helpful (however, ESR and C-reactive protein levels are usually elevated). A bone scan, indium scan, and aspiration are most helpful. Tissue biopsies at the time of débridement (with frozen section confirmation of >**5 PMNs/high-power field**) are also useful for diagnosing infection. Acute infections (within the first 12 weeks) are managed with irrigation and debridement (superficial only if not confirmed deep by aspiration of joint; posterolateral incision if infection in joint to allow better drainage), preservation of hardware if it is not loose, and IV antibiotics for 4–6 weeks followed by oral antibiotics for at least another 6 weeks. Close follow-up is necessary. Deep delayed infections (3–24 months postop) require removal of prosthesis and all cement as well as long-term antibiotics. Exchange arthroplasty for less virulent organisms should follow at least a several-week delay. Late hematogenous infections occur more than 2 years after surgery and can follow an infection elsewhere. Removal of components and all cement is required, and an extended delay should precede a decision to insert a replacement prosthesis. Recurrence following replantation may be as high as 13% and is **greatest with retained cement and in replantations within 1 year after component removal.** For virulent organisms such as *Pseudomonas,* a resection arthroplasty should be strongly considered. Antibiotic impregnated cement (vancomycin/gentamicin) is used for infected revisions and prophylactically in high-risk patients. Approximately 800 mg of antibiotic (gentamicin/tobramycin) is used for 40 grams of cement in order to preserve the strength and integrity of the cement. Local antibiotic mic's last 6–8 weeks.

j. Other Problems—Include nerve injury (sciatic > femoral > obturator—rare with good technique) and urinary retention (lowest with

TABLE 4–3. PROPHYLACTIC ANTIBIOTIC REGIMENS

DENTAL, ORAL, UPPER RESPIRATORY TRACT
Amoxicillin 3 grams PO 1° before procedure/1.5 grams PO 6° after procedure
Penicillin allergic:
Erythromycin 1 gram 1° before procedure/500 mg PO 6° after procedure
Clindamycin 300 mg 1° before procedure/150 mg PO 6° after procedure
Severe penicillin allergy
Vancomycin 1 gram IV 1° before procedure
Unable to take PO
Ampicillin 2 grams IV/IM 30 minutes before procedure/1 gram IV 6° after procedure
Clindamycin 300 mg IV/IM 30 minutes before procedure/150 mg IV 6° after procedure
GU/GI PROCEDURES
Ampicillin *and* gentamycin 1.5 mg/kg (~80 mg) 30 minutes before procedure; then; Amoxicillin 1.5 grams PO 6° after procedure
Penicillin allergic:
Vancomycin 1 gram IV before procedure and gentamycin 1.5 mg/kg (~80 mg); 1 ° before procedure; then;
Repeat 8° after procedure

preop and 24 hour postop indwelling catheters). Sciatic nerve injury, often transient, is the result of traction from excessive lengthening. Femoral nerve injury is usually secondary to excessive retraction of the psoas muscle.

7. Revision THA—Associated with less satisfactory results and increased operative time, dislocation rate, blood loss, infection, and other complications. Additionally, revisions are less durable. Painful prosthetic loosening is the major indication for revision, although impending femoral fracture, component malposition with recurrent dislocation, and wear of the polyethlyene acetabular cup are other indications. Removal of hardware and all previous cement is often followed by replacement of the existing component with a porous ingrowth or cemented prosthesis. The revision femoral stem length should be 1–3 cm longer than the original stem. **If there is femoral cortical disruption, the revision stem should extend two to three shaft diameters distal to the defect.** Bone grafting is often required, sometimes using allografts when host bone is severely deficient. Cemented revisions have a high failure rate of 10–30% after 5 years. Better cementing techniques may improve these results. Extensively porous coated implants have a re-revision rate of approximately 7% after 5 years. Impaction bone grafting (the Ling technique) where morselized allograft is packed tightly into the proximal femur followed by implantation of a cemented, smooth, wedge shaped implant, which is designed to subside into the cement mantle, is gaining popularity. The use of large bulk allografts in the acetabulum to support an acetabular component is controversial because migration and loosening of the acebabular cup can occur.
8. Special Problems
   a. Acetabular Defects (Fig. 4–4)—Can be classified as: I, segmented; II, cavitary; III, combined; IV, pelvic discontinuity; or V, arthrodesed. Special techniques are required to address these problems.
   b. Otto Pelvis (Arthrokatadysis)—Primary protrusio acetabuli characterized by progressive protrusio in middle-aged women. Can be bilateral in one-third of patients and causally related to osteomalacia. Large cortical-cancellous bone grafting may be required using the patient's femoral head in a primary arthroplasty as well as a large acetabular component.
9. Additional Points—**Childhood hip subluxation is the most common cause of hip DJD in patients younger than 40 years.** THA in hips with DDH (Fig. 4–5) has been based on anatomic reconstruction; however, studies suggest that proximal placement of acetabular components without lateralization may be superior to the use of large grafts. Both auto- and allografting of the acetabulum are associated with high (approximately 30%) failure rates at 5 years. Vertical alignment of the hardware may allow for "controlled collapse" and prevent catastrophic failure. Smaller pelvis size may make surgery difficult. Superolateral bone grafting is often required in severe cases. Other forms of childhood hip disease that commonly result in THA include Perthes disease and slipped capital femoral epiphysis (SCFE). Postoperative ROM is most dependent on the preoperative motion of the hip.

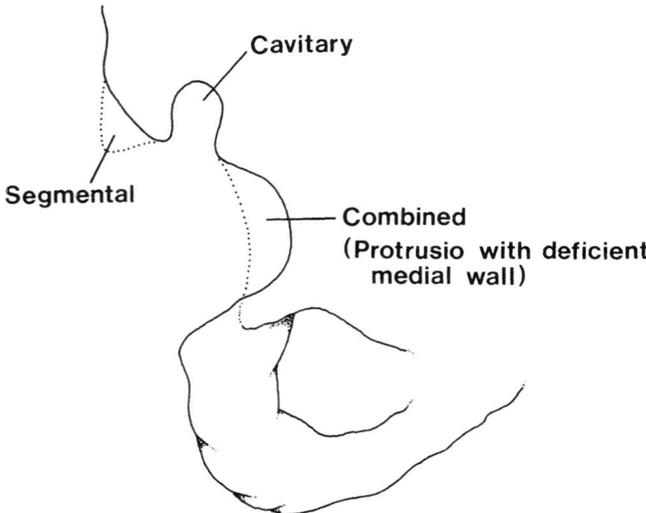

FIGURE 4–4. Acetabular defects (AAOS classification scheme). Pelvic discontinuity and hip arthrodesis are not shown.

II. Knee Reconstruction

A. Arthrodesis—Indicated in a patient with uncontrollable septic arthritis and complete joint destruction, in young patients with severe ligamentous and articular damage, in neuropathic joint disease, and in patients with failed total knee replacements. **Successful arthrodesis is possible in about 80% of failed condylar components but only 55% of failed hinged prostheses** (higher rates of fusion reported with intramedullary fixation). Fusion in 10–15 degrees of flexion and 0–7 degrees valgus is preferred. Complications include delayed, non-, or malunion.

B. Osteotomy—Indicated in selected cases of unicompartmental degenerative arthritis of the knee to transfer weight bearing load to an uninvolved tibiofemoral joint surface. Most commonly performed for medial compartment disease but can also be done for lateral compartment disease.

1. Medial Compartment Disease—Valgus osteotomy of the proximal tibia is indicated with medial tenderness only, **less than 15 degrees of fixed varus deformity,** and radiographically **intact lateral and patellofemoral compartments. Contraindications** also include **lateral subluxations** of the tibia on the femur >**1 cm** (which indicates articular incongruity), tibial subchondral bone loss, **flexion contracture > 15 degrees, limitation of flexion beyond 90 degrees,** peripheral vascular disease, and lateral thrust (high adductor moment). Full length radiographs are necessary preoperatively to correct the mechanical axis of the limb. A lateral closing wedge osteotomy held with staples (stepped Coventry or standard) and fibular shortening (or tibiofibular disarticulation) is the standard method. Overcorrection of the mechanical axis 2–3 degrees beyond neutral is ideal. Most favorable results are in young patients with good bone stock. Complications include **undercorrection (most common),** overcorrection, penetration of the articular surface, avascular necrosis (AVN) of the

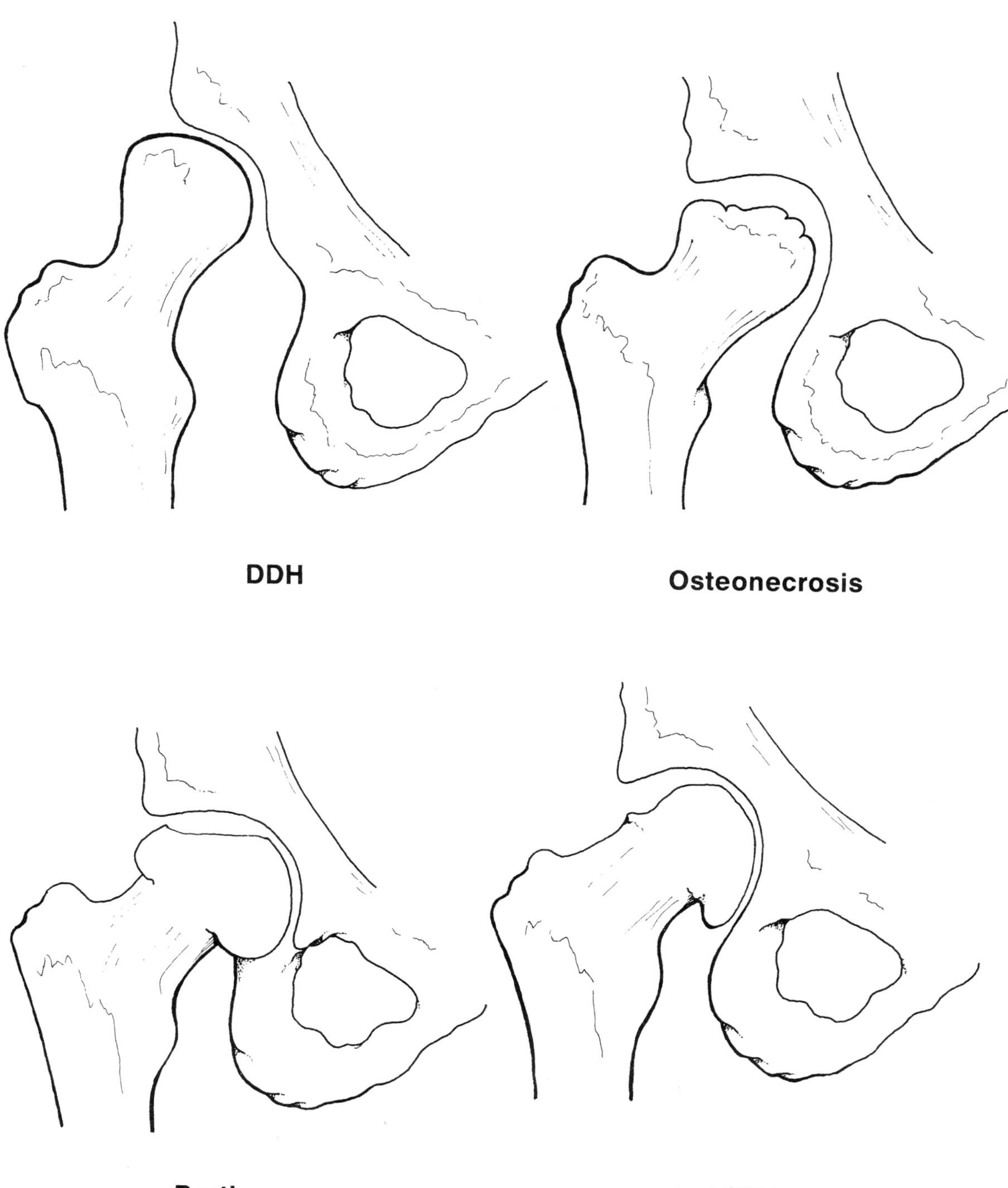

FIGURE 4–5. Common hip deformities producing early arthritis.

plateau, patella baja, peroneal nerve injuries, and anterior compartment syndrome. The most important factors influencing the long-term results of proximal tibial osteotomies is adequacy of correction of the angular deformity and patient body weight. Poor results are reported with patients older than age 60. A high tibial osteotomy is usually considered a temporizing procedure that will last 7–10 years prior to consideration for a total knee arthroplasty (TKA). A TKA may be more difficult after an upper tibial osteotomy but is possible. **Shortening** of the patellar tendon and subsequent patellar baja complicate conversion to TKA. Therefore, osteotomy is rarely indicated in a patient over 60 years.

2. Lateral Compartment Disease—Varus osteotomy; usually involves a medial closing wedge osteotomy of the distal femur (supracondylar region)

fixed with a plate. The femoral osteotomy is generally reserved for **valgus deformities of >12 degrees** and **>10 degrees deviation of the knee joint from the horizontal.** Preoperative ROM of at least 90 degrees, <15 degrees flexion contracture, and no associated instability are required. Medial displacement of the distal fragment helps maintain the mechanical axis of the limb in the center of the knee joint by restoring the axis of the femoral shaft to its preoperative position. Plate fixation of the distal femur is usually indicated.

C. Débridement—Débridement and drilling of subchondral bone may allow for formation of granulation tissue with metaplasia into fibrocartilage and has had some temporary success. This procedure which includes abrasion chrondroplasty, are typically done arthroscopically.

D. Arthroplasty—Includes noncompartmental arthroplasty and TKA, with separate indications.

1. Unicompartmental Arthroplasty—Reserved for patients with single compartment disease (DJD or osteonecrosis) who are not candidates for high tibial osteotomy (usually because of age). In comparison to TKA, there is usually a better ROM, preservation of cruciate ligaments and preservation of bone stock. Usually reserved for **older sedentary patients** who are not obese and contraindicated in significant fixed deformities, inflammatory arthritis, anterior cruciate ligament (ACL) insufficiency, young patients, active obese patients, dynamic instability, or severely decreased ROM. The technique is important, as the tibial implant must be placed at right angles to the mechanical axis of the tibia; overcorrection should be avoided. The overall mechanical axis should fall just over the implant. The most common complication is loosening.
2. Total Knee Arthroplasty (Table 4–4)

a. Indications—Disabling knee pain and decreased function due to arthritis/arthropathy that involves at least two compartments in a patient who has failed all non-operative treatment. **It is contraindicated with nonfunctioning knee extensors,** severe neuromuscular dysfunction, **active sepsis, prior surgical fusion,** and in a **neuropathic joint.**

b. Implant Design—Most commonly are "conforming" implants. Other types of implants are the "linked" prosthesis, which is fully constrained (tibial loosening, increased wear and high infection rates have limited their use to patients with markedly unstable knees, especially after failure of prior TKAs), and "resurfacing" implants, which retain both cruciate ligaments (also rarely used due to the exacting surgical technique and soft tissue balancing required). Conforming implants have condylar metallic femoral components and metal-backed polyethylene tibial components. All such implants sacrifice the ACL and some ("posterior stabilized") designs also sacrifice the posterior cruciate ligament. Although posterior stabilized designs are used routinely by some surgeons, they are often indicated for large fixed contractures that require removal of the PCL and in post-patellectomy knees. **PCL sacrifice may cause difficulty with climbing stairs** in some patients and may cause increased shear stress on the prosthesis. Posterior stabilization facilitates femoral rollback and improves stair climbing. The goals of TKA are to achieve (1) horizontal joint in stance phase of gait; (2) restoration of the anatomic and mechanical axes; (3) a flexion gap equal to the extension gap; (4) proper soft tissue balance; and (5) good patellar placement/alignment.

c. Range of motion—Range of motion postop closely relates to ROM preop. Continuous passive motion (CPM) and manipulations have no effect on long term ROM. At least 90 degrees of flexion is required to arise from a chair with ease.

Continuous Passive Motion:

The effects of CPM have been shown to increase the short-term range of motion and decrease the

TABLE 4–4. TKA COMPLICATIONS

COMPLICATION	RISK FACTORS	RECOMMENDATIONS/TREATMENT
Infection[a]		**Exchange arthroplasty**
Patella fracture	Sacrifice of lateral geniculate artery; thin/small patella; component malposition	Preserve artery Minimally **displaced** fracture; Immobilize in extension Displaced fracture; **removal** of component and patellectomy
Patella dislocation	Int rotated femoral component	Place femoral component in external rotation
Component loosening	Poor alignment	Careful preparation, aseptic technique, aspirations, R/O infection, then revise components
Tibial tray wear	Thin (<8 mm) components	Thicker trays/exchange
Peroneal nerve palsy	Flexion contracture/valgus knee	Flex knee postop
Supracondylar fracture	Anterior femoral notching rheumatoid arthritis, osteoporosis	Avoid notching; ORIF
Skin slough	Poor incisions, excessive raising of lateral flaps	Plan incisions accordingly
Decreased ROM	Poor rehabilitation; poor ROM	Manipulation under anesthesia (long term results unchanged)

[a] In infections with duration of >2 weeks the average success rate with just irrigation/débridement/antibiotics and *retention* of *implants* is about 25%.
ROM, poor presurgical range of motion.

TABLE 4–5. DEFORMITIES AND THEIR CORRECTION

DEFORMITY	CORRECTION
Fixed varus	Elevate medial capsular sleeve, resect medial osteophytes, deep MCL followed by superficial MCL
Lateral subluxation	Release popliteus tendon
Fixed valgus	Lateral approach, release IT band, LCL, posterolateral capsule
Fixed flexion	Remove anterior osteophytes, elevate capsule and PCL, release gastrocnemius, ± posterior capsulotomy
Limited flexion	Quadricepsplasty (V–Y) or patella tendon Z-plasty, or patellar tubercle osteotomy

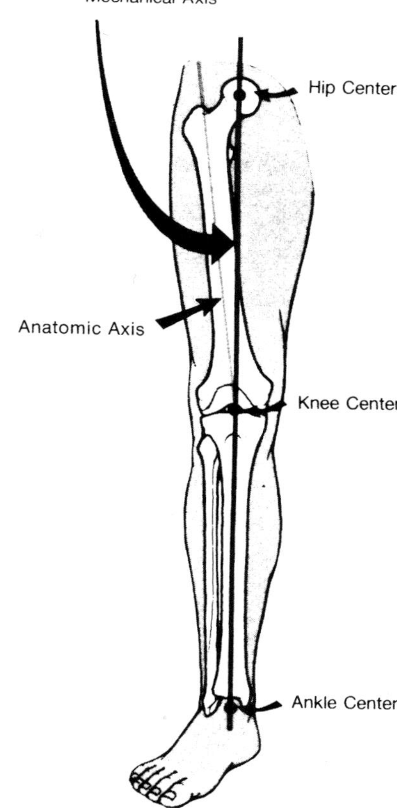

FIGURE 4–6. Knee axes. (From Rohr, W.L.: Primary total knee arthroplasty. In Chapman's Operative Orthopaedics, p. 718. Philadelphia, JB Lippincott, 1988; reprinted by permission.)

length of stay in primary total knee recipients. Few studies have shown significant increases in range of motion of those patients receiving CPM when measured against controls at one year. Most studies used early CPM between 0–40 degrees of flexion to avoid wound problems. (PO_2 saturation at the wound edges has been shown to decrease with early flexion beyond 40 degrees.) Recently, renewed interest has been generated by starting early, aggressive CPM (in flexion 70–100 degrees) in the recovery room, followed by 50–100 degrees Day 1, then 0–100 degrees Day 2, with significant increases in flexion at one year.

d. Surgical Technique—Correction of deformities is outlined in Table 4–5
Close attention to technique is essential. Special emphasis should be placed on resecting the tibial surface at 90 degrees, avoiding a notch of the anterior femoral surface, making proper cuts, and allowing proper tracking of the patella. Maximum coverage of the tibial plateau is essential. Correct alignment is best assured with the use of both extra- and intramedullary guides to achieve a normal mechanical axis (Fig. 4–6) (malalignment is the most common complication of Paget's disease of bone leading to failure). Lateral parapatellar incisions are best for severe valgus knees (>15 degrees). Additionally, appropriate trial components should be inserted prior to the final prosthesis to check for flexion and extension gaps and alignment (Fig. 4–7). An increased **flexion gap** (loose in flexion and tight in extension) is more common and can be corrected by resecting more of the distal femur. An increased **extension gap** (loose in extension and tight in flexion) is usually the result of a technical error and can be corrected by resecting the posterior sloping surface of the tibia. When the knee is tight in both flexion and extension, more proximal tibia should be resected. Excessive patellar thickness can also result in tightness with flexion and may require additional patellar resection. Close attention to patellar tracking is important, and the superolateral geniculate artery should be preserved. Bone grafting is indicated for defects involving >50% of the tibial plateau. In general, bone stock should be preserved whenever possible, and large defects should be replaced with allograft bone.

e. Patella—Controversy regarding patellar resurfacing has swung toward resurfacing in most cases (especially in all RA patients). The original patellar thickness should be restored. Resurfacing leads to less patellofemoral pain and better stair climbing ability. Patellar alignment is enhanced by placing the femoral component in slight external rotation. Less than 20 mm of patellar thickness is a relative contraindication for patellar resurfacing. Metal-backed patellar components have been uniformly unsuccessful, leading to wear fracture and metal debris in joints (related to decreased polyethylene thickness and increased stress).

f. Revision TKA—The key to successful revision surgery is restoration of the original joint line. Radiographs taken prior to the index procedure and of the opposite knee are helpful. The adductor tubercle, the tip of the fibula, and other landmarks are used to determine component position preoperatively. **The MCL must be intact to use a nonconstrained prosthesis.** Revision implants with more mechanical restraints are associated with higher failure rates secondary to implant loosening. (because of increased stresses at the bone–cement interface).

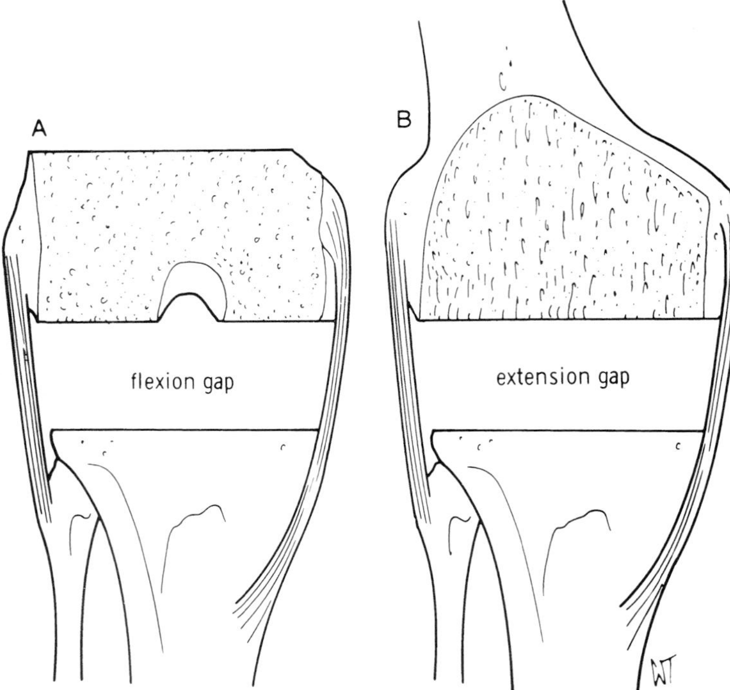

FIGURE 4–7. Flexion and extension gap in total knee arthroplasty. (From Scuderi, G.R., and Insall, J.N.: The posterior stabilized knee prosthesis. Orthop. Clin. North Am. 20(1):73, 1989; reprinted by permission.)

Selected Bibliography

Hip

Alberts, K.A., and Jervaeus, J.: Factors predisposing to healing complications after internal fixation of femoral neck fractures. Clin. Orthop. 257, 129–133, 1990.

Amstutz, H.C., Friscia, D.A., Dorey, F., and Carney, B.T.: Warfarin prophylaxis to prevent mortality from pulmonary embolism after total hip replacement. J. Bone Joint Surg. [Am.] 71:321, 1989.

Bucholz, H.W., Elson, R.A., Engelbrecht, E., et al.: Management of deep infection of total hip replacement. J. Bone Joint Surg. [Br.] 62:342–353, 1981.

Callaghan, J.J., Dysart, S.H., and Savory, C.G.: The uncemented porous-coated anatomic total hip prosthesis. Two-year results of a prospective consecutive series. J. Bone Joint Surg. [Am.] 70:337, 1988.

Canner, G.C., Steinberg, M.E., Heppenstall, R.B., and Balderston, R.: The infected hip after total hip arthroplasty. J. Bone Joint Surg. [Am.] 66:1393–1399, 1984.

Chandler, H.P., Reineck, F.T., Wixson, R.L., and McCarthy, J.C.: Total hip replacement in patients younger than 30 year old: A five-year follow-up. J. Bone Joint Surg. [Am.] 63:1426–1434, 1981.

Charnlely, J. and Cupix, Z.: The nine- and ten-year results of the low friction arthroplasty of the hip. Clin. Orthop. 95:9–25, 1973.

Dorr, L.D., Sakimura, I., and Mohler, J.G.: Pulmonary emboli followed total hip arthroplasty: Incidence study. J. Bone Joint Surg. [Am.] 61:1083–1087, 1979.

Elting, J.J., Aicat, B.A., Mikhail, M., et al.: Impaction Grafting, Preliminary Report of a New Method for Exchange Femoral Arthroplasty. Orthopedics, vol 18, No. 2, 107–112.

Engh, C.A.: Hip arthroplasty with a Moore prosthesis with porous coating: A five-year study. Clin. Orthop. 176:52–66, 1983.

Fackler, C.D.: Dislocation in Total Hip Arthroplasties. Clin Ortho 151:169, 1980.

Galante, J.O.: Current concepts in review. Causes of fractures of the femoral component in total hip replacement. J. Bone Joint Surg. [Am.] 62:670–673, 1980.

Garvin, K.L., Fitzgerald, R.H., Salvatti, S.A., et al.: Reconstruction of the infected total hip and knee with bentamycin impregnated palaios bone cement. Instructional Course Lectures, vol 42; 293–302, 1993.

Garvin, K.L., Pellicci, P.M., Windsor, R.E., et al.: Contralateral total hip arthroplasty or ipsilateral total knee arthroplasty in patients who have a long standing fusion of the hip. J. Bone Joint Surg. [Am.] 71:1355, 1989.

Gle, G.A., Linder, L., Ling, L.S.M., et al.: Impacted cancellous allografts and cement revision total hip arthroplasty. J. Bone Joint Surg. [Br.] 75-b, 14–21, 1993.

Goodman, S.B., Adler, S.J., Fyhrie, D.P., and Schurman, D.J.: The acetabular teardrop and its relevance to acetabular migration. Cyn. Otrho. 236:199, 1988.

Gruen, J.A., McNiece, G.M., and Amstutz, H.C.: Modes of failure of cemented stem-type femoral components. Clin. Orthop. 141: 17–27, 1979.

Harris, W.H., and White, R.E. Jr.: Advantages of metal-backed acetabular components for total hip replacement; A clinical assessment with a minimum 5-year follow-up. Hip 11:240–246, 1983.

Harris, W.H.: Advances in total hip arthroplasty; The metal-backed acetabular component. Clin. Orthop. 183:3–11, 1984.

Hastings, D.E., Parker, S.M.: Protrusio acetabuli in rheumatoid arthritis. Clin. Orthop. Rel. Res. 108:76, 1975.

Hill, E. Flaman, R., Maza, S.F., and Evrard, J.: Prophylactic cefazolin versus placebo in total hip replacement. Report of a multicenter double-blind randomized trial. Lancet 1; 1981.

Johnston, R.C., Brand, R.A., and Cronninshield, H.D.: Reconstruction of the hip—A mathematical approach to determine optimum geometric relationships. J. Bone Joint Surg. 61A July 1979.

Kavanagh, B.F., Dewits, M.A., Ilstrup, D.M., et al.: Charnley total hip arthroplasty with cement, fifteen-year results. J. Bone Joint Surg. [Am.] 71:1496, 1989.

Keating, E.M., Ritter, M.A., and Faris, P.M.: Structures at risk from medially placed acetabular screws. J. Bone Joint Surg. [Am.] 72: 45, 1990.

Lestrange, N.L.: Bipolar arthroplasty for 496 hip fractures. Clin. Orthop. Rel. Res.; 251, 1990, 7.

Lewinnek, G.E., Lewis, J.L., Rara, R., et al.: Dislocations after total hip replacement arthroplasties. J. Bone Joint Surg. 60:217, 1978.

Lewis, J.L., Asken, M.J., and Nixon, R.L.: The influence of prosthetic stem stiffness and a calcar collar on stresses in the proximal end of the femur with a cemented femoral component. J. Bone Joint Surg. 66A, 1984.

Liechti, R.: Hip arthrodesis and associated problems. Berlin, Springer-Verlag, 1978.

Ling, R.S.M.: Complications of total hip replacement. Edinburgh, Churchill Livingstone, 1984.

Lyons, W.W., Berquist, T.H., Lyons, J.C., et al.: Evaluation of radiographic findings in painful hip arthroplasties. Clin. Orthop. 195: 235–251, 1985.

Maloney, W.J., and Harris, W.H.: Comparison of a hybrid with an uncemented total hip replacement. A retrospective matched-pair study. J. Bone Joint Surg. [Am.] 72:1349, 1990.

McDonald, D.J., Fitzgerald, R.H. Jr., and Ilstrup, D.M.: Two-stage reconstruction of a total hip arthroplasty because of infection. J. Bone Joint Surg. 71:828, 1989.

McDonald, D.J., Fitzgerald, R.M. Jr., Ilstrup, D.M.: Two-stage reconstruction of a total hip arthroplasty because of infection. J. Bone Joint Surg. 71A, 828, 1989.

Neoblewski, B.M., Delsel, H.S.: Uretheral instrumentation and deep sepsis in total hip replacement. Clin. Orthop. 146, 1986.

Noo, R.Y.G., and Morrey, B.F.: Dislocations after total hip arthroplasty. J. Bone Joint Surg. 64A, 1982.

Pellicci, P.M., Wilson, P.D. Jr., Sledge, D.B., et al.: Revision total hip arthroplasty. Clin. Orthop. 170:34–41, 1982.

Perrin, T., Dorr, L.D., Perry, J., et al.: Functional evaluation of total hip arthroplasty with five to ten-year follow up evaluation. Clin. Orthop. 195:252–260, 1985.

Salvati, E.A., Wilson, P.D. Jr. Jolley, M.N., et al.: A ten-year follow-up study of our first 100 consecutive Charnley total hip replacements. J. Bone Joint Surg. [Am.] 63:753–767, 1981.

Sanford, J.P., Gilbert, D.N., Gerberding, J.L., and Sande, M.A.: Guide to Antimicrobial Therapy; 1994.

Sarmiento, A., Ebramzadel, E., Gogan, W.J., et al: Total hip arthroplasty with cement. A long-term radiographic analysis in patients who are older than fifty and younger than fifty years. J. Bone Joint Surg. [Am.] 72:1470, 1990.

Schutzer, S.F., and Harris, W.H.: Deep-wound infection after total hip replacement under contemporary aseptic conditions. J. Bone Joint Surg. [Am.] 70:724–727, 1988.

Sculco, T.P., and Ranawat, C.: The use of spinal anesthesia for total hip-replacement arthroplasty. J. Bone Joint Surg. [Am.] 57: 173–177, 1975.

Strathy, G.M., and Fitzgerald, R.H.: Total hip arthroplasty in the ankylosed hip. J. Bone Joint Surg. 70-A:963–966, 1988.

Weisman, B.N., Leland-Sosman, J., Braunstein, E.M., et al.: Total hip joint replacement in the United States. J.A.M.A. 248(15): 1817–1821, 1982. J. Bone Joint Surg. 66-A, No. 3, 443–450, March 1984.

Knee

Andriacchi, T.P., Galante, J.O., and Fermier, R.W.: The influence of total knee-replacement design on walking and stair climbing. J. Bone Joint Surg. [Am.] 64:1328–1335, 1982.

Bayley, J.C., Scott, R.D., Bnald, F.C., and Holmes, G.B.: Failure of the metal-backed patellar component after total knee replacement. J. Bone Joint Surg. 70A, July 1988.

Bayley, J.C., Scott, R.D., Ewald, F.C., and Holmes, G.B. Jr.: Failure of the metal-backed patellar component after total knee replacement. J. Bone Joint Surg. [Am.] 70:688, 1988.

Coventry, M.B.: Proximal tibial varus osteotomy for osteoarthritis of the lateral compartment of the knee. J. Bone Joint Surg. [Am.] 69:32–38, 1987.

Coventry, M.B.: Upper tibial osteotomy for gonarthrosis. Clin. Orthop. North Am. 10:191–210, 1979.

Coventry, M.B.: Upper tibial osteotomy for osteoarthritis. J. Bone Joint Surg. [Am.] 67:1136–1140, 1985.

Coventry, M.B.: Upper tibial osteotomy. Clin. Orthop. 182:46–52, 1984.

Dorr, L.D., and Boiardo, R.A.: Technical considerations in total knee arthroplasty. Clin. Orthop. 205:5–11, 1986.

Gable, G.T., Rand S.A., and Sim, F.H.: Total knee arthroplasty for osteoarthritis in patients who have past disease of bone at the knee. J. Bone Joint Surg. 73A, June 1991.

Goldberg, V.M., Figgie, M.P., Figgie, H.E. III, et al.: Use of a total condylar knee prosthesis for treatment of osteoarthritis. Long term results. J. Bone Joint Surg. [Am.] 70:802, 1988.

Holden, D.L., James, S.L., Larson, R.L., and Slocum, D.B.: Proximal tibial osteotomy in patient show are fifty years old or less, A long-term follow-up study. J. Bone Joint Surg. [Am.] 70:977, 1988.

Insall, J.N., and Kelly, M.: The total condylar prosthesis. Clin. Orthop. 205:43–48, 1986.

Insall, J.N., Hood, R.W., Flawn, L.B., and Sullivan, D.J.: The total condylar knee prosthesis in gonarthrosis: A five- to nine-year follow-up of the first one hundred consecutive replacements. J. Bone Joint Surg. [Am.] 65:619–628, 1983.

Johnson, M.B.: The effect of continuous passive motion on wound healing and joint mobility after knee arthroplasty. J. Bone Joint Surg. [Am.] 101.72-A No. 3, 4211–432, March 1990.

Jordan, L.R., Siegal, J.L., and Olivo, J.L.: Early flexion routine following total knee arthroplasty: An alternative method of continuous passive motion; personal communication—unpublished.

Kitziger, K.G., and Lotke, P.A.: Unicompartmental knee arthroplasty. Instructional course lectures, VA 43; 95–100, 1992.

Landy, M.M., and Walker, P.S.: Wear of ultra-high-molecular-weight polyethylene components of 90 retrieved knee prosthesis. J. Arthop. suppl., pp. S73–S85, 1988.

Lynch, A.F., Bourne, R.B., Rorabeck, C.H., et al: Deep-vein thrombosis and continuous passive motion after total knee arthroplasty. J. Bone Joint Surg. [Am.] 70:11–14, 1988.

Maloney, W.J., Schurman, D.J., Hagend, D., et al.: The influence of continuous passive motion on outcome in total knee arthroplasty. Clin. Orthop. 256:162–168, 1980.

Marquest, P.: Mechanics and osteoarthritis of the patellofemoral joint. Clin. Orthop. 144:70–73, 1979.

Picetti, G.D. III, McGann, W.A., and Welch, R.B.: The patellofemoral joint after total knee arthroplasty without patellar resurfacing. J. Bone Joint Surg. [Am.] 72:1379, 1990.

Rand, J.A., and Bryan, R.S.: Results of revision total knee arthroplasties using condylar prosthesis. A review of fifty knees. J. Bone Joint Surg. [Am.] 70:738, 1988.

Rand, J.A.: Alternatives to re-implantation for salvage of the total knee arthroplasty complicated by infection. Instructional course lectures, VA 42:341–347, 1993.

Rand, J.A., Peterson, L.F.A., Bryan, R.S., et al: Revision total knee arthroplasty. Instr. Course Lect. 35:305–318, 1986.

Rosenberg, T.D., Paulos, L.E., Parker, R.D., et al.: The forty-five degree posteroanterior flexion weight-bearing radiograph fo the knee. J. Bone Joint Surg. [Am.] 70:1479, 1988.

Schneider, R., Abenavoli, A.M., Soundry, M., and Install, J.: Failure of total condylar knee replacements; Correlation of radiographic, clinical, and surgical findings. Radiology 152:309–315, 1984.

Schoifet, D.S., and Morrey, B.F.: Treatment of infection after total knee arthroplasty by débridement with retention of the components. J. Bone Joint Surg. [Am.] 72:1383, 1990.

Schoifet, S.D., and Morrey, B.D.: Treatment of infection after total knee arthroplasty by débridement with retention of the components. J. Bone Joint Surg. 72A, 1990.

Schoifet, S.D., and Morrey, B.F.: Infected knee arthroplasty treated by débridement and retention of components. J. Bone Joint Surg. 72A, 1990.

Scott, R.D., and Santore, R.F.: Unicondylar unicompartmental replacement for osteoarthritis of the knee. J. Bone Joint Surg. 63A: 536–544, 1981.

Scott, W.N.: Symposium on total knee arthroplasty (foreword). Clin. Orthop. North Am. 13:1–249, 1981.

Shoji, H., Yoshino, S., and Kajino, A.: Patellar replacement in bilateral total knee arthroplasty. A study of patients who had rheumatoid arthritis and no gross deformity of the patella. J. Bone Joint Surg. [Am.] 71:853, 1989.

Stulberg, B.N., Insall, J.N., Williams, G.W., and Ghelman, B.: Deep-vein thrombosis following total knee replacement: An analysis of six hundred thirty-eight arthroplasties. J. Bone Joint Surg. [Am.] 666:194–201, 1984.

Wang, J., Kuo, K.N., Adriacchi, T.P., and Galante, J.O.: The influence of walking mechanics and time on the results of proximal tibial Osteotomy. JBJS 72A; 905–909, 1990.

Windsor, R.E., Insall, J.N., and Vince, K.E.: Technical consideration of total knee arthroplasty after proximal tibial osteotomy. J. Bone Joint Surg. 70A, April 1988.

Windsor, R.E., Insall, J.N., and Vince, K.G.: Technical considerations of total knee arthroplasty after proximal tibial osteotomy. J. Bone Joint Surg. [Am.] 70:547, 1988.

Miscellaneous

Bullough, P.G., DiCarlo, E.F., Jansraj, K.K., et al: Factors that influence the duration of satisfactory function. Clin. Orthop. 229:193, 1988.

Chapman, Michael, W., ed: Operative Orthopaedics. Philadelphia, J.B. Lippincott, 1988.

Haddad, R.J. Jr., Cook, S.D., and Thomas, K.A.: Biological fixation of porous-coated implants. J. Bone Joint Surg. [Am.] 69:1459–1466, 1987.

Matthews, L.S.: Pathologic studies of total joint replacement. Clin. Orthop. North Am. 19:611–625, 1988.

Rose, R.M., Crugnola, A., Ries, M., Cimino, W.R., et al.: On the origins of high in vivo wear rates in polyethylene components of total joint prostheses. Clin. Orthop. 145:277–286, 1979.

Walker, P.S.: Human joints and their artificial replacements. Springfield, IL, Charles C Thomas, 1977.

5

DISORDERS OF THE FOOT AND ANKLE

MARK S. MIZEL and MARK SOBEL

This chapter provides a review of adult foot and ankle deformities. Pediatric and congenital deformities are covered in Chapter 2.

I. Biomechanics of the Foot and Ankle

A. Gait Cycle—This brief review of biomechanics assumes a basic knowledge of anatomy of the lower extremity and specifically of the foot and ankle. Should the necessity for review exist, numerous anatomy textbooks are available for review. The center of mass of the human body displaces in a vertical plane during the gait cycle. It is necessary, as the distance between the floor and the center of mass must be greater when it passes over the extended leg during the midstance phase of gait than during transmission of body weight from one leg to the other. Horizontal body displacements occur with the rotatory movement of the pelvis as the leg advances. Lateral body displacements occur as the body is shifted slightly over the weight-bearing limb with each step. The total lateral displacement of the body is approximately 5 cm from side to side with each complete gait cycle. This distance can be increased by walking with the feet more widely separated. Ground forces for walking reach approximately 11/2 times body weight, and during jogging they reach almost three times body weight. The weight-bearing phase of the gait cycle for each leg is divided into multiple parts (Fig. 5–1), starting with heel strike, then going to foot flat, to heel off, to toe off. The next cycle of the same foot starts again with heel strike. It should be noted that the contralateral foot goes into toe off soon after foot flat and enters heel strike soon after the initial foot passes through heel rise. The lower extremity is considered to go through two phases: the stance phase, where it is bearing weight, and the swing phase, where it is being advanced. The stance phase constitutes approximately 62% and the swing phase 38% of the gait cycle. The stance phase itself consists of double limb support followed by a period of single limb support and then proceeding back to double limb support.

B. Ankle Axes of Rotation—The ankle axis is directed laterally and posteriorly. External rotation produces some lateral movement of the foot, and plantar flexion produces some medial movement of the foot (Fig. 5–2). The subtalar joint is a single axis joint that acts as a hinge joint connecting the talus and calcaneus. As the tibia internally rotates, the subtalar joint everts the calcaneus; and as the tibia externally rotates, the subtalar joint inverts and causes the calcaneus to go into a varus position.

C. Energy Absorption—The midtarsal articulation (Chopart's joint) consists of the calcaneocuboid joint and the talonavicular joint. With inversion of the hindfoot (subtalar joint), the midtarsal joints are not parallel, and this joint (Chopart's joint) is locked. As the subtalar joint everts, these joints (Chopart's joint) become parallel and allow motion (Figs. 5–3, 5–4, 5–5). This flexibility is important during the heel strike and the subsequent stance phase of gait, when the hindfoot is in valgus; it allows pronation of the foot, absorbing some of the energy from heel strike. From heel strike to foot flat, the anterior compartment of the leg (tibialis anterior) contracts eccentrically, thus lengthening, while the gastroc soleus is quiescent. During foot flat the gastroc soleus complex is contracting eccentrically, and the anterior tibialis is quiet. During heel rise the gastroc soleus complex contracts concentrically, and the tibialis anterior (anterior compartment) is quiescent. From heel strike to foot flat there is progressive eversion of the subtalar joint, which unlocks the transverse tarsal joint and causes internal rotation of the tibia. Heel rise is the opposite. The plantar aponeurosis originates on the plantar calcaneus and passes distally, inserting into the base of the flexor mechanism of the toes. It is primarily a medial structure. It functions as a windlass, increasing the arch as the toes dorsiflex during toe off. This is a passive function during heel rise and serves to bring about some inversion of the calcaneus, which results in some external rotation of the tibia and locking of the midtarsal joint, thereby providing a rigid lever arm. The main invertor of the subtalar joint during heel rise is the posterior tibial tendon, which initiates subtalar inversion. The Achilles tendon provides the motor for the heel rise phase of gait.

D. Mechanisms of Running—The difference between running and the normal walking gait cycle is that at one point during the running cycle the person is airborne and not bearing weight on

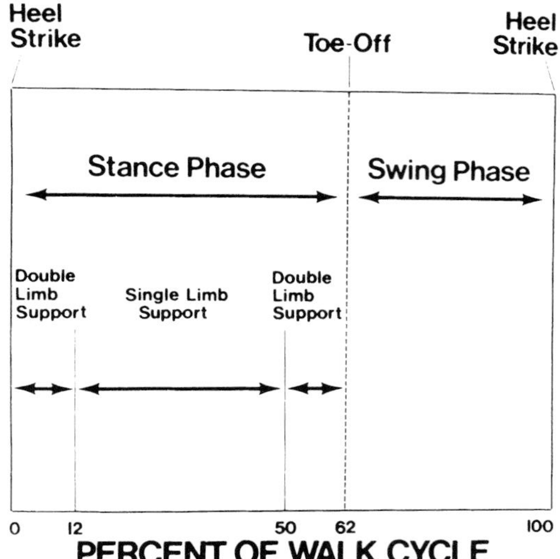

FIGURE 5–1. Phases of walking cycle. Stance phase constitutes approximately 62% and swing phase 38% of cycle. Stance phase is further divided into two periods of double limb support and one period of single limb support. (From Mann, R.A., and Coughlin, M.J., eds.: Surgery of the Foot and Ankle, 6th ed., vol. 1, p. 15. St. Louis, CV Mosby, 1993; reprinted by permission.)

either lower extremity. This considerably increases the force generated, from approximately 11/2 times body weight to almost 3 times body weight.

II. Physical Examination of the Foot and Ankle

A. Neurovascular, Muscle Strength, Tendon Competence—Neurovascular examination of every foot and ankle prior to further examination is mandatory. Pain in the foot or ankle can be caused by neurologic pathology, such as peripheral neuropathy, peripheral nerve entrapment, or possibly herniated nucleus pulposus. Vascular evaluation is critical, especially if elective surgery is contemplated. Ankle motors for dorsiflexion, plantar flexion, inversion, and eversion should all be checked. Bilateral comparison, inspection, and strength testing of right to left foot is essential. It is important when checking the posterior tibial muscle for its strength to invert that it be done from an everted position. The ankle should be plantar flexed to avoid recruitment of the tibialis anterior. In addition, asking the patient to stand on toes with repetitive single stance heel rise to assess the ability of the posterior tibial tendon to initiate heel rise of the inverted subtalar joint is important. When the ankle is in neutral or inverted, the anterior tibial muscle can function as

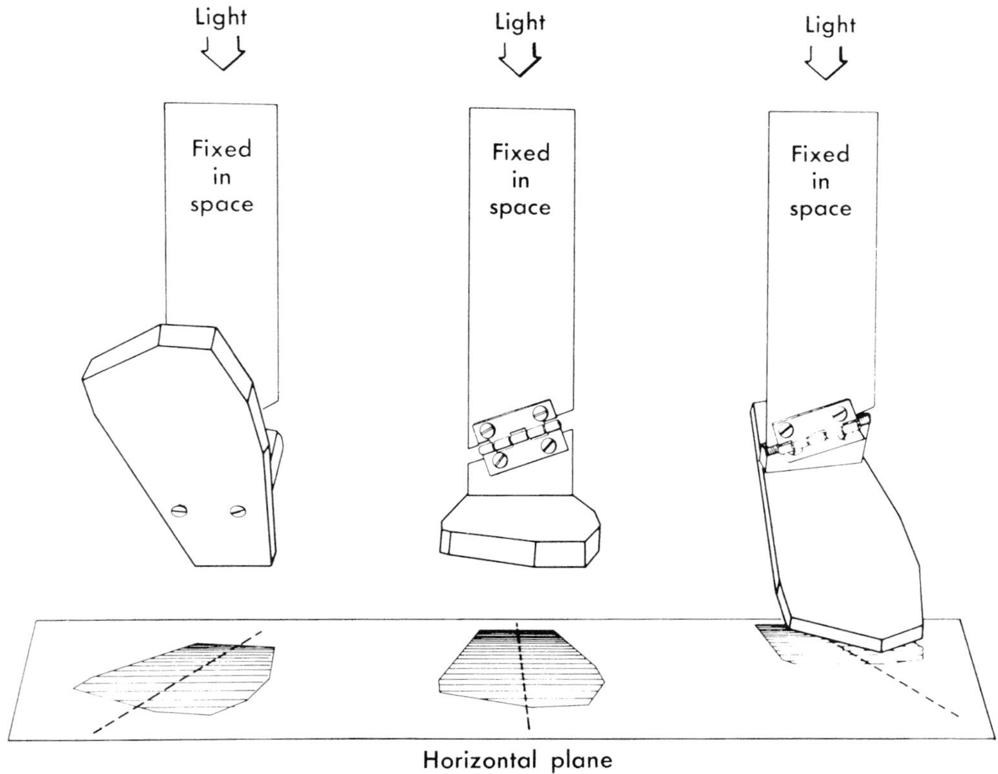

FIGURE 5–2. Effect of obliquely placed ankle axis on rotation of foot in horizontal plane during plantar flexion and dorsiflexion, with foot free. Displacement is reflected in shadows of foot. (From Mann, R.A., and Coughlin, M.J., eds.: Surgery of the Foot and Ankle, 6th ed., vol. 1, p. 17. St. Louis, CV Mosby, 1993; reprinted by permission.)

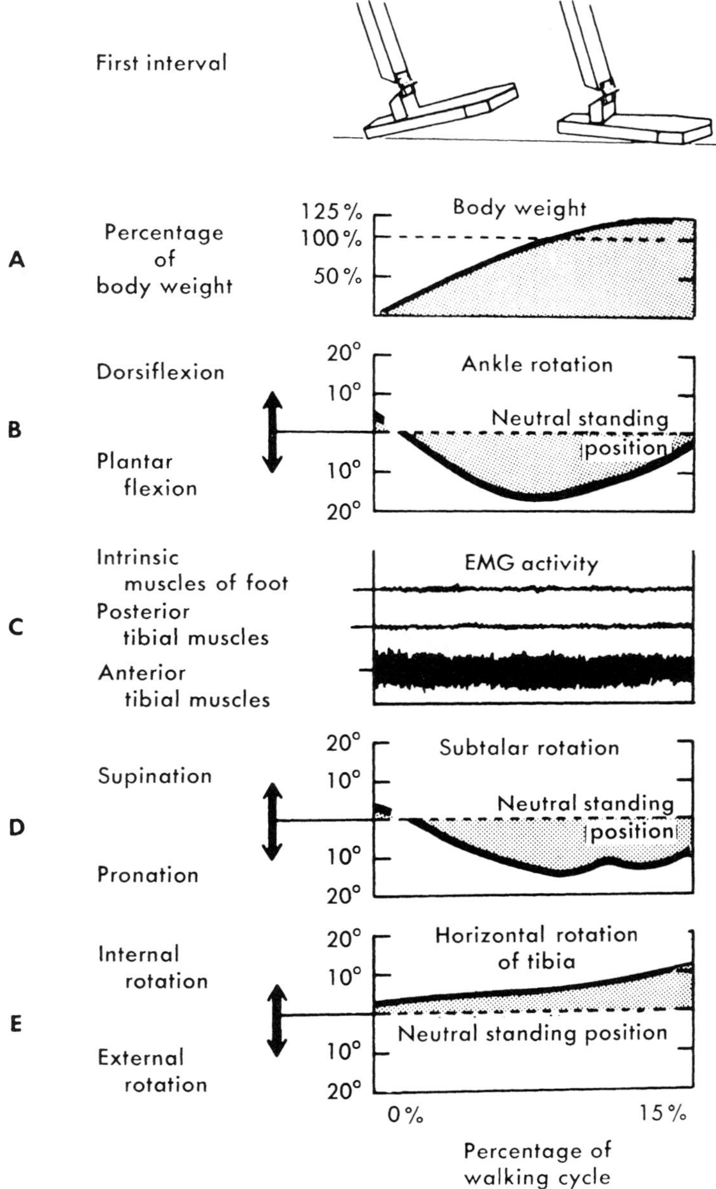

FIGURE 5–3. Events of first interval of walking, or period that extends from heel strike to foot flat. (From Mann, R.A., and Coughlin, M.J., eds.: Surgery of the Foot and Ankle, 6th ed., vol. 1, p. 29. St. Louis, CV Mosby, 1993; reprinted by permission.)

an inverter along with the posterior tibial muscle. From an everted position only the posterior tibial tendon functions as an invertor.

B. Joint Motion—Motion of the ankle, subtalar joint, and Chopart's joints should be checked and compared right to left. In a similar fashion, motion of Lisfranc's joints can be checked with a dorsiflexion/plantar flexion motion at the distal metatarsals. The MTP joints should be tested for ROM, for tenderness or swelling of the joints, and with careful palpation of the interdigital spaces. Competence of the MP joints can be tested with the drawer sign or looking for deviation of the second or third toe when the patient is standing due to insufficiency of the collateral ligament.

C. Palpation—Palpation of the ankle ligaments should be performed as well as inversion of the ankle in dorsiflexion (to stress the calcaneofibular ligament) and anterior drawer in plantar flexion (to stress the anterior talofibular ligament). The tarsal tunnel should be palpated and checked for a Tinel's sign to evaluate the posterior tibial nerve. However, the diagnosis of tarsal tunnel syndrome must be supported by EMG and nerve conduction studies prior to decompression.

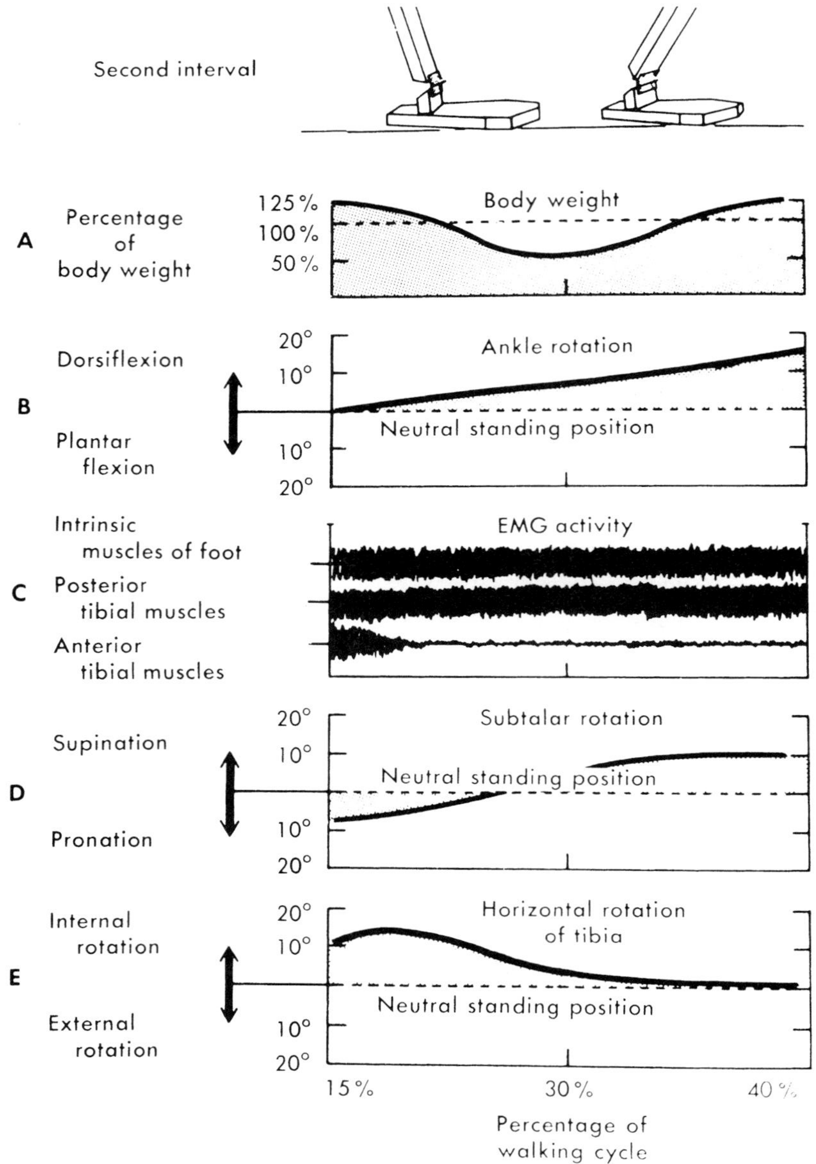

FIGURE 5–4. Events of second interval of walking, or period of foot flat. (From Mann, R.A., and Coughlin, M.J., eds.: Surgery of the Foot and Ankle, 6th ed., vol. 1, p. 30. St. Louis, CV Mosby, 1993; reprinted by permission.)

III. Adult Hallux Valgus

A. There are multiple intrinsic causes of hallux valgus, including heredity, pes planus, and metatarsus primus varus. Other causes of hallux valgus deformity include rheumatoid arthritis (RA) and other connective tissue diseases, neurologic disorders such as cerebral palsy, and the most common cause, poorly fitted shoewear (i.e., narrow, low toe box fashion shoes).

B. Pathophysiology—Hallux valgus deformity consists of the hallux being in a valgus position (Fig. 5–6). Multiple other anatomic deformities occur concurrently, including the first metatarsal shifting into a varus position and the sesamoid complex remaining in its same position, connected to the second metatarsal by the intermetatarsal ligament. As the first metatarsal shifts into a varus position, the sesamoid complex is shifted laterally relative to the first metatarsal. The lateral capsule contracts, as the medial capsule becomes more attenuated. The adductor insertion into the first metatarsal base and sesamoid complex contributes to this hallux valgus deformity. The alignment of the articular surface of the first metatarsal may contribute to the hallux valgus deformity. This finding is a radiographic parameter. Unlike a subluxed first MTP joint, it may lead to a similar degree of hallux valgus deformity but is secondary to an abnormally laterally sloped distal metatarsal articu-

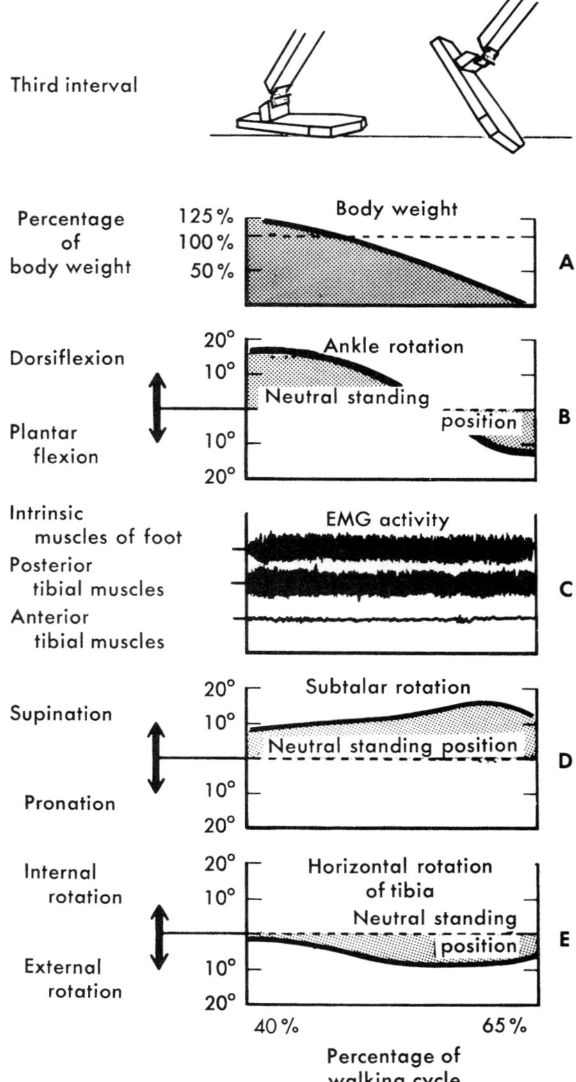

FIGURE 5–5. Composite of all events of third interval of walking, or period extending from foot flat to toe-off. (From Mann, R.A., and Coughlin, M.J., eds.: Surgery of the Foot and Ankle, 6th ed., vol 1, p. 31. St Louis, CV Mosby, 1993, reprinted by permission.)

lar angle (DMAA). Another cause of hallux valgus can be the proximal phalanx being abnormally laterally deviated through the shape of the bone itself (i.e., hallux valgus interphalangeus).

C. Conservative Treatment of Hallux Valgus—Hallux valgus deformities can be well treated with wide (high toe box) laced shoes. Should concurrent hammer toe or crossover toe deformities exist, extra-depth shoes may be helpful. Stretching the leather over the bunion region can also be helpful. This parameter is considered a guideline regarding evaluation of the patient and for deciding which procedure (or combination) is appropriate.

D. Surgical Treatment of Hallux Valgus—*Normal* MTP joint angle is 9 degrees on average but definitely less than 15 degrees. Intermetatarsal angle is considered abnormal when it is more than 9 degrees (Fig. 5–7).

1. Medial Eminence Resection (Silver)—It is good for elderly patients with a large medial exostosis. It is important that a minimal hallux valgus angle and minimal metatarsus primus varus exist.
2. Distal Soft Tissue Realignment—Modified McBride—This operation is good for a mild to moderate deformity with an intermetatarsal angle of less than 15 degrees and hallux valgus less than 35 degrees. It combines a medial exostectomy with release of the lateral capsule and soft tissues and plication of the medial capsule. Modified McBride means that the fibular sesamoid is *not* excised. The reason for this modification is that sesamoid excision can be associated with deviation of the hallux (i.e., fibular sesamoid excision can cause a hallux varus deformity); tibial sesamoid excision can cause a hallux valgus deformity; excision of both sesamoids can cause a cock-up deformity and decreased push-off power of the first MTP joint.
3. Distal V Osteotomy (Chevron)—This procedure is indicated for patients less than 50 years old with intermetatarsal angles of 15 degrees and hallux valgus angles less than 35 degrees. It is performed with a medial exostectomy as well as distal V osteotomy and lateral displacement of the metatarsal head. Trimming of prominent medial metaphysis and a capsulorrhaphy is also performed. An intermetatarsal angle of 16 degrees or more is a contraindication to the Chevron procedure.
4. Mitchell Osteotomy—Indicated for intermetatarsal angles of less than 20 degrees and hallux valgus angles of less than 40 degrees. It involves a medial incision and resection of the medial eminence as well as an osteotomy cut at a right angle to the long axis of the foot and displacement of the MT. It may be associated with significant shortening of the first MT with subsequent transfer metatarsalgia.
5. Keller Bunionectomy—Consists of removing the distal MT medial eminence and the proximal aspect of the proximal phalanx. It is stabilized for approximately 6 weeks postop as fibrous tissue forms. This procedure is indicated only for household ambulators. The common complications include cock-up deformity of the hallux, transfer metatarsalgia, and stress fracture of the lesser MTs, which are due to the lack of weight-bearing by the first MTP joint.
6. Proximal Metatarsal Osteotomy—Can be added to a distal soft tissue repair to increase the correction that is obtainable. An osteotomy is often necessary if the intermetatarsal angle is 14 degrees or more. A stiff first metatarsocuneiform joint is another indication. The most popular proximal MT osteotomy performed is a crescentic osteotomy.
7. First M-C Arthrodesis—Needed when the ligaments of this joint are lax. (Lapidus procedure).
8. Aiken Procedure—Closing wedge osteotomy of the proximal aspect of the proximal phalanx,

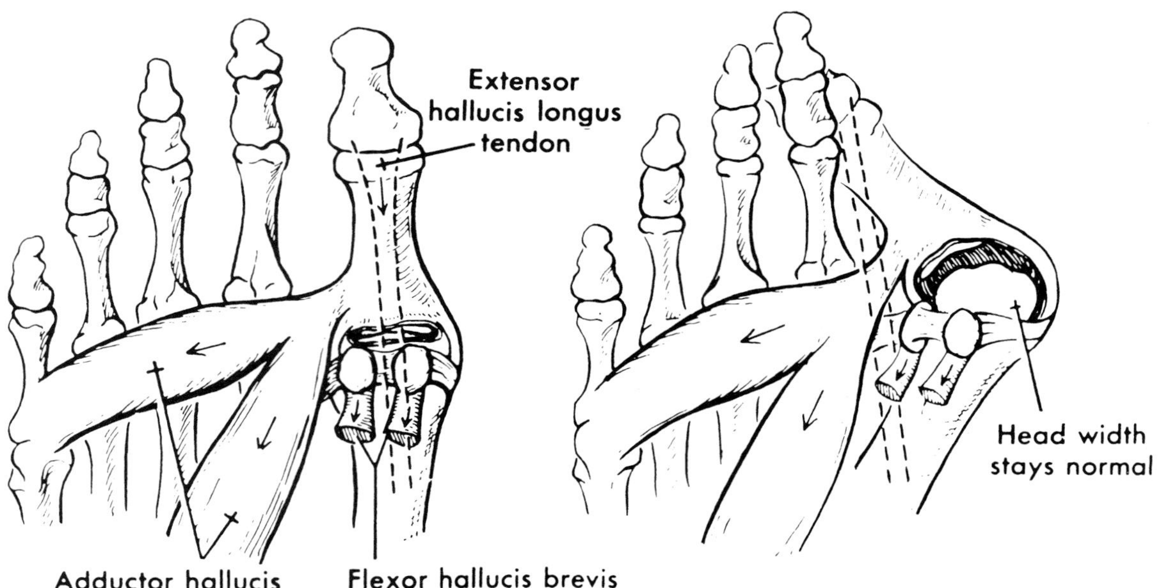

FIGURE 5–6. Pathophysiology of hallux valgus deformity. Normally, metatarsal head is stabilized within sleeve of ligaments and tendons, which provide stability to joint. As proximal phalanx deviates laterally it places pressure on metatarsal head, and deviates medially. It results in attenuation of medial joint capsule and contracture of lateral joint capsule. (From Mann, R.A., and Coughlin, M.J., eds.: Surgery of the Foot and Ankle, 6th ed., vol. 1, p. 184. St. Louis, CV Mosby, 1993; reprinted by permission.)

indicated for hallux valgus interphalangeus. It is also indicated for hallux valgus with a congruent joint with insufficient correction after a Chevron procedure.

E. Complications of Surgical Procedures
   1. Silver Bunionectomy—The disadvantages are a high rate of recurrence and limited applications. It has a low complication rate. If salvage is necessary, an Aiken procedure (closing wedge osteotomy of the proximal phalanx) or a modified McBride procedure can be considered. An arthrodesis can act as an effective salvage.
   2. Modified McBride—The disadvantage of a modified McBride is that soft tissue may stretch out and deformity can recur. Contraindications include connective tissue disorders, and complications include recurrence and hallux varus. It should be noted that the lateral sesamoid is no longer excised (it is the modification of the original procedure). Salvage can be done with an Aiken procedure or a redone McBride with a proximal MT osteotomy. Arthrodesis and the Keller procedure can also be considered. If hallux varus occurs, an extensor hallucis longus split transfer can be done; and if the deformity is long-standing, rigid, or associated with first MTP degenerative joint disease, an arthrodesis of the first MP joint, a soft tissue rebalancing procedure, can be done.
   3. Chevron Osteotomy—Disadvantages are limited correction of metatarsus primus varus. Pronation of the hallux cannot be corrected. Avascular necrosis can occur after a Chevron osteotomy and is a devastating complication. Other complications include shortening of the MT, hallux varus, excessive displacement, loss of position of the distal fragment, and nonunion. Salvage of a failed procedure can be performed with an Aiken procedure or a modified McBride with a proximal metatarsal osteotomy.
   4. Mitchell Osteotomy—Disadvantages include a high rate of avascular necrosis, first MT shortening, and loss of position of the osteotomy; moreover, it is a technically difficult operation. Contraindications include a short first MT or metatarsalgia. Complications include potential shortening and dorsal displacement of the MT head, along with transfer metatarsalgia.
   5. Keller Bunionectomy—Disadvantages include metatarsalgia due to lateral weight shifting and weakening of the plantar aponeurosis. Cock-up deformities and recurrence rates are relatively high. Transfer calluses and MT stress fractures can occur.
   6. Proximal Metatarsal Osteotomy—The possibility of malunion including the possibility of overcorrection leading to hallux varus exists along with dorsiflexion of the first MT, which would impair its ability to bear weight. Nonunion and delayed union in proximal metaphyseal bone are uncommon.
   7. First M-C Arthrodesis—Nonunion is the most common complication.
   8. Hallux varus—Can be caused by:
      a. Overplication of the medial capsule.
      b. Overcorrection of the intermetatarsal angle with an MT osteotomy.

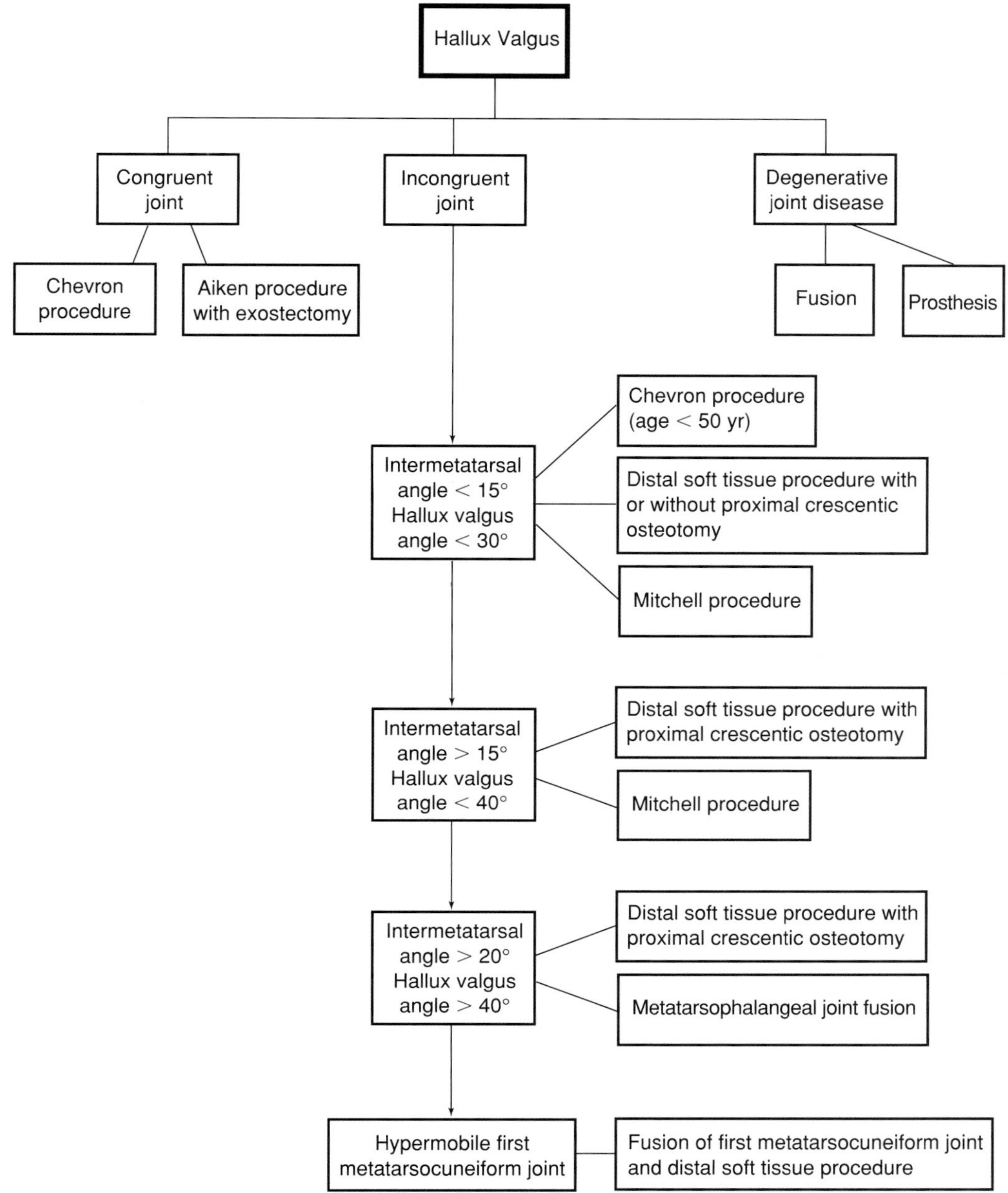

FIGURE 5–7. (From Mann, R.A., and Coughlin, M.J., eds.: The Video Textbook of Foot and Ankle Surgery, p. 152. St Louis, Medical Video Productions 1991; reprinted by permission.)

c. Overresection of too much of the medial aspect of the distal first MT.

9. Hallux varus can be treated with:
   a. Extensor tendon transfer (for supple deformity with satisfactory articular surface).
   b. Arthrodesis of the first MTP joint (Fig. 5–8).

IV. Lesser Toe Deformities

A. Hammer Toe—Deformity at the PIP of a lesser toe (Fig. 5–9). It can be fixed or flexible, with a flexible deformity reducible with ankle plantar flexion or dorsal pressure on the plantar surface of the involved lesser metatarsal.

1. A fixed deformity can be treated with a Duvries arthroplasty, which removes the distal condyles of the proximal phalanx, creating a fibrous joint. This should be fixed with a K-wire or bolster for approximately 2–3 weeks after surgery and then protected for another 3 weeks with taping the PIP joint in extension. Alternatively, arthrodesis of the joint can be accomplished, but it has a high incidence of nonunion.
2. Treatment of a flexible hammer toe must ad-

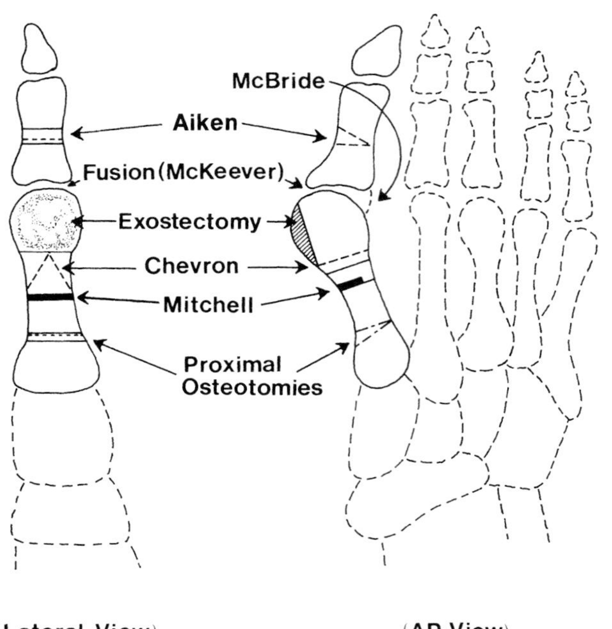

FIGURE 5–8. Common surgical procedures available for hallux valgus correction.

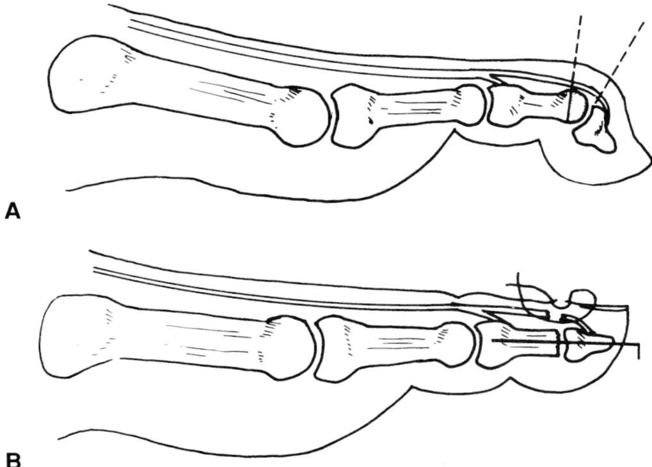

FIGURE 5–10. *A,* Proposed resection for mallet toe repair. *B,* Alternate means of fixation. Stabilization of toe using vertical mattress suture of 3-0 nylon incorporating two Telfa bolsters. (From Coughlin M.: Orthopedics 10:63–75, 1987 reprinted by permission.)

dress the contracture of the flexor digitorum longus (FDL) tendon, which is the presumed cause of this deformity. A standard Duvries arthroplasty of the PIP joint can be performed along with release of the FDL tendon through the same incision at the level of the PIP joint. Alternatively, a Girdlestone flexor tendon transfer can be performed, releasing the FDL tendon distally, splitting it longitudinally, and transferring the two tails to the dorsal extensor hood where they are attached.

B. Mallet Toe—Flexion deformity of the DIP (Fig. 5–10). It usually presents with pain or callus formation on the tip of the toe that is striking the ground or the dorsal DIP joint. If tightness of the FDL tendon is noted, the tendon can be released at the same time as removal of the distal condyles of the middle phalanx. Postoperative care is similar to that for hammer toe.

C. Claw Toe—This deformity is a combination of a hyperdorsiflexion deformity of the MP joint along with either a hammer toe or mallet toe deformity. It can be treated at the MP joint with an arthrotomy and release of the extensor tendon and dorsal capsule, as well as release of the medial and lateral collateral ligaments. A Girdlestone flexor tendon transfer can be performed if necessary, after which correction of the hammer toe or mallet toe deformity can be accomplished. If the MTP joint is dislocated and the deformity is longstanding and/or fixed, a Duvries resection arthroplasty of the MT head may be necessary. It involves excision of the distal 3–4 mm of the MT head.

D. Fifth Toe Deformities—The most common fifth toe deformity is an overlapping fifth toe, which is generally a congenital deformity. The pathology involves both dorsal and medial contracture of the capsule and extensor tendon, as well as of the dorsal skin. Surgical procedures involve release of the extensor tendon and capsule, as well as resolution of the skin contracture. A Duvries procedure consists of a longitudinal dorsal incision and joint and tendon release; when closure of the

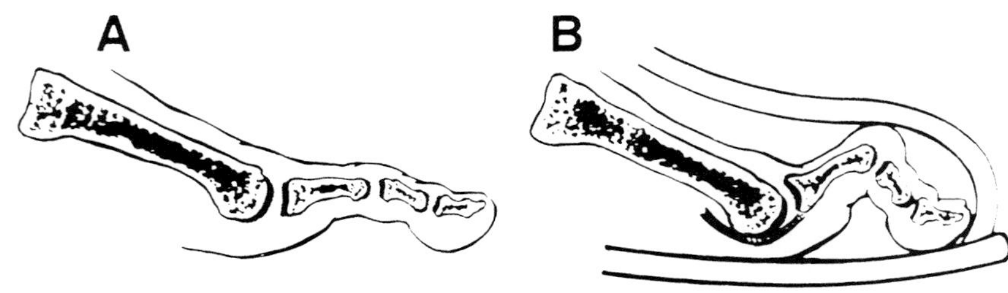

FIGURE 5–9. *A,* Phalanx extended to normal length. *B,* Buckling of phalanx caused by restriction of end of shoe. Interphalangeal joints and metatarsophalangeal joints become subluxed. Over time, dislocation may occur. (From Mann, R.A., and Coughlin, M.J., eds.: Surgery of the Foot and Ankle, 6th ed., vol. 1, p. 343. St. Louis, CV Mosby, 1993; reprinted by permission.)

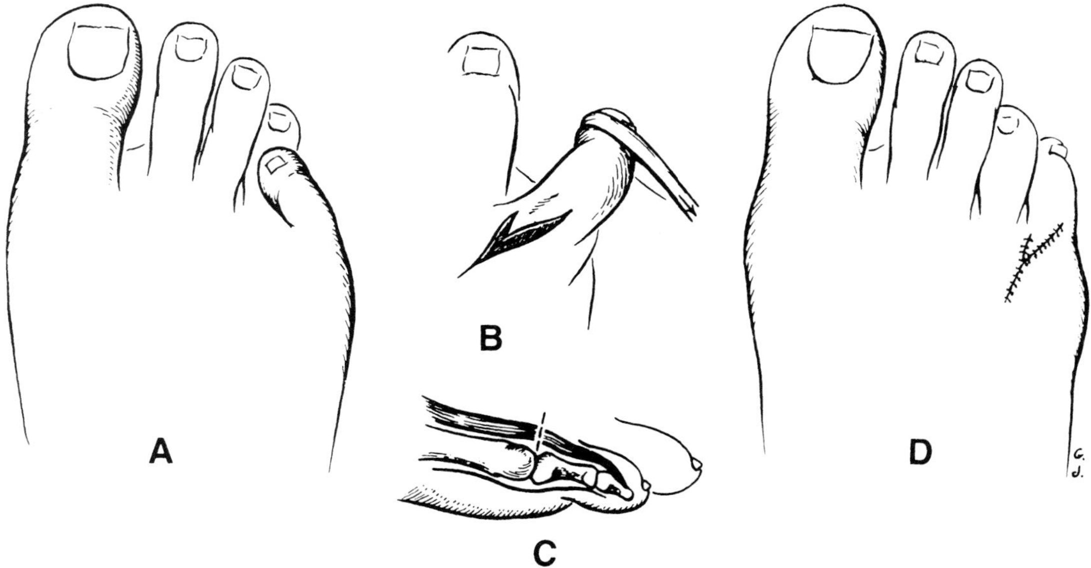

FIGURE 5–11. Wilson technique for correction of mild to moderate overlapping fifth toe. *A,* Preoperative appearance. *B,* Y-Shaped incision over fifth metatarsophalangeal joint. *C,* Sectioning of extensor tendon and dorsal capsule of metatarsophalangeal joint. *D,* Correction of deformity and suturing of skin. (From Mann, R.A., and Coughlin, M.J., eds.: Surgery of the Foot and Ankle, 6th ed., vol. 1, p. 397. St. Louis, CV Mosby, 1993; reprinted by permission.)

skin is performed, it is important to stretch the fibular margin distally and displace the tibial margin proximally. A Wilson V-Y plasty involves making a V-type incision centered over the medial aspect of the fifth toe and extending it into the fourth interspace (Fig. 5–11). After release of the extensor tendon and the dorsal and medial MP joint, the toe is plantar flexed and the V incision becomes Y-shaped skin flap. It is closed with the toe held in an overcorrected position.

E. Hyperkeratotic Pathology of the Lesser Toes
   1. Hard Corn—Hyperkeratotic skin reaction on the dorsolateral aspect of the fifth toe, usually at the PIP joint. It results from the condyle of the proximal phalanx of the fifth toe rubbing against the lateral side of the toe box, with a subsequent skin reaction. Nonsurgical treatment consists in a wider toe box or donut-type skin protectors and trimming the callus with a blade or pumice stone. Should this treatment be unsatisfactory, surgical intervention with removal of the distal condyles of the proximal phalanx is helpful.
   2. Soft Corn—Hyperkeratotic reaction of the skin between the toes that is a result of the pressure of one toe on another with subsequent skin reaction. Surgical treatment consists in a wider toe box in shoewear, lamb's wool or a foam insert between the toes, and trimming the callus. Should this treatment not be satisfactory, removal of the distal condyles of the offending proximal phalanx, as is done during a hammer toe repair, can be performed. If there is uncertainty as to which bony prominence is the offender, a lead marker can be placed over the soft corn and a radiograph obtained.

V. Hyperkeratotic Pathology of the Plantar Foot

A. Intractable Plantar Keratoses (IPKs)
   1. IPK is a hyperkeratotic skin reaction on the plantar surface of the foot. It is the result of excess pressure on a small area with subsequent skin reaction. It is sometimes confused with a plantar wart, which is the result of a virus. A plantar wart has pinpoint vessels when trimmed with a blade. An IPK, of necessity, is at a weight-bearing area, whereas a plantar wart is not necessarily so. There are several types of IPK.
      a. Discrete IPK
         1. Localized intractable plantar keratosis is sometimes found under a distal plantar MT condyle. They form focal or discrete IPKs. Nonsurgical options include pads or orthotics to relieve weight-bearing under the region; surgery, if necessary, can be performed to remove the plantar condyle. A "seed corn" IPK (Fig. 5–12) is another form of a focal or discrete IPK caused by invagination of epithelium over which a skin reaction occurs. They become narrower and deeper when trimmed with a blade and are usually cured after one or two trimmings after the "seed corn" is removed.
         2. If the focal or discrete lesion is under the first MT head, it may be due to a prominent fibular or tibial sesamoid. If refractory to trimming, padding, and so on, sesamoid shaving is the surgical approach.
         3. If the focal or discrete lesion is under the interphalangeal joint of the hallux

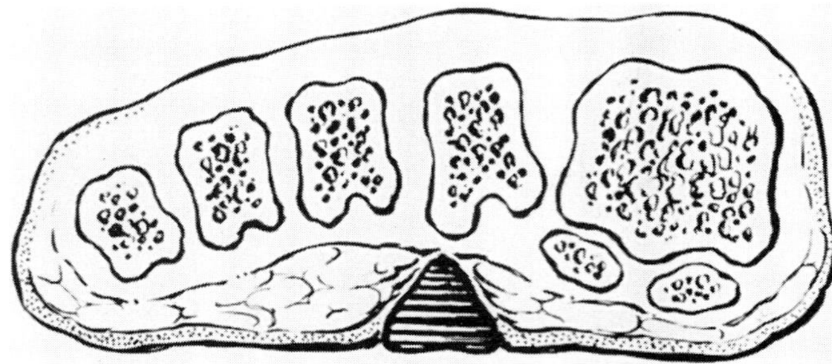

FIGURE 5–12. Location of a discrete plantar keratosis underneath the prominent fibular condyle. (From Mann, R.A., and Coughlin, M.J., eds.: Surgery of the Foot and Ankle, 6th ed., vol. 1, p. 420. St. Louis, CV Mosby, 1993; reprinted by permission.)

and midline, it may be due to a subhallux sesamoid in the flexor hallucis longus and removed if refractory to padding, trimming, and so on.

b. Diffuse IPK—Result of extra weight-bearing in an area of the foot, with a subsequent skin reaction. They are often treated nonsurgically with MT pads or orthotics. There are numerous causes, and the treatment can be specific to the problem. Most common causes are short first MT, long second MT, MT head resection, or dorsiflexed lesser MT.

B. Bunionette—This deformity (tailor's bunion) is characterized by a prominence on the lateral distal fifth MT head that is painful and causes a diffuse callus laterally and occasionally in a plantar direction. Constrictive shoewear and friction between the shoe and the underlying bony structure can lead to the hyperkeratotic reaction. Sometimes the fifth MT is deviated in a mild plantar position as well as laterally, resulting also in a plantar callus. They are generally of three types.

1. A large lateral condyle of the fifth MT head may be noted. Following conservative treatment, the lateral side of the head can be trimmed or Chevron-type osteotomy done of the fifth MT.
2. Laterally deviated fifth MT (normal 4–5 intermetatarsal angle averages 6 degrees) can be treated with a fifth MT osteotomy. Several variations have been described, including Chevon-type and shaft-type osteotomies. Proximal osteotomies at the metaphyseal–diaphyseal juncture are generally avoided because of poor healing.
3. When a plantar callus is present as well as a lateral callus, a diaphyseal osteotomy, oriented so as to shift the MT head medially and somewhat dorsally has been found to be associated with symptomatic relief.

VI. Sesamoids and Accessory Bones—Sesamoids under the MT heads are variable from foot to foot and from person to person. The most common constant is two sesamoids underneath the first MT heads. One or both can be bipartite. About 80% of bipartite sesamoids involve the tibial sesamoids; 25% of bipartite tibial sesamoids have an identical bipartite sesamoid on the contralateral side. The medial sesamoid is frequently divided into two, three, or four parts; the lateral sesamoid is rarely divided into more than two. The sesamoids are encased in the flexor digitorum brevis tendon and help to provide stability to the hallux. One rides on either side of the crista of the plantar first MT. The sesamoidal ligament interconnects the sesamoids, and the intermetatarsal ligament prevents subluxation of the sesamoids from their position in relation to the second MT. Differentiating a bipartite sesamoid that is inflamed from a sesamoid fracture can be difficult. Although they both remain tender with the great toe in dorsiflexion, the inflamed sesamoid tends to be significantly less tender during palpation with the hallux in plantar flexion. The regular, smooth cortex is consistent with a bipartite sesamoid.

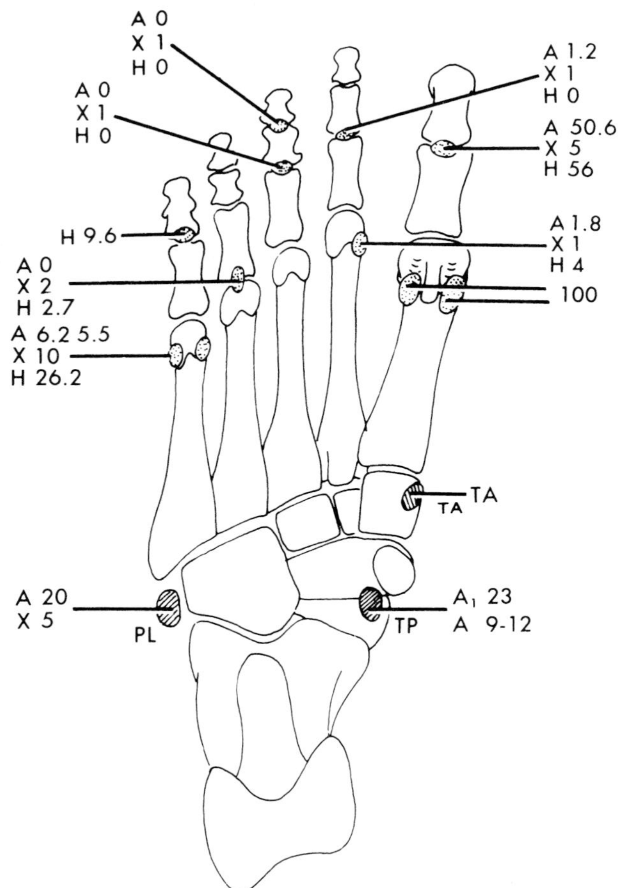

FIGURE 5–13. Sesamoids of the foot. Frequency of occurrence based on anatomic evaluation (A), histoembryologic investigation (H), and radiographic investigation (X). (From Mann, R.A., and Coughlin, M.J., eds.: Surgery of the Foot and Ankle, 6th ed., vol. 1, p. 500. St. Louis, CV Mosby, 1993; reprinted by permission.)

A. Accessory Bones—An accessory bone within the posterior tibial tendon is found by radiography approximately 10% of the time. It should be differentiated from an accessory navicular. An os peroneum in the peroneus longus is found in approximately 5% of feet by radiography. Osteochondritis dissecans of the os peroneum may occur and be quite painful (Fig. 5–13). Rupture

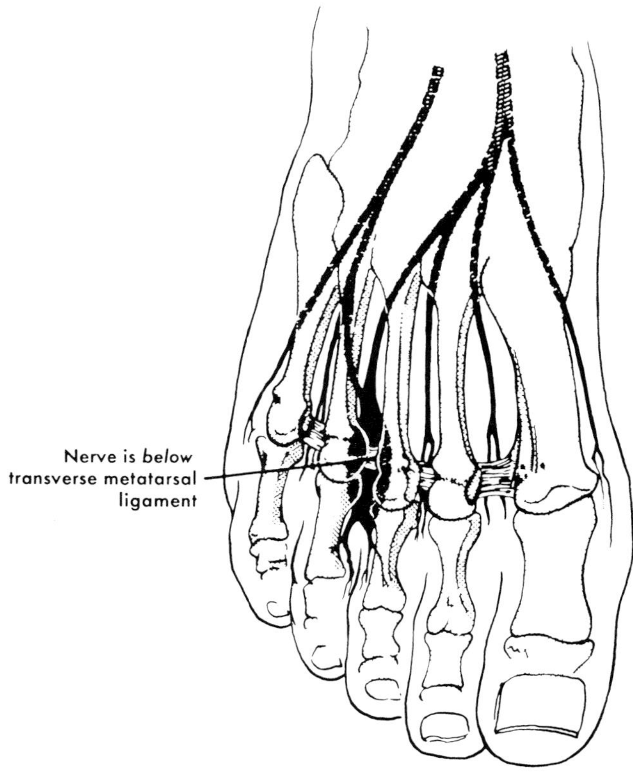

FIGURE 5–14. Third branch of medial plantar nerve. Note that it courses in a plantar direction, under the transverse metatarsal ligament. (From Mann, R.A., and Coughlin, M.J., eds.: Surgery of the Foot and Ankle, 6th ed., vol. 1, p. 546. St. Louis, CV Mosby, 1993; reprinted by permission.)

of the peroneus longus tendon can occur and be noted by proximal migration of the os peroneum on radiographs. An os trigonum can be found posterior to the talus and can cause posterior impingement, which presents with posterior ankle pain during extremes of ankle plantar flexion.

VII. Neurologic Disorders

A. Interdigital Plantar Neuroma—Morton's neuroma usually occurs in the second or third interdigital space (Fig. 5–14). It is rare in the first and fourth interdigital space. It is thought to probably be the result of continuous trauma in the region, although this concept is not certain. Positive physical findings include tenderness in the involved interdigital space and pain on compression of the MT heads. Differential diagnosis includes plantar fasciitis, tarsal tunnel syndrome, MT stress fracture, and synovitis of the MTP joint.
  1. Nonsurgical Treatment—MT pads, soft-soled wide-laced shoes, and local corticosteroid injection.
  2. Surgical Treatment—Excision of the nerve (80% successful). Most surgeons prefer a dorsal approach for a neuroma that has not previously been operated on.

B. Recurrent Neuromas—Can recur 1–4 years after the initial surgery. Clinical symptoms are similar to the initial preoperative pain, and nonsurgical treatment remains similar. Surgical excision of a recurrent neuroma involves a longer dorsal incision than an initial neuroma. Careful dissection proximally should be undertaken to enhance exposure and ensure removal of adequate nerve tissue. Many surgeons prefer a plantar incision and approach for recurrent neuromas, but plantar incisions have been associated with painful scars, often worse than the initial problem.

C. Tarsal Tunnel Syndrome—Involves compression of the posterior tibial nerve under the flexor retinaculum. Tarsal tunnel syndrome can be cause by trauma or swelling of any of the three tendons under the retinaculum (posterior tibial tendon, flexor digitorum longus tendon, flexor hallux longus tendon). It can also be caused by a ganglion of one of these tendon sheaths, a lipoma within the tarsal canal, an exostosis or bony fracture fragment, enlarged venous complex, or neurologic pathology such as a neurilemoma of the posterior tibial nerve. The diagnosis should be confirmed with a positive EMG and nerve conduction velocity (NCV) study prior to surgical release.

D. Incisional Neuromas
  1. A neuroma over the dorsum of the foot can be disabling, as there is so little soft tissue protection over this area. Shoewear can cause continuous pressure and pain in the region. The general anatomy of nerves on the dorsum of the foot has wide variability, and the surgeon must exercise great care because of this variation. The patient usually complains of well localized pain, sometimes radicular in nature. The patient is often comfortable when ambulating without shoes. Physical examination reveals a scar and a localized area of tenderness.
  2. Nonsurgical treatment consists in pads to protect the area of the tender neuroma. Resection of the nerve leaves an area of anesthesia and possibly dysesthesia, but this situation is often an improvement over the initial condition because the new nerve ending is in an area not continuously irritated by shoewear or ankle motion.

E. Central Nervous System Disorders
  1. Stroke
     a. Orthotic Management—Indicated for either stroke or a traumatic brain injury where weak plantar flexors of the ankle allow dorsiflexion during the stance phase of gait. A stiff ankle-foot orthosis (AFO) with the ankle in neutral can be helpful. Weak ankle dorsiflexion can also be helped with an AFO. Impaired proprioception in the ankle or knee can also often be helped with an AFO.
     b. Surgical Treatment—Surgical correction should not take place until the neurologic status has stabilized. In a patient injured by a cerebrovascular accident, variable recovery usually occurs over a 6-month period. With traumatic brain injury, improvement can continue for 18 months or more. An incomplete spinal cord injury can continue to improve for 12 months. Cerebral palsy does not progress. However, function problems and deformities may change because of growth of the affected limb, with changing soft tissue contractures or bony deform-

ities. Flexion deformities of the toes are not uncommon and can often be treated with flexor tendon release or Girdlestone-Taylor flexor tendon transfer. When contractures exist, release of the contracted tissues or decompression by resection of bone might be necessary. With an isolated equinus contracture, Achilles tendon lengthening may be enough to restore a plantar grade foot.

1. A relatively common deformity of gait following a stroke or traumatic brain injury is an equinovarus deformity during swing and stance. There are five muscles that can produce this deformity: anterior tibialis, flexor hallux longus, posterior tibialis, flexor digitorum longus, and gastroc-soleus complex. The posterior tibialis rarely is overreactive in the stance phase.
2. SPLATT—A split anterior tendon transfer can effectively enhance ankle dorsiflexion and balance the foot out of inversion to a more neutral position.

F. Charcot-Marie-Tooth Disease—Hereditary neurologic disorder characterized by weakness of the peroneal muscles and progress weakness of the intrinsic muscles of the foot, dorsiflexors of the foot and toes, and plantar flexors. The end presentation of this syndrome is usually clawing of the toes, forefoot and hindfoot varus and cavus deformity, and equinus of the ankle. Intrinsic weakness of the muscles of the hand is often associated.

1. The disease is inherited as a sex-linked recessive, autosomal dominant (AD), and autosomal recessive (AR) disorder. Males are affected more than females, and the age of onset of symptoms varies with the genetic etiology: The AR disorder presents early, usually before age 10 years. The AD variety presents during the third decade. The sex-linked recessive form usually presents during the second decade. The earlier the onset of symptoms, the more severe is the clinical presentation.
2. Treatment consists initially in orthotic management, supporting the foot in a plantargrade position. A plastic AFO might be sufficient. An important diagnostic point consists in evaluation as to whether the patient's symptomatology is hindfoot, forefoot, or both. With forefoot pathology sometimes plantar flexion of the first metatarsal is the primary symptom and sometimes plantar flexion of multiple rays. The pathology is usually obvious if present. The Coleman block test differentiates fixed from flexible hindfoot varus deformities. Procedures such as Achilles tendon lengthening, split anterior tibial tendon transfer, plantar fascia release, and claw toe procedures (as previously described) are often helpful. A Jones procedure (hallux IP arthrodesis and transfer of the extensor hallucis longus (EHL) tendon into the distal first MT) can be helpful early in the disease process. First MT dorsiflexing osteotomy is sometimes necessary. A Dwyer calcaneal osteotomy can be performed for fixed hindfoot varus. If the varus deformity is flexible, a tenodesis of the peroneus brevis to the longus can be performed.

G. Peripheral Nerve Injuries

1. Neuropraxia—Minor peripheral nerve injury involving a local conduction block with continuity of the axon. Prognosis for recovery is good.
2. Axonotmesis—More serious and involved loss of axonal continuity with an intact endoneural tube. There is good potential for reinnervation.
3. Neurotmesis—Complete severance of the nerve. Spontaneous regeneration does not occur.
4. The most common peripheral nerve injured in the lower extremity is the common peroneal nerve. If spontaneous function does not return during the 3–6 months after a compression injury, surgical exploration should be considered. Penetrating injuries can be explored approximately 1 month after injury, which allows for demarcation of the injury. Nonsurgical treatment consists in an AFO.
   a. Motor injury to the common peroneal usually results in paralysis of the anterior tibialis and the peroneus longus and brevis nerves.
   b. Sensory loss usually involves the dorsum of the foot and is not considered clinically important.
   c. The most common transfer for this motor deficiency is transfer of the posterior tibialis through the interosseous membrane to the dorsum of the foot.

H. Post-Polio Syndrome—Usually characterized by progressive weakness and fatigue of the muscle(s) affected by polio, often presenting approximately 30 years after the initial onset of infectious poliomyelitis. It is probably the result of excessive muscle action during walking due to chronic overuse of weakened muscles. Other theories include activation of latent polio virus in the anterior horn cells or progression of polio to a variation of amyotrophic lateral sclerosis. Treatment often consists in changes in life style to reduce demands on the symptomatic muscles. The use of equipment such as wheelchairs, crutches, walkers, or canes can also be helpful. In addition, AFOs with locked ankles or dorsiflexion or plantar flexion stops can be helpful.

VIII. Arthritic Disease

A. Crystal Disease

1. Gout—Systemic disease of altered purine metabolism with subsequent sodium urate crystal precipitation into synovial fluids. This results in an inflammatory response to the deposition of these crystals which can form into tophi. The tophi can cause periarticular destruction, which is often found as a manifestation of the chronic disease. The disease is more frequently seen in men than in women, and approximately 50–75% of the initial attacks occur in the great toe MTP joint. Diagnosis is often made by identifying sodium urate crystals, but it can be inferred on the basis of clinical examination, serum uric acid, or the response to the treatment with colchicine. Allopurinol can be used to prevent further at-

tacks. Approximately 10% of patients with untreated gout develop chronic tophaceous deposits in the soft tissues, followed by destruction of the joints. One of the distinguishing features of gouty arthritis is the destructive bony lesions remote from the articular surface. Treatment of an acute attack is symptomatic, with elevation and rest. Colchicine or NSAIDs are also helpful. Symptomatic tophi can be excised with curettage. Medical treatment sometimes results in dissolution of tophi.

2. Pseudogout—Also known as chondrocalcinosis, results from the deposition of calcium pyrophosphate. It becomes symptomatic when crystals are shed into a joint, where they can lead to phagocytosis and enzyme release by leukocytes. The resulting painful inflammatory response can cause significant pain. The talonavicular and subtalar joints are more often implicated in the foot, and the end result often resembles advanced degenerative arthritis. Treatment consists in anti-inflammatory medications. When joint destruction is significant, surgical treatments used for degenerative arthritis are indicated.

B. Seronegative Diseases—The three seronegative spondyloarthropathies—ankylosing spondylitis, Reiter syndrome, and psoriatic arthritis—have clinical and radiologic manifestations different from those of rheumatoid arthritis (RA). Radiologic differences are (1) intra-articular ankylosis; (2) calcification within the adventitia; and (3) the lack of osteopenia. Clinically, all of these problems can present with painful heel syndrome or Achilles tendinitis, whereas they do not appear in RA.

1. Psoriatic arthritis antedates the skin lesions of psoriasis by years in approximately 20% of patients. There is often symmetric involvement of hands and feet, and cuticle changes are not uncommon (splitting nails). Involvement of the distal interphlanageal joints and dorsal tuft resorption can also be seen. Destruction of the proximal phalanges can produce a "cup and saucer" appearance of a destroyed joint.
2. Reiter Syndrome—Consists of conjunctivitis, urethritis, and symmetric arthritis (possibly a painful heel). It is much more common in males and correlates often with a positive HLA-B27. Lower extremities are usually involved, and "sausage toes" are common. Radiographic changes can range from nothing to soft tissue swelling. Occasionally demineralization is noted at the PIP joints.
3. Ankylosing Spondylitis—Its main effect is on the axial skeleton. Manifestations within the foot and ankle are relatively minor compared to these effects and often involve attachments of tendons and ligaments to the calcaneus. Manifestations that are similar, but less intense, can be seen in the MTP joints.

C. Lyme Disease—Caused by the spirochete *Borrelia burgdorferi.* It is transmitted by an arthropod-borne tick (*Ixodes dammini*), which infects deer and other animals. Endemic areas include the northeastern part of the United States, Minnesota, Oregon, and California. The infection presents in stages, including a target-shaped skin rash, fever, and systemic disease, although these stages do no always occur. Late manifestations in the musculoskeletal system masquerade as tendinitis, internal derangement of the joint, or overuse syndrome. Symptoms are not helped by steroid injections, physical therapy, or arthroscopy. Positive blood studies for titers to the Lyme disease antibody comprise the method of diagnosis; a high level of suspicion in endemic areas is appropriate. Treatment with antibiotics results in alleviation or resolution of symptoms.

D. Degenerative Joint Disease (DJD)—Usually occurs in the middle-aged or elderly population, but it can follow trauma or osteochondritis dissecans. Obesity and high levels of physical activity are also found to correlate with this disease. The cause of the degenerative changes is uncertain, but biochemical changes within the articular cartilage have been noted. Nonsurgical treatment is aimed at stress reduction. Anti-inflammatory medications can be helpful, as can weight loss, activity modification, and properly fitted shoes. Orthotics can be helpful for removing stress from rigid or painful areas. An AFO is sometimes helpful. Surgical treatments are limited to patients with a great deal of pain, and techniques usually involve arthrodesis, excisional arthroplasty, or occasionally osteotomy. Implants within the foot and ankle have had disappointing results.

E. Rheumatoid Arthritis (RA)—Systemic disease affecting synovial tissues that is often symmetric in pattern but can be extra-articular. There is thought to be a predilection among those with HLA-DR4. Females are affected three times more often than males.

1. Diagnosis is based on clinical, laboratory, and roentgenographic findings. Approximately 17% of RA begins in the feet. The forefoot is involved more commonly than the hindfoot. Involvement may be asymmetric, but progression to symmetric involvement often occurs.
   a. Pathophysiology—Basic pathologic change is chronic synovitis, which invades and destroys the bone, capsular tissue, and ligamentous structures, causing loss of stability of the joint. Mechanical stresses applied to the weakened supporting structures result in deformity. The magnitude of the deformity is usually dependent on the length of time the disease has been present.
   b. Forefoot Changes—Approximately 90% of patients with RA have forefoot involvement, and approximately 15% of them first present with forefoot pain. As the MP joints lose their competence, the toes sublux dorsally and dislocate dorsally at the MTP joints, pulling the plantar fat pad distally with them so it becomes an anterior rather than an plantar structure. The hallux often deforms into a severe valgus deformity, helping to dorsally displace the lesser toes. Many RA forefoot deformities have interphalangeal joint hyperextension. Hallux varus is a less common deformity of the great toe.
   c. Midfoot Changes—The midfoot is not usually severely involved. Chronic synovitis

can occur with eventual loss of the joint space.

d. Hindfoot Changes—Hindfoot deformity is probably the result of destruction of the ligaments and soft tissues supporting the hindfoot. The subtalar joint collapses into valgus, and the talonavicular joint subluxes into abduction, creating a forefoot abduction deformity. Posterior tibial tendon destruction can also result in a flatfoot deformity.

e. Surgical Treatment—Soft tissue repairs tend to do poorly, and arthrodeses and bony resection are often necessary. The timing of surgery is highly variable among patients.

1. Hallux valgus deformities can be treated with arthrodesis, a Keller type procedure (excisional arthroplasty), or Silastic implant (fraught with problems). All the above, except for arthrodesis have a high recurrence rate.
2. Forefoot Reconstruction—The aim of forefoot reconstruction is to provide a stable medial post via arthrodesis of the first MTP joint. The other goal of forefoot reconstruction is to reduce the plantar fat pad to its proper plantar position. It is usually done with a Hoffman-type procedure, which involves resection of the MT heads. Extensor tenotomies or removal of the proximal aspect of the proximal phalanges help to decompress the area.
3. The hindfoot responds well to arthrodesis—isolated subtalar arthrodesis or triple arthrodesis—depending on the involvement of the talonavicular and calcaneocuboid joint.

F. Treatment for Specific Arthritic Joints

1. Interphalangeal Joint—Arthritis of the interphalangeal joint can be treated with a stiffened shoe to prevent motion or with arthrodesis of the joint.
2. First MP joint (Hallux Rigidus)—Degenerative arthritis of the first MTP joint usually produces a dorsal and/or lateral osteophyte. Dorsiflexion of the great toe, as in heel rise, produces pain from both the arthritis and the bone on bone bumping of the osteophytes. Limitation of motion of the MP joint is usually significant. A number of treatments are available.

a. Cheilectomy—Removes the dorsal and lateral osteophytes from the distal MT and proximal phalanx, allowing greatly increased motion. Degenerative arthritis continues to exist, but the bone-on-bone contact is resolved, which appears to satisfy most patients. If the aim is for 70 degrees dorsiflexion intraoperatively, approximately 50% of that is usually seen at 2 months.

b. Silastic implant can be helpful in resolving the degenerative arthritis pain but it involves all the pitfalls of a Silastic implant (transfer metatarsalgia, breakage, silicone synovitis, variable stability, cock-up toe, and stress fracture).

c. Arthrodesis of the first MP joint can resolve the pain of degenerative arthritis—but at the cost of the loss of motion and the loss of pivoting sports and the ability of wear high heels if desired.

d. Closing wedge osteotomy of the proximal phalanx can be performed to bring the toe into greater dorsiflexion.

3. First Metatarsal Cuneiform Joint—Can be treated with a steel shank stiffener to decrease the motion of the joint and anti-inflammatory drugs. If unsuccessful, arthrodesis of the joint can be accomplished. Rigid internal fixation is helpful for achieving fusion.
4. Talonavicular Joint—Nonsurgical treatment for arthritis in this joint consists of a UCBL-type insert or polypropylene AFO. If unsatisfactory, an isolated talonavicular arthrodesis is helpful in the RA patient or patients with a sedentary life style. For more active patients a double (talonavicular and calcaneocuboid) or triple arthrodesis is necessary.

IX. **Arthrodeses of the Foot and Ankle**—There are many arthrodesis techniques for the foot and ankle and many methods of internal fixation.

A. Ankle Arthrodesis—Indicated for arthritis that produces pain or deformity. Ankle arthrodesis should be in a neutral position regarding dorsiflexion and plantar flexion. Approximately 10 degrees of equinus is appropriate for a patient with osteomyelitis, polio, or other neurologic disease where the patient otherwise cannot stabilize the knee. Varus/valgus alignment should be approximately 5 degrees of valgus, and rotation should be similar to the contralateral limb, usually approximately 7 degrees of external rotation. A SACH heel may be a helpful hindfoot cushion. For failed total ankle arthrodesis, the patient may require a tibiocalcaneal arthrodesis positioned in 5–10 degree of dorsiflexion.

B. Subtalar Arthrodesis—For isolated subtalar arthritis, subtalar arthrodesis is an appropriate procedure. Subtalar arthrodesis should be placed in approximately 5 degrees of valgus. Up to 10 degrees is well tolerated but a greater amount can result in lateral impingement against the fibula. Varus alignment is poorly tolerated, as it locks Chopart's joint.

C. Talonavicular Arthrodesis—Arthrodesis of the talonavicular joint results in loss of motion of the calcaneocuboid joint and significant loss of motion in the subtalar joint. Talonavicular arthrodesis is usually satisfactory in sedentary patients, including those with RA. For a patient with a higher level of activity, a calcaneocuboid arthrodesis should be performed concurrently to add stability to the construct. The position of arthrodesis should be with the calcaneus in 5 degrees of valgus and the forefoot in a neutral position so the long axis of the talus is aligned with the long axis of the first MT.

D. Double Arthrodesis—Consists of arthrodesis of the calcaneocuboid joint and the talonavicular joint (Chopart's joint). The effect of this arthrodesis is the same as a triple arthrodesis, as it also restricts subtalar motion. Position of the heel is important when a double arthrodesis is performed, as there is little or no motion after it is performed. The subtalar joint should be placed in 5 degrees of valgus and Chopart's joint manipulated to provide a plantargrade foot (neutral) with respect to varus/valgus and abduction/adduction of the forefoot.

E. Triple Arthrodesis—Arthrodesis of the calcaneocuboid joint with the talonavicular joint and the subtalar joint. It prevents inversion, eversion, abduction, and adduction.

F. Tarsometatarsal Arthrodesis—Sometimes indicated for degenerative changes or after injury to the plantar MT cuneiform ligaments; if no deformity exists, in situ arthrodesis is appropriate. If there is deformity or subluxation, reduction of all planes should be carried out prior to arthrodesis.

G. Metatarsophalangeal Joint Arthrodesis—This procedure is indicated for repair of hallux valgus in a patient with RA or other significant soft tissue disease or neuromuscular disorder. It is also satisfactory for severe hallux valgus deformity or hallux rigidus or as a salvage procedure for failed bunion surgery. The great toe should be in approximately 10–20 degrees of valgus and 10–15 degrees of dorsiflexion relative to the plantar aspect of the foot and neutral rotation. Various means of internal fixation are used, including interfragmentary screws, dorsal plates, or a combination of the two. Steinman pin fixation is also used. Complications include nonunion and malunion.

H. Interphalangeal (IP) Joint Arthrodesis of the Hallux—Indications for arthrodesis of the IP joint of the hallux include arthritis, flexion deformity, or loss of competence of the EHL tendon. The joint should be arthrodesed in approximately 5 degrees of plantar flexion with neutral varus or valgus orientation.

X. Postural Disorders in Adults

A. Congenital Flatfoot

1. Congenital flatfoot is divided into two categories: flexible and fixed. Flexible flat feet are pronated with weight-bearing, but with non-weight-bearing they form a normal arch. They are almost always nonpathologic, although they can be caused by a tight heel cord. To examine for a tight heel cord the subtalar joint should be placed into inversion and the ankle then dorsiflexed.
2. Rigid flat feet are pronated regardless of whether bearing weight. They are pathologic, and etiologies include tarsal coalition, congenital vertical talus, and arthrogryposis.

B. Acquired Flatfoot—multiple etiologies in the adult. Posterior tibial tendon dysfunction, RA, and Charcot with subsequent collapse and primary DJD of the tarsometatarsal joints are most common. Severe trauma including calcaneus fractures, Lisfranc fracture-dislocations, acquired neuromuscular imbalance due to polio, peripheral nerve injury, or trauma to the muscles of the leg can also cause this deformity.

C. Pes cavus—Usually caused by neuromuscular pathology, although it can also be caused by congenital or traumatic entities. The patient with pes cavus should have a thorough neurologic evaluation including CT or MRI of the spine. The disease can affect the hindfoot, forefoot, or both. The Coleman block test can evaluate whether a hindfoot varus deformity is fixed or flexible.

1. Neuromuscular diseases causing pes cavus include muscle disease such as muscular dystrophy, peripheral and lumbosacral spinal nerve problems including Charcot-Marie-Tooth disease, spinal dysraphism, polyneuritis, and spinal tumor. Anterior horn cell disease such as poliomyelitis can cause muscular imbalance and central nervous system diseases such as Friedreich's ataxia, or cerebellar disease.
2. Congenital Causes—Residual clubfoot, arthrogroyposis, idiopathic causes.
3. Traumatic Causes—Residuals of compartment syndrome, crush injuries to the lower extremity, severe burns, malunion of foot fractures.

XI. Tendon Disorders

A. Achilles Tendon—The most common Achilles tendon pathology is a rupture. These injuries can be treated surgically or nonsurgically. Nonsurgically a long-leg cast in plantar flexion is necessary. There is controversy regarding surgical versus nonsurgical treatment. Ruptures that present late often need supplementation. The flexor digitorum longus tendon and flexor hallucis longus tendon have been used, along with the plantaris.

B. Peroneal Tendon—The common peroneal tendons can have traumatic dislocation or less commonly traumatic rupture. Attenuation of the superior peroneal retinaculum allows subluxation of the tendons around the posterior fibula region. Chronic subluxation can lead to longitudinal splitting of the peroneus brevis over the sharp posterior ridge of the fibula (Fig. 5–15). This tendon should be repaired if a laceration occurs. Any associated lateral ankle instability can also be addressed by a modified Brostrom repair.

C. Flexor Hallucis Longus (FHL)—This tendon should be repaired if lacerated.

D. Stenosing Tenosynovitis—Can result from swelling within the tendon, and the FHL is the most commonly involved tendon in the foot. It may present with triggering of the hallux. It usually occurs at the tarsal retinaculum posterior to the medial malleolus, and as the tendon passes through the sesamoids inserting into the distal phalanx of the hallux. Treatment consists in immobilization to reduce the inflammation, followed by physical therapy to stretch the hallux. The use of anti-inflammatory medications or possibly steroid injection can be helpful. If this treatment fails, surgery for decompression of the area can be carried out.

E. Extensor Tendons—Lacerations of the extensor tendons (EHL and EDL) should be surgically repaired. Extensor tendinitis can be diagnosed by producing pain with active dorsiflexion and passive plantar flexion of the toes.

F. Posterior Tibial Tendon—Incompetence of the posterior tibial tendon can produce a hindfoot in a valgus position and a forefoot in abduction. This problem gives rise to the "too many toes sign' that are visualized on the affected side when the patient is viewed from behind. Patients often complain about pain in the midfoot region, some-

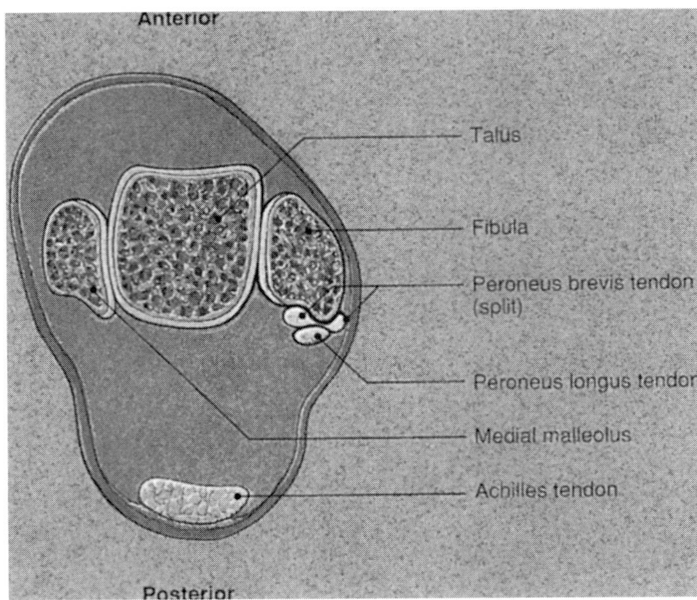

FIGURE 5–15. Cross section of the peroneal tendons at the level of the fibular groove showing the mechanism of injury. The peroneus brevis is compressed by the longus, which lies posterior, into the sharp edge of the fibula. Such compression results in splitting of the peroneus brevis tendon. The superior peroneal retinaculum is not shown. (From Yodlowski, M., and Mizel, M.: Reconstruction of peroneus brevis pathology. Op. Tech. Orthop. 4(3):147, 1994; reprinted by permission.)

times describing a weakness or instability in gait. Physical examination is remarkable for weakness in inversion from an everted position. In addition, patients have difficulty or are unable to stand on tiptoes on only the affected side. If they are capable of standing on tiptoes on the affected side, heel inversion does not occur. Nonsurgical treatment consists in a UCBL insert or an AFO that locks the hindfoot and midfoot. Surgical treatment consists in arthrodesis (a subtalar, double, or triple). Controversy exists as to the best treatment. Reconstruction of the posterior tibial tendon with the flexor digitorum longus tendon through a hole in the navicular is another surgical option and is indicated when the deformity is supple (i.e., no fixed forefoot varus and no limitation in hindfoot inversion).

XII. Heel Pain

A. Plantar Heel Pain—Has multiple causes.

1. Neurologic Causes—Tarsal tunnel syndrome, herniated nucleus pulposus, spinal stenosis. Entrapment or irritation of the medial or lateral branches of the posterior tibial nerves can cause heel pain. In addition, the nerve to the (Baxter) abductor digiti quinti can be irritated as it passes through the abductor hallucis. This problem is usually seen in the athletic population.
2. Bone Pathology—Stress fractures of the calcaneus due to overuse. Calcification at the base of the plantar fascia (heel spur) rarely causes pain, whereas a fracture at the base of a "heel spur" does.
3. Soft Tissue Problems—Such as plantar fasciitis or inflammation of the plantar heel pad can cause pain. Treatment includes a Visco heel, night splint, rigidly soled shoe, steel sole stiffener and rocker bottom, or cast immobilization.

B. Posterior Heel Pain

1. Posterior heel pain is also referred to retrocalcaneal bursitis, Haglund's disease, or insertional Achilles tendinitis. It presents pain and tenderness in the superoposterior portion of the calcaneus at the area of the insertion of the Achilles tendon.
2. Treatment—It can be treated nonsurgically with anti-inflammatory medications, a heel lift, or cast immobilization. Surgical procedures are not commonly necessary. Excision of the retrocalcaneal bursa and superior bony prominence is necessary in some cases.

XIII. Infections of the Foot and Ankle

A. Bacterial Infections

1. Soft Tissue Infections—Superficial lesions such as blisters or scratches are most commonly caused by *Staph. aureus* and β-hemolytic streptococci. Puncture wounds of the foot can cause osteomyelitis, osteochondritis, and septic arthritis. If a puncture wound causes an infection, evaluation and treatment should be aggressive, with a bone scan and possibly CT. If there is abscess formation or a septic joint, surgical débridement (through a dorsal approach) should be performed. If there is osteomyelitis of a sesamoid, it should be removed. Parenteral antibiotics should be administered. *Pseudomonas* is the most common organism

involved. *Staph. aureus* is the second most common. Cat and dog bites can result in an infection from *Pasteurella multocida.* Antibiotics should be administered if a pet bite occurs. This organism is usually covered by penicillin, but cephalosporins cover *P. multocida* as well as *Staph. aureus.*

2. Joint Infections—Usually caused by *Staph. aureus,* although in the young adult *Neisseria gonorrhoea* is also common. Treatment of joint infections is usually parenteral antibiotics and repeated aspirations. If it does not improve after several days, surgical intervention should be considered.
3. Bone Infections
   a. Diagnosis—Similar to that for infections elsewhere. Diagnostic studies, including bone scan, CT scan, and MRI, can be helpful.
   b. Treatment—Usually involves surgical débridement and parenteral antibiotics.
4. Infected Diabetic Foot—Infected feet in the diabetic population account for 15% of the admissions of diabetic patients. More than 5% of diabetics eventually require a below-the-knee amputation. The peripheral neuropathy they often develop prevents them from taking appropriate protective care of their limb, and the large and small vessel disease make healing more difficult. *Staph. aureus* is the most common bacterium, but polymicrobic infections are not uncommon. Wound culture from the surface may not be inaccurate, and if possible an aspiration or deep culture should be obtained. Parenteral antibiotics should be used unless the infection is relatively mild. Hyperbaric oxygen treatment has not been proved to be of additional benefit. Evaluation should include a vascular examination. Should profusion be poor, possible revascularization or amputation might be appropriate. Débridement and drainage should be carried out as would be done for a nondiabetic foot. Heel systolic pressure ratio of 0.45 or higher is a good prognostic indicator for healing.

B. Mycobacterial Infections
   1. Tuberculosis: Rare in the foot.
   2. Atypical Mycobacteria—Rare in the foot. *Mycobacterium avium-intracellulare* is seen in patients with AIDS. *Mycobacterium marinum* is found in patients exposed to infections with marine life.

C. Fungal Infections
   1. *Tinea pedis*—Common fungal infection of the skin and cuticles in the foot. It presents with scaling, itching, and blisters and is often found on the sole and in the interdigital spaces. Local skin infection can be treated with topical agents, and nail infection can be treated with oral griseofulvin, which can take 8 months to a year. Significant potential complications can occur with this medications. Because of these complications, treatment is often inappropriate given the low-level symptoms usually present.
   2. Mycetoma—This fungus infection can cause madura foot, a chronic foot infection. The condition is rare in developed countries.

XIV. Diabetic Foot

A. Pathophysiology—The primary cause of diabetic foot problems is peripheral neuropathy, which allows excess pressure to cause soft tissue pathology while undetected. The often coexisting circulatory impairment causes delayed or possibly no healing. In addition to peripheral neuropathy, diabetics suffer an earlier, more common, more severe arteriosclerotic disease than nondiabetics. In relation to the nondiabetic population it occurs earlier, is more diffuse, often affects both limbs, and affects a higher percentage of the diabetic population. The aorta and iliac and femoral arteries are often involved, and vascular evaluation for large-vessel disease should be carried out in diabetics with nonhealing ulcers or infection. Effects of neurologic pathology include lesser-toe deformities and dry, flaking skin.

B. Clinical Problems and Treatment—One of the main problems of diabetic foot is a nonhealing plantar ulcer that results from excess pressure. Treatment consists in relieving the pressure with orthotics, pads, braces, or a total contact cast. If nonsurgical treatment is not successful, removal of prominent condyles or resection of the offending bony structure can be considered. If osteomyelitis exists, excision of the infected bone or partial amputation should be performed as needed. If an ulcer is present under the heel and cannot be resolved, a partial calcanectomy can be helpful. A Symes amputation might be necessary, which has lower energy consumption during ambulation than a below-the-knee amputation.
   1. Infections fall into the general categories of cellulitis, abscess, and osteomyelitis. Cellulitis should be treated with parenteral antibiotics, and an abscess needs irrigation and débridement, as well as packing and appropriate wound care. Osteomyelitis in the foot, if it exists, requires excision of the infection bone. Partial amputation of a digit, ray, or part of the foot may be necessary for exposed bone or tendon. In the case of suspected infection in a diabetic foot, it is important to evaluate the foot for possible Charcot changes.
   2. Differential diagnosis between infection and Charcot joint may be difficult. Charcot joints (ankle, subtalar joint, midtarsal joint, and tarsometatarsal joints) are warm and erythematous, similar to an infection. Treatment may include a cast, total contact cast, or a wooden shoe depending on the deformity present. During the initial stages they are swollen and weight-bearing should be avoided. A biopsy is not indicated, and the differential diagnosis of a Charcot joint and an infectious process can be aided by a CBC, ESR, and possibly an MRI, which can reveal bony changes consistent with osteomyelitis. The goal of treatment is obtain a plantegrade foot that will probably need continued bracing.

XV. Amputations of the Foot and Ankle

A. Surgical Techniques
   1. Tourniquet—There is no contraindication to a tourniquet in diabetic patients.
   2. Wound Closure—For partial foot amputa-

tions, removal of slightly more bone than originally intended might be necessary to achieve wound closure. In the case of infection, delayed primary closure can be considered.

a. The amputation should be at a level that preserves as much viable bony architecture as is reasonable under the circumstances. Vascular evaluation of the large vessels of the extremity is appropriate, as improvement of enlarged blood vessels may allow a higher level of amputation.

B. Amputation Levels

1. Great Toe—With amputation of the great toe it is better to save the proximal aspect of the proximal phalanx if possible, as it helps preserve some function of the plantar fascia.
2. Lesser Toes—If part of a lesser toe can be preserved during amputation, it provides the advantage of a residual partial toe in place, which can prevent adjacent toes from drifting toward each other.
3. Ray amputation can be successful in the case of infection, gangrene, or trauma. Complications of this procedure occur with weight-bearing on the remaining metatarsals.
4. Transmetatarsal amputation is a solid amputation that allows good ambulation. The most common complication is ulceration of the stump.
5. Chopart's amputation, an amputation through the calcaneocuboid and talonavicular joint, must be accompanied by release of the Achilles tendon to prevent a plantar-flexion contracture. Ambulation requires an AFO.

XVI. Toenail Pathology

A. Systemic Nail Pathology

1. Psoriasis—Changes in the cuticles of a patient with psoriasis often look similar to those seen with fungal infection. Toenail changes include stippling and pitting.
2. Dermatitis—If chronic can result in maladies in the nail plate. Transverse ridging and scaling can occur along with discoloration. Etiologies include allergic reactions to solvents, dyes, nailpolish, detergents, and other chemicals. Pigmentation under the cuticle can be caused by malignant melanoma. Other causes of darkening under the cuticle include Addison's disease. Ingrown toenail (onychocryptosis) occurs when the border of the cuticle pierces the adjacent skin at the border of the cuticle. This soft tissue irritation leads to localized edema and often cellulitis or small abscess formation. Treatment is with antibiotics for any cellulitis or abscess. If the problem continues to recur, a Winograd procedure for permanent ablation of the border of the cuticle can be considered.

XVII. Ankle Sprains

A. Lateral Ankle Sprains—Account for 90% of all ankle sprains. The anterior talofibular ligament (ATFL) alone is involved in approximately two-thirds of ankle sprains and in another 25% with the calcaneofibular ligament (CFL).

1. Evaluation of the ATFL is done by palpating the sinus tarsi region and inversion of the ankle in plantar flexion. Evaluation of the CFL is done with inversion of the ankle in dorsiflexion. The anterior drawer sign is done with the ankle in mild plantar flexion, the tibia stabilized, and the hindfoot drawn forward. Anterior subluxation of the talus under the tibia is consistent with an incompetent ATFL.
2. Differential diagnosis of lateral ankle sprains includes osteochondral fractures of the talus, fracture at the base of the fifth MT, fracture of the lateral process of the talus, and fracture of the anterior process of the calcaneus. Fractures of the lateral malleolus and syndesmosis injuries can also produce significant lateral ankle pain.
3. Treatment of Acute Ankle Sprains
   a. Nonoperative Treatment—The treatment of choice for most ankle sprains. It is indicated for all mild or moderate injuries and most severe ankle sprains. Rest, immobilization, cold, and elevation (RICE) comprise the basics of treatment. Immobilization can range from an Ace bandage, UNA boot, or taping of the ankle (to prevent inversion) to an ankle brace (to prevent inversion) to a cast.
   b. Surgical treatment is controversial. It is recommended at this time only for young, athletic patients with severe injuries.
4. Chronic Lateral Ankle Sprains and Instability—Patients with chronic lateral ankle sprains or instability should be carefully evaluated to detect any occult bony tenderness or cartilaginous or neurologic pathology. Inversion stress views, in both dorsiflexion and plantar flexion, can be helpful. Bone scans can reveal unsuspected fractures. Arthroscopy should be considered in cases where débridement of soft tissue from the anterolateral ankle has relieved symptoms. Reconstruction using the peroneus brevis tendon or plantaris tendons and tightening of the ligaments (Brostrom procedure) have been successful. The anatomic Brostrom ligament repair appears to be the most mechanically stable and is now in favor.

XVIII. Arthroscopy of the Foot and Ankle

A. Indications and Contraindications—Indications include unexplained pain, instability, stiffness, popping, and osteochondral injury or bony impingement. Some fractures are fixed arthroscopically. Contraindications include active infection and vascular insufficiency. Ankle arthroscopy has been shown to be useful for synovitis or anterolateral soft tissue impingement. Arthroscopic ankle arthrodesis has been performed. Complications include injuries to a branch of the superficial peroneal nerve with the anterolateral portal.

B. Arthroscopic Portals—Anteromedial and anterolateral portals are commonly used. An anterocentral portal is sometimes used and is placed between the tendons of the extensor digitorum communis to decrease the potential injury to neurovascular structures. Posterolateral portals are sometimes indicated. Posteromedial portals are not used because of the potential for injury to the posterior tibial nerve.

XIX. Soft Tissue Trauma and Compartment Syndromes

A. Acute Compartment Syndrome—With numerous compartments made up of inelastic fascial structures, the foot is susceptible to compartment syndromes, as is the leg. They occur after an injury, with subsequent edema and an intracompartmental increase in pressure; crush injuries and fractures are frequent causes. Diagnosis often reveals a palpable dorsalis pedis and posterior tibial pulse. Pain caused by a compartment syndrome does not decrease with immobilization, and the pain can be exacerbated with passive dorsiflexion of the toes. During evaluation of the patient the foot should be kept elevated at the level of the heart. Pressure-measuring devices should be used to determine the intracompartmental pressure. Fasciotomy should be performed if the pressure is more than 30 mm Hg. Fasciotomy is often performed through two dorsal incisions, and the fascial compartments within the foot are released.

B. Chronic Compartment Syndrome—If an acute compartment syndrome is left untreated, intrinsic muscles suffer ischemia and necrosis. This process produces lesser-toe deformities with hyperdorsiflexion at the MP joint and hyperflexion deformities at the PIP and DIP joints, as the extrinsic muscles overcome the remaining power of the intrinsics. Sensory deficit results from local injury to nerves and is often present.

XX. Fractures and Dislocations of the Ankle

XX. Fractures and Dislocations of the Ankle—Ankle fractures were classified by Lauge-Hansen, who divided them into supination-adduction, supination-eversion, pronation-abduction, and pronation-eversion. The Weber classification, done by the AO group, is based on the level of the fibula fracture in relation to the plafond. Type A is at or level with the plafond; type B is a spiral fracture beginning at the level of the plafond and extending proximally; and type C is a fracture above the syndesmosis. Weber's B or C injuries require evaluation of the syndesmosis, as fixation may be necessary. If a Weber B fracture has more than 1 mm of displacement, it should be treated with open reduction/internal fixation.

XXI. Fractures and Dislocations of the Foot

A. Calcaneus Fractures—Evaluated radiologically using Bohler's angle, which ranges from 25 to 40 degrees, as well as the angle of Gissane, which normally ranges from 120 to 145 degrees. The subtalar joint can be evaluated with Broden's view, and the entire calcaneus is evaluated for possible surgical intervention using a CT scan in two planes.

1. Extra-articular Fractures—usually do well treated nonsurgically.
2. Anterior process of the calcaneus fractures—Usually do well when treated nonsurgically with cast immobilization. If pain persists, excision of the fragment is usually successful. Triple arthrodesis is considered a last step to relieve pain.
3. Tuberosity Fractures (Beak and Avulsion Fractures)—Displaced beak fractures (without Achilles tendon involvement) can often be reduced closed and immobilized. If there is a possibility of skin necrosis and an unsatisfactory closed reduction, open reduction should be considered. Displaced avulsion fractures (with involvement of the Achilles tendon) require reduction, with open reduction/internal fixation often necessary.
4. Fractures of the Sustentaculum Tali—usually do not need surgical intervention.
5. Fractures of the Body Involving the Posterior Facet—Often treated with open reduction/internal fixation. A lateral approach is popular at this time, but some authors prefer a medial approach and others a combined approach.

B. Talus Fractures

1. The potential complications for talus fractures include avascular necrosis and degenerative changes of the ankle and subtalar joints. Displaced talar neck fractures require open reduction/internal fixation. Nonunion and malunion are other complications.
2. Osteochondral fractures, if acute, are treated with either immobilization or excision and drilling depending on the severity of the fracture. For long-standing lesions, excision of the fragment and drilling are recommended. It can often be done arthroscopically.
3. Fractures of the lateral process of the talus can be treated with immobilization, open reduction/internal fixation, or excision, depending on the severity of the fracture, the size and displacement of the fragment, and the chronicity of the problem.

C. Metatarsal Fractures—When these fractures are displaced such that there is difficulty with the MT heads bearing weight because of significant displacement, they should be fixed with either closed reduction or open reduction and internal fixation. "Jones fractures," which occur at the proximal diaphysis of the fifth MT, are best treated closed if there is no significant displacement. They are treated with cast immobilization and non-weight-bearing. If a nonunion occurs, it may require late treatment with internal fixation and bone grafting. High performance athletes are sometimes treated directly with internal fixation.

D. Subtalar Dislocations—Involve dislocation of the subtalar joint and talonavicular joint. Open subtalar joint dislocations should be taken to the operating room and subjected to irrigation and débridement prior to reduction. These dislocations are classified as medial, lateral, anterior, and posterior. The latter two are rare.

1. Medial Dislocation—Involves an injury of the lateral ankle ligaments with the calcaneus dislocated medially. The talonavicular joint is dislocated so the talar head is dislocated laterally. Closed reduction may be impossible if the talar neck becomes entrapped by the extensor retinaculum or peroneal tendons or if there is impaction of the talus onto the lateral aspect of the navicular.
2. Lateral Dislocation—With the calcaneus dislocated laterally, the talar head and neck dislocate medially. Failure of closed reduction can be caused by the talar neck and head entangled in the posterior tibial tendon or flexor digitorum longus tendon or by a small fracture involving the head of the talus.

E. Lisfranc's Joint Injury—There is no ligament between the base of the first and second MTs. The second MT is attached obliquely to the first cuneiform by an interosseous ligament termed Lisfranc's ligament. These fracture-dislocations should be reduced and treated with screw fixation.

Selected Bibliography

Mann, R.A.: Biomechanics of the foot. In Atlas of Orthotics: Biomechanical Principles and Application, pp. 257–266. St. Louis, CV Mosby, 1975.

Anatomy

Sarraflan, S.K.: Functional Anatomy of the Foot and Ankle. In Anatomy of the Foot and Ankle, 2nd ed. Philadelphia, JB Lippincott, 1993.

Biomechanics

Buck, P., Morrey, B.F., and Chao, E.Y.S.: The optimum position of arthrodesis of the ankle: A gait study of the knee and ankle. J. Bone Joint Surg. [Am.] 69:1052–1062, 1987.

Inman, V.T.: The Joints of the Ankle. Baltimore, Williams & Wilkins, 1976.

Johnson, J.E.: Axis of rotation of the ankle. In Inman's Joints of the Ankle, Stiehl, J.B., ed. Baltimore, Williams & Wilkins, 1991.

Mann, R.A.: Biomechanics of the foot and ankle. In Surgery of the Foot and Ankle, vol. 1, pp. 3–43. St. Louis, Mosby 1993.

Nerves

Mann, R.A.: The tarsal tunnel syndrome. Orthop. Clin. North Am. 5:109, 1974.

Mann, R.A., and Reynold, J.: Interdigital neuroma: A critical analysis. Foot Ankle 3:238, 1983.

Diabetes

Wagner, F.W.: The dysvascular foot: A system for diagnosis and treatment. Foot Ankle 2:84–122, 1982.

Walker, S.R.: The contact casting and chronic diabetic neuropathic foot ulcerations: Healing rates by wound location. Arch. Phys. Med. Rehabil. 68:217–221, 1987.

Waters, R.L., Perry, J., Antonelli, E.E., and Hislop, H.: Energy cost of walking of amputee: The influence of level of amputation. J. Bone Joint Surg. [Am.] 58:42–46, 1976.

Arthritis—Forefoot

Mann, R.A., and Coughlin, M.J.: The rheumatoid forefoot: A review of the literature and method of treatment. Orthop. Rev. 8:105, 1979.

Mann, R.A., and Oates, J.C.: Arthrodesis of the first metatarsophalangeal joint. Foot Ankle 1:159, 1980.

Mann, R.A., and Thompson, F.M.: Arthrodesis of the first metatarsophalangeal joint for hallux valgus in rheumatoid arthritis. J. Bone Joint Surg. [Am.] 66:687, 1984.

Mann, R.A., and Clanton, T.O.: Hallux rigidus: Treatment by cheilectomy. JBJS Volume J. Bone Joint Surg. [Am.] 70A:400–406, 1988.

Shereff, M., and Jahss, M.: Complications of Silastic implant arthroplasty in the hallux. Foot Ankle 1:95, 1980.

Arthritis—Hindfoot/Ankle

Buck, P., Morrey, B.F., and Chao, E.Y.S.: The optimum position of arthrodesis of the ankle. J. Bone Joint Surg. [Am.] 69:1052–1062, 1987.

Elbaor, J.E., Thomas, W.H., Weinfeld, M.S., et al.: Talonavicular arthrodesis for rheumatoid arthritis of the hindfoot. Othop. Clin. North Am. 7:821–826, 1976.

Fogel, G.R., Katoh, Y., Rand, J.A., et al.: Talonavicular arthrodesis for isolated arthrosis: 9.5 Year results and gait analysis. Foot Ankle 3:105–113, 1982.

Iwata, H., Yasuhara, N., Kawashima, K., et al.: Arthrodesis of the ankle joint with rheumatoid arthritis: Experience with the transfibular approach. Clin. Orthop. 153:189–193, 1980.

Mann, R.A.: Surgical implications of biomechanics of the foot and ankle. Clin. Orthop. 146¸1–118, 1980.

Mazur, J.M., Schwartz, E., and Simon, S.R.: Ankle arthrodesis: Long-term follow-up with gait analysis. J. Bone Joint Surg. [Am.] 61: 964–975, 1979.

Bunions

Bordelon, R.L.: Evaluation and operative procedures for hallux valgus deformity. Orthopedics 10:37–44, 1987.

Coughlin, M.J.: Arthrodesis of the first metatarsophalangeal joint. Orthop. Rev. 19:177–186, 1990.

Coughlin, M.J., and Mann, R.A.: Arthrodesis of the first metatarsophalangeal joint as salvage for the failed Keller procedure. J. Bone Joint Surg. [Am.] 69:68–75, 1987.

Coughlin, M.J., and Mann, R.A.: The pathophysiology of the juvenile bunion. Instr. Course Lect. 36:123–136, 1987.

Mann, R.A.: Complications in surgery of the foot. Orthop. Clin. North Am. 7:851, 1976.

Mann, R.A.: Hallux valgus. Instr. Course Lect. XXXV:339–353, 1986.

Mann, R.A.: Treatment of the bunion deformity. Orthopedics 10: 49–56, 1987.

Mann, R.A., and Coughlin, M.J.: Hallux valgus—etiology, anatomy, treatment, and surgical considerations. Clin. Orthop. 157:31–41, 1981.

Mann, R.A., and Coughlin, M.J.: Hallux valgus and complications of hallux valgus. In: Surgery of the Foot, 5th ed., Mann, R.A., ed., pp. 66–130. St. Louis, CV Mosby, 1986.

Mann, R.A., and Oates, J.C.: Arthrodesis of the first metatarsophalangeal joint. Foot Ankle 1:159–166, 1980.

Mitchell, C.L., Fleming, J.L., Allen, R., Glenney, C., et al.: Osteotomy-bunlonectomy for hallux valgus. J. Bone Joint Surg. [Am.] 40:41, 1958.

Silver, D.: The operative treatment of hallux valgus. J. Bone Joint Surg. 5:225–232, 1923.

Lesser Toes

Coughlin, M.J.: Crossover second toe deformity. Foot Ankle 8:29–39, 1987.

Coughlin, M.J.: Second metatarsophalangeal joint instability in the athlete. Foot Ankle 14:309–319, 1993.

Coughlin, M.J.: Subluxation and dislocation of the second metatarsalphalangeal joint. Orthop. Clin. North Am. 20:535–551, 1989.

Coughlin, M.J., and Mann, R.A.: Lesser toe deformities. Instr. Course Lect. 36:137–159, 1987.

Coughlin, M.J., and Mann, R.A.: Lesser toe deformities. In Surgery of the Foot and Ankle, 6th ed., Mann, R.A., and Coughlin, M.J., eds. St. Louis, CV Mosby, 1993.

Mizel, M.S.: Correction of hammertoe and mallet toe deformities: Operative techniques. Orthopedics 2:188–194, 1992.

Sangeorzan, B.J., Benirschke, S.K., Mosca, V., Mayo, et al.: Displaced intra-articular fractures of the tarsal navicular. J. Bone Joint Surg. [Am.] 71:1504–1510, 1989.

Intractable Plantar Keratosis

Bordelon, L.R.: Orthotics, shoes and braces. Orthop. Clin. North Am. 20:751–757, 1989.

Brodsky, J.W., Kourosh, S., Stills, M., and Mooney, V.: Objective evaluation of insert material for diabetic and athletic footwear. Foot Ankle 9:111–116, 1988.

Holmes, G.B., and Timmerman, L.: A quantitative assessment of the effect of metatarsal pads on plantar pressures. Foot Ankle 11: 141–145, 1990.

Mann, R.A., and Coughlin, M.J., Keratotic disorders of the plantar skin. In: Surgery of the Foot and Ankle, Mann, R.A., and Coughlin, M.J., eds. Mosby-Yearbooks, 1993.

Mann, R.A., and Duvries, H.L.: Intractable plantar keratosis. Orthop. Clin. North Am. 4:67–73, 1973.

Mann, R.A., and Wapner, K.L.: Tibial sesamoid shaving for treatment of intractable plantar keratosis. Foot Ankle 13:196–198, 1992.

Tendon Injury

Hamilton, W.G.: Stenosing tenosynovitis of the flexor hallucis longus tendon and posterior impingement upon the os trigonum in ballet dancers. Foot Ankle 3:74–80, 1982.

Inglis, A.E., Scott, W.N., Sculo, T.P., et al.: Ruptures of the tendon Achillis: An objective assessment of surgical and non-surgical treatmeamt. J. Bone Joint Surg. [Am.] 52:990–993, 1976.

6

HAND

JAMES F. BRUCE

I. Anatomy and Pathophysiology (see also Chapter 11, Anatomy)

A. Dorsal Extensor Compartments of the Wrist

COMP	TENDONS	ASSOCIATED PATHOLOGIC CONDITIONS
1	EPB, APL	de Quervain's tenosynovitis
2	ECRL/B	Carpal boss
3	EPL	Rupture over Lister's tubercle
4	EDC, EIP	Extensor tenosynovitis
5	EDQ	Rupture in rheumatoids (Vaughn-Jackson syndrome)
6	ECU	Snapping at ulnar styloid

B. Joint Flexion and Extension

JOINT	FLEXION	EXTENSION
MCP	IO, lumbricals	EDC (sagittal bands)
PIP	FDS, FDP	Lumbricals (lateral bands), EDC (central slip)
DIP	FDP	EDC (terminal tendon), ORL (Landsmeer's ligaments)

C. Relationships

1. Extensor indicis proprius (EIP) and extensor digiti quinti (EDQ) are ulnar to extensor digitorum communis (EDC) tendons.
2. Cleland's and Grayson's ligaments cover the digital neurovascular bundles. Cleland's ligament is above (dorsal; ceiling) and Grayson's (volar; ground) is below the nerve.
3. There are four dorsal interosseous (IO) abductors (DAB) and three palmar IO adductors (PAD). The long finger is considered the central axis of the hand.
4. The lumbricals are the "workhorse of the hand" and insert radially into the extensor apparatus (lateral bands). The two radial lumbricals are supplied by the median nerve, and the two ulnar lumbricals are supplied by the ulnar nerve. Ulnar innervated muscles are multipenniform; median-innervated lumbricals are unipenniform. The **lumbrical** is the only muscle that **relaxes its own antagonist** (flexor digitorum profundus [FDP]).
5. The thenar and hypothenar abductors are superficial; the opponens muscles are deep. The flexor pollicis brevis (FPB) has a dual innervation (median supplies the superficial fibers, ulnar the deep fibers). The abductor pollicis brevis (APB), which is innervated by the median nerve, is the key thenar muscle involved in opposition.
6. The superficial arch is distal and is supplied by the ulnar artery; the deep arch is proximal and is fed by the radial artery. However, the classic complete arch (condominant) is present in only one-third of patients.
7. Digital arteries are volar to nerves in the palm but are dorsal to the digital nerves in the fingers.
8. Autogenous Zones of Sensory Nerves

NERVE	ZONE
Ulnar	Small finger pulp
Median	Index finger pulp
Radial	Dorsal first web space

9. Carpal Tunnel—Nine tendons in tunnel: eight finger flexors and flexor pollicis longus (FPL; most radial structure) in canal.

D. Pathophysiology

1. Intrinsic Minus or Claw Hand—**Hyperextension of MCPs and flexion of PIPs,** with a flattened metacarpal arch (Fig. 6–1); results from ulnar ± median nerve palsies or Volkmann's ischemic contracture. This condition has decreased grip strength, a weak pinch (positive Froment's sign), asynchronous movement, and loss of abduction and adduction. Operative treatment includes tendon transfers (Bunnell, Zancolli).
2. Intrinsic Plus or Tight Hand—Presents with **MCPs flexed and IP joints in extension.** It results from ischemia or fibrosis of the intrinsics and other causes such as rheumatoid arthritis (RA). It is associated with stiffness and weak grasp. Patients typically have more flexion of the PIP when the MCP is flexed than when it is extended (intrinsic tightness or Bunnell's test).
3. Lumbrical Plus Hand—Occurs when the lumbricals are tighter than the extrinsics. It can be caused by an FDP laceration distal to the lumbrical origin leading to the quadriga effect, loose tendon grafts, amputations. It presents

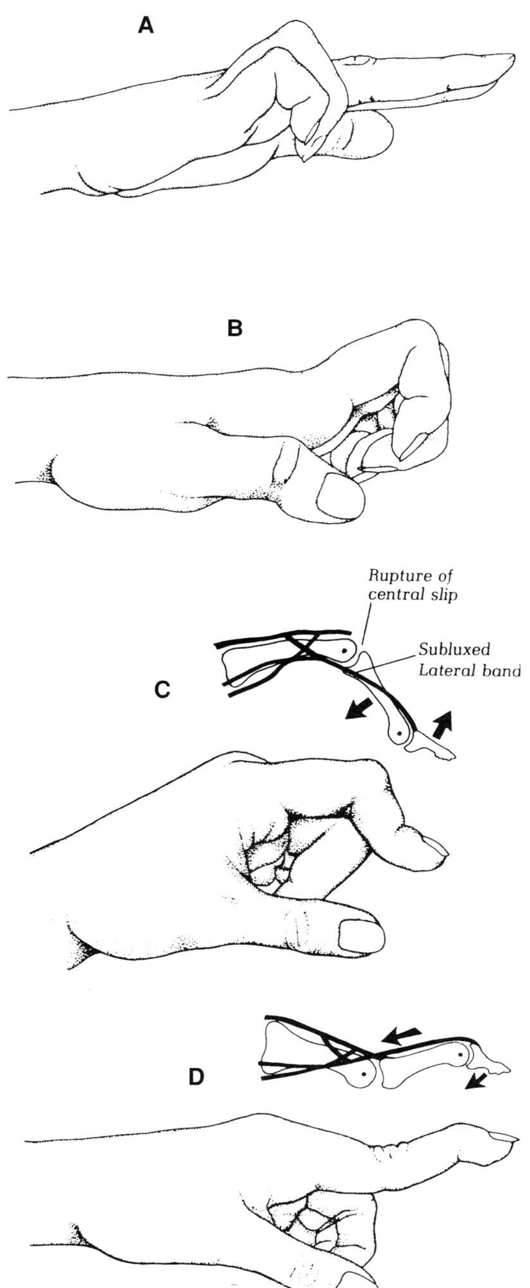

FIGURE 6–1. Anatomy of the hand. *A,* Ulnar claw hand. *B,* Ulnar and median claw hand. *C,* Boutonnière deformity. *D,* Swan neck deformity. (From The Hand, 2nd ed., pp. 67, 68, 69. Aurora, CO, American Society for Surgery of the Hand, 1983; reprinted by permission.)

with paradoxical extension: Active flexion of the MCP joint causes extension of the PIP joint.

4. Swan Neck Deformity—Results in PIP hyperextension and DIP flexion (Fig. 6–1). It is caused by dorsal subluxation of the lateral bands following flexor digitorum superficialis (FDS) rupture, or entrapment (i.e., trigger finger and rheumatoid nodules), volar plate injuries, extrinsic adhesions. Treatment must be individualized but includes central slip tenotomy (Fowler) or FDS tenodesis (Swanson).
5. Boutonnière Deformities—PIP flexion and DIP hyperextension (Fig. 6–1); result from volar subluxation of the lateral bands usually after an unrecognized central slip rupture. Early diagnosis of central slip rupture is important for avoiding this deformity. In addition to tenderness over the central slip, active extension of the DIP with the PIP stabilized on the edge of a table (Elson test) can help in making the diagnosis. Boutonnière deformities are classically defined in four stages (Table 6–1). For established flexible boutonnière deformities with hyperextended DIP joints, an extensor tenotomy distal to the PIP is favored. Late reconstruction efforts may require central slip advancement or lateral band transfer.
6. Quadrigia Effect—Occurs when FDPs act as a single unit (i.e., individual finger flexion is not possible). The effect is caused by affected individual FDP tendons that share a common muscle belly. It usually presents with loss of maximum active flexion and decreased grip strength in adjacent digits. May be seen after digital amputation where flexors are sutured to the extensors or any time an FDP is tenodesed or lacerated (e.g., in replants, poor flexor tendon repairs).

II. Compressive Neuropathies

A. Introduction—Compression neuropathies occur in predictable areas (Fig. 6–2), are evaluated in a similar manner, probably have a common pathophysiology involving localized ischemia due to mechanical pressure, and, unless severe or long-standing, resolve after release of the pressure on the nerve. The essentials of diagnosis are first to demonstrate neuropathy of a nerve trunk and second to localize that lesion along the peripheral nerve. Multiple pathophysiologic mechanisms have been described, including anatomic, postural, developmental, inflammatory, metabolic, neoplastic, iatrogenic, and idiopathic causes. Indications for surgical decompression include failure of nonsurgical treatment; acute, rapidly progressive symptoms; severe, chronic symptoms; recurrence; and the presence of motor weakness.

B. Median Nerve

1. Pronator Syndrome—Compression by the **ligament of Struthers,** lacertus fibrosis, pronator teres muscle, or proximal arch of the flexor digitorum superficialis. Symptoms include pain in volar forearm that increases with activity. Physical findings are similar to those of carpal tunnel syndrome, including weak thenar muscles and numbness in the radial three and one-half digits. Findings that differentiate this entity from carpal tunnel syndrome include a positive Tinel's sign in the forearm (rather than at the wrist), a negative Phalen's test, pain on resistance to pronation, and pain in the forearm on resistance to isolated flexion of the PIP joint of the long and ring fingers. The following provocative tests have been described.

TABLE 6–1. STAGES OF BOUTONNIÈRE DEFORMITY

STAGE	DESCRIPTION	PRESENTATION	TREATMENT
1	Acute injury	Immediate	Splint in extension
2	Passively correctable	<2	Splint in extension
3	Retinacular contracture	2–4	Casting/joint jack
4	Articular stiffness	>8	Splint → capsulectomy

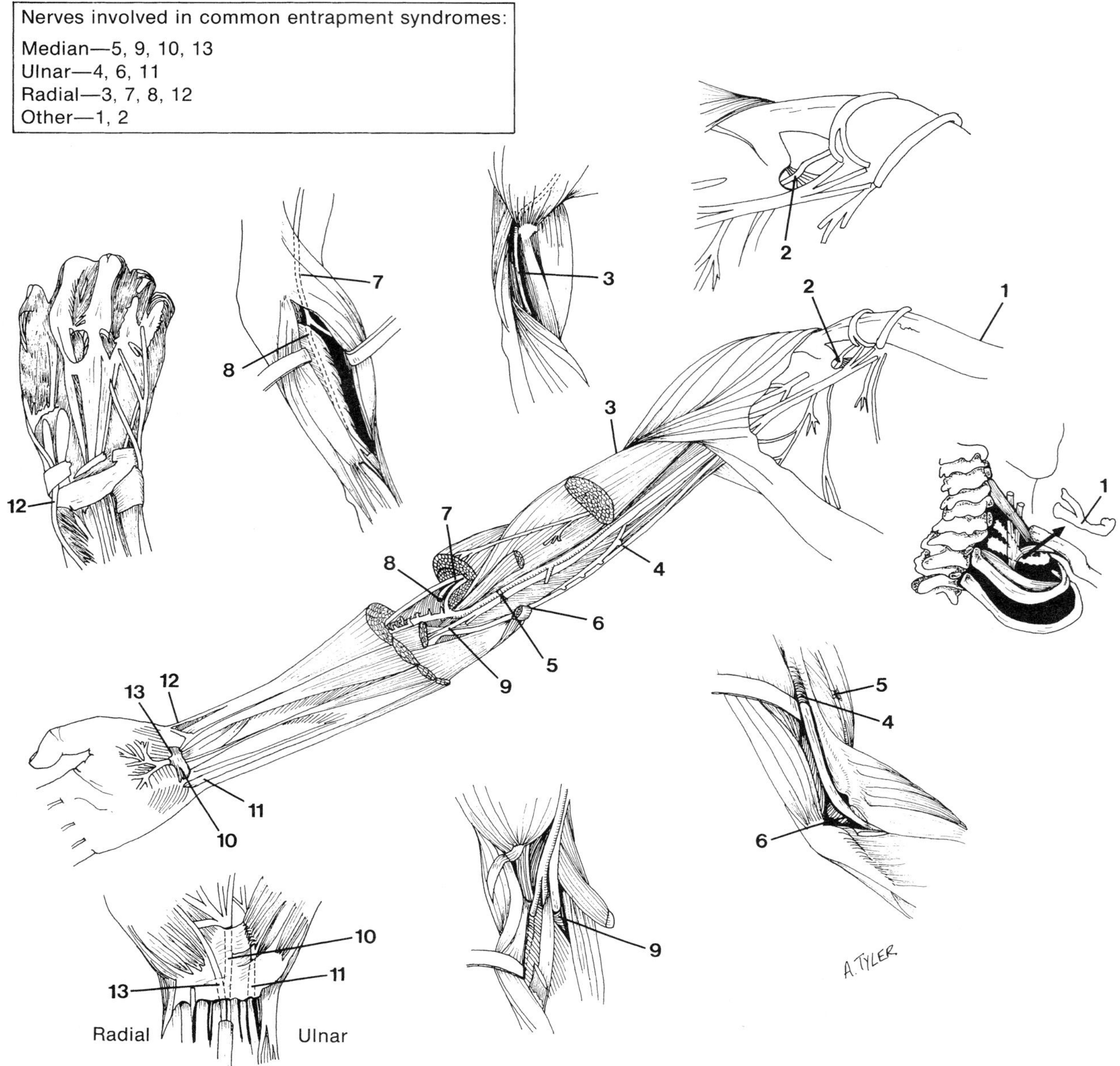

FIGURE 6–2. Upper extremity sites of nerve entrapment. 1, thoracic outlet syndrome (lateral cord entrapment); 2, suprascapular nerve entrapment; 3, proximal humerus (radial nerve entrapment); 4, arcade of Struthers (ulnar nerve entrapment); 5, ligament of Struthers (off supracondylar process) (median nerve entrapment); 6, cubital tunnel (ulnar nerve entrapment); 7, radial tunnel (radial nerve entrapment); 8, arcade of Froshe (posterior interosseous [deep radial] nerve entrapment); 9, pronator syndrome (median nerve entrapment); 10, carpal tunnel syndrome (median nerve entrapment); 11, Guyon's canal ulnar tunnel syndrome (ulnar nerve entrapment); 12, Wartenberg syndrome (superficial radial nerve entrapment); 13, flexor-retinaculum (palmar cutaneous branch of median nerve entrapment).

ENTRAPMENT LOCATION	PROVOCATIVE TEST
Lacertus/Struthers ligament	Elbow flexed 130°, resisted pronation
Pronator	Elbow extended, resisted supination
FDS arcade	Resisted flexion of middle finger FDS

EMGs are usually confirmatory. Treatment involves rest and splinting for 4–6 weeks and NSAIDs. Surgical treatment is indicated in cases unresponsive after 3 months of conservative therapy. Surgery includes exploration for compression by the ligament of Struthers, lacertus fibrosis, pronator muscle, or the arch of the superficialis muscle.

2. Anterior Interosseous Syndrome—Involves entrapment of this median nerve branch (usually at the origin of the deep head of the pronator teres), which supplies motor innervation to the radial FDP, FPL, and pronator quadratus, causing forearm pain and **loss of precise pinch** (unable to make "OK sign"). Early, the patient may present with a "signpost" hand with poor flexion of the thumb and index finger. There are no sensory branches of this nerve, and therefore there are **no sensory findings** with this syndrome. Important to rule out Mannerfelt syndrome (FPL rupture) in the differential diagnosis. Failure of 3 months of conservative treatment is an indication for surgical exploration and release of accessory muscles, aberrant vessels, or tendinous bands that may be entrapping the nerve.
3. Carpal Tunnel Syndrome—Most common nerve entrapment syndrome. It results from compression of the median nerve within the carpal canal (under the transverse carpal ligament). Can be associated with diabetes, thyroid disease, alcohol abuse, amyloidosis. Nerve compression most commonly is a result of flexor tenosynovitis. Diagnosis is confirmed with a classic history (e.g., night pain, paresthesias, clumsiness) as well as distribution of sensory complaints (median), APB weakness/atrophy, Tinel's sign, Phalen's sign, median nerve compression test, and diagnostic/therapeutic injections. As with all compressive neuropathies, nerve studies may be helpful (sensory conduction >3.5 ms) but are not always diagnostic. Activity modification, cock-up wrist splints, NSAIDs, and judicious use of steroid injections are often helpful. Carpal tunnel release using an ulnarly based incision to **avoid the palmar cutaneous branch** of the nerve is successful for treatment of refractory cases.

C. Ulnar Nerve

1. Cubital Tunnel Syndrome—Due to compression at the cubital tunnel (at the flexor carpi ulnaris [FCU] origin) at the elbow. Findings include a positive Tinel's sign over the ulnar nerve and reproduction of symptoms with full elbow flexion. Grip weakness may also be present. Nerve conduction velocity studies are helpful (change in velocity across elbow). Compression can be secondary to trauma, deformity (cubitus valgus), subluxation of the nerve, bony spurs, tumors, aberrant muscles. Activity modification and splinting are sometimes successful. Many procedures, including transposition, medial epicondylectomy, and procedures that bury the nerve, have been devised but are not always successful. External and internal neurolysis can disrupt the blood supply to the nerve. The **arcade of Struthers** is a bridge of fibrous tissue underneath the medial intermuscular septum and medial head of the triceps (8 cm above the medial epicondyle). It must be excised when the ulnar nerve is transposed.
2. Ulnar Tunnel Syndrome—Due to compression in Guyon's canal performed by the volar carpal ligament on the roof, by the hook of the hamate and insertion of the transverse carpal ligament on the lateral side, and by the pisiform and pisohamate ligament on the medial side. Usually secondary to repetitive trauma (hypothenar hammer syndrome); compression can be caused by ulnar artery thrombosis or aneurysm, ganglia, anomalous muscle or ligaments, and palmaris brevis hypertrophy. Symptoms include paresthesias, dysesthesias, local pain, weakness, and cold intolerance. Physical findings include hypesthesia in the ulnar two digits, intrinsic muscle atrophy, and lack of filling of the ulnar artery (Allen's test). Treatment involves rest, immobilization, and avoidance of repetitive trauma. Surgical treatment includes decompression and possible epineurolysis.

D. Radial Nerve

1. Proximal Entrapment—Rarely, the radial nerve is entrapped as it crosses the lateral intermuscular septum in the arm (between the brachialis and brachioradialis). This situation is most commonly associated with humerus fractures and is addressed in Chapter 10, Trauma.
2. Posterior Interosseous Nerve (PIN) Syndrome—Due to entrapment of this main radial nerve branch in the arcade of Frohse (proximal supinator); space-occupying lesions (ganglia, lipoma, fibroma) may contribute to nerve entrapment. Trauma secondary to radial head dislocations or iatrogenic causes due to proximal radius surgery or local injections. With the common presentation of "Saturday night" or "honeymoon" palsy from weight resting on the forearm, classically the patient gives a history of awakening with a wristdrop. The patient had increased pain with pronation and resisted supination of the forearm. The complete syndrome involves loss of extension for all digits and the extensor carpi ulnaris (ECU); dorsiflexion of the wrist results in radial deviation. The brachioradialis and extensor carpi radialis longus are spared owing to their proximal innervation. Distal PIN syndrome can cause dorsal wrist pain secondary to innervation of the dorsal wrist capsule from the terminal branch of this nerve. There is no sensory deficit present. The condition frequently resolves spontaneously, and treatment is observation. Surgical

release through a dorsal (Thompson) approach is indicated for persistent symptoms.

3. Radial Tunnel Syndrome—Due to compression of the radial nerve. The radial tunnel is bounded by the brachioradialis and brachialis and extends distally to the distal border of the supinator. The radial nerve can be compressed at four levels within this tunnel: under the fibrous bands proximal to the supinator, under the radial recurrent vessels (leash of Henry), underneath the arcade of Frohse, and under the extensor carpi radialis brevis (ECRB) origin. **There are no motor or sensory deficits,** and it is often confused with tennis elbow. Typically, the pain is localized to an area 5 cm distal to the lateral epicondyle and is aggravated by stressing the extended middle finger (ECRB insertion is at the base of the third metacarpal [MC]) or resisting forearm pronation. The mobile wad is intact and not affected by this syndrome. It may, in fact, be a mild PIN syndrome. Treatment includes activity modification, splinting, and often surgical exploration/release.
4. Superficial Radial Nerve Syndrome (Cheiralgia Paresthetica)—The superficial radial nerve can be compressed by tight fascial bands at the wrist as the nerve becomes superficial at the extensor carpi radialis longus (ECRL) and brachioradialis (BR) interval (Wartenberg syndrome), leading to sensory disturbances. Exploration may reveal a pseudoneuroma.

E. Other Compressive Neuropathies

1. Thoracic Outlet Syndrome—Due to the cervical ribs, anterior scalene muscle constriction, abnormal fibrous bands, or head of the sternocleidomastoid muscle compressing the lateral cord of the brachial plexus. Typically affects young or middle-age females. Deficit is similar to ulnar nerve compression at the elbow combined with neck pain and paresthesias that are increased with overhead activities. Adson's test and hyperabduction stress test (3 minutes required) may be helpful for making the diagnosis. Radiographs should be examined for cervical ribs, pancoast tumors, and other problems. Arteriography is occasionally indicated (aneurysms are associated with cervical ribs). MRI can also be useful to rule out spinal disorders or soft tissue abnormalities. EMG/NCS studies may also be helpful to rule out other problems. Nonoperative treatment includes weight reduction, bracing-type exercises, and exercises with weights below chest level. Rarely operative treatment is necessary and includes rib resection and/or scalenotomy.
2. Suprascapular Nerve—Entrapment of this nerve is uncommon and difficult to diagnose. Presents with deep diffuse pain in the posterolateral shoulder with radiation to the neck and arm. Weakness and atrophy of the supraspinatus and infraspinatus are common. Symptoms are aggravated with arm adduction and palpation of the suprascapular notch. EMGs may be helpful; decompression is occasionally needed. When associated with trauma, the nerve can recover spontaneously. After 3 months surgical decompression can be considered.

III. Tendon Injuries

A. Extensor Tendons—Pain may be the only symptom in proximal lacerations because junctura can function to extend digit. Partial lacerations (<50%) should not be repaired (actually weakens tendons). Treatment is based on zones (Fig. 6–3).

1. Zone I (Central Slip Insertion Distal)—Repair lateral bands if they are injured. Mallet injuries (disruption of terminal tendon) can usually be treated closed with splinting of the DIP only (full time for 6–10 weeks then nighttime only for another 4–6 weeks). Classification is as follows: I, closed; II, laceration; III, deep abrasion; IV, epiphyseal. If there is bony involvement and the joint is subluxed >30–50%, some advocate ORIF.
2. Zone II (MCP to Central Slip)—Roll stitch (later pulled out) favored, especially over the MCP joint. Unrecognized/untreated injuries to the central slip can result in the development of a boutonnière deformity. The lateral bands displace volarly and create a tenodesis effect. Early diagnosis is best made with the Elson test (have patient extend PIP over edge of table). Early, nonoperative treatment includes splinting or casting in extension and use of a "reverse knuckle bender" orthosis. The senior editor believes that the best results are obtained with full-time use of a Capner splint for 8 weeks.
3. Zone III (Extensor Retinaculum to MCP)—Permanent suture is acceptable in this zone.
4. Zone IV (Extensor Retinaculum)—Excise the overlying retinaculum after primary repair of the tendons. Some of the retinaculum should be left intact to prevent extensor tendon bowstringing.
5. Zone V (Proximal to Extensor Retinaculum)—Repair the musculotendinous unit.
6. Thumb Extensors—Treatment is similar. Late repair of the extensor pollicis longus (EPL) at the MCP joint may require rerouting the tendon around Lister's tubercle or EIP transfer.
7. Late repair of extensor tendon lacerations may require reconstruction. Tendon grafts using

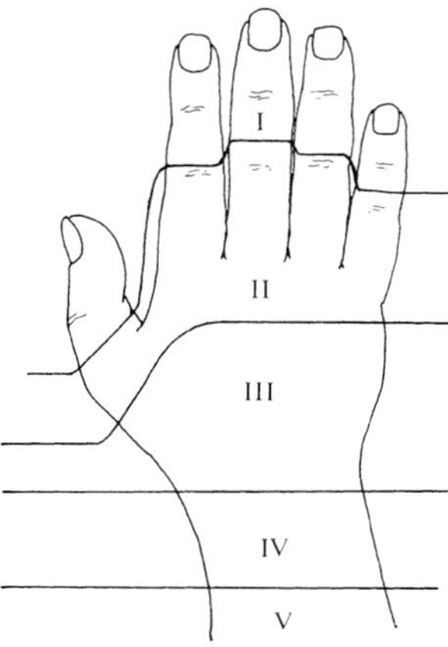

FIGURE 6–3. Extensor zones of the hand.

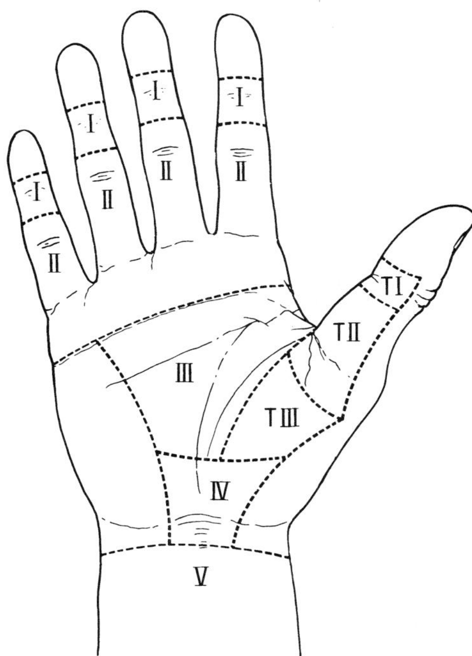

FIGURE 6–4. Flexor zones of the hand (refer to text). Note thumb zones (T). (From Tubiana, R.: The Hand, vol. 3, p. 172. Philadelphia, WB Saunders, 1986; reprinted by permission.)

palmaris longus, plantaris, or toe extensors may be required. Postoperative splinting should allow 30–40 degrees of MCP motion.

B. Flexor Tendon Injuries—Repair also based on zones (Fig. 6–4). The **A2** (base of proximal phalanx) **and A4** (base of middle phalanx) flexor **pulleys should be preserved** or reconstructed if they are involved with these injuries.

1. Zone I (Distal to FDS Insertion)—FDP avulsion is commonly seen with sports injuries (jersey finger—typically involves ring finger) and is best appreciated by having patients flex their distal phalanx over the edge of a hard, flat surface with the proximal joints immobilized. Direct repair is accomplished if possible; otherwise advance to bone with pull-out suture if less than 1 cm of tendon remains. Repair volar plate if injured and preserve A4 pulley. Zone I injuries can be repaired with a graft if recognized late (after 10 days) or retracted far in a young patient and if required for occupation (especially index finger). In older patients, DIP fusion is favored.
2. Zone II (Fibro-osseous Tunnel [MC Neck] to FDS Insertion)—"Bunnel's no man's land." Tendon lacerations are distal to the skin laceration and at different levels in an injury to a flexed hand (e.g., by grasping a knife). Successful repairs are more difficult owing to flexor sheath adhesion during healing. Repair both FDP and FDS and preserve both the A2 and A4 pulleys (over proximal and middle phalanges, respectively). At least 1 cm of tendon must be visible on each end for repair, which may require a distal window. With FDS be careful to recreate the normal anatomic spiral at Camper's chiasm. Late tenolysis is sometimes required.
3. Zone III (Transverse Carpal Ligament to Fibro-osseous Tunnel)—Repair all nerves and tendons through additional incisions if necessary. Late segmental grafting is helpful.
4. Zone IV (Transverse Carpal Ligament)—Although uncommon, repair through complete or incomplete transverse carpal ligament incision. Meticulous repair, Z-plasty, or step-cut release with repair of the carpal ligament may avoid bowstringing. Immobilize postop with wrist at neutral and MCP joints more acutely flexed.
5. Zone V (Musculotendinous Junctions to Transverse Carpal Ligament)—Accurate identification of the proximal and distal stump ["spaghetti wrist"] may be difficult. Look for hematoma in the tendon sheath or muscle belly. End-to-end repair is recommended.
6. Thumb—Similar guidelines apply, although cruciate pulleys are more important and should be preserved. Splint with 30 degrees of wrist flexion and 15 degrees of MCP and IP flexion.
7. Principles—Core sutures should be palmar to the central axis of the tendon to preserve the dorsal blood supply. Supplementation with a running (Lembert) suture improves function and minimizes extrinsic healing. The strongest tendon repair is the Pulvertaft weave; the strongest suture is the Kirihmayer, a grasping suture later described by Kessler. The Kessler-Tajima stitch is popular. Sheath repair may improve gliding and initial nutrition. Repair is weakest at 7–10 days. Adhesions are best avoided with atraumatic technique and a good postop program. Postoperatively only 5 mm of tendon excursion (passive) is required for 4 weeks. Begin active motion at this point; no full passive motion for 6 weeks. **Kleinert traction** allows controlled active extension and passive flexion in a dorsal protective splint with flexed wrist and MCPs, and rubber bands under a roller bar from fingertip to forearm for 4 weeks, with wrist band traction for an additional 2–3 weeks if early motion is excellent. The **Duran program** is based on controlled passive motion with a dorsal block splint with full passive motion for the first 4 weeks, then weaning of the splint over the next 2 weeks and addition of active motion to wrist and composite digits. Late reconstruction techniques include the use of Silastic (Hunter) or silicone rods (the latter are preferred by the senior editor because of less synovitis) followed by staged tendon transfer (>3 months after rod insertion and after full passive ROM achieved).

IV. Infections

A. Overview—Infections are uncommon in the hand because of its good blood supply, but risk factors such as diabetes and fight bites should cause a high index of suspicion. Most hand infections involve *Staph. aureus* species, but polymicrobial infections are also common. Anaerobic species can be isolated in 30–40% of infections. Examination should include palpation of lymph nodes. Epitrochlear nodes drain the ring finger and small finger. Axillary nodes drain the radial digits. Cellulitis resolves with antibiotics only, but pus under pressure requires surgical drainage (localized by the point of maximal tenderness). Initial IV antibiotics may resolve infection or localize area better.

B. Common Hand Infections—The following are some of the more common hand infections encountered.
   1. Paronychia/Eponychia—Infection of the nail bed, the most common infection of the hand (Fig. 6–5). Best treated with I&D to include partial nail removal, loose packing, soaks, and oral antibiotics. An eponychia involves the entire eponychium and lateral fold. *Staph. aureus* is the most common organism.
   2. Felon—Subcutaneous abscess of the distal pulp. I&D with lateral/dorsal incision and disruption of septae plus antibiotics (usually IV antibiotics should be considered) is the treatment regimen of choice. Avoid nerves, vessels, and flexor tendon sheath. Incisions should be placed lateral and ulnar (except in the thumb and small finger, where they should be radial).
   3. Human Bite—Infections can be serious and, if they involve bone or joints, require formal I&D. Most commonly involves third- and fourth-digit MCP joints. Although the most common organism involved is *Staph. aureus,* cover *Eikenella corrodens* (gram-negative, G−) with penicillin or Augmentin. Treat aggressively with IV antibiotics and I&D.

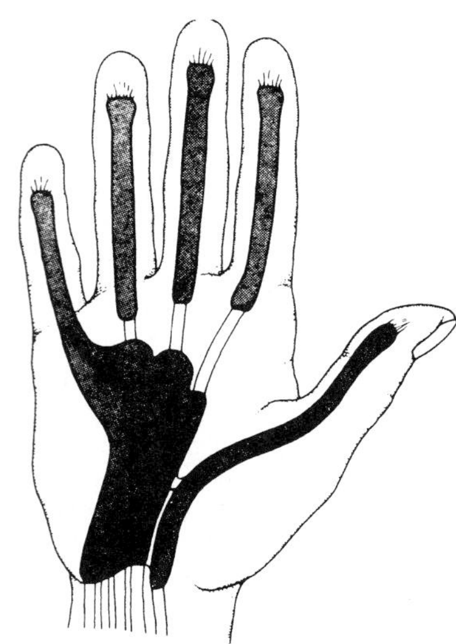

FIGURE 6–6. Tendon sheaths of the flexor tendon. Note communication of small finger sheath with ulna bursa. (From The Hand, 2nd ed., p. 96. Aurora, CO, American Society for Surgery of the Hand, 1983; reprinted by permission.)

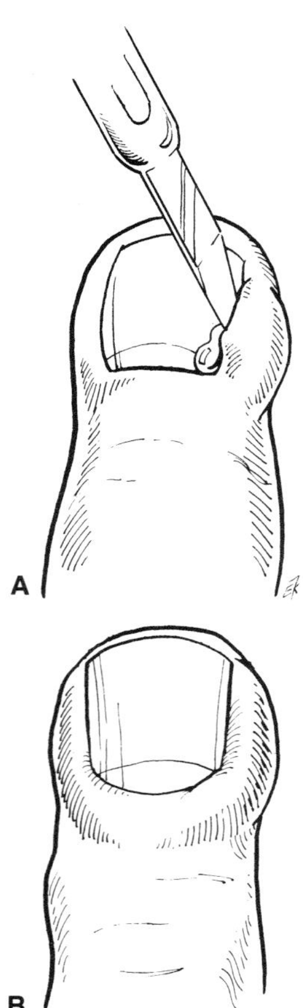

FIGURE 6–5. *A,* Paronychia, *B,* Eponychia. (From Bora, F.W.: The Pediatric Upper Extremity, pp. 362, 363. Philadelphia, WB Saunders, 1986; reprinted by permission.)

   4. Dog and Cat Bites—Can also be serious. Cover *Pasteurella multocida* (G− coccobacillus) with ampicillin (or, again, Augmentin). Early I&D is required with any joint or flexor sheath penetration.
   5. Suppurative Flexor Tenosynovitis—Infection of the flexor tendon sheath. If untreated, leads to tendon adhesions (decreased ROM) and necrosis. Presents classically with Kanavel's four cardinal signs: pain on passive extension (early), finger held in flexed position, ***severe tenderness along the tendon sheath,*** and symmetric swelling (sausage digit). Treat with IV antibiotics if less than 48 hours. Surgical treatment if no dramatic improvement in 24 hours or if presented after 48 hours. Open drainage through midlateral incision or closed sheath irrigation. Spread of infection into the deep spaces is as follows:

      Index finger, thumb → thenar space
      Middle, ring, small fingers → midpalmar space
      Small finger → ulnar bursa
   6. Radial and Ulnar Bursal Infections—FDP and FDS (small finger) sheath infection with proximal extensions. Proximal extension requires I&D of these respective bursae. Ulnar bursa connects to small finger flexor sheath (Fig. 6–6).
   7. Herpetic Whitlow—Seen especially in medical/dental personnel. Presents with pain, swelling, tenderness, and a vesicular rash. Usually involves thumb or index finger and may follow a viral illness. Splint, elevate, and

restrict patient contact—**do not treat with I&D** for risk of systemic dissemination. Self-limiting disease of 3 weeks' duration. May recur.

8. Deep Fascial Space Infections—Occur usually in the palm and may be limited to web space (**collar button** abscess). Treat with I&D both dorsally and volarly. Opening all deep spaces is required because the transverse MC ligament limits deep dissection; IV antibiotics to follow. With **midpalmar** infections (rare), there is loss of midline contour and pain on movement of the long, ring, and small fingers. With a **thenar space** infection there is thenar pain and pain on flexion of the thumb and index finger. Treatment for both includes I&D. Hypothenar space infections are rare.
9. Gangrene—**Necrotizing fasciitis** can be seen with streptococci (G+ cocci) (Meleny's) or with clostridia (G+ rod). Aggressive treatment is immediate I&D or amputation and hyperbaric oxygen in some cases.
10. Sporotrichosis—From roses; lymphatic spread causing discoloration and small bumps on skin of hand/forearm. Treat with potassium iodine supersaturated solution (KISS).
11. Atypical *Mycobacterium* Infections—Include *Mycobacterium marinum* (seen in fishermen or pool workers) and *Mycobacterium kansasii* (in farm workers). May present with chronic swelling and a nonhealing ulcer; biopsy and treat with appropriate antimicrobials. The specimens must be cultured at 30–32°C for identification. Oral rifampin and ethambutol or tetracycline are often successful. I&D may be required.
12. Insect Bites—Brown recluse spider bite can cause areas of local necrosis and requires early wide local excision.

V. Vascular Occlusion/Disease

A. Compartment Syndrome—Increased tissue pressure within a limited space leads to decreased blood flow and function. Caused by fracture, soft tissue injury (classically ringer injury), arterial injury, drug/IV fluid infusion, burns, crush injuries, among others. Symptoms/findings include the "five Ps": pain, pallor, pulselessness, paresthesias, and paralysis. Pain (accentuated by passive stretching) is the most important and reliable parameter. Subacute compartment syndrome may not have classic signs but may develop late sequelae (progressive contractures, weakness). Recurrent compartment syndrome can occur in athletes with repetitive activities. Diagnosis is aided by measurement of compartment pressures. Myoglobinuria can lead to renal failure in severe cases. Fasciotomy is required if compartment pressures exceed 30 mm Hg or if there is any question. Compartments in the hand and digits frequently also must be released. Muscle viability can be determined by the "four Cs": color, consistency, contractility, and capacity to bleed.

B. Volkmann's Contracture—End result of compartment syndrome from injury to the deep tissues, usually the volar compartment. Can follow supracondylar or forearm fracture in children. Three varieties of established Volkmann's exist.

TYPE	AFFECTED MUSCLES	TREATMENT
Mild	Wrist flexors	Dynamic split, therapy, tendon lengthening/slide
Moderate	FDP/FDS, FPL, FCR/FCU	Tendon slide, neurolysis (M&U), extensor transfer
Severe	Flexors and extensors	Débridement, release, salvage procedures

C. Occlusive Disorders—Vascular occlusion can be caused by many factors.

1. Embolic Phenomena—Unusual in the upper extremity but can involve the brachial artery from mural thrombi ± atrial septal defect.
2. Buerger's Disease—Paninflammatory arthritis in cigarette smokers characterized by development of tortuous digital arteries.
3. Hypothenar Hammer Syndrome—Ulnar artery spasm or thrombosis. Symptoms include pain, cold intolerance, numbness, and ulceration. Often seen in smokers, heavy alcohol users, and patients with hypertension, heart disease, or blood dyscrasias. It can be verified with Doppler studies ± angiography; treated with microvascular surgery (resection and grafting).
4. Frostbite—Can be treated with intra-arterial reserpine if warming is not sufficient.
5. Raynaud's
   a. ***Phenomenon***—Pallor of the digits, triple color changes (hyperemia, pallor, and cyanosis—red, white, and blue) with exposure to the cold.
   b. ***Syndrome***—When Raynaud's phenomenon occurs in conjunction with a disease such as a connective tissue disorder, neurologic disorder, occlusive disorder, or blood dyscrasia.
   c. ***Disease***—When Raynaud's phenomenon occurs without any underlying disease. Usually occurs in young females (often African-American) without clinical occlusion and peripheral arteries with ***distal*** trophic changes/gangrene.
   d. Treatment is based on addressing the underlying disease (if known), smoking cessation, avoiding cold weather, digital protection, calcium channel blockers, β-blockers, calcitonin or serotonin antagonists, and sympathetic blockade. Digital sympathectomy is sometimes indicated.

D. Reflex Sympathetic Dystrophy—Neurologic dysfunction following trauma, surgery, or disease characterized by intense/exaggerated burning pain, vasomotor disturbances, delayed functional recovery, and trophic changes of the extremity. Caused by sustained efferent activity from sympathetic fibers. If associated with a known nerve trunk injury it is termed "causalgia." Related to shoulder-hand syndrome.

1. Stages (Lankford and Evans)

STAGE	ONSET (months)	FINDINGS
1—Acute	0–3	Localized pain, swelling, warmth, decreased ROM, negative radiographs, positive triple-phase bone scan
2—Dystrophic	3–6	Change in pain, glossy skin, cool, atrophy, contracture
3—Atrophic	6–9+	Tight skin, flexion contractures, ↓ temp, diffuse osteoporosis on radiographs (Sudek's atrophy)

2. Diagnosis—Four cardinal signs (pain out of proportion, swelling, stiffness, discoloration), endurance testing, and relief with sympathetic blockade are diagnostic. ESR, thermography, radiographs, and triple-phase bone scan (increased during both early and late phases) are also helpful. Early diagnosis is critical to successful treatment.
3. Treatment—Splinting and physical therapy (TENS and fluidotherapy) are essential early. Later sympathetic block (stellate ganglion) can be curative. Sympathectomy considered if six to eight blocks provide initial relief but with recurrence of signs and symptoms. Sympatholytic medications (guanethidine and reserpine) and steroids are sometimes helpful. Prevention (protecting nerves, avoiding tight dressings and casts, early treatment) is most effective.

VI. Replantation and Microsurgery

A. Traumatic Amputation

1. Replantation—Reattachment of a body partly or totally severed from the body; requires revascularization to restore viability. Attempted for all thumb amputations, patients with multiple digits amputated, all children, all amputations proximal to digits, and single digits **distal to FDS insertion** (Fig. 6–7). Thumb amputations should be salvaged or reconstructed (index pollicization or toe transfer) whenever possible. Contraindicated for mangled/crushed digits, with other life-threatening injuries, for individual digits proximal to FDS, for prolonged warm ischemia time, for severe ring avulsion (degloving) injuries, with arteriosclerotic vessels, and in mental patients. Maximum warm ischemia time is 6 hours; maximum cold ischemia time is 12–18 hours. Later repairs can lead to renal damage due to muscle breakdown. High-volume diuresis and alkalization of urine (pH >6.5) helps. Sequence: Isolate nerves and vessels, débride, **shorten and fix bone, repair extensor tendon, repair flexor tendon, anastomose artery, then nerve repair, and finally anastomosis of veins [BEFANV].** Postop care includes anticoagulation, rest, monitoring (keep >30°C). Early failure is due to thrombosis, which usually responds only to vascular revision. Results are best in children (85% viable). Adults can usually expect 10–12 mm two-point discrimination, 50% total active motion (TAM), and cold intolerance for up to 2 years.
2. Ring Avulsion Injuries—Classified based on extent of injury (Urbaniak).

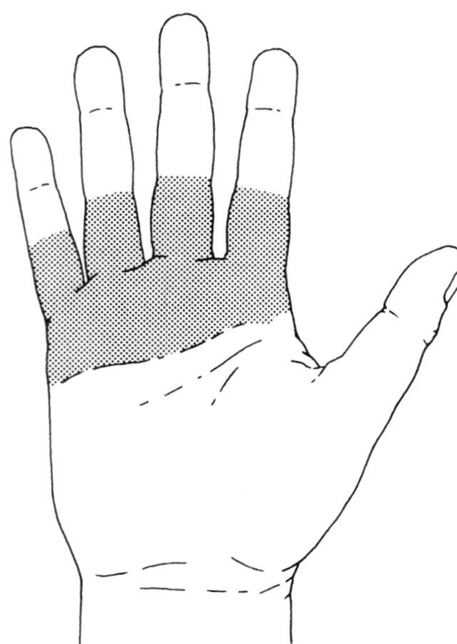

FIGURE 6–7. "No man's zone" is also a zone where single-digit replantation is not recommended. (From Magee, D.J.: Orthopedic Physical Assessment, p. 109. Philadelphia, WB Saunders, 1987; reprinted by permission.)

I Circulation intact
IIA Arterial compromise but no bone, tendon, or nerve injury
IIIB Arterial compromise and bone, tendon, and/or nerve injury
III Complete degloving or amputation

Treatment is selective. Types I and IIA can be salvaged, but types IIB and III may not be salvageable and, if so, should undergo skeletal shortening and closure (injury proximal to FDS—see above).

3. Fingertip Amputations—Usually require only rongeuring of the exposed distal phalanx and allowing the wound to heal by secondary intention.
Simple flaps (volar advancement flaps are useful for thumb tuft avulsions) and split-thickness skin grafting are alternative treatment options.

B. Elective Amputations—May be required because of infection, tumors, trauma, or other reasons. Function is of primary importance, but cosmesis should be considered. Distal tuft amputations can be managed with rongeuring of bone to allow soft tissue coverage and wound care to allow granulation tissue to cover the digit. Skin grafts may also be used. For more proximal amputations, contour the condyles, allow tendons to retract, and use generous volar flaps. For ray amputation, particularly with the long finger, suture the intermetacarpal ligaments or perform a transposition. Index ray amputations should include digital nerve transposition to lower the incidence of painful dysfunction. With crush injuries, bony defects should be stabilized before soft tissues are addressed. Late problems with digital amputations can be caused by adherence of tendons.

C. Microsurgery
   1. Vessels and Nerves—Repair is limited to structures >0.3 mm diameter. Reversed vein graft patency can be improved with papaverine (with cold heparinized blood), atraumatic technique, and controlled distention. Arterial repair with magnification requires exacting technique. Experimental mechanical coupling devices, thermic sleeves, and laser techniques may improve results in the future. Patency may be improved with topical agents (chlorpromazine [Thorazine]) and heparin infusion. Use of streptokinase is reserved for salvage procedures. Nerve repair should be primary when possible and done with 10-0 or 11-0 nylon suture under microscopic control. Poor prognosis is associated with intra-articular fractures, vascular impairment, and immediate precise loss of function. Other factors include patient age and condition, delay, level, and experience of the surgeon. Treatment should be delayed 4 months in the presence of intra-articular fractures and 9 months after gunshot wounds. Key areas for digital nerve repair are ulnar thumb and radial index finger (pinch) and ulnar small finger. Fascicular matching (electrically or histochemically) improves results. Tube grafts may have future use. Nerve grafting may be required if primary repair is not possible (e.g., under tension). The lateral (LABC) or medial (MABC) antibrachial cutaneous nerve can be used to fill a segmental defect in a digital nerve; sural nerve grafts are used for large defects. Again, best results are in young patients. Specific guidelines for some nerves follow.

NERVE	REPAIR
Superficial branch radial nerve	Resect proximally, avoiding a neuroma
Dorsal branch ulnar nerve	Can repair at wrist
Ulnar nerve at wrist	Match bundles for correct rotation
Median nerve at wrist	Resect proximal neuroma and distal glioma
Digital nerve	Primary repair using MABC nerve graft
Cranial nerve XI (iatrogenic)	Neurolysis early (6 mo), reconstruction (Eden Lange-rhomboid and levator transfer) late

   Differential motor and sensory staining may be of value when repairing chronic defects of mixed nerves.
   2. Monitoring—Done with transcutaneous oxygen monitors (requires precise temperature regulation and patient cooperation), tissue pH monitors (abrupt decline signifies arterial occlusion; slow decline is consistent with venous occlusion), or laser Doppler velocimetry (measures moving RBCs less effective).
   3. Flaps—If done for injury, they are usually best accomplished within 72 hours (less scar, infection, or necrosis) but can be effective up to 1 week postinjury. **Flaps can also be helpful for treating osteomyelitis after the wound is clean.** In the presence of dorsal hand burns, immediate escharotomy is preferred. The following types of skin flaps (Fig. 6–8) have been described.

TYPE	VESSELS	EXAMPLE
Random pattern cutaneous	Random vessel supply	Abdominal
Axial pattern cutaneous	A + V supply	Scapular
Fasciocutaneous	Vessels in fascia	Radial forearm
Myocutaneous (pedicle)	Muscle with A + V	Plantar island
Free	Reattach vessels	Latissimus dorsi

   Myocutaneous flaps can significantly reduce bacterial infection in tissues. Free muscle flaps, including latissimus dorsi and rectus abdominus muscles, have the advantage of being a one-stage procedure: They close the wound, enhance mobilization, and improve vascularity to the recipient area. The disadvantages of these flaps include the risk of flap loss, and they require extensive surgery. Local heel flaps include the instep flap (provides padding and innervation), FDB, abductor hallucis, and abductor digiti minimus flaps. **Gastrocnemius flaps are used for wounds in the proximal third of the leg (medial head for medial and *midline* defects, lateral head for lateral defects); soleus flaps for wounds in the middle third of the leg; and free myocutaneous (latissimus) flaps for the distal third of the leg and to cover large defects.** Expanded flaps have increased vascularity and may be useful. Newer indications for flaps include coverage of fourth-degree burns, peripheral vascular disease, and chronic osteomyelitis.
   4. Other Tissue Transfers—Include free bone as an osteomyocutaneous free flap (e.g., vascularized fibula grafts), vascularized nerve graft (sural vascularized graft under investigation), and free functional muscle graft (e.g., gracilis and pectoralis major). Temporoparietal free flaps, dorsalis pedis flaps, and back fascial flaps can also be used.
   5. Other Microsurgical Procedures in Hand Surgery—Include digital sympathectomy for digital ischemia that improves with local anesthetic block.

D. Reconstruction of Bony Defects
   1. Thumb

LOCATION	PROCEDURE
Proximal to MCP	Pollicization or toe transfer
Distal to MCP	Pollicization, toe transfer, or osteoplastic lengthening

   2. Joints—Reconstruction with second toe joint transfer may be an alternative in children.
   3. Bone—Allografts for metacarpal segmental defect may be useful.

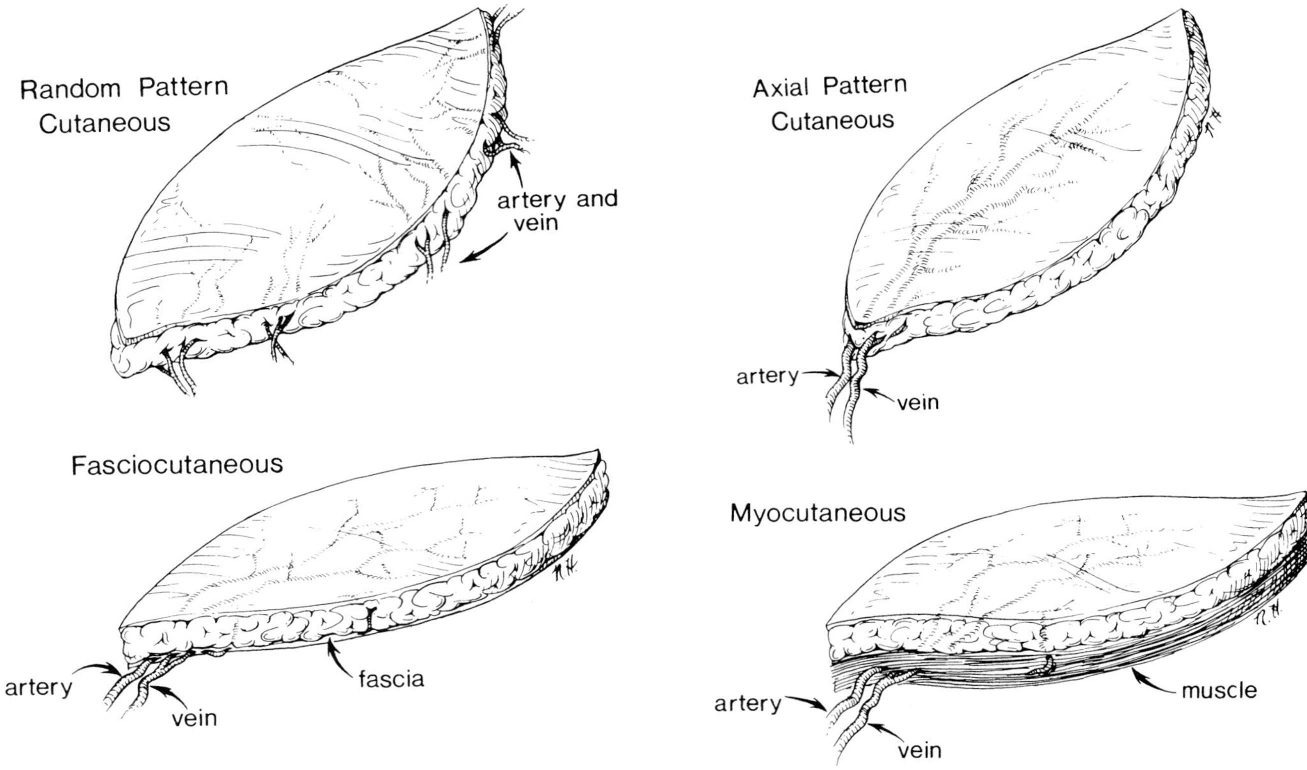

FIGURE 6–8. Skin flaps. (From Regional Review Course in Hand Surgery, pp. 11-7, 11-8, 11-9. Aurora, CO, American Society for Surgery of the Hand, 1990; reprinted by permission.)

VII. Wrist Pain/Instability

A. Introduction—Wrist instability often leads to wrist pain. Functional ROM of the wrist is 5 degrees of palmar flexion, 30 degrees of dorsiflexion, 10 degrees of radial deviation, and 15 degrees of ulnar deviation. Evaluation of wrist pain requires an accurate history, documentation of motion, and localization of pain. Key tools in this effort include a physical examination (PMT and provocative tests, e.g., Watson), diagnostic injections, plain radiographs, bone scan, cineradiograms (for carpal instability), polytomograms, arthrograms (ligament injection), CT (structural abnormalities), MRI (avascular necrosis, soft tissue tumors), and arthroscopy. The proximal row of carpal bones dorsiflex with ulnar deviation and palmar flex with radial deviation. The volar intercarpal ligaments (particularly the radioscaphocapitate and radioscapholunate) are important stabilizers of the wrist.

B. Wrist Instability—Many classifications have been developed, but most are based on the scapholunate angle (normal 30–60 degrees) (Linscheid and Dobyns). It may be further classified based on dissociation (presence or absence of separation [gap]).

1. Carpal Instability, Dissociative (CID)—Includes the following.

a. Dorsal Intercalated Segment Instability (DISI)—Can result from scaphoid fracture or scapholunate dissociation (usually secondary to disruption of the scapholunate interosseous and radioscaphoid ligaments, best seen with a PA clenched fist view showing a gap >3 mm [Terry Thomas sign]). The disorder is also characterized by an **increased scapholunate angle** on lateral radiographs (>60 degrees) and an abnormal radiolunate angle. Rotary subluxation of the scaphoid decreases contact area and increases pressure at the radioscaphoid articulation. Acute injuries (within 3–6 weeks) should be immobilized or (if ligaments are 100% torn) repaired through a dorsal approach and stabilized with K-wires. Late reconstruction (>6 weeks) usually results in a salvage procedure (limited fusion, scaphoid-trapezium-trapezoid [STT] or scaphocapitate, proximal row carpectomy, or wrist fusion). Late repair is unpredictable.

b. Volar Intercalated Segment Instability (VISI)—May result from disruption of the radial carpal ligaments on the ulnar side of the wrist and is characterized by a decreased scapholunate angle (<30 degrees). Examination should include a ballottement test (Reagan). Early treatment with closed reduction and casting (± percutaneous K-wires) may avert the need for difficult late ligamentous reconstruction or limited arthrodesis.

c. Other types of CID can involve the distal row or be a combination of proximal and distal rows.

2. Carpal Instability, Nondissociative (CIND)—Includes the following.
   a. Radiocarpal—Due to ligament injuries or deformity (e.g., Madelung's).
   b. Midcarpal (Triquetrohamate [TQH])—Disruption of this "helicoid" joint often presents with painful click (Lichtman) and ulnar tenderness. Triquetrohamate or four-bone arthrodesis may be indicated if conservative options fail.
   c. Combined Radiocarpal and Midcarpal—May result in wrist arthrodesis.
3. Limited Arthrodesis—May be successful in some disorders with severe decreases in ROM (55% decrease with radiocapitate fusion, 27% decrease with intercarpal fusion between rows).

C. Diagnosis Based on Location
1. Radial—Can be scaphoid (fracture, dissociation, arthritis, or avascular necrosis [AVN]), tendonitis, or other problems.
   a. Scaphoid Fracture—May not be seen on plain films until 10–21 days postinjury. Due to a precarious blood supply that enters the scaphoid predominantly distally; nonunion and AVN are common in fractures of the scaphoid. Most fractures involve the middle third; and if there is no displacement or carpal instability, they heal with nonoperative treatment >90% of the time. Treatment should proceed by assuming that a scaphoid fracture is present (with anatomic snuff box tenderness) until proved otherwise. Prolonged immobilization (up to 5 months) may be required. Displaced fracture requires ORIF and bone grafting. Bone grafting and internal fixation of nonunions is important to avoid progressive DJD. Silastic implants should be avoided because of late development of cystic lesions. Although controversial, some authors (Watson) suggest that silicone disease does not occur if the wrist is adequately stabilized. Bone scans may have a role in early diagnosis. Polytomography is also helpful.
   b. Proximal Scaphoid Avascular Necrosis (Preiser's Disease)—Can be a late result of a scaphoid fracture because the blood supply enters the scaphoid distally. MRI may be helpful, but the presence of punctuate bleeding when the proximal fragment is curetted is most prognostic. Russe' bone grafting provides the best results.
   c. Perilunar Instability/Scapholunate Dissociation—Findings include a history of injury (usually wrist extension and supination) and a positive Watson test (clunk [dorsal displacement of proximal pole with radial deviation] with passive radioulnar wrist movement when scaphoid is immobilized volarly). Radiographs may show widening of the scapholunate interval, scaphoid "ring" sign, and lack of parallelism on AP fist view; definitive study is wrist cinearthrogram with radial and ulnar deviation. Four stages have been described (Mayfield). See also Fig. 10–24.

STAGE	CHARACTERISTICS
I	Scapholunate diastasis
II	Perilunar dislocation
III	Lunotriquetral diastasis
IV	Lunate dislocation (volar)

   Treatment includes ligament reconstruction and pinning (early) or intercarpal arthrodesis (STT fusion [Watson]) proximal row carpectomy or fusion (late).
   d. Scapholunate Advanced Collapse (SLAC Wrist)—Can follow scaphoid fracture or scapholunate dissociation and is manifested by degeneration of the radioscaphoid and capitolunate joints (**radiolunate joint is spared**). Four stages are described (Fig. 6–9).

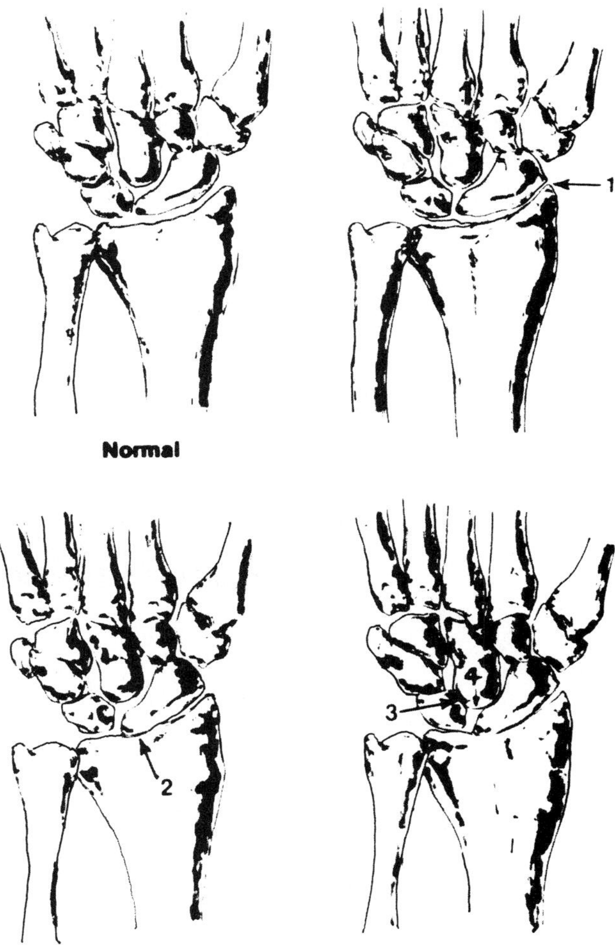

FIGURE 6–9. SLAC wrist. Note the four stages of progression to proximal migration of the capitate. (From Watson, H.K., and Ryu, J.: Evolution of wrist arthritis. Clin. Orthop. 202:61, 1986; reprinted by permission.)

STAGE	INVOLVEMENT
1	Radial styloid and scaphoid
2	Radioscaphoid articulation
3	Capitolunate ± scaphocapitate joint
4	Scapholunate dissociation and migration of the capitate proximally

Treatment options include scaphoid excisional arthroplasty with capitolunate fusion, proximal row carpectomy, and wrist fusion. The first two options preserve motion but are associated with pain and decreased grip strength. Fusion allows maximum grip strength and no pain, but at the sacrifice of motion. Proximal row carpectomy requires good lunate fossae of the radius and proximal capitate articular surfaces. Fusion available include dorsal fusion with iliac crest bone graft to second and fourth MC and AO plate (8–10 holes).

e. Triscaphe Degeneration (Trapezium-Trapezoid-Scaphoid)—Second most common degenerative pattern in the wrist. Treatment options include triscaphe (STT) fusion, trapeziectomy with soft tissue, or (rarely) silicone arthroplasty with trapezoid-scaphoid fusion and soft tissue interposition.
f. Lunotriquetral Sprain—Can be diagnosed with the "shear test" (Kleinman: shear force is applied at this joint while stabilizing the lunate dorsally and the pisotriquetral plane volarly). Shuck test (Reagan) is similar but less specific. The compression test (Linscheid) applies an axial load to this joint and is also less specific for lunotriquetral pathology. Treatment of lunotriquetral injuries is usually nonoperative. Occasionally, limited arthrodesis is required.
g. Tendonitis—Includes de Quervain's, tenosynovitis, flexor carpi radialis (FCR) tendonitis, and intersection syndrome.
   1. De Quervain's tenosynovitis involves the first dorsal wrist compartment. Most common in 30- to 50-year-old women engaged in repetitive actions. Diagnosis is confirmed with the Finkelstein test (ulnar deviation of wrist with passive flexion of thumb causes maximum pain). Rule out CMC DJD with the grind test and radiographs. Treatment includes injection, splinting, and first compartment release. Postoperative pain can be caused by neuromas of the superficial branch of the radial nerve (positive Tinel's sign, hypesthesias) or inadequate decompression of the involved tendons. (Extensor pollicis brevis [EPB] usually lies in a separate compartment and is often overlooked because both EPB and abductor pollicis longus [APL] can have several tendinous slips.)
   2. FCR Tendonitis—Similar to de Quervain's, with localized pain and tenderness on stretch. Splinting and injection are also helpful. Surgical treatment is rarely required.
   3. Intersection Syndrome—Caused by irritation at the intersection of the outrigger muscles (APL, EPB) and ECRL/ECRB. Supportive therapy, splinting, and injections are helpful.

2. Ulnar—Includes instability, tendonitis, abutment, pisiform pathology, and TFCC injuries.
   a. Ulnar—Carpal instability is less common but includes lunotriquetral instability CID (*VISI*) (point tenderness and positive ballottement test are diagnostic), and triquetral-hamate instability (CIND—midcarpal). Treatment may include lunotriquetral or triquetral-hamate fusion.
   b. Tendonitis—Involves ECU or FCU.
      1. ECU Subluxation—Can palpate snapping out of groove. Treatment involves operative stabilization.
      2. FCU Calcific Tendonitis—Represents a chemical process. Treatment is splinting and NSAIDs; aspiration/steroid injection is also useful. It is usually a self-limited process.
   c. Ulnar-Carpal Abutment—Diagnosed radiographically (lytic lunate ± triquetrum [chondromalacia] and ulnar plus variant) and with a positive bone scan. Treatment is ulnar shortening. This and other distal radioulnar problems may benefit from a "matched" distal ulna resection (Bower's hemiresection arthroplasty), which preserves the ulnar styloid and TFCC.
   d. Pisiform Pathology—Includes fractures (immobilize) and pisotriquetral DJD (inject or, if it persists, remove the pisiform).
   e. TFCC Tears—TFCC consists of the articular disc (triangular fibrocartilage), meniscus homologue (lunocarpal), ulnocarpal ligament, dorsal and volar radioulnar ligament, and ECU sheath. The TFCC is important for loading and stabilizing the distal radioulnar joint. History of a twisting injury with palmar rotation and a positive bone scan are helpful. May be associated with ulnar plus variance. Arthrogram demonstrate leakage of dye proximally. Treatment can be difficult but includes casting in supination, injections, joint leveling procedures, and arthroscopic débridement or repair.
3. Dorsal Wrist Problems—Includes AVN of the lunate and capitate (rare), distal PIN syndrome, occult ganglion, and abutment syndrome.
   a. Keinböck's Disease (AVN of the Lunate)—Associated with ulnar minus variance and is described as having four stages (Lichtman).

STAGE	RADIOGRAPHY	TREATMENT
I	Sclerosis	Conservative/splinting
II	Fragmentation	Joint leveling (radial shortening or ulnar lengthening)
III	Collapse	Controversial (most treat like stage II ± scaphocapitate or triscaphe (STT) and capitohamate fusion)
IV	Radiocarpal intercarpal DJD	Salvage (fusion or proximal row carpectomy)

Radiographs, bone scan (positive before plain radiograph), and MRI all may have a role in diagnosis.

b. AVN of the Capitate—Rare; can follow a transverse fracture. Treatment is curettage/fusion.

c. Distal PIN Syndrome—See Section II: Compressive Neuropathies.

d. Occult Ganglion—Can cause dorsal wrist pain. Ganglions result from cystic degeneration within the dorsal scapholunate ligament and may be related to scapholunate pathology.

4. Palmar Wrist Problems—Can include carpal tunnel syndrome (discussed in Section II: Compressive Neuropathies) and volar carpal ganglion, which arises from the scaphotrapezial ligament.

VIII. Arthritis—Pain relief and increasing function are the primary considerations when dealing with the arthritic hand. Many arthritides affect the hand; some of the more common forms are discussed in this section.

A. DJD—Typically females are affected more than males. Joints commonly involved include the CMC joint of the thumb (diagnose with grind test, decreased pinch strength, and characteristic radiographs), the DIP joints of the digits (Heberden's nodes and mucous cysts), and less commonly the PIP joints (Bouchard's nodes). Treatment includes splinting, therapy, paraffin (digits), injections (CMC), and NSAIDs. Surgical options include mucous cyst and osteophyte excision, arthroplasty (PIP), arthrodesis (DIP), and interposition arthroplasty (CMC). Occasionally, DJD of the radial sesamoid of the thumb can cause pain at the CMC joint with narrowing of the space between the radial sesamoid and radial condyle of the metacarpal and osteophytes. Excision is usually helpful. Wrist DJD is discussed in Section VII: Wrist Pain/Instability.

B. Rheumatoid Arthritis (RA)—Systemic and soft tissue disease that affects the bones secondarily. Hypertrophic synovitis, if not controlled adequately medically, can destroy cartilage, compress or rupture tendons, affect nerves, and result in erosion and often dislocation of joints. Compensatory deformities often develop. Joints of the wrist and the MCP joints are most often affected. PIP joints can be involved with Sjögren syndrome (associated with dry eyes/mouth). Synovitis can also lead to de Quervain's syndrome, carpal tunnel, trigger finger/thumb, and tendon ruptures.

STAGE	CLINICAL FINDINGS	TREATMENT
I	Early synovitis	Nonoperative medical management/splinting
II	Persistent synovitis	Synovectomy
III	Specific deformation	Reconstructive
IV	Severe crippling	Salvage

Splinting and therapy are important early. Surgery is often directed at correcting the specific problem (synovectomy—limited, use when isolated; preserve collateral ligaments). Surgical indications include pain, chronic synovitis not responsive to adequate medical therapy for 6 months, nerve entrapment, tendon rupture, and deformities resulting in decreased function. Tenosynovectomy is universally acceptable and prevents tendon rupture. It must be done early; however, because tenosynovitis is relatively painless, patients typically present late. A helpful axiom for surgical procedures in RA is to start proximally and work distally, alternating fusion with motion-sparing procedures. Begin with predictable procedures. Staged procedures are usually favored, but the thumb is frequently addressed (usually with fusion) at the same time as other procedures (e.g., MCP arthroplasties). Deformity alone is not an indication for surgery. The procedure must be tailored to the individual's needs. The simplest, most successful procedure should be tried first. Goals of treatment should be (1) pain relief, (2) improved function, (3) prevention of further damage, and (4) cosmesis. Severe, progressive deformities (arthritis mutilans, end-stage disease with a characteristic "opera-glass" hand) should be fused early to avoid progressive bone loss. Specific deformities and their management follow.

1. Intrinsic Plus Deformity—Results from intrinsic stiffness (diagnosed by Bunnel test—hold the MCP in extension and flex the PIP joint). Corrected with therapy or if that fails sometimes by intrinsic release/transfer (Littler distal, Zancolli proximal, especially later).
2. PIP Swan Neck Deformity—Dysfunctional disorder caused by muscle imbalance, (including FDS tenosynovitis), intrinsic tightness, and ligamentous/capsular relaxation at the PIP leading to hyperextension. Treatment includes splinting early, PIP synovectomy, mobilization of lateral bands ± intrinsic release, and lengthening of the central slip; or tenodesis of the FDS proximal to the PIP (Swanson). The MCP joint must be addressed at the same time (arthroplasty) to balance the extensor mechanism. There is a high incidence of recurrence.
3. PIP Boutonnière—Functional deformity caused by extensor imbalance at the MCP resulting in hyperextension or PIP synovitis, leading to volar subluxation of the lateral bands. Patients may be unable to actively flex their DIP joints. Treatment includes injection early, release or reconstruction of the lateral bands distal to the PIP (lateral bands can be transferred to the attenuated or ruptured central slip), and release of the terminal tendon at the DIP. Later, salvage procedures or fusions are used. Soft tissue procedures commonly fail and are indicated only if the DIP can be passively flexed. PIP arthroplasties fail frequently, so arthrodesis is often favored at this joint for severe deformities. Fusion should be at 25–50 degrees of flexion at the PIP (more flexion for ulnar digits).
4. MCP Ulnar Drift—Occurs at the MCPs due to stretching of soft tissues and ulnar shift of the extensor tendons (etiology is obscure). Nonsurgical treatment includes rest, injection, splinting, and synovectomy—results are unpredictable. Surgery includes realignment of extensor tendons and intrinsic balancing. If the deformity is severe (possibly including MCP dislo-

cation—arthritis multilans), MCP Silastic implants ± PIP fusion may be required. This measure often results in pain relief, improved function, cosmesis, and delayed progression. Patients should expect only limited improvement in motion and no change in grip strength. Complications include recurrence, implant failure, infection (rare), and Silastic synovitis (very rare).

5. Tendon Rupture—Can occur owing to tenosynovitis.
   a. **Vaughn-Jackson Syndrome—Rupture** of the **EDC of the ring finger and small finger** secondary to caput ulna. This disorder is an attritional rupture that must be differentiated from subluxation (patient can maintain extension achieved passively), PIN palsy (tenodesis effect present [not present with rupture]), and locked trigger finger (no passive movement possible). Prior to rupture, extensor tenosynovectomy and ulnar resection (Darrah) can be done when the symptomatic wrist is unresponsive to medical management. The "tuck sign" (synovitis tucks under the skin with movement) is helpful. Wrist prosthesis implantation after a Darrah is contraindicated. Primary tendon repair may be possible early (within 4–6 weeks). Later, grafting (EIP to EDQ and ring finger EDC to long finger) and synovectomy are possible, but tendon grafts may become adherent; therefore tendon transfer may be a better alternative.
   b. EPL—Related to avascularity of the tendon with subsequent rupture at Lister's tubercle. EPL rupture is best reconstructed with EPI transfer.
   c. **Mannerfelt Syndrome—FPL rupture** due to carpal irregularities, volar synovitis, or volar carpal subluxation at the carpal tunnel. Patients typically have passive but not active flexion of the thumb at the PIP joint. Treatment includes rerouting of the tendon or arthrodesis of the PIP joint and synovectomy after anterior interosseous nerve compression is first ruled out. FDP rupture is uncommon, and surgery is less successful.
6. Thumb Deformities—Classified by Nalebuff into six common types (although several less common types were also noted) (Table 6–2; Fig. 6–10). MCP thumb fusion is the single most helpful hand procedure for RA.
7. Synovitis—Usually controlled by appropriate rheumatologic management. Synovectomy is indicated if synovitis is uncontrolled after 6 months of excellent conservative management, including medications and splinting. Surgical synovectomy must be meticulous and remove all synovium from the affected joint. Synovium regenerates initially with normal synovium; however, it usually degenerates into rheumatoid synovium later. Tenosynovitis may present with difficulty with active PIP flexion, carpal tunnel symptoms, trigger finger, and de Quervain's; it is best managed with NSAIDs, splinting, selective injections, and ultimately release of the affected soft tissue. Persistent pain following de Quervain's release can be due to a neuroma of the superficial radial nerve (hypesthesias, positive Tinel's sign) or inadequate release of the EPB tendon (numerous tendinous slips of APL can be deceiving). Careful surgical technique can avert these complications. Flexor synovectomy, as on the extensor side, can be of benefit in patients with boggy flexor synovium. Unlike with conventional triggering, the A1 pulley should be preserved in RA patients. MCP/PIP synovectomy (combined with intrinsic release at MCP) and extensor relocation may allow temporary correction.
8. Wrist Involvement—Begins with synovitis at the distal ulna and can lead to dorsal subluxation of the ulna (supination of hand on wrist) and carpal shift. Resection of the distal ulna (Darrah) and soft tissue procedures may help initially. Indications include pain at the distal radioulnar joint ± tendon rupture. Distal ulna resection can lead to carpal migration and ulnar snapping; therefore some surgeons favor preserving the distal ulnar buttress and TFCC with a hemiresection arthroplasty or a Lauenstein procedure (distal arthrodesis with proximal resection). Later, arthrodesis (in neutral or slight dorsiflexion) or wrist arthroplas-

TABLE 6–2. TYPES OF THUMB DEFORMITY

TYPE	DEFORMITY	1MC	JOINT POSITION MCP	IP	INITIATING FEATURE	COMMENTS
I	Boutonnière	Abd.	Flex.	Hyperext.	MCP synovitis	Arthroplasty, *MCP* (or IP) *fusion,* ± extensor realignment
II	Boutonnière and swan neck	Add.	Flex.	Hyperext.	MCP and CMC synovitis	Same as type I uncommon
III	Swan neck	Add.	Hyperext.	Flex.	CMC synovitis, MCP volar plate attenuation	CMC arthroplasty
IV	Gamekeeper's	Add.	Abd.	—	Ulnocarpal ligament destruction	Ligament reconstruction/MCP fusion
V	—	Neutral	Hyperext.	Flex.	Stretching of MCP volar plate	MCP fusion
VI	Arthritis mutilans	Short	Unstable	Unstable	Bone destruction	Fusion

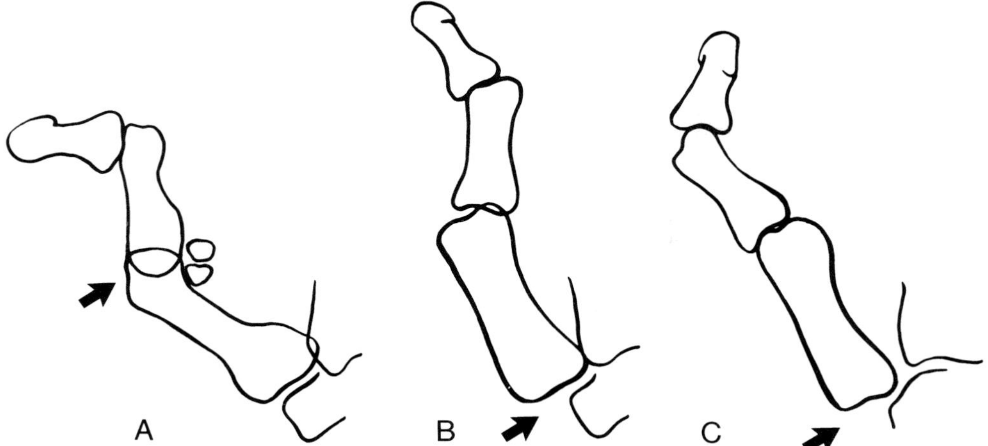

FIGURE 6–10. Nalebuff classification of common rheumatoid thumb disorders. *A,* Type I (boutonnière). *B,* Type II (boutonnière and swan neck). *C,* Type III (swan neck). (From Wiessman, B.N., and Sledge, C.B., eds.: Orthopaedic Radiology, p. 103. Philadelphia, WB Saunders, 1986; reprinted by permission.)

ties (Swanson's can be successful in RA, especially with the opposite side fused) are required. Fusion is often favored because of frequent failure of arthroplasties. The Nalebuff technique for wrist arthrodesis includes placing a Steinman pin through the third MC or interspace. AO fusion is preferred for younger patients. Concurrent distal ulnar resection is often necessary in RA patients.

9. Elbow—See Section XIII: Elbow.

C. Other Forms of Arthritis of the Hand—Include **systemic lupus erythematosus** (SLE), which causes ligamentous laxity affecting the MCPs, and **psoriasis,** which can involve the DIP joints with fusiform swelling of the digits and nail changes (it is also associated with a "gull wing" deformity). **Reiter syndrome** and **gout** more commonly affect the lower extremity. **Scleroderma** or progressive systemic sclerosis is associated with skin and GI manifestations and calcinosis; ulcerations can lead to spontaneous fingertip amputation.

IX. Dupuytren's Disease (Fig. 6–11)—Proliferative fibrodysplasia of subcutaneous palmar connective tissue; can lead to contractures due to nodules and cords that progressively develop. Usually seen in men between the ages of 40 and 60 years. Nodules are often painful when first noticed. The ring and little finger are most often involved, but the thumb web space can also be affected. The disease affects the palmar aponeurosis and its digital prolongations. The flexion contracture is most frequent at the MCP joint and can affect the PIP joint but rarely the DIP joint. Usually bilateral but more advanced in one hand. Other areas involved include the dorsum of the PIP joints (knuckle pads), dorsum of the penis (Peyronie's disease), and plantar fascia (Ledderhosen's disease). Can be associated with epilepsy, alcoholism, and diabetes. The disease represents a pathologic change in pre-existing normal fascia. In the palm, the pretendinous bands of the palmar aponeurosis cause MCP joint contracture. In the finger the superficial volar fascia, lateral digital sheet, spiral band, Grayson ligament, and retrovascular band alone or in combination produce PIP joint contracture. The pathognomonic sign is the nodule located at the distal palmar crease or over the proximal phalanx of the finger. Cords developed from new collagen laid down in pre-existing fascia and consist of increased percentages of type III collagen. These changes are not specific and are also seen in granulation tissue and scar. Nonsurgical treatment such as vitamin E, steroids, and allopurinol are not of proved value. Surgery is indicated

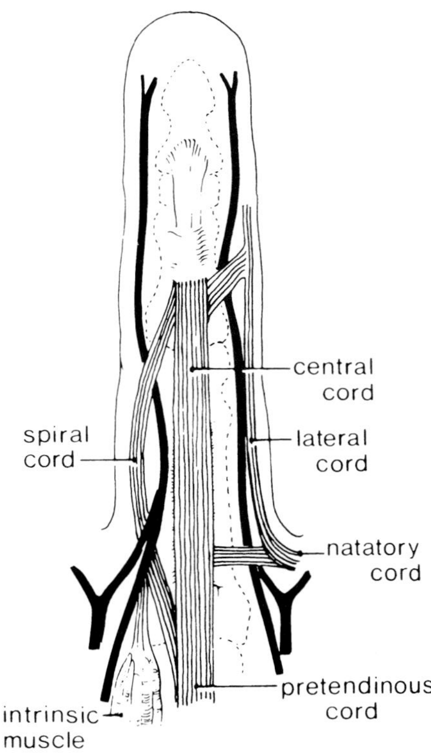

FIGURE 6–11. Pathoanatomy of Dupuytren's disease. (From Chiu, H.P., and McFarlane, R.M.: Pathogenesis of Dupuytren's contracture. J. Hand Surg. 3:9, 1978; reprinted by permission.)

for contractures of 30 degrees of the MCP or PIP joints. Painful nodules usually are transient and should be observed prior to considering surgery. Careful dissection of neurovascular structures is necessary to avoid injury, as the spiral cords can displace the neurovascular bundle. Subtotal palmar fasciectomy of the involved fascia is usually the procedure of choice. For advanced disease the incisions may be left open, especially in diabetics, and allowed to heal by secondary intention. Dermofasciectomy (Hueston) may be required for recurrent disease in which the overlying skin is excised with the fascia and the wound is closed with a full-thickness graft. PIP joint release for contracture is not often indicated and may cause loss of finger flexion. A 30 degree residual contracture of the PIP joint is acceptable after complete fascial excision. Therapy likely will alleviate the contracture. Extra-articular procedures of the PIP joint are best and are usually sufficient. Postoperative complications include recurrence, hematoma, skin loss, infection, joint stiffness, and occasionally reflex sympathetic dystrophy. Salvage options for severe PIP joint contractures include arthrodesis, skeletal shortening, arthroplasty, and amputation.

X. **Nerve Injury/Paralysis/Tendon Transfers**—Paralysis can be at any level and due to a variety of causes. Tendon transfers are helpful in allowing function when return of normal function has not occurred after the appropriate time period (classically nerves regenerate at about 1 mm/day or 1 inch/month after a 1-month latent period following an injury). Principles of tendon transfer include first correcting all contractures and ensuring that there is adequate power and amplitude in the transfer. Muscle expendability and a synergistic group of donor muscle are also important. Amplitude of tendons can generally be considered in four groups.

TENDONS	AMPLITUDE (mm)
Wrist flexors/extensors, EPB, APL	30
BR, lumbricals, thenar muscles	40
EDC, FPL, EPL	50
FDS, FPL	60–70

Muscle power can also be considered in groups.

MUSCLE(S)	RELATIVE POWER
FDP/FDS	4.5
FCU, BR, EDC	2.0
PT, FPL, ECU, ECRL	1.1
ECRB, FCU, FCR	0.9
PL, APL	0.1

One grade decrease of muscle strength with tendon transfer can be expected (5 = full, 4 = resistance, 3 = resistance against gravity, 2 = movement with gravity eliminated, 1 = trace of movement, 0 = no contraction). A straight line of pull for transferred tendons is best. Pulleys may be required if this is not possible. Synergistic muscle transfer and integrity (one transfer, one function) should be preserved if possible. Individual levels/nerves are considered below.

A. C-Spine Paralysis—Divided into three classes based on highest functional level.

CLASS	LEVEL	FUNCTIONING MUSCLES	TRANSFERS
1	C5	BR only	BR → wrist ext. (Moberg)
2	C6	BR, ECRB/L	ECRL → FDP, BR → FPL
3	C7	BR, ECRB/L, FCR	FCR → thumb opposition

As a general rule, surgery should follow a year of observation. With partial/incomplete quadriplegia, spasticity should be considered.

B. Brachial Plexus Injuries—Elbow flexion (biceps, C5 dysfunction) can be restored with latissimus dorsi flexeroplasty (Zancolli) or pectoralis major and minor transfer. Elbow extension can be restored with transfer of the posterior third of the deltoid to the trapezius. Free functioning muscle transfer (gracilis, pectoralis major, latissimus) is sometimes useful.

1. Anatomic Considerations—Root-level avulsion involves both anterior (plexus) and posterior (dorsal sensory) regions, whereas plexus injuries spare posterior areas. C4–7 nerve roots are well secured to their respective vertebrae and are less prone to avulsion injuries; C8 and T1 roots are not. T1-level preganglionic injuries often include a Horner syndrome because of disrupting the first sympathetic ganglion. Traction injuries are most common at C5 and C6 levels. Proximal cord lesions injure supraclavicular branches as well as the distal plexus and lead to winging of the scapula (long thoracic nerve).
2. Leffert Classification

CLASS	DESCRIPTION	
I	Open (usually from stabbing)	
II	Closed (usually from motorcycle accident)	
IIA	Supraclavicular	
	1. Preganglionic—Avulsion of nerve roots, usually from high-speed injuries with other injuries and loss of consciousness (LOC). No proximal stump, no neuroma formation (negative Tinel's sign), pseudomeningocele, denervation of dorsal neck muscles are common sequelae. Horner's sign (ptosis, miosis, anhydrosis).	
	2. Postganglionic—Roots remain intact; usually due to traction injuries. There are proximal stump and neuroma formation (positive Tinel's); deep dorsal neck muscles are intact; and pseudomeningocele does not develop.	
IIB	Infraclavicular—Usually involves branches from the trunks (suprascapular). Function is affected based on trunk involved.	
	Trunk Injured	*Functional Loss*
	Upper	Biceps, shoulder muscles
	Middle	Wrist and finger extension
	Lower	Wrist and finger flexion
III	Radiation therapy induced	
IV	Obstetric (see Chapter 2, Pediatric Orthopaedics)	
IVA	Erb's (upper root)—waiter's tip hand	
IVB	Klumpke (lower root)	
IVC	Mixed	

The nerve injury can be classified into five degrees (Sunderland) (Table 6–3; Fig. 6–12).

TABLE 6–3. DEGREES OF NERVE INJURY

DEGREE	DISCONTINUITY	DAMAGE	TREATMENT	PROGNOSIS
First	None; conduction block (neurapraxia)	Distal nerve fibers remain intact	Observation	Excellent
Second	Axon (axonotmesis)	Based on fibrosis	Observation	Good
Third	Axon and endoneurium	Based on fibrosis	Lysis	OK
Fourth	Axon, endoneurium, perineurium	Fibrotic connective tissue connects	Nerve grafts	Marginal
Fifth	Complete (neurotmesis)	Complete	Graft/transfer	Poor

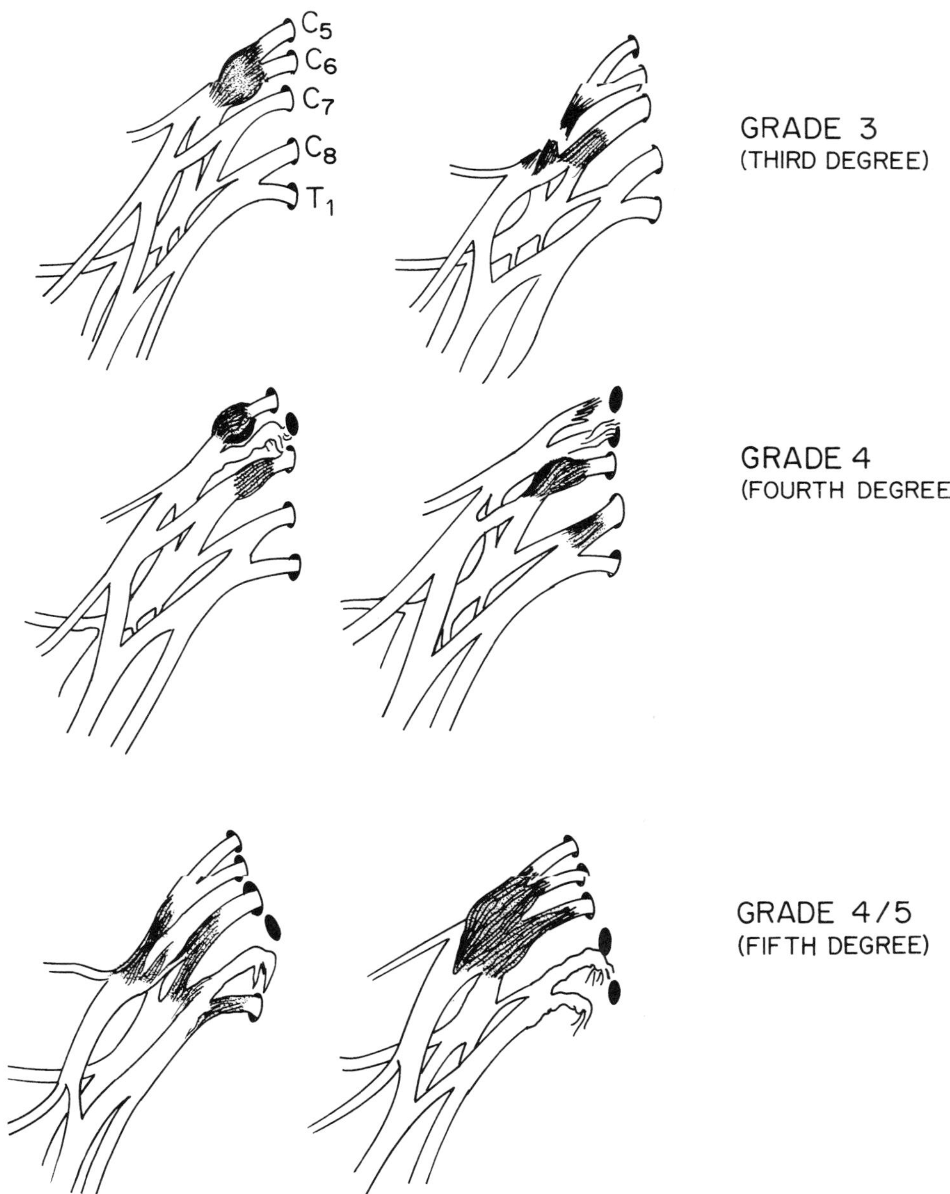

FIGURE 6–12. Classification of nerve injuries. Grades 1 and 2 (not shown) have no macroscopic changes. (From Bora, F.W.: The Pediatric Upper Extremity, p. 250. Philadelphia, WB Saunders, 1986; reprinted by permission.)

3. Treatment—Controversial, but most closed injuries are treated with observation, usually for 3 months with passive ROM and bracing. If no progress or halted progress is noted, neurolysis and nerve grafting may be indicated. Fibrosis, which is subclassified based on extent, is common; and treatment is based on overcoming this problem. Nerve transfer (usually with neurotization of intercostal nerves) and muscle/tendon transfers are also helpful in some cases. Prognosis is guarded but is better with C5, C6 injuries. Open injuries (especially from lacerations) should be repaired primarily.

C. Upper Extremity Peripheral Nerve Paralysis—**Tendon transfers** (Table 6–4) and fusions should be considered as the final step in the rehabilitation of the hand following maintenance of full passive ROM, adequate soft tissue coverage, appropriate bone work, and adequate sensation. FDS tendons are often used for transfers because they are the most important expendable tendons and are best for motion, opposition, and strength.

D. Cerebral Palsy (CP)—The hand in CP is usually palmar flexed and may have a thumb-in-palm deformity, a flexed elbow, and a pronated forearm. Patients may also demonstrate mirror movements of the upper extremities and poor sensation. Usually surgery is indicated only for those with spastic hemiplegia and a reasonable IQ. Nonoperative treatment includes splinting in extension and with thumb out of palm. Surgery includes early myotomies after age 7 (APB and FPB release); later tendon transfers (pronator teres for pronation deformities; FPL radial and proximal for thumb-in-palm; FCU to EDC for finger extension and release, or FCU to ECRB/L if finger extension is possible with an extended wrist—used in patients with a weak grasp); and finally arthrodesis (fuse wrist only if fingers can extend in fixed position and patient is at least 12 years old). Elbow flexion contractures may be present with normal pronation and supination. Early treatment is observation. Later, musculocutaneous neurectomy or biceps/brachialis release may be effective for contractures of <30 degrees caused by increased biceps tone.

E. Neuromas—Usually result from disorderly growth of resected nerves; become sensitive to mechanical stimulation and develop spontaneous activity.

TABLE 6–4. TENDON TRANSFERS

TRANSFER	LOSS	RECONSTRUCTION
Low radial	EDC	FCU → EDC
	EPL	PL—(reroute) → EPL
	APL	PT → APL
High radial (Jones)	EDC	FCU → EDC
	EPL	PL—(reroute) → EPL
	APL	
	ECRB/L	PT (insertion) → ECRB
	BR	
Low ulnar	Adductor pollicis	BR—reroute around third MC → add. pollicis (Boyes); or FDS → add. pollicis (Royle-Thompson, Brand)
	IO (and ulnar lumbricals)	Stabilize MCP (Zancolli capsulotomy, tenodesis, or bone block); or split transfers (e.g., FDS, EIP) to radial dorsal extensor apparatus
High ulnar	Adductor pollicis	BR—(reroute) → APL
	IO	As for low ulnar transfer
	FDS (RF, SF)	Suture to other tendons ±
	FCU	ECRL for power
Low median	Thumb opposition	FDS (ring finger) → FCU pulley → APB (Riordan); EIP → APB (opponensplasty); or muscle transfer (ADQ → APB) (Huber)
	Decreased sensation	Neurovascular island graft (ulnar ring finger → thumb)
	Radial first, second lumbricals	No significant deficit if ulnar nerve intact
High median	Pronation of forearm	
	Wrist flexion	
	Index and middle finger flexion	Suture to FDP of index and middle fingers ± ECRL transfer (adds power)
	Thumb flexion	BR → FPL
	Thumb opposition	EIP transfer to APB + EPL (Burkhalter)
	Decreased sensation	Neurovascslar island graft
Low median and ulnar	Palm sensation	Correct contractures, fuse IP if required
	Intrinsics	ECRB—tendon graft—intrinsics (Brand)
	Thumb opposition	FDS (ring finger) → FCU pulley → EPL (Riordan)
	Thumb adduction	EIP → adductor
High median and ulnar	Hand anesthesia	Arthrodesis of thumb MCP, (Zancolli)
	Flexors, intrinsics	Capsulodesis of MCP joints, ECRL → FDP, BR → FPL, ECU (with graft) → EPB

Usually responsive to treatment with anticonvulsants and local injection with local anesthetics ± steroids.

XI. Congenital Hand Disorders

A. Introduction—Genetic cause in 30%, nongenetic (environmental) in 10%, and unknown in 60%. Goals of surgery for these disorders are to preserve or improve function and appearance. Timing of surgery should be immediate if extremity is threatened (e.g., constriction band), within the first year if disorder has a tethering growth effect (e.g., clubhand), before age 3 if development patterns are influenced (e.g., pollicization), and delayed until past 4 years in cases that require cooperation of the child (e.g., tendon grafts).

B. Digits
1. Syndactyly (Joined Phalanges)—One of the most common congenital hand deformities; it is the most common anomaly in the United States. **More common in white males** and most frequently involves the ring and long fingers.

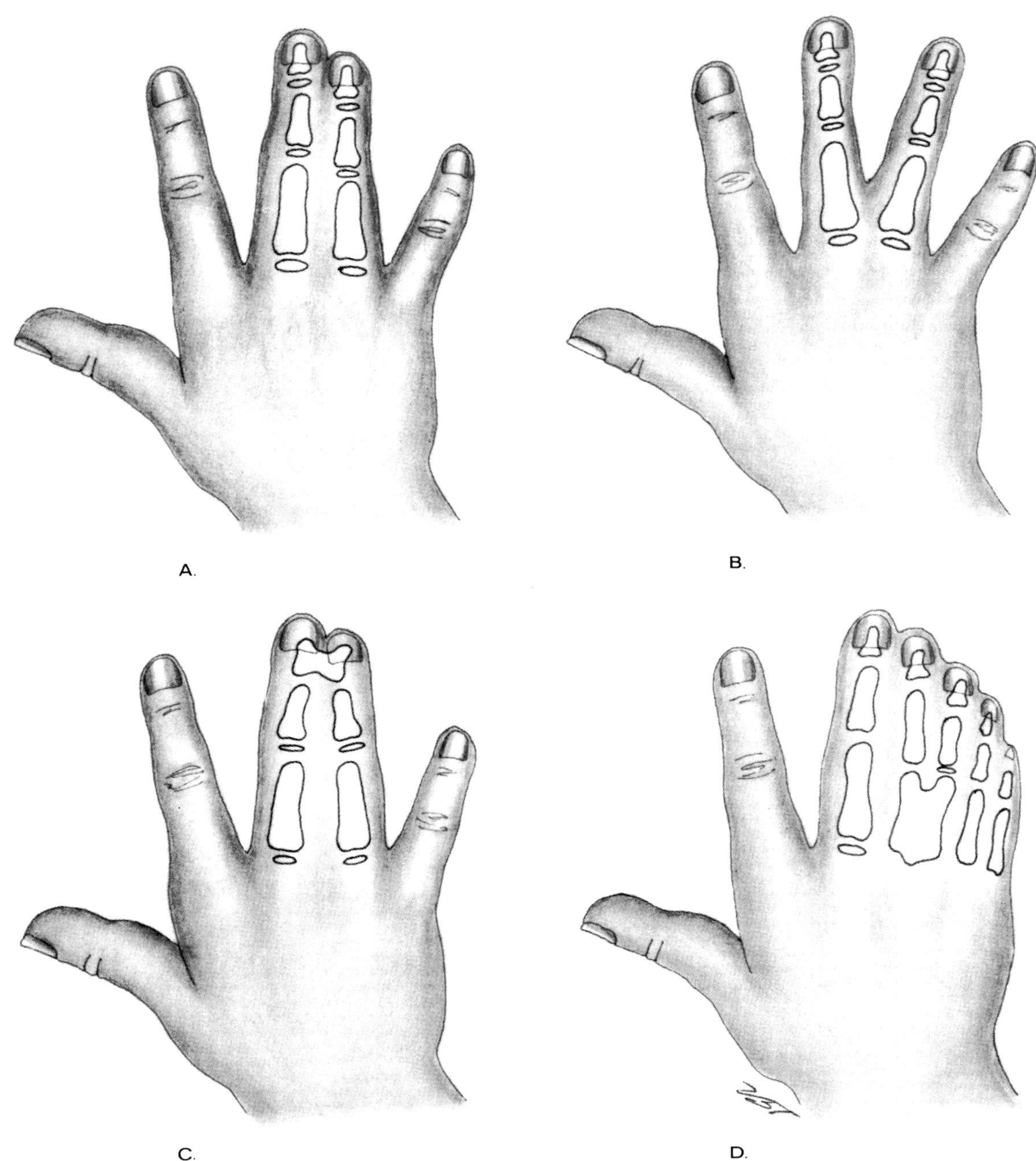

FIGURE 6–13. Classification of syndactyly. *A,* Complete simple syndactyly. *B,* Incomplete simple syndactyly. *C,* Complex syndactyly. *D,* Complex syndactyly and polydactyly. (From Tachdjian, M.O.: Pediatric Orthopaedics, 2nd ed., p. 223. Philadelphia, WB Saunders, 1990; reprinted by permission.)

Can be simple (skin only), complex (bony involvement), complete (entire length of digits), or incomplete/partial (Fig. 6–13). Release should be done at 18 months to 5 years and usually requires a skin graft. Can be associated with many anomalies, including Poland syndrome (also associated with chest wall anomalies), Streeter's dysplasia, and Apert syndrome. **Apert syndrome** (acrocephalosyndactyly) is a severe form of syndactyly that involves all of the digits; it has limited interphalangeal motion and sometimes is associated with mental retardation, visceral abnormalities, and grotesque facies. Surgery is indicated earlier in this case and should initially address the thumb and small finger. Web space contractures following release are common (decreased incidence with large zigzag incisions and dorsal flaps). Skin graft is required, and careful neurovascular dissection is necessary.

2. Polydactyly (Duplicated Phalanges)—Most common congenital hand abnormality; **more common in African-Americans.** Usually involves ulnar digits (postaxial), especially in African-Americans. Can be one of three types based on development: I, extra soft tissue only, can be treated in nursery with ligation; II, includes bone, tendon, and cartilage; and III, completely developed with own metacarpal (rare). Involvement of radial digits (preaxial), usually only the thumb, is more common in whites and is often associated with a generalized syndrome. Wassel classification (Fig. 6–14) is commonly used: I, bifid distal phalanx (DP); II, duplicated DP; III, bifid proximal phalanx (PP); IV, duplicated PP (most common type); V, bifid metacarpal (MC); VI, duplicated MC; VII, triphalangism. Surgical excision of the least developed digit (preserving the ulnar collateral ligament) or a combination of bifid portions (Bilhaut-Cloquet) is recommended. Postaxial (ulnar) is more common in African-Americans and Orientals and is isolated.
3. Brachydactyly (Short Digits)—Highly variable presentation. Amputation of useless tiny nubbins is recommended. If empty digital skin sleeve is of sufficient size, a nonvascularized toe proximal phalanx transfer to fill the skin sleeve and to create an MCP joint is favored prior to 12 months of age. Vascularized second toe transfer has limited indications.
4. Macrodactyly—Involves enlargement of all structures, especially the nerves of one or more digits. Can be isolated or **associated with** generalized disorders such as neurofibromatosis. Two types are based on proportionate increase with growth. Osteotomy or physeal arrest may be helpful. Digital nerve resection does not diminish growth.
5. Deviated Digits
   a. Clinodactyly—Skeletal abnormality with deviation in the lateral plane, usually involves the small finger at the joint; often seen in mentally retarded patients. It is usually caused by a trapezoid-shaped middle phalanx. Closing wedge osteotomy may be done but only for cosmesis.
   b. Camptodactyly—Familial soft tissue abnormality with deviation in the AP plane. May be secondary to aberrant lumbrical insertion, abnormal FDS, or an abnormal extensor apparatus. Commonly involves the small finger with a flexion contracture of the PIP joint and may be associated with a PIP flexion deformity. There are two peaks in presentation (ages 3 and 13 years). Passive stretching or static splinting may correct the deformity. Few good surgical options exist. FDS transfer to the extensor hood, if the deviated digit is passively correctable, is acceptable.
   c. Kirner's Deformity—In-curling of small finger DP in prepubertal girls. Treatment usually is observation. Hemiepiphysiodesis is required for early deformities, osteotomies are required late.
   d. Symphalangism—Stiff PIPs secondary to congenital ankylosis of the joint. Often associated with Apert syndrome and brachy-

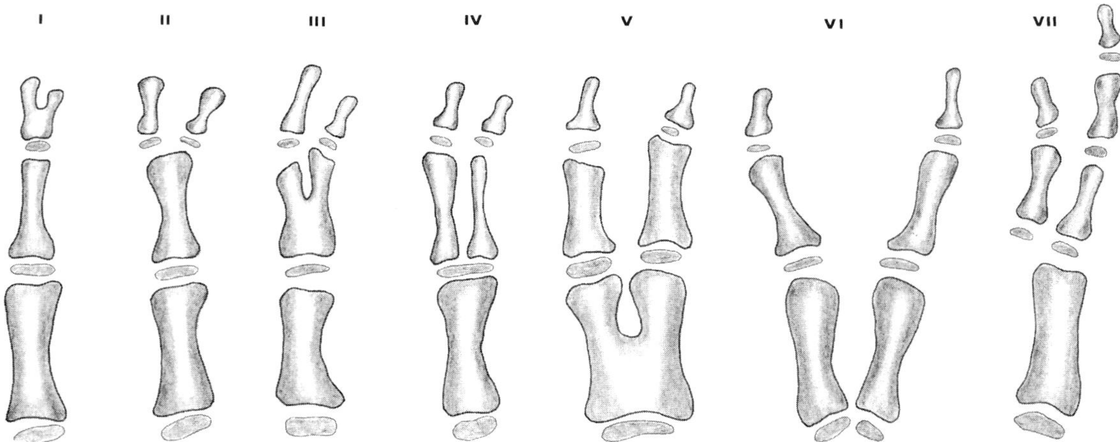

FIGURE 6–14. Wassel classification of thumb polydactyly. (From Tachdjian, M.O.: Pediatric Orthopaedics, 2nd ed., p. 243. Philadelphia, WB Saunders, 1990; reprinted by permission.)

dactyly. Treatment is observation, especially in children.

e. Delta Phalanx—Triangular phalanx and physis, usually the proximal phalanx of thumb and small finger with deviation toward the middle digit. Realignment procedures are indicated with severe deformation.

6. Thumb Anomalies (Hypoplastic Thumb)—Generally are best corrected at about 1 year of age and are classified as follows (Blauth).

GRADE	DESCRIPTION	TREATMENT
I	Short thumb, hypoplastic thenar muscles	Augment intrinsics
II	Like grade I with adducted thumb MCP	Soft tissue Z-plasty
III	Deficient metacarpal abducted thumb	Augment/bone graft or pollicization
IV	Floating thumb	Pollicization
V	Absent thumb	Pollicization

a. Congenital Flexion/Adduction of Thumb (Thumb-in-Palm or "Clasped Thumb" Disorder)—EPB weakness or absence, sex-linked recessive inheritance, usually bilateral. Passive correction early, EIP transfer late.

b. Anomalous FPL Insertion—Reroute insertion of FPL around APB for better function.

c. Congenital Hypoplasia of Thumb—Absent EPL and APL. Treated by tendon transfers (EIP to EPL, PL to APL) and MCP arthrodesis.

d. Floating Thumb—Attached to radial surface of the hand by a slender pedicle with skeletal support, usually containing a single neurovascular bundle and no intrinsic or extrinsic structures. Treatment is ablation of the pouce "flottant."

7. Congenital Trigger Finger/Thumb—Congenital stenosing tenosynovitis at A1 pulley. Often bilateral, with fixed flexion contractures at presentation. Up to 30% may resolve spontaneously by 1 year of age. Attempt splinting early and correct surgically before age 2–3 years to avoid permanent flexion contractures.

8. Constriction Band/Ring (Streeter's Dysplasia)—Most commonly involves digits, especially central fingers and toes, but can be more proximal. Fibrous amniotic bands can cause intrauterine constriction of extremities. Associated with syndactyly, club feet, and neurologic abnormalities. Treatment includes Z-plasties and avoidance of amniocentesis with future children.

9. Congenital Amputation—Can be due to constriction bands or failure of development. Most common form is very short below-elbow amputation, usually with radial head dislocation. Treatment can include lengthening of digits, toe transfers, index finger pollicization, or prosthesis if more proximal. **Passive terminal devices are indicated as early as 3–6 months** of age (when the child is able to sit upright) in the upper extremity. With complete absence of the hand, a Krukenberg procedure (creation of a radial-ulnar claw) may be indicated in blind children.

C. Hand, Wrist, Forearm

1. Clubhand (Hemimelia)

a. Radial Clubhand (Radial Aplasia [Preaxial])—Disorder of radial development leading to radial deviation of the hand, absent scaphoid, stiff fingers, and sometimes a hypoplastic thumb. It is most common in the right hand (bilateral in 50%) of males. Any radial deformity can be associated with concomitant heart or GI/GU abnormalities. These children usually have symptoms that can be discovered at the same time. Can be **associated with aplastic anemia** (Fanconi's syndrome, an autosomal recessive [AR] disorder with pancytopenia, brown skin pigment, aplastic thumb, hip dislocation, and poor prognosis); **thrombocytopenia** (TAR syndrome thrombocytopenia with absent radii, which is always bilateral, AR, and often lower limb anomalies, especially knee dysplasia); **heart anomalies** (Holt-Oram-Lewis); VATER (*v*ertebral anomalies, imperforate *a*nus, *t*racheo *e*sophageal aplasia, and *r*enal [and cardiac] anomalies); and chromosomal abnormalities (trisomy 17). Classified I–IV based on the amount of radius present (Bayne) (Table 6–5). The intercalary variety includes an absent radius with normal carpus and first ray; the longitudinal type has a normal ulna. Treatment initially may involve early splinting and manipulation ± soft tissue releases (median nerve may be radially displaced and immediately subcutaneous!). Later, centralization of the distal wrist/hand over the ulna with a "shish kebab" procedure within the first year of life is favored. Newer centralization procedures (radialization) do not disrupt the carpal bones and require less immobilization time. Contraindications to surgery include severe associated medical problems and stiff, nonfunctional elbow.

b. Ulnar Clubhand (Postaxial)—Much less common. Also classified into four subtypes (Miller).

TYPE	ULNA	ELBOW	TREATMENT
A	Anlage	Radial head dislocated	None
B	Absent	Radial head dislocated, cubital webbing	Radical release; amputation
C	Anlage	Synostosis	Humeral osteotomy
D	Neutral	Synostosis	None

Ulnar clubhand is not associated with systemic disorders, as is the radial hand, but can be associated with other musculoskeletal (especially digital) disorders. Treatment of digital disorders (syndactyly release, web deepening) often requires surgical intervention.

TABLE 6–5. CLASSIFICATION OF RADIAL CLUBHAND

TYPE	CHARACTERISTICS	RADIOGRAPHIC FINDINGS	CLINICAL FINDINGS	TREATMENT
I	Short distal radius	Delayed distal epiphyses	Hypoplastic thumb	Address thumb
II	Hypoplastic radius	Defective proximal and distal epiphyses, short radius, bowed ulna	Short forearm	Individualized
			—	
III	Partially absent radius	Usually medial/distal third; thick, bowed ulna	Short and bowed deviation	Centralization[b]
IV	Totally absent radius[a]	Radius absent, forearm deviated	Marked deviation, elbow stiffening	Centralization[b]

[a] Most common.
[b] Contraindicated with stiff elbow.

c. Central Deficiencies (Cleft Hand)—Often autosomal dominant (AD) and bilateral; may also have foot deformities. Classified as follows (Blauth and Falliner).

TYPE	CATEGORY	FEATURES	TREATMENT
I	Typical	Bilateral, familial, syndactyly	Close defect
II	Atypical	Severe, lobster claw	Krukenberg
III	Absent rays	Best function	Syndactyly release

2. Reduplication of the Ulna (Mirror Hand)—Ulna and carpus are reduplicated, leaving seven or eight digits and no thumb. Treatment includes removing the most abnormal digit and pollicization of a digit to create a five-digit hand and correct radial deviation of the hand.
3. Congenital Radial-Ulnar Synostosis—Union of the forearm bones, usually proximally, placing the forearm in pronation; most often bilateral. Associated with developmental dysplasia of the hip, clubfoot, and chromosomal abnormalities. Two types exist: (1) medullary canals of both bones are joined, creating a large radius with anterior bowing; and (2) proximal radius dislocation with less extensive fusion, usually unilateral. Both types are difficult to treat. Consider osteotomies for disabling pronation deformities. If bilateral, leave the dominant arm pronated and osteotomize the nondominant arm at the distal portion of the fusion mass, for 20–30 degrees of supination. Can be associated with fetal alcohol syndrome (associated also with bradydactyly and camptodactyly). Surgical release should be considered if motion, function, and potential growth of interconnected segments are interfered with. Classified based on the location of the synostosis and the position of the radial head.

TYPE	SYNOSTOSIS	RADIAL HEAD
I	Fibrous	Normal
II	Osseous	Normal
III	Osseous	Hyperplastic; posteriorly dislocated
IV	Short/osseous	Anteriorly dislocated

4. Congenital Dislocation of the Radial Head—Abnormally formed head on a long radius with a bowed ulna. Often associated with a connective tissue disorder. Abnormal shape of capitellum differentiates this condition from traumatic dislocations. Treatment includes therapy and late head resection (after growth is complete), which relieves pain but does not correct the abnormality or ROM.
5. Madelung's Deformity (AD, Female > Male)—Abnormal growth of the distal radial epiphysis with premature fusion of the ulnar half of the distal radius. Can cause progressive ulnar and volar angulation. Early treatment includes observation, especially in the asymptomatic patient. Operative treatment includes ulnar shortening ± dorsal radial closing wedge ostectomy for severe cases. Epiphysiolysis of the ulnar/palmar aspect of the radius may also be successful.
6. Congenital Pseudarthrosis of the Forearm—Rare disorder associated with neurofibromatosis. Can be cystic (leads to fractures and pseudarthrosis and is refractory to treatment) or associated with diaphyseal narrowing (more destructive with proliferative fibrous tissue). Vascularized bone graft may be helpful.
7. Lipofibromatous Hematoma of the Median Nerve—Rare enlargement of median nerve at the wrist; can present as progressive macrodactyly. Microvascular excision is difficult.
8. Congenital Webbing of the Elbow (Pterygium Cubitale)—Characterized by a broad skin web spanning the elbow, a flexion deformity, and pronated forearm. Can be associated with other webbing disorders and underlying muscle abnormalities (especially biceps and BR). Surgery is difficult and usually hazardous; and because it sometimes requires vessel and nerve lengthening, it may not be helpful.

XII. Hand Tumors (see also Chapter 8, Orthopaedic Pathology)

A. Benign Tumors

1. Giant Cell Tumor of the Tendon Sheath (Fibroxanthoma)—A benign but highly recurrent lesion that may originate in tendon sheaths or joint synovium. It is usually seen on the palmar surface of digits, especially at the PIP of index and long fingers. It is slow growing and recurs in 10% of excisions. Second most common

hand mass (next to ganglions). Prognosis is guarded with recurrence and on rare occasions requires amputation.

2. Vascular Tumors/Abnormalities
   a. False Aneurysm—Does not include all layers of the arterial wall. Can follow trauma late but may not have a bruit.
   b. True Aneurysms—May be difficult to differentiate; has all layers of the arterial wall on pathologic examination.
   c. A-V Fistula—May have thrill or bruit with decreased distal filling.
   d. Glomus Tumor—Tumor that frequently involves the nail bed with the classic triad of **pain, tenderness, and cold sensitivity.** Nail bed ridging ± a small blue spot at the base of the nail can be seen. Radiographs may show a shelled-out dorsal lesion. Treatment is excision; usually a normal nail matrix can be preserved. Excellent prognosis if entire tumor is removed.
   e. Kaposi's Sarcoma—Vascular tumor associated with AIDS.
3. Neural Tumors—Traumatic neuromas are usually iatrogenic, due to prior operative procedures. Treatment includes excision and transfer to a deeper, padded area. Neurofibromas are less common and rarely require excision (only if irritating). Neurolemomas are also uncommon but should be excised while protecting the involved nerve.
4. Enchondroma—Most destructive benign lesion of bone, usually in the proximal phalanx. Frequently a cause of pathologic fractures. Radiographs show a lytic lesion. Curettage and bone grafting may be required **after fracture healing.** Excellent prognosis.
5. Lipomas—Common in 30- to 60-year-old women; can be mistaken for ganglions. Mobile, nontender. Excision may be required. May produce nerve compression with motor deficit.

B. Tumorous Conditions
1. Ganglion—Most common hand mass. Usually dorsal carpal ganglion (over scapholunate ligament) but can be volar (from ST interval) or elsewhere. Lesions are soft, nontender, and transilluminant. Treatment includes aspiration or rupture and surgical excision (with a portion of the wrist capsule) if it recurs and is symptomatic. There is a significant incidence of recurrence.
2. Epidermoid (Inclusion) Cyst—Implantation of epithelioid tissues into deeper areas as a result of penetrating trauma. Mildly painful palmar bulboid deformity that does not transilluminate. Mass is nontender and subcutaneous. Radiographs may show a cystic lesion. Excision and curettage requires preserving very little overlying adherent skin. Low recurrence rate.
3. Mucous Cyst—Usually at the dorsal DIP joint in women, these cysts are actually ganglia that originate from the DIP joint. Frequently associated with Heberden's nodes; osteophytes that should be removed at surgery.
4. Volar Retinacular Cyst—Located at volar A1 pulley. They often disappear spontaneously. Treatment includes aspiration and removal of a window of the pulley if it recurs.
5. Foreign Body Granuloma—Firm, fibrous capsule and deep granuloma; resolves with resection.
6. Calcinosis—May be secondary to degeneration. Symptoms include pain, tenderness, and erythema. Commonly occurs near FCU insertion. Treatment includes heat, rest, injection/aspiration, and surgery for large deposits. Calcinosis circumscripta can be seen in SLE, RA, and scleroderma, usually in the fingers, and may be associated with Raynaud's phenomenon. Treatment may include partial excision.
7. Dejerine-Sottas Disease—Localized swelling of a peripheral nerve due to hypertrophic interstitial neuropathy. Usually involves the median nerve and may require carpal tunnel release. Resection of the lesion is not possible without resecting the nerve.
8. Turret Exostosis—Traumatic subperiosteal hemorrhage that follows trauma. Extracortical bone underneath the extensor mechanism can be excised after the bone matures.
9. CMC Boss—Bony growth at bases of second and third metacarpal. Special radiographs can demonstrate the osteophytes, which may be resected if symptoms warrant. Associated with ganglia at least 30% of the time and often associated with os styloideum (accessory ossicle).

C. Malignancies—Extremely rare in the hand. Most common primary malignancy of the hand is squamous cell carcinoma. This tumor in the hand requires aggressive treatment (usually amputation). The most common bony malignancy in the hand is chondrosarcoma. Most common metastasis in the hand is from lung (and may involve the DP). Epitheloid is the commonest soft tissue sarcoma.

XIII. Elbow

A. Introduction—The medial collateral ligament is a more important stabilizer than the lateral collateral ligament. Functional ROM of 30–130 degrees with 50 degrees of pronation and supination.

B. Distal Biceps Tendon Rupture—Rare. Presents with painful swollen elbow usually in a 30- to 50-year-old active man. If treated nonoperatively, supination and flexion strength are affected (35–40%), and patients complain of prolonged pain. Repair is with the two-incision approach (Boyd and Anderson anterior and posterior incisions) to decrease the incidence of radial nerve injury, but it may be associated with increased incidence of synostosis.

C. Tennis Elbow
1. Lateral Epicondylitis—Common degeneration at extensor origin, usually ECRB. Conservative treatment: strap, wrist extension stretching exercises, NSAIDs, injections (peritendinous, *not* intratendinous). Surgical treatment: release of origin (slide) or excision of fibrinous tissue at ECRB origin. This disorder is often difficult to distinguish from posterior interosseous nerve compression.
2. Medial Epicondylitis—Less common (10%) in tennis players; seen more commonly in golfers and baseball players. Usually responds to conservative treatment (e.g., injections, casting, bracing). It is commonly associated with ulnar nerve neurapraxia. Rarely, surgery (pathology usually localized to EDC origin) is indicated.

D. Rheumatoid Elbow—Three primary methods of treatment.
   1. **Synovectomy—With radial head excision** if secondary change present; useful if done early in the disease process. Radial head implant is not required. Also useful in hemophiliacs with refractory hemarthrosis. Arthrodesis rarely indicated because of increased incidence of failure.
   2. Total Elbow Arthroplasty—Greater constraint leads to loosening; lower constraint leads to instability. Has evolved to semiconstrained design. Increased complications (especially infection) with revisions.
   3. Excisional Arthroplasty with Interposition of Various Substances—Good motion but unstable (especially in RA patients).

E. Contractures—If arthrosis is absent, anterior capsulotomy is often effective to regain some extension in a posttraumatic patient.

Selected Bibliography

Allen, B.N., Frykman, G.K., Unsell, R.S., et al.: Ruptured flexor tendon tenorrhaphies in zone. II. Repair and rehabilitation. J. Hand Surg. [Am.] 12:18–21, 1987.

American Society for Surgery of the Hand: Regional Review Courses in Hand Surgery, San Antonio, TX, October 13–14, 1990.

Badalamente, M.A., Stern, L., and Hurst, L.C.: The pathogenesis of Dupuytren's contracture: Contractile mechanisms of the myofibroblasts. J. Hand Surg. 8:235–243, 1983.

Bayne, L.G., and Klug, M.S.: Long-term review of the surgical treatment of radial deficiencies. J. Hand Surg. [Am.] 12:169–179, 1987.

Beckenbaugh, R.D.: Total joint arthroplasty: The wrist. Mayo Clin. Proc. 54:513–515, 1979.

Bieber, E.J., Weiland, A.J., and Volenec-Dowling, S.: Silicone-rubber implant arthroplasty of the metacarpophalangeal joints for rheumatoid arthritis. J. Bone Joint Surg. [Am.] 68:206–209, 1986.

Bora, F.W.: The Pediatric Upper Extremity. Philadelphia, WB Saunders, 1986.

Brumfield, R.H., Jr., and Resnick, C.T.: Synovectomy of the elbow in rheumatoid arthritis. J. Bone Joint Surg. [Am.] 67:16–20, 1985.

Burke, F., and Flatt, A.: Clinodactyly: A review of a series of cases. Hand 11:269–280, 1979.

Chapman, M.W., ed.: Operative Orthopaedics. Philadelphia, J.B. Lippincott, 1988.

Chow, S.P., and Ho, E.: Open treatment of fingertip injuries in adults. J. Hand Surg. 7:470–476, 1982.

Cooney, W.P., Linscheid, R.L., Dobyns, J.H., et al.: Scaphoid nonunion: Role of anterior interpositional bone grafts. J. Hand Surg. [Am.] 13:635–650, 1988.

Crenshaw, A.H., ed.: Campbell's Operative Orthopaedics, 7th ed. St. Louis, CV Mosby, 1987.

Daniel, R.K., and May, J.W., Jr.: Free flaps: An overview. Clin. Orthop. 133:122–131, 1978.

Daniel, R.K., and Weiland, A.J.: Free tissue transfer for upper extremity reconstruction. J. Hand Surg. 7:66–76, 1982.

Dee, R., Mango, E., and Hurst, L.C.: Principles of Orthopaedic Practice. New York, McGraw-Hill, 1989.

Eaton, R.G., Glickel, S.Z., and Littler, J.W.: Tendon interposition arthroplasty for degenerative arthritis of the trapeziometacarpal joint of the thumb. J. Hand Surg. [Am.] 10:645–654, 1985.

Epps, C.H., ed.: Complications in Orthopaedic Surgery, 2nd ed. Philadelphia, JB Lippincott, 1986.

Ewald, F.C., and Jacobs, M.A.: Total elbow arthroplasty. Clin. Orthop. 182:137–142, 1984.

Failla, J.M., Amadio, P.C., and Morrey, B.F.: Post-traumatic proximal radio-ulnar synostosis: Results of surgical treatment. J. Bone Joint Surg. [Am.] 71:1208, 1989.

Fatti, J.F., Palmer, A.K., and Mosher, J.F.: The long-term results of Swanson silicone rubber interpositional wrist arthroplasty. J. Hand Surg. [Am.] 11:166–175, 1986.

Flatt, A.E.: The Care of Congenital Hand Anomalies. St. Louis, CV Mosby, 1977.

Gelberman, R.H., Van de Berg, J.S., Lundborg, G.N., and Akeson, W.H.: Flexor tendon healing and restoration of the gliding surface: An ultrastructural study in dogs. J. Bone Joint Surg. [Am.] 65: 70–80, 1983.

Gelberman, R.H., Wolock, B.S., and Siegal, D.B.: Current concepts review: Fractures and non-unions of the carpal scaphoid. J. Bone Joint Surg. [Am.] 71:1560, 1989.

Goldberg, V.M., Figgie, H.E., III, Inglis, A.E., and Figgie, M.P.: Current concepts review: Total elbow arthroplasty. J. Bone Joint Surg. [Am.] 70:778, 1988.

Green, D.P., ed.: Operative Hand Surgery, 2nd ed. New York, Churchill Livingstone, 1988.

Green, D.P.: Proximal row carpectomy. Hand Clin. 3:163–168, 1987.

Jaeger, S.H., Tsai, T., and Kleinert, H.E.: Upper extremity replantation in children. Orthop. Clin. North Am. 12:897–907, 1981.

Kleinert, H.E., Kutz, J.E., and Cohen, M.: Primary repaired zone 2 flexor tendon lacerations. AAOS Symposium on Tendon Surgery in the Hand, pp 115–124. St. Louis, CV Mosby, 1975.

Kleinert, J.M., Stern, P.J., Lister, G.D., and Kleinhans, R.J.: Complications of scaphoid silicone arthroplasty. J. Bone Joint Surg. [Am.] 67:422–427, 1985.

Kleinman, W.B., Steichen, J.B., and Strickland, J.W.: Management of chronic rotary subluxation of the scaphoid by scapho-trapezio-trapezoid arthrodesis. J. Hand Surg. 7:125–136, 1982.

Kudo, H., and Iwano, K.: Total elbow arthroplasty with a non-constrained surface-replacement prosthesis in patients who have rheumatoid arthritis. A long-term follow-up study. J. Bone Joint Surg. [Am.] 72:355, 1990.

Levinsohn, E.M., Palmer, A.K., Coren, A.B., et al.: Wrist arthrography: The value of the three compartment injection technique. Skeletal Radiol. 16:539–544, 1987.

Lichtman, D.M., Noble, W.H., and Alexander, C.E.: Dynamic triquetiolunate instability. J. Hand Surg. 9:185, 1984.

Linscheid, R.L., Dobyns, J.H., Beckenbaugh, R.D., Cooney, W.P.: Instability patterns of the wrist. J. Hand Surg. 8:682–686, 1983.

Lister, G.D., Kalisman, M., and Tsai, T.M.: Reconstruction of the hand with free microneurovascular toe-to-hand transfer: Experience with 54 toe transfers. Plast. Reconstr. Surg. 71:372–384, 1983.

McCash, C.R.: The open palm technique in Dupytren's contractions. Br. J. Plastic Surg. 17:271, 1964.

McFarlane R.M.: The current status of Dupytren's disease. J. Hand Surg. 8:703, 1983.

Mackinnon, S.E., and Holder, L.E.: The use of three-phase radionuclide bone scanning in the diagnosis of reflex sympathetic dystrophy. J. Hand Surg. [Am.] 9:556–563, 1984.

Miller, J.K., Wenner, S.M., and Kruger, L.M.: Ulnar deficiency. J. Hand Surg. 11A:822–829, 1986.

Morrey, B.F.: The Elbow and Its Disorders. Philadelphia, WB Saunders, 1985.

Morrey, B.F., and An, K.N.: Functional anatomy of the ligaments of the elbow. Clin. Orthop. 201:84–90, 1985.

Morrey, B.F., and Bryan, R.S.: Revision total elbow arthroplasty. J. Bone Joint Surg. [Am.] 69:523–532, 1987.

Nalebuff, E.A.: Surgical treatment of the swan neck deformity in rheumatoid arthritis. Orthop. Clin. North Am. 15:369, 1984.

Nirschl, R.P., and Pettrone, F.A.: Tennis elbow: The surgical treatment of lateral epicondylitis. J. Bone Joint Surg. [Am.] 61:832–839, 1979.

Omer, G.E., and Spinner, M., eds.: Management of Peripheral Nerve Problems. Philadelphia, WB Saunders, 1980.

Orthopaedic Knowledge Update Home Study Syllabus I, II, and III.

Chicago, American Academy of Orthopaedic Surgeons, 1984, 1987, 1990.
Palmer, A.K., and Werner, F.W.: The triangular fibrocartilage complex of the wrist: Anatomy and function. J. Hand Surg. 6:153–162, 1981.
Reagan, D.S., Linscheid, R.L., and Dobyns, J.H.: Lunotriquetral sprains. J. Hand Surg. 9:502–514, 1984.
Simmons, B.P., Southmayd, W.W., and Riseborough, E.J.: Congenital radioulnar synostosis. J. Hand Surg. 8:829–838, 1983.
Smith, R.J., ed.: Symposium on congenital deformities of the hand. Hand Clin. 1:371–596, 1985.
Smith, R.J., Atkinson, R.E., and Jupiter, J.B.: Silicone synovitis of the wrist. J. Hand Surg. [Am.] 10:47–60, 1985.
Strickland, J.W.: Flexor tendon repair. Hand Clin. 1:55–68, 1985.
Sunderland, S.: Nerves and Nerve Injuries, 2nd ed. Edinburgh, Churchill Livingstone, 1978.
Swanson, A.B., Swanson, G.D., and Tada, K.: A classification for congenital limb malformation. J. Hand Surg. 8:693–702, 1983.
Taleisnik, J.: Current concepts review. Carpal instability. J. Bone Joint Surg. [Am.] 70:1262, 1988.
Tolego, L.C., and Ger, E.: Evaluation of the operative treatment of syndactyly. J. Hand Surg. 4:556–564, 1979.
Upton, A.R.M., and McCames, A.J.: The double crush in nerve entrapment syndromes. Lancet 1:359, 1973.
Urbaniak, J.R., Evans, J.P., and Bright, D.S.: Microvascular management of ring avulsion injuries. J. Hand Surg. 6:25–30, 1981.
Urbaniak, J.R., Hansen, P.E., Beissinger, S.F., and Aitken, M.S.: Correction of post-traumatic flexion contracture of the elbow by anterior capsulotomy. J. Bone Joint Surg. [Am.] 67:1160–1164, 1985.
Urbaniak, J.R., Roth, J.H., Nunley, J.A., Goldner, R.D., et al.: The results of replantation after amputation of a single finger. J. Bone Joint Surg. [Am.] 67:611–619, 1985.
Vicar, A.J., and Burton, R.I.: Surgical management of the rheumatoid wrist: Fusion or arthroplasty. J. Hand Surg. [Am.] 11:790–797, 1986.
Watson, H.K., and Ballet, F.L.: The SLAC wrist: Scapholunate advanced collapse pattern of degenerative arthritis. J. Hand Surg. [Am.] 9:358–365, 1984.
Weiland, A.J., Kleinert, H.E., Kutz, J.E., and Daniel, R.K.: Free vascularized bone grafts in surgery of the upper extremity. J. Hand Surg. 4:129–144, 1979.
Weissman, B.N., and Sledge, C.B., eds.: Orthopaedic Radiology. Philadelphia, WB Saunders, 1986.
Wood, V.E.: Polydactyly and the triphalangeal thumb. J. Hand Surg. 3:436–444, 1978.
Zancolli, E.: Structural and Dynamic Basis of Hand Surgery, 2nd ed. Philadelphia, JP Lippincott, 1979.
Zancolli, E.A., and Zancolli, E.J.: Surgical management of the hemiplegic spastic hand in cerebral palsy. Surg. Clin. North Am. 61: 395–406, 1981.

7

SPINE

WILLIAM C. LAUERMAN and MICHAEL REGAN

I. Introduction

A. Anatomy—See Chapter 11, Anatomy

B. History and Physical Examination (Table 7–1)—A complete history is critical to fully assess complaints, including evaluation of localized pain (trauma, tumor, infection), mechanical pain (instability, discogenic disease), radicular pain (HNP versus stenosis), night pain (tumor), and associated symptoms such as fevers and weight loss (infection, tumor). The physical examination must be complete to evaluate both the spine and the neurologic function of the extremities. Localized hip and shoulder pathology may simulate spine disease and must also be evaluated. The examination must include the following.

EXAMINATION	FEATURES
Inspection	Overall alignment in sagittal and coronal planes, balanced posture
Gait	Wide-based (myelopathy), forward-leaning (stenosis), antalgic
Palpation	Localized posterior swelling (trauma), acute gibbus deformity, tenderness
Range of motion	Flexion/extension, lateral bend, full vs. limited
Neurologic assessment	Motor, sensory, reflexes, long tract signs (Fig. 7–2, 7–4)
Special tests	Straight-leg raise, Spurling's test, Waddell's signs of inorganic pathology

C. Objective Tests—Plain radiographs after 6 weeks and occasionally dynamic flexion/extension views (instability). CT scans with fine cuts ± myelographic dye (bony anatomy), and MRI scan (soft tissue, tumor, infection) are excellent for further imaging. Bone scan helpful to evaluate metastatic disease, may be negative with multiple myeloma. Laboratory evaluation: CRP and ESR for infection, metabolic screen, SPEP/UPEP for myeloma, CBC (often normal WBCs with infection, anemia with myeloma).

D. Back Pain—Ubiquitous complaint, second only to URI as cause of office visits, with 60–80% lifetime prevalence. Standard work-up, beginning with history taking (most important) and progressing to physical examination (Table 7–1). Radiographic and laboratory studies can help in diagnosis. Some important considerations in the evaluation of back pain are presented below.

1. Age—Children may be affected by congenital or, more commonly, developmental disorders, infection, or primary tumors. Young adults are more likely to suffer from disc disease, spondylolisthesis, or acute fractures. In older adults, spinal stenosis, metastatic disease, and osteopenic compression fractures are more common.
2. Radicular Signs and Symptoms—Often associated with disc herniation or spinal stenosis. Intraspinal pathology or other entities associated with cord or root impingement may be responsible. Herpes zoster is a rare cause of lumbar radiculopathy with pain preceding the skin eruption.
3. Systemic Symptoms—Careful history taking can lead to the diagnosis of metabolic disease, ankylosing spondylitis, tumor, or infection (confirmed with laboratory studies). Associated signs and symptoms may be essential to the diagnosis (e.g., ophthalmologic symptoms with spondyloarthropathies; other joint involvement with rheumatoid arthritis [RA] or osteoarthritis [OA]). Metastatic tumor should be suspected in patients with a history of cancer, pain at rest, or unexplained weight loss, or in those over age 50.
4. Referred Pain—"Back pain" can often be viscerogenic, vascular, or related to other skeletal areas (especially with hip arthritis). Careful history and physical examination are essential.
5. Psychogenic—Psychological disturbances play an important role in some patients with chronic low back disorders. Evidence of secondary gain (especially compensation or litigation) and inappropriate (Waddell) signs and symptoms can help identify these patients. Nevertheless, one must be wary of real pathology, even in such patients.
6. History of Back Pain—Perhaps the most important risk factor for future pain, especially with frequent disabling episodes and short intervals between episodes. Compensation work situations, smoking, and age >30 years are also associated with development of persistent disabling lower back pain. The incidence of disabling pain actually declines after age 60.

II. Cervical Spine

A. Cervical Spondylosis—Chronic disc degeneration and associated facet arthropathy. Resultant syndromes include **discogenic neck pain** (mechanical pain), **radiculopathy** (root compromise), **myelopathy** (cord compression), or combination. Cervical spondylosis typically begins at age 40–50, is seen in men > women, and most commonly occurs at the C5–C6 > C6–C7 levels. Risk factors include frequent lifting, cigarette smoking, and a history of excessive driving.

TABLE 7–1. DIFFERENTIAL DIAGNOSIS OF DISORDERS IN THE L-SPINE

EVALUATION	BACK STRAIN	HNP	SPINAL STENOSIS	SPONDYLO-LISTHESIS/ INSTABILITY	TUMOR	SPONDYLO-ARTHROPATHY	METABOLIC	INFECTION
Predominant pain (leg versus back)	Back	Leg	Leg	Back	Back	Back	Back	Back
Constitutional symptoms				+	+		+	
Tension sign		+						
Neurologic examination		+	+ After stress					
Plain x-ray studies			+	+	±	+	+	±
Lateral motion x-ray studies				+				
CT scan		+	+		+			+
Myelogram		+	+					
Bone scan					+	+	+	+
ESR					+	+		+
Ca/P/alk phos					+			

From Weinstein, J.N., and Wiesel, S.W.: The Lumbar Spine, p. 360. Philadelphia, WB Saunders, 1990; reprinted by permission.

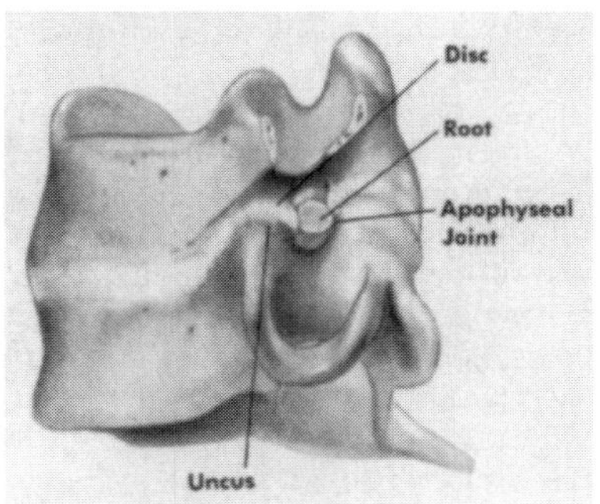

FIGURE 7–1. Cervical root impingement. (From Rothman, R.H., and Simeon, F.A.: The Spine, 2nd ed., p. 452. Philadelphia, WB Saunders, 1982; reprinted by permission.)

1. Pathoanatomy—Involves the disc and four other articulations (Fig. 7–1): two facets joints and two false uncovertebral joints (of Luschka). The cervical cord becomes compromised when the diameter of the canal (normally about 17 mm) is reduced to less than 13 mm. With neck extension the cord is pinched between the degenerative disc and spondylotic bar anteriorly and the hypertrophic facets and infolded ligamentum flavum posteriorly. With neck flexion the canal dimension increases slightly to relieve pressure on the cord. Progressive collapse of the cervical discs results in loss of normal lordosis of the cervical spine and chronic anterior cord compression across the kyphotic spine/anterior chonro-osseous spurs. Spondylotic changes in the foramina primarily from chondro-osseous spurs of the joints of Luschka may restrict motion and may lead to nerve root compression. Soft disc herniation is usually posterolateral, between the posterior edge of the uncinate process and the lateral edge of the posterior longitudinal ligament, resulting in acute radiculopathy. Anterior herniation may cause dysphagia. Myelopathy may be seen with large central herniation, or spondylotic bars with a congenitally narrow canal. Ossification of the posterior longitudinal ligament (OPLL), resulting in cervical stenosis and myelopathy, is common in Asians but may also be seen in non-Asians.
2. Signs and Symptoms—Degenerative **discogenic neck pain** may present with the insidious onset of neck pain without neurologic signs or symptoms, exacerbated by excess vertebral motion. Occipital headache is common. **Radiculopathy** can involve one or multiple roots, and symptoms include neck, shoulder, and arm pain, paresthesias, and numbness. Findings may overlap because of intraneural intersegmental connections of sensory nerve roots. Mechanical stress, such as excessive vertebral motion, may exacerbate these symptoms. The lower nerve root at a given level is usually affected (Table 7–2). **Myelopathy** may be characterized by weakness (upper > lower extremity), ataxic broad-based shuffling gait, sensory changes, spasticity, and rarely urinary retention. "Myelopathy hand" and the "finger escape sign" (small finger spontaneously abducts because of weak intrinsics) suggest cervical myelopathy. Upper motor neuron findings such as hyperreflexia, Hoffmann's sign, inverted radial reflex (ipsilateral finger flexion with elicitation of the brachioradialis reflex), clonus, or Babinski's sign may be present. Additionally, the upper extremities may have radicular (LMN) signs along with

TABLE 7–2. FINDINGS IN NERVE ROOT COMPRESSION

LEVEL	ROOT	MUSCLES AFFECTED	SENSORY LOSS	REFLEX
C3–C4	C4	Scapular	Lateral neck, shoulder	None
C4–C5	C5	Deltoid, biceps	Lateral arm	Biceps
C5–C6[a]	C6	Wrist extensors, biceps, triceps (supination)	Radial forearm	Brachioradialis
C6–C7	C7	Triceps, wrist flexors (pronation)	Middle finger	Triceps
C7–C8	C8	Finger flexors, interossei	Ulnar hand	None
C8–T1	T1	Interossei	Ulnar forearm	None

[a] Most common.

the myelopathic signs. Funicular pain, characterized by central burning and stinging ± Lhermitte's phenomenon (radiating lightning-like sensations down the back with neck flexion) may also be present with myelopathy.

3. Diagnosis—Largely based on history and physical. Plain radiographs, including oblique views, should be studied for changes in Luschka and facet joints, osteophytes (bars), and disc space narrowing. However, radiographic changes of the degenerated cervical spine may not correlate with symptoms. CT-myelography or MRI demonstrates neural compressive pathology well, although false-positive MRI scans are common; therefore correlation with history and physical examination is critical. MRI is also useful for detecting intrinsic changes in the spinal cord, as well as disc degeneration. Discography is controversial and is rarely used for cervical spine disorders. Electrodiagnostic studies have a high false-negative rate but may be helpful in select cases for differentiating peripheral nerve compression from more central compression and diseases such as amyotrophic lateral sclerosis.
4. Treatment—NSAIDs, exercises, use of a cervical collar, cervical traction, and pain clinic modalities are helpful in most cases of discogenic neck pain and radiculopathy. Indications for surgery include myelopathy with motor/gait impairment or radiculopathy with persistent disabling pain and weakness. Surgery for discogenic neck pain is less rewarding. Anterior Smith Robinson discectomy and block fusion is preferred over the Cloward dowel for involvement of one or two interspaces. Posterior foraminotomy is useful for single-level radiculopathy with a lateral soft disc herniation. For multilevel spondylosis and myelopathy, more extensive decompression is necessary. The anterior approach involves excision of osteophytes and multiple vertebrectomies with a strut graft fusion. Posterior approaches include canal-expansive laminoplasty (commonly used for OPLL), which can help decrease the incidence of instability associated with multilevel laminectomy. Overall alignment must be lordotic for this approach to be successful. Multilevel laminectomy may fail owing to failure to adequately relieve anterior compression or secondary to progressive kyphosis, which may require anterior decompression and fusion with a strut graft for salvage. Complications of the anterior approach include neurologic injury (<1%), pseudarthrosis (treated with posterior wiring or plating and arthrodesis), upper airway obstruction after multilevel corpectomy, or injury to other neck structures, including the recurrent laryngeal nerve if the right-side approach is used. Complications of laminectomy include subluxation if facets are sacrificed, leading to a swan neck deformity, muscle ischemia, and direct spinal cord injury with quadriparesis. Radicular symptoms may be alleviated after decompression, but gait changes may not.

B. Cervical Stenosis—May be congenital or acquired (traumatic, degenerative). Absolute (AP canal diameter <10 mm) or relative (10–13 mm diameter) stenosis predisposes the patient to the development of radiculopathy, myelopathy, or both owing to relatively minor soft or hard disc pathology or trauma. Pavlov's ratio (canal/vertebral body width) should be 1.0. A ratio <0.80 or a sagittal diameter of <13 mm is considered a significant risk factor for later neurologic involvement. Minor trauma such as hyperextension may lead to a central cord syndrome, even without overt skeletal injury. In relative stenosis, radicular symptoms usually predominate. CT scan and MRI (including flexion and extension studies) are helpful. Evaluation may include somatosensory evoked potentials, which help identify cord compromise in absolute stenosis. Surgery may serve a prophylactic function but is usually reserved for patients who develop myelopathy or radiculopathy. Surgical approaches are similar to those described above.

C. Rheumatoid Spondylitis—Cervical spine involvement is common in RA (up to 90%) and is more common with long-standing disease and multiple joint involvement. Neck pain, decreased ROM, crepitation, or occipital headaches are the most common complaints. Neurologic impairment in patients with RA usually occurs gradually (weakness, decreased sensation, hyperflexia) and is often overlooked or attributed to other joint disease. Surgery may not be successful in reversing significant neurologic deterioration, especially if a tight spinal canal is present. Therefore it is essential to look for subtle signs of early neurologic involvement and to assess the space available for the cord (SAC). Indications for surgical stabilization include instability, pain, neurologic deficit due to neural compression, impending neuro deficit (based on objective studies), or some combination of the above.

1. Atlantoaxial Subluxation—Most common, 50–80% of cases. Usually a result of pannus formation at the synovial joints between the dens and the ring of C1, resulting in destruction of the transverse ligament, the dens, or both. Anterior subluxation of C1 on C2 is most common, but posterior and lateral subluxation can also occur. Findings on examination may include limitation of motion, upper motor neuron signs, and detection of a "clunk" with neck flexion (Sharp and Purser sign [not recommended]). Plain radiographs to include patient-controlled **flexion and extension views** are evaluated to determine the anterior atlantodens interval (ADI) as well as the SAC, which is the posterior atlantodens interval. Instability is present with a 3.5 mm ADI difference on flexion and extension views, although radiographic instability in RA is common and is not an indication for surgery. A 7 mm difference may imply disruption of the alar ligaments. A difference of >9–10 mm or SAC of <14 mm is associated with an increase risk of neurologic injury and usually requires surgical treatment. Progressive neurologic impairment or progressive instability are also indications for surgical stabilization, usually a posterior C1–C2 fusion and wiring with halo vest stabilization. Transarticular screw fixation across C1–C2 has been described and may eliminate the need for halo immobilization. Atlantoaxial subluxation that is not reducible may require removal of the posterior arch of C1 for cord decompression followed by occiput–C2 fusion. Neurologic impairment with RA has been classified by Ranawat.

GRADE	CHARACTERISTICS
I	Subjective paresthisias
II	Subjective weakness; UMN findings
III	Objective weakness; UMN findings (A = ambulatory; B = nonambulatory)

Surgery is less successful in patients with severe (Ranawat IIIB) neurologic deficits. Complications include pseudarthrosis (20%) and recurring myelopathy. The pseudarthrosis rate may be lessened by extending the fusion to the occiput with wire fixation. An ADI of >7–10 mm or a posterior space of <13 mm is a relative contraindication to surgery in other areas, and the spine should be stabilized first.

2. Cranial Settling (Basilar Invagination)—Least common. Cranial migration of the dens from erosion and bone loss between the occiput and C1/C2. Measurement techniques are shown in Fig. 7–2. Landmarks may be difficult to identify, with Ranawat's line probably the most easily reproducible. Progressive cranial migration (>5 mm) or neurologic compromise may require operative intervention (occiput–C2 fusion). SSEPs may be helpful in evaluation. When brain stem compromise is significant with functional impairment, transoral or anterior retropharyngeal odontoid resection may be required.
3. Lower Cervical Spine—Occurs in 20% of cases. Because the joints of Luschka and facet joints are affected by RA, subluxation may occur at multiple levels. Lower cervical spine involvement is more common in males, with steroid use, with seropositive RA, in patients with rheumatoid nodules, and in those with severe RA. Posterior fusion and wiring is sometimes required for subluxation >4 mm with intractable pain and neurologic compromise.

D. Cervical Spine and Cord Injuries

1. Introduction—Spinal cord injuries (SCIs) occur most commonly in young males involved in motor vehicle accidents, falls, and diving accidents. Gunshot wounds are an increasing etiology. Findings may be subtle; the significant morbidity and mortality associated with missed injuries has led to current emphasis on cervical spine protection after polytrauma. Missed cervical spine injuries are most common in the presence of decreased level of consciousness, alcohol/drug intoxication, head injury, or in patients with multiple injuries. Facial injuries, hypotension, and localized tenderness or spasm should be sought. Careful neurologic examination to document the lowest remaining functional level and to assess for the possibility of sacral sparing, or sparing of posterior column function indicating an incomplete SCI, is essential. Neurologic level by ASIA standards is defined as the most caudal level with normal motor and sensory function bilaterally. Initial treatment with large doses of methylprednisolone (30 mg/kg initially and 5.4 mg/kg per hour for the next 23 hours) has been shown to improve neurologic recovery if initiated within the first 8 hours after injury. **Spinal shock** usually involves a 24- to 72-hour period of paralysis, hypotonia, and areflexia. At its conclusion the progressive onset of spasticity, hyperreflexia, and clonus develops over days to weeks. The return of the **bulbocavernosus reflex** (BCR: anal sphincter contraction in response to squeezing the glans penis or tugging on the Foley catheter) signifies the end of spinal shock, and for complete injuries further neurologic improvement is minimal. Prognosis with incomplete SCI is unaffected by the BCR. Injuries below the thoracolumbar level (conus or cauda equina) may permanently interupt the bulbocavernosus reflex. Neurogenic shock (secondary to loss of sympathetic tone) can be differentiated from hypovolemic shock based on the presence of relative bradycardia in neurogenic shock, in contrast to the presence of tachycardia and hypotension with hypovolemic shock. Swan-Ganz monitoring is helpful in this setting as neurogenic and hypovolemic shock often occur concurrently. Hypovolemic shock is treated with fluid resuscitation, whereas selective vasopressors are effective in neurogenic shock.

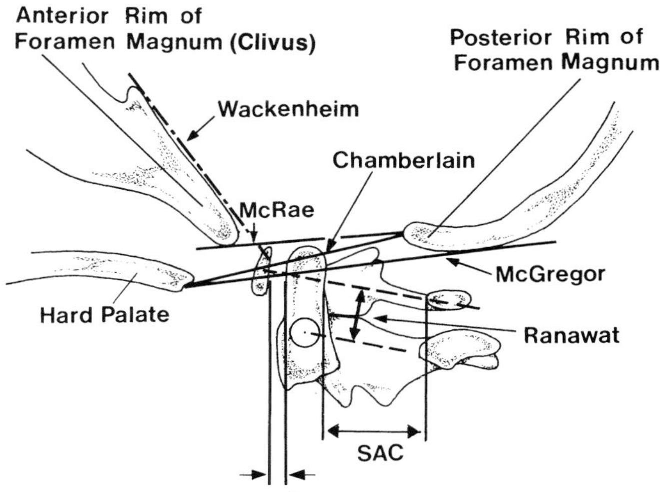

FIGURE 7–2. Common measurements in C1–C2 disorders.

2. Prognosis—The Frankel classification is useful when considering functional recovery from spinal cord injury.

FRANKEL GRADE	FUNCTION
A	Complete paralysis
B	Sensory function only below injury level
C	Incomplete motor function (grade 1–2/5) below injury level
D	Fair to good motor function (grade 3–4/5) below injury level
E	Normal function (grade 5/5)

3. Radiographic Evaluation—Includes complete cervical spine series (C1–T1, multiple-level injuries are common [10–20%]), obliques (facet subluxation, dislocations, factures), and tomograms (dens fractures and facet joint injuries) may be helpful. CT scanning is useful for evaluating C1 fractures and assessing bone in the canal but may

miss an axial plane fracture (type II odontoid). Myelography may be used in patients with an otherwise unexplained neurologic deficit. MRI has advantages for demonstrating posterior ligamentous disruption, disc herniation, canal compromise, and the status of the spinal cord.

4. Cord Injuries—May be complete (no function below a given level) or incomplete (with some sparing of distal function). With complete injuries an improvement of one nerve root level can be expected in 80% of the patients, and approximately 20% recover two additional function levels. Several categories of incomplete lesions exist. These syndromes are classified based on the area of the spinal cord that has been the most severely damaged. The **central cord** syndrome is the **most common** and is usually seen in patients with preexisting cervical spondylosis who sustain a hyperextension injury. The cord is compressed by osteophytes anteriorly and by the infolded ligamentum flavum posteriorly. The cord is injured in the central gray matter, which results in proportionately greater loss of motor function to the upper extremities than the lower extremities, with variable sensory sparing. The second most common cord injury is the **anterior cord** syndrome, in which the damage is primarily in the anterior two-thirds of the cord, sparing the posterior columns (proprioception and vibratory sensation). These patients demonstrate greater motor loss in the legs than the arms. CT scan may demonstrate bony fragments compressing the anterior cord. The anterior cord syndrome has the worst prognosis. The rare **Brown-Séquard** syndrome damages half of the cord, causing ipsilateral motor loss and position/proprioception loss and contralateral pain and temperature loss (usually two levels below the insult). This injury carries the best prognosis. The **posterior cord** syndrome spares only a few tracts anteriorly (with only crude touch sensation remaining). It is very rare; in fact some authors do not believe that it exists. **Single-root** lesions can occur at the level of the fracture, most commonly C5 or C6, leading to deltoid or biceps weakness; and they are usually unilateral. A summary of the syndromes is presented in Table 7–3.
5. Specific Cervical Spine Injuries—The reader is referred to Chapter 10, Trauma, for classification and treatment of cervical spine injuries.
6. Treatment—Discussed in Chapter 10, Trauma. It basically includes immobilization (collar for undispaced, stable fractures; skeletal traction, halo vest, or surgery for unstable fractures) and immediate application of skeletal traction to realign the spine in the presence of a displaced fracture with or without neurologic injury. Skeletal traction requires the placement of Gardner-Wells tongs (pins parallel to the external auditory meatus) and the addition of 5–10 pounds initially with 5–7 pounds per cervical level with sequential radiographs between the addition of weight. If necessary, anterior decompression for incomplete injuries with persistent cord compression (can lead to improvement of one to three levels, even with complete injuries) and stabilization may be indicated. Late decompression for up to 1 year may be effective in improving root return. Laminectomies are contraindicated except in the rare case of posterior compression from a fractured lamina. Gunshot wounds are treated nonoperatively except with esophageal perforation.
7. Complications—Numerous and include neurologic injury, nonunion, and malunion. **Autonomic dysreflexia** can follow cervical and upper thoracic spinal cord injuries. Is commonly related to bladder overdistention or fecal impaction and manifests with pounding **headache (from severe hypertension), anxiety, profuse head and neck sweating, nasal obstruction, and blurred vision.** Urinary catheterization or rectal disimpaction and supportive treatment usually relieve symptoms. If not, nifedipine (10 mg) is given sublingually immediately, followed by phenoxybenzamine (Dibenzylene) (10 mg) administered daily for prophylaxis. Instability in the cervical spine can occur late and is associated with >3.5 mm of subluxation and >11 degrees difference in angulation between adjacent motion segments.

E. Other Cervical Spine Problems—Ankylosing Spondylitis (AS) and neuromyopathic conditions can cause severe flexion deformities of the cervical spine. Patients with AS must be carefully evaluated for silent fractures because of the problem of pseudarthrosis and progressive kyphotic deformity. Severe chin-on-chest deformity in AS, with the inability to look straight ahead, occasionally represents a major functional limitation and is often associated with severe hip flexion contractures as well as a flexion deformity of the lumbar spine. Treatment usually begins by addressing the hip and lumbar pathology first but may ultimately require cervicothoracic laminectomy, osteotomy, and fusion for correction of the neck deformity. This procedure is performed under local anesthesia with brief general anesthesia, and immobilization postoperatively is carried out in a halo cast. Traction, surgical release of contracted sternocleidomastoid muscles, and posterior fusion are sometimes required for severe neuromyopathic conditions.

TABLE 7–3. SPINAL CORD INJURY SYNDROMES

SYNDROME	MOI/PATHOLOGY	CHARACTERISTICS	PROGNOSIS
Central	Age >50, extension injuries	Affects upper > lower extremities, motor and sensory loss	Fair
Anterior	Flexion-compression (vertebral A)	Incomplete motor and some sensory loss	Poor
Brown-Séquard	Penetrating trauma	Loss of ipsilateral motor function, contralateral pain and temperature sensation	Best
Root	Foramina compression/herniated nucleus pulposis	Based on level—weakness	Good
Complete	Burst/canal compression	No function below injury level	Poor

III. Thoracic/Lumbar Spine

A. Herniated Nucleus Pulosus (HNP)

1. Introduction—Disc degeneration with aging includes loss of water content, annular tears, and myxomatous changes, resulting in herniation of nuclear material. Changes in proteoglycan metabolism, secondary immunologic factors, and structural factors also play a role. Discs can **protrude** (bulging nucleus, intact annulus), **extrude** (through the annulus but confined by the posterior longitudinal ligament [PLL]), or be **sequestrated** (disc material free in canal) (Fig. 7–3). HNP is usually a disease of young and middle-age adults, as the disc nucleus desiccates and is less likely to herniate in older patients.
2. Thoracic Disc Disease—Relatively uncommon (<1% of all HNPs), it usually involves the mid to lower thoracic levels and is divided between central and lateral herniations. Thoracic HNP usually presents with the onset of back or chest pain that may progress to radicular symptoms (band-like chest or abdominal discomfort, numbness, paresthesias, leg pain), and/or myelopathy (sensory changes, paraparesis, bowel/bladder/sexual dysfunction). Physical findings may be difficult to elicit but may include localized tenderness, sensory pinprick level, upper motor neuron signs with leg hyperreflexia, weakness, and abnormal rectal examination. Radiographs may show disc narrowing and calcification or osteophytic lipping. Underlying Scheuermann's disease may predispose patients to develop HNP. Myelo-CT or MRI should demonstrate thoracic HNP. MRI is useful for ruling out cord pathology, but there is a high false-positive rate, requiring close clinical correlation. Immobilization, analgesics, and nerve blocks are sometimes helpful for radiculopathy. Surgery, usually through an anterior transthoracic approach or costotransversectomy (including anterior discectomy and hemicorpectomy as needed), is recommended in the presence of myelopathy or persistent unremitting pain with documented pathology. Posterior approach to a thoracic HNP is contraindicated because of the high rate of neurologic injury.
3. Lumbar Disc Disease—Major cause of increased morbidity and financial impact in the United States. Most often involves the L4–L5 disc (the "backache disc"), followed closely by L5–S1. Most herniations are posterolateral (where the PLL is the weakest) and may present with back

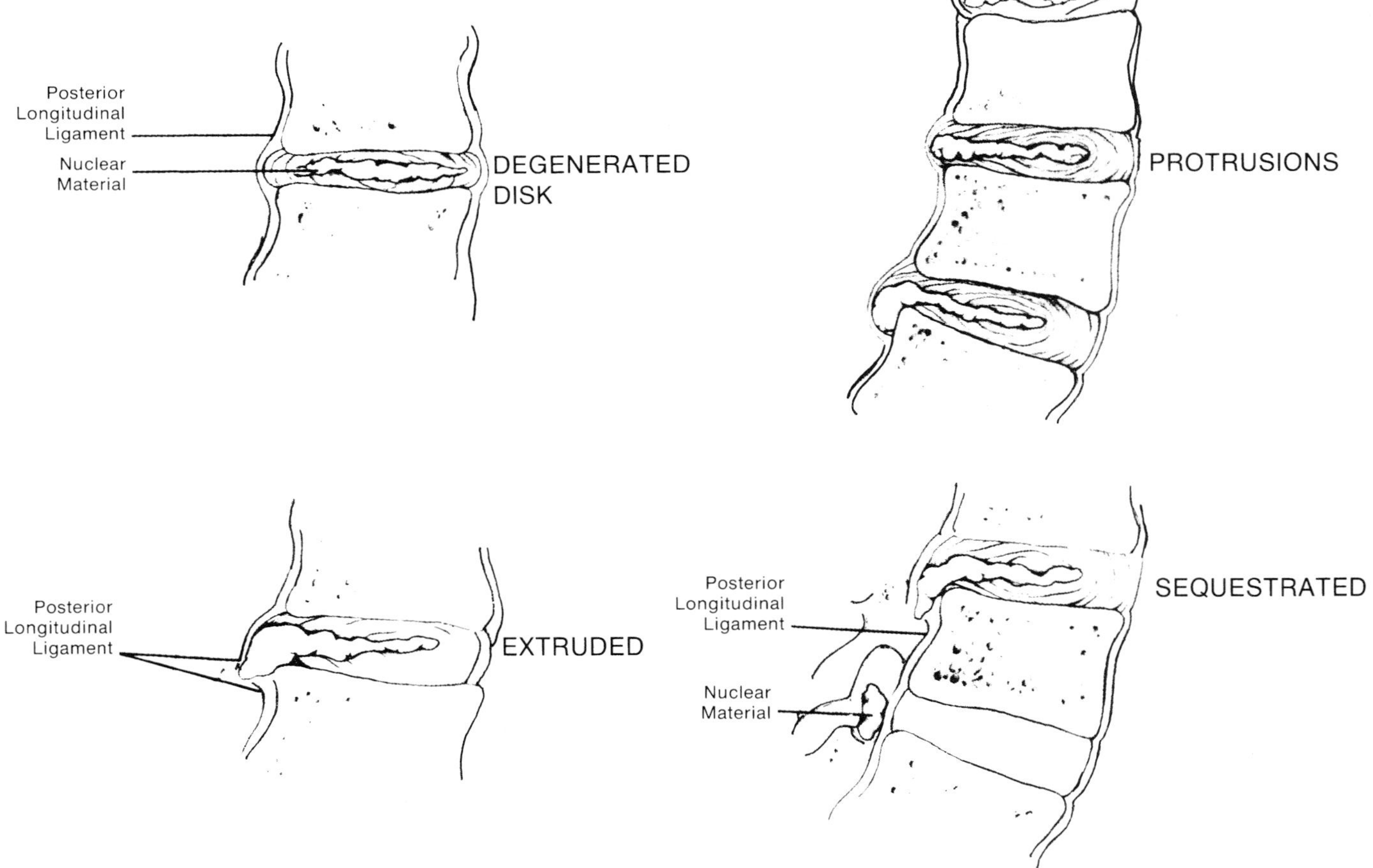

FIGURE 7–3. Nomenclature for disc pathology. (From Wiltse, L.L.: Lumbosacral spine reconstruction. In Orthopaedic Knowledge Update I, p. 247. Chicago, American Academy of Orthopaedic Surgeons, 1984; reprinted by permission.)

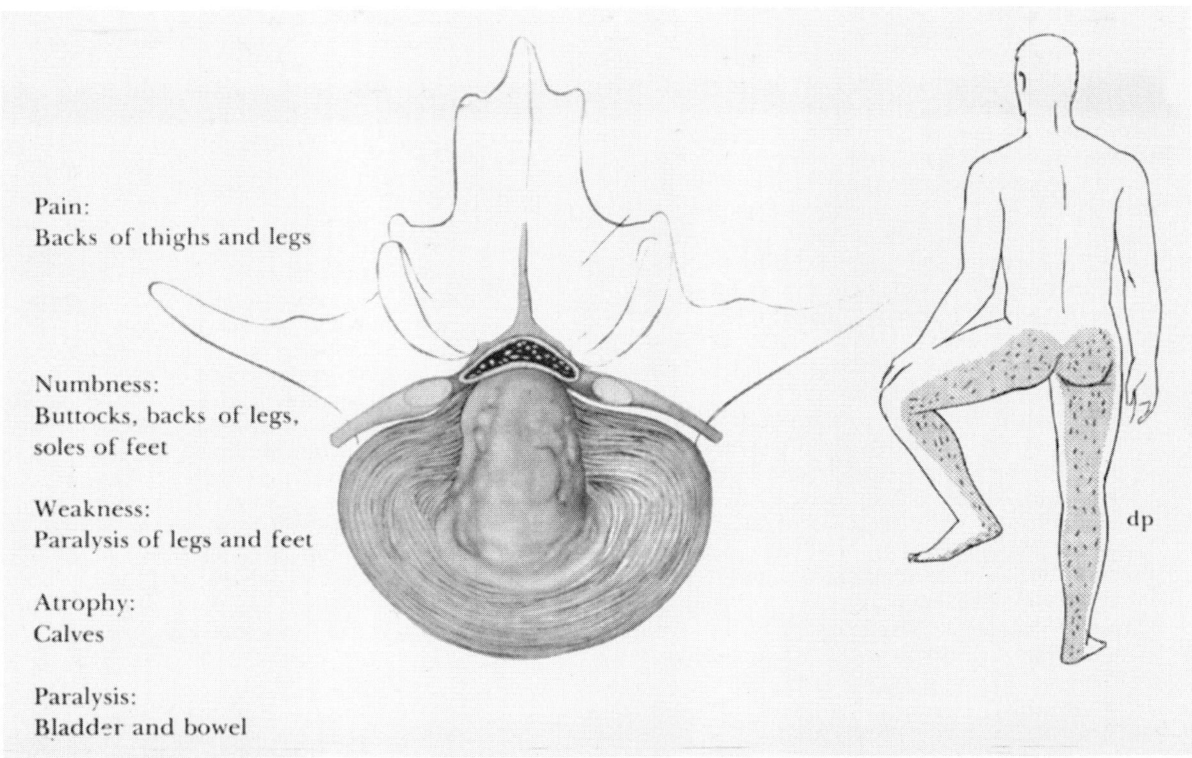

FIGURE 7–4. Cauda equina syndrome. (From DePalma, A.F., and Rothman, R.H.: The Intervertebral Disc, p. 194. Philadelphia, WB Saunders, 1970; reprinted by permission.)

pain and nerve root pain/sciatica involving the lower nerve root at that level. Central prolapse is usually associated with back pain only; however, acute insults may precipitate a **cauda equina compression syndrome** (Fig. 7–4). This syndrome is a surgical emergency that most commonly presents with bilateral buttock and lower extremity pain as well as bowel or bladder dysfunction (usually urinary retention), saddle anesthesia, and varying degrees of loss of lower extremity motor or sensory function. Digital rectal examination and evaluation of perianal sensation is important for the immediate diagnosis. Immediate myelography (or MRI) and surgery (if the tests are positive) are indicated to arrest progression of neurologic loss.

a. History and Physical Examination—An acute injury or precipitating event should be sought; and the location of symptoms (especially pain radiating to the extremity), character of pain, postural changes (neurogenic claudication), effect of increased intrathecal pressure, and a complete review of symptoms (including psychiatric history) should be elicited. Occupational risks, such as a jobs requiring prolonged sitting and repetitive lifting, are also important factors. Intradiscal pressure is lowest when lying supine and highest when sitting, flexed forward with weights in hands. Referred pain in mesodermal tissues of the same embryologic origin, often to the buttocks or posterior thighs, must be differentiated from true radicular pain due to nerve root impingement, with symptoms that typically reach distal to the knee. Psychosocial evaluation, pain drawings, and psychological testing are helpful in some cases. The finding of an "inverted V" triad of hysteria, hypochondriasis, and depression on MMPI has been identified as a significant adverse risk factor in lumbar disc surgery. Physical examination should include observation (change in posture, gait); palpation of the posterior spine (spasm, localized tenderness); measurement of ROM (decreased flexion); hip examination; vascular evaluation (distal pulses); abdominal and rectal examination; and neurologic evaluation—all are important. Tension signs such as straight-leg-raising or the bowstring sign (L4–L5 or L5–S1) and the femoral nerve stretch test (L2–L3 or L3–L4) are important findings that suggest HNP and are essential when considering a patient for discectomy. A positive contralateral straight-leg-raising test is most specific for HNP. Specific findings, by level are presented in Table 7–4. A large central disc herniation at one level may impringe on more than one nerve root. Inappropriate signs and symptoms (Waddell) are also important to note. Inappropriate symptoms include pain at the tip of the "tailbone," pain plus numbness, or giving way of the whole leg. Nonorganic physical signs include tenderness with light touch in nonanatomic areas, light axial loading, distraction testing, pain with pelvic rotation, negative sitting (and positive supine) straight-leg-raising test, regional nonanatomic disturbances, and overreaction.

TABLE 7–4. FINDINGS IN LUMBAR DISC DISEASE

LEVEL	NERVE ROOT	SENSORY LOSS	MOTOR LOSS	REFLEX LOSS
L1-L3	L2, L3	Anterior thigh	Hip flexors	None
L3-L4	L4	Medial calf	Quadriceps, tibialis anterior	Knee jerk
L4-L5	L5	Lateral calf, dorsal foot	EDL, EHL	None
L5-S1	S1	Posterior calf, plantar foot	Gastrocnemius/soleus	Ankle jerk
S2-S4	S2, S3, S4	Perianal	Bowel/bladder	Cremasteric

b. Diagnostic Tests—Plain radiographs are indicated before proceeding with special tests to rule out other pathology, such as isthmic defects. However, most plain radiographic findings are nonspecific, and plain radiography can usually be deferred for 6 weeks. Myelography, CT, or MRI are effective when used as a confirming study. CT is noninvasive and helpful for demonstrating bony stenosis and identifying lateral pathology. Combined with myelography (invasive), imaging of neural compression may be improved. MRI is superior for identifying cord pathology, neural tumors, and far lateral discs. It is noninvasive, involves no ionizing radiation, and gives a "myelogram" effect on the T2 images. Multiplanar views allow imaging of central, foraminal, and extraforaminal stenosis. In addition, it demonstrates the state of hydration of the discs and visualizes the marrow of the vertebral bodies, thus representing an excellent modality to screen for tumor or infection. False-positive MRI scans are common (35% of those <40 years old; 93% of those >60 years old) and therefore require correlation with the history and physical examination. EMG studies (which demonstrate fibrillations 3 weeks after nerve root pressure) are not usually helpful and rarely provide more information than a good physical. Thermography does not have proved efficacy in the evaluation of disc disease.

c. Treatment—Short-term bed rest (2 days) with support underneath the knees and neck, NSAIDs or aspirin, and progressive ambulation are successful in returning most patients to their normal function. More than half of patients who present with low back pain recover in 1 week and 90% recover within 1–3 months. One-half of patients with sciatica recover in 1 month. This treatment is followed by back rehabilitation and fitness programs Aerobic conditioning and education are the most important factors in avoiding missed work days due to disc disease and in returning patients to work. Instruction should include avoiding rotation and flexion due to increased disc pressure associated with these activities. If patients fail to improve within 6 weeks of conservative care, further evaluation is indicated. Those patients with predominantly low back pain should undergo a bone scan and medical work-up (to rule out spinal tumors or infection). If these studies are normal, back rehabilitation is continued. In patients failing conservative therapy who have predominantly leg pain (sciatica), a trial of lumbar epidural steroids may be helpful, although it has not been proved effective in controlled studies. Additional studies (CT [± myelogram] or MRI) are undertaken in patients who after 6–12 weeks continue to be symptomatic with pain, neurologic deficit, or positive nerve tension signs. These studies are, as a rule, preoperative tests and should be done to confirm clinical suspicions. Patients with positive studies, neurologic findings, tension signs, and predominantly sciatic symptoms without mitigating psychosocial factors are the best candidates for surgical discectomy. Standard partial laminotomy and discectomy are most commonly performed. Operative positioning requires the abdomen to be free to decrease pressure on the inferior vena cava and consequently on the epidural veins. With proper indications, 95% of patients have initially good or excellent results, although as many as 30% of patients have significant backache on long-term follow-up. Microdiscectomy decreases visualization of herniated or extruded disc fragments and lateral root stenosis, and some authors report a high complication rate. Percutaneous discectomy currently has limited indications in the treatment of lumbar disc disease, with no long-term follow-up studies proving its efficacy. It is contraindicated in the presence of a sequestered fragment or spinal stenosis. Intradiscal enzyme therapy has fallen out of favor because of its questionable efficacy and serious complications (anaphylaxis and transverse myelitis). Indications for its use for disc herniations are similar to those for surgery (leg pain, tension signs, neurologic deficits, positive studies).

d. Complications—Fortunately rare but can be devastating.
   1. Vascular Injury—May occur during attempts at disc removal if curettes are allowed to penetrate the anterior longitudinal ligament. Intraoperative pulsatile bleeding due to deep penetration is treated with rapid wound closure, IV fluids and blood, repositioning the patient, and a transabdominal approach to find and stop the source of bleeding. Mortality may exceed 50%. Late sequelae of vascular injuries may include delayed hemorrhage, false aneurysm, or A-V fistula formation.
   2. Nerve Root Injury—More common with anomalous nerve roots. Dural tears should be repaired primarily when they occur to avoid the developmental of a pseudomen-

ingocele or spinal fluid fistula. Adequate exposure, as well as hemostasis, lighting, magnification, and careful surgical technique, are important for diminishing the incidence of the "battered root syndrome."

3. Failed Back Syndrome—Often the result of poor patient selection, but other causes include recurrent herniation (usually acute recurrence of signs/symptoms following 6- to 12-month pain-free interval), herniation at another level, discitis (occurs 3–6 weeks postoperatively with rapid onset of severe back pain), unrecognized lateral stenosis (may be most common), or vertebral instability. Epidural fibrosis occurs at about 3 months postoperatively, and there may associated leg pain. It is related to hemorrhage and surgical trauma and responds poorly to re-exploration. Scar can best be differentiated from recurrent HNP with a gadolinium-enhanced MRI.
4. Dural Tear—More common during revision surgery and should be repaired immediately if it is recognized. Fibrin adhesive sealant may be a useful adjunct for effecting dural closure. Bed rest and subarachnoid drain placement is advocated if CSF leak is suspected postoperatively.
5. Infection—Similar to infection elsewhere. Increased risk in diabetics. I&D and removal of loose graft may be required.
6. Cauda Equina Syndrome—Secondary to extruded disc, surgical trauma, hematoma. Suspect with postop urinary retention; digital rectal examination is used to diagnose initially. Further imaging may be necessary.

B. Lumbar Segmental Instability—Present when normal loads produce abnormal spinal motion. The most common symptom is mechanical back pain, although "dynamic" stenosis can occur, leading to leg symptoms. The most consistent clinical sign is the "instability catch" (sudden, painful snapping with extension from flexed position). Degenerative lumbar disc disease is indicated by disc space narrowing. A combination of annulus damage and disc space narrowing may cause reduction in the disc's ability to resist rotatory forces. Continuing degeneration or facet subluxation may then lead to instability. Radiographically, traction spurs (horizontal and below disc margin [versus syndesmophyte], angular changes > 10 degrees (20 degrees at L5–S1) on flexion films, and translatory motion > 3–4 mm (6 mm at L5–S1) with flexion-extension views are all characteristic of lumbar instability but are difficult to quantify and may not correlate with clinical symptoms. Iatrogenic instability can occur after removal of one or more facet joints during surgery. Surgical treatment options do not have clearly defined indications but include posterolateral fusion, posterior lumbar interbody fusion (PLIF—graft is "keyed" into the intervertebral space), and anterior interbody fusion. PLIF is associated with a high incidence of pseudarthrosis and neurologic injury. Internal fixation, utilizing pedicle screw fixation in rod or plate constructs, is gaining popularity as an adjunct in lumbar spine fusion surgery; but the efficacy of these implants, particularly when the added cost and potential complications are considered, remains unproved.

C. Spinal Stenosis
1. Introduction—Spinal stenosis is narrowing of the spinal canal or neural foramina producing nerve root compression, root ischemia, and a variable syndrome of back and leg pain. Central stenosis produces compression of the thecal sac, whereas lateral stenosis involves compression of individual nerve roots either in the subarticular (lateral) recess (by the medial overgrowth of the superior articular facet at a given facet joint) or in the intervertebral foramen. Stenosis usually does not become symptomatic until patients reach late middle age; it affects men twice as often as women.
2. Central Stenosis
   a. Introduction—Can be congenital (idiopathic or developmental in achondroplasic dwarfs) or acquired. Acquired stenosis, the most common type, is usually degenerative owing to enlargement of osteoarthritic facets with medial encroachment, but it can be secondary to degenerative spondylolisthesis, posttraumatic, postsurgical, or due to various disease processes (e.g., Paget's, fluorosis). Preexisting "trefoil" canal shapes, a congenitally narrow canal, or medially placed facets may limit the ability to tolerate minor acquired encroachment (Fig. 7–5). Central stenosis represents

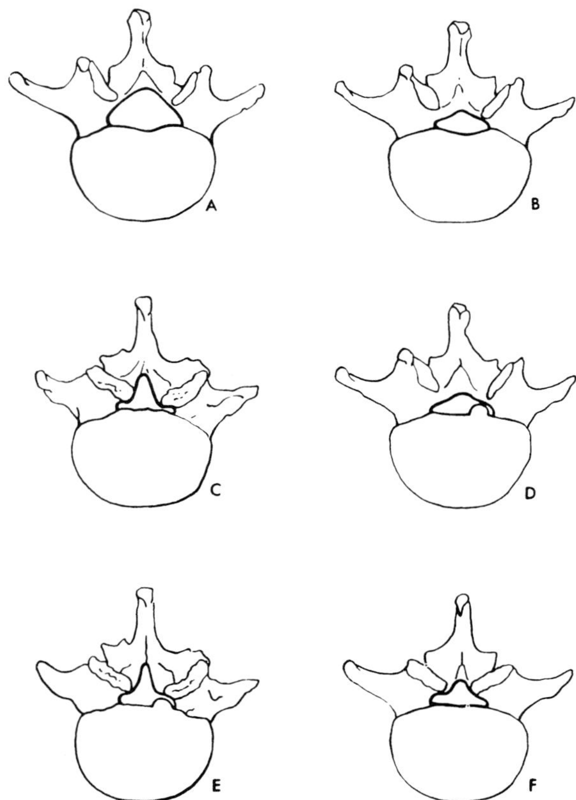

FIGURE 7–5. Spinal stenosis. *A,* Normal. *B,* Congenital stenosis. *C,* Degenerative stenosis. *D,* Congenital stenosis with disc herniation. *E,* Degenerative stenosis with disc herniation. *F,* Congenital and degenerative stenosis. (From Arnoldi, C.C., et al.: Lumbar spinal stenosis and nerve root entrapment syndromes. Clin. Orthop. 115: 4, 1976; reprinted by permission.)

compression of the thecal sac, with absolute stenosis defined as a cross-sectional area of <100 mm or <10 mm of AP diameter as seen on CT cross section. Soft tissue (ligamentum flavum and disc) may contribute as much as 40% to thecal sac compression. Central stenosis is more common in men because their spinal canal is smaller at the L3–L5 levels than is that of women.

b. Symptoms—Include insidious pain and paresthesias with ambulation and extension, relieved by lying supine or with flexion of the spine. Patients commonly complain of lower extremity pain, numbness, or "giving way." A history of radiating leg pain in a dermatomal distribution, although typical in patients with HNP, is relatively uncommon in those with spinal stenosis. Neurogenic claudication, which occurs in fewer than half of patients with stenosis, usually can be differentiated from vascular claudication by history.

ACTIVITY	VASCULAR CLAUDICATION	NEUROGENIC CLAUDICATION
Walking	Distal-proximal pain, calf pain	Proximal-distal thigh pain
Uphill walking	Symptoms develop sooner	Symptoms develop later
Rest	Relief with standing	Relief with sitting or bending
Bicycling	Symptoms develop	Symptoms do not develop
Lying flat	Relief	May exacerbate symptoms

Physical examination is also important. Patients with stenosis may have pain with extension, typically have normal pulses, and may have neurologic findings. Abnormal neurologic findings, however, or positive tension signs are seen in fewer than one-half of patients. Neurologic findings not otherwise obvious are sometimes demonstrated with a "stress test" (walking until symptoms occur).

c. Imaging—Further work-up may include plain radiographs on which disc degeneration, interspace narrowing, medially placed facets, and flattening of the lordotic curve are commonly seen; subluxation and degenerative changes of the facet joints may be seen. Plain CT, postmyelo-CT, and MRI are standard imaging modalities. Careful inspection of these studies is necessary to assess lateral nerve root entrapment by medial hypertrophy of the superior facet, the tip of the superior facet, osteophyte formation off the posterior vertebral body (uncinate spur), or a combination of these problems. Central stenosis is a diminution in the area of the thecal sac and is produced by thickening of the ligamentum flavum and/or posterior protrusion of the disc, in combination with enlarged facet joints. Simply looking for the "bony" measurements results in underestimating the degree of stenosis; soft tissue contribution to thecal sac narrowing must be considered. Bone scan or MRI may help to rule out malignancy. EMGs or SSEPs may be used, but sensitivity is variable and depends on the examiner.

d. Treatment—Rest, isometric abdominal exercises, pelvic tilt, Williams' flexion exercises, NSAIDs, and weight reduction are important in management of patients with stenosis. Lumbar epidural steroids may be helpful for short-term relief but have not shown efficacy in controlled studies. Surgery is indicated in patients with positive studies and persistent, unacceptably impaired quality of life. Adequate decompression of the identified pathology should include laminectomy and partial medial facetectomy, which can usually be done without destabilizing the spine, thus avoiding fusion. Fusion is indicated in patients with surgical instability (removal of one facet or more), neural arch defects (including postsurgical) with disc disease, symptomatic radiographic instability, degenerative or isthmic spondylolisthesis, and degenerative scoliosis.

3. Lateral Stenosis—Impingement of nerve roots lateral to the thecal sac, as they pass through the lateral recess and into the neural foramen. Often associated with facet joint arthropathy (superior articular process enlargement) and disc disease (Fig. 7–6). The three-joint complex (disc and both facets) must be considered when evaluating lateral stenosis. Nerve root compression can occur at more than one level and must be completely decompressed to relieve symptoms. Compression can be subarticular (lateral recess stenosis), which consists of compression between the medial aspect of a hypertrophic superior articular facet and the posterior aspect of the vertebral body and disc. Hypertrophy of the ligamentum flavum and/or joint capsule and vertebral body osteophyte/disc exacerbates the stenosis. Foraminal stenosis can be produced by intraforaminal disc protrusion, impingement of the tip of the superior facet, uncinate spurring, or a combination. Subarticular stenosis, which is more common, af-

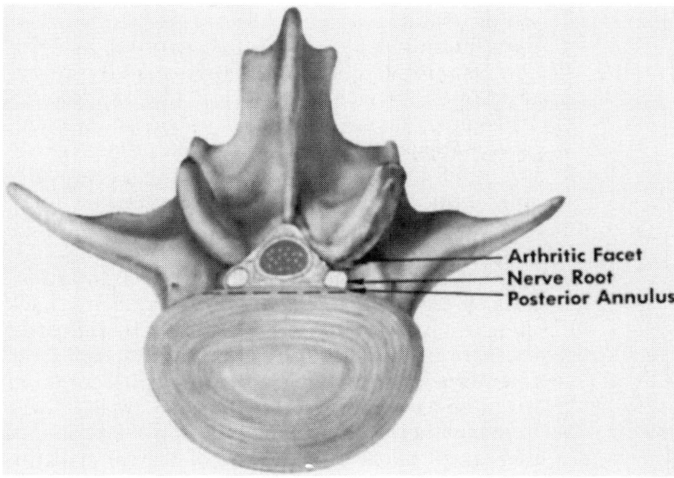

FIGURE 7–6. Lateral stenosis. Note nerve root entrapment laterally on the right by arthritic facet and bulging posterior annulus. (From Rothman, R.H., and Simeon, F.A.: The Spine, 2nd ed., p. 520. Philadelphia, WB Saunders, 1982; reprinted by permission.)

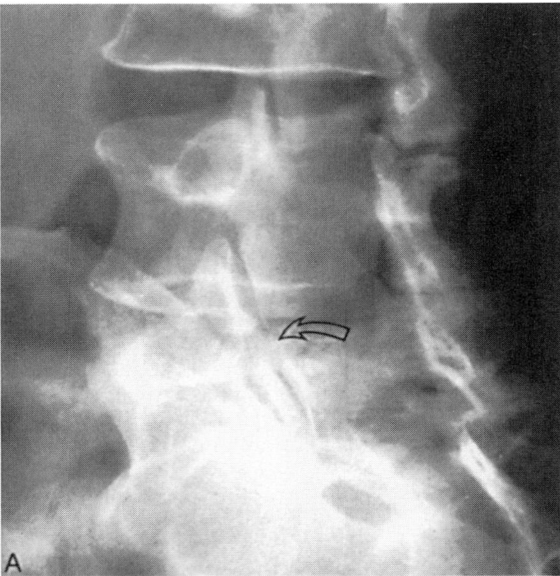

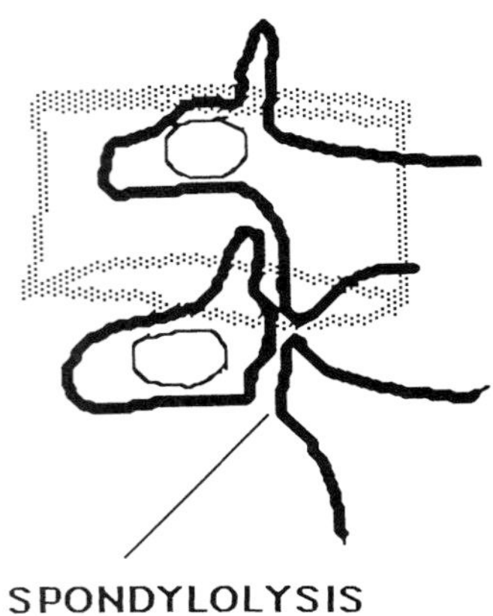

A B

FIGURE 7–7. Spondylolysis. Note disruption of "collar" on Scottie dog. (From Helms, C.A.: Fundamentals of Skeletal Radiology, p. 101. Philadelphia, WB Saunders, 1989; reprinted by permission.)

fects the traversing (lower) nerve root, whereas foraminal stenosis affects the exiting (upper) root at a motion segment. Lateral stenosis is most frequently seen in combination with central stenosis but can appear as an isolated entity usually involving middle-aged or even young adults with symptoms of radicular pain unrelieved by rest and without tension signs. Lower lumbar areas are most commonly involved because the foramina size decreases as the nerve root size increases. Pain may be the result of intraneural edema and demyelination. Substance P may be released as a response to spinal nerve root irritation. After failure of nonoperative treatment, decompression of the hypertrophied lamina and ligmentum flavum and partial facetectomy are usually successful. Fusion may be necessary if instability is present or created.

4. Extraforaminal Lateral Root Compression ("Far Out Syndrome" ([Wiltse])—Involves L5 root impingement between the sacral ala and the L5 transverse process. It is usually seen in degenerative scoliosis, isthmic spondylolisthesis, or extraforaminal herniated discs. It must be specifically sought on special radiographs (25-degree caudocephalic [Ferguson] view) or CT.

D. Spondylolysis and Spondylolisthesis

1. Spondylolysis—Defect in the pars interarticularis. It is the most common cause of low back pain in children and adolescents. The defect in the pars is thought to be a fatigue fracture from repetitive hyperextension stresses (most common in gymnasts, football linemen), to which there may be a hereditary predisposition. Plain lateral radiographs demonstrate 80% of lesions, with another 15% visible on oblique radiographs, which show a defect in the "neck" of the 'Scottie dog' as described by Lachapelle (Fig. 7–7). CT, bone scan, and more recently SPECT scanning may be helpful in identifying subtle defects; increased uptake is more compatible with acute lesions that have the potential to heal. Bracing or casting (a single thigh pantaloon spica) has been advocated for acute lesions, but treatment is usually aimed at symptomatic relief rather than fracture healing and includes activity restriction, flexion exercises, and bracing. Nonunion is common and may have normal scans.

2. Spondylolisthesis—Forward slippage of one vertebra on another. Can be classified into six types (Newman, Wiltse, McNab) (Table 7–5; Figs. 7–8, 7–9). Severity of slip in spondylolisthesis is based on the amount or degree (as compared to S1 width); I, 0–25%; II, 25–50%; III, 50–75%; IV, >75%; V, >100% (spondyloptosis). Other measurements, including the sacral inclination (normally >30%) and the slip angle (normally >0 degrees), are also useful for quantifying lumbopelvic deformity, which affects cosmesis as well as prognosis (Fig. 7–10).

TABLE 7–5. TYPES OF SPONDYLOLISTHESIS

CLASS	TYPE	AGE	PATHOLOGY/OTHER
I	Congenital	Child	Congenital dysplasia of S1 superior facet
II	Isthmic[a]	5–50	Predisposition leading to elongation/fracture of pars (L5-S1)
III	Degenerative	Older	Facet arthrosis leading to subluxation (L4-L5)
IV	Traumatic	Young	Acute fracture/other than pars
V	Pathologic	Any	Incompetence of bony elements
VI	Postsurgical	Adult	Excessive resection of neural arches/facets

[a] Most common.

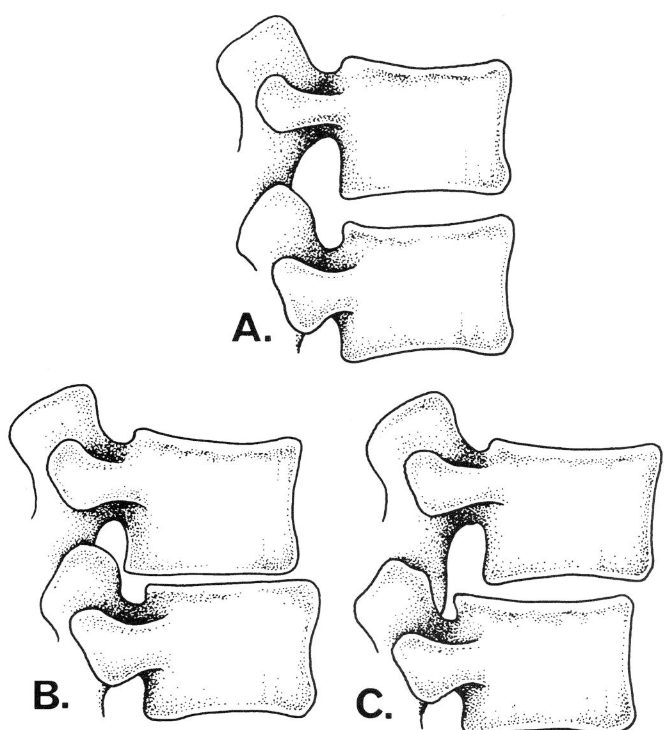

FIGURE 7–8. Degenerative spondylolisthesis. *A,* Normal. *B,* Retrolisthesis—disc narrowing is greater than posterior joint degeneration. *C,* Anterolisthesis—posterior joints are more degenerated than the disc. (From Weinstein, J.N., and Wiesel, S.W.: The Lumbar Spine, p. 84. Philadelphia, WB Saunders, 1990; reprinted by permission.)

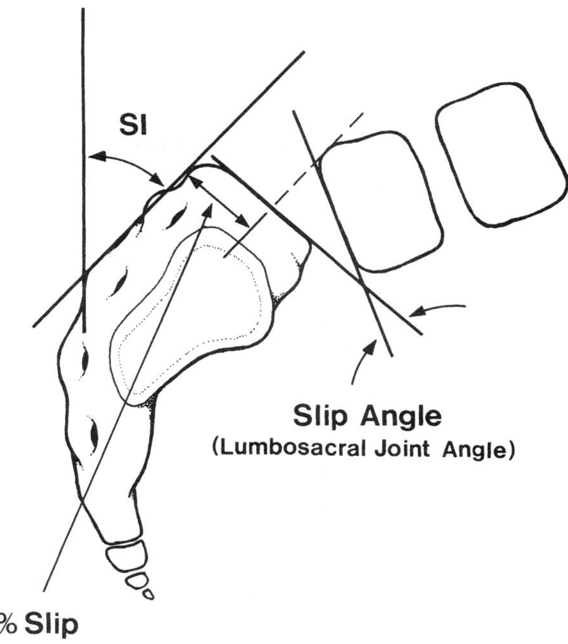

FIGURE 7–10. Measurements used for evaluation of spondylolisthesis. (Modified from Wiltse, L.L., and Winter, R.B.: Terminology and measurement of spondylolisthesis. J. Bone Joint Surg. [Am.] 65: 768–772, 1983; reprinted by permission.)

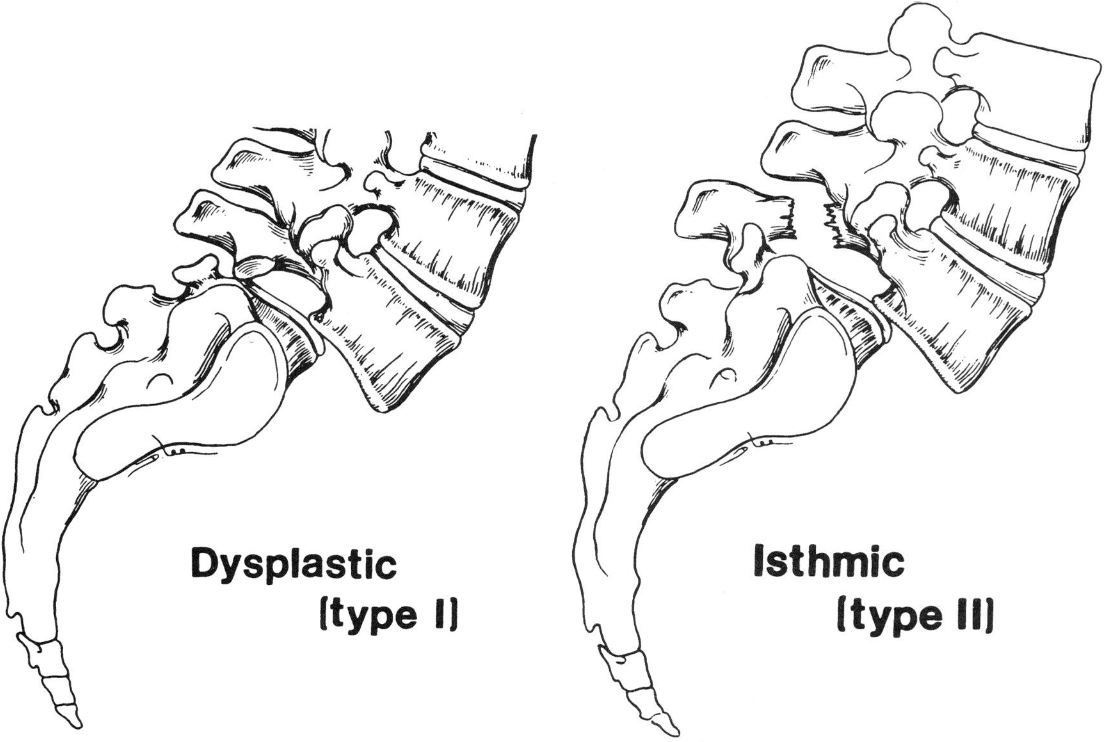

FIGURE 7–9. Spondylolisthesis. (From Rothman, R.H., and Simeon, F.A.: The Spine, 2nd ed., p. 264. Philadelphia, WB Saunders, 1982; reprinted by permission.)

3. Childhood Spondylolisthesis—Usually at L5–S1, is typically type II, and usually presents with back pain (instability), hamstring tightness, deformity, or alteration in gait ("pelvic waddle"). Although the onset of symptoms may occur at any time in life, screening studies identify the occurrence of the slippage as being most common at 4–6 years. Spondylolisthesis is most common in whites, boys, and youngsters involved in hyperextension activities; and it is remarkably common in Eskimos (>50%). It is thought to result from shear stress at the pars interarticularis associated with repetitive hypertension. Severe slips are rare and are associated with radicular findings (L5), cauda equina dysfunction, kyphosis of the lumbosacral junction, and a "heart-shaped" buttocks. Spina bifida occulta, thoracic kyphosis, and Scheuermann's disease are associated with spondylolisthesis.
   a. Low Grade Disease (<50% Slip)—Spondylolysis or mild spondylolisthesis may require bone scan or CT for diagnosis and usually responds to nonoperative treatment consisting of activity modification and exercise. Adolescents with a grade I slip may return to normal activities, including contact sports, once they are asymptomatic. Those with asymptomatic grade II spondylolisthesis are restricted from activities such as gymnastics or football. Progression is uncommon, but risk factors include young age at presentation, female sex, a slip angle of >10 degrees (Fig. 7–10), a high grade slip, and a domed-shaped or significantly inclined sacrum (>30 degrees beyond vertical). Furthermore, patients with type I or congenital spondylolisthesis are at higher risk for slip progression and the development of cauda equina dysfunction because the neural arch is intact. Surgery for patients with a low grade slip generally consists of L5–S1 posterolateral fusion in situ and is usually reserved for those with intractable pain who have failed nonoperative treatment or those demonstrating progressive slippage. Wiltse has popularized a paraspinal splitting approach to the lumbar transverse process and sacral alae that is frequently utilized in this setting. L5 radiculopathy is uncommon in children with low grade slips and rarely if ever requires decompression. Repair of the pars defect utilizing a lag screw (Buck) or tension band wiring (Bradford) with bone grafting has been reported. It may be indicated in young patients with slippage less than 25% and a pars defect at L4 or above.
   b. Grades III and IV Spondylolisthesis and Spondyloptosis (Grade V)—Commonly causes neurologic abnormalities. L5–S1 isthmic spondylolisthesis causes an L5 radiculopathy (contrast with S1 radiculopathy in L5–S1 HNP). Prophylactic fusion is recommended in children with slippage of more than 50%. It often requires bilateral posterolateral fusion in situ, usually at L4–S1 (L5 is too far anterior to effect L5–S1 fusion) without instrumentation. Nerve root exploration is controversial but is usually limited to children with clear-cut radicular pain or significant weakness. Reduction of spondylolisthesis has been associated with a 20–30% incidence of L5 root injuries and should be utilized cautiously. A cosmetically unacceptable deformity or L5–S1 kyphosis so severe that the posterior fusion mass from L4 to the sacrum would be under tension without reversal of the kyphosis are the most common cited indications. Close neurologic monitoring should be done during the procedure and for several days afterward to identify postoperative neuropathy. Posterior decompression, fibular interbody fusion, and posterolateral fusion without reduction has been reported with excellent long-term results (Bohlman). "Spondylolisthesis crisis" is seen in patients with severe slips, increasing pain, and hamstring tightness. The Gill procedure, consisting of removal of the loose elements without fusion, is contraindicated in children and is rarely performed in adults.
4. Degenerative Spondylolisthesis—More commonly involves African-Americans, diabetics, and women over age 40; it is most common at the L4–L5 level (Fig. 7–8). It is reported to be more common in patients with transitional L5 vertebrae. Degenerative spondylolisthesis frequently causes L5 radiculopathy owing to root compression in the lateral recess between the hypertrophic and subluxated inferior facet of L4 and the posterosuperior body of L5. The operative treatment of degenerative spondylolisthesis involves decompression of the nerve roots and stabilization by posterolateral fusion.
5. Adult Isthmic Spondylolisthesis—Although the significance of isthmic spondylolisthesis in an adult is controversial, it remains a common indication for surgery. Nonoperative treatment includes rest, corset, NSAIDs, and flexion exercises. It is essential to assess for other common sources of back pain before assuming that spondylolisthesis is the cause; MRI scanning is a useful tool in this setting. Isthmic L5–S1 spondylolisthesis frequently causes radicular symptoms in the adult, resulting from compression of the exiting L5 root in the L5–S1 foramen; compression may involve hypertrophic fibrous repair tissue at the pars defect, uncinate spur formation off the posterior L5 body, and bulging of the L5–S1 disc. Operative treatment is favored in the presence of radicular symptoms and usually involves thorough foraminal decompression and fusion, with or without pedicular screw fixation. Compromised results in workers' compensation patients have been reported.

E. Thoracolumbar Injuries
1. Introduction—Although the classification and treatment of these injuries is included in Chapter 10, Trauma, some points need to be emphasized here. The upper thoracic spine (T1–T10) is stabilized by the ribs and the facet orientation, as well as the sternum, and is less susceptible to trauma. At the thoracolumbar junction, however, there is a fulcrum of increased motion, and this area is more commonly affected by spinal trauma. Two anatomic points also bear noting: (1) the middle T-spine is a vascular "watershed" area, and vascular insult can lead to cord ischemia; and (2) the spinal cord ends and the cauda equina begins at

the level of L1–L2, so lesions below the L1 level carry a better prognosis because nerve roots, not cord, are affected.

2. Stable Versus Unstable Injuries—The three-column system (Denis) has been proposed for evaluating spinal injuries and determining which are stable or unstable. The anterior column is composed of the anterior longitudinal ligament and the anterior two-thirds of the annulus and vertebral body. The middle column consists of the posterior third of the body and annulus and the posterior longitudinal ligament. The posterior column is comprised of the pedicles, facets, spinous processes, and posterior ligaments, including the interspinous and supraspinous ligaments, ligamentum flavum, and facet capsules. Disruption of the middle column (seen as widening of the interpedicular distances on AP radiographs or a change in height of the posterior cortex of the body on lateral views) suggests in an unstable injury that may require operative fixation. In addition, disruption of the posterior ligamentous complex in the face of anterior fracture or dislocation is a strong indication of instability and of the potential need for surgical stabilization. Exceptions may include the upper thoracic spine, which is inherently more stable, and bony Chance fractures. Compression fractures of three sequential vertebrae lead to an increase in risk of posttraumatic kyphosis.
3. Treatment—May be either operative or nonoperative (bracing or casting) for stable fractures, with a well aligned spine with less than 20–30 degrees of kyphosis and no neurologic compromise. Operative intervention includes decompression for progressive neurologic deficit (emergency) or for incomplete neurologic deficit. May be accomplished anteriorly via vertebrectomy and stabilization or posteriorly via a transpedicular route. Posterior instrumentation with restoration of height and sagittal alignment may decompress the canal by repositioning the "posterolateral complex." Historically, posterior instrumentation and fusion have extended three levels above and two levels below the injury to stabilize the fracture. A recent alternative is the "rod-long, fuse short" technique, allowing fusion across only two motion segments but requiring implant removal. Constructs are created either in compression (fracture-dislocations, Chance fractures, or shear fractures) or in distraction (burst fractures) to reduce and stabilize the injury. Newer, more rigid segmental systems with multiple hooks, wires, and screws or rod-sleeve constructs have supplanted the standard Harrington system and allow maintenance of the normal sagittal contour of the spine. Pedicle screw systems are available that purport to limit instrumentation levels to one above and one below the injury. High rates of screw breakage have been reported, and the concepts regarding fusion levels and constructs are in evolution. The goals of surgery include stabilization of the fracture and preservation or improvement of neural function in all patients, as well as more rapid entry into rehabilitation and a shorter hospital stay for patients with complete injuries. Rehabilitation following spinal cord injury is discussed more fully in Chapter 9.
4. Complications—The most common long-term complication of a thoracolumbar fracture, treated with or without surgery, is pain. Unfortunately, the relationship between chronic pain and "stability," deformity, pseudarthrosis, and many other factors is unclear. Various types of posttraumatic deformity are noted, including scoliosis caudal to a complete injury (an age-related phenomenon with 100% occurrence in those <10 years old) and progressive kyphosis (common with unrecognized posterior ligamentous injury). Symptomatic flat back of the lumbar spine results in forward flex posture and easy fatigue (occurs with uncontoured distraction instrumentation). Other complications include late progressive neurologic loss and pain due to the development of posttraumatic syringomyelia. Late development of a neuropathic spine with gross bony destruction and bony spicules in the soft tissue has also been described.

F. Other Thoracolumbar Disorders

1. Destructive Spondyloarthopathy—Seen in hemodialysis patients with chronic renal failure. Typically involves three adjacent vertebrae with two intervening discs. Changes include subluxation, degeneration, and narrowing of the disc height. Although the process may resemble infection, it probably represents crystal or amyloid deposition.
2. Facet Syndrome—Inflammation or degeneration of the lumbar facet joints. May cause pain that is characteristically in the low back with radiation down one or both buttocks and posterior thighs that is worse with extension. Selective injections of local anesthetic can be helpful in the diagnosis of this condition, but anesthetic/steroid injections into the facet joint as a treatment modality are less effective (<20% with excellent pain relief). The significance of the facet syndrome is debated, and no widely accepted treatment regimen exists. There is no proof that surgery (facet rhizotomy or fusion) is beneficial.
3. Diffuse Idiopathic Skeletal Hyperostosis (DISH)—Also known by the eponym Forestier's disease, this entity is defined by the presence of nonmarginal syndesmophytes (differentiated from ankylosing spondylitis, which has marginal syndesmophytes [Fig. 7–11]) at three successive levels. DISH can occur anywhere in the spine but is most common in the T-spine and is more often seen on the right side. DISH is associated with chronic lower back pain and is more common in patients with diabetes and gout. The prevalence of DISH has been found to be as high as 28% in autopsy specimens. Although there appears to be no relationship between DISH and spinal pain, DISH is associated with extraspinal ossification at several joints, including an increased risk of heterotopic ossification following total hip surgery.
4. Ankylosing Spondylitis—HLA-B27-positive patients are usually young men who present with insidious onset of back and hip pain during the third or fourth decade. Sacroiliac joint obliteration and marginal syndesmophytes allow radiographic differentiation from DISH. Ankylosing spondylitis may result in fixed cervical, thoracic, or lumbar hyperkyphosis. It occasionally causes

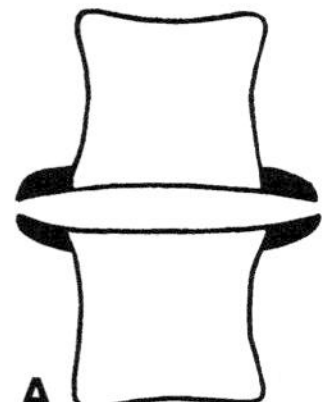

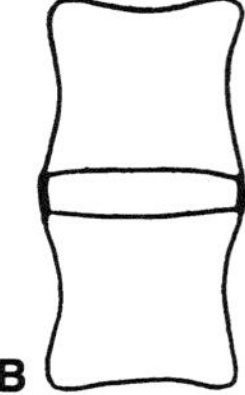

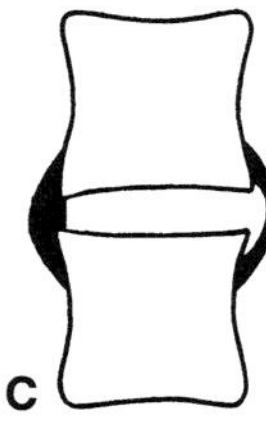

FIGURE 7–11. Differential diagnoses of *A*, osteophytes (DJD); *B*, marginal syndesmophytes (ankylosing spondylitis); and *C*, nonmarginal syndesmophytes (DISH). (From Rothman, R.H., and Simeon, F.A.: The Spine, 2nd ed., p. 924. Philadelphia, WB Saunders, 1982; reprinted by permission.)

marked functional limitation, primarily due to the inability of affected patients to face forward. Extension osteotomy and fusion of the lumbar spine with compression instrumentation can successfully balance the head over the sacrum. Assessment for hip flexion contractures or cervicothoracic kyphosis is mandatory. The cervical spine may be corrected by a C7–T1 osteotomy and fusion under local anesthesia. Complications of osteotomies include nonunion, loss of correction, and neurologic and aortic injury.

5. Adult Scoliosis—Usually defined as scoliosis in patients over age 20, it is more symptomatic than its childhood counterpart (discussed in Chapter 2, Pediatric Orthopaedics). Etiology is usually idiopathic but can also be neuromuscular, senescent (secondary to degenerative disease or osteoporosis), posttraumatic, or postsurgical. Curves are usually thoracic (secondary to unrecognized adolescent scoliosis) or lumbar/thoracolumbar (senescent). Although the association between pain and scoliosis is controversial, back pain is the most common presenting complaint and appears to be related to curve severity and location (lumbar curves more painful). Pain usually begins in the convexity of the curve and later moves to the concavity, reflecting a more refractory condition. Radicular pain and stenosis can occur and may require surgical decompression. Other complaints include cosmetic deformity, cardiopulmonary problems (thoracic curves >60–65 degrees may alter PFTs; curves >90 degrees may affect mortality), and neurologic symptoms (secondary to stenosis). There is no demonstrated association between curve progression and pregnancy. Progression is unlikely in curves <30 degrees. Right thoracic curves >50 degrees are at highest risk for progression (usually 1 degree/year) followed by right lumbar curves. Myelography with CT or MRI is useful for the evaluation of nerve root compression in stenosis. MRI, facet injections, and/or discography may be utilized to evaluate symptoms in the lumbar spine. Nonoperative treatment includes NSAIDs, weight reduction, back school, muscle strengthening, facet joint injections, and orthotics (used with activity). The uncertain correlation between adult scoliosis and back pain makes conservative management, including a thorough evaluation for other common causes of back pain, essential. Surgery is usually reserved for symptomatic curves >50–60 degrees in young adults and up to 90 degrees and beyond in older patients, for progressive curves, for patients with cardiopulmonary compromise (worsening PFTs in severe curves), and for patients with refractory spinal stenosis. Operative risk is high (up to 25% complication rate in older patients); and complications include pseudarthrosis (15% with posterior fusion only), UTI, instrumentation problems, infection (up to 5%), and neurologic deficits. Additionally, long convalescence is usually required. Combined anterior release and fusion and posterior fusion and instrumentation may be beneficial for large (>70 degrees), more rigid curves (as determined on side-bending films) or curves in the lumbar spine. Preservation of normal sagittal alignment with fusion is critical. Fusion to the sacrum is associated with more complications (pseudarthrosis, instrumentation failure, loss of normal lordosis, and pain) and should be avoided when possible. Achieving a successful result, including fusion to the sacrum, is enhanced by combined anterior and posterior fusion. The ideal implant for instrumentation in these cases has not been found; commonly used instrumentation for sacral fixation includes Galveston fixation and sacral pedicle or alar screw constructs.
6. Postlaminectomy Deformity—Progressive deformity (usually kyphosis) due to a prior wide laminectomy. Laminectomy in children is followed by a high risk (90%) deformity. Fusion plus internal fixation may be considered prophylactic for young patients who require extensive decompression. Fusion utilizing pedicular screw fixation is best for reconstruction in the adult lumbar spine.

G. Kyphosis

1. Introduction—Kyphosis in adults may be idiopathic (old Scheuermann's), posttraumatic, secondary to trauma or ankylosing spondylitis, or a result of metabolic bone disease. Progressive kyphosis secondary to multiple osteoporotic compression fractures (occur secondary to loss of vertical trabeculae in vertebral body) is usually treated with exercises, bracing, and medical management of the underlying bone disease. Surgical attempts at correction and stabilization are marked by high complication rate. An underlying malignancy as a cause of the osteopenia should be considered; evaluation with MRI is sensitive for determining the presence of tumor.
2. Nontraumatic Adult Kyphosis—Severe idiopathic or congenital kyphosis may be a source of back pain in the adult, particularly when present in the thoracolumbar or lumbar spine. When the symptoms fail to respond to nonoperative management (see Adult Scoliosis, above), posterior instrumentation and fusion of the entire kyphotic segment, utilizing a compression implant, may be indicated. Anterior fusion in conjunction is performed for curves not correcting to 55 degrees or less on hyperextension lateral radiographs.
3. Posttraumatic Kyphosis—May be seen following fractures of the thoracolumbar spine treated nonoperatively, particularly when the posterior ligamentous complex has been disrupted, fractures treated by laminectomy without fusion, and fractures for which fusion has been performed unsuccessfully. Progressive kyphosis may produce pain at the fracture site, with radiating leg pain and/

or neurologic dysfunction if there is associated neural compression. Operative options include posterior fusion with compression instrumentation for milder deformities; combined anterior and posterior osteotomies, instrumentation, and fusion for more severe deformities; and anterior spinal cord or cauda equina decompression combined with posterior instrumentation and fusion for cases involving neurologic dysfunction.

IV. Sacrum and Coccyx

A. Sacroiliac Joint Pain—Elicited with the patient lying on the affected side without support (Gaenslen's test), direct compression, or flexion, abduction, and external rotation (FABER or Patrick test). Local injections may have a diagnostic and therapeutic role. Orthotic management (trochanteric cinch) can be helpful. Fusion is not indicated unless an infection is present.

B. Idiopathic Coccygodynia—Painful coccyx is frequently associated with psychological conditions. Four types have been identified (Postacchini and Massobrio).

TYPE	COCCYX MORPHOLOGY	COCCYGODYNIA
I	Slight forward curve, apex dorsal	Rare
II	Marked curve, apex ventral	Common
III	Sharp angulation between coccyx segments	Common
IV	Ventral subluxation of segments (sacrococcygeal or coccycoccygeal)	Common

Treatment of coccygodynia should be conservative, with a donut pillow and NSAIDS. Local steroid injection is occasionally utilized for resistant cases. Complete or partial coccygectomy may relieve symptoms of type III or IV disorder but is a last resort and is associated with a high complication and failure rate.

C. Sacral Insufficiency Fracture—Occurs in older patients with osteopenia often without a history of trauma. Complaints include low back and groin pain. Diagnosed with technetium bone scan (H-shaped uptake pattern is diagnostic) or CT scan. Treatment is nonoperative with rest, analgesics, and ambulatory aids until symptoms resolve.

V. Spine Tumors and Infections

A. Introduction—The spine is a frequent site of metastasis, and certain tumors with a predilection for the spine have unique manifestations in vertebrae. Tumors of the vertebral body include histiocytosis X, giant cell tumor, chordoma, osteosarcoma, hemangioma, metastatic disease, and marrow cell tumors. Tumors of the posterior elements include aneurysmal bone cysts, osteoblastoma, and osteoid osteoma. Radiographic changes include absent pedicle, cortical erosion or expansion, and vertebral collapse. Bone scans can be helpful in cases of protracted back pain or night pain. MRI is also useful: Malignant tumors have decreased T1 and increased T2 intensity, the sensitivity of which is increased with use of gadolinium. Malignant tumors occur more commonly in lower (lumbar > thoracic > cervical) spinal levels and in the vertebral body. Complete surgical excision is difficult and usually consists of tumor debulking and stabilization. Adjuvant therapy is essential. For more details on these tumors, refer to Chapter 8, Orthopaedic Pathology.

B. Metastasis—Most common tumors of the spine, with spread to the vertebral body first and later to the pedicles. "Red flags" for spinal metastasis include a history of cancer, recent unexplained weight loss, night pain, and age >50 years. Most tumors are osteolytic and are not demonstrated on plain films until >30% destruction of the vertebral body has occurred. Breast, lung, and prostate metastases are most common, the latter being blastic. CT-guided needle biopsy is often possible, and surgery for diagnosis can be avoided. Poor prognosis is associated with neurologic dysfunction, proximal lesions, long duration of symptoms, and rapid growth. Radiation therapy and chemotherapy are the mainstays of treatment unless the tumor is destabilizing and progressive or causes spinal cord or cauda equina dysfunction. Radiosensitivity varies among primary tumor types: Prostate and lymphoid tumors are quite radiosensitive; breast cancer is 70% sensitive, 30% are resistant; GI and renal cell tumors are quite radioresistant. Surgical indications include progressive neurologic dysfunction unresponsive to radiation therapy, persistent pain despite radiation therapy, need for a diagnostic biopsy, or pathologic fracture-dislocation. In cases of neurologic deficit and/or spinal instability, anterior decompression and stabilization (preserving intact posterior structures) have a role and may result in recovery of neurologic function. Posterior stabilization or a circumferential approach is indicated in cases with multiple levels of destruction, involvement of both anterior and posterior columns, or translational instability. Life expectancy should play an important role as to whether surgical treatment is performed. Methylmethacrylate may be useful as an anterior strut but should only be utilized as an adjunct because of the high complication rate. Iliac crest graft is favored if life expectancy is > 6 months. Anterior internal fixation may be indicated to maximize immediate stability and rehabilitation.

C. Primary Tumors

1. Osteoid Osteoma and Osteoblastoma—Common in the spine. May present with painful scoliosis in a child. Scoliosis (the lesion is typically at the apex of the convexity) resolves with early resection (within 18 months) in a child <11 years of age. Osteoblastomas typically occur in the posterior elements in older patients, with neurologic involvement in more than half. This presentation typically requires resection and posterior fusion.
2. Aneurysmal Bone Cyst (ABC)—May represent degeneration of other, more aggressive tumors. ABCs typically occur during the second decade of life. They occur in the posterior elements but may also involve the anterior elements. Treatment is excision and/or radiation therapy.
3. Hemangioma—Typically seen in asymptomatic patients. Symptomatic patients over age 40 may present after small spinal fractures. Classically has "jailhouse striations" on plain films and "spikes of bone" demonstrated on CT. Vertebrae are typically normally sized and not expanded (as in Paget's disease). Treatment is observation or radiation therapy in cases of persistent pain after

pathologic fracture. Anterior resection and fusion are reserved for refractory cases or pathologic collapse and neural compression, but massive bleeding may be encountered.

4. Eosinophilic Granuloma—Seen more often in the thoracic spine; may present with progressive back pain. Classically causes vertebral flattening (vertebra plana—Calve's disease) seen on lateral radiographs. Biopsy may be required for diagnosis unless the radiographic picture is classic or histiocytosis has already been diagnosed. Chemotherapy is useful for the systemic form. Bracing may be indicated in children to prevent progressive kyphosis. Low dose radiation therapy may be indicated in the presence of neurologic deficits; otherwise symptoms are usually self-limited. At least 50% reconstitution of vertebral height may be expected.
5. Giant Cell Tumor—Destroys the vertebral body. Surgical excision and bone grafting comprise the usual recommended treatment. High recurrence rate is reported. Radiation therapy should be avoided because of the possibility of malignant degeneration of the tumor.

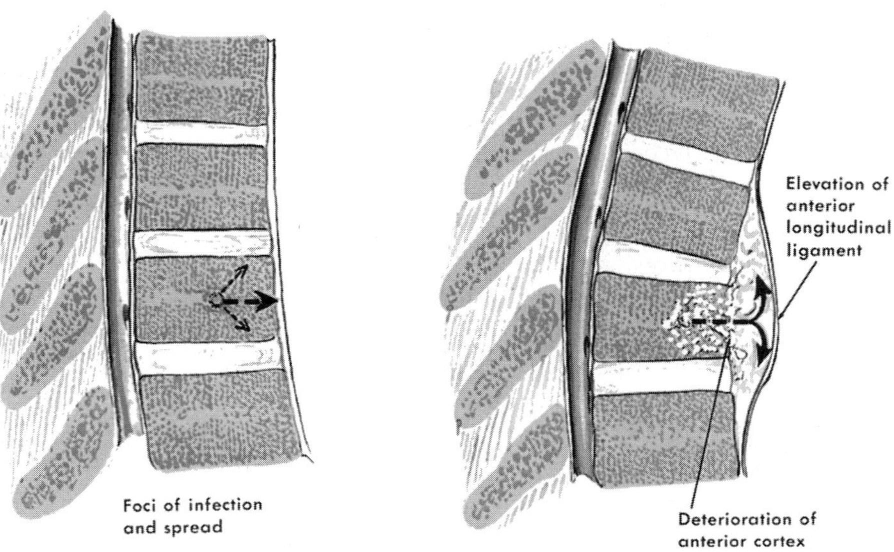

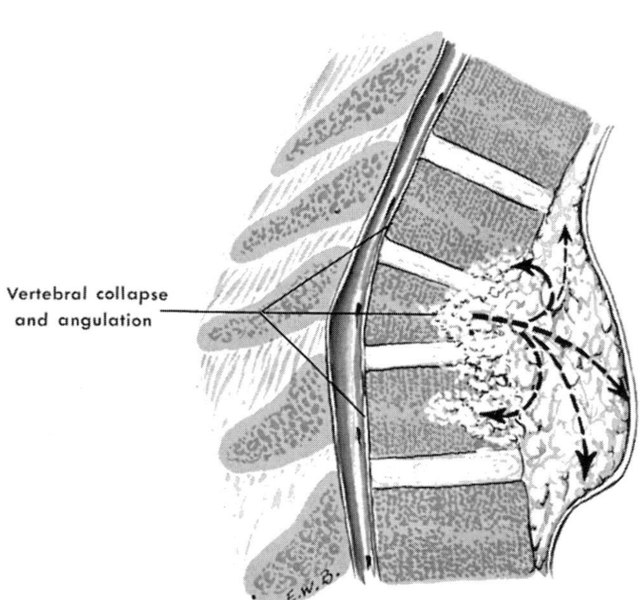

FIGURE 7–12. Pathogenesis of spinal tuberculosis. (From Tachdjian, M.O.: Pediatric Orthopaedics, 2nd ed., p. 1450. Philadelphia, WB Saunders, 1990; reprinted by permission.)

6. Plasmacytoma/Multiple Myeloma—Also common in the spine, causing osteopenic, lytic lesions. Pain, pathologic fractures, and diffuse osteoporosis are common. Increased calcium and decreased hematocrit are common, as well as abnormal protein studies. Treatment is radiation therapy (3000–4000 cGy ± chemotherapy. Surgery is reserved for instability and patients with refractory neurologic symptoms.
7. Chordoma—Classically a slow-growing lytic lesion in the midline of the anterior sacrum. May occur in other vertebrae (cervical most common). These tumors may present with intra-abdominal complaints and a presacral mass. Radiation therapy and surgery are favored. Surgical excision can include up to half of the sacral roots (i.e., all roots on one side) and still maintain bowel and bladder function. Recurrence rate is high, but aggressive attempts at surgical excision are indicated. Although a "cure" is rare, patients typically survive 10–15 years after diagnosis.
8. Osteochondroma—Arises in the posterior elements. It is seen commonly in the cervical spine. Treatment is excision, which may be necessary to rule out sarcomatous changes.
9. Neurofibroma—Can present with enlarged intervertebral foramina seen on oblique radiographs.
10. Malignant Primary Skeletal Lesions—Osteosarcoma, Ewing's sarcoma, and chondrosarcoma are uncommon in the spine. When they do occur they are associated with a poor prognosis. Chemotherapy and irradiation are the mainstays of treatment, but aggressive surgical excision may have a role. Lesions may actually be metastases, which are treated palliatively.
11. Lymphoma—Can present with "ivory" vertebrae. Usually associated with a systemic disease, lymphoma is treated after histologic diagnosis by irradiation and/or chemotherapy.

D. Spinal Infections
   1. Disc Space Infection—Osteomyelitis of the vertebral end plates can secondarily invade the disc space in children. *Staph. aureus* is the most common offender, but gram-negative organisms are common in older patients. Children (mean age 7, although all age groups are affected) commonly present with inability to walk, stand, or sit; back pain/tenderness; and restricted spine ROM. Laboratory studies may be normal except for an elevated ESR and WBC count. Radiographic finding include disc space narrowing and end plate erosion; but these findings do not occur until 10 days to 2 weeks, and their absence is unreliable. MRI scan is the diagnostic test of choice, although bone scan is also useful in the diagnosis. Treatment includes bed rest (traction, however, is contraindicated), immobilization, and antibiotics.
   2. Pyogenic Vertebral Osteomyelitis—Seen with increasing frequency but still associated with a significant (6–12 week) delay in diagnosis. Older debilitated patients and IV drug addicts are at increased risk. A history of pneumonia, UTI, skin infection, or immunologic compromise is common. The organism is usually hematogenous in origin. A history of unremitting spinal pain at any level is characteristic; and tenderness, spasm, and loss of motion are seen. Neurologic deficits are seen in 40% and are increased in older patients, with infections at higher levels in the spine, in patients with debilitating systemic illness (diabetes or RA), and with a marked delay in diagnosis. Plain radiographic findings include osteopenia, paraspinous soft tissue swelling (loss of psoas shadow), erosion of the vertebral end plates, and disc destruction. Disc destruction, seen on plain radiographs or MRI, is atypical of neoplasms. Bone scanning is sensitive for a destructive process. MRI is both sensitive for detecting infection and specific in differentiating infection from tumor. Gadolinium enhances sensitivity. Tissue diagnosis via blood cultures or aspirate of the infection is mandatory; when made, 6–12 weeks of IV antibiotics is the treatment of choice. Bracing may be used adjunctively. Open biopsy is indicated when a tissue diagnosis has not been made, and anterior approaches or costotransversectomy are utilized. Anterior débridement and strut grafting are reserved for refractory cases, typically associated with abscess formation, or cases involving neurologic deterioration, extensive bony destruction, or marked deformity.
   3. Spinal Tuberculosis (TB; Pott's Disease)—The most common extrapulmonary location of TB is in the spine. Originating in the metaphysis of the vertebral body and spreading under the anterior longitudinal ligament, spinal TB can cause destruction of several contiguous levels or can result in skip lesions (15%) or abscess formation (50%) (Fig. 7–12). About two-thirds of patients have abnormal chest radiographs, and 20% have a negative PPD test or are anergic. Severe kyphosis, sinus formation, and (Pott's) paraplegia are late sequelae. Spinal cord injury may occur secondary to direct pressure from the abscess, bony sequestra (good prognosis), or rarely meningomyelitis (poor prognosis). Radical anterior débridement of the infection followed by autogenous strut grafting (Hong Kong procedure) is the accepted surgical treatment in most centers. Advantages include less progressive kyphosis, earlier healing, and decrease in sinus formation. Adjuvant chemotherapy beginning 10 days before surgery is recommended. In cases without severe kyphosis or neurologic deficit, adjuvant chemotherapy and bracing remain a viable treatment option, particularly in centers not equipped for major anterior spinal surgery.

Selected Bibliography

All references marked with an asterisk are required reading.

General Information

*Boden, S.D., Davis, D.O., Dina, T.S., et al.: Abnormal magnetic-resonance scans of the lumbar spine in asymptomatic subjects. J. Bone Joint Surg. [Am.] 72:403, 1990.

Boden, S.D., McCown, P.R., Davis, D.O., et al.: Abnormal MRI scans of cervical spine in asymptomatic subjects: A prospective investigation. J. Bone Joint Surg. [Am.] 72:1178–1184, 1990.

Cervical Spine Research Society: The Cervical Spine, 2nd ed. Philadelphia, JB Lippincott, 1989.

Dommisse, G.F.: The blood supply of the spinal cord. J. Bone Joint Surg. [Br.] 56:225, 1974.

Garfin, S.R., ed.: Complications of Spine Surgery. Baltimore, Williams & Wilkins, 1989.

Garfin, S.R., Bottle, M.J., Walters, R.L., and Nickel, V.L.: Complications in the use of the halo fixation device. J. Bone Joint Surg. [Am.] 68:320, 1986.

Macnab, I.: The blood supply of the lumbar spine and its application to the technique of intertransverse lumbar fusion. J. Bone Joint Surg. [Br.] 53:628, 1971.

Orthopaedic Knowledge Update Home Study Syllabus I, II, III, and IV. Chicago, American Academy of Orthopaedic Surgeons, 1984, 1987, 1990, 1994.

White, A.A., III, Johnson, R.M., Panjabi, M.M., et al.: Biomechanical analysis of clinical stability in the cervical spine. Clin. Orthop. 109:85–96, 1975.

Wiesel, S.W., Tsourmas, N., Feffer, H.L., et al.: A study of computer-assisted tomography: The incidence of positive CAT scans in an asymptomatic group of patients. Spine 9:549, 1984.

Wiltse, L.L., Bateman, J.G., Hutchinson, R.H., and Nelson, W.E.: The paraspinal sacrospinalis-splitting approach to the lumbar spine. J. Bone Joint Surg. [Am.] 50:919, 1968.

Back Pain

Andersson, G.B., Jr.: Epidemiologic aspects of low-back pain in industry. Spine 6:53–60, 1981.

*Deyo, R.H., Diehl, A.K., and Rosenthal M.: How many days of bed rest for acute low back pain? A randomized clinical trial. N. Engl. J. Med. 315:1064–1070, 1986.

Deyo, R.A., and Tsui-Wu, Y.J.: Descriptive epidemiology of low back pain and its related medical care in the United States. Spine 12: 264–268, 1987.

Frymoyer, J., Pope, M., Costanza, M., et al.: Epidemiologic studies of low-back pain. Spine 5:419–423, 1980.

Frymoyer, J.W., Pope, M.H., Clements, J.H., et al.: Risk factors in low-back pain: An epidemiological survey. J. Bone Joint Surg. [Am.] 65:213–218, 1983.

Frymoyer, J.W.: Back pain and sciatica. N. Engl. J. Med. 318: 291–300, 1988.

Jensen, M.E., et al.: MRI of the lumbar spine in people without back pain. N. Engl. J. Med. 331:69, 1994.

Kirkaldy-Willis, W.H., and Hill, R.J.: A more precise diagnosis for low back pain. Spine 4:102, 1979.

Nachemson, A.L.: The lumbar spine: An orthopaedic challenge, Spine 1:59, 1976.

Nachemson, A.: Work for all: For those with low back pain as well. Clin. Orthop. 179:77–85, 1983.

Cervical Spondylosis, Stenosis

*Bernhardt, M., Hynes, R.A., Blume, H.W., and White, A.A.: Cervical spondylotic myelopathy. J. Bone Joint Surg. [Am.] 75:119, 1993.

*Bohlman, H.H., Emery, S.E., Goodfellow, D.B., and Jones, P.K.: Robinson anterior cervical diskectomy and arthrodesis for cervical radiculopathy. J. Bone Joint Surg. [Am.] 75:1298–1307, 1993.

Cervical Spine Research Society: Cervical spondylotic myelopathy. Spine 13:828–880, 1988.

Emery, S.E., Smith, M.D., and Bohlman, H.H.: Upper-airway obstruction after multilevel cervical corpectomy for myelopathy. J. Bone Joint Surg. [Am.] 73:544–551, 1991.

Fielding, J.W., Hensinger, R.N., and Hawkins, R.J.: Os odontoideum. J. Bone Joint Surg. [Am.] 62:376, 1980.

Gore, D.R., and Sepic, S.B.: Anterior cervical fusion for degenerated or protruded discs: A review of one hundred forty-six patients. Spine 9:667–671, 1984.

Gore, D.R., Sepic, S.B., Gardner, G.M., et al.: Neck pain: a long-term follow-up of 205 patients. Spine 12:1–5, 1987.

Herkowitz, H.N., Kurz, L.T., and Overholt, D.P.: Surgical management of cervical soft disk herniation: A comparison between anterior and posterior approach. Spine 15:1026–1030, 1990.

Hirabayashi, K., and Satomi, K.: Operative procedure and results of expansive open-door laminoplasty. Spine 13:870–876, 1988.

Hirabayashi, K., Watanabe, K., Wakano, K., et al.: Expansion open-door laminoplasty for cervical spinal stenotic myelopathy. Spine 8:693, 1983.

Nurick, S.: The normal history and results of surgical treatment of the spinal cord disorder associated with cervical spondylosis. Brain 95:101–108, 1972.

Robinson, R.A., and Smith, G.W.: Anterior lateral cervical disc removal in interbody fusion for cervical disc disease. Bull. Johns Hopkins Hosp. 96:223–224, 1955.

*Smith, G.W., and Robinson, R.A.: The treatment of certain cervical spine disorders by anterior removal of the intervertebral disk and interbody fusion. J. Bone Joint Surg. [Am.] 40:607–623, 1958.

Zdeblick, T.A., and Bohlman, H.H.: Cervical kyphosis and myelopathy: Treatment by anterior corpectomy and strut-grating. J. Bone Joint Surg. [Am.] 71:170, 1989.

Rheumatoid Spondylitis

*Boden, S.D., Dodge, L.D., Bohlman, H.H., and Rechtine, G.R.: Rheumatoid arthritis of the cervical spine: A long term analysis with predictors of paralysis and recovery. J. Bone Joint Surg. [Am.] 75: 1282, 1993.

Brooks, A.L., and Jenkins, E.B.: Atlanto-axial arthrodesis by the wedge compression method. J. Bone Joint Surg. [Am.] 60:279, 1978.

*Clark, C.R., Goetz, D.D., and Menezes, A.H.: Arthrodesis of the cervical spine in rheumatoid arthritis. J. Bone Joint Surg. [Am.] 71:381–392, 1989.

Kraus, D.R., Peppleman, W.C., Agrwal, A.K., et al.: Incidence of subaxial subluxation in patients with generalized rheumatoid arthritis who have had previous occipital cervical fusions. Spine 16S: 486–489, 1991.

Pellicci, P.M., Ranawat, C.S., Tsairis, P., and Beyan, W.J.: A prospective study of the progression of rheumatoid arthritis of the cervical spine. J. Bone Joint Surg. [Am.] 63:342, 1981.

Rana, N.A.: Natural history of atlanto-axial subluxation in rheumatoid arthritis. Spine 14:1054–1056, 1989.

Ranawat, C.S., O'Leary, P., Pellicci, P., et al.: Cervical spine fusion in rheumatoid arthritis. J. Bone Joint Surg. [Am.] 61:1003, 1979.

Santavirta, S., Slatis, P., Kankaanpaa, U., Sandelin, J., and Laasonen, E.: Treatment of the cervical spine in rheumatoid arthritis. J. Bone Joint Surg. [Am.] 70:658, 1988.

Slatis, P., Santavirta, S., Sandelin, J., et al.: Cranial subluxation of the odontoid process in rheumatoid arthritis. J. Bone Joint Surg. [Am.] 71:189, 1989.

Zoma, A., Sturrock, R.D., Fisher, W.D., et al.: Surgical stabilization of the rheumatoid cervical spine: A review of indications and results. J. Bone Joint Surg. [Br.] 69:8–12, 1987.

Cervical Spine Injury

Allen, B.L., Jr., Ferguson, R.L., Lehmann, T.R., et al.: A mechanistic classification of closed, indirect fractures and dislocation of the lower cervical spine. Spine 7:1–27, 1982.

*Anderson, L.D., and D'Alozono, R.T.: Fractures of the odontoid process of the axis. J. Bone Joint Surg. [Am.] 56:1663, 1974.

Anderson, P.A., and Bohlman, H.H.: Anterior decompression and arthrodesis of the cervical spine: Long-term motor improvement. Part II. Improvement in complete traumatic quadraplegia. J. Bone Joint Surg. [Am.] 74:683–692, 1992.

*Bohlman, H.H.: Acute fractures and dislocations of the cervical spine: An analysis of 300 hospitalized patients and review of the literature. J. Bone Joint Surg. [Am.] 61:1119–1142, 1979.

Bohlman, H.H.: The pathology and current treatment concepts of cervical spine injuries: A critical review of 300 cases. J. Bone Joint Surg. [Am.] 54:1353, 1972.

*Bohlman, H.H., and Eismont, F.J.: Surgical techniques of anterior decompression and fusion for spinal cord injuries. Clin. Orthop. 154:57, 1981.

*Bohlman, H.H., and Anderson, P.A.: Anterior decompression and arthrodesis of the cervical spine: Long term motor improvement. Part I. Improvement in incomplete traumatic quadraparesis. J. Bone Joint Surg. [Am.] 74:671–682, 1992.

Bosch, A., Stauffer, E.S., and Nickel, V.L.: Incomplete traumatic quadriplegia: A ten-year review. J.A.M.A. 216:473, 1971.

Carroll, C., McAfee, P.C., and Riley, L.H., Jr.: Objective findings for diagnosis of "whiplash." J. Musculoskel. Med. 3:57, 1986.

Cattell, H.S., and Filtzer, D.L.: Pseudosubluxation and other normal variations of the cervical spine in children: A study of 160 children. J. Bone Joint Surg. [Am.] 47:1295, 1965.

*Clark, C.R., and White, A.A., III: Fractures of the dens: A multicenter study. J. Bone Joint Surg. [Am.] 67:1340–1348, 1985.

*Eismont, F.B., Rena, M.J., and Green, B.A.: Extrusion of an intervertebral disk associated with traumatic subluxation and dislocation of cervical facets: Case report. J. Bone Joint Surg. [Am.] 73: 1555–1556, 1991.

Fielding, J.W., and Hawkins, R.J.: Atlanto-axial rotatory fixation: Fixed rotatory subluxation of the atlanto-axial joint. J. Bone Joint Surg. [Am.] 59:37, 1977.

Gallie, W.E.: Fractures and dislocations of the cervical spine. Am. J. Surg. 46:495, 1939.

Johnson, R.M., Hart, D.L., Simmons, E.F., et al.: Cervical orthoses: A study comparing their effectiveness in restricting cervical motion in normal subjects. J. Bone Joint Surg. [Am.] 59:332, 1977.

Kang, J.E., Figgie, M.P., and Bohlman, H.H.: Sagittal measurements of the cervical spine in subaxial fractures and dislocations: An analysis of two hundred eighty-eight patients with and without neurologic deficits. J. Bone Joint Surg. [Am.] 76:1617–1628, 1994.

*Levine, A.M., and Edwards, C.C.: The management of traumatic spondylolisthesis of the axis. J. Bone Joint Surg. [Am.] 67: 217–226, 1985.

Levine, A.M., and Edwards, C.C.: Treatment of injuries in the C1–C2 complex. Orthop. Clin. North Am. 17:31–44, 1986.

Lucas, J.T., and Ducker, T.B.: Motor classification of spinal cord injuries with mobility, morbidity and recovery indices. Am. Surg. 45:151–158, 1979.

*Stauffer, E.S.: Diagnosis and prognosis of acute cervical spinal cord injury. Clin. Ortho. 112:9–15, 1975.

Stauffer, E.S.: Wiring techniques of the posterior cervical spine for the treatment of trauma. Orthopaedics 11:1543, 1988.

Torg, S., Pavlov, H., Genuario, S.E., et al.: Neuropraxia on the cervical spinal cord with transient quadraplegia. J. Bone Joint Surg. [Am.] 68:1354–1370, 1986.

Disc Disease

Albrand, O.W., and Corkill, G.: Thoracic disc herniation: Treatment and prognosis. Spine 4:41–46, 1979.

Bell, G.R., and Rothman, R.H.: The conservative treatment of sciatica. Spine 9:54–56, 1984.

*Bohlman, H.H., and Zdeblick, T.A.: Anterior excision of herniated thoracic discs. J. Bone Joint Surg. [Am.] 70:1038, 1988.

Cloward, R.B.: The treatment of ruptured lumbar intervertebral discs by vertebral body fusion. I. Indications, operative technique, after care. J. Neurosurg. 10:154, 1953.

Crawshaw, C., Frazer, A.M., Merriam, W.F., et al.: A comparison of surgery and chemonucleolysis in the treatment of sciatica: A prospective randomized trial. Spine 9:195–198, 1984.

*Eismont, F.J., and Currier, B.: Current concepts review: Surgical management of lumbar intervertebral-disc disease. J. Bone Joint Surg. [Am.] 71:1266, 1989.

Ethier, D.E., Cain, J.E., Yaszemski, M.J., et al.: The influence of annulotomy selection on disc competence: A biomechanical, radiographic, and histologic analysis. Spine 19:2071–2076, 1994.

Hanley, E.N., and Shapiro, D.E.: The development of low back pain after excision of a lumbar disk. J. Bone Joint Surg. [Am.] 71: 719–721, 1989.

Konnberg, M.: Erythrocyte sedimentation rate following lumbar discectomy. Spine 11:766, 1986.

*Kostuik, J.P., Harrington, I., Alexander, D., Rand, W., and Evans, D.: Cauda equina syndrome and lumbar disc herniation. J. Bone Joint Surg. [Am.] 68:386, 1986.

Mixter, W.J., and Barr, J.S.: Rupture of the intervertebral disc with involvement of the spinal canal. N. Engl. J. Med. 211:210, 1934.

Nachemson, A.L., and Rydevik, B.: Chemonucleolysis for sciatica: A critical review, Acta Orthop. Scand. 59:56, 1988.

Waddell, G., Kummell, E.G., Lotto, W.M., et al.: Failed lumbar disk surgery and repeat surgery following industrial injuries. J. Bone Joint Surg. [Am.] 61:201–207, 1979.

*Weber, H.: Lumbar disc herniation: A controlled, prospective study with ten years of observation. Spine 8:131, 1983.

Lumbar Stenosis

Epstein, J.A., Carras, R., Ferrar, J., et al.: Conjoined lumbosacral nerve roots. J. Neurosurg. 55:585, 1981.

Hall, S., Bartleson, J.D., Onbrio, B.M., et al.: Lumbar spinal stenosis; clinical features, diagnostic procedures, and results of surgical treatment in 68 patients, Ann. Intern. Med. 103:271–275, 1985.

Kirkaldy-Willis, W.H.: The relationship of structural pathology to the nerve root. Spine 9:49–52, 1984.

Kirkaldy-Willis, W.H., Wedge, J.H., Yong-Hing, K., and Reilly, J.: Pathology and pathogenesis of lumbar spondylosis and stenosis. Spine 4:319, 1978.

*Spengler, D.M.: Current concepts review: Degenerative stenosis of the lumbar spine. J. Bone Joint Surg. [Am.] 69:305, 1987.

Spondylolisthesis

Boxall, D., Bradford, D.S., Winter, R.B., and Moe, J.H.: Management of severe spondylolisthesis in children and adolescents. J. Bone Joint Surg. [Am.] 61:479, 1979.

Bradford, D.S.: Closed reduction of spondylolisthesis and experience in 22 patients. Spine 13:580, 1988.

Bradford, D.S., and Boachie-Adjei, O.: Treatment of severe spondylolisthesis by anterior and posterior reduction and stabilization: a long-term follow-up study. J. Bone Joint Surg. [Am.] 72:1060, 1990.

Farfan, H.: The pathological anatomy of degenerative spondylolisthesis: A cadaver study. Spine 5:412–418, 1980.

*Frederickson, B.W., Baker, D., McHolick, W.J., et al.: The natural history of spondylolysis and spondylolisthesis. J. Bone Joint Surg. [Am.] 66:699–707, 1984.

Gill, G.G., Manning, J.G., and White, H.L.: Surgical treatment of spondylolisthesis without spine fusion. J. Bone Joint Surg. [Am.] 37:493, 1955.

Harris, I.E., and Weinstein, S.D.: Long-term follow-up of patients with grade III and IV spondylolisthesis: Treatment with and without posterior fusion. J. Bone Joint Surg. [Am.] 69:960–969, 1987.

*Hensinger, R.N.: Current concepts review: Spondylolysis and spondylolisthesis in children and adolescents. J. Bone Joint Surg. [Am.] 71:1098, 1989.

*Herkowitz, H.N., Kurz, L.T.: Degenerative lumbar spondylolisthesis with spinal stenosis: A prospective study comparing decompression with decompression and intertransverse process arthrodesis. J. Bone Joint Surg. [Am.] 73:802–808, 1991.

Kirkaldy-Willis, W.H., Wedge, J.H., Yong-Hing, K., and Reilly, J.: Pathology and pathogenesis of lumbar spondylosis and stenosis. Spine 4:319, 1978.

Lehmann, T.R., Spratt, K.F., Tozzi, J.R., et al.: Long term follow-up of lower lumbar spine fusion patients. Spine 12:97–104, 1987.

Macnab, I.: Spondylolisthesis with an intact neural arch-the so-called pseudospondylolisthesis. J. Bone Joint Surg. [Br.] 32:325, 1950.

Ogilvie, J.W., and Sherman, J.: Spondylolysis in Scheuermann's disease. Spine 12:251–253, 1987.

Osterman, K., Lindholm, T.S., and Laurent, L.E.: Late results of removal of the loose posterior element (Gill's operation) in the treatment of lytic lumbar spondylolisthesis. Clin. Orthop. 117:121, 1976.

Peek, R.D., Wiltse, L.L., Reynolds, J.B., et al.: In situ arthrodesis without decompression for grade III or IV isthmic spondylolisthesis in adults who have severe sciatica. J. Bone Joint Surg. [Am.] 71:62, 1989.

Saraste, H: The etiology of spondyloysis: A retrospective radiographic study. Acta Orthop. Scand. 56:253, 1985.

Wiltse, L.L., and Winter R.B.: Terminology and measurement of spondylolisthesis. J. Bone Joint Surg. [Am.] 65:768–772, 1983.

Wiltse, L.L., Guyer, R.D., Spencer, C.W., et al.: Alar transverse process impingement of the L5 spinal nerve: The far-out syndrome. Spine 9:31, 1984.

*Wiltse, L.L., Newman, P.H., and Macnab, I.: Classification of spondylolysis and spondylolisthesis. Clin. Orthop. 117:23, 1976.

Wiltse, L.L., Widell, E.H., Jr., and Jackson, D.W.: Fatigue fracture: The basic lesion in isthmic spondylolisthesis. J. Bone Joint Surg. [Am.] 57:17, 1975.

*Zdeblick, T.: A prospective randomized study of lumbar fusion. Spine 18:983–991, 1993.

Thoracolumbar Injury

An, H.S., Vaccaro, A., Cotler, J.M., et al.: Low lumbar burst fractures: Comparison among body cast, Harrington rod, Luque rod, and Steffee plate. Spine 16:S440–S444, 1991.

*Bohlman, H.H.: Current concepts review: Treatment of fractures and dislocations of the thoracic and lumbar spine. J. Bone Joint Surg. [Am.] 67:165, 1985.

Bohlman, H.H., and Eismont, F.J.: Surgical techniques of anterior decompression and fusion for spinal cord injuries. Clin. Orthop. 154:57, 1981.

*Bracken, M.B., Shepard, M.J., Collins, W.F., et al.: A randomized, controlled trial of methylprednisolone or naloxone in the treatment of acute spinal cord injury. N. Engl. J. Med. 322:1405, 1990.

Cain, J.E., DeJung, J.T., Divenberg, A.S., et al.: Pathomechanical analysis of thoracolumbar burst fracture reduction: A calf spine model. Spine 18:1640–1647, 1993.

Cammissa, F.P., Jr., Eismont, F.J., and Green, B.A.: Dural laceration occurring with burst fractures and associated laminar fractures. J. Bone Joint Surg. [Am.] 71:1044–1052, 1989.

*Denis, F.: The three column spine in its significance in the classification of acute thoracolumbar spinal injuries. Spine 8:817–831, 1983.

*Ferguson, R.L., and Allen, B.L., Jr.: A mechanistic classification of thoracolumbar spine fractures. Clin. Orthop. 189:77, 1984.

*Holdsworth, F.W.: Fractures, dislocations, and fracture-dislocations of the spine. J. Bone Joint Surg. [Am.] 52:1534, 1970.

Holdsworth, F.W.: Fractures, dislocations, and fracture-dislocations of the spine. J. Bone Joint Surg. [Br.] 45:6, 1963.

Kaneda, K., Abumi, K., and Fujiya, M.: Burst fractures with neurologic deficits of the thoracolumbar-lumbar spine: Results of anterior decompression and stabilization with anterior instrumentation. Spine 9:788, 1984.

McAfee, P.C., Bohlman, H.H., and Yuan, H.A.: Anterior decompression of traumatic thoracolumbar fractures with incomplete neurologic deficit using a retroperitoneal approach. J. Bone Joint Surg. [Am.] 67:89–104, 1985.

McAfee, P.C., Yuan, H.A., Frederickson, B.E., and Lubicky, J.P.: The value of computed tomography in thoracolumbar fractures. J. Bone Joint Surg. [Am.] 64:461, 1983.

Mumfred, J., Weinstein, J.N., Spratt, K.F., and Goel, V.K.: Thoracolumbar burst fractures: The clinical efficacy and outcome of nonoperative management. Spine 18:955–970, 1993.

Stauffer, E.S., Wood, R.W., and Kelly, E.G.: Gunshot wounds of the spine: The effects of laminectomy. J. Bone Joint Surg. [Am.] 61: 389, 1979.

Transfeldt, E.E., White, D., Bradford, D.S., and Roche, B.: Delayed anterior decompression in patients with spinal cord and cauda equina injuries of the thoracolumbar spine. Spine 15:953, 1990.

Deformity

*Allen, B.L., Jr., and Ferguson, R.L.: The Galveston technique of pelvic fixation with L-rod instrumentation of the spine. Spine 9: 388, 1984.

*Bradford, D.S.: Adult scoliosis: Current concepts of treatment. Clin. Orthop. 229:70, 1988.

Bradford, D.S., Ganjavian, S., and Antonious, D.: Anterior strut-grafting for the treatment of kyphosis: Review of experience with forty-eight patients. J. Bone Joint Surg. [Am.] 64:680, 1982.

Bradford, D.S., Moe, J.H., Montalvo, F.J., and Winter, R.B.: Scheuermann's kyphosis and roundback deformity: Results of Milwaukee brace treatment. J. Bone Joint Surg. [Am.] 56:740, 1974.

Hall, J.E.: The anterior approach to spinal deformities. Orthop. Clin. North Am. 3:81, 1972.

Herring, J.A., and Wenger, D.R.: Segmental spine instrumentation. Spine 7:285, 1982.

Hibbs, R.A.: An operation for progressive spinal deformities. N. Y. Med. J. 93:1013, 1911.

Jackson, R.P., Simmons, E.H., and Stripinis, D.: Incidence and severity of back pain in adult idiopathic scoliosis. Spine 8:749, 1983.

Lauerman, W.C., Bradford, D.S., Ogilvie, J.W., and Transfeldt, E.E.: Results of lumbar pseudarthrosis repair. J. Spinal Disord. 5: 128–136, 1992.

Lauerman, W.C., Bradford, D.S., Transfeld, E.E., and Ogilvie, J.W.: Management of pseudarthrosis after arthrodesis of the spine for idiopathic scoliosis. J. Bone Joint Surg. [Am.] 73:222–236, 1991.

*Luque, E.R.: Segmental spinal instrumentation of the lumbar spine. Clin. Orthop. 203:126–134, 1986.

Murray, P.M., Weinstein, S.L., and Spratt, K.F.: The natural history and long term follow-up of Scheuerman's kyphosis. J. Bone Joint Surg. [Am.] 75:236–248, 1993.

Nachemson, A.: Adult scoliosis and back pain. Spine 4:513–517, 1979.

*Sponseller, P.D., Cohen, M.S., Nachemson, A.L., et al.: Results of surgical treatment of adults with idiopathic scoliosis. J. Bone Joint Surg. [Am.] 69:667–675, 1987.

Swank, S., Lonstein, J.E., Moe, J.H., et al.: Surgical treatment of adult scoliosis: A review of two hundred and twenty-two cases. J. Bone Joint Surg. [Am.] 63:268, 1981.

*Weinstein, S.L., and Ponseti, I.V.: Curve progression in idiopathic scoliosis. J. Bone Joint Surg. [Am.] 65:447–455, 1983.

Winter, R.B., Lonstein, J.E., and Denis, F.: Pain patterns in adult scoliosis. Orthop. Clin. North Am. 19:339, 1988.

Sacrum

*Denis, F., Davis, S., and Comfort T.: Sacral fractures: An important problem retrospective analysis of 236 cases. Clin. Orthop. 227: 67–81, 1988.

Newhouse, K.E., El-Khoury, G.Y., and Buckwalter, J.A.: Occult sacral fractures in osteopenic patients. J. Bone Joint Surg. [Am.] 75: 1472–1477, 1992.

Postacchini, F., and Massobrio, M.: Idiopathic coccygodynia: Analysis of fifty-one operative cases and a radiographic study of the normal coccyx. J. Bone Joint Surg. [Am.] 65:1116–1124, 1983.

Infections, Tumors

Allen, A.R., and Stevenson, A.W.: A ten-year follow-up of combined drug therapy and early fusion in bone tuberculosis. J. Bone Joint Surg. [Am.] 49:1001, 1967.

Batson, O.B.: The function of the vertebral veins and their role in the spread of metastases. Ann. Surg. 112:138–149, 1940.

Bohlman, H.H., Sachs, B.L., Carter, J.R., et al.: Primary neoplasms of the cervical spine: Diagnosis and treatment of twenty three patients. J. Bone Joint Surg. [Am.] 68:483, 1986.

Constans, J.P., Devitiis, E.D., Donzelli, R., et al.: Spinal metastases with neurological manifestations: review of 600 cases, J. Neurosurg. 59:111, 1983.

*Eismont, F.J., Bohlman, H.H., Soni, P.L., et al.: Pyogenic and fungal vetebral osteomyelitis with paralysis. J. Bone Joint Surg. [Am.] 65: 19–29, 1983.

Emery, S.E., Chan, D.P.K., and Woodward, H.R.: Treatment of hematogenous pyogenic vertebral osteomyelitis with anterior debridement and primar bone grafting. Spine 14:284, 1989.

Frederickson, B., Yuan, H., and Olans, R.: Management and outcome of pyogenic vertebral osteomyelitis. Clin. Orthop. 131:160, 1978.

Heusner, A.P.: Nontuberculous spinal epidural infection. N. Engl. Med. J. 239:845, 1948.

Hodgson, A.R., Stock, F.E., Fang, H.S.Y., and Ong, G.B.: Anterior spinal fusion: The operative approach and pathological findings in 412 patients with Pott's disease of the spine. Br. J. Surg. 48: 172, 1960.

Kostulk, J.P., Errica, T.J., Gleason, T.F., and Errico, C.C.: Spinal stabilization of vertebral column tumors. Spine 13:250, 1988.

McAfee, P.C., and Bohlman, H.H.: One-stage anterior cervical decompression and posterior stabilization with circumferential arthrodesis: A study of twenty-four patients who had a traumatic or neoplastic lesion. J. Bone Joint Surg. [Am.] 71:78, 1989.

Paus, B.: Tumor, tuberculosis and osteomyelitis on the spine: Differential diagnostic aspects. Acta Orthop. Scand. 44:372, 1973.

Roca, R.P., and Yoshikawa, T.T.: Primary skeletal infections in heroin users: A clinical characterization, diagnosis and therapy. Clin. Orthop. 144:238, 1979.

*Siegal, T., Tiqva, P., and Siegal, T.: Vertebral body resection for epidural compression by malignant tumors: Results of forty-seven consecutive operative procedures. J. Bone Joint Surg. [Am.] 67: 375–382, 1985.

Smith, A.D.: Tuberculosis of the spine: Results in 70 cases treated at the New York Orthopaedic Hospital from 1945 to 1960. Clin. Orthop. 58:171, 1968.

*Weinstein, J.N., and MacLain, R.F.: Primary tumors of the spine. Spine 12:843–851, 1987.

Complications

*Deyo, R.A., Cherkin, D.C., Loeser, J.D., et al.: Morbidity and mortality in association with operation on the lumbar spine. J. Bone Joint Surg. [Am.] 74:536, 1992.

Eismont, F.J., Wiesel, S.W., and Rothman, R.H.: The treatment of dural tears associated with spinal surgery. J. Bone Joint Surg. [Am.] 63:1132, 1981.

Farey, I.D., McAfee, P.C., Davis, R.F., et al.: Pseudarthrosis of the cervical spine after anterior arthrodesis: Treatment by posterior nerve-root decompression, stabilization and arthrodesis. J. Bone Joint Surg. [Am.] 72:1171, 1990.

Flynn, J.C., and Price, C.T.: Sexual complications of anterior fusion of the lumbar spine. Spine 9:489, 1984.

Graham, J.J.: Complications of cervical spine surgery: A five-year report on a survey of the membership of the Cervical Spine Research Society by the morbidity and mortality committee. Spine 14:1046–1050, 1989.

*Grarfin, S.R., Botte, M.J., Waters, R.L., and Nickel, V.L.: Complications in the use of the halo fixation device. J. Bone Joint Surg. [Am.] 68:320, 1986.

Kitchel, S.H., Eismont F.J., and Green B.A.: Closed subarachnoid drainage for management of cerebral spinal fluid leakage after an operation on the spine. J. Bone Joint Surg. [Am.] 71:984–987, 1989.

Klink, B.K., Thurman, R.T., Wittpen, G., et al.: Muscle flap closure for the salvage of complex back wounds. Spine 19:1467–1470, 1994.

Kraus, D.R., and Stauffer, E.S.: Spinal cord injury as a complication of elective anterior cervical fusion. Clin. Orthop. 112:130, 1975.

Kurz, L.T., Garfin, S.F., and Both, R.E.: Harvesting autologous iliac bone grafts: A review of complications and techniques. Spine 14: 1324–1331, 1989.

McAfee, P.C., Bohlman, H.H., Ducker, T., and Eismont, F.J.: Failure of stabilization of the spine with methylmethacrylate. J. Bone Joint Surg. [Am.] 68:1145, 1986.

*Nash, C.L., Jr., and Brown, R.H.: Current concepts review: Spinal cord monitoring. J. Bone Joint Surg. [Am.] 71:627, 1989.

Simpson, J.M., Silveri, C.P., Balderston, M.D., et al.: The results of operation on the lumbar spine in patients who have diabetes mellitus. J. Bone Joint Surg. [Am.] 75:1823–1829, 1993.

Other

Detwiler, K.N., Loftus, C.M., Godersky, J.C., and Menezes, A.H.: Management of cervical spine injuries in patients with ankylosing spondylitis. J. Neurosurg. 72:210, 1990.

Graham, B., and Can Peteghem, P.K.: Fractures of the spine in ankylosing spondylitis: Diagnosis, treatment, and complications. Spine 14:803–807, 1989.

Simmons, E.H.: Flexion deformities of the neck and ankylosing spondylitis. J. Bone Joint Surg. [Br.] 51:193, 1969.

Simmons, E.H.: Kyphotic deformity of the spine in ankylosing spondylitis. Clin. Orthop. 128:65–77, 1977.

8

ORTHOPAEDIC PATHOLOGY

FRANK J. FRASSICA and EDWARD F. MCCARTHY, Jr.

I. Introduction

A. Nomenclature—Primary bone lesions can be broadly classified into three types: malignant bone tumors (sarcomas), benign bone tumors, and lesions that simulate bone tumors (reactive and miscellaneous conditions). Common lesions that occur in bone but are not of mesenchymal origin include metastatic bone disease, myeloma, and lymphoma. A common classification system for bone tumors is shown in Table 8–1. Sarcomas are malignant neoplasms of connective tissue (mesenchymal) origin. Sarcomas generally exhibit rapid growth in a centripetal fashion and invade adjacent normal tissues. High grade malignant bone tumors tend to destroy the overlying cortex and spread into the soft tissues. Low grade tumors generally are contained within the cortex or a surrounding periosteal rim. Sarcomas primarily metastasize via the hematogenous route with the lungs being the most common site. Benign bone tumors may be small and have a limited growth potential or may be large and destructive. Tumor simulators and reactive conditions are processes that occur in bone but are not true neoplasms (e.g., osteomyelitis, aneurysmal bone cyst, bone island).

B. Staging—Staging systems may be useful for developing evaluation strategies, planning treatment, and predicting prognosis. For musculoskeletal lesions the staging system of The Musculoskeletal Tumor Society (also called the Enneking system) is the most popular and useful. There are two systems: one for malignant lesions and one for benign lesions. For malignant lesions, the system is based on knowing the histologic grade of the lesion (low or high), the anatomic features (intracompartmental or extracompartmental), and the absence (M_0) or presence of metastases (M_1).

1. Grade—Most malignant lesions are high grade (G_2) (potential for distant metastases is >25%). Low grade malignant (G_1) lesions are less common, with less than 25% chance of distant metastases. Grading of tumors requires a morphologic range, and most grading systems are based on four grades: grade 1, well differentiated; grade 2, less well differentiated; grades 3 and 4, poorly differentiated. Grading can be difficult and is based on anaplasia (degree of loss of structural differentiation), pleomorphism (variations in size and shape), and nuclear hyperchromasia (increased nuclear staining). Commonly graded lesions are shown in Table 8–2.
2. Tumor Site—The plain radiographs and special studies, such as CT and MRI scans, are studied to determine whether the tumor is situated within the bone compartment (intracompartmental, or T_1) or has left the confines of the bone (extracompartmental, or T_2).
3. Metastases—For most lesions a chest radiograph and CT scan of the chest are performed to search for pulmonary lesions. A technetium bone scan is used to exclude the presence of other bone lesions.
4. The staging system can be synthesized into six distinct stages (Table 8–3).

C. Evaluation

1. Clinical Presentation—Most patients with bone tumors present with musculoskeletal pain. The pain is similar whether the bone destruction is secondary to a primary mesenchymal tumor (e.g., osteosarcoma, chondrosarcoma) or due to metastatic bone disease, myeloma, or lymphoma. The pain is typically deep-seated and dull and may resemble a toothache. Initially, the pain may be intermittent and related to activity, a work injury, or a sporting injury. The pain usually progresses in intensity and becomes constant. Many patients experience pain at night. As the pain progresses, it is not relieved by NSAIDs or gentle narcotics.
2. Physical Examination—Patients with suspected bone tumors should be carefully examined. The affected site is inspected for soft tissue masses, overlying skin changes, adenopathy, and general musculoskeletal examination. When metastatic disease is suspected, the thyroid gland, abdomen, prostate, and breasts should be examined as appropriate.
3. Radiography—Plain radiographs in two planes are the first radiographic examinations to be performed. When the clinician suspects malignancy and the radiographs are normal, selected studies may follow. Technetium bone scans are an excellent modality to search for occult malignancies. In patients with myeloma where the scans may be negative, a skeletal survey is more sensitive. MRI is an excellent modality for screening the spine for occult metastases, myeloma, or lymphoma. A chest radiograph should be obtained in all age groups when the clinician suspects a

TABLE 8–1. CLASSIFICATION OF PRIMARY TUMORS OF BONE[a]

HISTOLOGY TYPE	BENIGN	MALIGNANT
Hematopoietic		Myeloma Lymphoma
Chondrogenic	Osteochondroma Chondroma	Primary chondrosarcoma Secondary chondrosarcoma
	Chondroblastoma	Dedifferentiated chondrosarcoma
	Chondromyxoid fibroma	Mesenchymal chondrosarcoma Clear cell chondrosarcoma
Osteogenic	Osteoid osteoma Benign osteoblastoma	Osteosarcoma Parosteal osteosarcoma Periosteal osteosarcoma
Unknown origin	Giant cell tumor	Ewing's tumor
	(Fibrous) histiocytoma	Malignant giant cell tumor Adamantinoma
Fibrogenic	Fibroma Desmoplastic fibroma	Fibrosarcoma Malignant fibrous histiocytoma
Notochordal		Chordoma
Vascular	Hemangioma	Hemangioendothelioma Hemangiopericytoma
Lipogenic	Lipoma	
Neurogenic	Neurilemoma	

[a] Classification is based on that advocated by Lichtenstein, L.: Classification of primary tumors of bone. Cancer 4:335–341, 1951.

TABLE 8–3. STAGING SYSTEM OF THE MUSCULOSKELETAL TUMOR SOCIETY (ENNEKING SYSTEM)

STAGE	GTM	DESCRIPTION
I-A	$G_1T_1M_0$	Low grade Intracompartmental No metastases
I-B	$G_1T_2M_0$	Low grade Extracompartmental No metastases
II-A	$G_2T_1M_0$	High grade Intracompartmental No metastases
II-B	$G_2T_2M_0$	High grade Extracompartmental No metastases
III-A	$G_{1/2}T_1M_1$	Any grade Intracompartmental With metastases
III-B	$G_{1/2}T_2M_1$	Any grade Extracompartmental With metastases

Grade system (G): low grade (G_1) and high grade (G_2). High-grade lesions are intermediate in grade between low grade, well differentiated tumors and high grade, undifferentiated tumors.
Tumor site (T): Determined using specialized procedures, including radiography, tomography, nuclear studies, CT, and MRI. Compartments are used to describe the tumor site. Usually compartments are easily defined based on fascial borders in the extremities. Of note, the skin and subcutaneous tissues are classified as a compartment, and the periosseous potential space between cortical bone and muscle is often considered as a compartment as well. T_0 lesions are confined within the capsule and within its compartment of origin. T_1 tumors have extracapsular extension into the reactive zone around it, but both the tumor and the reactive zone are confined within the compartment of origin. T_2 lesions extend beyond the anatomic compartment of origin by direct extension or otherwise (e.g., trauma, surgical seeding). Tumors that involve major neurovascular bundles are almost always classified as T_2 lesions.
Metastases (M): Regional and distal metastases both have an ominous prognosis; therefore the distinction is simply between no metastases (M_0) or the presence of metastases (M_1).

malignant lesion. The radiographs must be inspected carefully in order to formulate a working diagnosis. The working diagnosis then guides the clinician during further evaluation and treatment. Formulation of the differential diagnosis is based on several clinical and radiographic parameters.

a. Age of the Patient—Knowledge of common diseases in defined age groups is the first step. Certain diseases are uncommon in certain particular age groups (Table 8–4).
b. Number of Bone Lesions—Is the process monostotic or polyostotic? If there are multiple destructive lesions in the middle to older age patients (ages 40–80), the most likely diagnosis is metastatic bone disease, multiple myeloma, or lymphoma. In the young patient (ages 15–40), multiple lytic and oval lesions are most likely a vascular tumor (hemangioendothelioma). In children below age 5, multiple destructive lesions may represent metastatic

TABLE 8–2. TYPICAL LOW GRADE AND HIGH GRADE BONE AND SOFT TISSUE TUMORS

LOW GRADE	HIGH GRADE
Bone	
Parosteal osteosarcoma	Intramedullary (classic) osteosarcoma
Primary chondrosarcoma	Postradiation sarcoma
Secondary chondrosarcoma	Paget's sarcoma
Hemangioendothelioma	Fibrosarcoma
Chordoma	Malignant fibrous histiocytoma
Adamantinoma	
Soft Tissue	
Myxoid liposarcoma	Malignant fibrous histiocytoma
Lipoma-like liposarcoma	Pleomorphic liposarcoma
Angiomatoid malignant fibrous histiocytoma	Synovial sarcoma
	Rhabdomyosarcoma
	Alveolar cell sarcoma

TABLE 8–4. AGE DISTRIBUTION OF VARIOUS BONE LESIONS

AGE	MALIGNANT	BENIGN
Birth to 5 Years	Leukemia	Osteomyelitis
	Metastatic neuroblastoma	Osteofibrous dysplasia
	Metastatic rhabdomyosarcoma	
10–25 Years	Osteosarcoma Ewing's tumor Leukemia	Eosinophilic granuloma Osteomyelitis Enchondroma Fibrous dysplasia
40–80 Years	Metastatic bone disease Myeloma Lymphoma Paget's sarcoma Postradiation sarcoma	Hyperparathyroidism Paget's disease Mastocytosis

neuroblastoma or Wilms' tumor. Histiocytosis X may also lead to multiple lesions in the young patient. Fibrous dysplasia and Paget's disease may present with multiple lesions in all age groups.

c. Anatomic Location Within Bone—Certain lesions have a predilection for occurring within a certain bone or a particular location. Adamantinoma is a malignant tumor that most commonly occurs in the tibia in young patients. Chondroblastoma and giant cell tumors most commonly occur within the epiphysis of long bones. Ewing's tumor, in many cases, involves the diaphysis. Osteogenic sarcoma most commonly occurs in the metaphysis of the distal femur and proximal tibia but occurs within the diaphysis in about 7% of patients with long-bone lesions.

d. Effect of the Lesion on Bone—High grade malignant lesions generally spread rapidly through the medullary cavity. Cortical bone destruction occurs early, and the process spreads into the adjacent soft tissues. Low grade malignant lesions tend to spread slowly, but they can also destroy the cortical bone and produce a soft tissue mass.

e. Response of the Bone to the Lesion—With high grade lesions, there is often little ability of the host bone to contain the process; the result is rapid destruction of cortical bone and the presence of a soft tissue mass. In contrast with low grade lesions, the host bone often can contain the lesion with a thickened cortex or rim of periosteal bone. With benign or low grade lesions, there is often a thick periosteal response about the lesion.

f. Matrix Characteristics—If the lesion produces a matrix, it is helpful to determine whether the matrix is cartilage calcification or mineralization of osteoid. Cartilage calcification often appears stippled or may show arcs or rings; osteoid mineralization is often cloud-like.

4. Laboratory Studies—They are often nonspecific. There are a set of routine studies that should be obtained for all patients when there is not an obvious diagnosis (Table 8–5). The studies can be grouped into those for young patients (up to age 35) and those for older patients (36–80 years).

5. Biopsy—It is generally performed after complete evaluation of the patient. It is of great benefit to both pathologist and surgeon to have a narrow working diagnosis, as it allows accurate interpretation of the frozen section analysis and allows definitive treatment of some lesions based on the frozen section. There are several surgical principles to which the clinician must adhere.

a. The orientation and location of the biopsy tract is critically important. If the lesion proves to be malignant, the entire biopsy tract must be removed with the underlying lesion. Transverse incisions should be avoided (Fig. 8–1).

b. The surgeon must maintain meticulous hemostasis to prevent hematoma formation and subcutaneous hemorrhage. When possible, biopsies are done through muscles so the muscle layer can be closed tightly. Tourniquets are utilized to obtain tissue and then are released so bleeding points can be controlled. Avitene, Gelfoam, and Thrombostat sprays are used as necessary. If hemostasis cannot be achieved, a small drain should be brought out of the corner of the wound to prevent hematoma formation. A compression dressing is routinely used on the extremities.

c. A frozen section analysis is done on all biopsies to ensure that adequate diagnostic tissue is obtained. Prior to biopsy, the surgeon should review the radiographs with the pathologist to plan the biopsy site. When possible, the soft tissue component should be sampled, rather than the bony component.

d. It is an important tenet to remember that all biopsy samples should be submitted for bacteriologic analysis. Antibiotics should not be delivered until the cultures are obtained.

e. Needle biopsy is an excellent method to

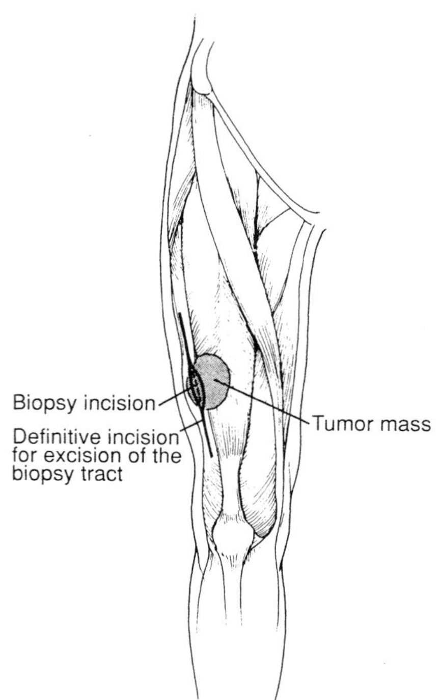

FIGURE 8–1. Lesion in the lateral aspect of the quadriceps mechanism. A short longitudinal incision is made over the lesion. Prior to incising the skin a second incision line should be drawn to demonstrate how the biopsy tract can be removed at the time of the definitive surgery. (From Sim, F.H., Frassica, F.J., and Frassica, D.A.: Soft tissue tumors: diagnosis, evaluation and management. AAOS 2(4):209, 1994; reprinted by permission.)

TABLE 8–5. LABORATORY EVALUATIONS FOR YOUNG AND MIDDLE-AGED PATIENTS

Age 5–30 Years
Complete blood count with differential
Peripheral blood smear
Erythrocyte sedimentation rate
Age 40–80 Years
Complete blood count with differential
Erythrocyte sedimentation rate
Chemistry group: calcium and phosphate
Serum or urine protein electrophoresis
Urinalysis

achieve a tissue diagnosis and provide for minimal tissue disruption. However, open biopsy remains the most reliable technique to avoid incorrect diagnoses. When the nature of the lesion is obvious based on the radiographic features and adequate tissue can be obtained with needle biopsy, the needle biopsy technique can be safely utilized. The pathologist must be experienced and comfortable with the small sample of tissue.

6. Surgical Procedures—The goal of treatment of malignant bone tumors is to remove the lesion with minimal risk of local recurrence. Limb salvage is performed when two essential criteria are met: (1) local control of the lesion must be at least equal to that of amputation surgery; and (2) the limb that has been saved must be functional. A wide surgical margin (a cuff of normal tissue around the tumor) is the surgical goal. Surgical procedures are graded according to the system of The Musculoskeletal Tumor Society (Fig. 8–2).
   a. Intralesional—The plane of dissection goes directly through the tumor. When dealing with malignant mesenchymal tumors, an intralesional margin results in 100% local recurrence.
   b. Marginal—A marginal line of resection goes through the reactive zone of the tumor; the reactive zone contains inflammatory cells, edema, fibrous tissue, and satellites of tumor cells. When resecting malignant mesenchymal tumors, a plane of dissection through the reactive zone will probably result in a local recurrence rate of 25–50%.
   c. Wide—A wide surgical resection is accomplished when the entire tumor is removed with a cuff of normal tissue. The local recurrence rate drops below 10% when such a surgical margin is achieved.

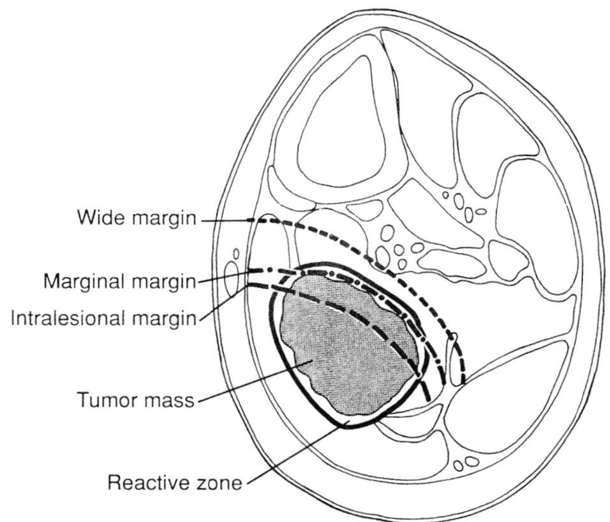

FIGURE 8–2. Types of surgical margin. An intralesional line of resection enters the substance of the tumor. A marginal line of resection travels through the reactive zone of the tumor. A wide surgical margin removes the tumor with a cuff of normal tissue. (From Sim, F.H., Frassica, F.J., and Frassica, D.A.: Soft tissue tumors: diagnosis, evaluation and management. AAOS 2(4):209, 1994; reprinted by permission.)

   d. Radical—A radical margin is achieved when the entire tumor and its compartment (all surrounding muscles, ligaments, and connective tissues) are removed.

7. Adjuvant Therapy
   a. Chemotherapy—Multiagent chemotherapy has a significant impact on both the efficacy of limb salvage and disease-free survival for osteogenic sarcoma and Ewing's tumor. Most protocols utilize preoperative regimens (called neoadjuvant chemotherapy) for 8–12 weeks. Patients are then restaged, and if appropriate limb salvage is performed. Patients then undergo maintenance chemotherapy for 6–12 months. Patients who present with localized disease have up to a 60–70% long-term disease-free survival with the combination of multiagent chemotherapy and surgery.
   b. Radiation Therapy—External beam irradiation is utilized for local control of Ewing's tumor, lymphoma, myeloma, and metastatic bone disease. It is also utilized as an adjunct for the treatment of soft tissue sarcomas, where it is used in combination with surgery. The role of surgery in the treatment of Ewing's tumor is evolving. In some centers chemotherapy and surgery are the major forms of treatment, whereas in others traditional chemotherapy and external beam irradiation are preferred.
      1. Postirradiation sarcoma is a devastating complication in which a spindle sarcoma occurs within the field of irradiation for a previous malignancy (e.g., Ewing's tumor, breast cancer, Hodgkin's disease). The histology is usually that of an osteosarcoma, fibrosarcoma, or malignant fibrous histiocytoma. Postirradiation sarcomas are probably more frequent in patients who undergo intensive chemotherapy (especially with alkylating agents) and irradiation.
      2. Late stress fractures also may occur in weight-bearing bones to which high-dose irradiation has been applied. The subtrochanteric region and the diaphysis of the femur are common sites.

II. Soft Tissue Tumors

A. Introduction—Soft tissue tumors are common. Patients may present with small lumps or large masses. Soft tissue tumors can be broadly classified as benign, malignant (sarcomas), or reactive tumor-like conditions (Table 8–6). Lesions are classified according to the direction of differentiation of the lesion—whether the tumor is tending to produce collagen (fibrous lesion), fat, or cartilage.
   1. Benign Soft Tissue Tumors—They may occur in all age groups. The lesions vary in their biologic behavior, from tumors that are asymptomatic and self-limited (Enneking stage 1—inactive) to growing and symptomatic (Enneking stage 2—active). Occasionally, benign lesions grow rapidly and invade adjacent tissues (Enneking stage 3—aggressive).
   2. Malignant Soft Tissue Tumors (Sarcomas)—Sarcomas are rare tumors of mesenchymal origin. In the United States each year there are approximately 5000 new cases of soft tissue sarcomas.

TABLE 8–6. CLASSIFICATION OF SOFT TISSUE TUMORS

Tumors and Tumor-Like Lesions of Fibrous Tissue

BENIGN

- Fibroma
- Nodular fasciitis
- Proliferative fasciitis

FIBROMATOSES

- Superficial fibromatoses
  - Palmar and plantar fibromatosis
  - Knuckle pads
- Deep fibromatoses (extraabdominal fibromatoses)

MALIGNANT

- Adult fibrosarcoma
- Postradiation fibrosarcoma

Fibrohistiocytic Tumors

BENIGN

- Fibrous histiocytoma
- Atypical fibroxanthoma

INTERMEDIATE (DERMATOFIBROSARCOMA PROTUBERANS)

MALIGNANT (MALIGNANT FIBROUS HISTIOCYTOMA)

- Storiform–pleomorphic
- Myxoid (myxofibrosarcoma)
- Giant cell (malignant giant cell tumor of soft parts)
- Inflammatory (malignant xanthogranuloma, xanthosarcoma)
- Angiomatoid

Tumors and Tumor-Like Conditions of Adipose Tissue

BENIGN

- Lipoma (cutaneous, deep, and multiple)
- Angiolipoma
- Spindle cell and pleomorphic lipoma
- Lipoblastoma and lipoblastomatosis
- Intramuscular and intermuscular lipoma
- Hibernoma

MALIGNANT

- Liposarcoma
  - Well differentiated (lipoma-like, sclerosing, inflammatory)
  - Myxoid
  - Round cell (poorly differentiated myxoid)
  - Pleomorphic
  - Dedifferentiated

Tumors of Muscle Tissue

SMOOTH MUSCLE

- Benign
  - Leiomyoma (cutaneous and deep)
  - Angiomyoma (vascular leiomyoma)
- Malignant (leiomyosarcoma)

STRIATED MUSCLE

- Benign (adult rhabdomyoma)
- Malignant (rhabdomyosarcoma—predominantly embryonal [including botryoid], alveolar, pleomorphic, and mixed)

Tumors and Tumor-Like Conditions of Blood Vessels

BENIGN

- Hemangioma
- Deep hemangioma (intramuscular, synovial, perineural)
- Glomus tumor

INTERMEDIATE (HEMANGIOENDOTHELIOMA)

MALIGNANT

- Hemangiosarcoma
- Malignant hemangiopericytoma

Tumors of Lymph Vessels

BENIGN (LYMPHANGIOMA)

- Cavernous
- Cystic (cystic hygroma)

MALIGNANT

- Lymphangiosarcoma
- Postmastectomy lymphangiosarcoma

Tumors and Tumor-Like Lesions of Synovial Tissue

BENIGN

- Giant cell tumor of tendon sheath
  - Localized (nodular tenosynovitis)
  - Diffuse (florid synovitis)

MALIGNANT

- Synovial sarcoma (malignant synovioma), predominantly biphasic (fibrous or epithelial) or monophasic (fibrous or epithelial)
- Malignant giant cell tumor of tendon sheath

Tumors and Tumor-Like Lesions of Peripheral Nerves

BENIGN

- Traumatic neuroma
- Morton's neuroma
- Neurilemoma (benign schwannoma)
- Neurofibroma, solitary
- Neurofibromatosis (von Recklinghausen's disease)
  - Localized
  - Plexiform
  - Diffuse

MALIGNANT

- Malignant schwannoma
- Peripheral tumors of primitive neuroectodermal tissues

Tumors and Tumor-Like Lesions of Cartilage and Bone-Forming Tissues

BENIGN

- Panniculitis ossificans
- Myositis ossificans
- Fibrodysplasia (myositis) ossificans progressiva
- Extraskeletal chondroma
- Extraskeletal osteoma

MALIGNANT

- Extraskeletal chondrosarcoma
  - Well differentiated
  - Myxoid (choroid sarcoma)
  - Mesenchymal
- Extraskeletal osteosarcoma

Tumors and Tumor-Like Lesions of Pluripotential Mesenchyme

- Benign mesenchymoma
- Malignant mesenchymoma

Tumors and Tumor-Like Conditions of Disputed or Uncertain Histogenesis

BENIGN

- Tumoral calcinosis
- Myxoma (cutaneous and intramuscular)

MALIGNANT

- Alveolar soft-part sarcoma
- Epithelioid sarcoma
- Clear cell sarcoma of tendons and aponeuroses
- Extraskeletal Ewing's sarcoma

Unclassified Soft Tissue Tumors and Tumor-Like Lesions

Adapted from Enzinger, F.M., and Weiss, S.W.: Soft Tissue Tumors, pp. 6–7. St. Louis, CV Mosby, 1983; reprinted by permission.

Patients often present with an enlarging painless or painful soft tissue mass. Most sarcomas are large (>5 cm), deep, and firm in character. In some instances they are small and may be present for a long time prior to recognition. Lesions that may be initially small include synovial sarcoma, epithelioid sarcoma, and clear cell sarcoma. Initial radiographic evaluation begins with plain radiographs in two planes. MRI scans are the best imaging modality to define the anatomy and to help characterize the lesion. When a mass is judged to be indeterminate, an open incisional or needle biopsy is performed. Radiation therapy is an important adjunct to surgery in the treatment of soft tissue sarcomas. The ionizing irradiation can be delivered preoperative, perioperatively with brachytherapy after-loading tubes, or postoperatively. Treatment regimens are often designed to use combinations of the three former types.

B. Tumors of Fibrous Tissue—Fibrous tumors are common, and there is a wide range, from small self-limited benign conditions to aggressive, invasive benign tumors. The malignant fibrous tumors are fibrosarcoma and malignant fibrous histiocytoma.

1. Calcifying Aponeurotic Fibroma—This entity presents as a slowly growing, painless mass in the hands and feet in children and young adults, ages 3–30 (Enzinger). Radiographs may reveal a faint mass with stippling. Histologic examination shows a fibrous tumor with centrally located areas of calcification and cartilage formation. Local excision often results in recurrence (in up to 50% of cases); however, the condition appears to resolve with maturity.
2. Fibromatosis
   a. Palmar (Dupuytren's) and Plantar (Ledderhosen) Fibromatosis—These disorders consist of firm nodules of fibroblasts and collagen that develop in the palmar and plantar fascia. The nodules and fascia hypertrophy, producing contractures.
   b. Extra-abdominal Desmoid Tumor—It is the most locally invasive of all benign soft tissue tumors. It commonly occurs in adolescents and young adults. On palpation, the tumor has a distinctive "rock hard" character. Multiple lesions may be present in the same extremity. Histologically, the tumor consists of well differentiated fibroblasts and abundant collagen. The lesion infiltrates adjacent tissues. Surgical treatment is aimed at resecting the tumor with a wide margin. Local recurrence is common. Radiotherapy has been used as an adjunct to prevent recurrence and progression. The behavior of the tumor is capricious in that recurrent nodules may remain dormant for years or grow rapidly for some time and stop growing.
3. Nodular Fascitis—It is a common reactive lesion that presents as a painful, rapidly enlarging mass in a young person (age 15–35 years). Half of the cases occur in the upper extremity. Histologically, the lesion is characterized by short, irregular bundles and fascicles, a dense reticulum network, and only small amounts of mature collagen. Mitotic figures are common, but atypical mitoses are never seen. Treatment consists in excision with a marginal line of resection.
4. Malignant Fibrous Soft Tissue Tumors—Malignant fibrous histiocytoma (MFH) and fibrosarcoma are the two malignant fibrous lesions. They have a similar clinical and radiographic presentation and are treated in a similar manner. Patients are generally between the ages of 30 and 80 years. The most common presentation is an enlarging, rather painless mass. When the mass reaches a substantial size (>10 cm) the patient often experiences symptoms. Plain radiographs are usually normal, except in advanced cases where there may be bone erosion or destruction. MRI often shows a deep-seated inhomogeneous mass. Histologically, the two lesions may be similar, but there are distinctive features. In MFH the spindle and histiocytic cells are arranged in a storiform (cartwheel) pattern. There are short fascicles of cells and fibrous tissue that appear to radiate about a common center around slit-like vessels (Enzinger). Chronic inflammatory cells may also be present. With fibrosarcoma, there is a fasciculated growth pattern with fusiform or spindle-shaped cells, scanty cytoplasm, and indistinct borders; and the cells are separated by interwoven collagen fibers (Enzinger). In some cases, the tissue is organized into a herringbone pattern, which consists of intersecting fascicles where the nuclei in one fascicle is viewed transversely, whereas in an adjacent fascicle they are viewed longitudinally. Treatment is wide local excision. Radiation therapy is employed in many cases when the size of the tumor exceeds 5 cm. A common scenario is to deliver radiation preoperatively (5000–5500 cGy) followed by resection of the lesion. A final radiation boost (2000 cGy) is then given postoperatively or perioperatively with brachytherapy afterloading tubes.
5. Dermatofibrosarcoma Protuberans (DFSP)—DFSP is a rare, nodular, cutaneous tumor that occurs in early to midadult life (Enzinger). The lesion is intermediate in grade. It has a tendency to recur locally, but it only rarely metastasizes, often after repeated local recurrences (Enzinger). In 40% of the cases it occurs on the upper or lower extremities (Enzinger). The tumor grows slowly but progressively. The central portion of the nodules show uniform fibroblasts arranged in a storiform pattern around an inconspicuous vasculature. Wide resection is the best form of treatment.

C. Tumors of Fatty Tissue—There is a wide spectrum of benign and malignant tumors of fat origin. Each has a particular biologic behavior, which guides evaluation and treatment.

1. Lipomas—Lipomas are common benign tumors of mature fat. They may occur in a subcutaneous, intramuscular, or intermuscular location. Patients often describe a long history of a mass and sometimes a mass that was only recently discovered. Most are not painful. Plain radiographs may show a radiolucent lesion in the soft tissues. CT or MRI shows a well demarcated lesion with the same signal characteristics as mature fat on all sequences. If the patient experiences no symptoms and the radiographic features are diagnostic of lipoma, no treatment is necessary. If the mass is growing or causing symptoms, excision with a marginal line of resection is all that is necessary. Local recurrence is uncommon. There are several variants of which the surgeon must be aware.

a. Spindle Cell Lipoma—This entity commonly occurs in male patients (age 45–65 years). The tumor presents as a solitary, painless, growing, firm nodule. Histologically, one sees a mixture of mature fat cells and spindle cells. There is a mucoid matrix with a varying number of birefringement collagen fibers (Enzinger). Treatment is excision with a marginal margin.

b. Pleomorphic Lipoma—This lesion is common in middle-aged patients and presents as a slowly growing mass. Histologically, there are lipocytes, spindle cells, and scattered bizarre giant cells. The lesion may be confused with different types of liposarcoma. Treatment is excision with a marginal margin.

2. Liposarcoma—Liposarcomas are sarcomas in which the direction of differentiation is toward fatty tissue. They comprise a heterogeneous group of tumors, having in common the presence of lipoblasts (signet ring-type cells) in the tissue. Liposarcomas are classified into several types.

Well differentiated liposarcoma
- Lipoma-like
- Sclerosing
- Inflammatory
- Dedifferentiated

Myxoid liposarcoma
- Round cell liposarcoma
- Pleomorphic liposarcoma

Liposarcomas range in biologic behavior from very low grade tumors (well differentiated) to very high grade tumors (poorly differentiated). Well differentiated liposarcomas can be difficult to distinguish from benign lipomas. The name well differentiated lipoma, like liposarcoma, attests to this difficulty (grade 1 liposarcoma). Grade 1 liposarcomas virtually never metastasize. Other authors believe these lesions are benign and classify them as an "atypical lipoma." High grade liposarcomas behave similarly to other high grade sarcomas, with a propensity for local recurrence and metastasis. Low grade lesions are treated with wide local resection. Radiotherapy is utilized as an adjunct depending on the adequacy of the surgical margin. High grade liposarcomas are treated with both wide excision and radiotherapy for large lesions (>5 cm).

D. Tumors of Neural Tissue—The two benign neural tumors are neurilemoma and neurofibroma. Their malignant counterpart is neurofibrosarcoma.

1. Neurilemoma (Benign Schwannoma)—This lesion is a benign nerve sheath tumor. It occurs in the young to middle-aged adult (20–50 years) and is usually asymptomatic except for the presence of the mass. The tumor grows slowly and may wax and wane in size (cystic change). MRI studies demonstrate an eccentric mass arising from a peripheral nerve. Histologically, the lesion is composed of Antoni A and B areas.

a. Antoni A—Compact spindled cells, usually having twisted nuclei, indistinct cytoplasm, and occasionally clear intranuclear vacuoles. When the lesion is highly differentiated there may be nuclear palisading, whorling of cells, and Verocay bodies.

b. Antoni B—Less orderly and cellular, the cells are arranged haphazardly in the loosely textured matrix (with microcystic change, inflammatory cells, and delicate collagen fibers); large irregularly spaced vessels.

c. When the lesion is predominantly cellular, (Antoni A), the tumor may be confused with a sarcoma.

Treatment consists in removing the eccentric mass while leaving the nerve intact.

2. Neurofibroma—It may be solitary or multiple (neurofibromatosis). Most are superficial, grow slowly, and are painless. When they involve a major nerve, they may expand it in a fusiform fashion. Histologically, there are interlacing bundles of elongated cells with wavy, dark-staining nuclei. The cells are associated with wire-like strands of collagen (Enzinger). Small to moderate amounts of mucoid material separate the cells and collagen. Treatment consists in excision with a marginal margin. Neurofibromatosis (von Recklinghausen's disease) is an autosomal dominant (AD) trait, with both a peripheral and central form of the disease. In addition to neurofibromas, patients have café au lait spots and variable skeletal abnormalities (nonossifying fibromas, scoliosis, and long-bone bowing). Malignant change occurs in 5–30% of patients.

3. Neurofibrosarcoma—These lesions are rare tumors that arise de novo or in the setting of neurofibromatosis. Neurofibrosarcomas are high grade sarcomas and are treated in similar fashion to other high grade sarcomas.

E. Tumors of Muscle Tissue—They are uncommon tumors ranging from benign leiomyoma and rhabdomyoma to the malignant entities of leiomyosarcoma and rhabdomyosarcoma. The benign entities seldom occur on the extremities.

1. Leiomyosarcoma—It may present as a small nodule or a large extremity mass. The lesions may or may not be associated with blood vessels. They may be either low or high grade and are treated as other low and high grade sarcomas.

2. Rhabdomyosarcoma—This highly malignant tumor is most common in young patients (<20 years of age). The tumor is the most common sarcoma in young patients and may grow rapidly. Histologically, the lesion is composed of spindle cells in parallel bundles, multinucleated giant cells, and racquet-shaped cells. The histologic hallmark is the appearance of cross striations within the tumor cells (rhabdomyoblasts). Rhabdomyoblasts may be difficult to find. Rhabdomyosarcomas are sensitive to multiagent chemotherapy. Wide surgical resection is performed after induction chemotherapy. External beam irradiation plays a prominent role in this tumor.

F. Vascular Tumors—Hemangiomas and glomus tumors are the two principal benign entities, and hemangiopericytoma and angiosarcoma are the less common malignant entities.

1. Hemangioma—This soft tissue tumor is commonly seen in children and adults. The lesion may occur in a cutaneous, subcutaneous, or intramuscular location. Patients with large tumors complain of symptoms of vascular engorgement (aching, heaviness, swelling). MRI scans demonstrate a heterogeneous lesion with numerous small blood vessels and fatty infiltration. The plain radiograph may reveal small phleboliths.

Nonoperative treatment is chosen if local measures adequately control discomfort: NSAIDs, vascular stockings, and activity modification. Wide surgical resection is utilized for resistant cases, but the local recurrence rate is high.

2. Hemangiopericytoma—This rare tumor of the pericytes of blood vessels appears in benign and malignant forms. Within the malignant group there is a morphologic range from intermediate to high grade malignancy. Patients present with a slowly enlarging painless mass. Treatment is based on the grade of the lesion.
3. Angiosarcoma—In these rare tumors the tumor cells resemble the endothelium of blood vessels. Treatment depends on the grade and location of the lesion.

G. Synovial Disorders—These entities include benign conditions, such as ganglia, and synovial proliferative disorders, such as pigmented villonodular synovitis (PVNS) and synovial chondromatosis.

1. Ganglia—It presents as an outpouching of the synovial lining of an adjacent joint. The most common locations include the wrist, foot, and knee. The cyst is filled with gelatinous, mucoid material. Histologically, the cyst wall is made up of paucicellular connective tissue without a true epithelial lining.
2. Pigmented Villonodular Synovitis—This reactive condition (not a true neoplasm) is characterized by an exuberant proliferation of synovial villi and nodules. The process may occur locally within a joint or diffusely. The knee is most commonly affected, followed by the hip and shoulder. Patients present with pain and swelling in the affected joint. Arthrocentesis demonstrates a bloody effusion. Cystic erosions may occur on both sides of the joint. Histologically, there are highly vascular villi lined with plump, hyperplastic synovial cells, hemosiderin-stained multinucleated giant cells, and chronic inflammatory cells. Treatment is aimed at complete synovectomy. Local recurrence is common.
3. Giant Cell Tumor of Tendon Sheath—This benign, nodular tumor occurs along the tendon sheaths of the hands and feet. Histologically, the lesion is moderately cellular (sheets of rounded or polygonal cells). There are hypocellular collagenized zones (Enzinger). Multinucleated giant cells are common, as are xanthoma cells. Treatment consists in resection with a marginal margin.
4. Synovial Chondromatosis—This lesion may occur within a joint, ranging in appearance from metaplasia of the synovial tissue to firm nodules of cartilage. The lesion typically affects young adults who present with pain, stiffness, and swelling. Radiographs may demonstrate fine stippled calcification. Treatment consists in removing the loose bodies and synovectomy.
5. Synovial Sarcoma—This highly malignant tumor occurs in close proximity to joints but rarely arises from an intra-articular location. The tumor may be present for years or present as a rapidly enlarging mass. Radiographs may show mineralization within the lesion (in up to 25% of cases). Histologically, the tumor is biphasic, with an epithelial component and a spindle cell component. The epithelial component may show epithelial cells that form glands or nests, or they may line cyst-like spaces. Regional lymph nodes may be involved. All synovial sarcomas are high-grade lesions. Wide surgical resection with adjuvant radiotherapy is the most common method of treatment.

H. Other Rare Sarcomas

1. Epithelioid Sarcoma—This rare nodular tumor commonly occurs in the hands of young adults. It may also occur about the buttock/thigh, knee, or foot. The lesion may ulcerate and mimic a granuloma or rheumatoid nodule. Lymph node metastases may occur. Histologically, the cells range from ovoid to polygonal with deeply eosinophilic cytoplasm (Enzinger). Cellular pleomorphism is minimal. The lesions are often misdiagnosed as benign processes. Wide surgical resection is necessary to prevent local recurrence.
2. Clear Cell Sarcoma—This tumor presents as a slowly growing mass associated with tendons or aponeuroses. The lesion most commonly occurs about the foot and ankle but may also involve the knee, thigh, or hand. Microscopically, it is characterized by compact nests or fascicles of rounded or fusiform cells with clear cytoplasm (Enzinger). Multinucleated giant cells are common. Wide surgical resection with adjuvant irradiation is the treatment of choice.
3. Alveolar Cell Sarcoma—It presents as a slowly growing, painless mass in young adults (age 15–35 years). It most commonly occurs in the anterior thigh. Microscopically, it appears as dense fibrous trabeculae dividing the tumor into an organoid or nest-like arrangement (Enzinger). Cells are large and rounded and contain one or more vesicular nuclei with small nucleoli. Vascular invasion is prominent. Treatment is wide surgical resection, with adjuvant irradiation in selected cases.

I. Posttraumatic Conditions

1. Hematoma—Hematomas may occur after trauma to the extremity. The lesions organize and resolve with time.
2. Myositis Ossificans (Heterotopic Ossification)—It occurs after single or repetitive episodes of trauma. Occasionally, patients cannot recall the traumatic episode. The most common locations are over the diaphyseal segment of long bones (in the midaspect of the muscle bellies). As maturation progresses, radiographs show peripheral mineralization with a central lucent area. In most cases the lesion is not attached to the underlying bone; but in some cases it may become fixed to the periosteal surface. Histologically, there is a zonal pattern with mature, trabecular bone at the periphery and immature tissue in the center. When the diagnosis is apparent, nonoperative treatment is all that is necessary.

III. Bone Tumors

A. Introduction—All bone lesions can be subdivided into three groups: benign bone neoplasms, malignant bone neoplasms, and nonneoplastic lesions (also called tumor-like conditions, tumor simulators, and reactive conditions). One can further subclassify lesions into processes that begin in the bone (intramedullary lesions) and processes that clearly begin outside the intramedullary cavity (surface lesions).

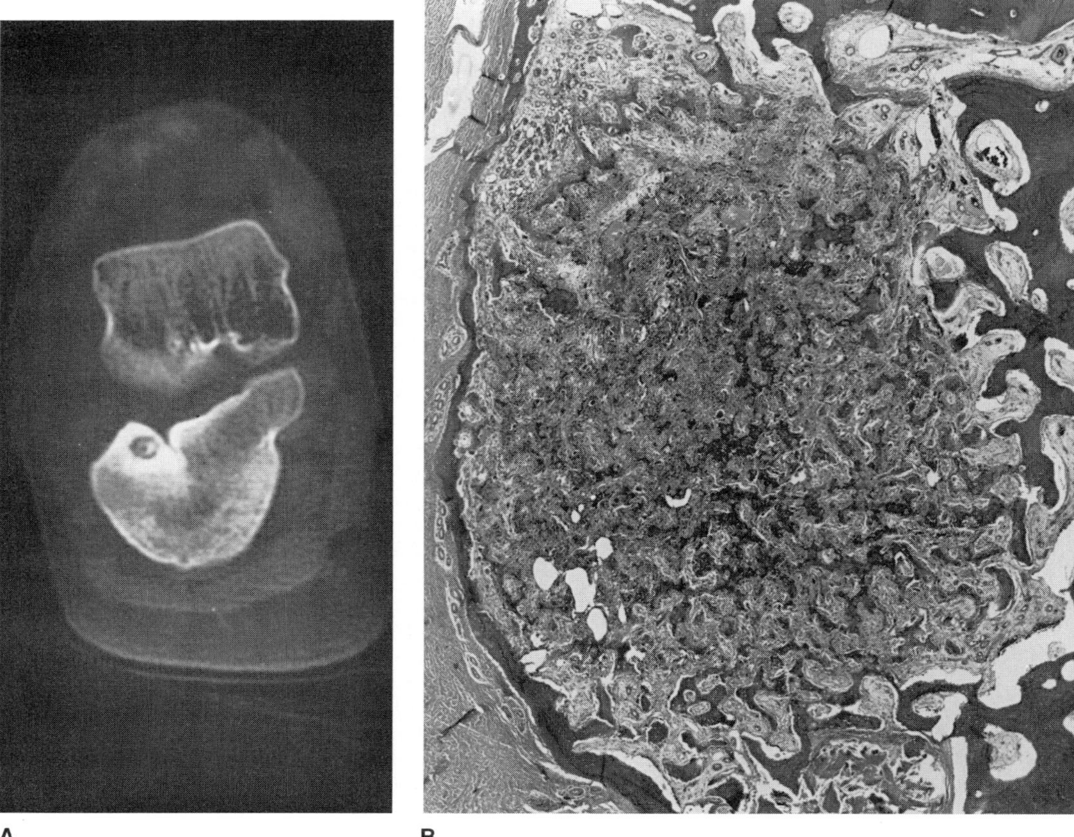

A B

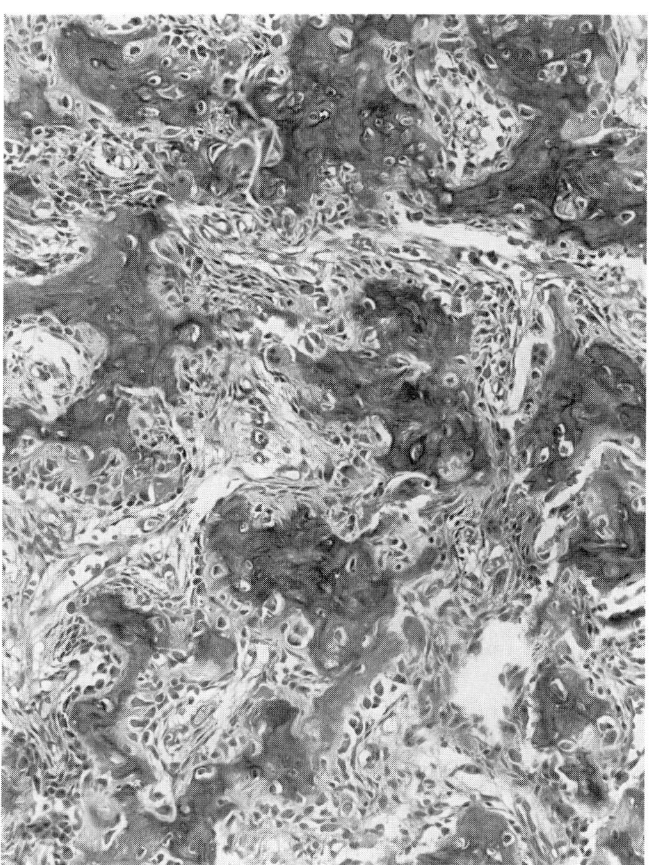

C

FIGURE 8–3. Osteoid osteoma of the calcaneus. *A*, Radiograph shows a well circumscribed lytic lesion with dense surrounding bone and a central nidus. *B*, Low power photomicrograph (×25) shows the nidus. *C*, Higher power photomicrograph (×160) shows mineralizing new bone with a loose fibrovascular stroma.

B. Bone-Producing Lesions—There are only three lesions where the tumor cells produce osteoid: osteoid osteoma, osteoblastoma, and osteosarcoma.

1. Osteoid Osteoma (Fig. 8–3)—This self-limited benign bone lesion produces pain in young patients (ages 5–30 years, although all age groups may be affected). Patients present with pain that increases with time. Most patients have pain at night, which may be strikingly relieved by salicylates. The pain may be referred to an adjacent joint; and when the lesion is intracapsular, it may simulate arthritis. The tumor may produce painful scoliosis, growth disturbances, and flexion contractures. The radiographs usually show intensely reactive bone and a radiolucent nidus. It may be possible to detect the lesion only with special studies, such as tomograms or CT or MRI scans, because of the intense sclerosis. The nidus is by definition always <1.5 cm, although the area of reactive bone sclerosis may be quite long. Technetium bone scans are always positive and show intense focal uptake. Microscopically, there is a distinct demarcation between the nidus and the reactive bone. The nidus consists of an interlacing network of osteoid trabeculae with variable mineralization. The trabecular organization is haphazard, and the greatest degree of mineralization is in the center of the lesion. Treatment consists in complete removal of the nidus (en bloc excision) or curettage of the nidus with hand and power instruments.
2. Osteoblastoma (Fig. 8–4)—This rare bone-producing tumor can attain a large size and is not self-limited as is osteoid osteoma. Patients present with pain; and when the lesion involves the spine, neurologic symptoms may be present. Radiographically, there is bone destruction with or without the characteristic reactive bone formation seen with osteoid osteoma. The bone destruction occasionally has a moth-eaten or permeative character simulating a malignancy. Histologically, the lesions shows regularly shaped nuclei containing little chromatin but with abundant cytoplasm (Dahlin). The tissue is loosely arranged with numerous blood vessels. The lesion does not permeate the normal trabecula bone but, rather, merges with them. Treatment consists in excision with at least a marginal line of resection.
3. Osteosarcoma—Spindle cell neoplasms that produce osteoid are arbitrarily classified as osteosarcomas. There are many types of osteosarcoma (Table 8–7). The lesions that must be recognized (in order to have a reasonable grasp on the entity osteosarcoma) include high grade intramedullary osteosarcoma (ordinary or classic osteosarcoma), parosteal osteosarcoma, periosteal osteosarcoma, osteosarcoma occurring with Paget's disease, and osteosarcoma following irradiation.
   a. High Grade Intramedullary Osteosarcoma (Fig. 8–5)—Also called ordinary or classic osteosarcoma, it is the most common type of osteosarcoma and most commonly occurs about the knee in children and young adults. Other common sites include the proximal humerus, proximal femur, and pelvis. Patients present primarily with pain. More than 90% of intramedullary osteosarcomas are high grade and penetrate the cortex early to form a soft tissue mass (stage II-B lesion). About 10–20% of patients have pulmonary metastases at presentation. Plain radiographs demonstrate a lesion in which there is both bone destruction and bone formation. Occasionally, the lesion is purely sclerotic or lytic. MRI or CT scans are useful for defining the anatomy of the lesion in regard to intramedullary extension, involvement of neurovascular structures, and muscle invasion. Histologically, two criteria are utilized: (1) the tumor cells produce osteoid; and (2) the stroma cells are frankly malignant. The lesions may be highly heterogeneous in appearance, with some lesions being predominantly chondroblastic, osteoblastic, or fibroblastic. Other lesions may contain large numbers of giant cells or predominantly small cells rather than spindle cells. Telangiectatic osteosarcoma is a type in which the lesional tissue can be described as a bag of blood with few cellular elements. The cellular elements present are highly malignant in appearance. The radiographic features of telangiectatic osteosarcoma are those of a destructive, lytic, expansile lesion. The historical treatment of osteosarcoma was amputation. Historically, long-term studies show a survival of only 10–20%, with the pulmonary system being the most common site of failure. Multiagent chemotherapy has dramatically improved long-term survival and the potential for limb salvage. It effectively destroys the malignant cells, and in many patients there is total necrosis of the tumor. The response both kills the micrometastases that are present in 80–90% of the patients at presentation and sterilizes the reactive zone around the tumor. Preoperative chemotherapy is delivered for 8–12 weeks, followed by resection of the tumor. Staging studies are performed at the end of chemotherapy to ensure that the lesion is resectable. Maintenance chemotherapy is then given for 6–12 months. Long-term survival is approximately 60–70% with these regimens.
   b. Parosteal Osteosarcoma (Fig. 8–6)—This low grade osteosarcoma occurs on the surface of the metaphysis of long bones. Patients often complain of a painless mass. The most common sites are the posterior aspect of the distal femur, proximal tibia, and proximal humerus;

TABLE 8–7. CLASSIFICATION OF OSTEOSARCOMA

High grade central osteosarcoma
Low grade central osteosarcoma
Telangiectatic osteosarcoma
Surface osteosarcomas
Parosteal osteosarcoma
Periosteal osteosarcoma
High grade surface osteosarcoma
Osteosarcoma of the jaw
Multicentric osteosarcoma
Secondary osteosarcomas
Osteosarcoma in Paget's disease
Postradiation osteosarcoma
Dedifferentiated chondrosarcoma
Osteosarcoma derived from benign precursors

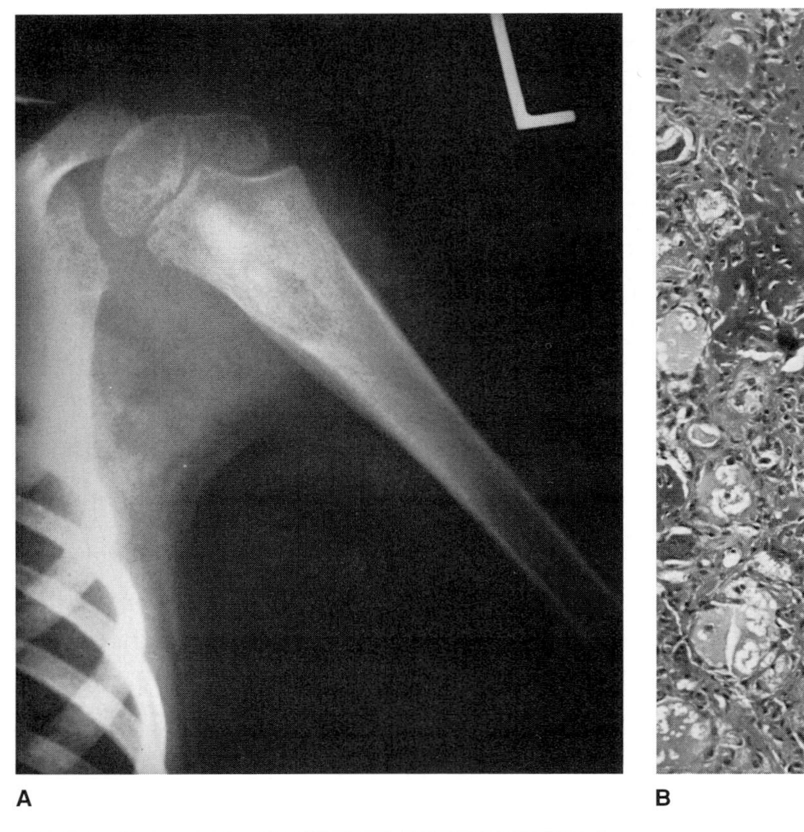

A

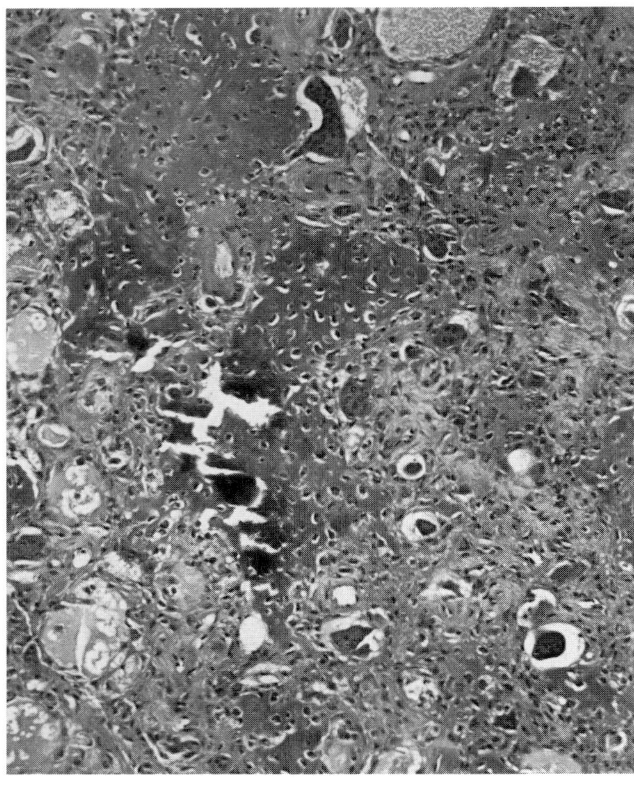

B

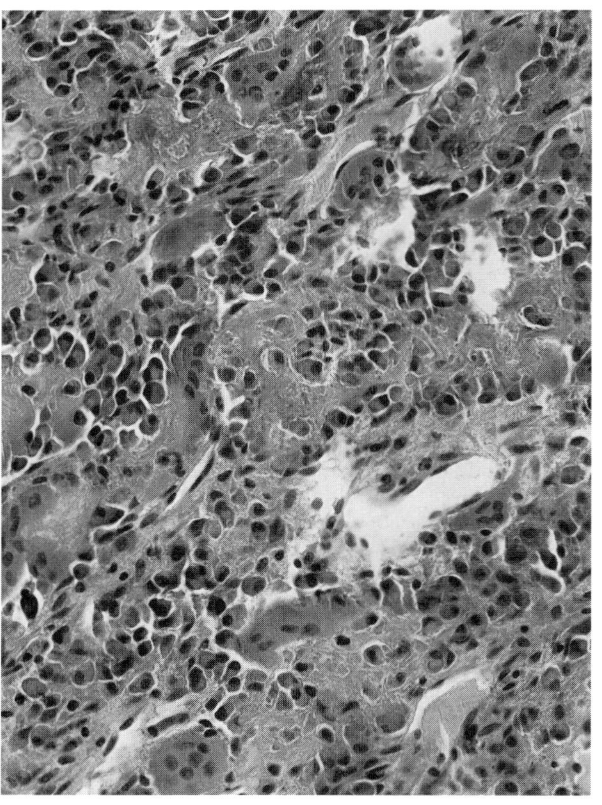

C

FIGURE 8–4. Osteoblastoma of the proximal humerus. *A*, Radiograph shows a well circumscribed lytic lesion in the proximal humerus. *B*, Low power photomicrograph (×100) shows abundant sheets of mineralizing osteoid. *C*, Higher power photomicrograph (×250) shows seams of osteoid and plasmacytoid osteoblasts.

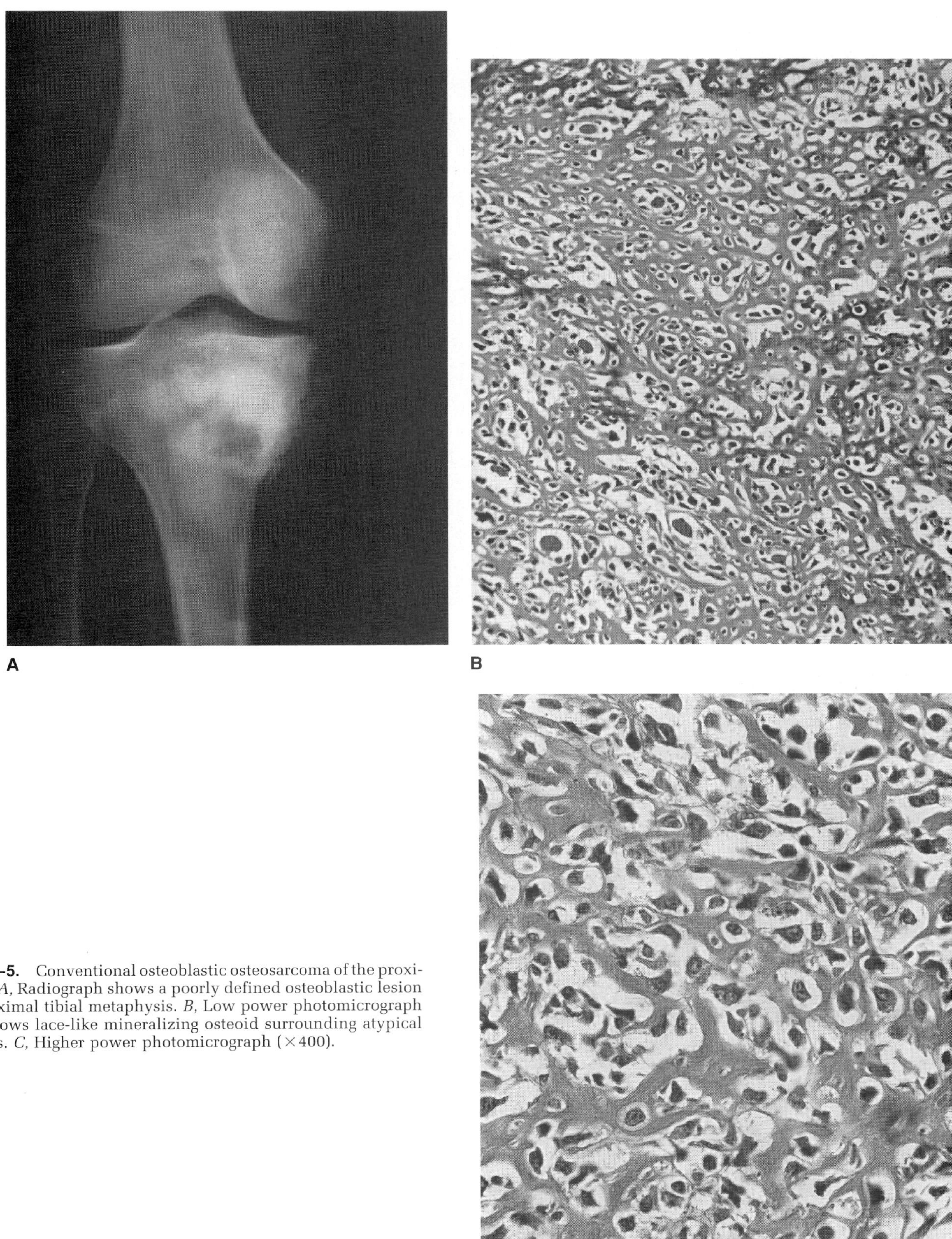

FIGURE 8–5. Conventional osteoblastic osteosarcoma of the proximal tibia. *A*, Radiograph shows a poorly defined osteoblastic lesion in the proximal tibial metaphysis. *B*, Low power photomicrograph (×160) shows lace-like mineralizing osteoid surrounding atypical osteoblasts. *C*, Higher power photomicrograph (×400).

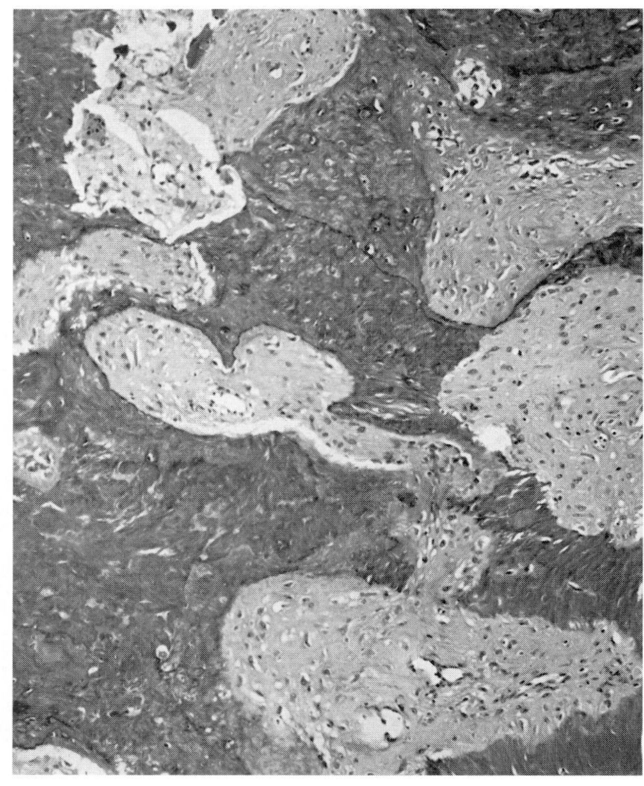

A

B

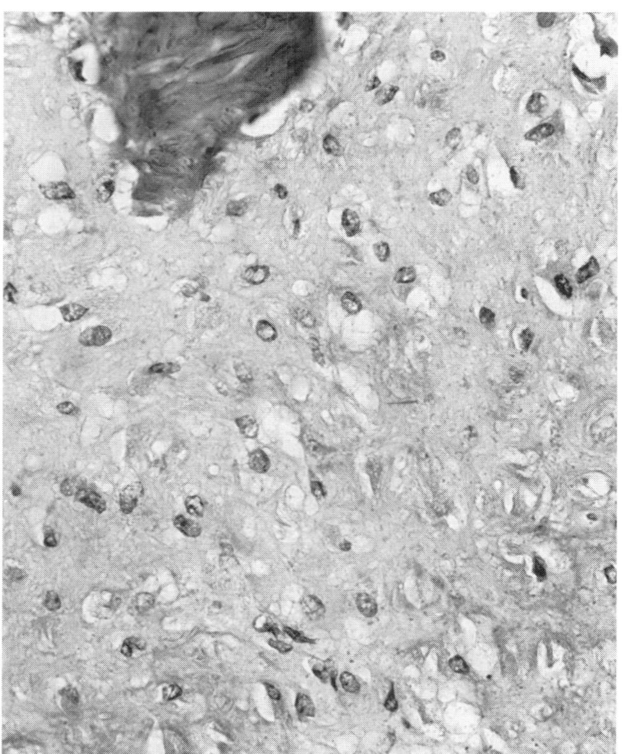

C

FIGURE 8–6. Parosteal osteosarcoma of the distal femur. *A*, Radiograph shows an exophytic bony mass in the posterior distal femur. *B*, Low power photomicrograph (×160) shows plates of new bone in a fibrous matrix. *C*, Higher power photomicrograph (×400) shows a fibrous stroma with atypical cells.

the lesion is more common in females than males. The radiographic appearance is characteristic in that it demonstrates a heavily ossified, often lobulated mass arising from the cortex. Histologically, the most prominent feature is regularly arranged osseous trabeculae (Dahlin). Between the nearly normal trabeculae are slightly atypical spindle cells. At the periphery of the tumor are spindle cells, which typically invade skeletal muscle. Interestingly, cartilage is frequently present and may be arranged as a cap over the lesion. Treatment of parosteal osteosarcoma is wide surgical resection, which is usually curative. In approximately one-sixth of the lesions that radiographically appear to be parosteal osteosarcoma, there is a high grade component. In this setting the lesion is called a dedifferentiated parosteal osteosarcoma. For typical low grade parosteal osteosarcomas chemotherapy or irradiation are not needed; however, the prognosis is much worse for dedifferentiated parosteal osteosarcomas, and multiagent chemotherapy is an important component of therapy.

c. Periosteal Osteosarcoma (Fig. 8–7)—This rare surface form of osteosarcoma occurs most commonly in the diaphysis of long bones (typically the femur or tibia). The radiographic appearance is fairly constant; a sunburst type lesion rests on a saucerized cortical depression. Histologically, the lesion is predominantly chondroblastic, and the grade of the lesion is intermediate (grade 2 or 3). Highly anaplastic regions are not found. The prognosis for periosteal osteosarcoma is intermediate between parosteal osteosarcoma (very low grade) and high grade intramedullary osteosarcoma. Preoperative chemotherapy, wide surgical resection, and maintenance chemotherapy comprise the preferred treatment.

C. Chondrogenic Lesions—The principal benign cartilage lesions are chondromas, osteochondroma, chondromyxoid fibroma, and chondroblastoma. The common malignant cartilage tumors are intramedullary chondrosarcoma and dedifferentiated chondrosarcoma. Clear cell chondrosarcoma and mesenchymal chondrosarcoma are rare forms.

1. Chondromas (Fig. 8–8)—These benign cartilage tumors may occur in the medullary cavity or on the surface of the bone (periosteal chondroma). Enchondromas are benign cartilage lesion that are most commonly localized in the metaphysis of long bones. They are common in the hand, where they usually occur in the diaphysis (Dahlin). Pathologic fractures in the hand are common. Involvement of the epiphysis is rare. Most enchondromas are asymptomatic. Radiographically, in long bones there may be a prominent stippled or mottled calcified appearance. Occasionally, active lesions are purely lytic without evidence of mineralization. Most enchondromas require no treatment other than observation. Histologically, they are composed of small cells that lie in lacunar spaces. The lesion is usually hypocellular, and the cells have a bland appearance (no pleomorphism, anaplasia, or hyperchromasia). In contrast, lesions in the hand may be hypercellular and display worrisome histologic features. When lesions are not causing pain, serial radiographs are obtained to ensure that the lesions are inactive (not growing). Radiographs are obtained at 3 months and 1 year after presentation. In contrast, periosteal chondromas occur on the surface of long bones (Fig. 8–9). Usually, there is a well demarcated cortical defect and a slight overhang of the cortical edges. The lesion usually demonstrates a mineralized cartilaginous matrix, although some lesions have no apparent mineralization. When surgical treatment is necessary, enchondromas are treated by curettage and bone grafting. Periosteal chondromas are usually excised with a marginal margin. Enchondromas may be multiple in the same extremity. When there are many lesions, when the involved bones are dysplastic, and the lesions tend to unilaterality, the diagnosis of multiple enchondromatosis, or Ollier's disease, is made. If soft tissue angiomas are also present, the patient has Maffucci syndrome. Chondrosarcomas virtually never occur in the setting of a previous enchondroma; however, patients with multiple enchondromatosis are at increased risk (Ollier's disease, 30%; Maffucci syndrome, 100%). Patients with multiple enchondromatosis also have an increased risk of visceral malignancies, such as astrocytomas, and gastrointestinal malignancies.
2. Osteochondroma (Fig. 8–10)—These benign surface lesions probably arise secondary to aberrant cartilage on the surface of bone (Dahlin). Patients usually present with a painless mass or, incidentally, when a radiograph is obtained for another reason. The characteristic appearance is a surface lesion in which the cortex of the lesion and the underlying cortex is continuous; the medullary cavity of the host bone also flows into (is continuous) with the osteochondroma. The osteochondroma may have a narrow stalk (pedunculated) or a broad base (sessile). These lesions typically occur at the site of tendon insertions, and the affected bone is abnormally wide (Dahlin). Histologically, the underlying cortex is covered by a thin cap of cartilage. Grossly, the cartilage cap is usually only 2–3 mm thick. In a growing child the cap may exceed 1–2 cm. Histologically, the chondrocytes are arranged in linear clusters with an appearance resembling that of the normal physis. When asymptomatic, these lesions are treated with observation only. Patients may experience pain secondary to muscle irritation, mechanical trauma (contusions), or an inflamed bursa over the lesion. In this scenario, excision is a logical alternative. Pain in the absence of mechanical factors is a warning sign of malignant change. The development of a sarcoma in an osteochondroma is rare, far less than 1%. The plain radiograph must be carefully inspected to exclude malignant change. Destruction of the subchondral bone, mineralization of a soft tissue mass, and an inhomogeneous appearance are radiographic changes of malignant transformation. When a malignant change occurs, a low grade chondrosarcoma is usually present, although a dedifferentiated chondrosarcoma may rarely occur.
3. Chondroblastoma (Fig. 8–11)—This benign cartilage tumor is centered in the epiphysis in young

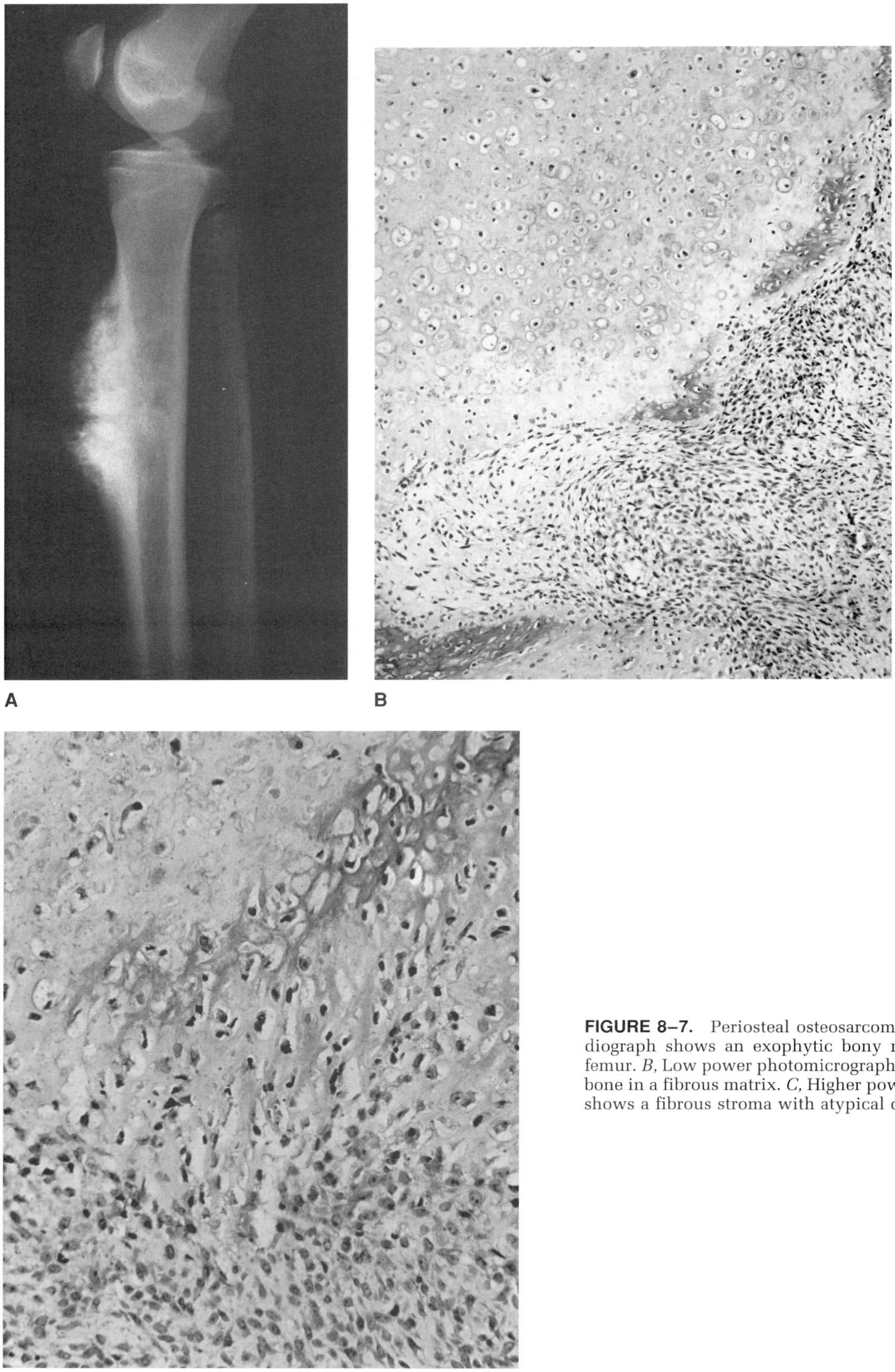

A B

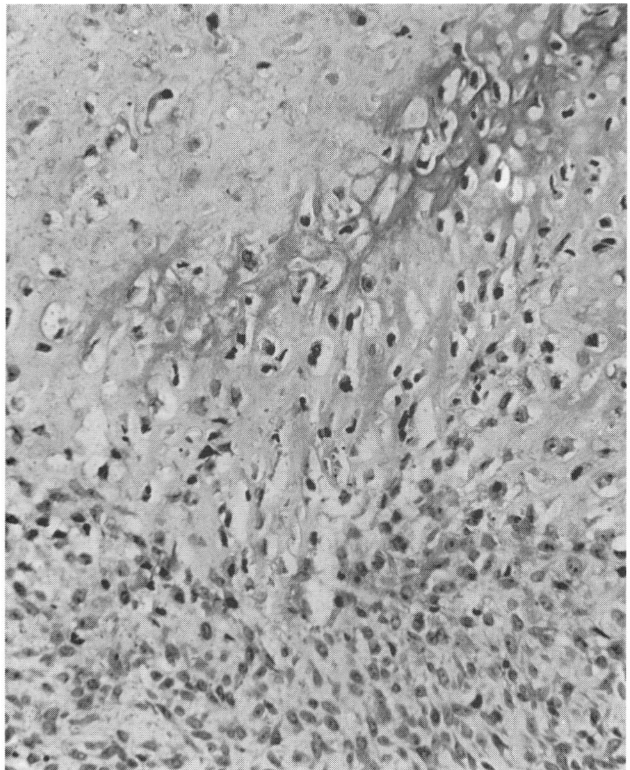

C

FIGURE 8–7. Periosteal osteosarcoma of the distal femur. *A,* Radiograph shows an exophytic bony mass in the posterior distal femur. *B,* Low power photomicrograph (×160) shows plates of new bone in a fibrous matrix. *C,* Higher power photomicrograph (×400) shows a fibrous stroma with atypical cells.

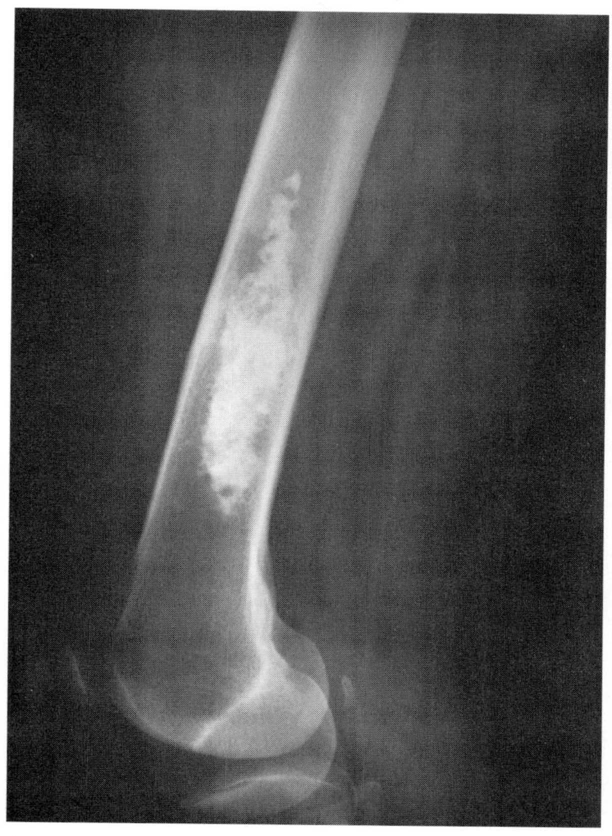

A

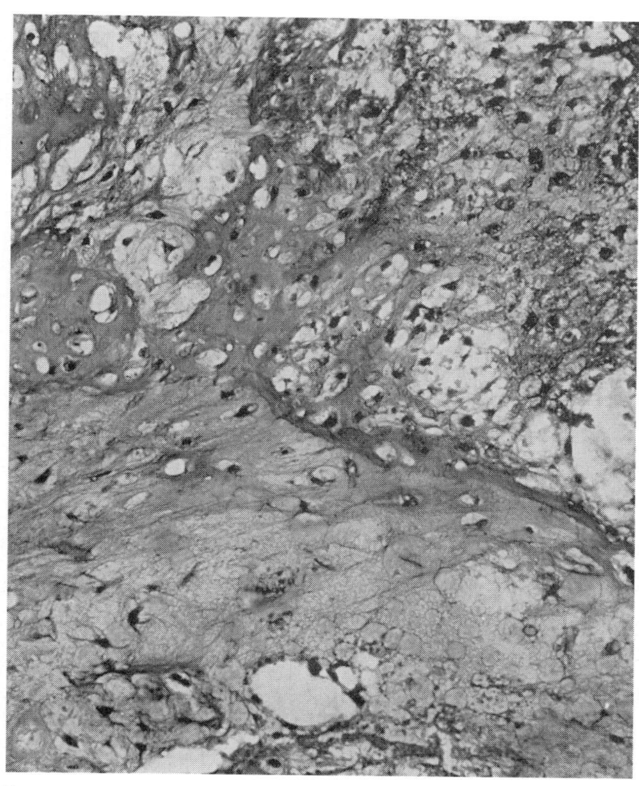

B

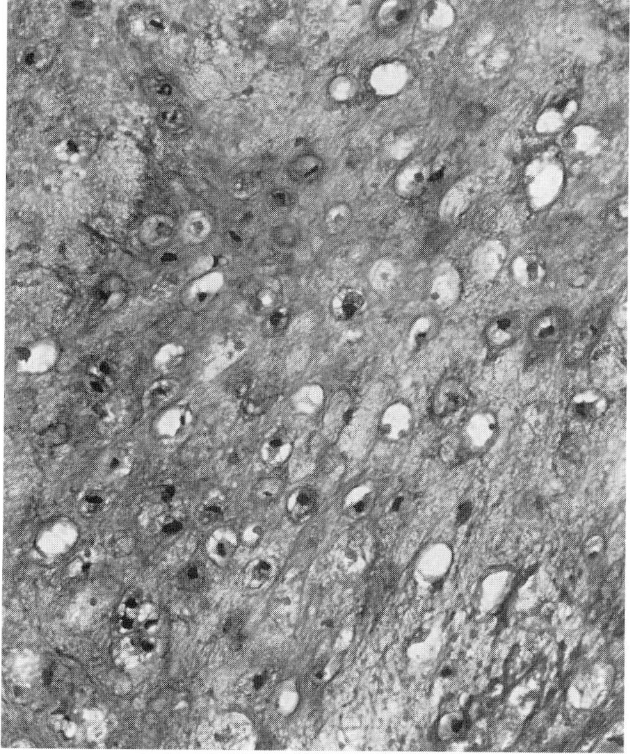

C

FIGURE 8–8. Enchondroma of the distal femur. *A*, Radiograph shows densely mineralized medullary lesion. *B*, Low power (×160) photomicrograph shows mineralized hyaline cartilage. *C*, Higher power (×250) photomicrograph shows bland chondrocytes in lacunae.

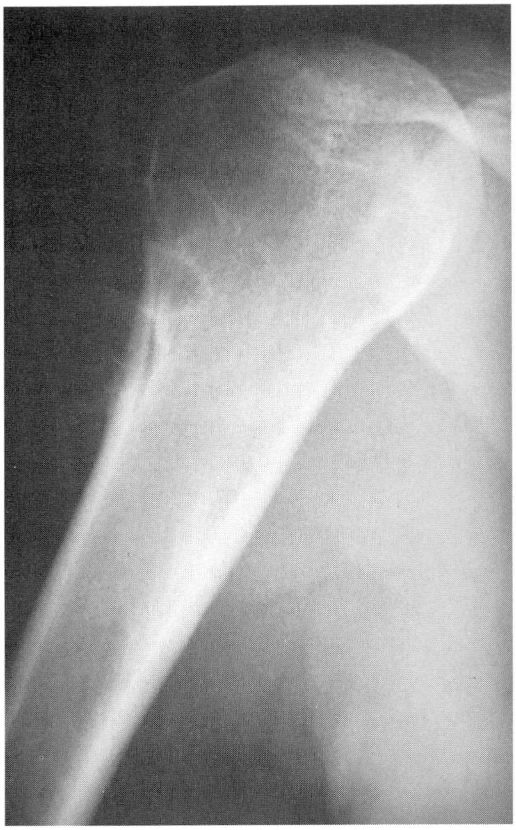

A

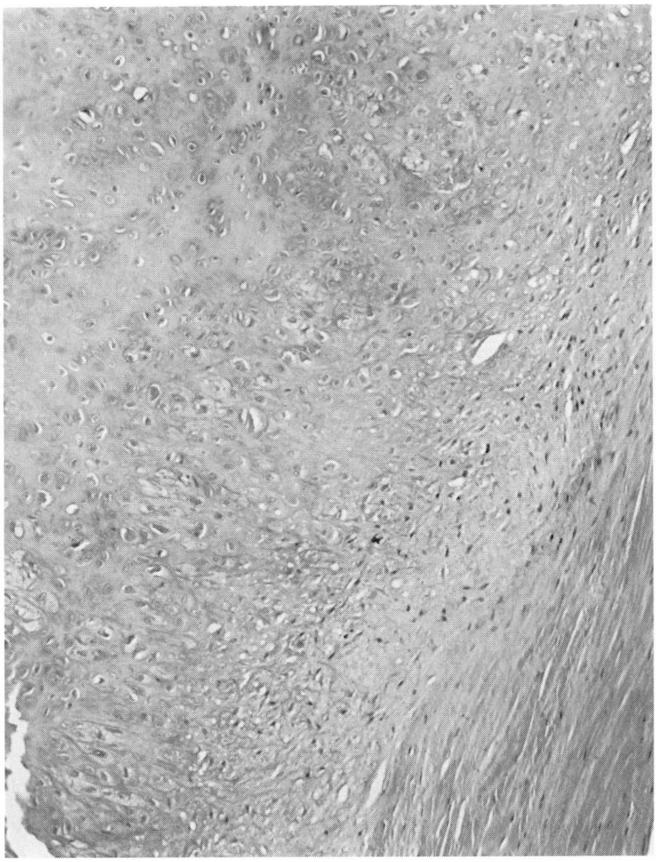

B

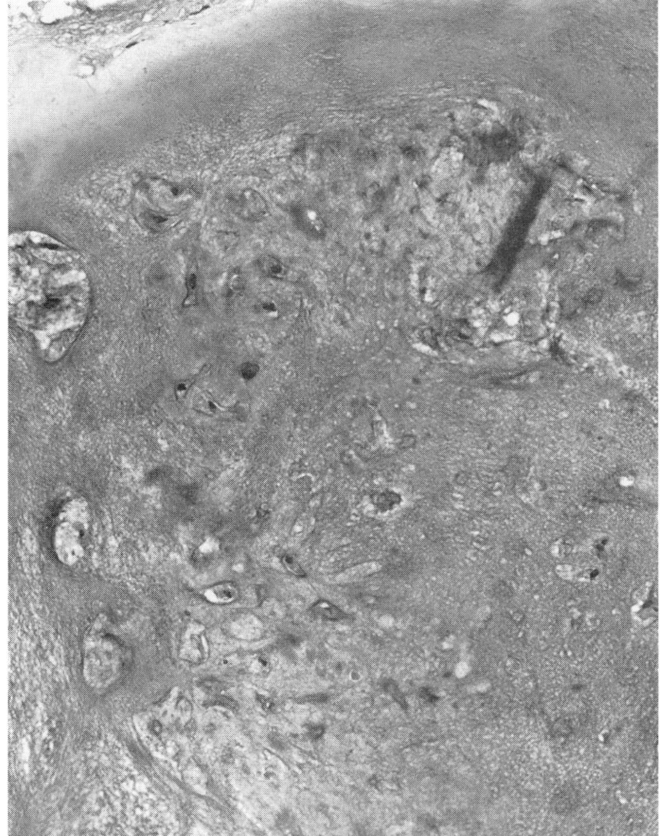

C

FIGURE 8–9. Periosteal chondroma of the proximal humerus. *A,* Radiograph shows surface lesion with stippled calcifications scalloping the cortex. *B,* Low power photomicrograph (×100) shows bland hyaline cartilage. *C,* High power photomicrograph (×250).

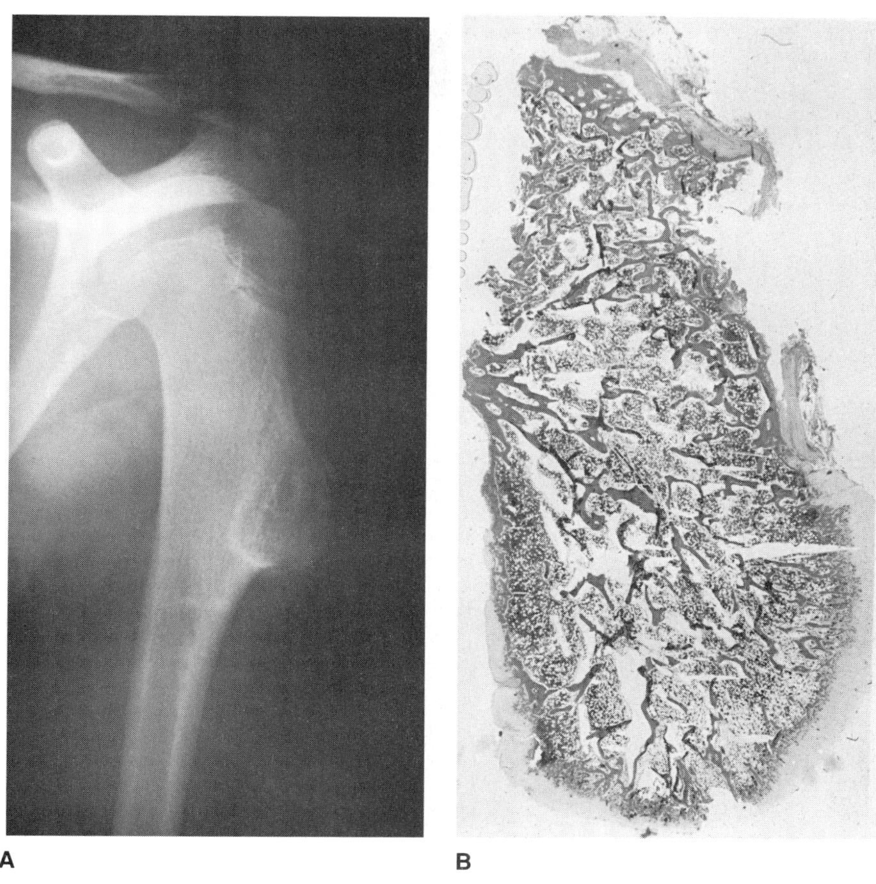

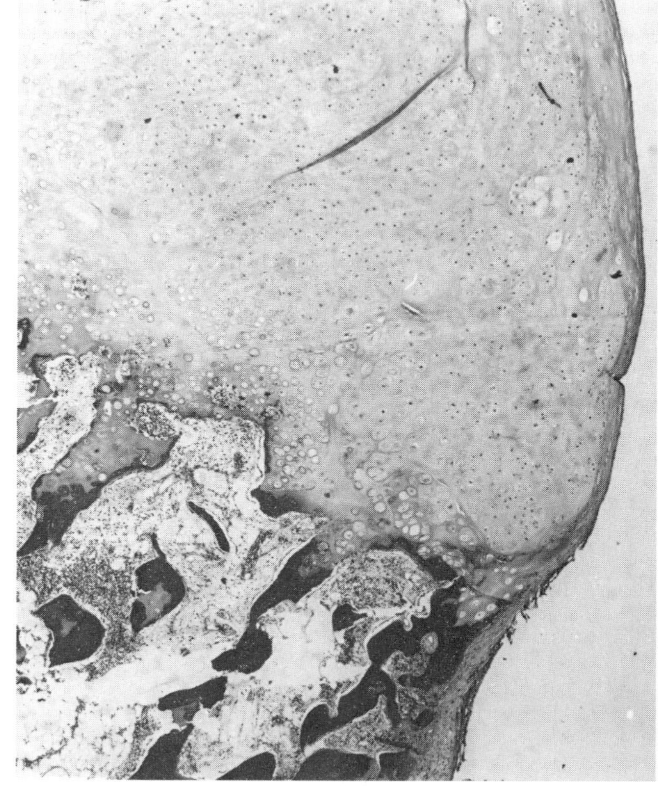

FIGURE 8–10. Osteochondroma of the proximal humerus. *A,* Radiograph showing sessile osteochondroma of the proximal humerus. *B,* Photomicrograph (×6) shows the osteochondroma with a cartilagenous cap. *C,* Higher power photomicrograph (×25) shows the cartilage cap, which is undergoing endochondral ossification.

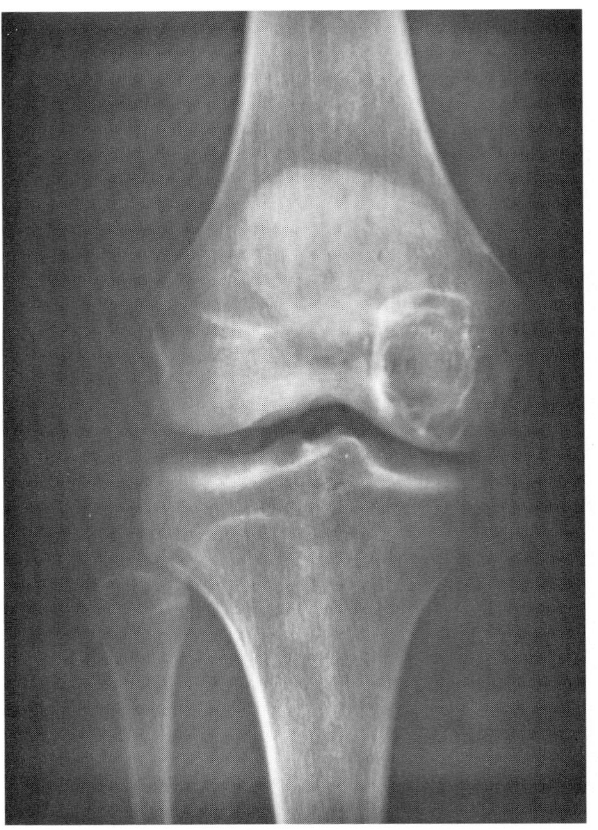
A

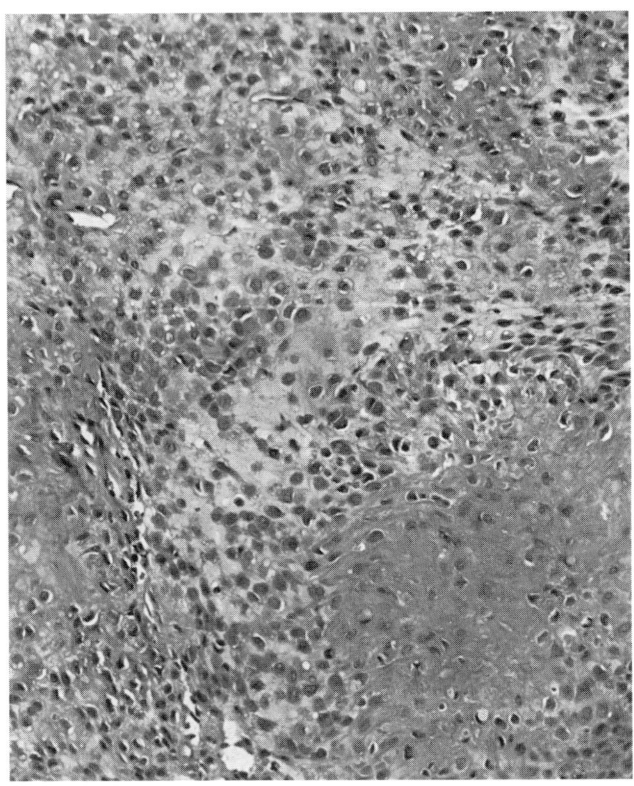
B

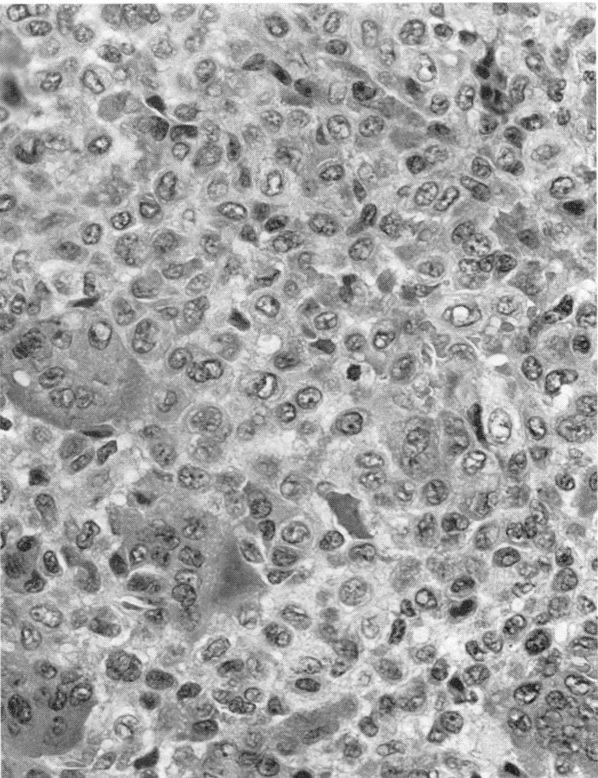
C

FIGURE 8–11. Chondroblastoma of the distal femur. *A*, Radiograph shows a well circumscribed lytic lesion with a sclerotic rim in the distal femoral epiphysis. *B*, Low power photomicrograph (×160) shows cellular stroma in a chondroid matrix. *C*, Higher power photomicrograph (×400) shows rounded stromal cells with multinucleated giant cells.

patients (most have open physes). The most common locations are the distal femur, proximal tibia, and proximal humerus. Although the lesion is usually in the epiphysis, it may also occur in an apophysis. Another common location is the triradiate cartilage of the pelvis. Patients usually present with pain referable to the involved joint. Radiographically, there is a central region of bone destruction that is usually sharply demarcated from the normal medullary cavity by a thin rim of sclerotic bone (Dahlin). There may or may not be mineralization within the lesion. Histologically, the basic proliferating cells are thought to be chondroblasts. There are scattered multinucleated giant cells throughout the lesion and zones of chondroid substance. Mitotic figures may be found. Treatment consists in curettage (marginal margin) and bone grafting. About 2% of benign chondroblastomas metastasize to the lungs.

4. Chondromyxoid Fibroma (Fig. 8–12)—This rare benign cartilage tumor contains variable amounts of chondroid, fibromatoid, and myxoid elements. The lesion is more common in males and tends to involve long bones (especially the tibia). Patients present with pain of variable duration (months to years). Radiographically, there is a lytic, destructive lesion that is eccentric and sharply demarcated from the adjacent normal bone. Usually no matrix mineralization is seen radiographically. The tumor grows in lobules, and there is often a condensation of cells at the periphery of the lobules. The chondroid element may vary from small to heavy concentrations. Treatment is resection with a marginal line of resection.
5. Intramedullary Chondrosarcoma (Fig. 8–13)—This common malignant neoplasm of cartilage cells occurs in adults and the older age groups. The most common locations include the shoulder and pelvic girdles, knee, and spine. Patients may present with pain or a mass. Plain radiographs are usually diagnostic, with bone destruction, thickening of the cortex, and mineralization consistent with cartilage within the lesion. A soft tissue mass is often present in patients who have had symptoms for a long time. It may be extremely difficult to differentiate malignant cartilage based on histologic features alone. The clinical, radiographic, and histologic features of a particular lesion must be combined to avoid incorrect diagnoses. The criteria for the diagnosis of malignancy are difficult: (1) many cells with plump nuclei; (2) more than an occasional cell with two such nuclei; and (3) especially giant cartilage cells with large single or multiple nuclei with clumps of chromatin (Dahlin). Chondromas of the hand, lesions in patients with Ollier's disease and Maffucci syndrome, and periosteal chondromas may have atypical histopathologic features; however, their behavior is that of a benign cartilage lesion and hence they are not malignant lesions. More than 90% of chondrosarcomas are grade 1 or 2 lesions. Grade 4 lesions do not occur; and when this degree of malignancy is observed the lesion is most likely a chondroblastic osteosarcoma. Treatment consists of wide surgical resection. For typical low grade (grades 1 and 2), chondrosarcoma there is no role for chemotherapy or irradiation.
6. Dedifferentiated Chondrosarcoma (Fig. 8–14)—This lesion is the most malignant cartilage tumor. It has a bimorphic histologic and radiographic appearance. Histologically, there is a low grade cartilage component that is intimately associated with a high grade spindle cell sarcoma (osteosarcoma, fibrosarcoma, malignant fibrous histiocytoma). Radiographically, in more than 80% of the lesions there is a typical chondrosarcoma with a superimposed highly destructive area. Patients present with a picture similar to that of low grade chondrosarcoma, including pain and decreased function. The prognosis is poor; and long-term survival is less than 10%. Wide surgical resection and multiagent chemotherapy are the principal methods of treatment.

D. Fibrous Lesions—Truly fibrous neoplasms of bone are not common and number only three: metaphyseal fibrous defect (fibroma), desmoplastic fibroma, and fibrosarcoma.

1. Metaphyseal Fibrous Defect (Fig. 8–15)—This is a common lesion occurring in young patients. Most of these lesions resolve spontaneously and are probably not true neoplasms. Common names for this lesion include fibroma, myxoma, nonosteogenic fibroma, cortical desmoid, fibromatosis, and xanthoma. Metaphyseal fibrous defect is the most descriptive form. The most common locations are the distal femur, distal tibia, and proximal tibia. Most patients are asymptomatic, and the lesion is discovered incidentally. The radiographic appearance is characteristic, with the lytic lesion that is metaphyseal, eccentric, and surrounded by a sclerotic rim. The cortex may be slightly expanded and thinned. Histologically, there is a cellular, fibroblastic connective tissue background with the cells arranged in whorled bundles (Dahlin). There are numerous giant cells, lipophages, and various amounts of hemosiderin pigmentation. Treatment is observation if the radiographic appearance is characteristic and there is not an excessive risk of pathologic fracture. If more than 75% of the cortex is involved and the patient is symptomatic, curettage and bone grafting are performed.
2. Desmoplastic Fibroma—These lesions are rare low grade malignant fibrous tumors of bone. Wide surgical resection is the treatment.
3. Fibrosarcoma (Fig. 8–16)—This malignant tumor of bone has a presentation and localization similar to that of osteosarcoma. The tumor affects primarily an older age group but does occur during all decades of life. Patients present with pain and swelling as with any other malignant bone tumor. Radiographically, one sees bone destruction that is typically in a permeative pattern. The histologic features are the same as soft tissue fibrosarcoma, with spindle cells, variable collagen production, and a herringbone pattern. Treatment consists in wide surgical resection. Although the prognosis is poor, the role of chemotherapy has not been fully defined; effective regimens for the older patient have not been adequately explored.

E. Histiocytic—Histiocytic lesions of bone are uncommon. Benign and malignant forms may be encountered.

1. Benign and Atypical Histiocytoma of Bone—These lesions are rare. Patients present with pain,

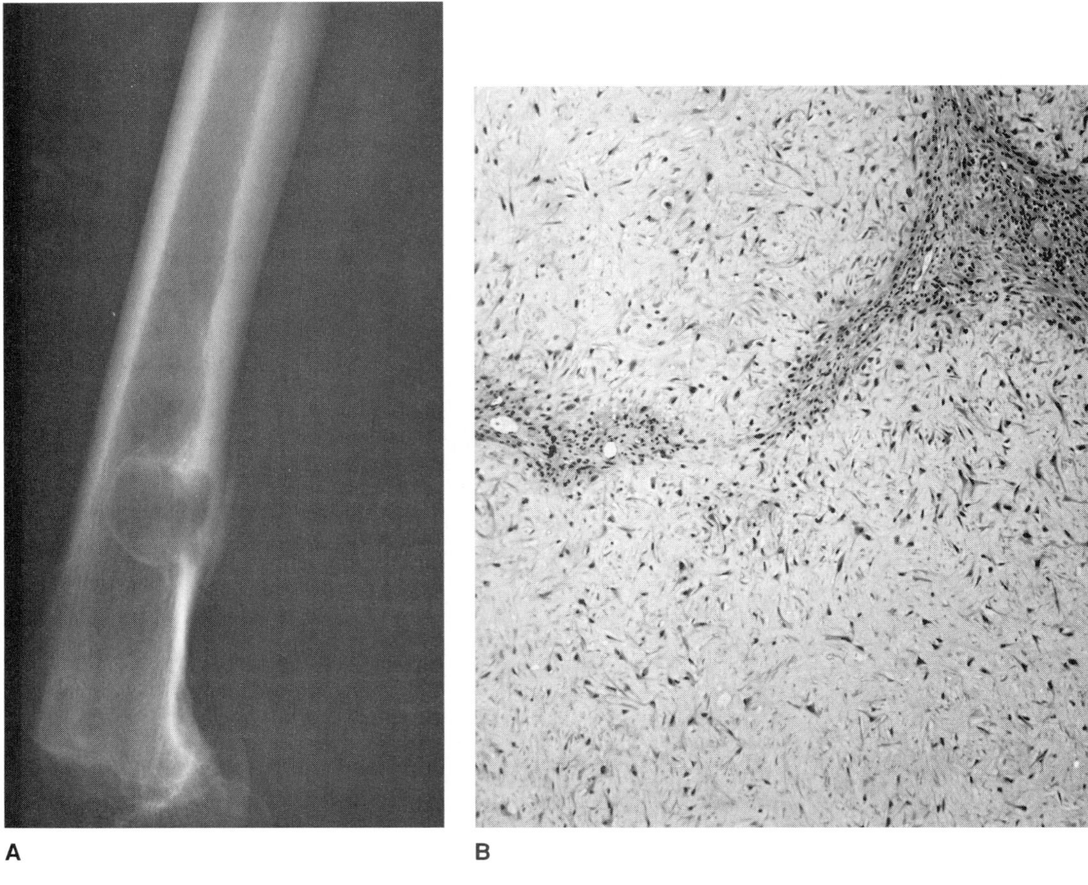

A B

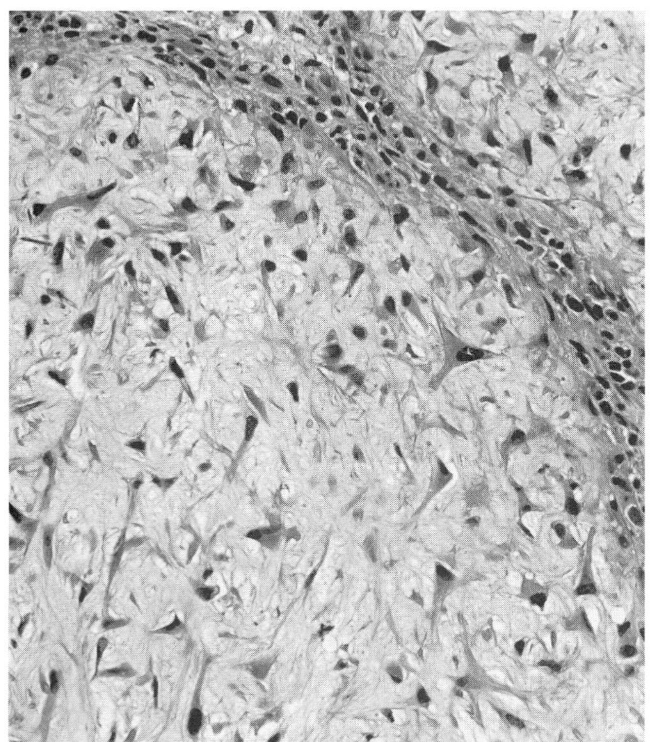

C

FIGURE 8–12. Chondromyxoid fibroma of the femur. *A*, Radiograph shows well circumscribed lytic lesion in the distal femur with a rim of sclerotic bone. *B*, Low power photomicrograph (×100) shows lobules of fibromyxoid tissue. *C*, Higher power photomicrograph (×250) shows myxoid stroma with stellate cells.

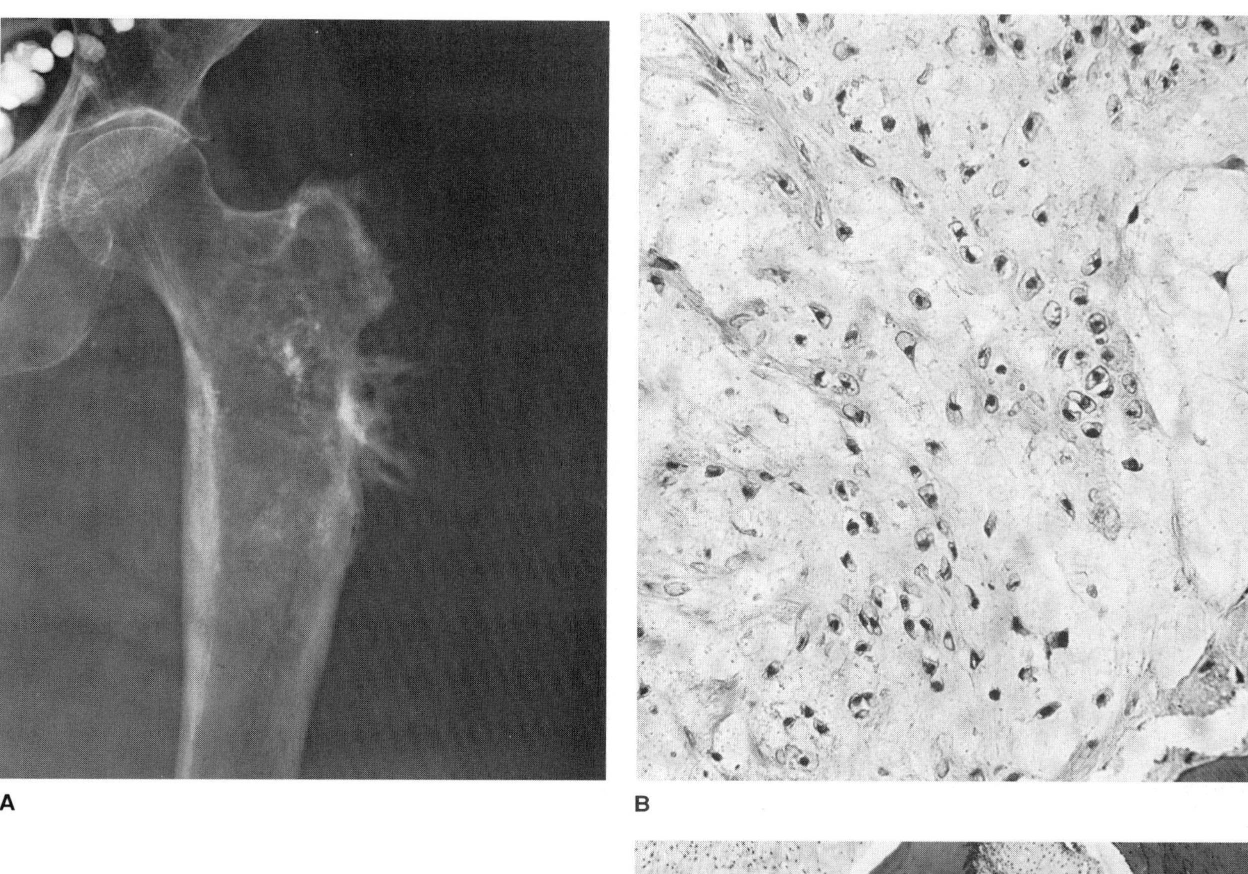

A

B

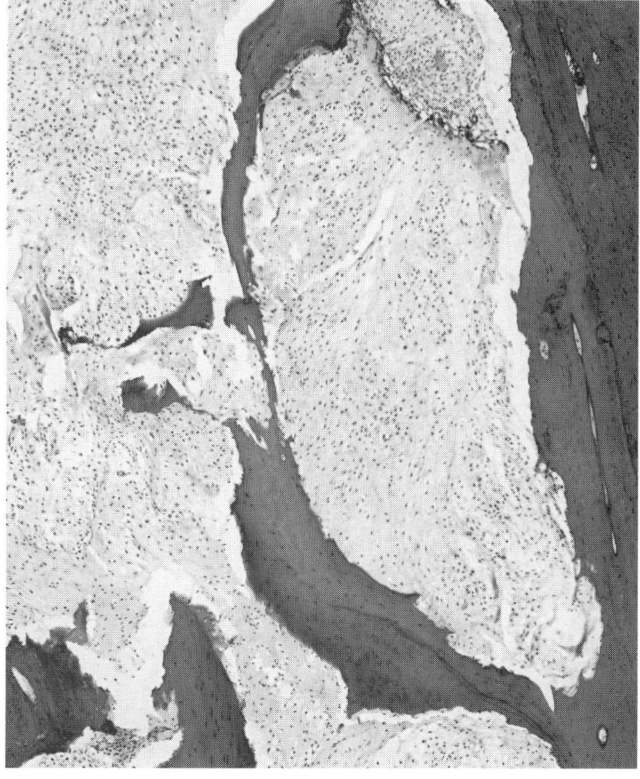

C

FIGURE 8–13. Central chondrosarcoma of the proximal femur. *A*, Radiograph shows an expansile lytic lesion in the proximal femur with stippled calcifications. *B*, Low power photomicrograph (×40) shows cartilage with a permeative growth pattern. *C*, Higher power photomicrograph (×250) shows cellular cartilage.

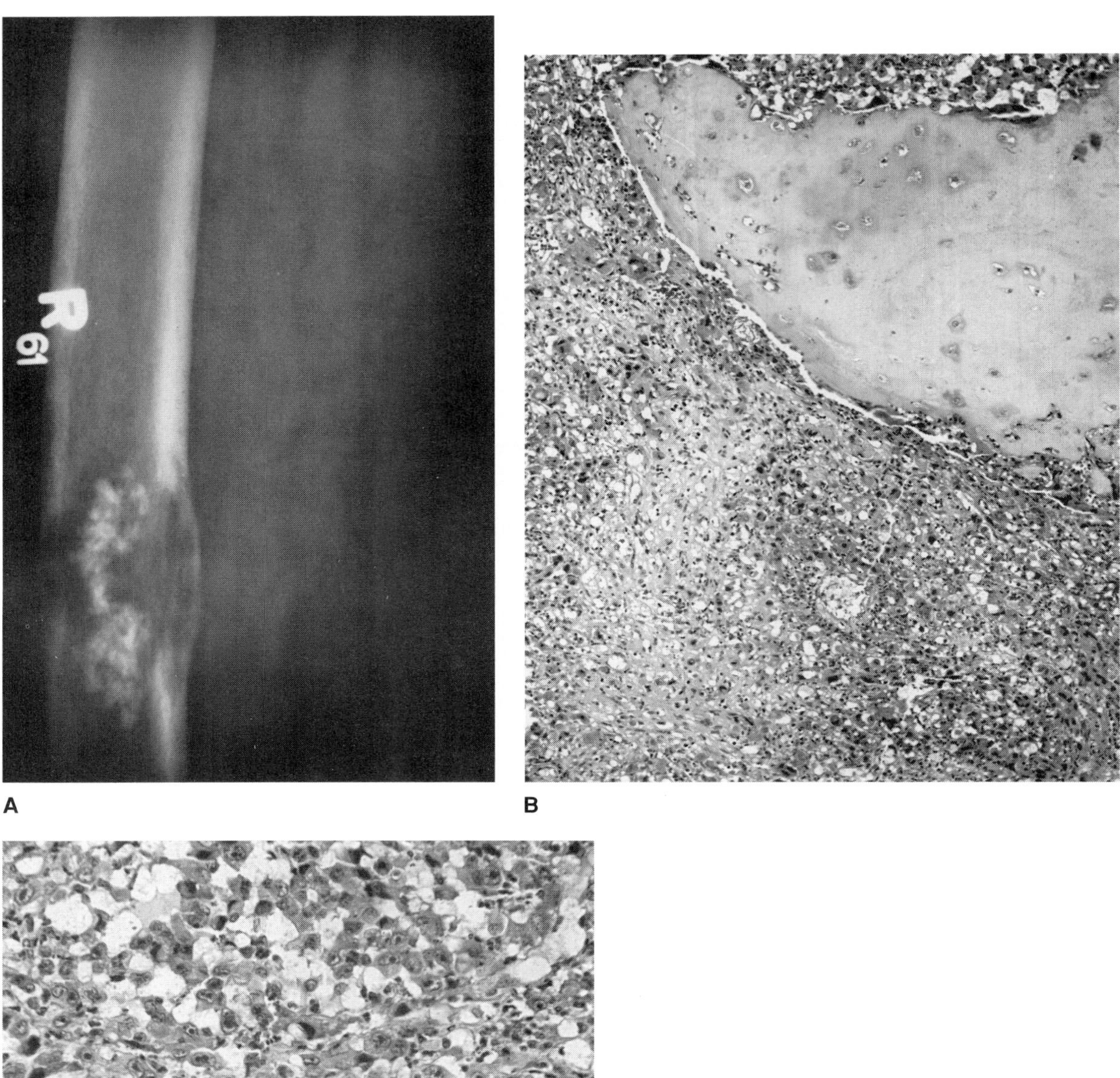

A

B

C

FIGURE 8–14. Dedifferentiated chondrosarcoma of the femur. *A,* Radiograph shows focal dense mineralization surrounded by a poorly defined lytic lesion. *B,* Low power photomicrograph (×100) shows an island of hyaline cartilage surrounded by a cellular neoplasm. *C,* Higher power photomicrograph (×250) shows hyaline cartilage adjacent to pleomorphic rounded cells.

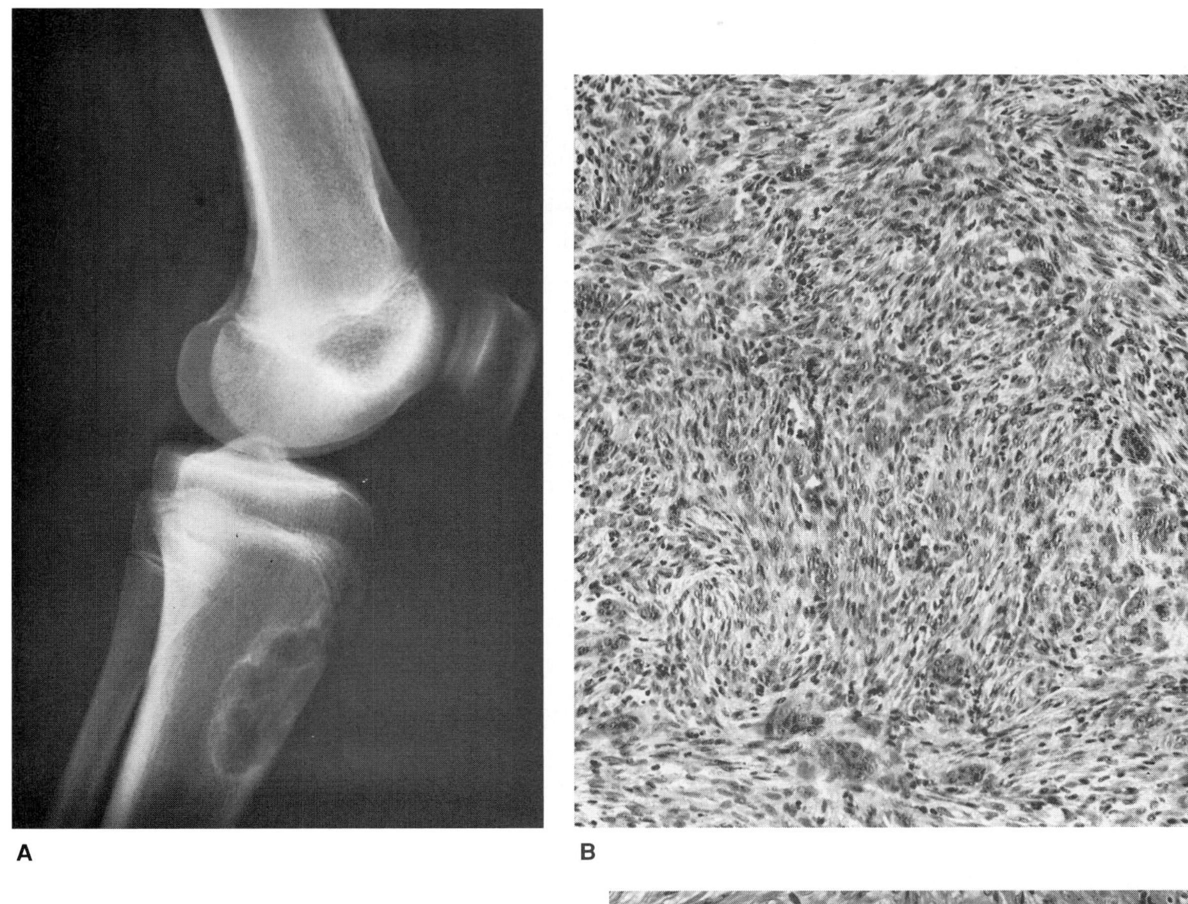

A

B

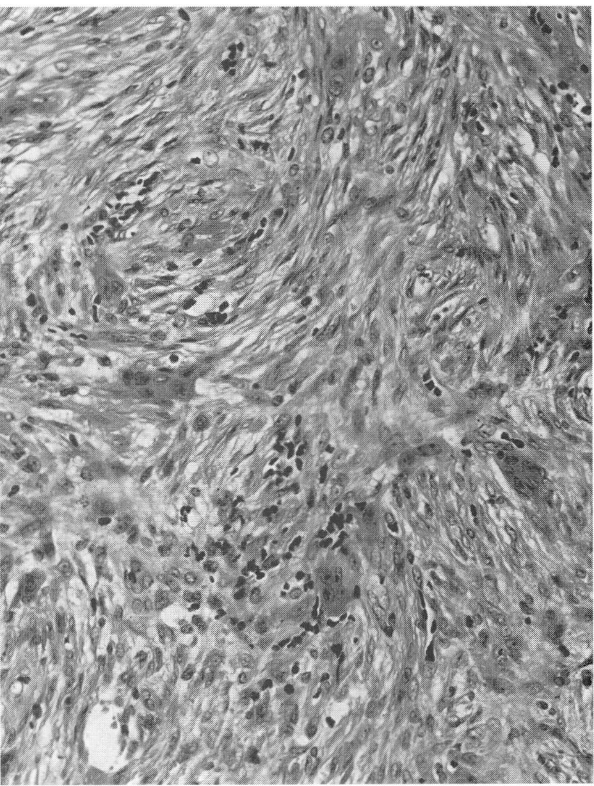

C

FIGURE 8–15. Nonossifying fibroma of the proximal tibia. *A,* Radiograph shows a scalloped, well circumscribed lesion with a sclerotic rim in the proximal tibial metaphysis. *B,* Low power photomicrograph (×160) showing spindle cells in a storiform pattern and occasional multinucleated giant cells. *C,* High power photomicrograph (×250).

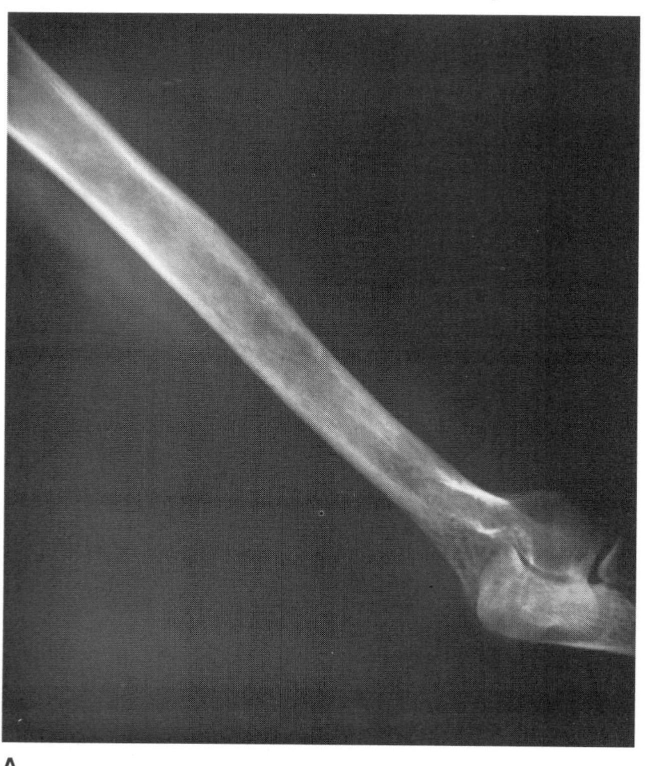

A

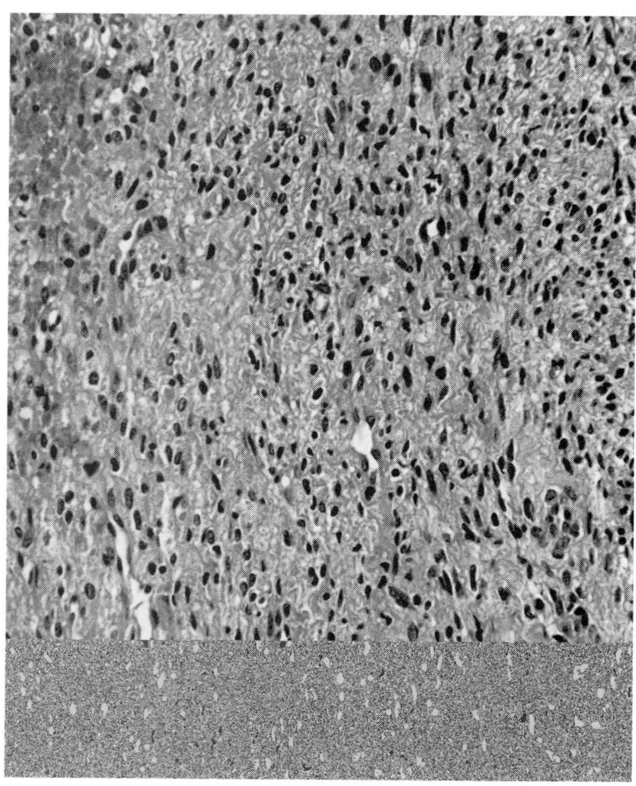

B

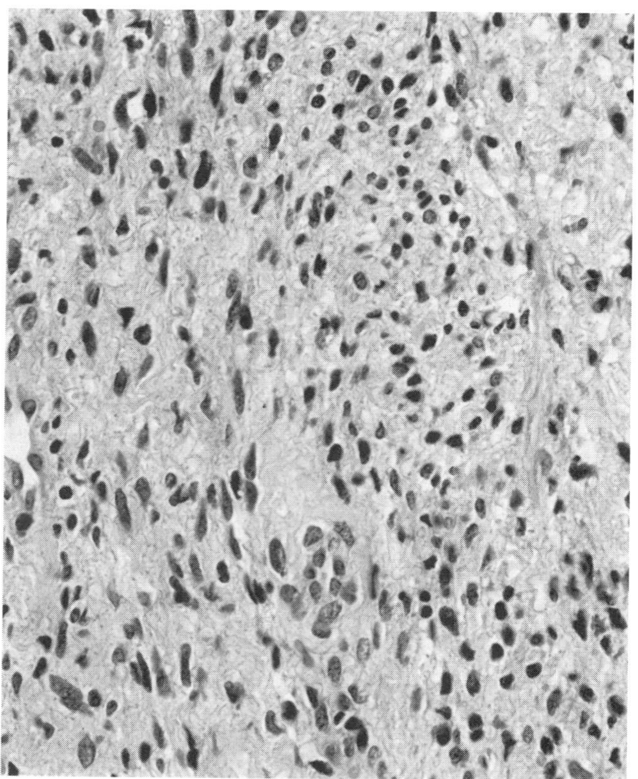

C

FIGURE 8–16. Fibrosarcoma of the humerus. *A*, Radiograph shows a permeative lesion in the midshaft of the humerus. *B*, Low power photomicrograph (×250) shows atypical spindle cells. *C*, High power photomicrograph (×400).

and the radiographs show bone destruction. Histologically, the lesions have nuclei that are indented or grooved, giving a histiocytic appearance. Little is known of the true behavior of these lesions because they are so uncommon. Wide surgical resection is the treatment of choice.

2. Malignant Fibrous Histiocytoma (Fig. 8–17)—This malignant bone tumor has proliferating cells with a histiocytic quality. The nuclei are often indented; the cytoplasm is usually abundant and may be slightly foamy; the nucleoli are often large; and multinucleated giant cells are usually a prominent feature (Dahlin). There may be variable amounts of fibrous tissue found within the lesion, and the fibrogenic areas have a storiform, or cartwheel, appearance. Chronic inflammatory cells are frequently found. Patients present with pain and swelling. Radiographs usually demonstrate a destructive lesion with either purely lytic bone destruction or a mixed pattern of bone destruction and formation. Treatment is wide surgical excision. Most patients are candidates for multiagent chemotherapy, although few studies have shown chemotherapy to be efficacious for this tumor.

F. Notochordal Tissue (Fig. 8–18)—Chordoma is a malignant neoplasm in which the cell of origin derives from primitive notochordal tissue. This lesion occurs predominantly at the ends of the vertebral column (spheno-occipital region and sacrum). About 10% of chordomas occur in the vertebral bodies (cervical, thoracic, and lumbar regions). Patients present with an insidious onset of pain. Lesions in the sacrum may present as pelvic pain, low back pain, hip pain, or with primarily GI symptomatology (obstipation, constipation, loss of rectal tone). In the vertebral bodies there may be a wide variation in neurologic symptoms due to nerve compression. Patients with a long-standing history of undiagnosed pelvic or low back pain should undergo a rectal examination in that more than half of sacral chordomas are palpable with digital examination. Plain radiographs often do not reveal the true extent of sacrococcygeal chordomas. The sacrum is difficult to evaluate on plain radiographs because of overlying bowel gas and fecal material. In addition, the anteroposterior pelvic view reveals bone destruction only at the sacral cortical margins and neural foramina; these areas are not typically involved early. CT scans show midline bone destruction and a soft tissue mass. The sacrum is often expanded, and the soft tissue mass may show irregular mineralization. In the vertebral bodies one often sees areas of both bone formation and bone destruction. The tumor grows in distinct lobules. The chordoma cells sometimes have a vacuolated appearance and are called physaliferous cells. The chordoma cells often are in strands in a mass of mucus. Treatment is resection with a wide surgical margin. Radiation therapy may be added if a wide margin is not achieved. Chordomas may metastasize, in about 30–50% of cases, and they often take the patient's life because of local extension.

G. Vascular Tumors—Vascular tumors of bone represent a very heterogeneous group of disorders. Benign conditions include hemangioma, lymphangioma, and perhaps vanishing bone disease (Gorham's disease or massive osteolysis). Malignant entities include hemangioendothelioma or hemangiosarcoma and hemangiopericytoma.

1. Hemangiomas (Fig. 8–19)—These tumors most commonly occur in vertebral bodies. Patients may present with pain or pathologic fracture. Vertebral hemangiomas have a characteristic appearance, with lytic destruction and vertical striations or a coarsened honeycombed appearance (Dahlin). Occasionally, patients have more than one bone involved. Histologically, there are numerous blood channels. Most lesions are cavernous in nature, although some may be a mixture of capillary and cavernous blood spaces.

2. Hemangioendothelioma (Hemangiosarcoma)—Malignant vascular tumors of bone are rare. Patients may be in any age group and present with pain. Approximately one-third of patients have multifocal lesions. Radiographs show a predominantly lytic lesion with no reactive bone formation. The low grade lesions often have residual trabecular bone. Histologically, the tumor cells form vascular spaces. The lesions range from very well differentiated (easily recognizable vascular spaces) to very undifferentiated tumors (difficult to recognize the vasoformative quality of the tumor). Surgical resection with or without radiotherapy is the treatment. Low-grade multifocal lesions may be treated with radiation alone.

H. Hematopoietic Tumors—Lymphoma and myeloma are the two malignant hematopoietic tumors.

1. Lymphoma (Fig. 8–20)—Lymphoma of bone is common and occurs in three scenarios: (1) as a solitary focus (primary lymphoma of bone); (2) in association with other osseous sites and nonosseous sites (nodal disease and soft tissue masses); and (3) as metastatic foci (Dahlin). Malignant lymphoma affects individuals at all decades of life. Patients generally present with pain. Large soft tissue masses may be present. The radiographs often show a lesion that involves a large portion of the bone (long lesion). Bone destruction is common and often has a mottled appearance. Reactive bone formation and cortical bone destruction are common. The cortex may be thickened. When lymphoma involves bone, there is a diffuse pattern rather than a nodular pattern (Dahlin). A mixed cell infiltrate is usually present. Treatment centers around multiagent chemotherapy and irradiation. Surgery may be used in selected cases to achieve local control.

2. Myeloma—Plasma cell dyscrasias represent a wide range of conditions, ranging from benign monoclonal gammopathy (Kyle's disease) to multiple myeloma. There are three plasma cell dyscrasias with which the orthopaedist must be familiar: multiple myeloma, solitary myeloma, and osteosclerotic myeloma.

   a. Multiple Myeloma (Fig. 8–21)—This plasma cell disorder commonly occurs in patients between 50 and 80 years of age. Patients usually present with bone pain, most commonly in the spine and ribs, or a pathologic fracture. Fatigue is a common complaint secondary to the associated anemia. Symptoms may be related to complications such as renal insufficiency, hypercalcemia, and the deposition of amyloid. Serum creatinine levels are elevated in about 50% of patients. Hypercalcemia is present in about one-third. The classic radiographic appearance is punched-out lytic lesions. The in-

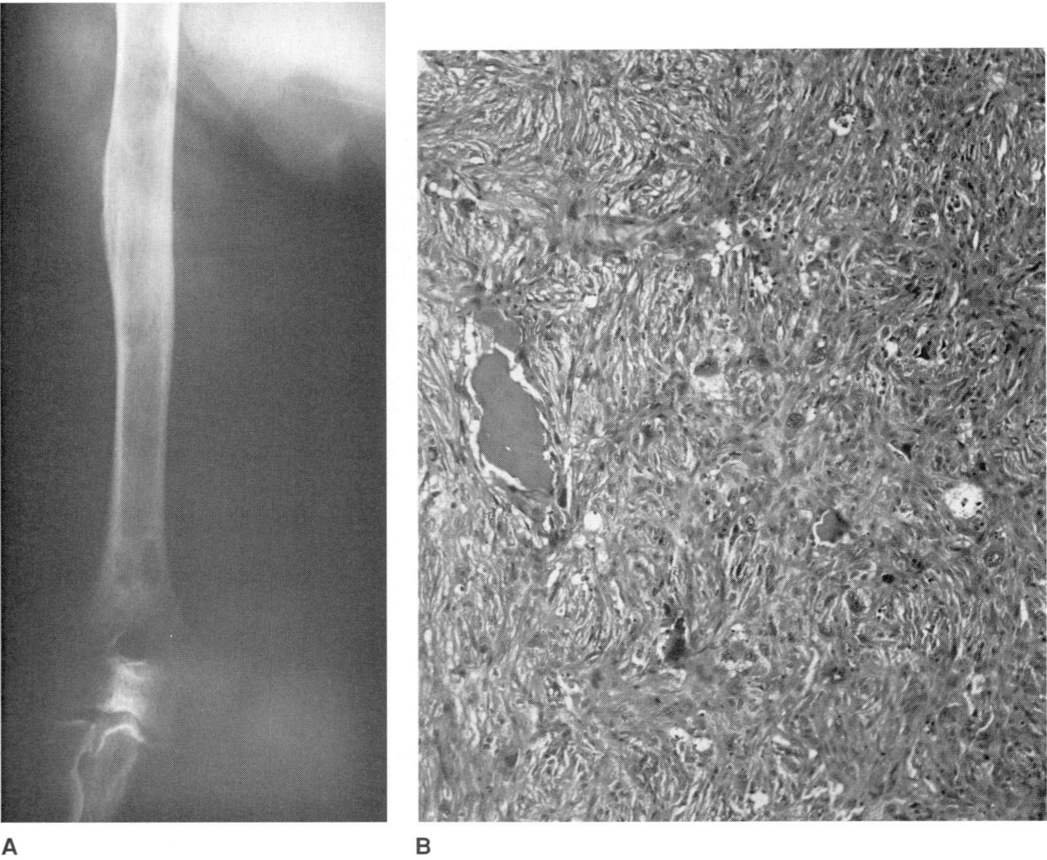

A B

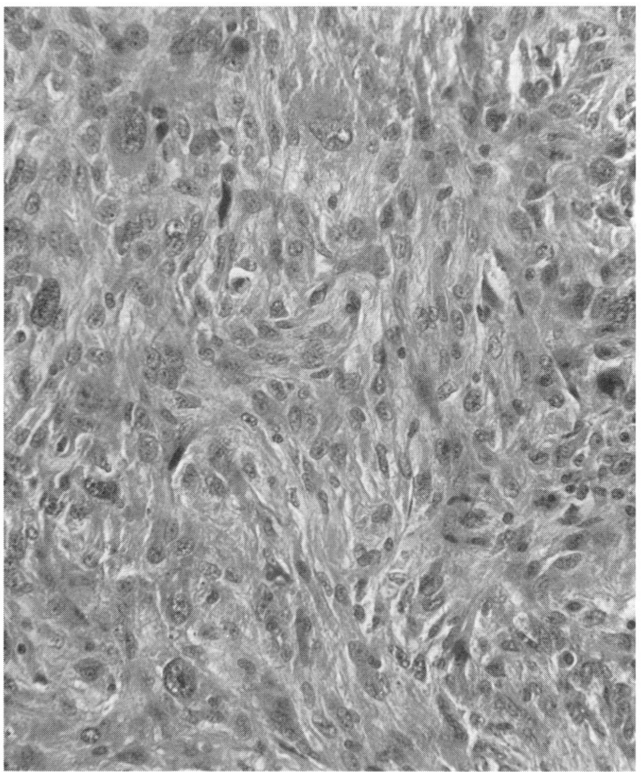

C

FIGURE 8–17. Malignant fibrous histiocytoma of the humerus. *A*, Radiograph shows poorly defined lytic lesions in the proximal and distal humerus. *B*, Low power photomicrograph (×200) shows spindle cells arranged in a storiform pattern. *C*, Higher power photomicrograph (×400) shows a uniform population of pleomorphic cells.

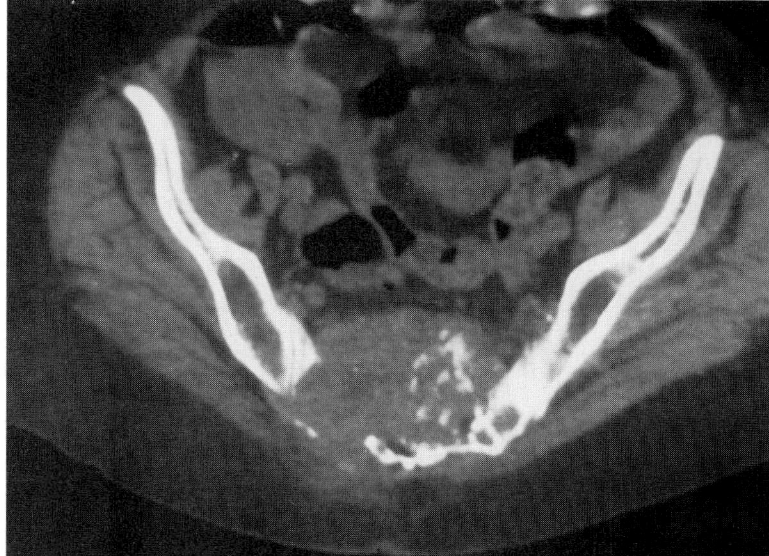

A

FIGURE 8–18. Chordoma of the sacrum. *A,* CT scan shows a destructive lesion in the sacrum. *B,* Low power photomicrograph (×100) shows a lobular arrangement of tissue. *C,* Higher power photomicrograph of (×250) shows nests of physaliferous cells.

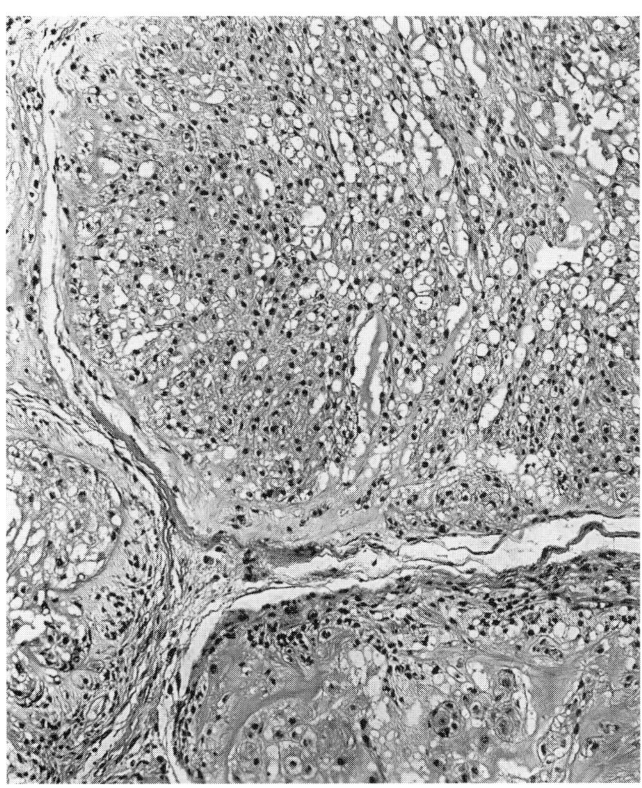

B

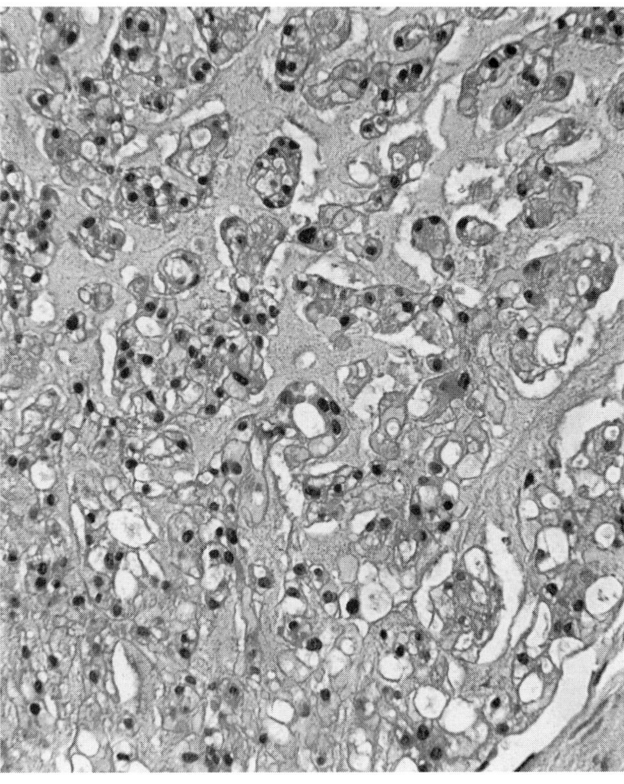

C

volved bone may show expansion and a "ballooned" appearance. Osteopenia may be the only finding. Histologically, the classic appearance is sheets of plasma cells. Well differentiated plasma cells have an eccentric nucleus and a peripherally clumped chromatic "clock face" (Fig. 8–22). There is a perinuclear clear zone (halo) that represents the Golgi apparatus. In contrast, undifferentiated tumors lack some or all of these features, and the cells are anaplastic. The treatment of myeloma is multiagent chemotherapy; surgical stabilization with irradiation is used for impending and complete fractures. Prognosis is related to the stage of disease, with an overall median survival of 18–24 months.

b. Solitary Myeloma—It is important to differentiate solitary myeloma from multiple myeloma because of the more favorable prognosis in patients with the former. Diagnostic criteria in-

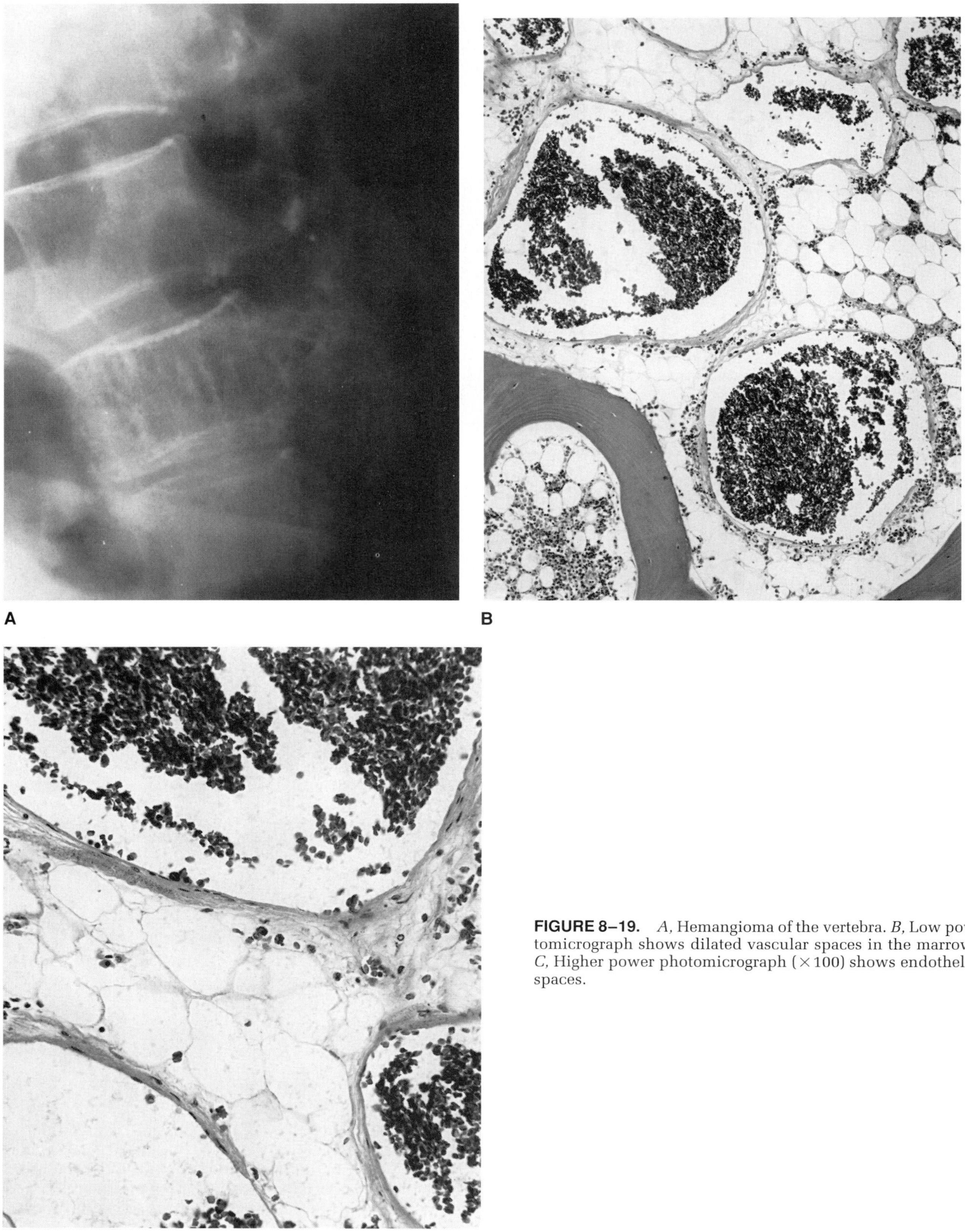

A

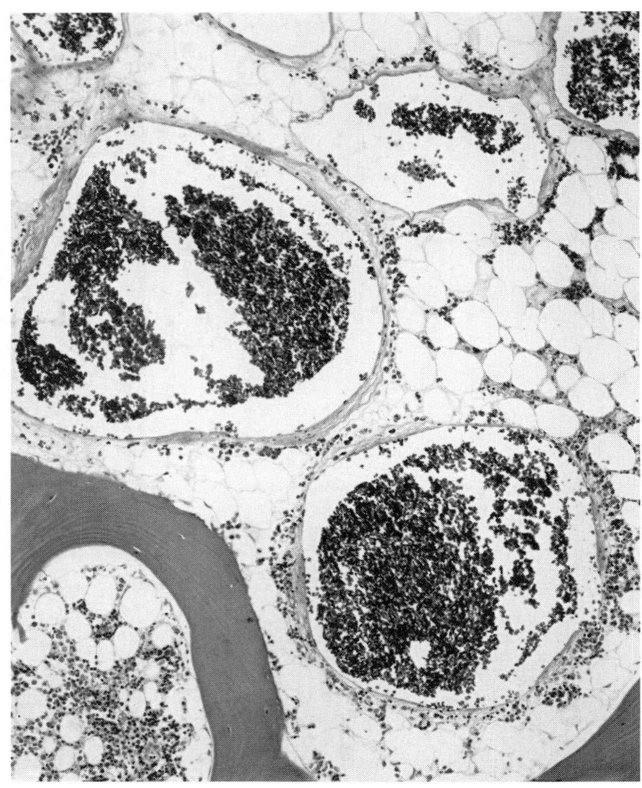

B

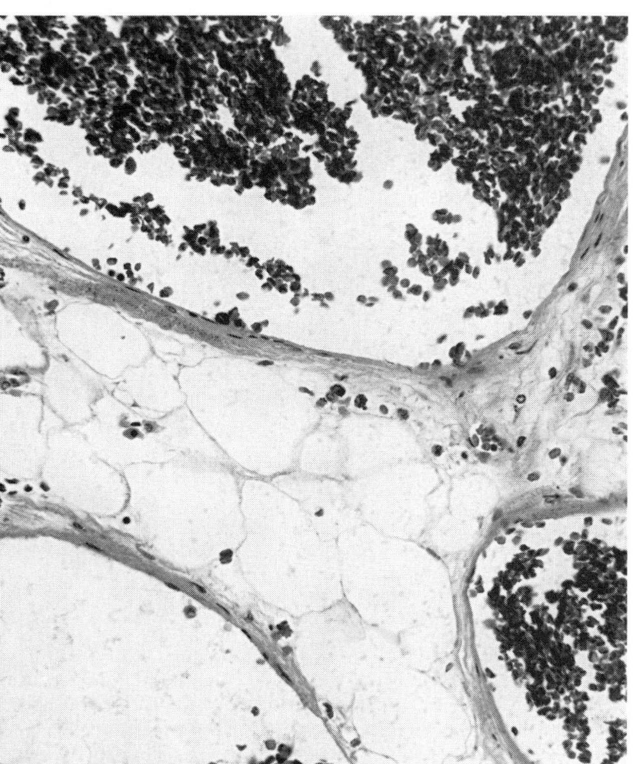

C

FIGURE 8–19. *A,* Hemangioma of the vertebra. *B,* Low power photomicrograph shows dilated vascular spaces in the marrow (×50). *C,* Higher power photomicrograph (×100) shows endothelial-lined spaces.

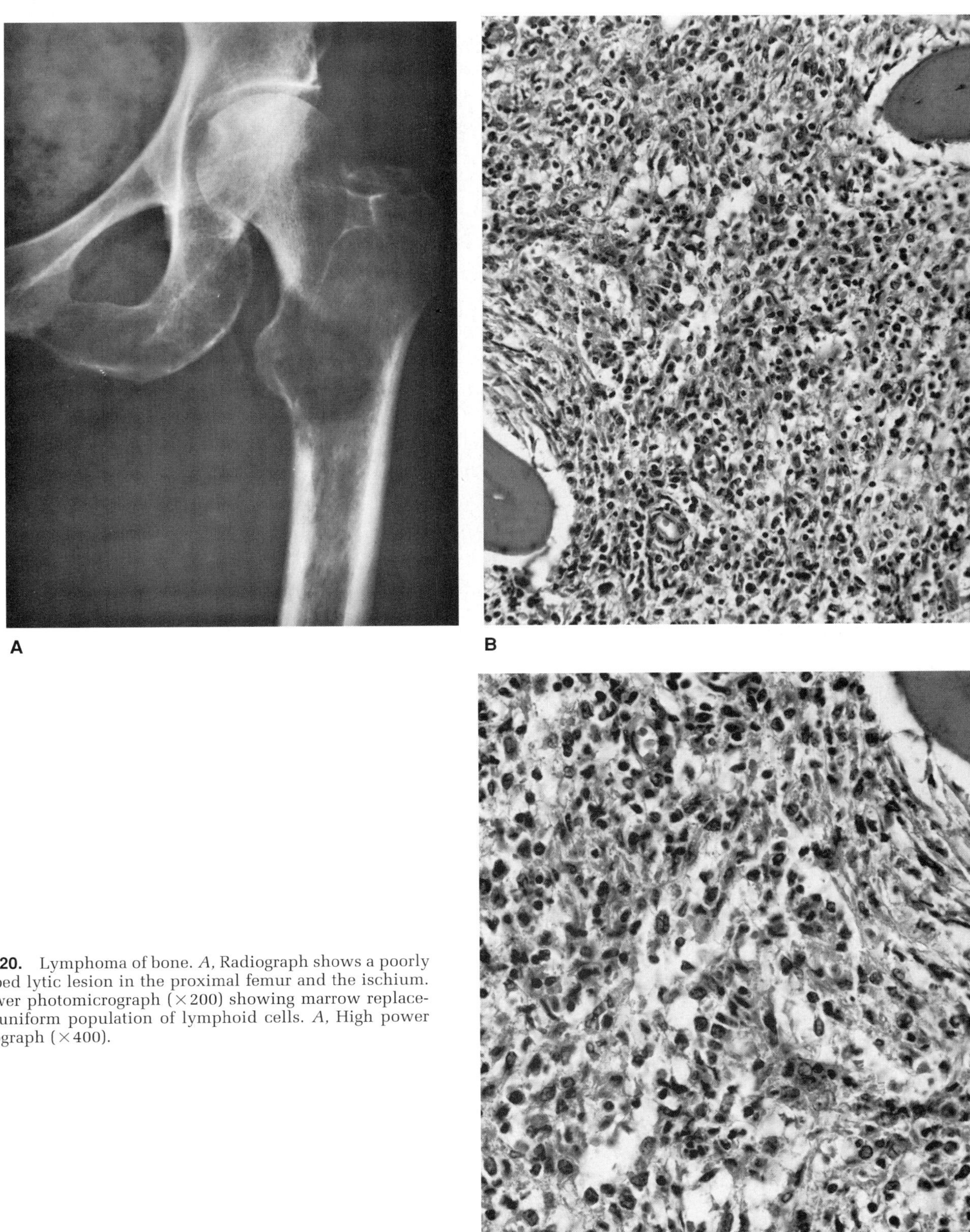

FIGURE 8–20. Lymphoma of bone. *A*, Radiograph shows a poorly circumscribed lytic lesion in the proximal femur and the ischium. *B*, Low power photomicrograph (×200) showing marrow replacement by a uniform population of lymphoid cells. *A*, High power photomicrograph (×400).

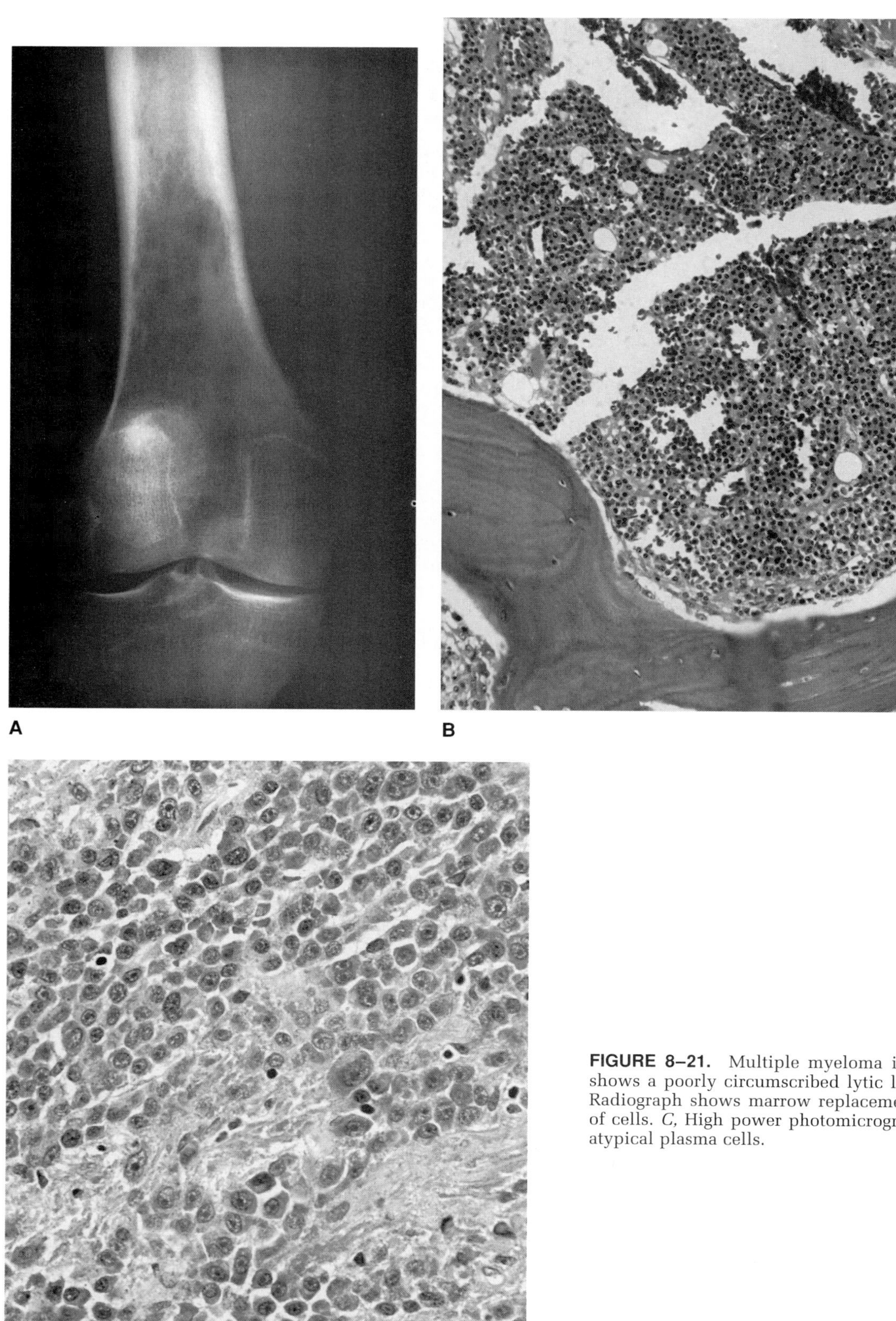

FIGURE 8–21. Multiple myeloma in the femur. *A,* Radiograph shows a poorly circumscribed lytic lesion in the distal femur. *B,* Radiograph shows marrow replacement by a uniform population of cells. *C,* High power photomicrograph (×400) shows sheets of atypical plasma cells.

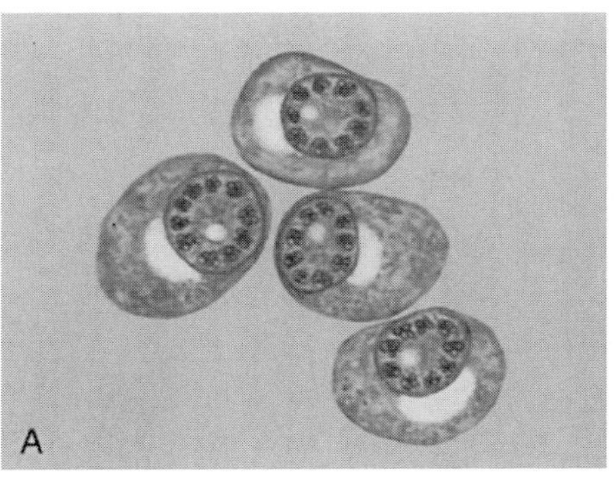

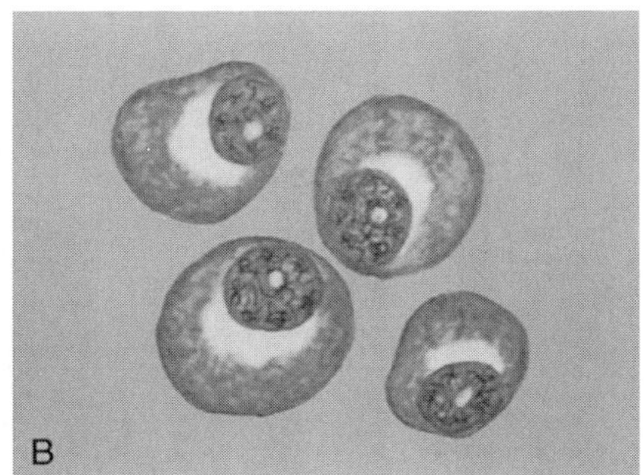

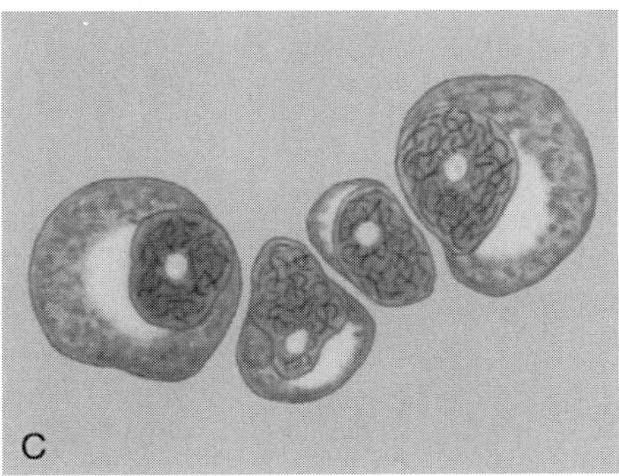

FIGURE 8–22. Myeloma cells. *A*, Plasma cells from a well differentiated case of myeloma that resemble plasma cells seen in benign inflammatory cases. *B*, Plasma cells of intermediate maturity. *C*, Plasma cells that are immature and less well differentiated. (From Frassica, F.J., Frassica, D.A., and Sim, F.H.: Myeloma of bone. In Stauffer, R.N., ed. Advances in Operative Orthopaedics, vol. 2, p. 362. St. Louis, Mosby-Year Book, 1994; reprinted by permission.)

clude (1) solitary lesion on skeletal survey; (2) histologic confirmation of plasmacytoma; (3) bone marrow plasmacytosis of 10% or less. Patients with serum protein abnormalities and Bence Jones proteinuria of less than 1 g/24 hours at presentation are not excluded if they meet the above criteria. The radiographic and histologic features are the same as for multiple myeloma. Treatment is external beam irradiation to the lesion (4500 cGy); when necessary, prophylactic internal fixation is performed.

c. Osteosclerotic Myeloma—This form is a rare variant in which bone lesions are associated with a chronic inflammatory demyelinating polyneuropathy. Generally, the diagnosis of osteosclerotic myeloma is not made until the polyneuropathy is recognized and evaluated. Sensory symptoms (tingling, pins and needles, coldness) are noted first, followed by motor weakness. Both the sensory and motor changes begin distally, are symmetric, and proceed proximally. Severe weakness is common, but, bone pain is not characteristic. Radiographic studies may show a spectrum from purely sclerotic to a mixed pattern of lysis and sclerosis. The lesions usually involve the spine, pelvic bones, and ribs; the extremities are generally spared. Patients may have abnormalities outside the nervous system and have a constellation of findings termed the POEMS syndrome (polyneuropathy, organomegaly, endocrinopathy, M protein, and skin changes). Treatment is difficult, with radiotherapy being the primary modality. The neurologic changes may not improve with treatment.

I. Tumors of Unknown Origin—The three principal tumors of unknown origin are giant cell tumor, Ewing's tumor, and adamantinoma.

1. Giant Cell Tumor (Fig. 8–23)—This distinctive neoplasm has poorly differentiated cells (Dahlin). The lesion is a benign but aggressive process. Further confusion results from the fact that this benign tumor may rarely (<2% of the time) metastasize to the lungs (benign metastasizing giant cell tumor). Unlike most bone tumors, which occur more commonly occur in males, giant cell tumor is more common in females. The lesion is uncommon in children with open physes. The lesion is most common in the epiphysis of long bones, and about 50% of lesions occur about the knee; the vertebra and sacrum are involved in about 10% of cases. Multicentricity occurs in fewer than 1% of patients; and when multiple lesions occur, hyperparathyroidism should be excluded. Patients present with pain that is usually referable to the joint involved. Radiographs show a purely lytic destructive lesion in the metaphysis; during the early symptomatic phase the radiographs may appear normal, as a small lytic focus is difficult to detect. The basic proliferating cell has a round

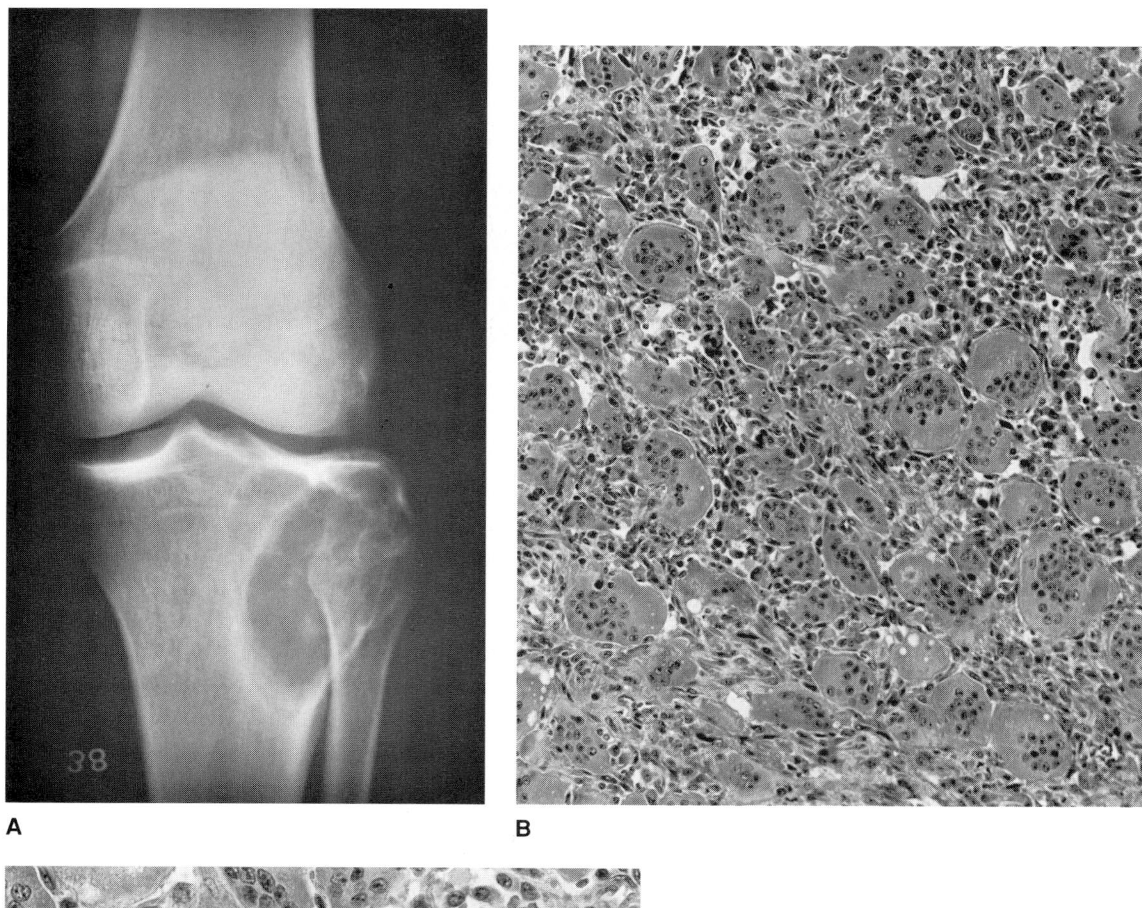

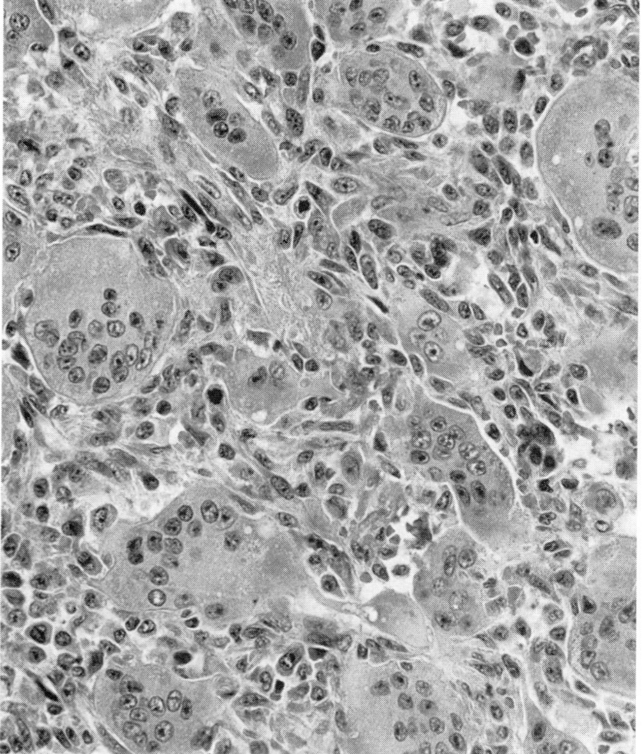

C

FIGURE 8–23. Giant cell tumor of the proximal tibia. *A*, Radiograph shows a well circumscribed lytic lesion in the proximal tibia involving both the epiphysis and the metaphysis. *B*, Low power photomicrograph (×160) shows sheets of multinucleated giant cells. *C*, High power photomicrograph (×300).

to oval or even spindle-shaped nucleus (Dahlin). The giant cells appear to have the same nuclei as the proliferating mononuclear cells. Mitotic figures may be numerous. Treatment is aimed at removing the lesion with preservation of the involved joint. Extensive exteriorization (removal of a large cortical window over the lesion), curettage with hand and power instruments, and chemical cauterization with phenol are performed. The large resulting defect is usually reconstructed with subchondral bone grafts and methylmethacrylate. Local control using this treatment regimen ranges between 80% and 90%.

2. Ewing's Tumor (Fig. 8–24)—This distinctive, small, round-cell sarcoma occurs most commonly in children and young adults; most children are older than 5 years. When a small blue cell tumor is found in a child less than 5 years old, metastatic neuroblastoma and leukemia should be excluded. In patients older than 30 years of age, metastatic carcinomas must be excluded. Patients generally present with pain, and fever may be present. Laboratory tests may show an elevated ESR, leukocytosis, anemia, and an elevated WBC count. Radiographs often show a large, destructive lesion that often involves the metaphysis and diaphysis; the lesion may be purely lytic or have variable amounts of reactive new bone formation. The periosteum may be lifted off in multiple layers, giving the characteristic, but uncommon, onion-skinned appearance. There is often a large soft tissue component. Treatment involves a multimodality approach with: (1) multiagent chemotherapy; (2) irradiation; and (3) surgical resection. Traditionally most lesions have been treated with chemotherapy and irradiation, but the role of surgery is becoming more prominent. Long-term survival with multimodality treatment may be as high as 60–70%.
3. Adamantinoma (Fig. 8–25)—This rare tumor of long bones contains epithelial-like islands of cells. The tibia is the most common site, although rarely other long bones are involved (fibula, femur, ulna, radius). Most patients are young adults and present with pain of months' to years' duration. The typical radiographic appearance is that of multiple, sharply circumscribed, lucent defects of different sizes, with sclerotic bone interspersed between the zones and extending above and below the lucent zones (Dahlin). Typically, one of the lesions in the midshaft is the largest and is associated with cortical bone destruction. Histologically, the cells have an epithelial quality and are arranged in a palisading or glandular pattern; the epithelial cells occur in a fibrous stroma. Treatment of this low grade malignant lesion is wide surgical resection. The lesion may metastasize either early or after multiple failed attempts at local control.

J. Tumor-like Conditions—There are many lesions that simulate primary bone tumors and must be considered in the differential diagnosis (Table 8–8). These lesions range from metastases to reactive conditions.

1. Aneurysmal Bone Cyst (Fig. 8–26)—This non-neoplastic reactive condition may be aggressive in its ability to destroy normal bone and extend into the soft tissues. The lesion may arise in bone primarily or be found in association with other tumors, such as giant cell tumor, chondroblastoma, chondromyxoid fibroma, and fibrous dysplasia. It may also occur within a malignant tumor. Three-fourths of patients with an aneurysmal bone cyst are <20 years of age. Patients present with pain and swelling, which may have been present months to years. The characteristic radiographic finding is an eccentric, lytic, expansile area of bone destruction in the metaphysis; in classic cases there is a thin rim of periosteal new bone surrounding the lesion. The plain radiograph may demonstrate the periosteal bone if it is mineralized, and the MRI scan usually shows the periosteal layer going all around the lesion. The essential histologic features are cavernous blood-filled spaces without an endothelial lining (Dahlin). There are thin strands of bone present in the fibrous tissue of the septae. Benign giant cells may be numerous. Treatment is careful curettage and bone grafting. Local recurrence is common, possibly as high as 25%.
2. Unicameral Bone Cyst (Fig. 8–27)—This lesion occurs most commonly in the proximal humerus and is characterized by cystic, symmetric expansion with thinning of the involved cortices; other common sites are the proximal femur and distal tibia. The cause is unknown, but it probably results from some disturbance of the physis. Patients generally present with pain, usually after a fracture due to minor trauma (e.g., sporting event, throwing a baseball, wrestling). The radiographic picture is characteristic, with a central lytic area and thinning of the cortices symmetrically. The bone is often expanded; however, the width of the bone generally is no greater than the width of the physis. The lesion often appears trabeculated.

TABLE 8–8. TUMOR-LIKE CONDITIONS (TUMOR SIMULATORS)

Young Patient
Eosinophilic granuloma
Osteomyelitis
Avulsion fractures
Aneurysmal bone cyst
Fibrous dysplasia
Osteofibrous dysplasia
Hetertopic ossification
Unicameral bone cyst
Giant cell reparative granuloma
Exuberant callus
Adult
Synovial chondromatosis
Pigmented villonodular synovitis
Stress fracture
Heterotopic ossification
Ganglion cyst
Older Adult
Metastatic bone disease
Mastocytosis
Hyperparathyroidism
Paget's disease
Bone infarcts
Bone islands
Ganglion cyst
Cyst secondary to joint disease
Epidermoid cyst

A

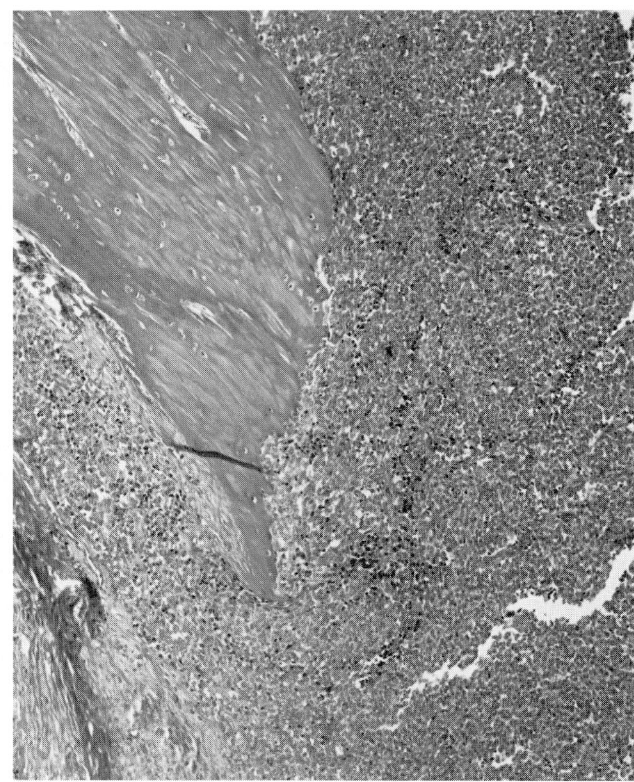

B

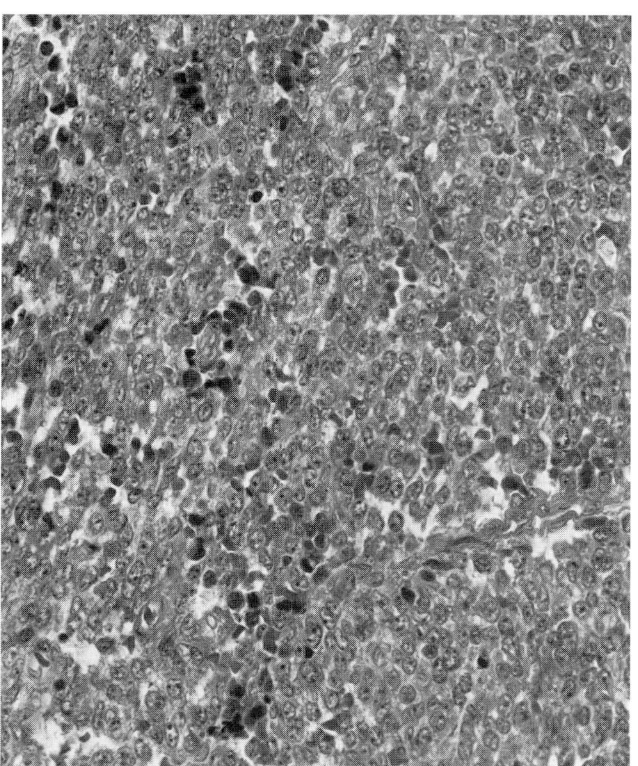

C

FIGURE 8–24. Ewing's sarcoma of the proximal radius. *A*, Radiograph shows a destructive expansile lesion in the proximal radius. *B*, Low power photomicrograph (×100) shows bone surrounded by a highly cellular neoplasm. *C*, High power photomicrograph (×400) shows sheets of round cells.

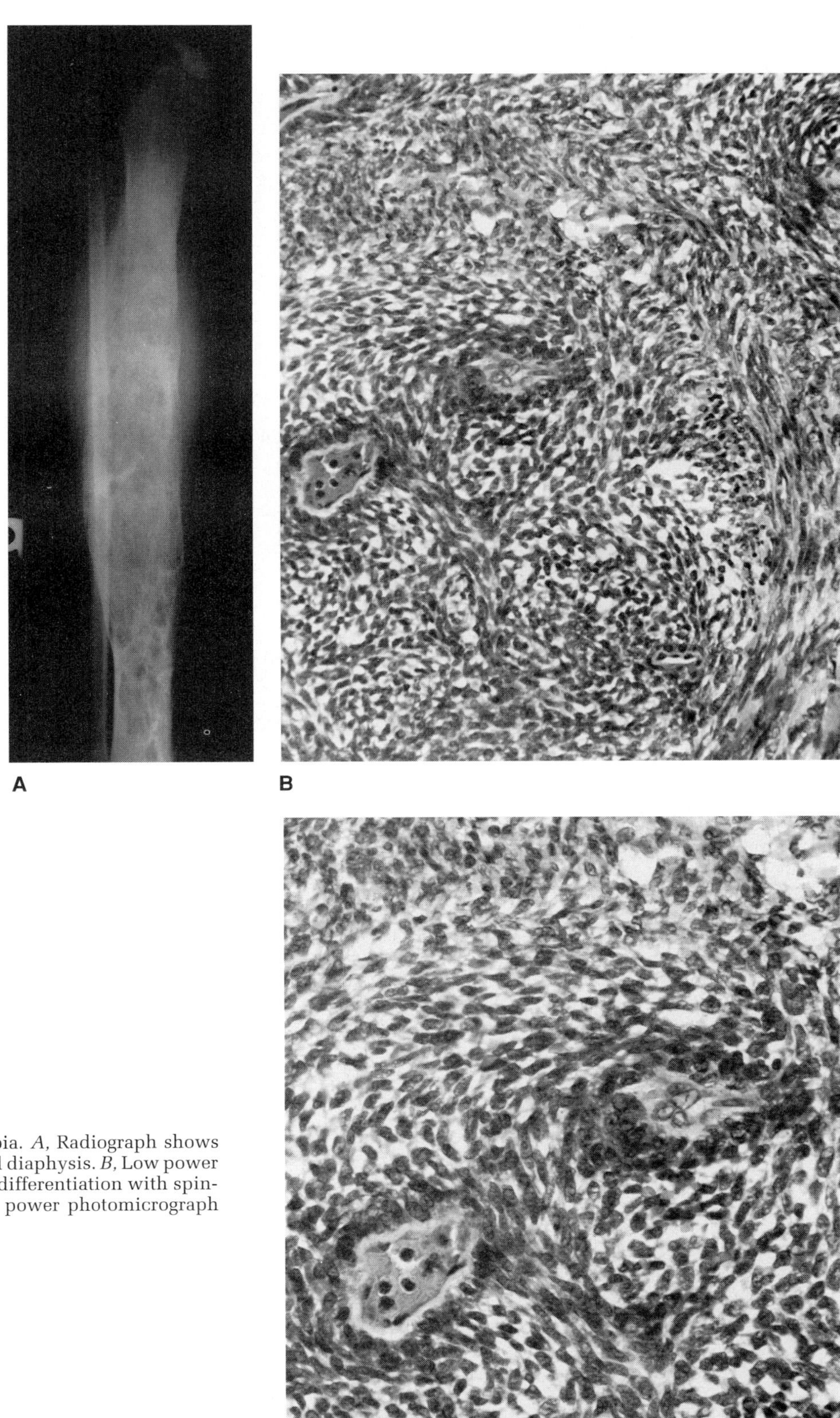

FIGURE 8–25. Adamantinoma of the tibia. *A,* Radiograph shows a bubbly symmetric lytic lesion in the tibial diaphysis. *B,* Low power photomicrograph (×250) shows biphasic differentiation with spindle cells and epithelioid cells. *C,* Higher power photomicrograph (×400).

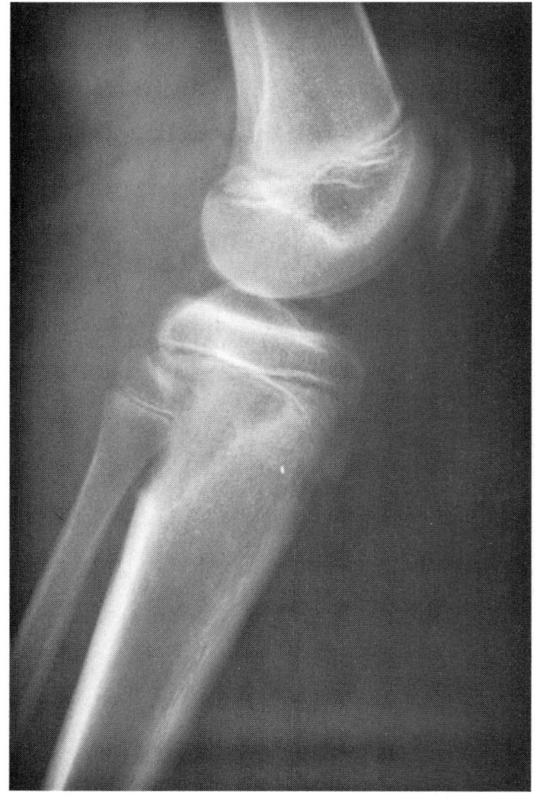

A

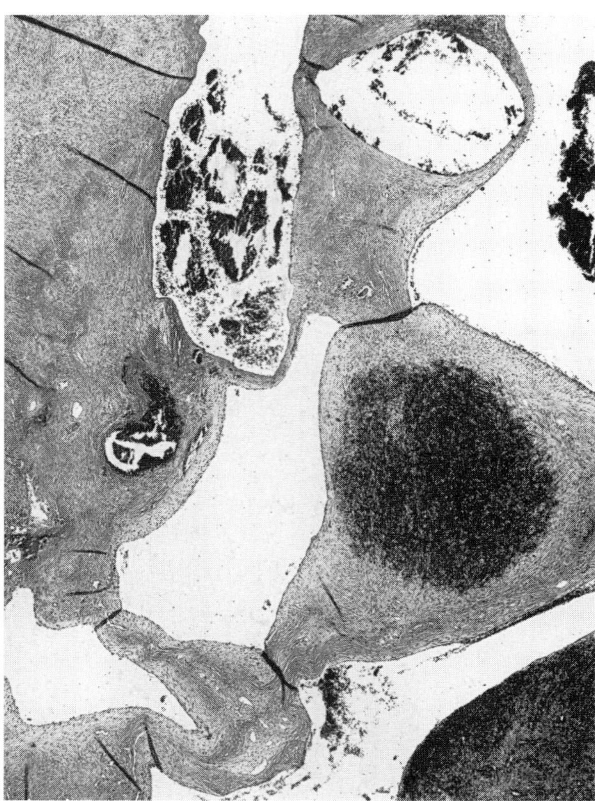

B

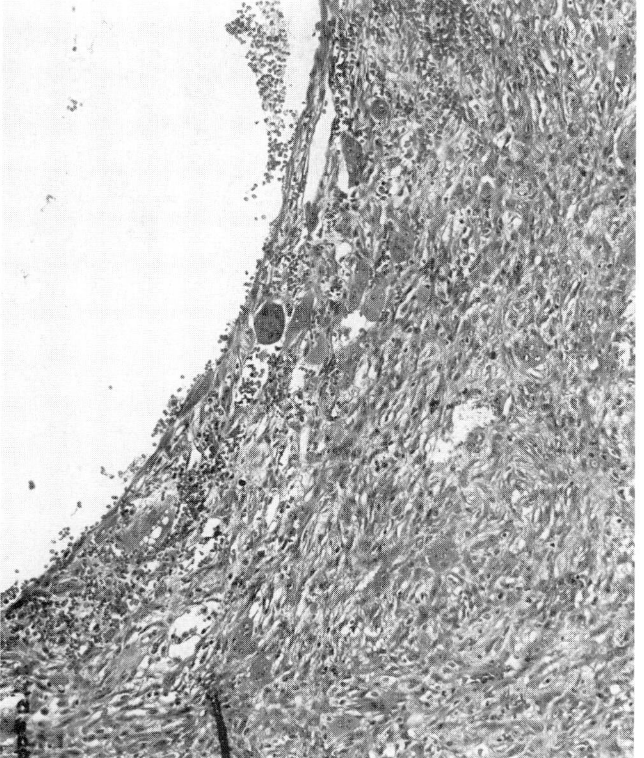

C

FIGURE 8–26. Aneurysmal bone cyst of the proximal tibia. *A,* Radiograph shows a well defined lytic lesion in the posterior tibial metaphysis. *B,* Low power photomicrograph (×25) shows blood-filled lakes. *C,* Higher power photomicrograph (×50) shows the wall of the cyst with fibroblasts and occasional multinucleated giant cells.

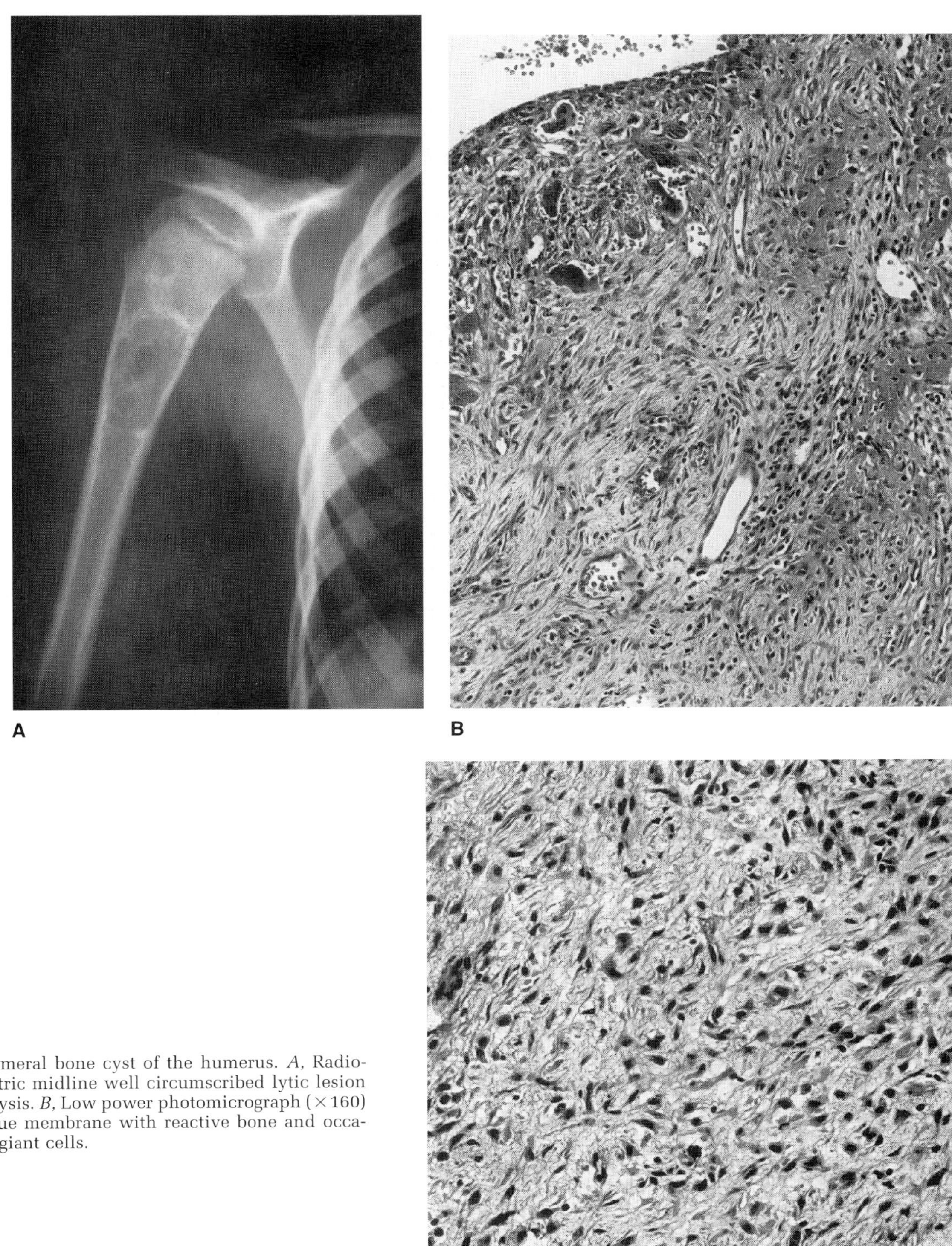

FIGURE 8–27. Unicameral bone cyst of the humerus. *A,* Radiograph shows a symmetric midline well circumscribed lytic lesion in the humeral metaphysis. *B,* Low power photomicrograph (×160) shows the fibrous tissue membrane with reactive bone and occasional multinucleated giant cells.

When the cyst abuts the physeal plate, the process is called "active"; when there is normal bone intervening, the cyst is termed "latent." Histologically, the cyst has a thin fibrous lining; the lining of the cyst contains fibrous tissue, giant cells, hemosiderin pigment, and a few chronic inflammatory cells (Dahlin). Treatment of unicameral bone cyst begins with aspiration to confirm the diagnosis followed by methylprednisolone acetate injection. Curettage and bone grafting are reserved for recalcitrant lesions, especially in the proximal femur where pathologic fractures can lead to severe hip disability.

3. Histiocytosis X (Fig. 8–28)—This disease of the reticuloendothelial system may manifest in a range from eosinophilic granuloma (usually in a single bone and self-limited) to Letterer-Siwe disease (which is a fulminant fatal form). Eosinophilic granuloma of bone is the most common manifestation where only a single bone or occasionally multiple bones are involved. Patients present with pain and swelling. The radiographs often show a highly destructive lesion with a well defined margination. The cortex may be destroyed with periosteal reaction, and there may be a soft tissue mass simulating a malignant bone tumor. There may be expansion of the involved bone. Any bone may be involved. Histologically, the proliferating histiocyte with an indented or grooved nucleus is the characteristic cell. The cytoplasm is eosinophilic, and the nuclear membrane has a crisp border. Mitotic figures may be common. Eosinophilic granuloma is a self-limited process, and several forms of treatment have been successful, including low dose irradiation (600–800 cGy), curettage and bone grafting, and observation. When the articular surface is in jeopardy or an impending fracture is a possibility, curettage and bone grafting comprise a logical choice. Low dose irradiation is effective for most lesions and is associated with low morbidity. Hand-Schüller-Christian disease is characterized by both bone lesions and visceral involvement; the classic triad, which occurs in fewer than one-fourth of patients, includes (1) exophthalmus; (2) diabetes insipidus; and (3) lytic skull lesions. Letterer-Siwe disease occurs in young children and usually runs a fatal course.
4. Fibrous Dysplasia (Fig. 8–29)—This developmental abnormality of bone is characterized by monostotic or polyostotic involvement. Yellow or brown patches of skin may accompany the bone lesions (Dahlin). When, in addition to the skin abnormalities, there are endocrine abnormalities (especially precocious puberty) with multiple bone lesions, the condition is called Albright syndrome. Virtually any bone may be involved, with the proximal femur being the most common. Radiographs may show a variable appearance with a highly lytic or ground-glass appearance; there is often a well defined rim of sclerotic bone around the lesion. The major histologic feature is proliferation of fibroblasts, which produce a dense, collagenous matrix (Dahlin). There is often trabeculae of osteoid and bone within the fibrous stroma. Cartilage may be present in variable amounts. The bone fragments are present in a disorganized fashion and have been likened to "alphabet soup" and "Chinese letters." Treatment of fibrous dysplasia is symptomatic. Internal fixation and bone grafting are used in areas of high stress where nonoperative treatment would not be effective; most patients do not need surgical treatment.
5. Osteofibrous Dysplasia—This rare variant of fibrous dysplasia primarily involves the tibia and is usually confined to the cortices. Bowing may occur. The lesion typically presents in young children below age 10. Nonoperative treatment is preferred until the child reaches maturity.
6. Paget's Disease—This condition is characterized by abnormal bone remodeling. The disease is most commonly diagnosed during the fifth decade of life. The process may be monostotic or polyostotic. Patients usually present with pain. Radiographs demonstrate coarsened trabeculae and remodeled cortices; the coarsened trabeculae give the bone a blastic appearance. Histologically, the characteristic features are irregular, broad trabeculae, reversal or cement lines, osteoclastic activity, and fibrous vascular tissue between the trabeculae (Dahlin). Medical treatment of Paget's disease is aimed at retarding the activity of the osteoclasts; agents used include diphosphonates, calcitonin, and methotrexate. The older diphosphonates (e.g., didronel) stopped both osteoclastic activity and new bone formation; didronel may cause osteomalacia and cannot be used for more than 6 months. Pamidronate, which can only be used intravenously, does not inhibit bone formation and has become one of the most useful agents in the diphosphonate class of medications. Patients may present with degenerative joint disease, fracture, or neurologic encroachment; joint degeneration is common in the hip and knee. Prior to replacement, arthroplasty patients should be treated to decrease bleeding at the time of surgery. Fewer than 1% of patients with Paget's disease develop malignant degeneration with the formation of a sarcoma within a focus of Paget's disease; the symptoms of a Paget's sarcoma are the abrupt onset of pain and swelling. The radiographs usually demonstrate cortical bone destruction and the presence of a soft tissue mass. Paget's sarcomas are deadly tumors with a poor prognosis (long-term survival is <20%).
7. Metastatic Bone Disease (Fig. 8–30)—This tumor is the most common entity that destroys the skeleton in the older patient. When a destructive bone lesion is found in a patient over age 40, metastases must be considered first; the five carcinomas that are most likely to metastasize to bone are breast, lung, prostate, kidney, and thyroid. The most common locations are the pelvis, vertebral bodies, ribs, and proximal limb girdles. The radiographs most commonly demonstrate a destructive lesion that may be purely lytic, a mixed pattern of bone destruction and formation, or a purely sclerotic lesion. The histologic hallmark is epithelial cells in a fibrous stroma; the epithelial cells are often arranged in a glandular pattern. Treatment of metastatic bone disease is aimed at controlling pain and maintaining the independ-

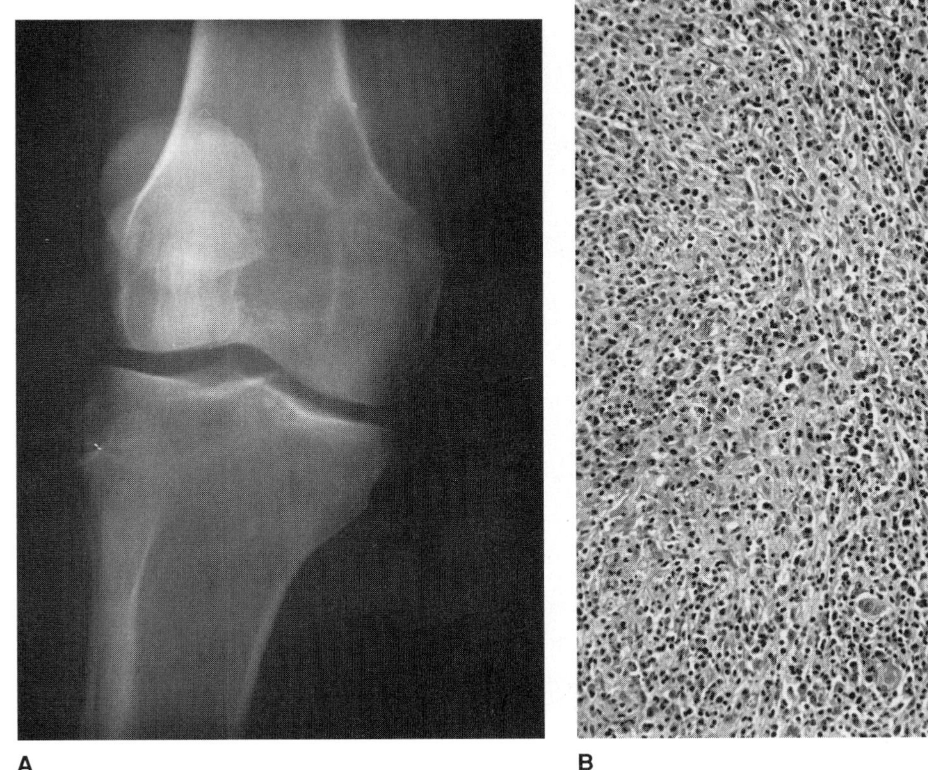

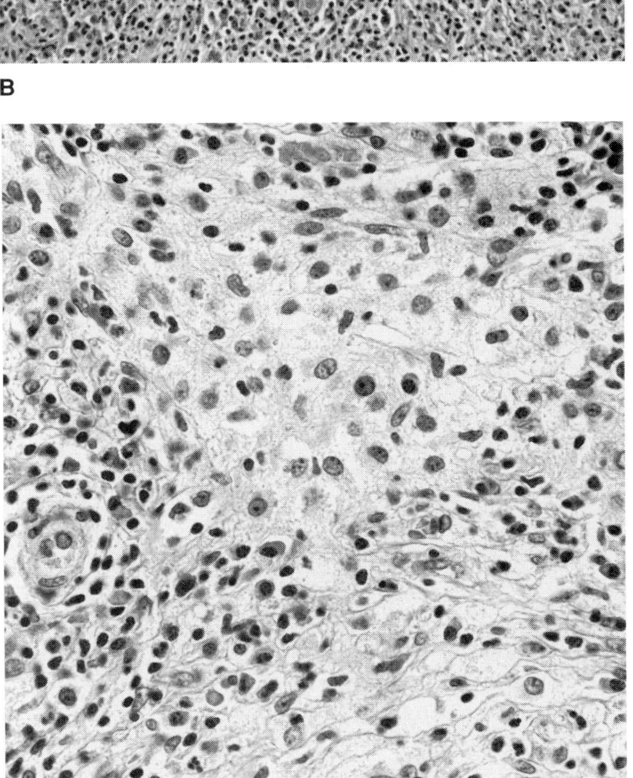

FIGURE 8–28. Eosinophilic granuloma of the distal femur. *A*, Radiograph shows a well circumscribed lesion with a sclerotic rim in the femoral metaphysis. *B*, Low power photomicrograph (×160) shows a heterogeneous population of inflammatory cells with an aggregation of histiocytes. *C*, Higher power photomicrograph (×400) shows nests of Langhans' histiocytes.

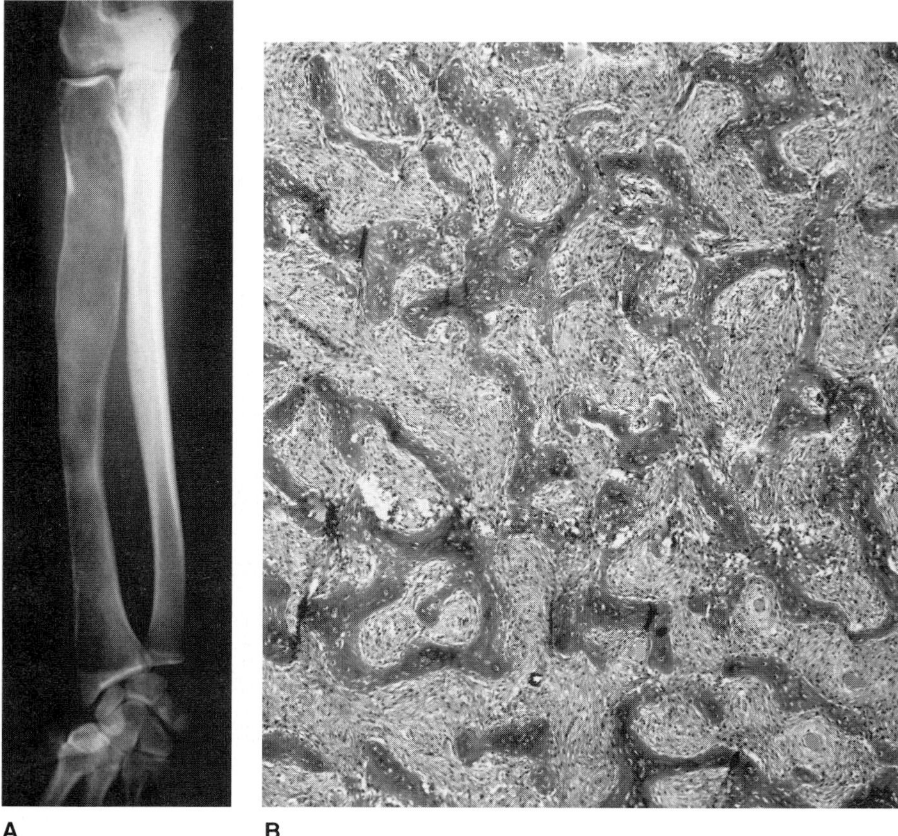

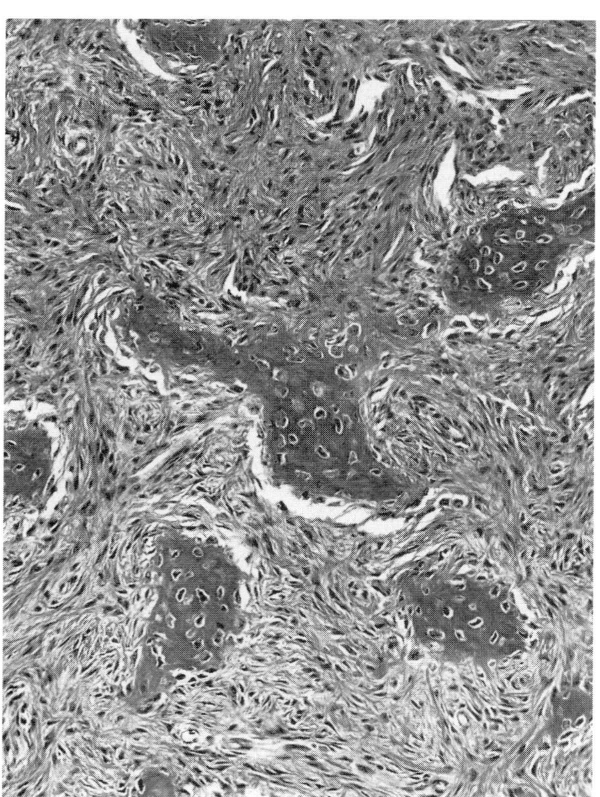

FIGURE 8–29. Fibrous dysplasia of the radius. *A,* Radiograph shows a long, symmetric, ground-glass lytic lesion of the radius. *B,* Low power photomicrograph (×50) shows seams of osteoid in a fibrous background. *C,* Higher power photomicrograph (×160) shows osteoid surrounded by bland fibrous tissue.

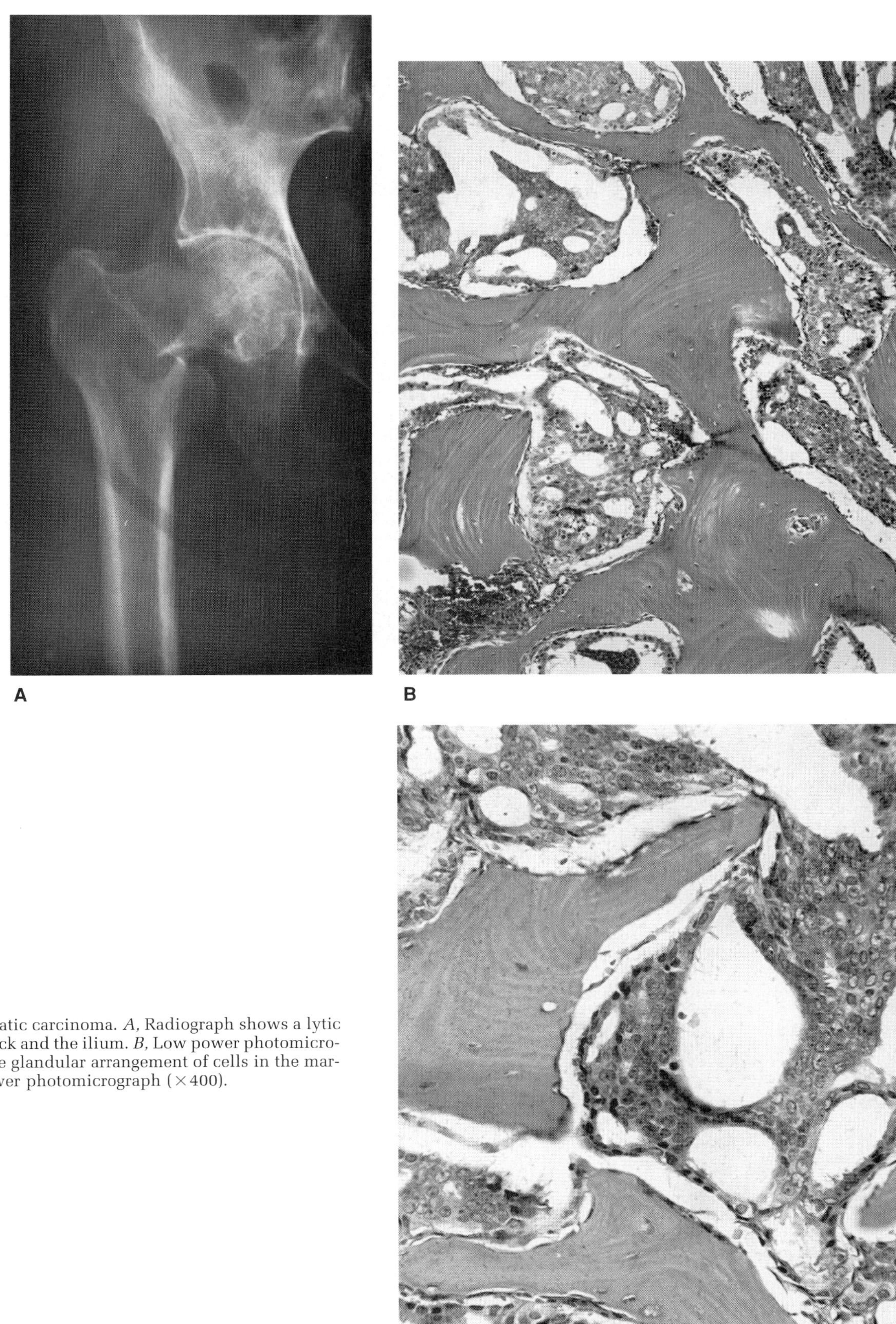

FIGURE 8–30. Metastatic carcinoma. *A*, Radiograph shows a lytic lesion in the femoral neck and the ilium. *B*, Low power photomicrograph (×100) shows the glandular arrangement of cells in the marrow space. *C*, High power photomicrograph (×400).

ence of the patient. Prophylactic internal fixation is performed when impending fracture is present. There are many criteria for fixation. Conditions that put the patient most at risk are the following.

a. More than 50% destruction of the diaphyseal cortices
b. Permeative destruction of the subtrochanteric femoral region
c. More than 50–75% destruction of the metaphysis
d. Persistent pain following irradiation

Patients over age 40 with a single destructive bone lesion without a known primary must still be considered to have metastatic disease. Simon outlined a diagnostic strategy that identifies the primary lesion in up to 80–90% of patients (Table 8–9).

8. Osteomyelitis—Bone infections often simulate primary neoplasms. Occult infections may occur in all age groups. Patients may present with fever, chills, and bone pain; most commonly, though, patients present with bone pain without systemic symptoms. The radiographs may be nonspecific. Bone destruction and bone formation are usually the characteristic findings of chronic infections; acute infections often produce cortical bone destruction and periosteal elevation. Serpiginous tracts and irregular areas of bone destruction suggest infection rather than neoplasm. Histologically, the lesion is usually apparent with: (1) edema of the granulation tissue; (2) numerous new blood vessels; and (3) a mixed cell population of inflammatory cells, plasma cells, polymorphonuclear leukocytes, eosinophils, lymphocytes, and histiocytes. Occasionally, a chronic infection is complicated by a squamous cell carcinoma. One should always biopsy material that has been sent for culture and culture material that has been sent for biopsy. The treatment of osteomyelitis is removal of all dead tissue and appropriate antibiotic therapy.

TABLE 8–9. EVALUATION OF THE OLDER PATIENT WITH A SINGLE BONE LESION AND SUSPECTED METASTASES OF UNKNOWN ORIGIN

Plain radiographs in two planes of the affected limb
Technetium bone scan to detect multiple lesions
Radiographic studies to search for occult neoplasms
  Chest radiograph and CT of the chest (to search for occult lung cancer)
  CT of the abdomen or ultrasonography of the abdomen (to detect renal cell cancer *or lymphoma*)
  Skeletal survey (if myeloma is suspected)
Screening laboratory studies
  Complete blood count with differential
  Erythrocyte sedimentation rate
  Chemistry group: liver function test, calcium, phosphorus, alkaline phosphatase
  Serum or urine immunoelectrophoresis

Selected Bibliography

Bell, R.S., O'Sullivan, B., Liu, F.F., et al.: The surgical margin in soft tissue sarcoma. J. Bone Joint Surg. [Am.] 71:370, 1989.

Berrey, B.H., Jr., Lord, C.F., Gebhardt, M.C., et al.: Fractures of allografts: Frequency, treatment, and end results. J. Bone Joint Surg. [Am.] 72:825, 1990.

Chapman, M.W., ed.: Operative Orthopaedics. Philadelphia, JB Lippincott, 1988.

Crenshaw, A.H., ed.: Campbell's Operative Orthopaedics, 7th ed. St. Louis, CV Mosby, 1987.

Dahlin, D.C., and Unni, K.K.: Bone Tumors: General Aspects and Data on 8542 Cases, 4th ed. Springfield, IL, Charles C Thomas, 1986.

Dee, R., Mango, E., and Hurst, L.C.: Principles of Orthopaedic Practice. New York, McGraw-Hill, 1989.

Dollahite, H.A., Tatum, L., Moinuddin, S.M., et al.: Aspiration biopsy of primary neoplasms of bone. J. Bone Joint Surg. [Am.] 71: 1166, 1989.

Eilber, F.R., Eckhardt, J., and Morton, D.L.: Advances in the treatment of sarcomas of the extremity—current status of limb salvage. Cancer 54:2695–2701, 1984.

Enneking, W.F.: Clinical Musculoskeletal Pathology, 3rd rev. ed. Gainesville, University of Florida Press, 1990.

Enneking, W.F., Eady, J.F., and Burchardt, H.: Autogenous cortical bone grafts in the reconstruction of segmental skeletal defects. J. Bone Joint Surg. [Am.] 62:1039–1058, 1980.

Enneking, W.F., Spanier, S.S., and Goodman, M.A.: A system for the surgical staging of musculoskeletal sarcoma. Clin. Orthop. 153: 106–120, 1980.

Enneking, W.F., Spanier, S.S., and Malawer, M.M.: The effect of the anatomic setting on the results of surgical procedures for soft parts sarcoma of the thigh. Cancer 47:1005–1022, 1981.

Enzinger, F.M., and Weiss, S.W.: Soft Tissue Tumors. St. Louis, Mosby-Yearbook, 1983.

Enzinger, F.M., and Weiss, S.W.: Soft Tissue Tumors, 2nd ed. St. Louis, CV Mosby, 1987.

Gitellis, S., Bertoni, F., Picci, P., and Campanacci, M.: Chondrosarcoma of bone—the experience at the Istituto Ortopedico Rizzoli. J. Bone Joint Surg. [Am.] 63:1248–1257, 1981.

Goldenberg, R.R., Campbell, C.J., and Bonfiglio, M.: Giant cell tumor of bone—an analysis of 218 cases. J. Bone Joint Surg. [Am.] 52: 619–663, 1970.

Goorin, A.M., Abelson, H.T., and Frei, E., III: Osteosarcoma—fifteen years later. N. Engl. J. Med. 313:1637–1643, 1985.

Goorin, A.M., Frei, E., III, and Abelson, H.T.: Adjuvant chemotherapy for osteosarcoma—a decade of experience. Surg. Clin. North Am. 61:1379–1389, 1981.

Heare, T.C., Enneking, W.F., and Heare, M.J.: Staging techniques and biopsy of bone tumors. Orthop. Clin. North Am. 20:273, 1989.

Levy, R.N.: Symposium on metastatic disease of bone. Clin. Orthop. 169:15–114, 1982.

Madewell, J.E., Ragsdale, B.D., and Sweet, D.E.: Radiologic and pathologic analysis of solitary bone lesions. Part I. Internal margins. Radiol. Clin. North Am. 19:715–748, 1981.

Mankin, H.J., Doppelt, S.H., Sullivan, T.R., and Tomford, W.W.: Osteoarticular and intercalary allograft transplantation in the management of malignant tumors of bone. Cancer 50:613–630, 1982.

Mankin, H.J., Lange, T.A., and Spanier, S.S.: The hazards of biopsy in patients with malignant primary bone and soft tissue tumors. J. Bone Joint Surg. [Am.] 64:1121–1127, 1982.

Medsger, T.A., Jr., et. al.: Twenty-fifth rheumatism review—Paget's disease. Arthritis Rheum. 26:281–283, 1983.

Merkow, R.L., and Lane, J.M.: Current concepts of Paget's disease of bone. Orthop. Clin. North Am. 15:747–764, 1984.

Miller, M.D., Yaw, K.M., and Foley, H.T.: Malpractice maladies in the management of musculoskeletal malignancies. Contemp. Orthop. 23:577–584, 1991.

Mindell, E.R.: Chordoma. J. Bone Joint Surg. [Am.] 63:501–505, 1981.

Mirra, J.H.: Bone Tumors—Clinical, Radiographic, and Pathologic Correlations. Philadelphia, Lea & Febiger, 1989.

O'Connor, M.I., and Sim, F.H.: Salvage of the limb in the treatment of malignant pelvic tumors. J. Bone Joint Surg. [Am.] 71:481, 1989.

Orthopaedic Knowledge Update Home Study Syllabus I, II, III. Chicago, American Academy of Orthopaedic Surgeons, 1984, 1987, 1990.

Pritchard, D.J., Lunke, R.J., Taylor, W.F., Dahlin, D.C., and Medley, B.E.: Chondrosarcoma—a clinicopathologic and statistical analysis. Cancer 45:149–157, 1980.

Ragsdale, B.D., Madewell, J.E., and Sweet, D.E.: Radiologic and pathologic analysis of solitary bone lesions. Part II. Periosteal reactions. Radiol. Clin. North Am. 19:749–783, 1981.

Rougraff, B.T., Kneisl, J.S., and Simon, M.A.: Skeletal metastases of unknown origin: A prospective study of a diagnostic strategy. J Bone Joint Surg [Am.] 75:1276, 1993.

Schajowicz, F.: Tumors and Tumor-like Lesions of Bone and Joints. New York, Springer-Verlag, 1981.

Sim, F.H., Beauchamp, C.P., and Chao, E.Y.S.: Reconstruction of musculoskeletal defects about the knee for tumor. Clin. Orthop. 221:188–201, 1987.

Simon, M.A.: Biopsy of musculoskeletal tumors. J. Bone Joint Surg. [Am.] 64:1253–1257, 1982.

Simon, M.A.: Current concepts review—limb salvage for osteosarcoma. J. Bone Joint Surg. [Am.] 70:307–310, 1988.

Simon, M.A., and Nachman, J.: The clinical utility of pre-operative therapy for sarcomas. J. Bone Joint Surg. [Am.] 68:1458–1463, 1986.

Springfield, D.S., Schmidt, R., Graham-Pole, J., et al.: Surgical treatment for osteosarcoma. J. Bone Joint Surg. [Am.] 70:1124–1130, 1988.

Stauffer, R.N., Ehrlich, M.G., Fu, F.H., et al.: Advances in Operative Orthopaedics. St. Louis, Mosby-Yearbook, 1994.

Sung, H.W., Kuo, D.P., Shu, W.P., et al.: Giant cell tumor of bone—analysis of 208 cases in Chinese patients. J. Bone Joint Surg. [Am.] 64:755–761, 1982.

Sweet, D.E., Madewell, J.E., and Ragsdale, B.D.: Radiologic and pathologic analysis of solitary bone lesions. Part III. Matrix patterns. Radiol. Clin. North Am. 19:785–814, 1981.

Teper, J., Glaubiger, D., Lichter, A., et al.: Local control of Ewing's sarcoma of bone with radiotherapy and combination chemotherapy. Cancer 46:1969–1973, 1980.

Uhthoff, H.K., ed.: Current Concepts of Diagnosis and Treatment of Bone and Soft Tissue Tumors. New York, Springer-Verlag, 1984.

Wold, L.E., McLeod, R.A., Sim, F.H., and Unni, K.K.: Atlas of Orthopaedic Pathology. Philadelphia, WB Saunders, 1990.

Wuisman, P., and Enneking, W.F.: Prognosis for patients who have osteosarcoma with skip metastasis. J. Bone Joint Surg. [Am.] 72: 60, 1990.

Yaw, K.M., and Wurtz, D.: Resection and reconstruction for bone tumor in the proximal tibia. Orthop. Clin. North Am. 22:133–148, 1991.

Zimmer, W.D., Berquist, T.H., McLeod, R.A., et al.: Bone tumors—magnetic resonance imaging versus computerized tomography. Radiology 155:709–718, 1985.

9

REHABILITATION: GAIT, AMPUTATIONS, PROSTHETICS, ORTHOTICS

MICHAEL S. PINZUR

I. Gait

A. Human Locomotion—The process of moving from one location to another. Walking is a cyclic, energy-efficient pattern of accomplishing that task. Walking requires that one foot be in contact with the ground at all times, with a period when both limbs are in contact with the ground. Running requires a period when neither limb is in contact with the ground. Prerequisites for normal gait include stance phase stability, swing phase ground clearance, preposition of the foot just prior to initial loading (i.e., heel strike), and energy-efficient step length and speed. Stance phase generally occupies 60% of the cycle initiated with heel strike and progresses through periods described as foot flat, heel off, and toe off. Swing phase starts at toe off and proceeds with limb acceleration to midswing, when the limb decelerates just prior to heel strike of the next cycle.

B. Determinants of Gait—Six elements of gait attempt to make the process energy-efficient by lessening excursion of the center of body mass from its standing position just anterior to S2.

1. Pelvic Rotation—The pelvis rotates about a vertical axis alternately to the left and right of the line of progression, lessening the center of mass deviation in the horizontal plane and reducing impact at initial floor contact.
2. Pelvic List—The non-weight-bearing side drops 5 degrees, lessening the superior deviation.
3. Knee Flexion at Loading—The stance phase limb is flexed 15 degrees to dampen the impact of initial loading.
4. Foot and Ankle Motion—Through the subtalar joint, allows damping of the loading response, stability during midstance, and propulsion efficiency at push-off.
5. Knee Motion—acts as a caliper with the foot and ankle to lessen necessary limb motion.
6. Lateral Pelvic Motion—The motion is 5 cm over the weight-bearing limb, narrowing the base of support and increasing stance phase stability (Fig. 9–1).

C. Muscle Action—Agonist and antagonist muscle groups work in concert during the gait cycle to effectively advance the limb through space. The hip flexors advance the limb forward during swing phase and are opposed during terminal swing prior to heel strike by the decelerating action of the hip extensors. Muscle activity can be concentric, where the muscle shortens to move a joint through space. Eccentric contraction occurs while the muscle is lengthening, which allows an antagonist muscle to dampen the activity of an agonist and act as a "shock absorber" (Fig. 9–2).

D. Gait Nomenclature—The **gait cycle** includes all activity between initial loading (i.e., heel strike) on one limb and the succeeding initial loading on the same limb. The **step** or **stride** is the distance between toe off and heel strike of the same limb. **Velocity** is a function of cadence (steps per unit time) and stride length. **Stance phase** of a limb is the period of time when that limb is in contact with the ground. **Swing phase** is the period when that limb is not in contact with the ground. **Double limb support** is the period of the cycle when both limbs are in contact with the ground. During running there is a period of time when neither limb is in contact with the ground (Fig. 9–3).

E. Pathologic Gait—Abnormal gait patterns can be caused by multiple factors. Muscle weakness or paralysis decreases the ability to normally move a joint through space. A characteristic walking pattern develops based on the specific muscle or muscle group involved and the ability of the individual to achieve a substitution pattern to replace that muscle's action. Neurologic conditions act to alter gait by producing muscle weakness, loss of balance, loss of coordination between against and antagonist muscle groups (i.e., spasticity), and late joint contracture. Pain in a limb creates an antalgic gait pattern where the individual has a shortened stance phase to lessen the time that the painful limb is loaded. Joint abnormalities alter gait by changing the motion of that joint or by producing pain.

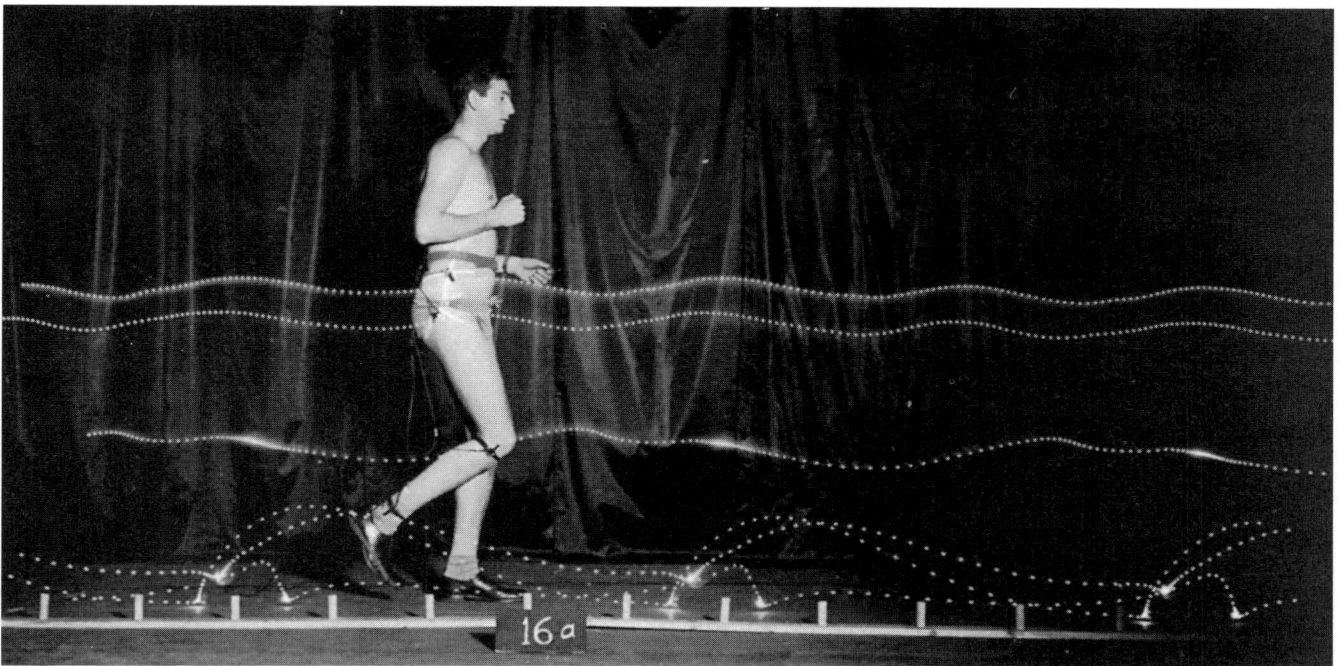

FIGURE 9–1. Interrupted light studies. The photograph was obtained by having a subject walk in front of the open lens of a camera while carrying small light bulbs located at the hip, knee, ankle, and foot. A slotted disc was rotated in front of the camera producing a series of white dots at equal time intervals. Note that the curve of displacement at the hip is a smooth curve but is not sinusoidal. This is due to the differences in phase of the two legs. (From Eberhart, H. D., and Inman, V. T. An evaluation of experimental procedures used in a fundamental study of human locomotion. Ann. N. Y. Acad. Sci. 51:1213, 1951. Inman, V.T., Ralston, H., and Todd, F.: Human Walking, p. 12. Baltimore, Williams & Wilkins, 1981, reprinted by permission.)

II. **Amputations**—Amputation of all or part of a limb is performed for trauma, peripheral vascular disease, tumor, infection, or congenital anomaly. It is often accomplished as a reasonable alternative to limb salvage. Because of the psychological implications and the alteration of body self-image, a multidisciplinary team approach should be taken to return the patient to maximum level of independent function. The process should be considered the first step in the rehabilitation of the patient, in contrast to a failure of treatment.

A. Metabolic Cost of Amputation—The metabolic cost of walking is increased with proximal level amputations, being inversely proportional to the length of the residual limb and the number of joints preserved. With more proximal amputation, patients have a decreased self-selected, and maximum, walking speed. Oxygen consumption is also increased with more proximal level amputation—so much so that the transfemoral peripheral vascular disease amputee uses virtually maximum energy expenditure during normal self-selected velocity walking (Fig. 9–4).

B. Load Transfer—The soft tissue envelope acts as an interface between the bone of the residual limb and the prosthetic socket. Ideally, it is composed of a mobile, nonadherent muscle mass covering the bone end and full-thickness skin that tolerates the direct pressures and pistoning within the prosthetic socket. It is rare for the prosthetic socket to achieve a perfect intimate fit. A nonadherent soft tissue envelope allows some degree of mobility, or "pistoning," of the bone within the soft tissue envelope, thus eliminating the shear forces that produce tissue breakdown and ulceration. Load transfer (i.e., weight-bearing) is accomplished by either direct or indirect load transfer. Direct load transfer (i.e., end weight-bearing) is accomplished with knee disarticulation, through-knee amputation, or through-ankle (Syme's) amputation. Intimacy of the prosthetic socket is necessary only for suspension. When the amputation is performed through a long bone (i.e., transfemoral or transtibial) the terminal residual limb must be unloaded and the load transferred indirectly by the total contact method. This process requires an intimate prosthetic socket fit and 7–10 degrees of flexion of the tibia below or adduction of the femur above the knee joint (Fig. 9–5).

C. Amputation Wound Healing—It is not solely dependent on vascular inflow. Patients with malnutrition or immune deficiency have a high rate of wound failure or infection. The general surgery literature has accepted a serum albumin level below 3.5 g/dl as a benchmark level for the malnourished patient. The hematology literature has accepted a total (absolute) lymphocyte count below 1500/mm^3 as its benchmark for immune deficiency. If possible, patients with stable gangrene should have amputation surgery delayed until these values can be improved by nutritional support, usually in the form of oral hyperalimentation. In severely affected patients, nasogastric or percutaneous feeding tubes are sometimes essential. When infection, infected gangrene, or severe ischemic pain dictates urgent surgery, open I&D or open amputation at the most distal viable level followed by open wound management can

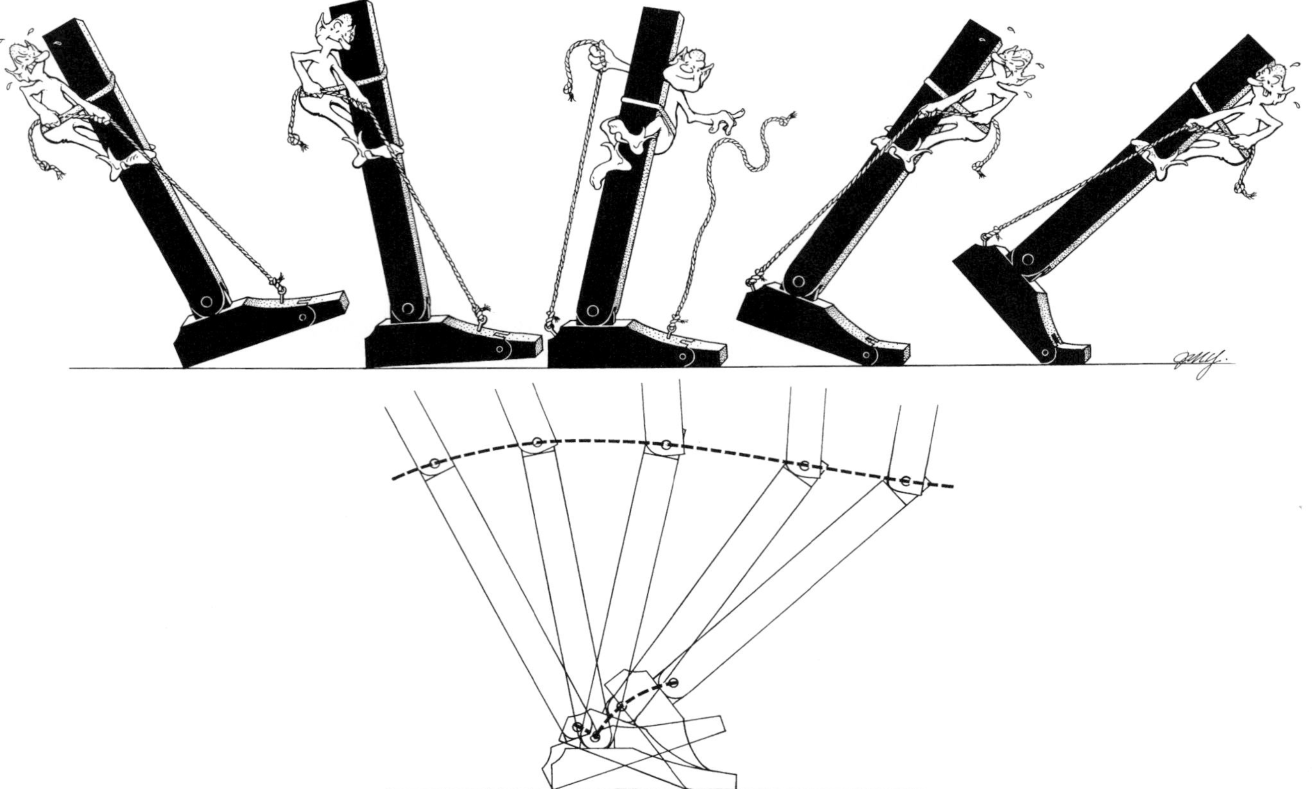

FIGURE 9–2. Effect of ankle motion, controlled by muscle action, on pathway of knee. The smooth and flattened pathway of the knee during stance phase is achieved by forces acting from the leg on the foot. Foot slap is restrained during initial lowering of the foot; afterward, the plantar flexors raise the heel. (From Inman, V.T., Ralston, H., and Todd, F.: Human Walking, p. 11. Baltimore, Williams & Wilkins, 1981, reprinted by permission.)

be accomplished until wound healing potential can be optimized. Oxygenated blood is a prerequisite for wound healing. Amputation wounds generally heal by collateral flow, so arteriography is rarely a useful tool for predicting wound healing. Doppler ultrasonography has historically been used as the measure of vascular inflow to predict wound healing in the ischemic limb. An absolute Doppler pressure of 70 mm Hg was originally described as the minimum inflow to support wound healing. The ischemic index is the ratio of the Doppler pressure at the level being tested to the brachial systolic pressure. It is generally accepted that patients require an ischemic index of 0.5 at the surgical level to support wound healing. The ischemic index at the ankle (i.e., the ankle-brachial index [ABI]) has evolved as the gold standard for assessing adequate inflow to the ischemic limb.

Standard Doppler ultrasonography measures arterial pressure. In the normal limb, the area under the Doppler waveform tracing is a measure of flow. These values are falsely elevated and nonpredictive in at least 15% of patients with peripheral vascular disease because of the noncompressibility and noncompliance of calcified peripheral arteries. The transcutaneous partial pressure of oxygen ($TcpO_2$) is the present "gold standard" measure of vascular inflow. It records the oxygen-delivering capacity of the vascular system to the level of contemplated surgery. Values of 20–30 mm Hg are correlated with acceptable wound-healing rates without the false-positive values seen in noncompliant peripheral vascular diseased vessels.

D. Pediatric Amputation—Pediatric amputations are typically the result of congenital limb deficiencies, trauma, or tumors. The old method for congenital amputations is based on the premise that the limb (or limb segment) was lost before birth, in contrast to the concept of failure of formation. The present system is based on the original work of a 1961 Conference of the International Society for Prosthetics and Orthotics (ISPO). Deficiencies are either longitudinal or transverse, with the potential for intercalary deficits (Fig. 9–6). Amputation is rarely indicated in the case of a congenital upper limb deficiency; even rudimentary appendages can be functionally useful. In the lower limb, amputation of an unstable segment may allow direct load transfer and enhanced walking. In the growing child, disarticulations should be performed whenever possible to maintain maximal residual limb length and to prevent terminal bony overgrowth. Such overgrowth occurs most commonly in the humerus, fibula, tibia, and femur, in that order; it is most commonly seen in diaphyseal amputations. Numerus surgical procedures have been described to resolve this problem, but the best method is surgical revision of the residual limb with adequate resection of

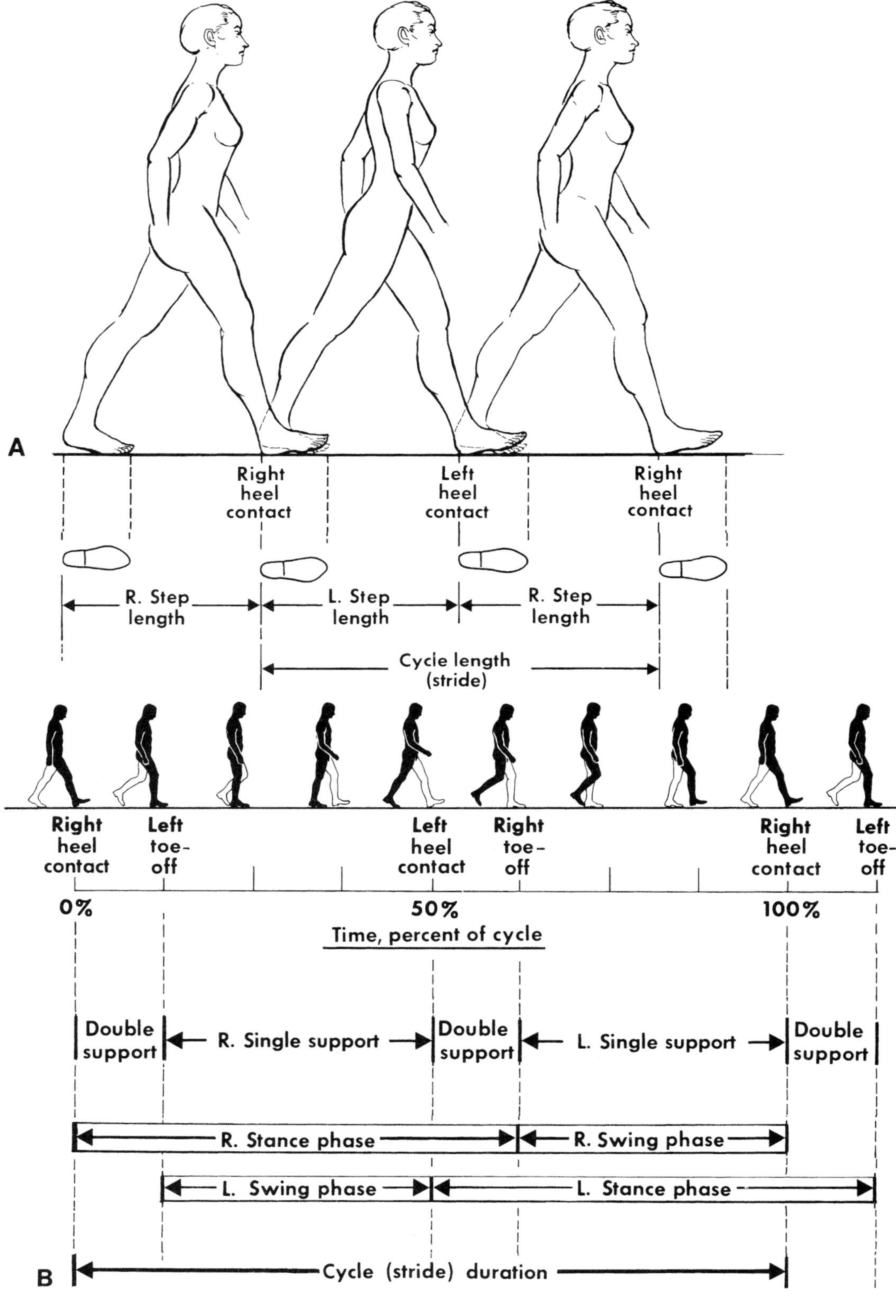

Time Dimensions of Walking Cycle

FIGURE 9–3. Distance and time dimensions of walking cycle. *A,* distance (length). *B,* time. (From Inman, V.T., Ralston, H., and Todd, F.: Human Walking, p. 26. Baltimore, Williams & Wilkins, 1981, reprinted by permission.)

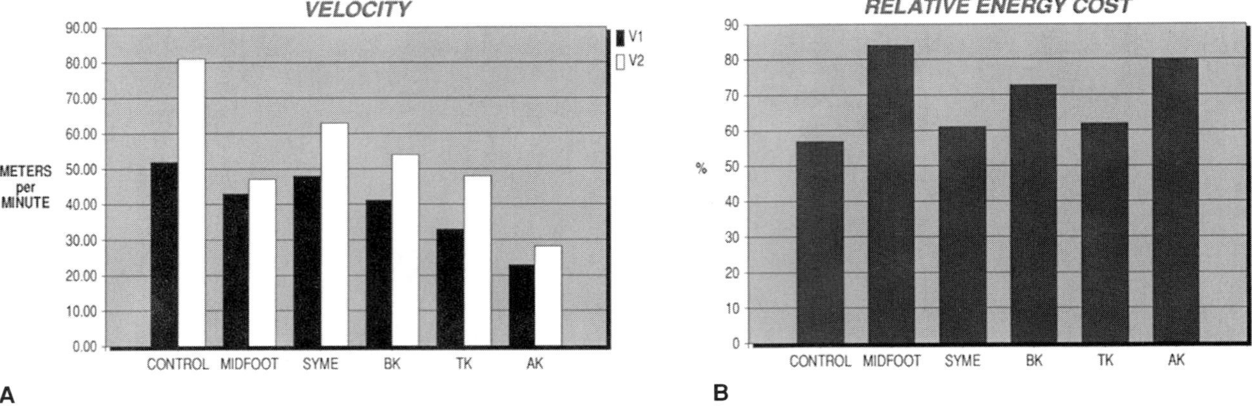

FIGURE 9–4. *A,* Walking velocity related to amputation level. *B,* Net energy cost. Ratio of oxygen consumed per meter walked to resting oxygen consumption. (From Pinzur, M., Gold, J., Schwartz, D., and Gross, N.: Energy demands for walking in dysvascular amputees as related to the level of amputation. Orthopaedics 15: 1033, 1992, reprinted by permission.)

bone or autogenous osteochondral stump capping (Fig. 9–7).

E. Trauma—The absolute indication for amputation after trauma is an ischemic limb with nonreconstructable vascular injury. Recent studies of severe open tibial fractures reveal that limb salvage is often associated with high mortality and morbidity due to sepsis, increased energy expenditure for ambulation, and decreased potential to return to work. Early amputation in the appropriate patient may prevent emotional, marital, financial, and addictive disasters. Guidelines for immediate or early amputation

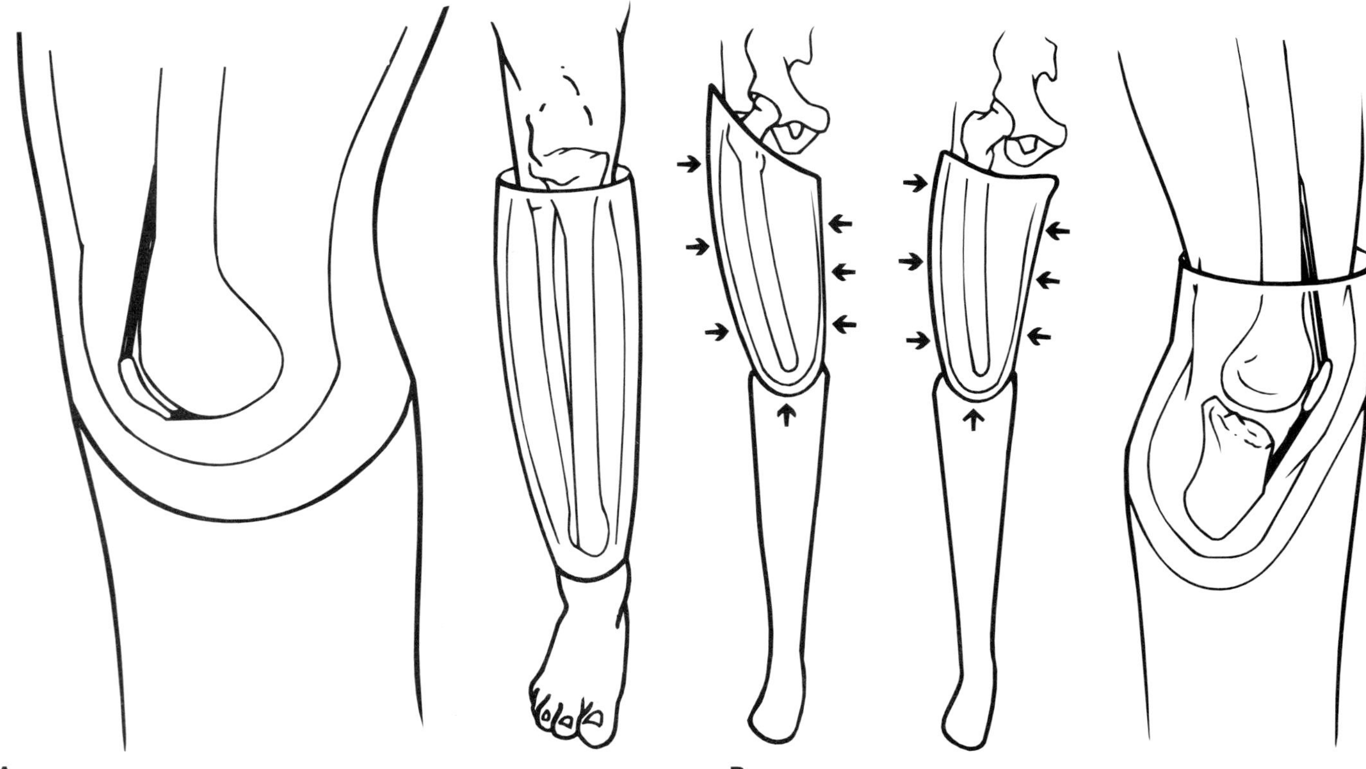

FIGURE 9–5. *A,* Direct load transfer is accomplished in the (left) through-knee and (right) Syme's ankle disarticulation amputations. *B,* Indirect load transfer is accomplished in above-knee amputations with either (left), a standard quadrilateral socket or (center) an adducted narrow medial-lateral socket. The below-knee amputation (right) transfers weight indirectly with the knee flexed approximately 10 degrees. (From Pinzur, M.: New concepts in lower limb amputation and prosthetic management. Instr. Course Lect. 39:361, 1990, reprinted by permission.)

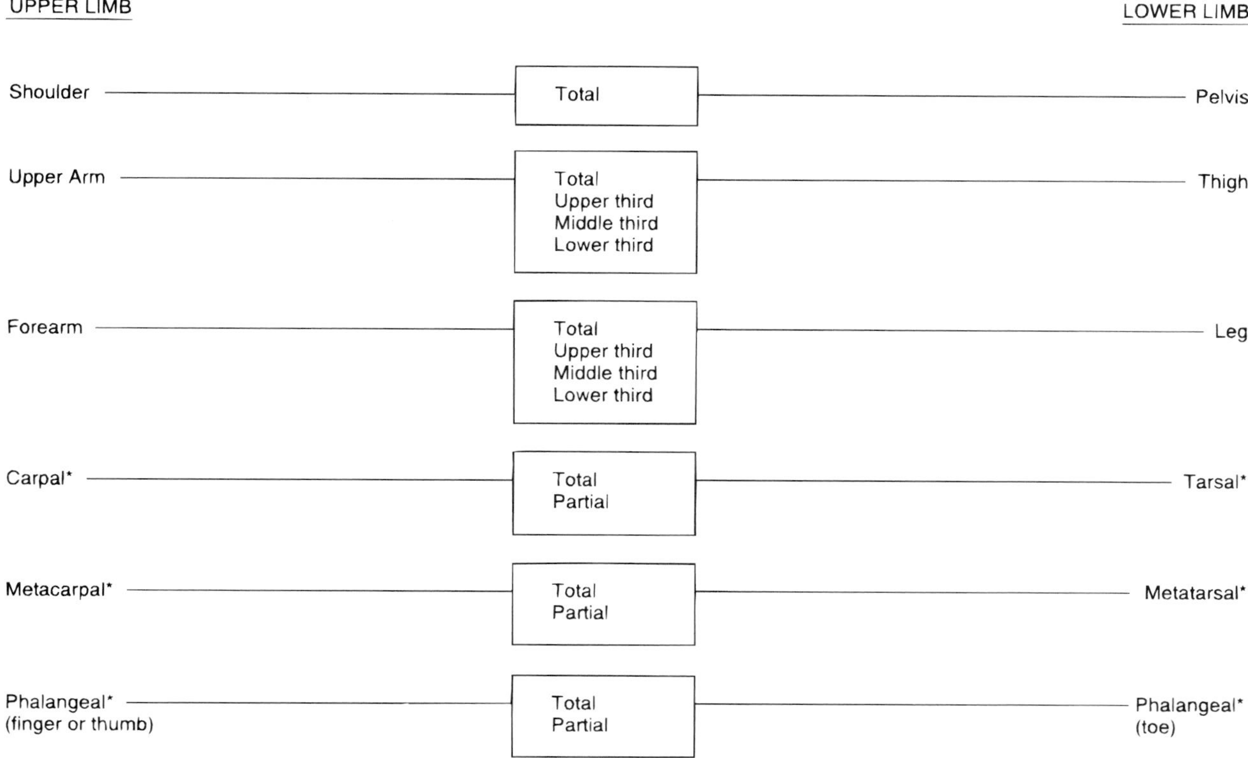

FIGURE 9–6. *A,* Designation of levels of transverse deficiencies of upper and lower limbs. Note that the skeletal elements marked with an *asterisk* are used as adjectives in describing transverse deficiencies, e.g., transverse carpal total deficiency. A total absence of the shoulder or hemipelvis (and all distal elements) is a transverse deficiency. If only a portion of the shoulder or hemipelvis is absent, the deficiency is of the longitudinal type. *B,* Description of longitudinal deficiencies of the upper limb. The *asterisk* indicates that the digits of the hand are sometimes referred to by name: 1 = thumb; 2 = index; 3 = middle; 4 = ring; 5 = little (or small). For the purpose of this classification such naming is deprecated because it is not equally applicable to the foot. (From Pinzur, M.S.: Knee disarticulation. In Atlas of Limb Prosthetics, Bowker, J., and Michael, J., eds., pp. 744–745. St. Louis, Mosby-Year Book, 1992, reprinted by permission.) *Illustration continued on following page*

of mangled limbs differs between upper and lower limbs. When a salvaged upper limb remains sensate and maintains prehensile function, it may well outperform a prosthesis. Sensation is not as crucial in the lower limb, where current prostheses more closely approximate normal function. The salvaged lower extremity with an insensate plantar weight-bearing surface is unlikely to provide a durable limb for stable walking and is likely a source of early or late sepsis. The grading scales for evaluating mangled extremities are not absolute predictors but act as a reasonable guideline for determining whether salvage is appropriate.

F. Peripheral Vascular Disease—In order for patients to learn to walk with a prosthesis and care for their residual limb and prosthesis, they must possess certain cognitive capacities: (1) memory; (2) attention; (3) concentration; and (4) organization. Patients with cognitive deficits or psychiatric disease have a low likelihood of becoming successful prosthesis users. Half of the patients are diabetic with inherent immune deficiency. Many are malnourished. If these patients have peripheral vascular disease of sufficient magnitude to require amputation, they likely have vascular disease in their coronary and cerebral vasculature. Appropriate consultation with physical therapy, social work, and psychology departments is valuable to determine rehabilitation potential. Medical consultation can determine cardiopulmonary reserve. The vascular surgeon should determine if vascular reconstruction is feasible or appropriate. The **biologic amputation level** is the most distal functional amputation level with a high probability of supporting wound healing. This level is determined by the presence of adequate viable local tissue to construct a residual limb capable of supporting weight-bearing, an adequate vascular inflow, and serum albumin and total lymphocyte count capable of supporting surgical wound healing. Amputation level selection is determined by combining the biologic amputation level with the rehabilitation potential to determine the amputation level that maximizes ultimate functional independence.

G. Musculoskeletal Tumors—Advances in chemotherapy and allograft or prosthetic reconstruction have made limb salvage a viable option in extremity sarcomas. The primary goal of musculoskeletal oncologic surgery is to provide adequate surgical margins. If adequate margins can be achieved with limb

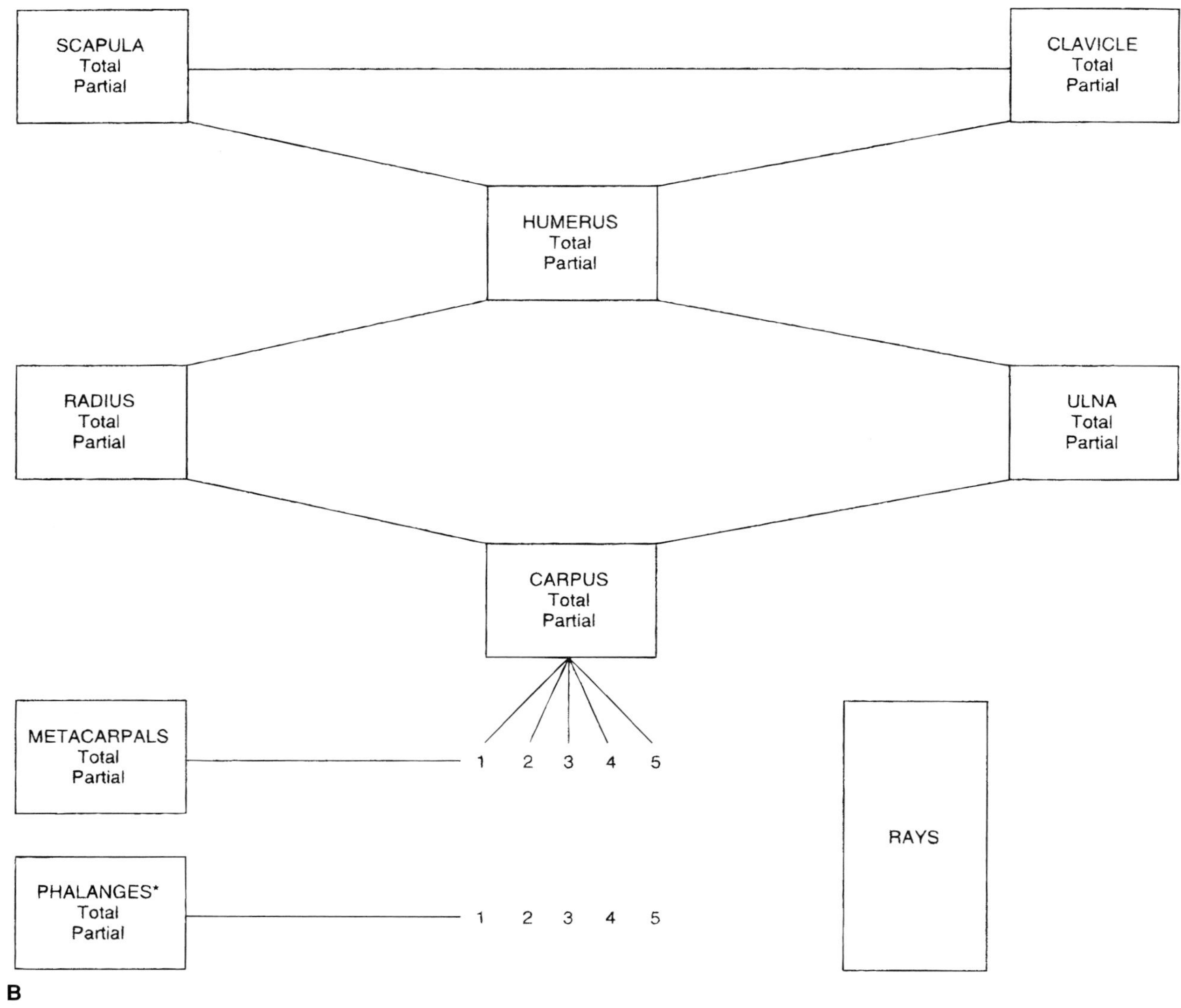

FIGURE 9–6. *Continued*

salvage, the decision can then be based on expected functional outcome. Significant controversy exists in the literature when limb salvage is compared to amputation regarding energy expenditure to ambulate and quality of life measures. Expected functional outcome should include the psychosocial and body image values associated with limb salvage. These concerns should be balanced with the apparent improved task performance and decreased worry of late mechanical injury associated with amputation and prosthetic limb fitting.

H. Gas Gangrene—There are three types of gas-forming extremity infection. Clostridial myonecrosis is the classic. Patients are acutely critically ill with sepsis and pain, and they are disoriented. There is a typical brownish discharge from their wounds and crepitus of the soft tissues when examined. Treatment requires open amputation above the level of infection. Adjunctive treatment is with penicillin and hyperbaric oxygen. Streptococcal myonecrosis is a tissue plane infection. Development is slower, and patients are not as quite as septic. Treatment requires excision of the involved compartments combined with open wound management and penicillin. Anaerobic gas-forming infections caused by gram-negative bacilli are common in diabetics. They rarely require emergency surgery.

I. Upper Limb Amputations (Fig. 9–8)—Reconstruction to obtain prehension can be accomplished with pollicization, ray transposition, central ray resection, or toe-to-hand transfer. Functional static partial hand prostheses can provide a stable post for opposition from remaining digits or the palm. Cosmetic partial hand prostheses may be psychologically beneficial to retain body image. Wrist disarticulation has two advantages over transradial amputation: (1) preservation of more forearm rotation due to preservation of the distal radioulnar joint; and (2) improved prosthetic suspension due to the flare of the distal radius. It provides challenges to the prosthetist that may outweigh its benefits. Cosmetically, the prosthetic limb is longer than the contralateral limb; and if myoelectric components are used, the motor and battery cannot be hidden

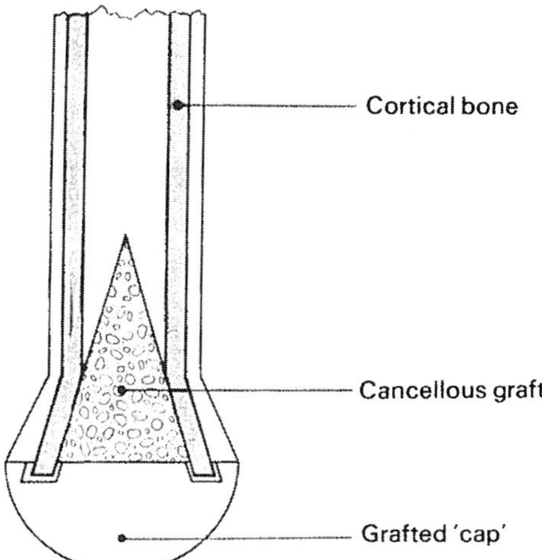

FIGURE 9–7. Diagram of the stump capping procedure. The bone end has been split longitudinally. (From Bernd, L., Blasius, K., Lukoschek, M., et al.: The autologous stump plasty: Treatment for bony overgrowth in juvenile amputees. J. Bone Joint Surg. [Br.] 73: 203–206, 1991, reprinted by permission.)

within the prosthetic shank. High levels of function can be obtained at this level of amputation. Forearm rotation and strength are directly related to the length of the transradial (i.e. below-elbow) residual limb. The optimum length is the junction of the middle and distal thirds of the forearm, where the soft tissue envelope can be constructed with adequate muscle myoplasty or myodesis, and the components of a myoelectric prosthesis can be hidden within the prosthetic shank. Because function at this level is accomplished prosthetically only by opening and closing the terminal device, elbow joint retention is essential. When the residual forearm is so short as to preclude an adequate lever arm for driving the prosthesis through space, supracondylar suspension (Munster socket) and step-up hinges can be used to augment function. Elbow disarticulation and transhumeral (i.e., above-elbow) amputations both require two acts to develop prehension, making both levels significantly less efficient and the prosthesis heavier than it is after amputation at the transradial level. The length and shape of elbow disarticulation provides improved suspension and lever arm capacity. The drawback is cosmetic, where the elbow is too far distal and the forearm shank too short for the limbs to be of equal length. This situation can be mimicked by 30 degree distal humeral osteotomy. Prosthetically, the best function with the least weight at the lowest cost is provided by hybrid prosthetic systems combining myoelectric, traditional body-powered, and body-driven switch components. These levels provide minimal function, as the patient must sequentially control two joints and a terminal device. When the lever arm capacity of the humerus is lost in proximal transhumeral or shoulder disarticulation amputations, limited function can be achieved with a manual universal shoulder joint positioned by the opposite hand, combined with lightweight hybrid prosthetic components. When not due to Raynaud's or Buerger's diseases, gangrene of the upper limb represents end-stage disease, especially in the diabetic patient. These patients are unlikely to survive 24 months after diagnosis. Localized amputations are unlikely to heal. When surgery becomes necessary, amputation should be performed at the transradial level to achieve wound healing during the final months of the patient's life.

J. Lower Limb Amputations (Fig. 9–8)—The great toe primarily and the lesser toes act as stabilizers during the stance phase. Ischemic patients generally ambulate with an propulsive gait pattern, so they suffer little disability from toe amputation. Traumatic amputees lose some late stance phase stability with toe amputation. The great toe should be amputated distal to the insertion of the flexor hallucis brevis. Isolated second toe amputation should be amputated just distal to the proximal phalanx metaphyseal flare to act as a buttress, preventing late hallux valgus. Single outer (first or fifth) ray resection functions well in standard shoes. Resection of more than one ray leaves a narrow forefoot that is difficult to fit in shoes and often develops a late equinus deformity. Central ray resections are complicated by prolonged wound healing and rarely outperform midfoot amputation.

1. Transmetatarsal and Lisfranc Tarsal-Metatarsal Amputation—There is little functional difference between these two. The long plantar flap acts as a myocutaneous flap and is preferred to fish-mouth dorsal-plantar flaps, which are performed if the available tissue dictates. Transmetatarsal amputation can be performed in the distal shaft to retain lever arm length or through the proximal metaphyses to prevent late plantar pressure ulcers under the residual bone ends. Percutaneous tendoachilles lengthening should be performed with the Lisfranc amputation to prevent the late development of equinus or equinovarus. Late varus can be corrected with lateral transfer of the tibialis anterior tendon. These patients rarely require the stability of "high-topped shoes," as they are generally sufficiently stable with oxford tie shoes. Some authors have reported reasonable functional outcomes with hindfoot amputation (i.e., Chopart's or Boyd's), but most experts recommend avoiding these levels if possible. Although children have been reported to function reasonably well, adults retain an inadequate lever arm and are prone to develop nonaccommodatable equinus.
2. Ankle Disarticulation (i.e., Syme's) Amputation—A durable amputation level that allows direct load transfer and is rarely complicated by late residual limb ulcers or tissue breakdown. It provides a stable gait pattern that rarely requires prosthetic gait training after surgery. Wagner has popularized performing the surgery in two stages; however, recent data suggest that it can be performed in one stage, even in ischemic limbs with insensate heel pads. The malleoli and metaphyseal flares should be removed from the tibia and fibula, but the remaining tibial articular surface should be retained to provide a resilient residual limb. The heel pad should be secured to the tibia either anteriorly through drill holes or posteriorly through securing the tendoachilles.
3. Transtibial (i.e., Below-Knee) Amputation—Should be performed with a long posterior myocutaneous flap as the preferred method of creating a soft tissue envelope. Optimal bone length

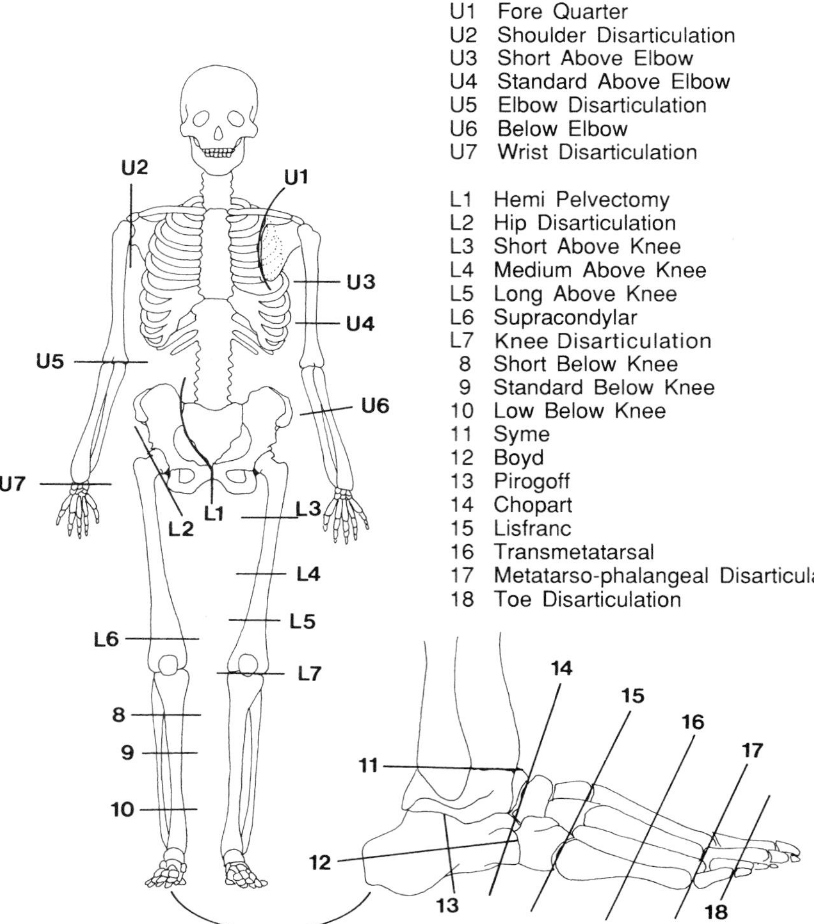

FIGURE 9–8. Composite illustration of common amputation levels.

is 12–15 cm below the knee joint or longer if adequate gastrocnemius or soleus can be used to construct a durable soft tissue envelope. Posterior muscle should be secured to the beveled anterior tibia by myoplasty or myodesis. Rigid dressings are preferred during the early postoperative period, and weight-bearing should be initiated 5–21 days after surgery if the residual limb is capable of transferring load. Young, active transtibial amputees seem to reap the greatest benefit from the new technology, including flexible sockets, silicone liner "suction" suspension, and dynamic response feet.

4. Knee Disarticulation (i.e., Through-Knee) Amputation—Presently performed using sagittal skin flaps and covering the end of the femur with gastrocnemius to act as a soft tissue envelope end pad. This level is generally performed in the nonwalker who can support wound healing at the transtibial, or distal, level. Knee disarticulation is muscle-balanced, provides an excellent weight-bearing platform for sitting, and a lever arm for transfer (Fig. 9–9). When performed in a potential walker, it provides a direct load transfer residual limb that can take advantage of the intrinsically stable polycentric four-bar linkage prosthetic knee joint.
5. Transfemoral (i.e., Above-Knee) Amputation—Creates significant problems in energy cost for walking as well as suspension of the prosthesis. Peripheral vascular disease transfemoral amputees are unlikely to become good walkers, so salvaging the limb at the knee disarticulation, or transtibial level, is critical to maintaining functional walking independence. With greater length, the lever arm, suspension, and limb advancement are optimized. The optimal transfemoral bone length is 12 cm above the knee joint to accommodate the prosthetic knee. Adductor myodesis is now thought to be essential for maintaining femoral adduction during the stance phase to allow optimum prosthetic function (Fig. 9–10). Rigid dressings are difficult to apply and maintain at this level. Elastic compression dressings must not stop short of the groin in order to prevent production of an adductor roll and should be suspended about the opposite iliac crest. Infrequently performed, few hip disarticulation amputees become meaningful walkers because of the high energy cost. Posttrauma or tumor patients occasionally use the prosthesis for limited activity. These patients sit in their prosthesis and must use their torso to achieve momentum to "throw" the limb forward to advance it.

III. Prosthetics

A. Upper Limb—The shoulder provides the center of the radius of the functional sphere of the upper limb.

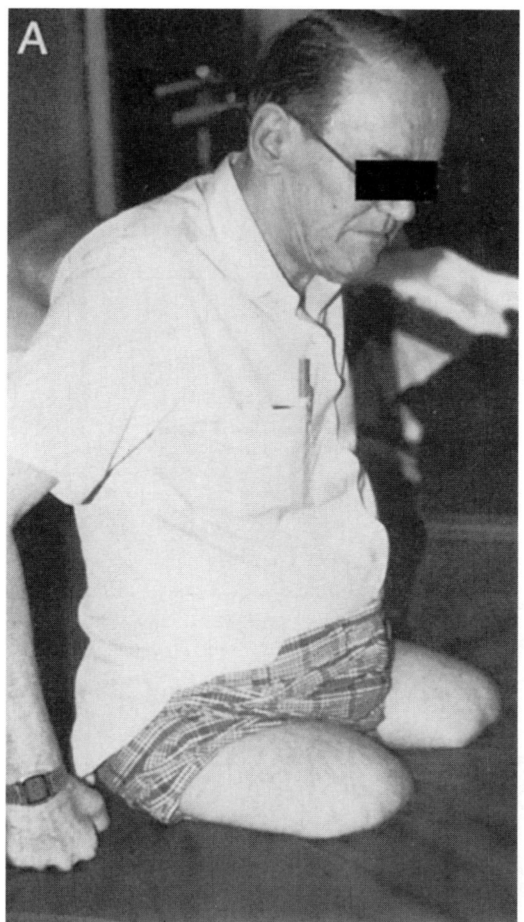

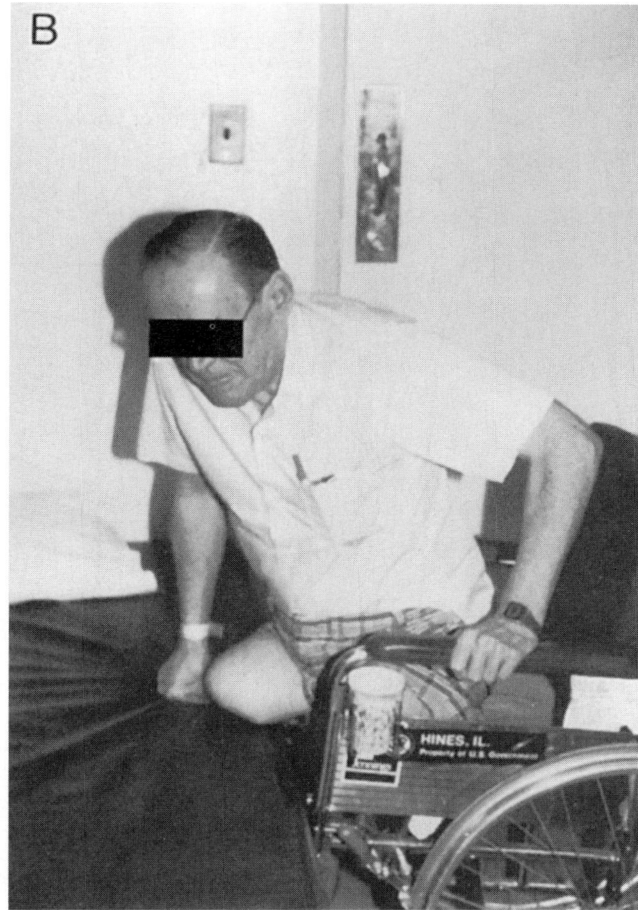

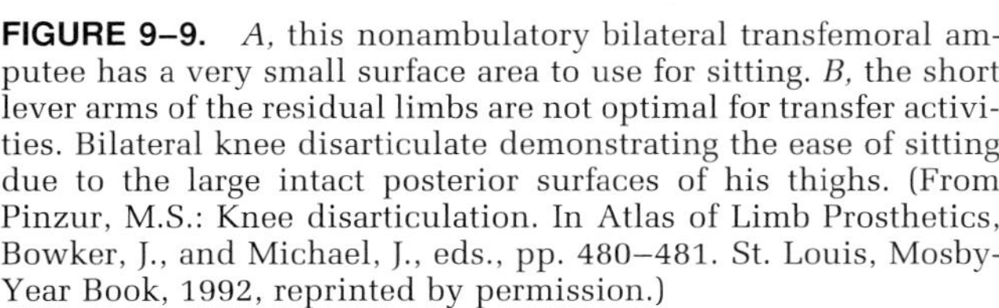

FIGURE 9–9. *A,* this nonambulatory bilateral transfemoral amputee has a very small surface area to use for sitting. *B,* the short lever arms of the residual limbs are not optimal for transfer activities. Bilateral knee disarticulate demonstrating the ease of sitting due to the large intact posterior surfaces of his thighs. (From Pinzur, M.S.: Knee disarticulation. In Atlas of Limb Prosthetics, Bowker, J., and Michael, J., eds., pp. 480–481. St. Louis, Mosby-Year Book, 1992, reprinted by permission.)

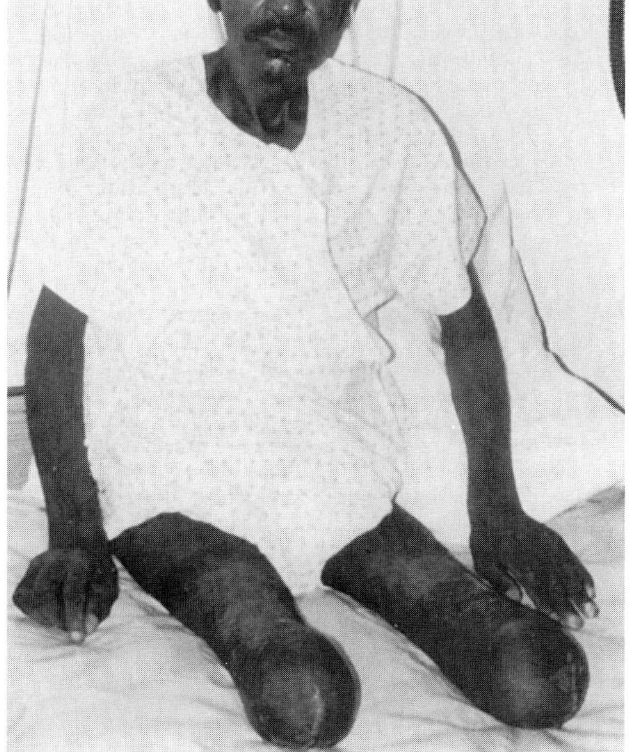

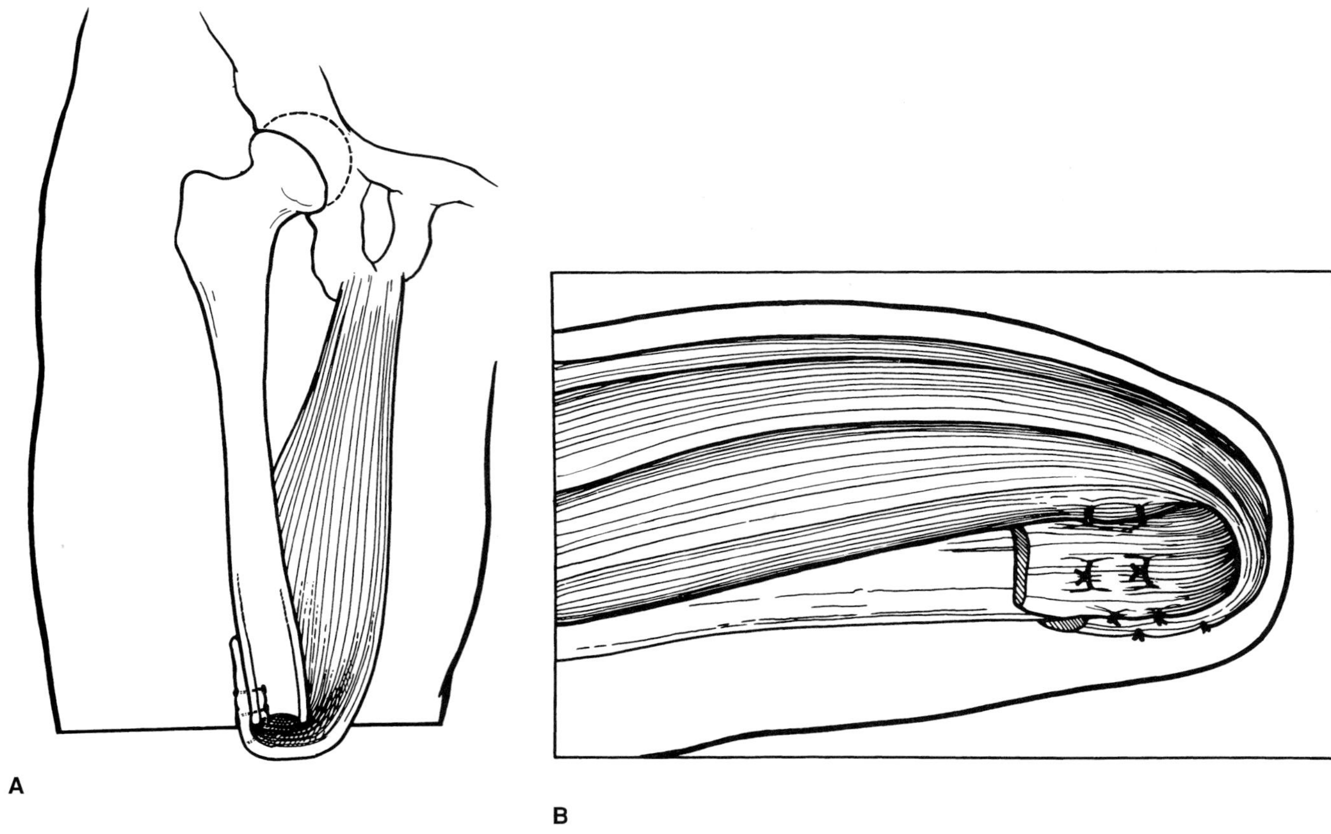

FIGURE 9–10. *A,* Diagram to show attachment of the adductor magnus to the lateral part of the femur. *B,* Diagram depicting attachment of the quadriceps over the adductor magnus. (From Pinzur, M.S.: Knee disarticulation. In Atlas of Limb Prosthetics, Bowker, J., and Michael, J., eds., pp. 479–486. St. Louis, Mosby-Year Book, 1992, reprinted by permission.)

The elbow acts as the caliper to position the hand at a workable distance from that center to perform tasks. We normally perform multiple joint segment tasks simultaneously, whereas upper limb prostheses perform these same tasks sequentially; thus joint and residual limb length salvage are directly correlated with functional outcome. Motion at the retained joints is essential to maximize that function. Residual limb length is valuable for both prosthetic socket suspension and providing the lever arm necessary to "drive" the prosthesis through space. Limb salvage is more critical for the upper limb, where sensation is critical to function. An insensate prosthesis provides less function than a partially sensate, partially functional salvaged limb. This situation is in contradistinction to the retained lower limb, where function is not as dependent on sensation. When amputation is chosen, prosthetic fitting should be initiated as soon as possible, even before the wound is secure. Outcomes of prosthetic limb use vary from 70% to 85% when prosthetic fitting is initiated within 30 days of amputation, in contrast to <50% when initiated late. Myoelectric prostheses are exciting but are slow to perform tasks. Increased speed and power requires increased weight for the motor and battery pack. They appear to be most successful in the midlength transradial amputee, where only the terminal device needs to be controlled. As more tasks are required to be performed by the prosthesis, improved function appears to be obtained with the use of a hybrid prosthesis, where myoelectric components are combined with body-powered and electrically switched components.

B. Lower Limb—Advances in lower limb prosthetics are related to socket design, socket fabrication, prosthetic–residual limb interface materials, prosthetic suspension, and dynamic response feet. New plastics allow sockets to be lighter and more flexible—and hence more comfortable. Computer-assisted design and fabrication allow more efficient fabrication with the newer materials. The standard quadrilateral prosthetic socket for transfemoral amputees is gradually being replaced by the newer ischial containment socket designs, which more efficiently transfer load by total contact. Ischial containment sockets improve comfort and suspension, but waist belts of various types are frequently necessary. Rigid outer frames can be lined with more flexible plastic liners to enhance weight distribution and improve patient comfort. Although suction remains the primary mode of suspension in transfemoral amputation prostheses, silicone liners, much like those used for transtibial amputation, are beginning to show promise. When silicone sheaths are used to provide prosthetic suspension, they provide an intimate prosthetic fit and eliminate pistoning and shear, the "enemy" of the amputation residual limb. A metal bolt can be attached to the end of the sleeve, which can lock to the prosthesis. This device has been used increasingly in young, active transtibial amputees, and most recently it has been adapted for use after transfemoral amputation. Dynamic response feet now provide "spring" to amputee walking in addition to decreasing the energy demands for walking or running. The prototype Seattle foot has a delrin plastic keel that deforms upon weight-bearing. During push-off, the Delrin "remembers" its resting shape, providing the dynamic response at "push-off." Carbon fiber has been incorporated in the keel of the prosthetic foot and is carried all the way up to the prosthetic socket attachment. The most dynamic of these prosthetic feet is the flex-foot, where carbon fiber is used to fabricate a foot–pylon unit. Prosthetic fitting for growing children is challenging, as frequent adjustments must be performed. Prosthetic fitting should be initiated to closely coincide with normal skill development. In the upper limb it begins at the time of sitting balance, usually 4–6 months of age. Initially, a passive rubberized terminal device with blunt, rounded edges is used. Active cable control and a voluntary opening terminal device are added when the child exhibits initiative in placing objects in the terminal device, usually during the second or third year of life. Myoelectric prostheses are not usually prescribed until the child has mastered body-powered components. In the lower limb, prosthetic fitting usually coincides with crawling and pulling to stand at 8–12 months of age. Knee control at the transfemoral level cannot be expected until the child demonstrates proficiency in walking with a locked knee. Children have unusual gait patterns, and formal gait training should be delayed until age 5–6.

IV. Orthoses

A. Introduction—The primary function of an orthosis is control of motion of certain body segments. Orthoses are used to protect long bones or unstable joints, support flexible deformities, and occasionally substitute for a functional task. Orthoses can be static, dynamic, or a combination. **With few exceptions, orthoses are not indicated for correction of fixed deformities or for spastic deformities that cannot be easily controlled manually.** Orthoses are named based on the joint(s) they control and the method used to obtain/maintain that control (i.e., a short-leg, below-the-knee brace is called an ankle–foot orthosis [abbreviated AFO]).

B. Shoe-Based Orthoses—Specific shoewear can be used by themselves or in conjunction with orthotics (shoe orthoses). The diabetic uses an extra-depth shoe with a high toe box to dissipate local pressures over bony prominences. The plantar surface of his/her insensate foot is protected by use of a pressure-dissipating orthotic made of pressure-dissipating materials. A paralytic, or flexible, foot deformity can be controlled with more rigid orthotics. SACH heels absorb the shock of initial loading and lessen the transmission of force to the midfoot as the foot passes through the stance phase. A rocker-bottom can lessen the bending forces on an arthritic, or limited motion capability, midfoot during midstance as the foot changes from accepting the weight-bearing load to pushing off.

C. Ankle–Foot Orthosis (AFO)—This most commonly prescribed lower limb orthosis acts to control the ankle joint. It can be fabricated with metal bars attached to the shoe or thermoplastic plastic. It can be rigid, preventing ankle motion, or can allow free, or spring-assisted motion, in either plane.

D. Knee–Ankle–Foot Orthosis (KAFO)—This orthosis extends from the upper thigh to the foot. It is generally used to control an unstable or paralyzed knee joint. It provides mediolateral stability with prescribed amounts of flexion or extension control. A subset of KAFOs are designated KOs. Knee orthoses can be made of elastic for treatment of patellar pathology or of metal and plastic in the case of anterior cruciate ligament instability.

E. Hip–Knee–Ankle–Foot Orthosis (HKAFO)—This orthosis provides hip and pelvic stability. Although it can be used for the adult paraplegic, it is rarely used because of the cumbersome nature of the orthosis and the magnitude of effort in achieving minimal gains. Experimentally, it is being used in conjunction with implanted electrodes and computerized functional stimulation of paraplegics. In children with upper level lumbar myelomeningocele, the reciprocating gait orthoses are modified HKAFOs that can be used for standing and simulated walking.

F. Shoulder Orthoses (SO)—Because of the multiple planes of motion required for normal shoulder activity, shoulder orthoses have not be successful for treating instabilities. They are usually used for post-operative immobilization after shoulder or rotator cuff surgery. The clavicular depression orthoses used for treating acromioclavicular separations have generally been discarded owing to the high incidence of pressure sores that have developed over the clavicle during treatment.

G. Elbow Orthoses—Hinged elbow orthoses provide minimal stability in the treatment of ligament instabilities. Dynamic spring-loaded orthoses have been successfully used in the treatment of flexion or extension contracture.

H. Wrist and Hand Orthoses (WHO)—The most common use of wrist and hand orthoses today is for post-operative care following injury or reconstructive surgery. These devices might be static or dynamic. The opponens splint is successful in prepositioning the thumb but has the detraction of impairing tactile sensation. Wrist-driven hand orthoses can be used in lower cervical quadriplegics. They can be body-powered by tenodesis action or motor-driven. Weight and cumbersomeness are the major limiting factors.

I. Fracture Braces—Fracture bracing remains a valuable treatment option for isolated fractures of the tibia and fibula. Prefabricated fracture orthoses can be used in simple foot and ankle fractures, ankle sprains, and simple hand injuries.

J. Pediatric Orthoses—Many dynamic orthoses are used in children to control motion without total immobilization. The Pavlik harness has become the mainstay for early treatment of congenital dislocation of the hip. Several dynamic orthoses have been used for containment in Perthes disease.

K. Spine (TLSO or CTLSO)

1. CTLSO—The prototype CTLSO is the Milwaukee brace used for scoliosis.
2. Cervical Spine—Numerous orthoses are used to immobilize the cervical spine. Effective immobilization ranges from the various types of collars, to posted orthoses that gain purchase about the

shoulders and under the chin, to the halo vest, which achieves the most stability by the nature of its fixation into the skull.

3. Thoracolumbar—Orthoses used for stabilizing mechanical back pain rely on increasing body cavity pressure. Three-point orthoses achieve their control by the length of their lever arm and the subsequent limitation of motion.

V. **Surgery for Stroke and Closed Head Injury**—The orthopaedic surgeon can play a role in the early management of adult-acquired spasticity secondary to stroke or closed head injury when the spasticity interferes with the rehabilitation program. Interventional modalities may include orthotic prescription, serial casting, or motor point nerve blocks with short-acting (bupivacaine HCl) or long-acting (phenol 3–4% in glycerol) agents. Splinting a joint (e.g., the ankle) at neutral is not sufficient to prevent the development of an equinus contracture. When functional joint ranging is insufficient to control deformity, intervention is often indicated. Anesthetic nerve blocks of the posterior tibial or sciatic nerve prior to casting relieves pain and allows for maximum correction of the deformity. Open nerve blocks may be warranted to avoid injecting mixed nerves with large sensory contributions. Irreversible surgical intervention in adult-acquired spasticity is delayed until the patient achieves maximum spontaneous motor recovery (6 months for stroke and 12–18 months for traumatic brain injury). When patients reach a plateau in functional progress or when their deformity impedes further progress, intervention can be entertained. Invasive procedures in this population should be an adjunct to a standard functional rehabilitation program, not an alternative. When surgery is considered for the goal of improving function, patients should be screened for cognitive deficits, motivation, and body image awareness. Patients should be out of a confusional state and possess short-term memory and the capacity for new learning. In addition to specific cognitive strengths, motivation is necessary for patients to utilize functional gains and participate in their rehabilitation program. Body image awareness is essential for surgical intervention to become meaningful and potentially beneficial. Patients who do lack the awareness of a limb (i.e., neglect) or its position in space should undergo therapy directed toward improving these deficits before entertaining surgical intervention.

A. Lower Limb—Balance is the best predictor of a patient's ability to ambulate following acquired brain injury. The mainstay of treatment for the dynamic ankle equinus component of this gait deviation is to achieve ankle stability in neutral position during initial floor contact (i.e., heel strike and stance) as well as floor clearance during swing phase. An adjustable AFO with available ankle dorsiflexion and a plantar flexion stop at neutral is often used during the recovery period, followed by a rigid AFO once the patient has plateaued in his/her recovery. When the dynamic equinus overpowers the holding power of the orthosis and patients "walk out" of their brace, motor balancing surgery is indicated. The equinus deformity is treated by percutaneous tendoachilles lengthening. The dynamic varus-producing force in adults is the result of out-of-phase tibialis anterior muscle activity during the stance phase. This dynamic varus deformity is corrected either by split or complete lateral transfer of the tibialis anterior muscle.

B. Upper Limb—There is a paucity of literature dealing with acquired spasticity in the upper limb. Invasive intervention can be considered for functional and nonfunctional goals. Surgical release of static contracture is generally performed to assist nursing care or hygiene when the fixed contracture ± spasticity component produces skin maceration or breakdown. A functional use of static contracture release is to improve upper extremity "tracking" (i.e., arm swing) during walking. Most upper extremity surgery performed in this patient population has the goal of increasing prehensile hand function. The goal may be simply to improve placement, enabling use of the hand as a "paperweight," or to achieve improved fine motor control. In patients with prehensile potential, surgery may be entertained to make the "one-handed" patient "two-handed" by increasing involved hand function from no function to assistive, or from assistive to independent. When the goal of surgery is to improve function, patients must first be screened for cognitive capacity, motivation, and body image awareness. Patients must have the cognitive skills and learning capability to participate in their therapy after surgery and to functionally make use of their newly acquired skills at the completion of their rehabilitation program. If they are not motivated, they will not participate in the prolonged effort necessary to achieve meaningful functional improvement. Patients with poor stereognosis or neglect (i.e., poor body image awareness) find that their involved hand "drifts" in space and is not "available" for use if they have not been carefully trained in visual compensation techniques. Once it has been determined that the patient has the potential to make functional upper extremity gains with surgery, he or she is graded on the basis of hand placement, proprioception and sensibility, and voluntary motor control. Dynamic EMG is utilized when delineation of phasic motor activity is essential. Muscle unit lengthening, by fractional musculotendinous or step-cut methods, of the agonist deforming muscle units is combined with motor-balancing tendon transfers of the antagonists to achieve muscle balance and improved prehensile hand function.

VI. **Spinal Cord Injury (SCI)**—The functional level in a spinal cord-injured patient is determined by the most distal intact functional dermatome (sensory level) and the most distal motor level where most of the muscles at that level function at least at a "fair" motor grade.

A. Mobility—SCI level determines mobility. C4 and higher levels require high back and head support. At C5, mouth-driven accessories can control a motorized wheelchair. Various body-powered or motor-driven orthoses can assist functional prehension. C6 levels can operate manual wheelchairs. Transfers are dependent at C4, assisted at C5, and dependent at C6.

B. Activities of Daily Living (ADL)—C6 levels can groom and dress themselves. C7 can cut meat. Bowel and bladder function can be controlled via rectal stimulation and intermittent catheterization.

C. Psychosocial Factors—Men may be impotent but can often achieve a reflex erection.

D. Autonomic Dysreflexia—This potentially catastrophic hypertensive event can occur with injuries above T5. It is usually caused by an obstructed urinary catheter or fecal impaction.

E. Surgery—Spinal fusion is frequently used to expedite rehabilitation and prevent the late development of pain or deformity at the fracture level. Spasticity and contracture can produce problems in hygiene or the development of pressure ulcers. Percutaneous, or open, motor nerve blocks with phenol can be used to treat these deformities. When the deformity is a static contracture, muscle release or disarticulation may improve sitting or transfer potential. Tendon transfers can be used in the upper limb to eliminate the need for an orthosis or allow the patient to achieve function with an orthosis.

VII. **Postpolio Syndrome**—The postpolio syndrome is probably not a reactivation of the polio virus. It is likely an aging phenomenon. These patients use a high proportion of their capacity for normal ADLs. With aging and the drop-off of muscle units, they no longer have the reserves to perform their daily activities. Treatment comprises prescribed limited exercise combined with periods of rest, so muscles are maintained but not overtaxed. Standard polio surgeries, combining contracture release, arthrodesis, and tendon transfer, are indicated when deformity overcomes functional capacity.

Selected Bibliography

Gait

Gage, J.R.: An overview of normal walking. Instr. Course Lect. 39: 291, 1990.

Inman, V.T., Ralston, H., and Todd, F.: Human Walking. Baltimore, Williams & Wilkins, 1981.

Ounpuu, S.: The biomechanics of running: A kinematic and kinetic analysis. Instr. Course Lect. 39:305, 1990.

Perry, J.: (1) Gait analysis in sports medicine. (2) Pathologic gait. Instr. Course Lect. 39:319, 325, 1990.

Amputations

Bernd, L., Blasius, K., Lukoschek, M., et al.: The autologous stump plasty: Treatment for bony overgrowth in juvenile amputees. J. Bone Joint Surg. [Br.] 73:203–206, 1991.

Bowker, J., and Michael, J., ed.: Atlas of Limb Prosthetics. St. Louis, Mosby-Year Book, 1992.

Day, H.: The ISO/ISPO classification of congenital limb deficiency. In Atlas of Limb Prosthetics, Bowker, J., and Michael, J., eds. St. Louis, Mosby-Year Book, 1992.

DeHaven, K., and Evarts, J.: Gas gangrene. J. Trauma 11:983, 1971.

Gottschalk, F., Kourosh, S., Stills, M., et al.: Does socket configuration influence the position of the femur in above-knee amputation? J. Prosthet. Orthot. 2:94–102, 1989.

Kay, H.: The Proposed International Terminology for the Classification of Congenital Limb Deficiencies, the Recommendations of a Working Group of ISPO. London, Spastics International Medical Publications, Heinemann Medical Books; Philadelphia, JB Lippincott, 1975.

Lagaard, S., McElfresh, E., and Premer, R.: Gangrene of the upper extremity in diabetic patients. J. Bone Joint Surg. [Am.] 71:257, 1989.

Pinzur, M.: New concepts in lower limb amputation and prosthetic management. Instr. Course Lect. 39:361, 1990.

Pinzur, M., Gold, J., Schwartz, D., and Gross, N.: Energy demands for walking in dysvascular amputees as related to the level of amputation. Orthopaedics 15:1033, 1992.

Pinzur, M., Sage, R., Stuck, et al.: Transcutaneous oxygen tension as a predictor of wound healing in amputations of the foot and ankle. Foot Ankle 11:394, 1990.

Pinzur, M.S.: Knee disarticulation. In Atlas of Limb Prosthetics, Bowker, J., and Michael, J., eds., pp. 479–486. St. Louis, Mosby-Year Book, 1992.

Wagner, F.: A classification and treatment program for diabetic, neuropathic, and dysvascular foot problems. Instr. Course Lect. 28: 143, 1979.

Waters, R.L., Perry, J., Antonelli, D., et al.: Energy cost of walking of amputees: The influence of level of amputation. J. Bone Joint Surg. [Am.] 58:42, 1976.

Wyss, C., Harrington, R., Burgess, and Matsen, F.: Transcutaneous oxygen tension as a predictor of success after an amputation. J. Bone Joint Surg. [Am.] 70:203, 1988.

Prosthetics

Bowker, J., and Michael, J., eds.: Atlas of Limb Prosthetics. St. Louis, Mosby-Year Book, 1992.

Light, T.: Kinesiology of the upper limb. In Atlas of Orthotics, Bunch, W., ed., pp. 126–138. St. Louis, CV Mosby, 1985.

Orthotics

Bunch, W., ed.: Atlas of Orthotics. St. Louis, CV Mosby, 1985.

Stroke and Closed Head Injury

Braun, R.: Stroke and brain injury. In Operative Hand Surgery, Green, D., ed., pp. 227–254. New York, Churchill Livingstone, 1988.

Braun, R., Vise, G., and Roper, B.: Preliminary experience with superficialis-to-profundus tendon transfer in the hemiplegia upper extremity. J. Bone Joint Surg. [Am.] 56:466–472, 1974.

Pinzur, M.: Surgery to achieve dynamic motor balance in adult acquired spastic hemiplegia: A preliminary report. J. Hand Surg. 10A:547–553, 1985.

Pinzur, M., Sherman, R., Dimonte-Levine, P., et al.: Adult-onset hemiplegia: Changes in gait after muscle-balancing procedures to correct the equinus deformity. J. Bone Joint Surg. [Am.] 68: 1249–1257, 1986.

10

TRAUMA

THOMAS E. SHULER

SECTION 1
Adult Trauma

I. **Introduction**—Fractures may be classified based on location (e.g., proximal, middle, distal thirds), direction (transverse, spiral, oblique, comminuted, segmental), alignment (angulation [apex], displacement [of distal fragment], articular involvement), and associated factors (e.g., open fractures, dislocations). Many factors come into play in the description and ultimate management of fractures. The mechanism of injury is important because it provides important clues to the nature of the injury. For example, traction injuries result in avulsion fractures, compression forces yield angulated or T-type fractures, and rotational forces cause spiral fractures. The mechanism of injury may also be used in classification schemes for certain injuries (e.g., ankle and spine fractures).

II. **Open Fractures**

A. Introduction—Open fractures, whether obvious or subtle, always communicate with the environment. Therefore contamination and soft tissue envelope disruption mandate that these injuries be handled with special consideration. Formal radical débridement and irrigation (ideally within 4–8 hours of the injury), IV antibiotics (consisting of a first or second generation cephalosporin and an aminoglycoside [and penicillin for barnyard or *Clostridium* infections]) for 48 hours and after each subsequent procedure, appropriate immobilization and fixation, and careful wound management help reduce the risk of acute infection. Early flap coverage (48 hours to 1 week after injury) has also been shown to reduce risk of chronic infections.

B. Classification—Based on the size of the wound and amount of soft tissue injury (Gustilo).

TYPE	SIZE (cm)	OTHER FACTORS
I	<1	Low energy
II	<10	Moderate energy
III	>10	High energy; high-velocity gunshot wounds, close range shotgun wounds, barnyard injuries, segmental fractures, neurovascular injury, open >8 hours

Type III fractures are further classified as follows.

SUBCLASS	DESCRIPTION
IIIA	Adequate soft tissue coverage
IIIB	Massive soft tissue destruction, bony exposure
IIIC	Fractures associated with repairable vascular injury

C. Gunshot Wounds (GSWs)—Soft tissue and bony destruction is based on the velocity of the missile (KE $= \frac{1}{2} mv^2$). Low velocity GSWs (<2000 ft/sec—most handguns) cause less soft tissue destruction, and treatment usually consists of entry/exit wound débridement. High velocity GSWs (>2000 ft/sec—military rifles) can cause massive soft tissue destruction and require two-stage débridement of the entire missile tract. Partially jacketed (dum-dum), unjacketed, and hollow point bullets cause greater soft tissue destruction. Shotgun wounds, especially at short range, often result in type III wounds because of extensive soft tissue injury. The wadding has a high potential for contamination of wounds and must be sought at the time of débridement. Intra-articular missiles should be removed because of the potential for lead intoxication. Nerve injuries associated with GSWs are often temporary (neurapraxia) and are caused by the blast effect of missiles traversing the tissue. Arterial injuries may present with decreased or absent pulses, an expanding hematoma, a thrill, or massive blood loss. Arteriograms should be used liberally if there is any question of an arterial injury.

III. **General Treatment Principles**

A. ATLS Guidelines—Treatment of orthopaedic injuries must follow adequate stabilization of the patient (life before limb). ATLS guidelines should be rigidly followed. An adequate airway should be secured before checking for pulses and bleeding. **Nasotracheal intubation** is recommended in **breathing patients with cervical spine injuries; oral endotracheal intubation** with in-line traction is favored **for all nonbreathing patients.** A chest radiograph should be checked for mediastinal widening and pneumo- or hemothorax. C-spine radiograph should include the top of T1. ATLS principles practiced at trauma centers have decreased preventable death from 14% to 3%. The trauma score (based on respiratory, cardiovascular, and neurologic parameters) is predictive of injury severity and prognosis. The most common abdominal injuries include rupture of the spleen followed by liver injuries. Diagnostic peritoneal lavage (DPL) and CT can be utilized for abdominal assessment. **False positive** DPL results can be seen in patients with **pelvic fractures.** Therefore DPL should be performed above the umbilicus in patients with pelvic fractures. Pericardial tamponade should be suspected with a narrow pulse pressure and an elevated diastolic blood pressure. IVP studies are indicated for gross hematuria only. Head injuries are the most common cause of early death with trauma (Glasgow Coma Scale score <8 being severe). Hemorrhage can result from ruptured viscera and is also commonly seen with pelvic fractures. The orthopaedist plays a key role in the latter injuries with early application of external fixation to select pelvic fractures and in guiding the trauma team regarding the placement of suprapubic tubes, incisions, and colostomies. Poor placement may preclude an approach to fixation of certain pelvic and acetabular fractures. Once stabilized, neurodynamically the patient should be carefully assessed for extremity injuries, which must be reduced and stabilized. Determining the mechanism of injury, careful physical examination, and obtaining appropriate radiographs should be done in every trauma patient.

B. Reduction—Reduction can be closed (manipulation or traction) or open (usually combined with internal fixation). Manipulative reduction usually involves exaggeration of the mechanism of injury followed by reversal of these forces. Traction, often applied to the femur or cervical spine through weights and skeletal fixation, may be temporary or prolonged. Open reduction, either primarily or after failure of other methods, should restore the fracture to as near anatomic alignment as possible. Joint surface involvement demands near-an-atomic reduction (≤ 2 mm). Age, function, and physiologic stability of the patient are important in considering the goals for reduction.

C. Immobilization—Used to prevent displacement or angulation, to decrease movement at the fracture site, or to relieve pain. Immobilization can be through casting, splinting, orthotics, traction, external fixation, or internal fixation. Internal fixation is indicated when closed methods have failed, when experience dictates it to be necessary (e.g., Galeazzi fractures of the forearm), for displaced intra-articular fractures, with tumors, with associated vascular injuries, and in multiply injured patients for mobilization.

D. Preservation of Function—Rehabilitation during and after fracture treatment is essential for good results. Judicious use of physical and occupational therapy often improves eventual fracture outcome. Lower extremity intra-articular fractures should be fixed anatomically, and affected patients should be kept non-weight-bearing with early range of motion for best results.

E. Fracture Healing (See Chapter 1, Basic Sciences)—Optimal conditions for fracture healing are an adequate vascular supply, minimal necrosis, anatomic reduction, immobilization, the presence of physiologic stress, and the absence of infection.

IV. Radiography

A. Introduction—Standard AP and lateral radiographs, to include the joint above and below the fracture level, are the minimal requirement for most fractures. Poor quality radiographs should be repeated. For severely displaced or comminuted fractures, traction radiographs may be useful. For periarticular fractures, internal and external oblique views as well as views centered on the fracture can provide additional detail.

B. Special Views—The radiographs listed in Table 10–1 are helpful for ascertaining fracture patterns of particular areas/injuries.

C. Additional Studies—Tomograms are useful for evaluating sternoclavicular injuries, tibial plateau fractures, and some carpal and tarsal fractures. CT scans are vital for evaluating complex spinal, pelvic, calcaneal, sternoclavicular, and other fractures. MRI is also becoming helpful, particularly for diagnosing soft tissue injuries. Nuclear medicine studies are useful for finding stress fractures and subtle wrist injuries.

V. Complications

A. Introduction—Complications occur commonly after trauma and can be a direct result of the injury (intrinsic) or can be associated with other organ systems (extrinsic). General complications are discussed in this section; specific complications unique to individual fractures/dislocations are listed in Tables 10–2 through 10–5 (following Part 1).

B. Bone Healing Abnormalities—Can include delayed union, nonunion, malunion, and avascular necrosis. These problems are more common with high-energy injuries and occur more frequently in bones with limited blood supply/healing potential.

1. Delayed Union/Nonunion—Although the distinction is not always clear, fractures that still allow free movement of the bone ends at 3–4 months after injury demonstrate delayed union, and if it persists (usually for more than 6 months) a diagnosis of nonunion can be made. Too much or too little motion at the fracture site, excessive space between fracture fragments, inadequate fixation, infection, soft tissue interposition, inadequate blood supply, and many other factors can lead to delay in bone healing. Nonunions are classified as hypervascular (hypertrophic) or avascular (atrophic) based on their capability of biologic reaction (vitality of the bone ends) and are classified as follows (Weber and Cech) (Fig. 10–1).

NONUNION	TYPE	COMMON CAUSE
Elephant foot	Hypervascular	Insecure fixation
Horse hoof	Hypervascular	Unstable fixation—plate and screws
Oligotrophic	Hypervascular	Displacement/distraction
Torsion wedge	Avascular	Intermediate fragment heals only on one side
Comminuted	Avascular	Necrotic intermediate fragment
Defect	Avascular	Sequestrum
Atrophic	Avascular	Intervening scar tissue

Delayed and nonunions can be seen in such bones as the tibia, ulna, proximal scaphoid, femoral neck, talus, and other areas with limited soft

TABLE 10–1. SPECIAL RADIOGRAPHIC VIEWS FOR SPECIFIC INJURIES

INJURY/LOCATION	EPONYM/DESCRIPTION	TECHNIQUE
Hand and Wrist		
Hand injuries		AP/lat./obl., digit: dental film
4th & 5th MC	Reverse obl.	Hand placed 45 degrees tilted
MC head	Brewerton	30 Degrees pronated from full supination
Gamekeeper's thumb	Robert	Stress view (with anesthesia); AP hypersupinated (dorsum on cassette)
1st MC-trapezium	Burnam	Robert with 15-degree cephalic tilt
Hamate hook/CT	CT view	Tangential through carpal tunnel
Dorsal carpal chip	Dorsal tangential	Tangential of dorsal carpus
Wrist—ulnar var.	Zero rotation	AP, shoulder and elbow at 90 degrees
Carpal instability	Motion	Cineradiography
Radial wrist	Pronation oblique	AP with 45 degrees' pronation
Ulnar wrist	Bura	Sup. obl.; AP with 35 degrees' supination
Scaphoid	Series	PA/lat./obl. fist, PA in ulnar deviation
Forearm and Elbow		
Forearm	Tuberosity	AP elbow with 20-degree tilt to olecranon
Radial head		45-Degree lateral of elbow, magnification
Elbow		Check fat pad, ant. humeral line, radius-capitellum
Elbow contracture	AP/lateral	AP humerus, AP forearm
Shoulder		
Shoulder	Trauma	True AP (scapula—45 degrees obl.), scapular lat. (Y)
Shoulder	Axillary lateral	Through axilla with arm abducted
Tuberosities	AP ER/IR	AP with arm in full extension and internal rotation
Impingement	Caudal tilt	AP with 30-degree caudal tilt
Impingement	Supraspinatus outlet	Scapula lat. with 10-degree caudal tilt
Hill Sachs	Stryker notch	Supine, hand on head, 10-degree cephalic tilt
Bankart	West Point	Prone axillary lat. with 25-degree lat. and post. tilt
Bankart	Garth	Apical obl. with 45-degree caudal and AP tilt
AC injury	Stress	AP both AC (large cassette) with 10 pounds **hanging** weight
AC injury	Alexander	Scapular lat. with shoulders forward
AC arthritis	Zanca	10-Degree cephalic tilt of AC
SC injury	Hobbs	PA, patient leans over cassette
SC injury	Serendipity	40-Degree cephalic tilt center on manubrium
Clavicle		AP 30-degree cephalic tilt
Spine		
C-spine	Series	AP/lat./obl., open-mouth odontoid
C7	Swimmers' view	Lat. through maximally abducted arm
Instability	Flex/Ext	AP with flexion and extension
L-spine	Series	AP/lat./obl. (foramina), L5/S1 spot lat.
Pelvis and Hip		
Pelvic injury	Inlet	45–50 Degrees caudad (assess AP displacement)
Pelvic injury	Outlet	45 Degrees cephalad (assess SI superior displacement)
Pelvic injury—Judet	Iliac obl.	Oblique on ilium **(post. column, ant. acetabulum)**
Pelvic injury—Judet	Obturator obl.	Oblique on obturator **(ant. column, post. acetabulum)**
Pelvic injury	Push-pull	Outlet view with stress (assess stability)
SI injury		Judet views centered on SI joints
Hip	Surgical lat.	Lat. from opposite side with that hip flexed
Femoral neck		AP with 15 degrees' internal rotation
Knee		
Knee AP & lat.		AP with 5 degrees' flexion, lat. with 30 degrees' flexion
Osteochondral Fx	Notch	Prone 45 degrees from vertical
Knee DJD	Rosenberg	Weight-bearing PA with 45 degrees' flexion
Patella	Merchant	45 Degrees' flexion, cassette perpendicular to tibia
Tibial plateau		AP with 10-degree caudal tilt
Tibial plateau		Internal and external obl. views
Foot and Ankle		
Ankle	Mortise	AP with 15 degrees internal rotation
Ankle	Stress	AP with lat. stress, lat. with drawer
Foot	Weight bearing	AP and lat. weight bearing
Midfoot		Include obliques
Talus	Canale	AP with 75-degree cephalic tilt, pronate 15 degrees
Talar neck		AP with 15 degrees' pronation
Subtalar	Broden	45-Degree rotation lat. with varying tilts
Calcaneus	Harris	AP standing, 45-degree tilt
Sesamoid		Tangentials with dorsiflexed toes

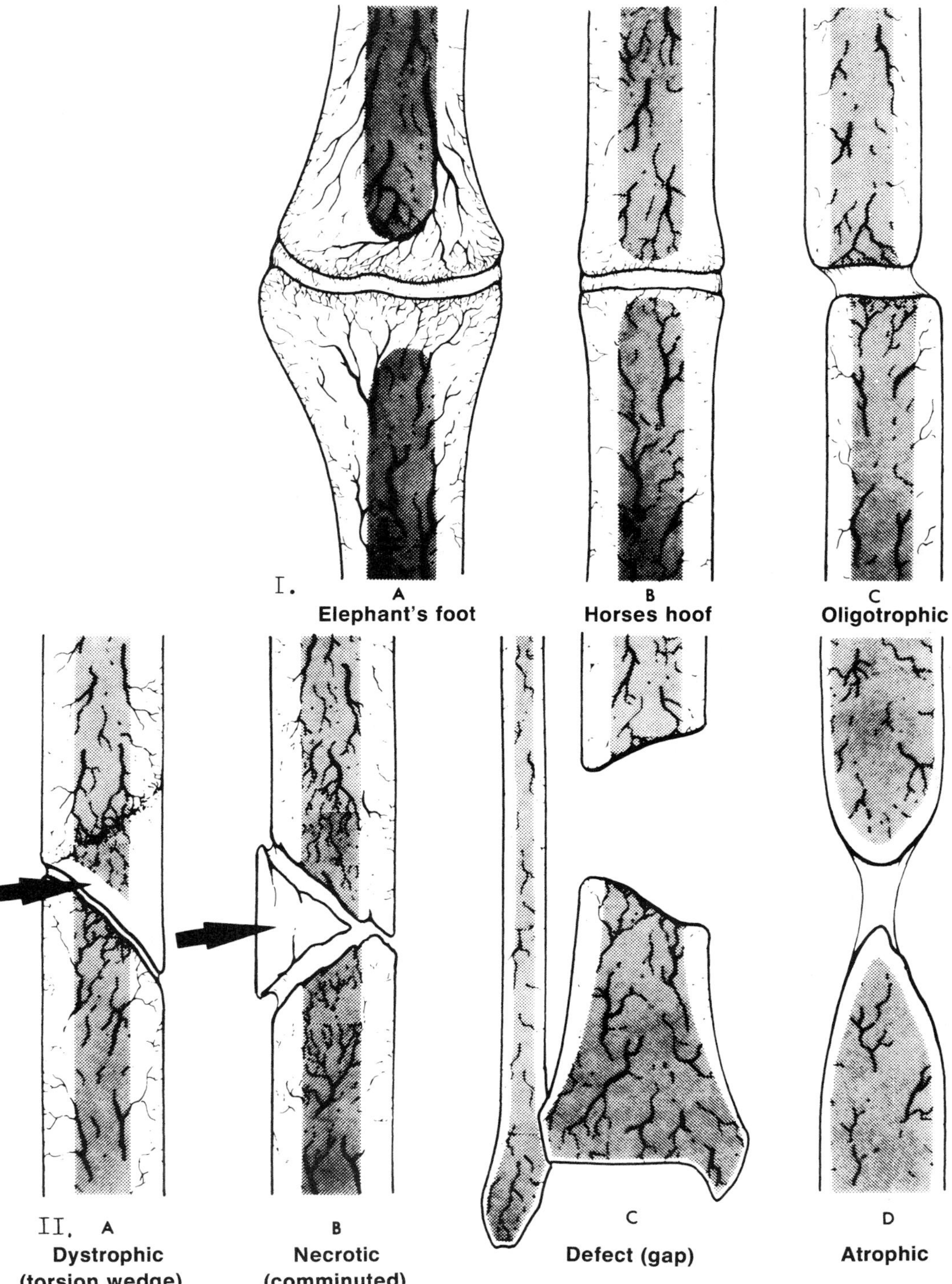

FIGURE 10–1. Types of nonunion. I—Hypervascular: *A,* Elephant foot. *B,* Horse hoof. *C,* Oligotrophic. II—Avascular: *A,* Torsion wedge. *B,* Comminuted. *C,* Defect. *D,* Atrophic. (From Weber, B.G., and Brunner, C.: The treatment of nonunions without electrical stimulation. Clin. Orthop. 161:25, 1981; reprinted by permission.)

tissue cover or blood supply. Treatment includes allowing compression at the fracture site, surgical excision of intervening tissue, more secure internal fixation, electrical stimulation, bone grafting, injection of marrow or other materials with osteogenic potential, and prosthetic replacement. Three types of electrical stimulation are available.

TYPE	APPLICATION
Direct current	Electrode placed at fracture site, subcutaneous battery
Inductive coupling	External coil with external power source required
Capacitive coupling	External coil with portable battery source required

Contraindications to electrical stimulation include inadequate fixation, poor alignment, pseudarthrosis, and nonviability of mesenchymal cells. Many methods of bone grafting have been described. The **Phemister** technique involves bone grafts placed in a healing granulation bed. Tibia fractures can be grafted posterolaterally to avoid the actual fracture site. With the increased use of intramedullary (IM) nails, revision reamed IM nailing (with/or without internal bone grafting) can be performed. It has been recommended that bone grafting be performed at the time of fixation for highly comminuted fractures with comminution involving more than one-third of the diameter of the bone to help avoid future problems with delayed bone healing.

2. Malunion—Union in a clinically significant imperfect position. Initial fracture care is critical to help avoid this result, but it often cannot be avoided. Treatment, if necessary, is directed at correcting the anatomic abnormality. Malunion may cause shortening (with overlap); or shortening may result from bone loss or growth plate injuries (see Section 2: Pediatric Trauma). Shortening is rarely a problem in the upper extremity.
3. Avascular Necrosis—Caused by disruption of the blood supply and can lead to nonunion, osteoarthritis, collapse, and other problems. It is more common with intra-articular fractures, especially of the femoral head/neck, femoral condyles, proximal scaphoid, proximal humerus, and talar neck. It is often recognized some time after injury when relative osteodensity in the affected area is noted in comparison to the relative osteopenia of normal bone. Excision of the avascular fragment, arthroplasty, or arthrodesis may be required in advanced cases. Osteonecrosis, which is the general term for all conditions causing bone death, is discussed in greater detail in Chapter 1, Basic Sciences.

C. Infection—Usually is a complication of open fractures and can lead to osteomyelitis (often chronic). Involvement of joints leads to persistent pain, stiffness, and progressive concentric joint space narrowing. Soft tissue infections may produce soft tissue air on radiographs from gangrene (*Clostridium*—a gram-positive anaerobe) and gas-producing gram-negative organisms. The most critical factor in avoiding infection in open injuries is adequate débridement and open wound care with adequate soft tissue cover within 1 week of injury. Prophylactic antibiotics for grade III open fractures should include a first generation cephalosporin, penicillin, *and* an aminoglycoside. Tetanus (caused by *Clostridium tetani*) can lead to devastating systemic complications and requires early treatment with boosters and toxoid for susceptible injuries. Recommended treatment includes 0.5 mg tetanus toxoid for patients with current immunizations and the addition of 250 units of tetanus immune globulin (in the opposite arm) for patients with unknown immunization history or whose immunizations have lapsed. Fight bites often are not appreciated early because of inaccurate patient histories and can cause significant infections with organisms such as *Eikenella corrodens* (an anaerobic gram-negative rod). Dog and cat bites are often infected with *Pasteurella multocida* (a gram-negative coccobacillus). Toxic shock syndrome, caused by gram-positive bacteria superinfection, can occur in an otherwise benign-appearing wound following internal fixation. Necrotizing fasciitis can cause severe, life-threatening infections following streptococci contamination of wounds. Osteomyelitis, other infections, and appropriate antibiotic coverage are discussed in Chapter 1, Basic Sciences.

D. Soft Tissue Injuries—Include direct injuries to vessels, nerves, and soft tissues as well as indirect compromise of these tissues. The functional status of the soft tissues often has a major bearing on ultimate outcome.
   1. Arterial Injury—Injuries to major arteries with fractures and dislocations are rare, but the consequences can be severe. A high index of suspicion is required, particularly with shoulder dislocations, supracondylar elbow fractures, and severe knee injuries/dislocations. Immediate diagnosis (with arteriograms if necessary) and repair (within 6 hours of injury) are essential. Although controversial, fracture fixation usually is helpful to protect vascular repairs. Fasciotomy, discussed below, is also necessary in most cases.
   2. Compartment Syndrome—Increased pressure within enclosed soft tissue compartments of the extremities can lead to serious sequelae. Elevated compartment pressures commonly follow significant injuries to the forearm and leg and should be diagnosed early with careful patient monitoring. Risk is also increased with prolonged use of pneumatic antishock garments. If used longer than 90 minutes, pressure should not exceed 20 mm Hg. **Pain** (especially with passive extension of the digits) is the **earliest** and **most reliable** indicator, but pallor, paralysis, paresthesia, and pulselessness are also indicative of elevated pressures. Compartment pressures should be measured with a Whitesides or indwelling catheter device for any suspected compartment syndrome and for patients who are unable to adequately feel pain (e.g., paralysis, intoxication). Compartment pressures >30 mm Hg or within 10–30 mm Hg of the diastolic blood pressure are highly suggestive of the diagnosis. Fasciotomy within 4 hours of onset usually prevents muscle necrosis (Fig. 10–2). Generous skin incisions should be utilized. The "mini" incision and "blind" releases should be avoided in the acute trauma setting. Concomitant muscle débride-

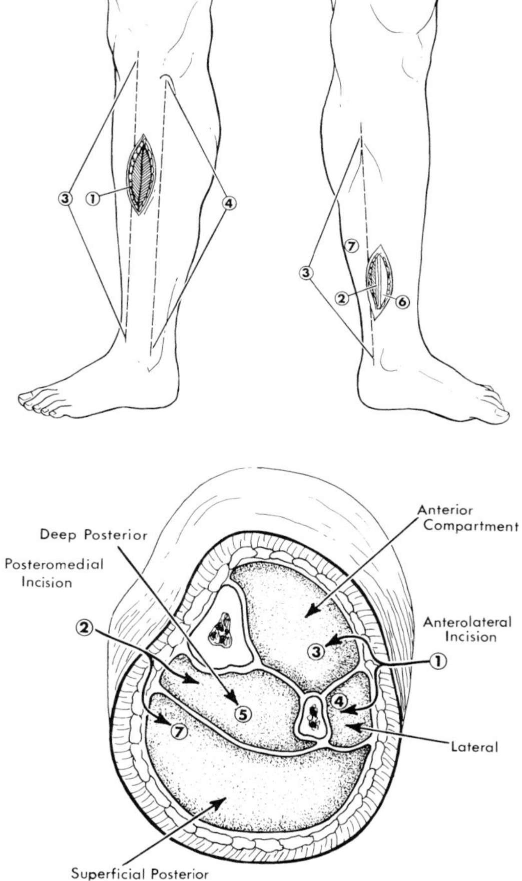

FIGURE 10–2. Fasciotomy for compartment syndrome of the leg. Note anterolateral and posteromedial incisions. (From Connolly, J.F., ed.: Depalma's The Management of Fractures and Dislocations, an Atlas, 3rd ed., p. 68. Philadelphia, WB Saunders 1981; reprinted by permission.)

ment is necessary for any ischemic muscle (lacking normal color, consistency, contraction, and capacity to bleed). Irreversible nerve injury may follow in >12 hours.

3. Nerve Injuries—Acute nerve injury is relatively uncommon but is more often associated with fractures than arterial injuries. Most injuries are neurapraxias from stretch, and 70% resolve in a few weeks. Common nervous system injuries with trauma include those of the spinal cord and cauda equina (spine fractures), axillary nerve (shoulder fractures and dislocations), radial nerve (humerus fractures), ulnar nerve (medial epicondyle fracture), posterior interosseous nerve (radial head and monteggia fractures), sciatic nerve (hip dislocation, acetabular fractures), and common peroneal nerve (lateral knee injuries). Nerve injury and repair are discussed in Chapter 1, Basic Sciences, and Chapter 6, Hand.

E. Pulmonary Complications
   1. Adult Respiratory Distress Syndrome (ARDS)—Pulmonary edema and decreased function commonly follow severe trauma. ARDS can be a result of direct (e.g., aspiration, inhalation), or indirect (e.g., sepsis, shock) insults. It is exacerbated by prolonged hypovolemia and decreased left ventricular function. ARDS is characterized by increased intrapulmonary shunting and decreased pulmonary compliance and functional reserve capacity. ABG measurements are best for diagnosing ARDS and after therapy (ventilation with PEEP). Hypoxic changes in the hypothalamus and/or cellular humeral mediators (including complement factors) may initiate the process.
   2. Fat Emboli Syndrome (FES)—A form of ARDS that follows major long bone fractures (0.5–2.0% of patients with multiple fractures). FES may be a result of systemic release of bone marrow fat and/or changes in chylomicron stability and conversion to free fatty acids in the lung parenchyma. It classically presents 24–72 hours after injury with tachycardia, hyperthermia, tachypnea, and hypoxia. Mental status changes, oliguria, and upper torso/conjunctival petechiae are also commonly seen. Early treatment is based on stabilization of long bone fractures (within 24 hours) and pulmonary support. Steroids have been shown to have a prophylactic role only.
   3. Pulmonary Embolism—Thromboembolic disease is the most common complication following surgery on the extremities. This subject is covered in detail in Chapter 1, Basic Sciences. The use of intermittent pneumatic compression, low-molecular-weight heparin warfarin (Coumadin) can be useful in appropriately selected trauma patients.

F. Bleeding Disorders—Excessive bleeding from injuries can cause hypovolemic shock and disseminated intravascular coagulation (DIC). Shock is a manifestation of decreased blood flow to the tissues and may present with tachycardia, oliguria, and pale, cool extremities. Treatment includes immediate whole blood, IV fluids, and sometimes dextran solutions. Albumin should be avoided. DIC is caused by microvascular thrombi that consume platelets and initiate a vicious cycle. Diagnosis involves recognition of symptoms in the appropriate setting and laboratory values showing decreased antithrombin III and fibrinogen and increased values of PT/PTT and fibrin split products. Treatment should be directed at the underlying cause, and judicious use should be made of heparin, platelets, and DDAVP. DIC or excessive anticoagulation can lead to excessive bleeding into soft tissues. Deep muscle hematomas can compress neurovascular structures (e.g., **iliacus hematoma can compress the femoral nerve**). Conservative treatment of these hematomas is usually best. Thrombotic thrombocytopenic purpura can occur in a trauma setting and is treated with IV steroids.

G. GI Complications—Can be a result of the trauma itself (the **spleen** is the **most commonly injured** organ with blunt trauma, followed by the liver) or can be a late complication. Stress ulcers are common in the ICU setting and are usually treated with appropriate antacids and H_2 blockers. **Cast syndrome** is a common orthopaedic complication and is a result of **compression of the second portion of the duodenum** by the superior mesenteric artery. It may present with postoperative small bowel obstruction with projectile vomiting. Cast syndrome can occur after placing spine fractures in plaster or children in hip spica casts. Diagnosis is usually made by a UGI series. Treatment includes removing the constrictive device and decompression (nasogotic tube).

H. Reflex Sympathetic Dystrophy (RSD)—Can follow trauma or surgery for local systemic disease and is characterized by pain, swelling, discoloration, and stiffness of the affected extremity. It is a result of vasomotor dysfunction of the sympathetic nervous system. A "vicious cycle" of pain, immobility, edema, tissue reaction, and vasospasm is influenced by noxious stimuli, abnormal sympathetic reflexes, and "personality diathesis." Three stages are defined (Lankford).

STAGE	DESCRIPTION	FEATURES
1	Acute	Pain, dusky/mottled smooth skin
2	Dystrophic	Max. pain, stiff, nail changes, edema
3	Atrophic	Atrophy, contractures, demineralization (Sudeck's atrophy)

A triple-phase bone scan showing uptake during the third phase and relief with a sympathetic block is diagnostic of this disorder. Treatment includes PT (early), NSAIDs, psychological aids, and sympathetic blockade (interrupts cycle). Sympathetic blockade is obtained with long-acting anesthetic injection of the sympathetic ganglia upper extremity (UE) or epidural injection lower extremity (LE). Prognosis is guarded.

I. Late Complications—Can be systemic or involve local soft tissue, bones, and joints. **Myositis ossificans** can follow injuries with large hematomas. It is common after elbow fractures/dislocations and soft tissue trauma in the thigh. Histologically, the peripheral areas are more mature than the center ("zoning phenomenon"). Conservative therapy is best, but late excision (6–9 months after the injury) of symptomatic areas is sometimes required. **Posttraumatic osteoarthritis** commonly follows intraarticular fractures that are not anatomically reduced. Treatment is similar to other forms of osteoarthritis discussed in Chapter 4, Adult Reconstruction. **Immobilization hypercalcemia** is an unusual disorder characterized by nausea, vomiting, abdominal pain, acute personality changes, and other symptoms. It occurs most commonly in children and patients with Paget's disease. Heterotopic ossification (HO) is often seen after acetabular fracture repairs. Rates appear to be highest with extended iliofemoral approaches and lowest with ilioinguinal approaches. Indomethacin and irradiation (600 rad—one dose) appear to decrease the incidence of HO.

VI. Soft Tissue Trauma

A. Introduction—Many of the important concepts have been discussed elsewhere, but other injuries are discussed in this section.

B. Snake Bites—Can cause extensive soft tissue destruction and may lead to compartment syndrome. Venomous snakes are most commonly pit vipers (e.g., Crotalids—rattlesnakes, copperheads). These snakes have a triangular head and a pit below their eyes. Elapids (e.g., coral snake) are less common, but their venom includes hemo-, cyto-, and neurotoxins. Systemic symptoms (nausea and vomiting, neurologic dysfunction, bleeding) can be severe. Local symptoms with snake bites include swelling, ecchymosis, and bullae formation. Treatment includes first aid (tourniquet, suction) and hospitalization. Monitoring, use of antibiotics, checking compartment pressures, and administration of antivenin are appropriate. At least five bottles of antivenin are required for moderate-sized bites, and this treatment can cause serum sickness (sometimes requiring systemic steroids to combat it). Fasciotomies are sometimes needed for compartment syndrome.

C. Thermal Injuries

1. Freezing Injuries—The most common cause of bilateral upper and lower extremity amputations. Injury may be direct (freezing of tissues with ice crystals in the extracellular space) or indirect (vascular damage). Treatment is based on restoring core body temperature, rapid rewarming of the extremity, débridement, physical therapy, and sometimes anticoagulation and sympathectomy. Psychosocial factors often are important.
2. Heat Injuries—Burns require close management. Treatment is based on burn depth.

DEGREE	DEPTH	FINDINGS	TREATMENT
First	Epidermis	Edema, erythema	Symptomatic
Second	Dermis	Blisters, blanching	Topical antibiotics, splint, ROM
Third	Subcutaneous	Waxy, dry	Excision, splint-thickness skin graft
Fourth	Deep	Exposed tissues	Amputation/flap/reconstruction

Burns can also result in compartment syndrome and sometimes require escharotomy/fasciotomy. Contractures are common and often require Z-plasties or releases. Infection is also common.

3. Electrical Injuries—Include ignition (burns at sites of direct contact), conductant (tunnels along neurovascular structures; the number one cause of bilateral high upper extremity amputations), and arc (high-voltage current jumps across flexor surfaces of joints, leading to late contractures). AC current is more dangerous than DC. Current density zones resulting from electrical burns are as follows.

ZONE	TISSUE CHARACTERISTICS
Charred	Unrecognizable tissue
Gray-white	Tissue necrosis
Red	Thrombosis

Treatment involves initial débridement of all necrotic muscle and tissue, fasciotomy (when indicated), second-look débridement at 2–3 days, and finally definitive flap coverage or amputation. Acute amputation may be required.

4. Chemical Burns—Follow exposure to noxious agents. Severity is based on concentration, duration of contact, penetrability, amount, and mechanism of action. The mainstay of treatment is co-

pious irrigation. Hydrofluoric acid burns can be successfully treated with calcium gluconate. White phosphorus burns are treated with a 1% copper sulfate solution.

5. Chemotherapeutic Extravasation—Early débridement and secondary coverage is important to reduce the high risk of soft tissue and skin necrosis.

D. High-Pressure Injection Injuries—Occur from accidental injections by paint or grease guns. They usually involve the hand. Paint gun injuries are more common and are more severe because they lead to soft tissue necrosis (grease gun injuries cause fibrosis). A seemingly innocuous entry wound may cover an area of extensive soft tissue destruction. Treatment includes IV antibiotics, thorough I&D, and occasionally steroids.

VII. Principles of Internal Fixation

A. Basic Principles—AO/ASIF technique should be practiced as taught in AO basic and advanced courses. The following fixation devices (Figs. 10–3 to 10–10) are commonly used.

DEVICE	FUNCTION	USE
Compression plate	Increases the stiffness of bone-implant unit; tension band	Obl. diaphyseal fractures
Neutralization plate	Artificial cortex; prevents rotation	Obl. diaphyseal fractures
Tension device	Tension band wiring	Patella, olecranon
Buttress plate	Supports/shores up intact side	Metaphysis
Strut plate	Maintains alignment/ length	Bone loss
Intramedullary	Mechanical stability, soft tissue conserved	Femur/tibia
External fixation	Avoids internal hardware	Infection and selected open fractures

With all devices, preoperative planning is critical, especially with complex fracture patterns.

B. Plates and Screws

1. Lag Screws—Allow compression of the fracture surface by overdrilling the proximal cortex or by using partially threaded screws and "drawing up" the distal cortex. Often used in conjunction with compression plating and forms the basis for AO technique. Screws are placed in a "compromise" of the best position to counteract shear forces (i.e., perpendicular to the applied load) and the optimum position for compression (i.e., perpendicular to the fracture).

2. Compression Plates—Used on the **tension side** of transverse or short oblique fractures. They provide stability (especially versus shear forces) and act as a **load-sharing device.** The dynamic compression plate (DCP) is designed for self-compression by the use of offset drill guides and contoured plate holes. The sequence of screw placement is as follows (Fig. 10–3).

1—Neutral (green) guide used to attach plate
2—Offset (gold) guide used to compress fracture
3—Offset (gold) guide used to further compress fracture after screw 2 loosened
4–6—Screws placed with neutral guide
7—Interfragmentary screw in different plane

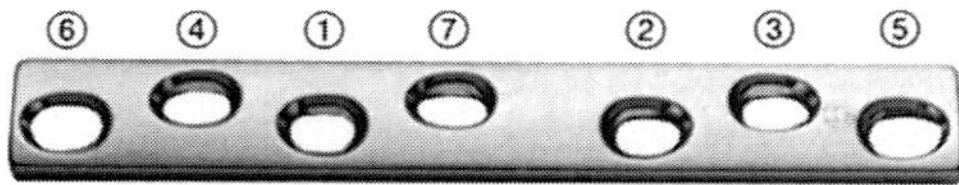

FIGURE 10–3. AO/ASIF dynamic compression plate. (Courtesy of Synthes, Ltd. [USA].)

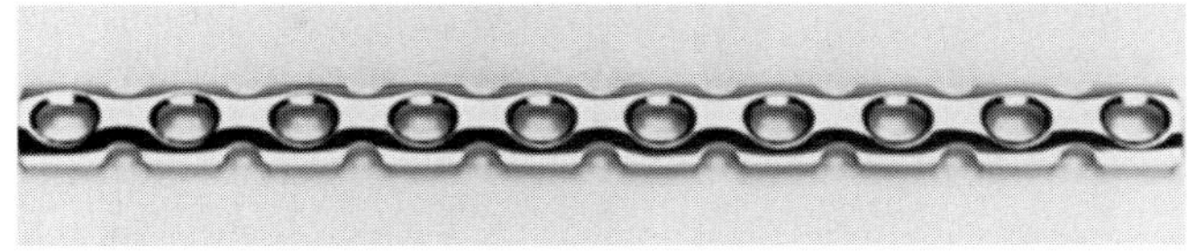

FIGURE 10–4. AO/ASIF reconstruction plate. (Courtesy of Synthes, Ltd. [USA].)

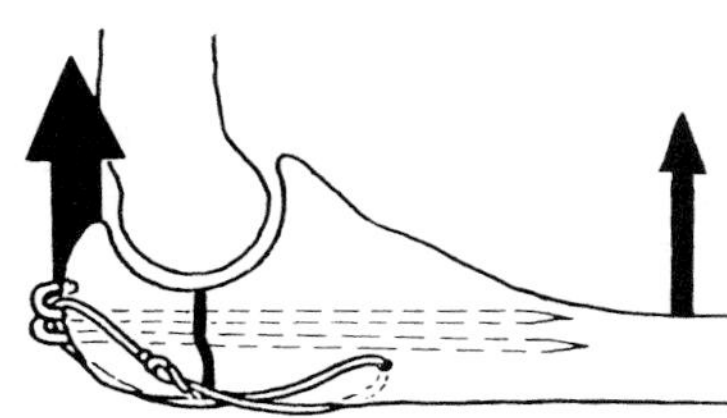

FIGURE 10–5. Tension band wiring. (From Sequin, F., and Texhammer, R.: AO/ASIF Instrumentation, p. 161. New York, Springer-Verlag, 1981; reprinted by permission.)

A total of **six or more cortices** on each side of the fracture is required for fixation of **forearm fractures** and **at least eight cortices** are required for fixation of **lower extremity and humerus fractures.** Plates are left in place but can be removed for contact sport participation, metal allergies, with prominent hardware, and occasionally in patients with psychological maladaptation to hardware, usually about 1–11/ 2 years after insertion. Extremities must be protected after plate removal.

3. Reconstruction Plates (Fig. 10–4)—Are more pliable and allow positioning for use as a neutralization plate not only in the pelvis but also in distal humerus fractures and other locations.

C. Tension Band Wiring (Fig. 10–5)—Commonly used for fixation of olecranon, patella, and sometimes ankle fractures. This method allows fixation on the tension side and relies on motion to allow union on the compression side. Parallel K-wires are placed closer to the outer cortex than the articular surface to take advantage of this design, and wire is placed under the K-wires, usually in figure-of-8 fashion, before it is tightened.

D. Intramedullary Fixation (Fig. 10–6)—Allows superior fixation for fractures in the diaphyses of weight-bearing bones. Advantages include proper axial alignment, early weight-bearing (load-sharing device), and that it can be placed in a "closed" fashion (does not open the fracture site). Disadvantages include the fact that the canal diameter can limit the size of nail used, there is less rotational control (improved with interlocking nails), there is disruption of the endosteal blood supply, and it is sometimes technically difficult. Nevertheless, it is a popular

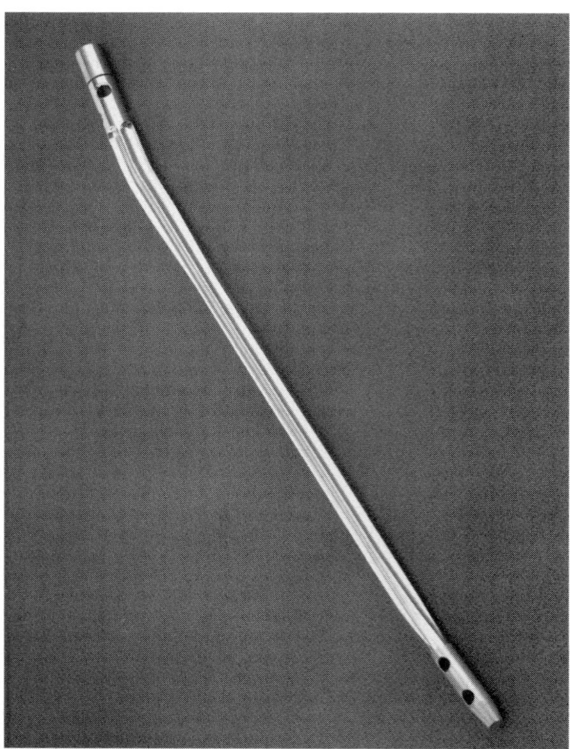

FIGURE 10–6. True-Flex intramedullary tibial nail. (Courtesy of Applied Osteo Systems, Inc., Walnut Creek, CA.)

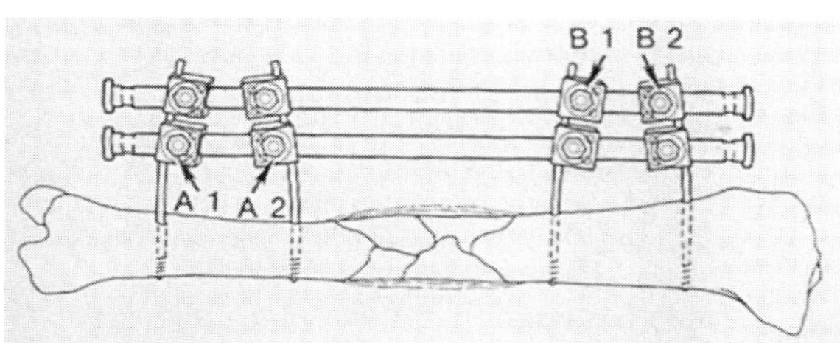

FIGURE 10–7. External fixation of an open comminuted tibial fracture. (Courtesy of Synthes, Ltd. [USA].)

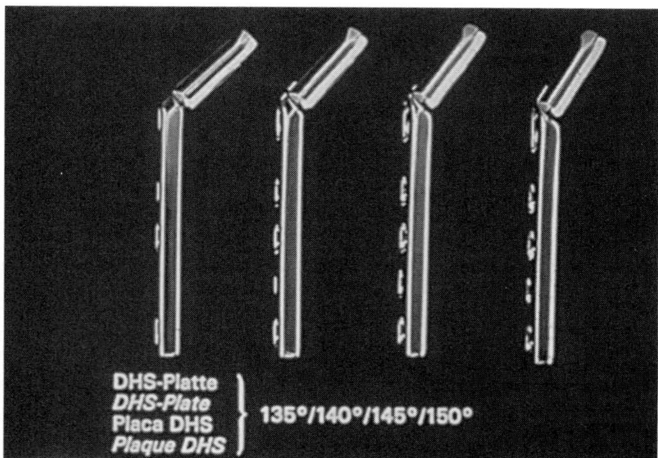

FIGURE 10–8. Side plate component of the dynamic hip screw for stabilization of intertrochanteric hip fractures. (Courtesy of Synthes, Ltd. [USA].)

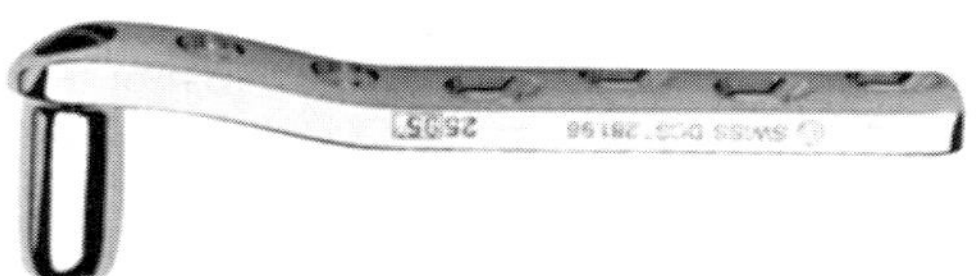

FIGURE 10–9. AO/ASIF dynamic condylar screw sideplate. (Courtesy of Synthes, Ltd. [USA].)

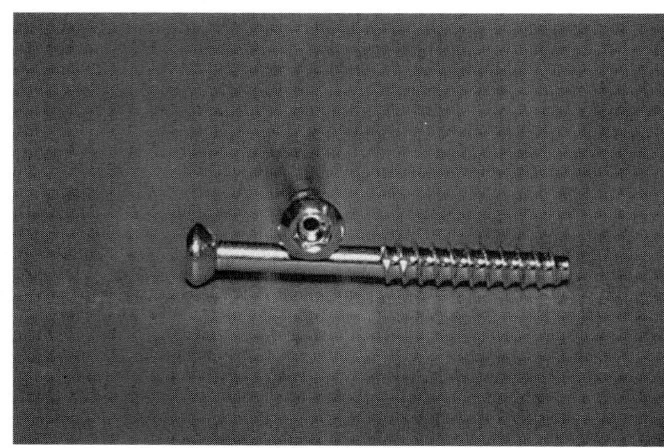

FIGURE 10–10. AO/ASIF small cannulated screws. (Courtesy of Synthes, Ltd. [USA].)

and successful method for fixation of lower extremity diaphyseal fractures. The surgeon should wait at least 1–1½ years prior to hardware removal if it is to be performed. There should be clinical and radiographic correlation of solid union as well.

E. External Fixation (Fig. 10–7)—Useful for management of grade III open fractures with high risk of infection. Allows access to these wounds while stabilizing fractures. Other uses include stabilization of anterior disruptions of the pelvis, management of comminuted distal radius fractures, and spacing in areas with segmental bone loss. A thorough understanding of local anatomy, injury characteristics, and mechanical demands is essential prior to placement.

F. Special Devices—Numerous and include the following.
   1. Sliding Hip Screw (Fig. 10–8)—A load-sharing device that allows fixation of intertrochanteric hip fractures with screw insertion that can be placed at variable angles.
   2. Sliding Condylar Screw (Fig. 10–9)—Best used for distal femur fractures 4–9 cm proximal to the joint. It can also be used proximally for some unstable subtrochanteric fractures.
   3. Cannulated Screws (Fig. 10–10)—Excellent for femoral neck fractures and becoming popular for fixation of a variety of fractures. Placement of small K-wires prior to insertion of large screws provides an alternative with less risk of iatrogenic neurovascular injuries after adequate closed or open reduction.

TABLE 10–2. ADULT TRAUMATIC ORTHOPAEDIC INJURIES—UPPER EXTREMITY

INJURY	EPONYM	CLASSIFICATION	TREATMENT	COMPLICATIONS
HAND—FRACTURES				
Distal phalangeal Fx		Longitudinal, comminuted, transverse	Splint DIP 3–4 weeks; evacuate hematoma and repair nail bed with fine absorbable suture	Nail bed injury
EDL avulsion (Fig. 10–11).	Mallet finger	Ext. tendon stretch Ext. tendon torn Bony mallet	Volar/stack splint 6 wk + 4 wk nights Bony—splint; ORIF volar subluxation	Deformity, nail bed injury (with ORIF), subluxation
FDP avulsion (Fig. 10–12)	Jersey finger	Leddy: I—tendon to palm II—tendon to PIP	Repair within 7–10 days Repair within 3 mo	Can lead to lumbrical plus finger (late) missed diagnosis (therapy or fuse DIP late)
		III—tendon to A4 pulley	Keep A4 pulley intact with repair	
		(Smith) IV—bony fragment DP base	Early fixation of bony fragments and tendon	
Proximal and middle phalanges		Extra-articular stable	Buddy tape	Decreased ROM, contractures, malunion/ malrotation (may require osteotomy), lateral deviation, volar angulation (osteotomy), nonunion, tendon adherence
		Extra-articular unstable	Reduce and immobilize (PCP or ORIF if irreducible ex. fix. comminuted Fxs)	
		Intra-articular undisplaced	Buddy tape, early ROM, close on follow-up	
		Intra-articular condylar	Reduce and PCP, ORIF and restore articular surface if >2 mm displacement	
		Intra-articular PP base	Small/nondisplaced—Buddy tape Large/displaced—ORIF	
	Boutonnière	Intra-articular MP base (D)	Splint PIP (extension) 6 wk, ORIF if large bony fragment	
		Intra-articular comminuted	Traction, ex. fix.	
MC		Head	ORIF large piece, early motion comminuted fractures	Soft tissue injury, malunion (rotation); prominent MC head in palm (affects grip); loss of reduction (no volar buttress); nonunion, contractures of intrinsics
	Boxer's	Neck—4th and 5th	20–40° Angulation OK, reduce/ splint	
		—2nd and 3rd	Usu. requires PCP pin to adjacent MC or ORIF	
		Shaft—transverse	Closed reduction, immobilize or PCP; accept 50–70° angulation IV and V 20° angulation II and III, ORIF if irreducible	
		—oblique	ORIF if >5 mm shortening or rotated—K-wire, AO screws	
		—comminuted	Nondisplaced splint, displaced PCP to adjacent MC or ORIF	
		Base of 5th MC	Most stable; if not, pin to adjacent MC	
1MC (Fig. 10–13) Base	Bennett's	I—Intra-articular volar lip	Attempt closed reduction and PCP MC to trapezium; ORIF if irreducible	Displaced by APL
	Rolando's	II—Intra-articular "Y" (volar and dorsal) III—Extra-articular (transverse or oblique)	Large frags ORIF comminuted—ex. fix. or early motion; closed reduction spica 4 wk	DJD
5MC	"Baby Bennett"	Base	PCP or ORIF	Displaced by ECU
HAND—DISLOCATIONS				
DIP		*Dorsal	Closed reduction, immobilize 2 weeks, late Dx or irreducible—open reduction	
		Collateral ligament injury	Sprain—buddy tape 3–6 wk Tear—repair RCL IF, RF, MF; UCL SF (of dominant hand)	
PIP		*Dorsal (volar plate [VP] disruption):		
		I—hyperextension; VP avulsion	Buddy tape or ext. block splint	Stiffness, contractures (Rx with VP arthroplasty)
		II—dislocation major ligamentous injury	Extension block splint	
		III—proximal dislocation (middle phalanx MP Fx)	If >4 mm displacement reduce; ORIF if required	

Table continued on following page

TABLE 10–2. *Continued*

INJURY	EPONYM	CLASSIFICATION	TREATMENT	COMPLICATIONS
HAND—DISLOCATIONS *cont.*	Boutonnière (Fig. 10–14)	Volar (central slip)	Closed reduction, splint (full extension 4–6 wk) if congruous	Late recognition: ORIF or VP arthroplasty
		Rotatory	ORIF if irreducible or incongruous	
		Dorsal Fx-dislocation	Extension block splint if congruous, ORIF or VP arthroplasty if incongruous	
MCP		Collateral ligament injury	Splint in 50° MCP flexion 3 wk Open if >2–3 mm displacement of fragments or 20% of joint	Late recognition—injection, splinting, operate late
		*Dorsal (Fig. 10–15) —simple	Closed reduction, 7–10 days immobilization	Failure to recognize complex dislocation
		—complex	Soft tissue volar plate interposition (pucker, sesamoid in joint and parallelism of MC and PP on radiographs) requires open reduction volar approach	Stiffness, contractures, neurovascular injury (open)
		Volar	Rare; requires open reduction	
CMC			Closed reduction, PCP; open reduction—4CMC dislocations and open dislocations	
1MCP (Fig. 10–16)	Gamekeeper's thumb	*UCL injury	Sprain—does not open >35–45° with stress thumb spica cast; rupture—open repair (interposition of adductor aponeurosis—Stener)	Unrecognized Stener lesion, chronic pain, instability
		RCL injury	Nonoperative: splint or PCP	
		Dorsal—simple	Reduce and immobilize 3 wk	
		—complex	Open after one attempt closed (VP ± FPL interposed)	
1CMC Dislocation (Fig. 10–17)			Hyperpronation and PCP, immobilize 6–10 wk	
Hamatometocarpal Fx-dislocation		Cain: IA—ligamentous injury	Reduce—If stable cast; if unstable PCP	Delay in Dx (pronation oblique films required)
		*IB—dorsal hamate Fx	Reduce—If stable cast; if unstable ORIF	
		II—Comminuted dorsal hamate Fx	ORIF, restore dorsal buttress	
		III—Coronal hamate Fx	ORIF, restore congruent joint surface	
WRIST—FRACTURES				
Radius	Colles' (dorsal displacement)	Frykman (I–VIII; even no. = ulna Fx; I extra-articular, III R-C, V R-U, VII R-C and R-U) (Fig. 10–18) Melone: 4 parts (shaft, radial styloid, dorsomedial, palmar medial): I—min. displacement, II—carpus displacement, III—volar spike, IV—volar fragment rotated (Fig. 10–19)	Distract, manipulate, splint 15° palmar flexion and ulnar deviation, ext. fix., and/or ORIF if comminuted/unstable; ext. fix. for severe comminution, ORIF large fragments with >15° DF, >1–2 mm articular displacement; bone graft comminuted Fxs	Loss of reduction, nonunion, malunion, median N neuropathy, weakness, tendon adhesion, instability, EPL rupture, DISI (>15° DF), ulnar side pain (shortening), RSD, Volkman's ischemic contracture
	Smith's (volar displacement)	Thomas (not used) Intra- vs. extra-articular	Distract, manipulate, splint supination, flexion; PCP; open red. if needed	Missed Dx, and as for Colles' Fx
Dorsal rim	Dorsal Barton's (Fig. 10–20)		Reduce, pronation, ORIF if needed	Similar to Colles' Fx
Radial styloid (Fig. 10–21)	Chauffeur's		Reduce, PCP or cann. screw, immobilize in ulnar deviation	Similar to Colles' Fx, associated perilunate injury (ORIF)
Volar rim	Volar Barton's (Fig. 10–22)		Reduce, supination, PCP or ORIF common (volar buttress plate)	Similar to Colles' Fx
Distal R-U		Based on ulna displacement	Dorsal—reduce, full supination LAC 6 wks Volar—reduce (may require open reduction) LAC pronation	Osteochondral fracture, TFCC injury, ulnar nerve compression, instability

Table continued on page 364

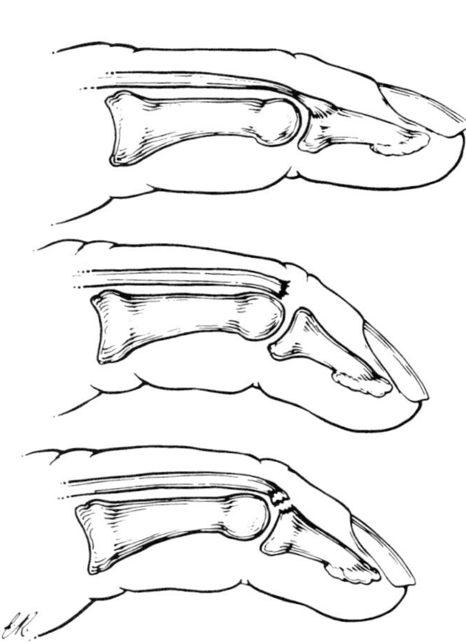

FIGURE 10–11. Mallet finger. *Top to bottom,* Extensor tendon stretch, extensor tendon rupture, bony avulsion. (From Green, D.P., and Rowland, S.A.: Fractures and dislocations in the hand. In Fractures in Adults, Rockwood, C.A., and Green, D.P., eds., 2nd ed., p. 319. Philadelphia, JB Lippincott, 1984; reprinted by permission.)

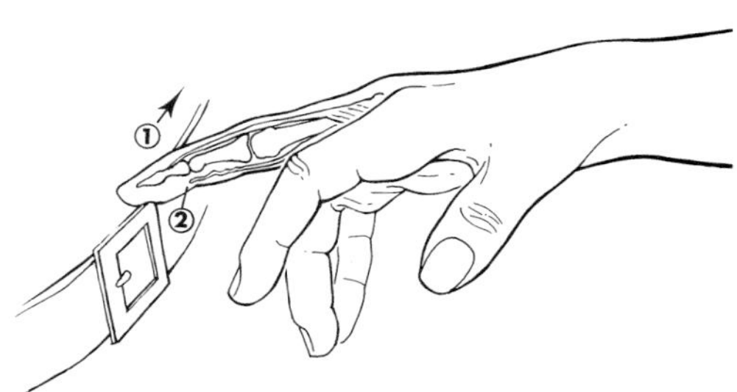

FIGURE 10–12. Avulsion of the flexor digitorum profundus. (From Connolly, J.F., ed.: Depalma's The Management of Fractures and Dislocations, an Atlas, 3rd ed., p. 1149. Philadelphia, WB Saunders, 1981; reprinted by permission.)

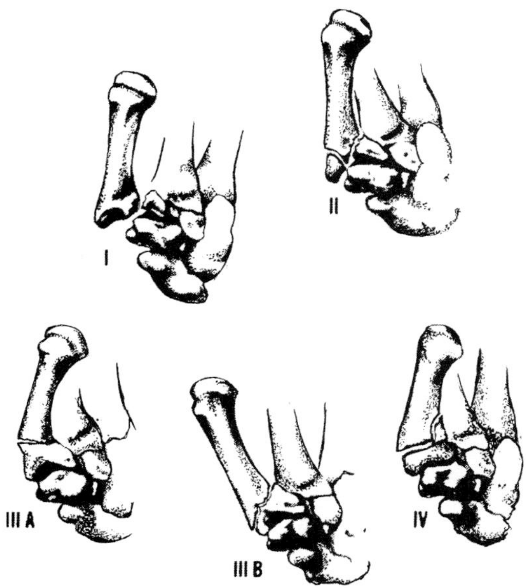

FIGURE 10–13. Classification of first metacarpal base fractures. *I,* Bennett's fracture. *II,* Rolando's fracture. *IIIA,* Transverse extra-articular fracture. *IIIB,* Oblique extra-articular fracture. *IV,* SH II epiphyseal fracture (pediatric). (From Green, D.P.,and O'Brien, E.T.: Fractures of the thumb metacarpal. South. Med. J. 65:807, 1972; reprinted by permission.)

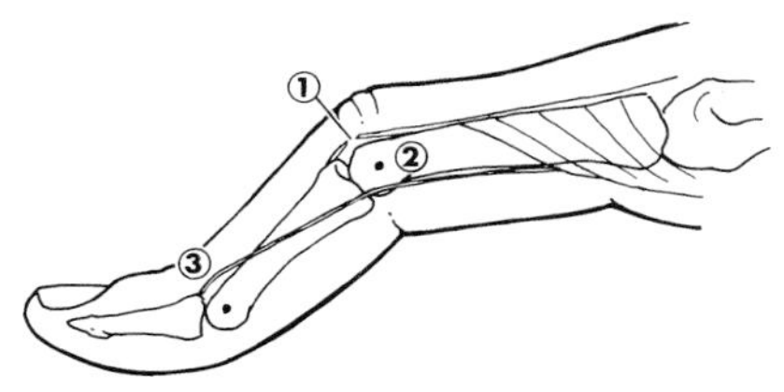

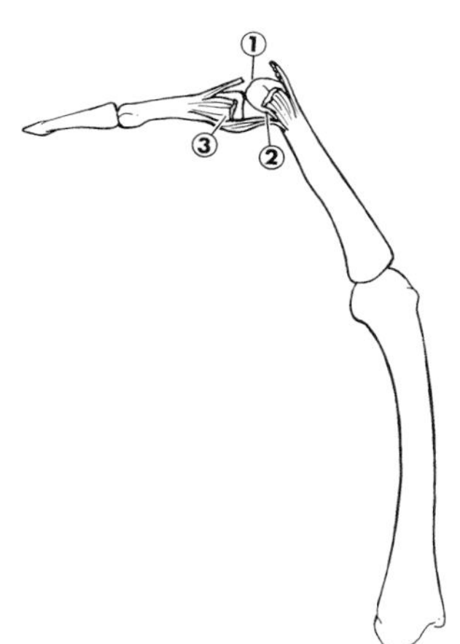

FIGURE 10–14. Boutonnière deformity, an injury to the central slip with volar subluxation of lateral bonds. (From Connolly, J.F., ed.: Depalma's The Management of Fractures and Dislocations, an Atlas, 3rd ed., p. 1149. Philadelphia, WB Saunders, 1981; reprinted by permission.)

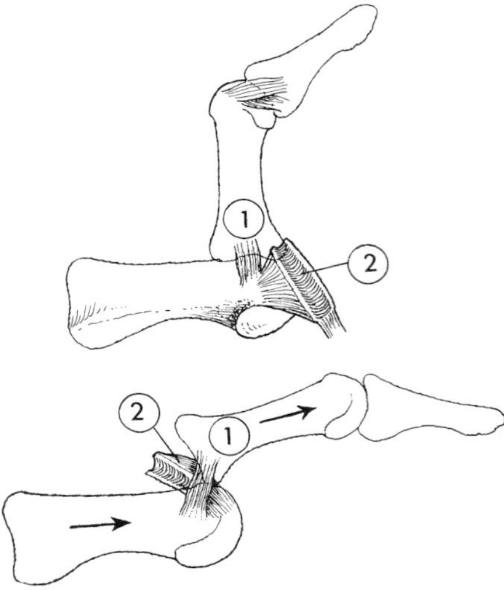

FIGURE 10–15. Thumb MCP dislocation. *Top,* Simple. *Bottom,* Complex; note interposition of volar plate. (From Connolly, J.F., ed.: Depalma's The Management of Fractures and Dislocations, an Atlas, 3rd ed., p. 1152. Philadelphia, WB Saunders, 1981; reprinted by permission.)

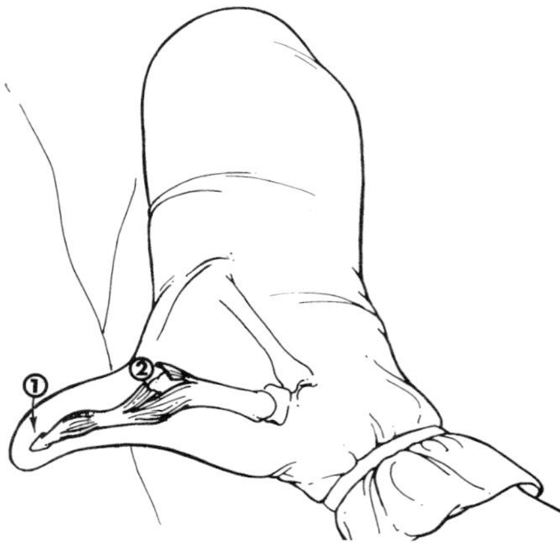

FIGURE 10–16. Gamekeeper's thumb (UCL injury). (From Connolly, J.F., ed.: Depalma's The Management of Fractures and Dislocations, an Atlas, 3rd ed., p. 1151. Philadelphia, WB Saunders, 1981; reprinted by permission.)

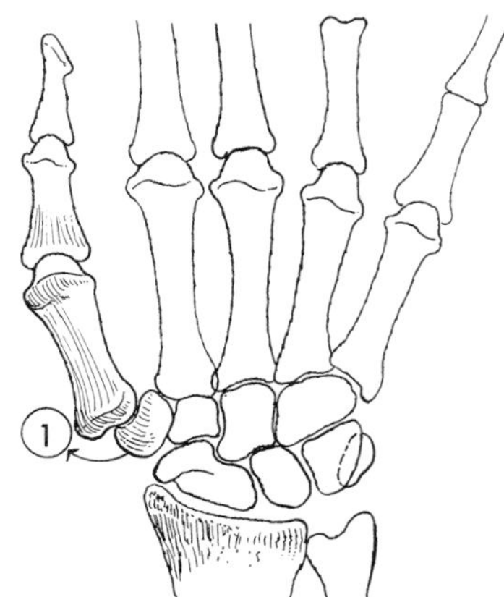

FIGURE 10–17. Subluxation/dislocation of the thumb carpometacarpal joint. (From Connolly, J.F., ed.: Depalma's The Management of Fractures and Dislocations, an Atlas, 3rd ed., p. 1165. Philadelphia, WB Saunders, 1981; reprinted by permission.)

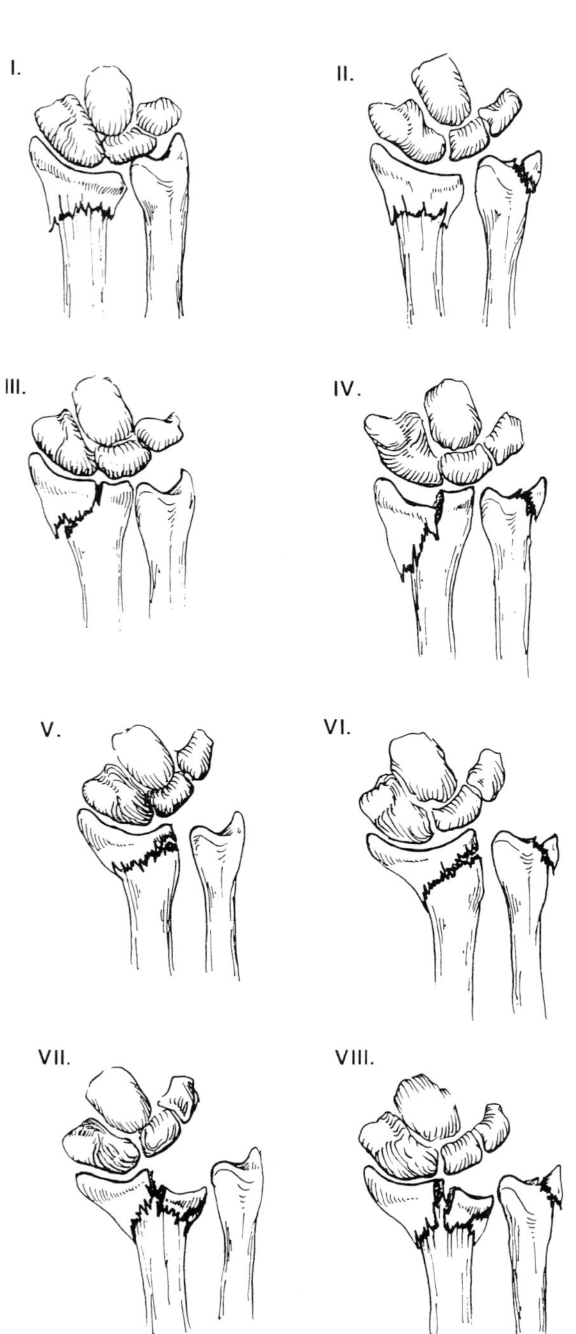

FIGURE 10–18. Frykman classification of distal radius fractures. Note even numbers with ulnar styloid involvement. (From Kozin, S.H., and Berlet, A.C.: Handbook of Common Orthopaedic Fractures, pp. 17, 19. West Chester, PA, Medical Surveillance, 1989; reprinted by permission.)

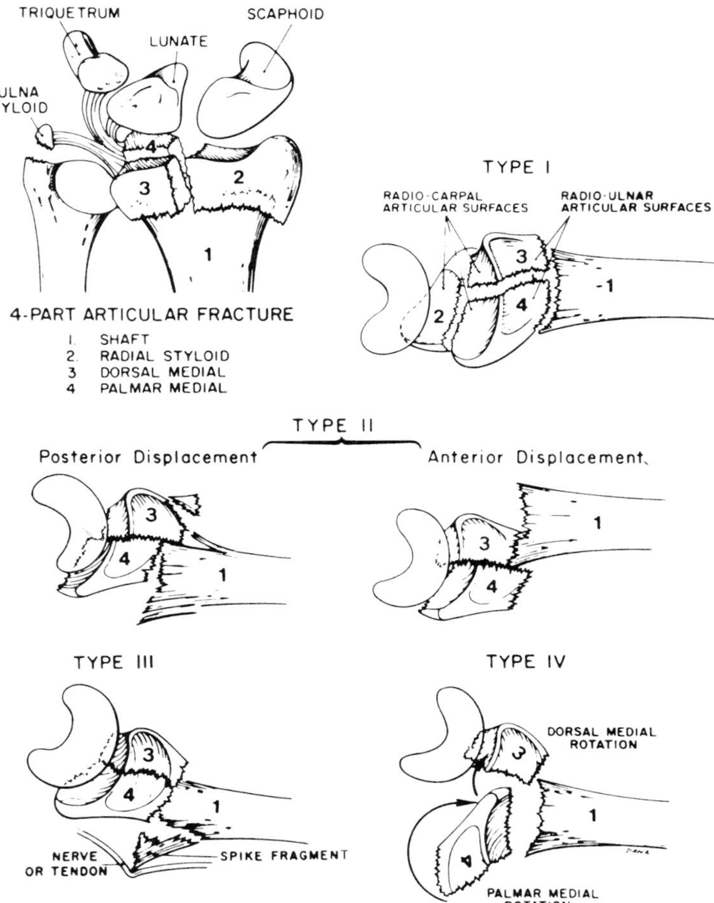

FIGURE 10–19. Melone classification of distal radius fractures. (From Melone, C.P., Jr.: Open treatment for displaced articular fractures of the distal radius. Clin. Orthop. 202:104, 1986; reprinted by permission.)

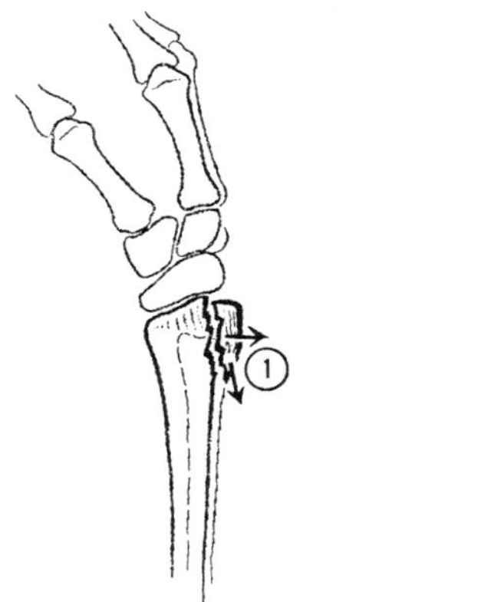

FIGURE 10–20. Dorsal Barton's fracture. (From Connolly, J.F., ed.: Depalma's The Management of Fractures and Dislocations, an Atlas, 3rd ed., p. 1032. Philadelphia, WB Saunders, 1981; reprinted by permission.)

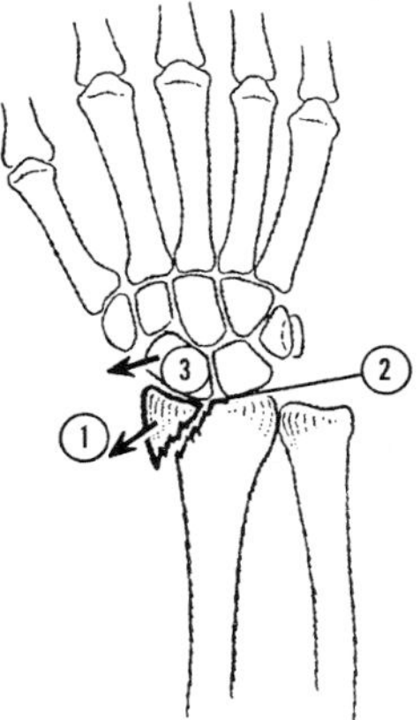

FIGURE 10–21. Radial styloid fractures. (From Connolly, J.F., ed.: Depalma's The Management of Fractures and Dislocations, an Atlas, 3rd ed., p. 1033. Philadelphia, WB Saunders, 1981; reprinted by permission.)

TABLE 10–2. *Continued*

INJURY	EPONYM	CLASSIFICATION	TREATMENT	COMPLICATIONS
*Scaphoid (Fig. 10–23)		Based on anatomic location	Thumb spica, LAC; ORIF displacement and nonunion	Nonunion (tomographic/CT evaluation, Russe bone graft), instability, refracture, nerve injury, RSD, DJD, pain, missed Fx (bone scan helpful)
Dorsal chip		*Triquetrum	SAC 6 weeks	
Perilunate dislocation (±scaphoid Fx)		Mayfield (Fig. 10–24) I—scapholunate disassociation II—lunocapitate disruption III—lunotriquetral disruption IV—lunate dislocation	Early (6–8 wk)—open (dorsally), ligament repair and ORIF scaphoid Fx (if present) Late—triscaphe fusion, proximal row carpectomy or wrist fusion	Rotatory instability of scaphoid, median N palsy, late flexor rupture
Rotatory lunate disassociation	Terry Thomas sign	>3 mm Sap on AP vs. opposite side	Closed—reduction, immobilization, ORIF if scaphoid Fx displaced; open—repair of ligaments (volar and dorsal)	Late DJD
Lunate	Kienböck's	(Osteonecrosis—late)	Ulnar lengthening/radial shortening/resection	Disorganization, disintegration
Carpal instability		*DISI (dorsal scapholunate angle >70°) (Fig. 10–25) VISI (volar scapholunate angle <35°)	Attempt closed reduction of acute injuries; open ST reconstruction for failed reduction or late	
Hook of hamate		Based on size of fragment	Excise small fragment for chronic pain	Missed on plain films (CT view required)
RADIAL/ULNAR SHAFT FRACTURES/DISLOCATIONS				
Radius and ulna	Both bone	Undisplaced Displaced	LAC neutral ORIF 6 hole DCP; external fixation for type III open Fx, bone graft if $>\frac{1}{3}$ (shaft) comminution	Mal/nonunion, vascular injury, PIN injury, compartment syndrome, synostosis, infection, refracture (after plate removal)
Ulna	Nightstick	Undisplaced Displaced (>10° ang, >50° disp)	LAC, ORIF if displaces ORIF—look for wrist/elbow injury	
Proximal ulna and radial head	Monteggia (Fig. 10–26)	Bado: *I—radial head ant. II—radial head post. III—radial head lat. IV—radial head ant. (and both bone Fx)	 ORIF (DCP), closed reduction head, cast 110° flexion ORIF (DCP), closed reduction head, cast 70° flexion ORIF (DCP), closed reduction head, cast 110° flexion ORIF (R + U), closed reduction head, cast 110° flexion	PIN injury (usu. spontaneously resolves), redislocation/subluxation (inadequate reduction)
Proximal radius		Undisplaced Displaced	LAC supination, close follow-up Prox $\frac{1}{5}$ closed, $\frac{1}{5}$–$\frac{2}{3}$ ORIF	
Distal radius and R-U dislocation	Galeazzi/ Piedmont (Fig. 10–27)	Supination/pronation	ORIF (volar), closed reduction ± PCP R-U if unstable	Angulation, distal subluxation, malunion, nonunion; displaced by gravity, PQ, BR, EHL/AHL
ELBOW FRACTURES/DISLOCATIONS				
Supracondylar (Figs. 10–28, 10–29)	Malgaigne	*Extension Flexion	Undisplaced—immobilize 1–2 wk Displaced—ORIF (double plating) bone graft if comminuted Reduce in flexion, PCP if needed	Neurovascular injury, nonunion, malunion, contracture, pain, decreased ROM (fibrosis, bony block)
Transcondylar	Kocher	Intra-articular (post. fragment)	Reduce PCP if required	$\downarrow$ROM
	Posadas	Intra-articular (ant. fragment)	ORIF may be required	

Table continued on opposite page

TABLE 10–2. *Continued*

INJURY	EPONYM	CLASSIFICATION	TREATMENT	COMPLICATIONS
Bicolumn (Fig. 10–30)		Jupiter 1—T pattern (a. high, b. low) 2—Y pattern 3—H pattern 4—Lambda pattern (a. medial, b. lateral)	Immobilize 2 wk to gentle motion ORIF (post. approach: fix condyles first then epitrochlear ridge to humeral metaphysis) Arthroplasty—elderly	Stiffness, heterotopic ossification, infection, ulnar neuropathy (Rx transposition)
Condylar (Fig. 10–31)		Milch (lat. $\gg$ med.): I—Lat. trochlear ridge intact	Undisplaced—immobilize in supination (lat condyle), pronation (med condyle) Displaced—closed reduction ± PCP	C. valgus (lat.), C. varus (med.), ulnar N neurapraxia, DJD
		II—Fx thru lat. trochlear ridge	ORIF	
Capitellar (Fig. 10–32)	Hahn-Steinthal	I—large trochlea piece	Splint 2–3 wk if nondisplaced, ORIF displaced fragment	
	Kocher-Lorenz	II—Min. subchondral bone	Splint 2–3 wk if nondisplaced, excise displaced fragment	
		III—Comminuted Fx	Excise if displaced	
Trochlea	Laugier	Rare	Splint nondisplaced 3 wk, ORIF displaced	
Epicondylar	Granger	Med. $\gg$ Lat.	Manipulation, immobilization 10–14 days	Painful, unsightly fragment or ulnar N symptoms—late excision
Olecranon		Cotton (modified): I. Undisplaced (<2 mm)	Immobilization 45–90° flexion 3 wk, elderly less	↓ROM, DJD, nonunion, ulnar N neurapraxia, instability (with removal of >80%)
		II. Displaced A. Avulsion Fx	ORIF tension band wiring or excise small fragment	
		B. Oblique/transverse Fx	Oblique—bicortical screw; transverse—tension band	
		C. Comminuted Fx	Excision, reattach triceps (up to 50%) if coronoid intact	
		D. Fracture-dislocation	ORIF, no early excision	
Coronoid	Regan & Morrey	I, tip avulsion; II, <50%; III, >50%	I, II—early motion; III—reduction/ fixation	Instability (MCL) and DJD
Radial head (Fig. 10–33)		Mason (and Johnston): I—undisplaced	Nonoperative, early motion ± aspiration	PIN injury; intraosseous membrane rupture; distal R-U disruption; Silastic synovitis; prosthesis for type IV, Monteggia, Essex Lopresti (distal R-U disruption)
		II—marginal with displacement	Excise/ORIF >30°, 3 mm, $\frac{1}{3}$ (McLaughlin)	
		III—comminuted	Early excision	
		IV—with elbow dislocation	Reduce dislocation, then address fracture	
Sideswipe			Traction, external fixation, soft tissue coverage, ORIF, amputation (hand key)	
Dislocation		*Posterior	Closed, reduction, check ROM/ stabilize splint 2–7 days then gentle active ROM; open reduce unstable/interposed soft tissue	Irreducibility, median and ulnar N injury, brachial A injury, flexion contracture, myositis ossificans, Fxs (medial epicondyle, radial head, coronoid)
Fractures of the Humerus Shaft				
Humerus shaft		Based on location/Fx pattern	Coaptation or cast brace, ORIF: segmental, pathologic Fx, distal spiral with nerve injury (Holstein-Lewis) or with forearm Fxs (floating elbow), obesity, ipsilateral thoracic trauma	Malunion (20° ant. and 30° V/V shortening and 3 cm short OK); radial N injury (5–10% incidence; observe unless follows reduction or open Fx, or persists 3–4 mo); nonunion (overdistraction) vascular injury

Table continued on page 369

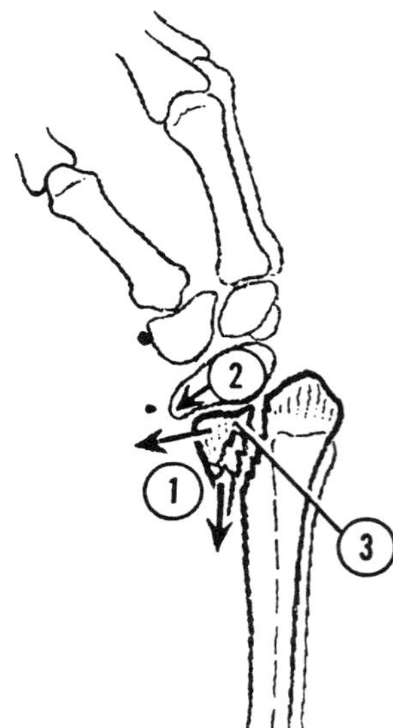

FIGURE 10–22. Volar Barton's fracture. (From Connolly, J.F., ed.: Depalma's The Management of Fractures and Dislocations, an Atlas, 3rd ed., p. 1028. Philadelphia, WB Saunders, 1981; reprinted by permission.)

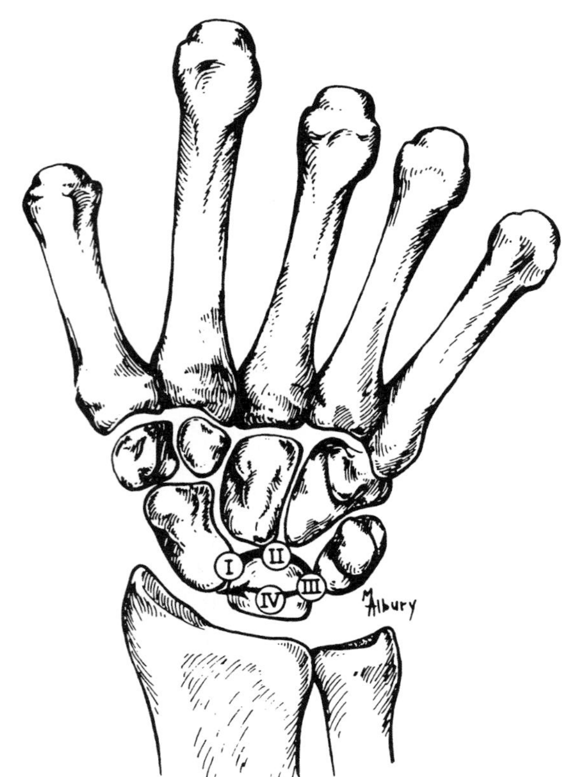

FIGURE 10–24. Perilunar instability—stages. *I,* Scapholunate. *II,* Capitolunate, *III,* Triquetrolunate. *IV,* Dorsal radiocarpal (leading to lunate dislocation). (From Mayfield, J.K.: Mechanism of carpal injuries. Clin. Orthop. 149:50, 1980; reprinted by permission.)

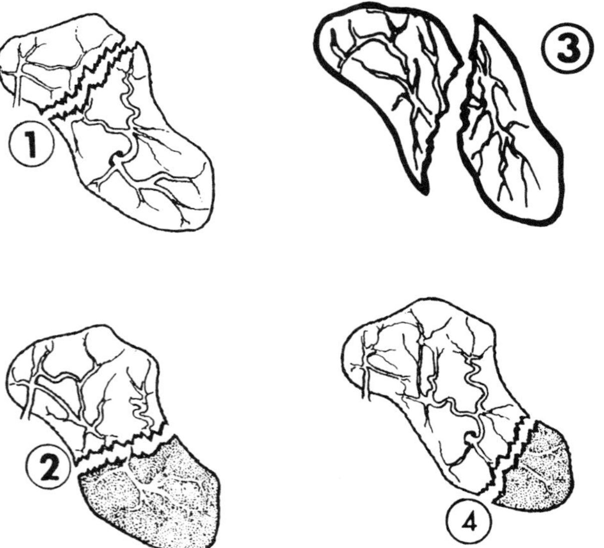

FIGURE 10–23. Classification of scaphoid fractures. *1,* Neck. *2,* Waist. *3,* Body. *4,* Proximal pole. Note progressive risk of avascular necrosis with proximal transverse fractures. (From Wiessman, B.N., and Sledge, C.B.: Orthopedic Radiology, p. 1060. Philadelphia, WB Saunders, 1986; reprinted by permission.)

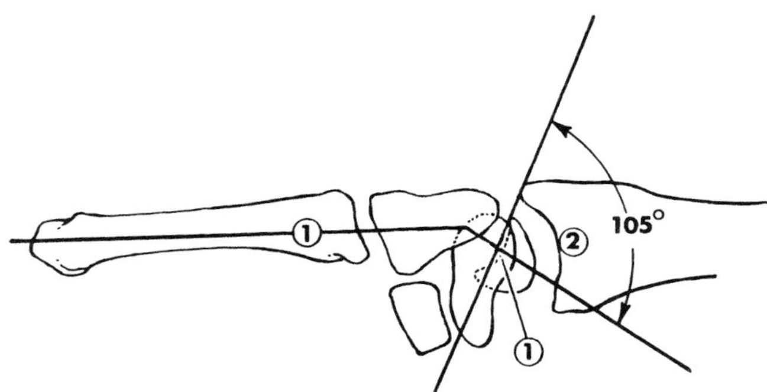

FIGURE 10–25. Dorsal intercalary segmental instability (DISI). Note scapholunate angle >70 degrees, consistent with a DISI pattern. (From Connolly, J.F., ed.: Depalma's The Management of Fractures and Dislocations, an Atlas, 3rd ed., p. 1085. Philadelphia, WB Saunders, 1981; reprinted by permission.)

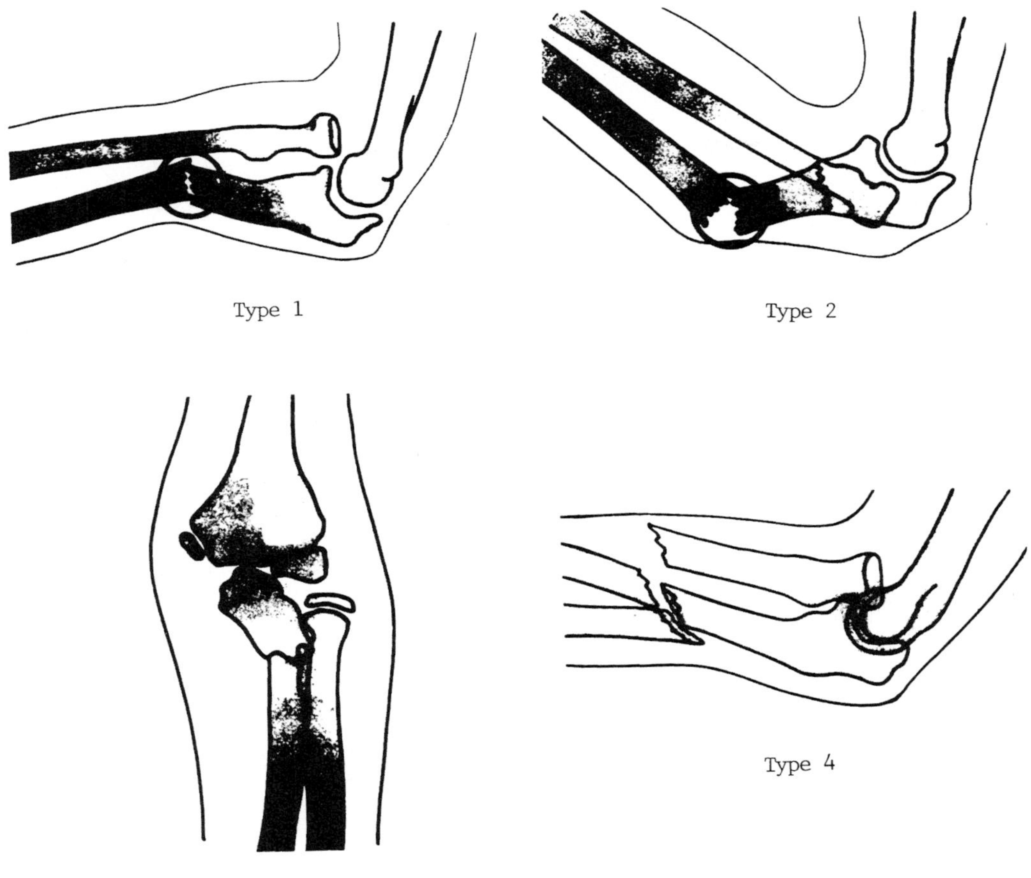

FIGURE 10–26. Classification of Monteggia fractures. (From Reckling, F.W., and Cordell, L.D.: Unstable fracture-dislocations of the forearm. Arch. Surg. 96:1004, 1968; reprinted by permission. Copyright 1968 American Medical Association.)

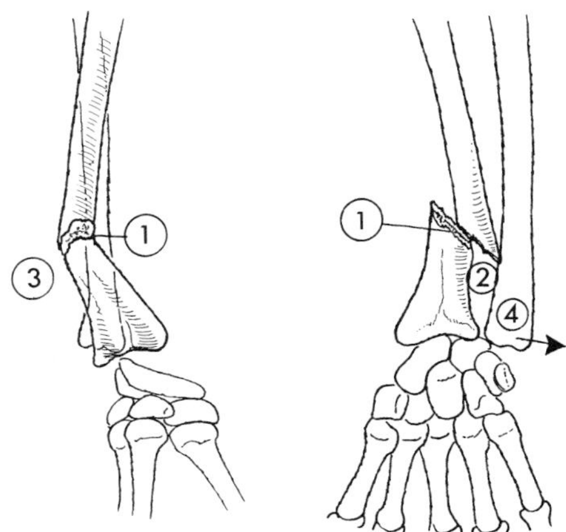

FIGURE 10–27. Galeazzi fractures. (From Connolly, J.F., ed.: Depalma's The Management of Fractures and Dislocations, an Atlas, 3rd ed., p. 927. Philadelphia, WB Saunders, 1981; reprinted by permission.)

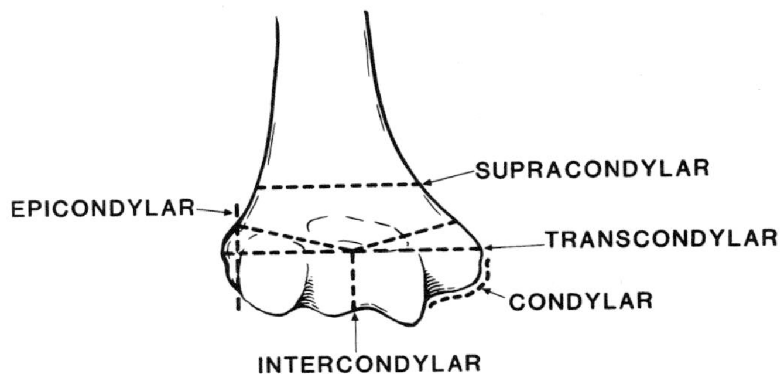

FIGURE 10–28. Distal humerus fractures. (From Gelman, M.I.: Radiology of Orthopedic Procedures, Problems and Complications, vol. 24, p. 54. Philadelphia, WB Saunders, 1984; reprinted by permission.)

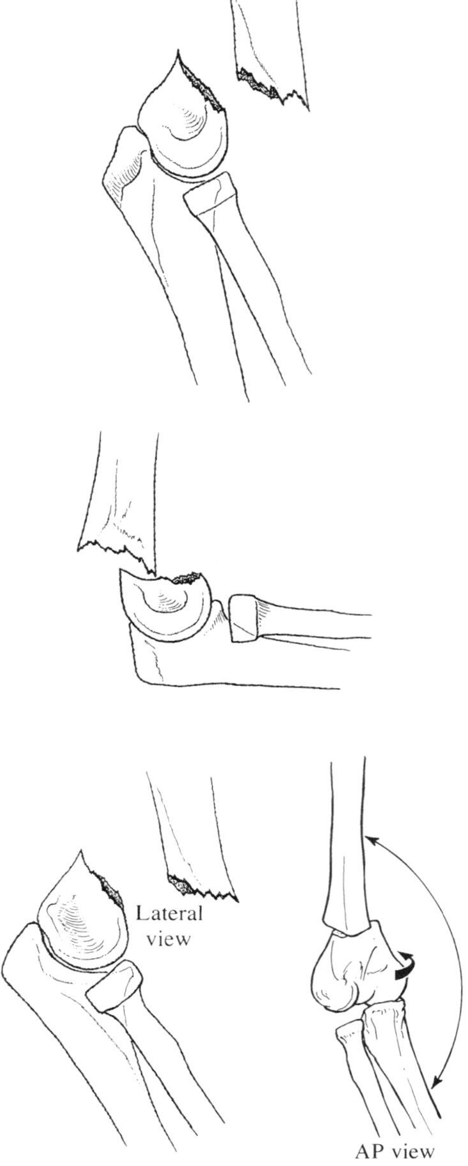

FIGURE 10–29. Supracondylar humerus fractures. *Top,* Extension. *Middle,* Flexion. *Bottom,* Note rotational component. (From Connolly, J.F., ed.: Depalma's The Management of Fractures and Dislocations, an Atlas, 3rd ed., p. 743. Philadelphia, WB Saunders, 1981; reprinted by permission.)

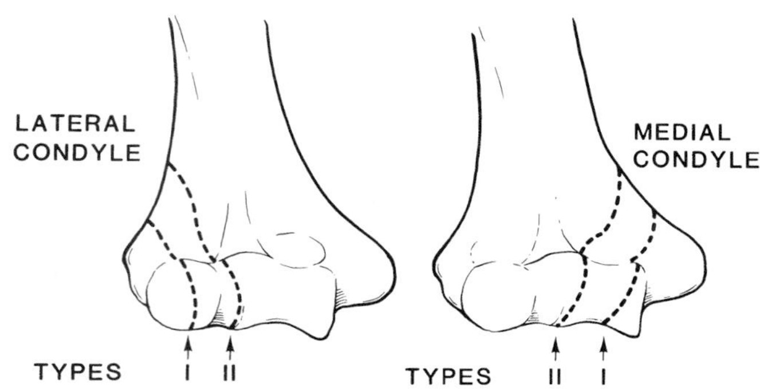

FIGURE 10–31. Humeral condyle fractures. (From Gelman, M.I.: Radiology of Orthopedic Procedures, Problems and Complications, Vol. 24, p. 56. Philadelphia, WB Saunders, 1984; reprinted by permission.)

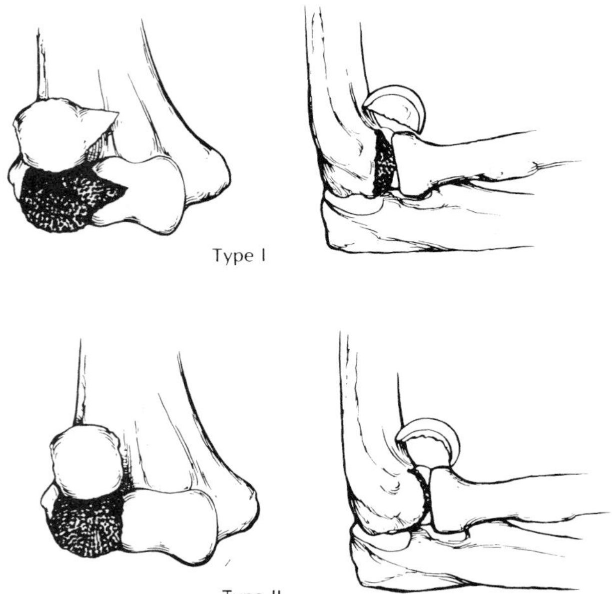

FIGURE 10–32. Capitellar fractures. Note presence of subchondral bone in type I fracture. (From DeLee, J.C., Green, D.P., and Wilkins, K.E.: Fractures and dislocations of the elbow. In Fractures in Adults, Rockwood, C.A., and Green, D.P., eds., 2nd ed., p. 591. Philadelphia, JB Lippincott, 1984; reprinted by permission.)

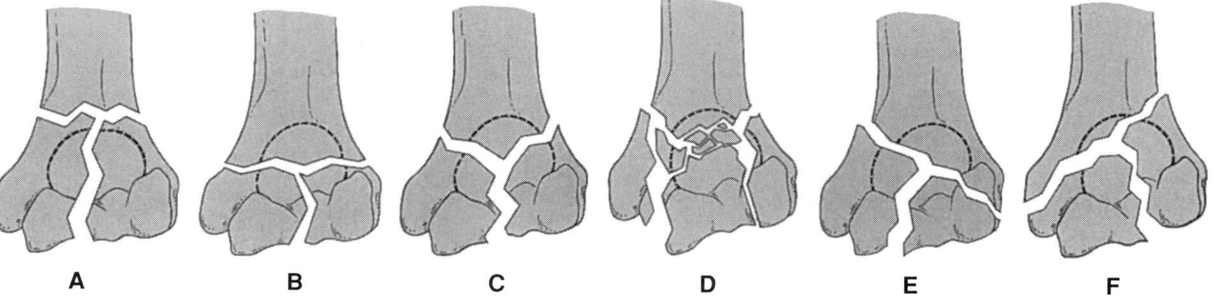

FIGURE 10–30. Bicolumn distal humerus fractures. *A,* High T. *B,* Low T. *C,* Y Pattern. *D,* H Pattern. *E,* Medial lambda. *F,* Lateral lambda. (From Jupiter, J.: Skeletal Trauma, vol. 2,pp. 1159–1163. Philadelphia, WB Saunders, 1992; reprinted by permission.)

TABLE 10–2. *Continued*

INJURY	EPONYM	CLASSIFICATION	TREATMENT	COMPLICATIONS
Shoulder Fractures				
Proximal humerus (Fig. 10–34)		Neer (parts >1 cm or 45° displacement):		Missed dislocation, adhesive capsulitis (moist heat, gentle ROM), malunion (reconstruction or TSA required), AVN (TSA required), nonunion (surgical neck, tuberosity Fxs: ORIF), disrupted rotator cuff
		*One-part	Early motion; isometrics → progressive resistance.	
		Two-part	Closed reduction unless articular segment (ORIF), shaft (impacted and angulated—traction, Velpeau; unimpacted—closed reduction, PCP or ORIF), greater tuberosity (repair cuff) tuberosity with block to med. rotation (ORIF)	
		Three-part	ORIF younger, prosthesis in older	
		Four-part	Prosthesis; nonoperative in elderly/diabetes/impacted 4-part valgus pattern	
Proximal humerus	Fx-Dislocation	Ant. (greater tuberosity displacement)	If >1 cm after reduction, open repair	As above plus axillary N or plexus injury, myositis ossificans, (wait >1 yr to excise heterotopic bone)
		Post. (lesser tuberosity displacement)	Closed reduction, ORIF if 3-part	
Impression	Hill-Sach	Stable (<20% articular surface)	Closed treatment	AVN, DJD (TSA)
		Unstable (20–50%)	Transfer lesser tuberosity → defect (McLaughlin)	
		Unstable (>45%)	Prosthesis vs. rotational osteotomy	
Head splitting			Prosthesis	
Clavicle		*Middle ⅓	Shoulder spica, sling	Vascular injury/ pneumothorax/other injury; skin necrosis; malunion (osteotomize young active patient); nonunion (ORIF and bone graft), nerve injury (rare); muscle fatigue/weakness, DJD (if articular)
		Distal ⅓ (Neer):		
		I—min. displacement interligamentous (CC-AC)		
		II—Fx medial to CC ligaments:		
		IIA—both ligaments attached to distal fragment	ORIF	
		IIB—conoid torn, trapezoid attached to distal fragment (Fig. 10–35)	ORIF	
		III—AC joint	Closed treatment, late excision arthroplasty if required	
		Proximal ⅓	Closed treatment	
Scapula		Zdravkovic and Damholt:		Associated injuries (clavicle, rib, pneumo), axillary artery injury, plexus palsy, pressure symptoms, vascular and plexus injuries
		I—body	Most treated conservatively	
		II—coracoid and acromion	Assoc. injury common (clavicle rib, pneumo), ORIF large displaced fragments	
		III—neck and glenoid	ORIF large unstable fractures (glenoid with displaced clavicle Fx)	
Glenoid		Ideberg		
		I—Ant avulsion Fx	>25° of surface—ORIF if head is subluxed with major fragment	
		II—Transverse/oblique Fx-inf glenoid free		
		III—Upper ⅓ glenoid + coracoid		
		IV—Horizontal glenoid through body		
		V—combination of II–IV		
Scapulothoracic dissociation		(Seen on scapular lateral or chest radiograph)	Closed reduction	Vascular and plexus injuries Associated clavicular fracture

Table continued on following page

TABLE 10–2. *Continued*

INJURY	EPONYM	CLASSIFICATION	TREATMENT	COMPLICATIONS
SHOULDER DISLOCATIONS/LIGAMENTOUS INJURIES				
*Ant. dislocation (Fig. 10–36)		Subcoracoid > subglenoid (subclavicular and intrathoracic)	Reduce, immobilize (young patient 4 wk, old patient 2 wk); passive → active rehab (Rockwood 7)	Axillary N neurapraxia, axillary A injury, cuff injury (>40 yo), recurrence (85% in <20 yo), bone injury (head, greater tuberosity, glenoid)
Ant. subluxation		Atraumatic	Conservative (vol-psych; nonoperative)	Dead arm syndrome (nerve impingement with subluxation), recurrent subluxation
		Traumatic	Rehab—Rockwood 7	
Recurrent	Ant. dislocation/ subluxation		Rockwood 7 for 6–12 mo; if fails, consider surgery:	
			Repair[a] — ***Technique***	***Complications***
			Bankart — Ant. capsule → ant. rim	Late instability
			Staple capsulorrhaphy — Capsule → glenoid	Late DJD, migration
			Putti-Platt — Subscapularis embrication	Late DJD, ↓ ER
			Magnuson-Stack — Subscapularis → lesser tuberosity	Late DJD, ↓ ER
			Bone block — Crest graft ant.	↓ROM, migration
			Bristow — Coracoid transfer	Nonunion, ↓ER, migration
			Capsular shift — Redundant capsule advanced	Min., procedure of choice with MDI
Post. dislocation (Fig. 10–37)		*Subacromial (seizures and shocks)	Reduce, immobilize 4 wk; operate if recurrent (glenoid osteotomy, bone block, post. capsule shift)	Lesser tuberosity fracture Late recognition (may require advancement or lesser tuberosity into defect or TSA [place in less retroversion]); avoid by checking axillary view
Inf. glenohumeral	Luxatio erecta (Fig. 10–38)		Reduce and immobilize	Neurovascular injury resolves after reduction; axillary A thrombosis
AC injury (Fig. 10–39)		I—AC sprain	7–10 Days rest/immobilization	Joint stiffness, deformity, CC ligament and soft tissue calcification, AC DJD, associated Fxs, distal clavicle osteolysis
		II—AC tear, CC sprain	Sling 2 wk, rehab, late excision arthroplasty if required	
		III—AC and CC tear	Conservative vs. repair (athletes, laborers)	
		IV—clavicle through trapezius posteriorly	Reduce and repair	
		V—clavicle 100–300% elevated	Reduce and repair	
		VI—clavicle inferior to caracoid	Reduce and repair	
SC injury (Fig. 10–40)		Anterior dislocation	Closed reduction with traction	Bump (cosmetic), DJD, mediastinal impingement, hardware migration (with operative treatment)
		Posterior dislocation	Closed reduction towel clip or open	
		Spontaneous atraumatic subluxation	Nonoperative	

* Most common.

PCP, percutaneous pin fixation; RCL, radial collateral ligament; LCL, lateral collateral ligament; UCL, ulnar collateral ligament; VP, volar plate; SAC, short arm cast; LAC, long arm cast; MC, metacarpal; PP, proximal phalanx; MP middle phalanx; DP, distal phalanx; MCP, metacarpal phalangeal joint; PIP, proximal interphalangeal joint; DIP, distal interphalangeal joint; IF, index finger; RF, ring finger; MF, middle finger; SF, small finger. Fx, fractive; ORIF, open reduction and lateral fixation; ROM, range of motion; EDL, extensor digitorum longus; FDP, flexor digitorum profundus; ECU, extensor carpii ulnaris; APL, adductor pollicis longus; PIN, posterior interosseous nerve; AVN, avascular necrosis; DJD, degenerative joint disease; TSA, total shoulder arthroplasty; Ex fix, external fixation.

[a] Note: Bankart and capsular shift are preferred among this group.

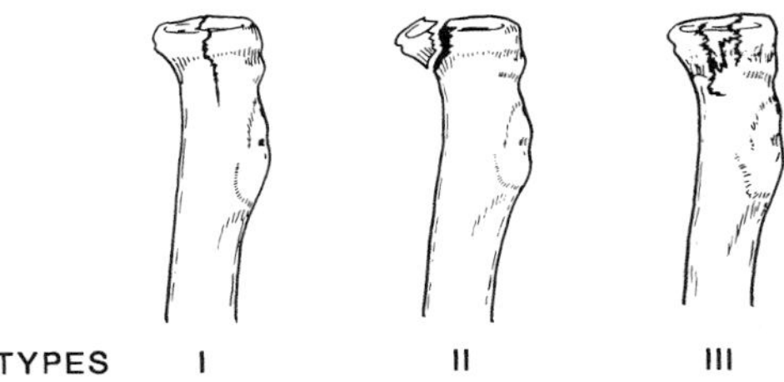

FIGURE 10–33. Classification of radial head fractures. (From Gelman, M.I.: Radiology of Orthopedic Procedures, Problems and Complications, Vol. 24, p. 59. Philadelphia, WB Saunders, 1984; reprinted by permission.)

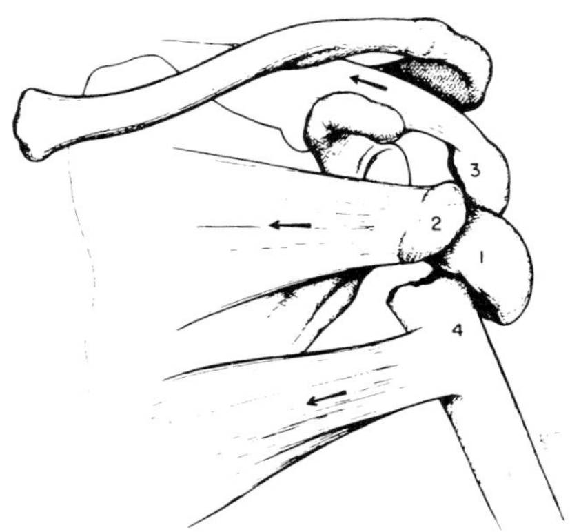

FIGURE 10–34. Proximal humeral fracture. Four parts: *1,* head; *2,* lesser tuberosity; *3,* greater tuberosity; *4,* humeral shaft. (From Neer, C.S., and Rockwood, C.A.: Fractures and dislocations of the shoulder. In Fractures in Adults, Rockwood, C.A., and Green, D.P., eds., 2nd ed., p. 696. Philadelphia, JB Lippincott, 1984; reprinted by permission.)

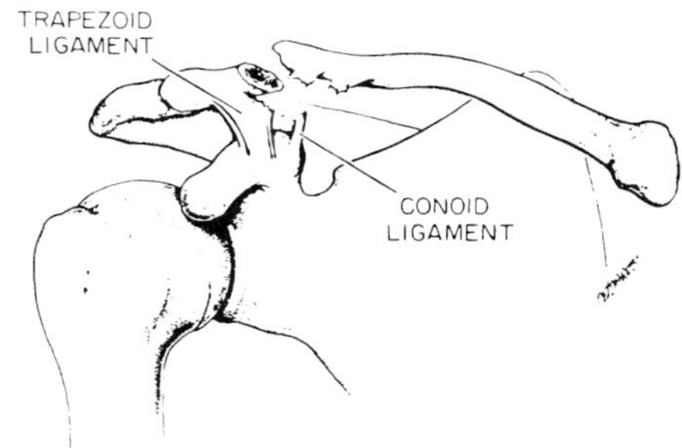

FIGURE 10–35. Neer type IIB fracture of the distal clavicle. (From Neer, C.S., II: Fracture of the distal clavicle with detachment of the coracoclavicular ligaments in adults. J. Trauma 3:101, 1963; reprinted by permission. Copyright © 1968 by Williams & Wilkins.)

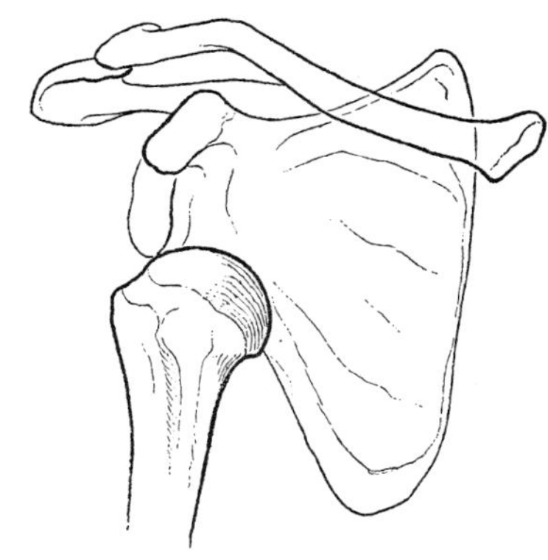

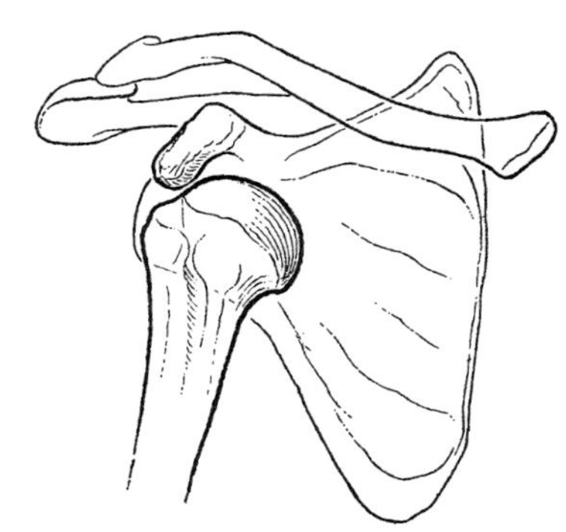

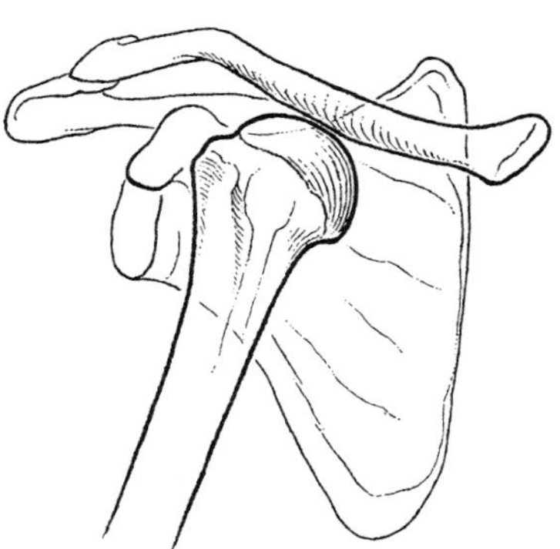

FIGURE 10–36. Anterior shoulder dislocation. *Top,* Subglenoid. *Middle,* Subcoracoid. *Bottom,* Subclavicular. (From Connolly, J.F., ed.: Depalma's The Management of Fractures and Dislocations, an Atlas, 3rd ed., p. 617. Philadelphia, WB Saunders, 1981; reprinted by permission.)

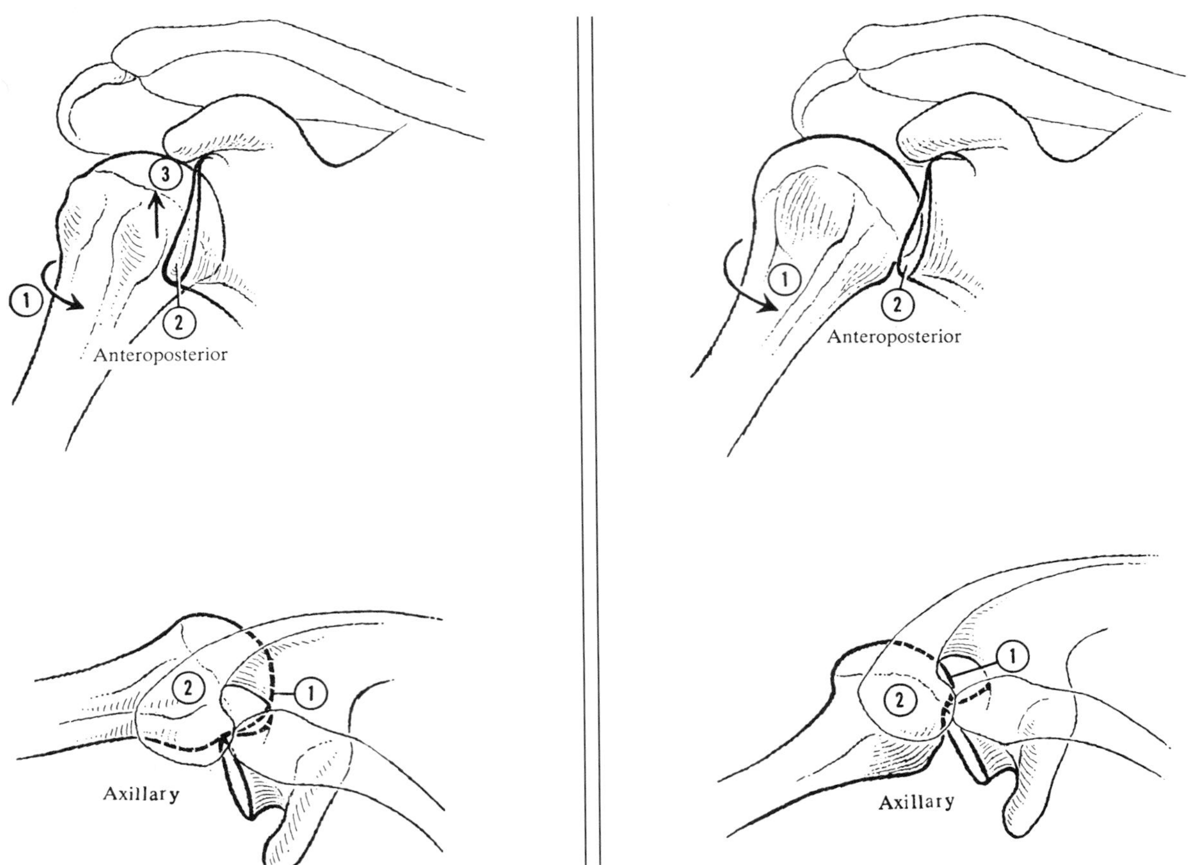

FIGURE 10–37. Posterior shoulder dislocation. *Left,* Subacromial. *Right,* Subcoracoid. (From Connolly, J.F., ed.: Depalma's The Management of Fractures and Dislocations, an Atlas, 3rd ed., p. 633. Philadelphia, WB Saunders, 1981; reprinted by permission.)

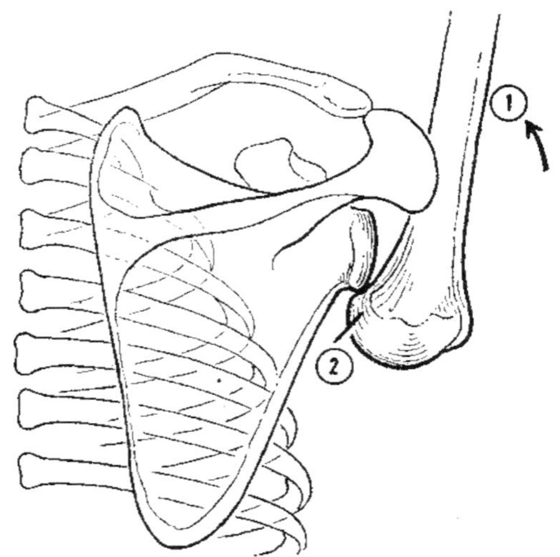

FIGURE 10–38. Luxatio erecta. (From Connolly, J.F., ed.: Depalma's The Management of Fractures and Dislocations, an Atlas, 3rd ed., p. 622. Philadelphia, WB Saunders, 1981; reprinted by permission.)

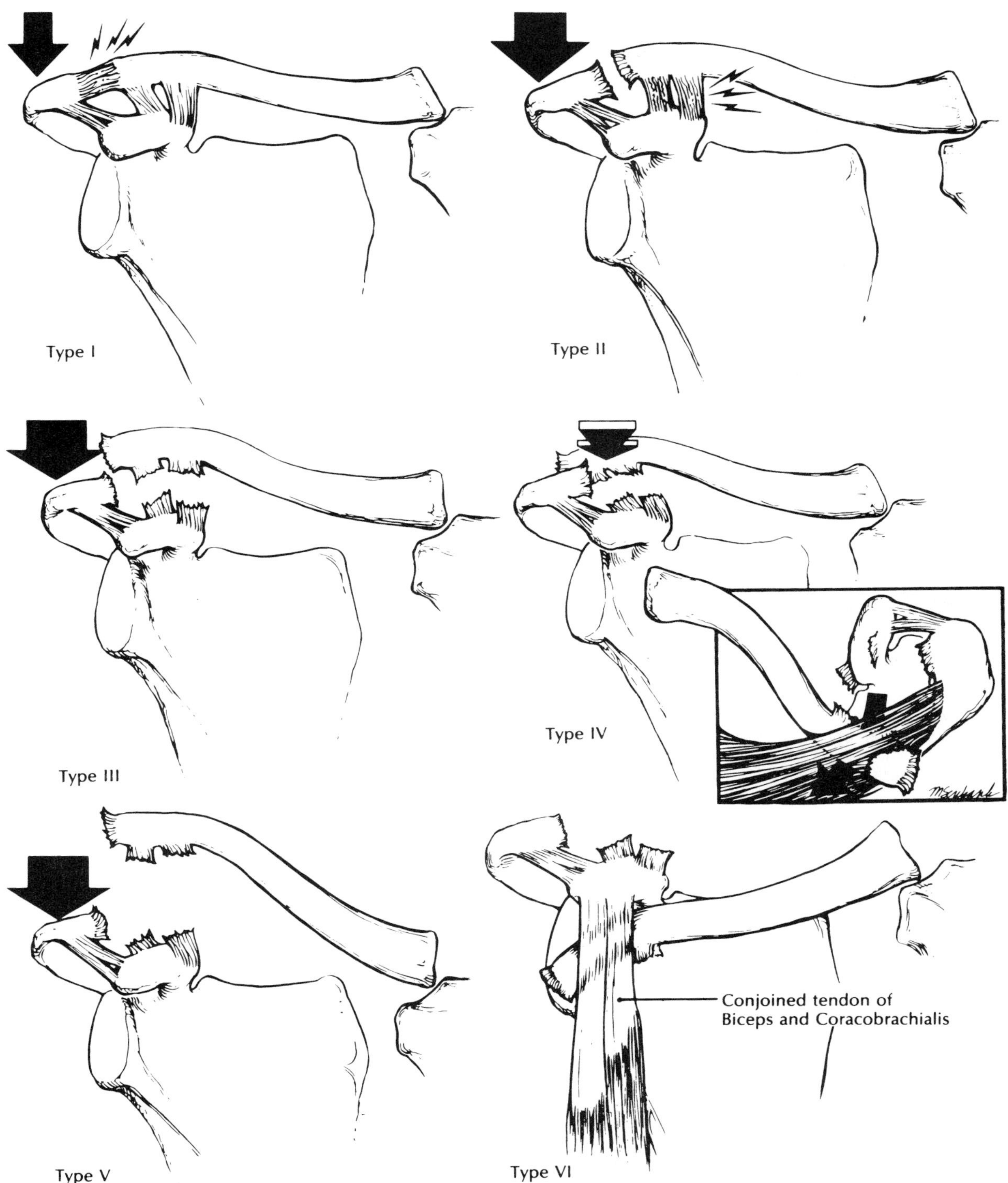

FIGURE 10–39. Classification of acromioclavicular injuries. (From Neer, C.S., and Rockwood, C.A.: Fractures and dislocations of the shoulder. In Fractures in Adults, Rockwood, C.A., and Green, D.P., eds., 2nd ed., p. 871. Philadelphia, JB Lippincott, 1984; reprinted by permission.)

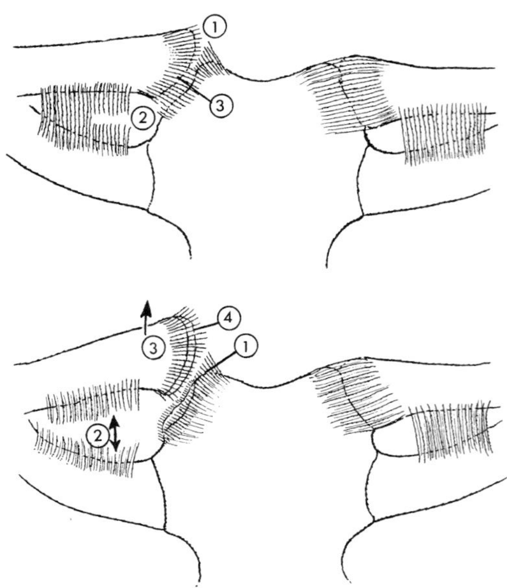

FIGURE 10–40. Sternoclavicular dislocations. *Top,* Partial injury. *Bottom,* Complete sternoclavicular dislocation. (From Connolly, J.F., ed.: Depalma's The Management of Fractures and Dislocations, an Atlas, 3rd ed., p. 560. Philadelphia, WB Saunders, 1981; reprinted by permission.)

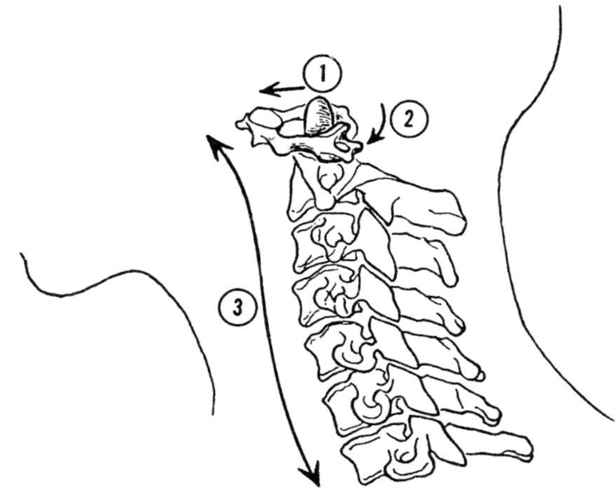

FIGURE 10–42. Rotatory subluxation of C1–C2. (From Connolly, J.F., ed.: Depalma's The Management of Fractures and Dislocations, an Atlas, 3rd ed., p. 287. Philadelphia, WB Saunders, 1981; reprinted by permission.)

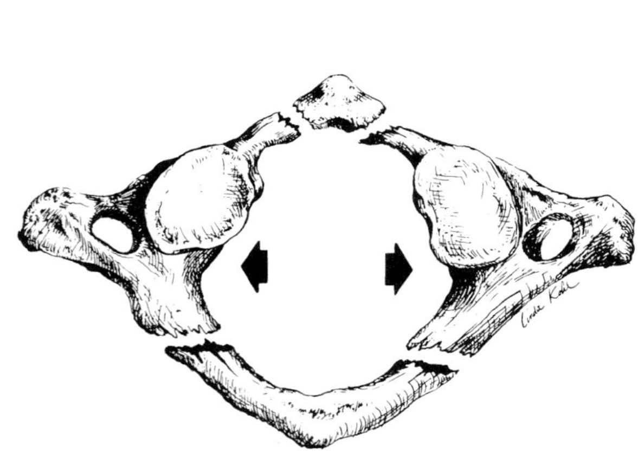

FIGURE 10–41. Jefferson fracture. (From Urbaniak, J.R.: Fractures of the spine. In Davis-Christopher Textbook of Surgery, Sabiston, D.C., Jr., ed., p. 1528. Philadelphia, WB Saunders, 1977; reprinted by permission.)

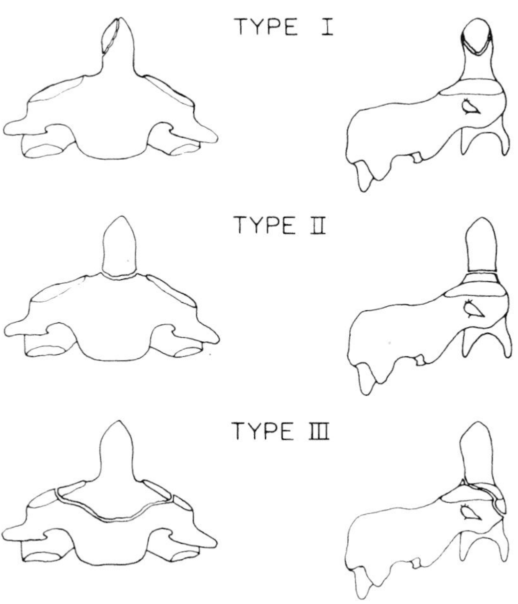

FIGURE 10–43. Odontoid fracture classification. (From Anderson, L.D., and D'Alonzono, R.T.: Fractures of the odontoid process of the axis. J. Bone Joint Surg. [Am.] 56:1664, 1974; reprinted by permission.)

TABLE 10–3. ADULT TRAUMATIC ORTHOPAEDIC INJURIES—CERVICAL SPINE

INJURY	EPONYM	MOI	CLASSIFICATION	TREATMENT	NEURO INJURY	COMPLICATIONS/ OTHER
Occiput–C1 dislocation		Distraction or translation	Anterior or posterior	Halo + occiput–C2 fusion	Usually fatal!	Overdistraction (avoid traction)
C1 Fx		Axial; + extension	Posterior	Usu. stable—orthosis (50% with other C-spine injuries)	Rare	Vertebral A injury (unilateral = Wallenberg's; Rx with heparin), CN VIII injury; diastasis of lat. masses (may require fusion late)
		Axial + flexion	Anterior	Halo, fusion if marked atlantoaxial sublux.		
	Jefferson (Fig. 10–41)	Axial load	Poster and anterior	Halo traction, C1–C2 fusion for mal/nonunion or instability (>5 mm atlantoaxial sublux.)		
			Lateral mass compression Fx	Orthosis		
C1–C2 subluxation/ dislocation		Transverse ligament rupture	Increased atlantodens interval	C1–C2 fusion		
			Ant. ± Fx	Reduction (traction)—orthosis	Ant. common	AP x-ray—"wink" sign (overlap of C1–C2 lat. masses)
			Post. ± Fx	Usu. requires post. fusion (recurrence)		
	"Cock robin"		Rotatory (Fig. 10–42)	Requires traction → halo or fusion (C_1C_2)		
C2 Fx odontoid (Fig. 10–43)		Flexion, extension, rotation	Anderson and D'Alonzo		Rare	Nonunion
			I—upper tip	Orthosis		
			II—at junction of odontoid and C2 body	PSF C1–C2 if >5 mm, post. displacement, imperfect reduction		Post. displaced Fxs require post. bone block
			III—through C2 body	Halo × 12 wk		
C2 isthmus FX	Hangman's (Fig. 10–44)	Hyperextension + axial	Levine		Uncommon	Follow for loss of reduction, often assoc. w/other lower C-spine injuries
			I—vertical fracture line, no angulation	→Philadelphia collar		Flexion-distraction variant: displacement in traction
			II—disc disrupted; >3 mm translation, angulation	→ halo ×6 wk		
			IIA—posterior fracture, almost horizontal	→halo traction, gentle manipulation		
			III—vertical fracture, bilateral facet dislocation	→open reduction		
C3–C7 facet dislocation	"Jumped" facet (Fig. 10–45)	Flexion-distraction/ rotation	Unilateral (<25% body) Bilateral (25–50% body)	Traction—sequential weight addition (10 lb + 5 lb/level); open reduction post. fusion if fails or unstable	Common (incr. risk with greater displacements)	Neuro injury, disc herniation with traction → paralysis MRI prior to closed or open reduction of disc herniation suspected
C3–C7 Fx			Translation	>3.5 mm vs. other levels → fusion		
			Angular displacement	>11° vs. other levels → fusion		
C3–C7 compression (Fig. 10–46)	Burst/crush		Canal compression (post. elements)	<25% compression with intact posterior wall → nonoperative Rx		
				Stable—halo; unstable or neuro injury—ant. strut with postop orthosis; post. elements—ant. + post. fusion; AS—laminectomy (only indication)	Common	Post-traumatic kyphosis
C3–C7 spinous processes	Clay shoveler's		Spinous process avulsion	Symptomatic		

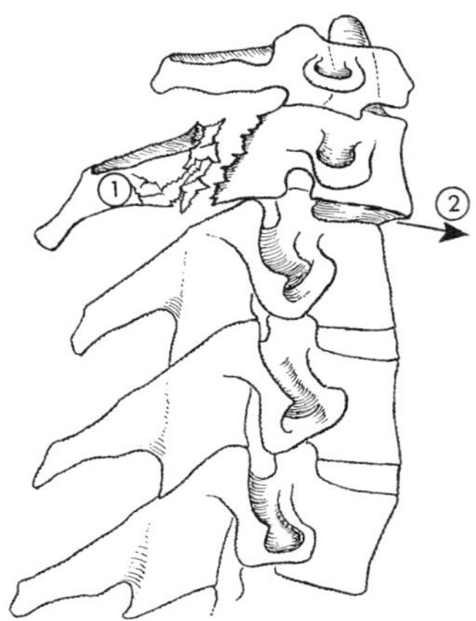

FIGURE 10–44. Hangman's fracture. (From Connolly, J.F., ed.: Depalma's The Management of Fractures and Dislocations, an Atlas, 3rd ed., p. 312. Philadelphia, WB Saunders, 1981; reprinted by permission.)

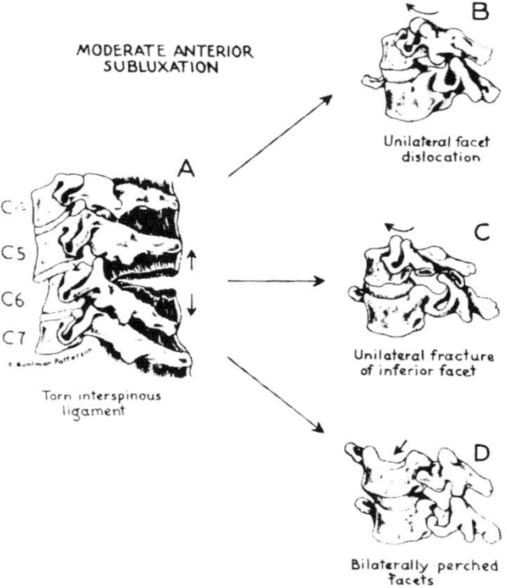

FIGURE 10–45. Jumped facet. Note 25% displacement with unilateral dislocation and 50% displacement with bilateral dislocation. (From Bohlman, H.H.: Fractures and dislocations of the cervical spine. J. Bone Joint Surg. [Am.] 61:1136, 1979; reprinted by permission.)

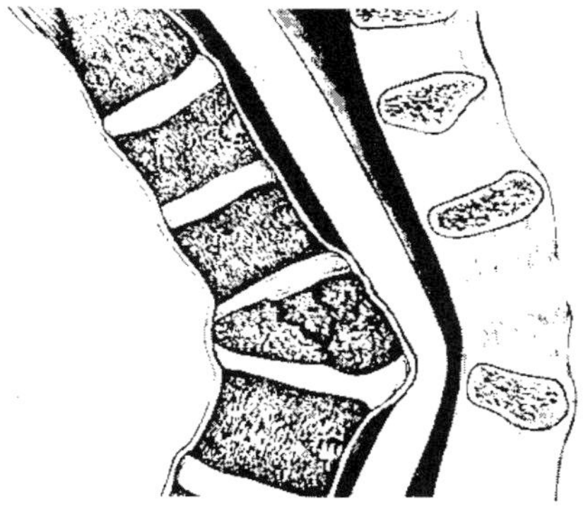

FIGURE 10–46. Crush fracture. (From Bohlman, H.H.: Fractures and dislocations of the cervical spine. J. Bone Joint Surg. [Am.] 61:1131, 1979; reprinted by permission.)

TABLE 10–4. ADULT TRAUMATIC ORTHOPAEDIC INJURIES—THORACIC AND LUMBAR SPINE (FERGUSON-ALLEN)

INJURY	EPONYM	COMMON FORCES[a] ANT.	MID.	POST.	CLASSIFICATION	TREATMENT	NEURO INJURIES	COMPLICATIONS/ OTHER
Compression Flexion	Wedge (Fig. 10–47)	C+	D	D	Stage I—<50% decrease ant. height	Bed rest acute, orthosis	Rare	Progression (rare for type I but incr. for type III > II if not stabilized)
Flexion-distraction		C+	D+	D	Stage II—SP separated ± facet Fx/dislocation	Posterior fusion (compression)	Occasional	
	Blowout	C+	D+	D+	Stage III—canal impingement (superior vertebral body)	Posterior fusion (compression) ± decompression for neuro injury	More common	
Flexion-distraction	Chance (seat belt) (Fig. 10–48)	D+	D+	D	Bony Ligamentous Bony and ligamentous	Bed rest/orthosis (hyperext.) Posterior fusion (compression) Posterior fusion (compression)	Occasional (based on trans)	
Lateral flexion		C+	C+	C±	Ipsilateral compression ± contralateral facet Fx-dislocation	Based on middle and post. column disruption (fuse concave—distraction convex—compression)	Occasional (ipsilateral)	
Translational	Shear (Fig. 10–49)	T+	T+	T+	Based on position of displacement (ant., post., lat.)	If >25%, segmental instrumentation (Luque rods)	Very common	
Flexion-rotation	Slice (Fig. 10–50)	DC+	D±	DT+	Facet Fx-dislocation, superior vertebral body → ant.	Most unstable! Segmental fixation favored	Very common	Usu. in lower T-spine
Vertical compression	Burst (Fig. 10–51)	C+	C+	C±	Based on canal compromise (CT)	Post. ± ant. decompression/fusion if increased canal compression (>50% or neuro injury), otherwise extended bed rest, then orthosis	Occasional	Progression? Dural tear, herniated roots (with laminar Fx)
Extension-distraction	Teardrop (Fig. 10–52)	D+		C+	Often spontaneously reduces	Nonoperative	Rare	

[a] C, compression; D, distraction; T, translation; R, rotation; +, likely disrupted; ±, may or may not be disrupted.

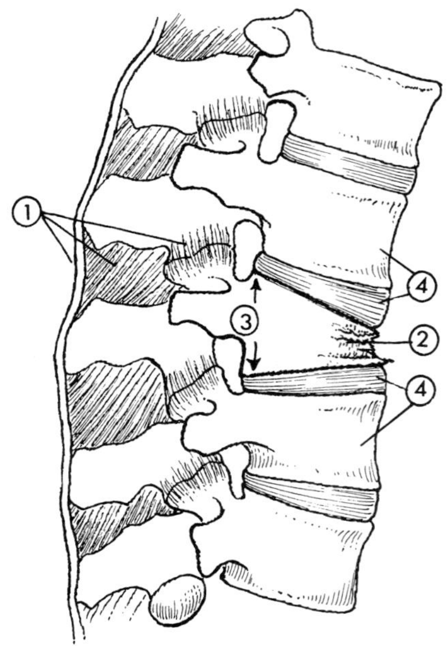

FIGURE 10–47. Wedge fracture. (From Connolly, J.F., ed.: Depalma's The Management of Fractures and Dislocations, an Atlas, 3rd ed., p. 407. Philadelphia, WB Saunders, 1981; reprinted by permission.)

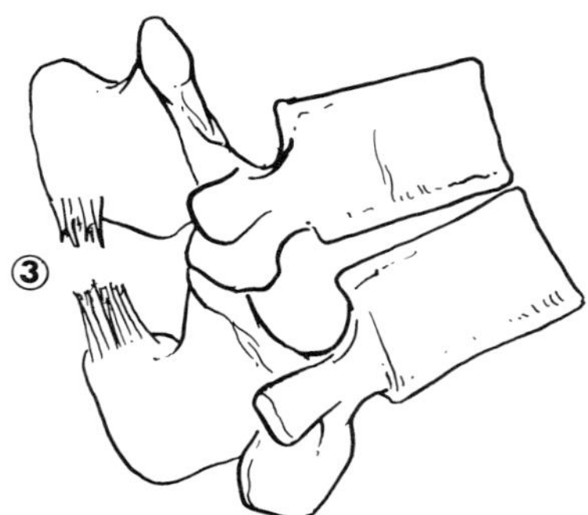

FIGURE 10–48. Chance fracture (ligamentous). (From Connolly, J.F., ed.: Depalma's The Management of Fractures and Dislocations, an Atlas, 3rd ed., p. 413. Philadelphia, WB Saunders, 1981; reprinted by permission.)

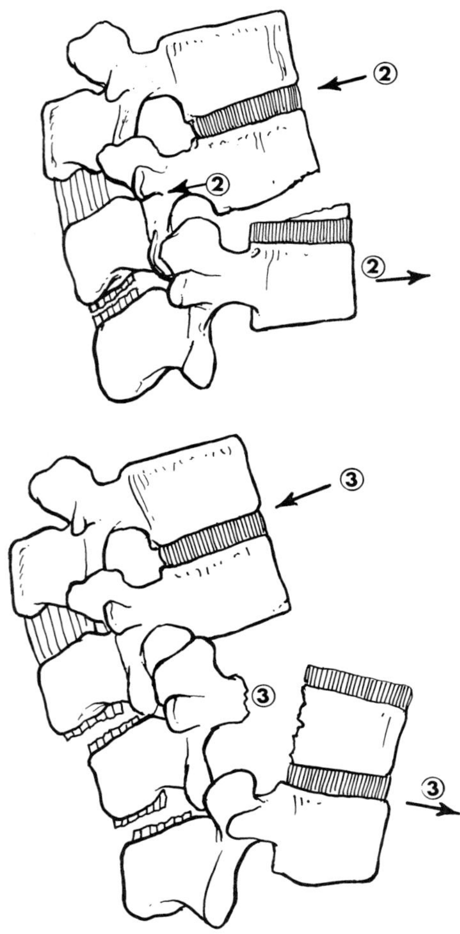

FIGURE 10–49. Shear fracture. *Top,* Stable. *Bottom,* Unstable. (From Connolly, J.F., ed.: Depalma's The Management of Fractures and Dislocations, an Atlas, 3rd ed., p. 412. Philadelphia, WB Saunders, 1981; reprinted by permission.)

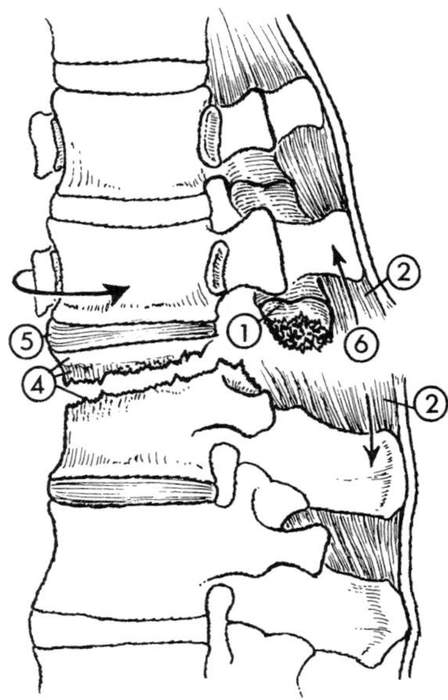

FIGURE 10–50. Slice fracture. (From Connolly, J.F., ed.: Depalma's The Management of Fractures and Dislocations, an Atlas, 3rd ed., p. 410. Philadelphia, WB Saunders, 1981; reprinted by permission.)

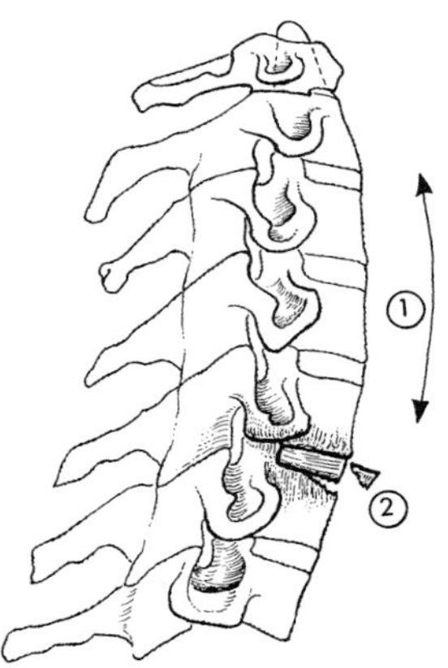

FIGURE 10–52. Teardrop fracture. (From Connolly, J.F., ed.: Depalma's The Management of Fractures and Dislocations, an Atlas, 3rd ed., p. 363. Philadelphia, WB Saunders, 1981; reprinted by permission.)

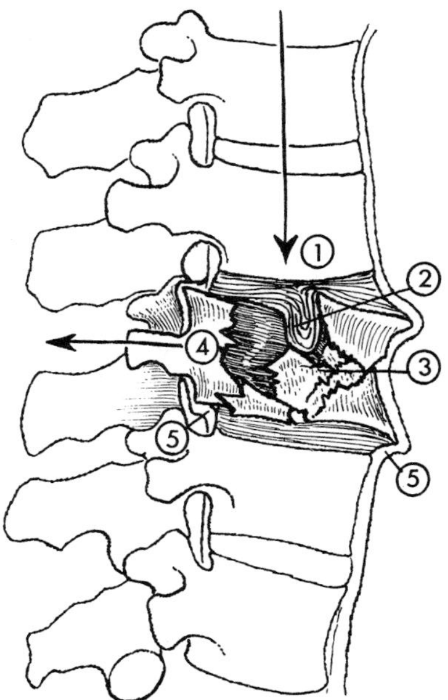

FIGURE 10–51. Burst fracture. Note retropulsion of bony fragments into spinal canal. (From Connolly, J.F., ed.: Depalma's The Management of Fractures and Dislocations, an Atlas, 3rd ed., p. 409. Philadelphia, WB Saunders, 1981; reprinted by permission.)

TABLE 10–5. ADULT TRAUMATIC ORTHOPAEDIC INJURIES—LOWER EXTREMITY

INJURY	EPONYM	CLASSIFICATION	TREATMENT	COMPLICATIONS
PELVIC FRACTURES				
Pelvis (Fig. 10–53)		Young *Lateral compression* (LC): *I—I/L or C/L ramii (transverse) and I/L sacral compression	 Bed rest	Post. skin slough, life-threatening hemorrhage, GI injury, GU injury (bladder, urethra, impotency), neuro injury, nonunion, DJD, pain, loss of reduction, sepsis, thrombophlebitis, malunion (leg-length discrepancy, sitting problems), heterotopic bone, vascular injuries (incl. aortic rupture), SI pain. APC III highest rate of associated injury.
		II—I/L or C/L ramii and I/L post. iliac	Bed rest or delayed ORIF	
		III—I/L or C/L ramii and LC I/II & C/L APC	Based on C/L injury	
		Anteroposterior compression (APC): I—symphysis (<2 cm) or ramii (vertical) & ant. SI ligament stretched	 Bed rest	
		II—symphysis or ramii and ant. SI ligament torn	Acute external fixation/ant. ORIF if concurrent laparotomy	
		III—symphysis or ramii and ant. and post. SI ligament torn	Acute external fixation/ant. ORIF if concurrent laporotomy, post. SI ORIF	
	Malgaigne	*Vertical shear* (VS): ant. and post. vertical displacement	Acute external fixation/ant. ORIF if concurrent laparotomy, post. SI ORIF	
		Combined mechanical (CM): combination of other injuries	Based on injuries, ORIF if posterior SI displaced	
Acetabulum (Fig. 10–54)		Tile Undisplaced Displaced I—posterior ± posterior dislocation A—posterior column B—posterior wall 1—associated with post. column 2—associated with transverse Fx II—anterior ± anterior dislocation A—anterior column B—anterior wall C—associated ant. and transverse Fx III—anterior ± central dislocation A—pure transverse B—"T" fractures C—assoc. transverse and acetabular wall Fxs D—double-column fractures	Nonoperative: less than 2 mm displacement in the acetabular dome, low ant. column Fxs, low transverse Fxs, associated both column Fxs with secondary congruence. Operative: incongruous or unstable joint: posterior column/wall use Kocher-Langenbach approach; anterior column/wall use ilioinguinal approach; both columns use extended iliofemoral or combined Kocher-Langenbach/ilioinguinal	Nerve injury (sciatic 16–33%, femoral, sup. gluteal), vascular injury (subgluteal A) heterotopic ossification (3–69%—consider XRT or Indocin), avascular necrosis (with posterior injury), chondrolysis, DJD
HIP FRACTURES				
Femoral neck		Garden (Fig. 10–55): I—incomplete/valgus impaction II—complete, undisplaced III—complete, partially displaced IV—complete, totally displaced	CRIF with 3 screws or sliding compression hip screw with derotation screw; prosthesis for elderly (>70 yo physio), sick, pathologic Fx, Parkinson's, RA, Dilantin Tx with displaced fractures (Garden III or IV); bipolar prosthesis for more active patients, THA for acetabular DJD (cement often indicated)	Malunion (accept <15° valgus and 10° AP displacement); AVN (25% at 12 hr, 30% at 24 hr, 40% at 24–48 hr, 100% at 1 wk); nonunion (incr. with sliding screws); infection; PE; mortality (35% at 1 yr; incr. with advanced age, medical problems, and in males)
Neck stress		Devas: Compression or transverse (distraction)	 Distraction type increased propensity to displace	
		Blickenstaff and Morris I—callus	 Bed rest → progressive weight bearing	 Completed fracture, as above
		II—nondisplaced	Fixation	
		III—displaced	CRIF 6 wks = ORIF ± bone graft	

Table continued on opposite page

TABLE 10–5. *Continued*

INJURY	EPONYM	CLASSIFICATION	TREATMENT	COMPLICATIONS
Intertrochanteric (Fig. 10–56)		Boyd and Griffin I—nondisplaced *II—displaced III—reverse obliquity IV—subtrochlear spike Evans (stable, unstable)	CRIF with sliding compression hip screw most reliable; unstable Fx (B&G III, or posteriomedial comminution) may require a fixation of posteromedial buttress before internal fixation in younger patients; calcar replacing arthroplasty for patients with osteopenia and metastatic disease	Varus deformity (esp. with nonrigid fixation [Ender's nails]); pin migration; nail cutout; loss of fixation (incr. with superolateral screws); joint penetration (screw ideally placed centrally) mortality, infection
Greater trochanter		Separation	>1 cm sep ORIF in younger patient	
Lesser trochanter		Separation	>2 cm sep ORIF in young athlete	
Subtrochanteric		Seinsheimer (I–V) (Fig. 10–57)		Refracture (note assoc. with Zickel nail removal); other complications similar to other hip fractures. No IM device if Fx propagates into piriformis fossa
		I—non/min. displaced	Locked intramedullary nail	
		II—two-part	Locked intramedullary nail	
		III—three-part	Recon nail or condylar plate/screw	
		IV—comminuted	Recon nail or condylar plate/screw	
		V—subtrochanteric-intertrochanteric	Sliding compression hip screw with long side plate (old patient), condylar blade plate (young patient)	
Hip Dislocations				
Hip dislocation		*Ant.* (Epstein) (Fig. 10–58) I—superior A—no Fx B—head Fx C—acetabular Fx II—inferior A—no Fx B—head Fx C—Acetabular Fx	In general, treatment of ant. hip dislocations includes closed reduction, with open reduction if needed (irreducible or interspersed fragments, or with instability [unstable exam/ <⅓ post. rim intact]) and ORIF of fractures or prosthetic replacement as indicated	Associated with increased energy trauma and often associated with other injuries; femoral A/N injuries (ant. dislocation), sciatic N (peroneal division) injuries; osteonecrosis (esp. with post. dislocation in elderly patients, delayed reduction; can present up to 5 yr after injury); posttraumatic DJD (esp. with retained fragments [CT required with type I dislocation to rule out fragments); instability (with 30–40% of post. wall Fxs); incr. complications w/instability after closed reduction
		Post. (Thompson and Epstein) (Fig. 10–59)		Unrecognized femoral neck Fx, AVN, instability, nonunion, malunion, posttraumatic DJD
		I—no/min. Fx	Closed reduction, abduction pillow or Pouch's Fx	
		II—post. acetabular rim III—comminuted rim IV—acetabular floor V—Femoral head Fx Pipkin subdivided these into	Closed reduction, open if necessary, ORIF if possible	
		I—head caudad	Closed reduction, excise loose frag., ORIF if large displ.	
		II—head cephalad	Closed reduction, excise loose frag. if large displ.	
		III—femoral head and neck Fx	ORIF (young pt) hemiarthroplasty/THA (older pt)	
		IV—associated acetabular Fx	ORIF (incongruous joint in young pt), THA (incongruous joint in older pt)	

Table continued on page 386

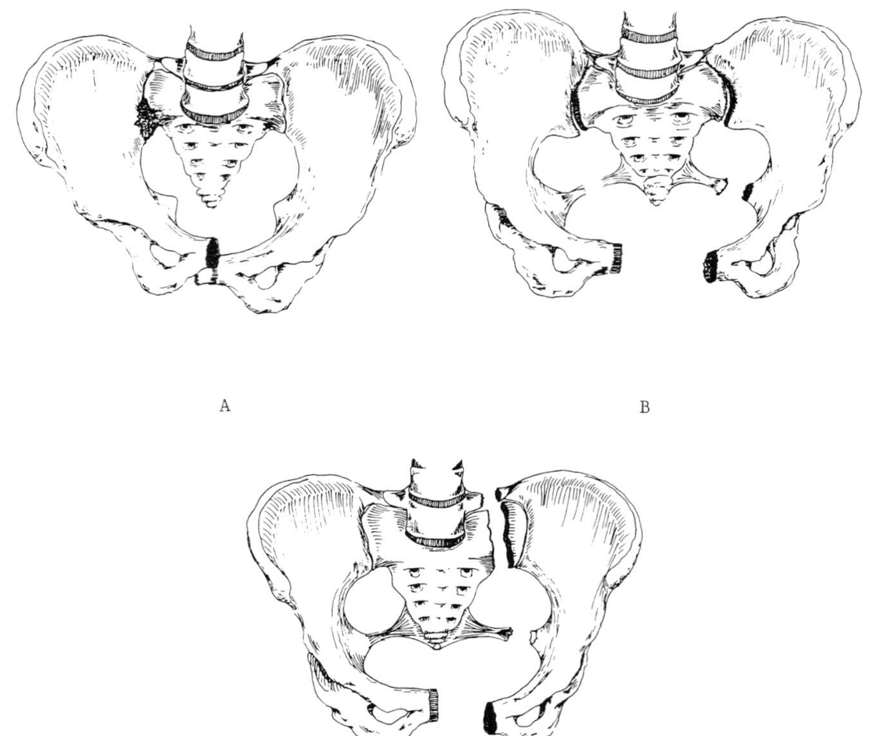

FIGURE 10–53. Young classification of pelvic fractures. *A,* Lateral compression. *B,* Anteroposterior compression. *C,* Vertical shear. (From Kozin, S.H., and Berlet, A.C.: Handbook of Common Orthopaedic Fractures, pp. 79, 83. West Chester, PA, Medical Surveillance, 1989; reprinted by permission.)

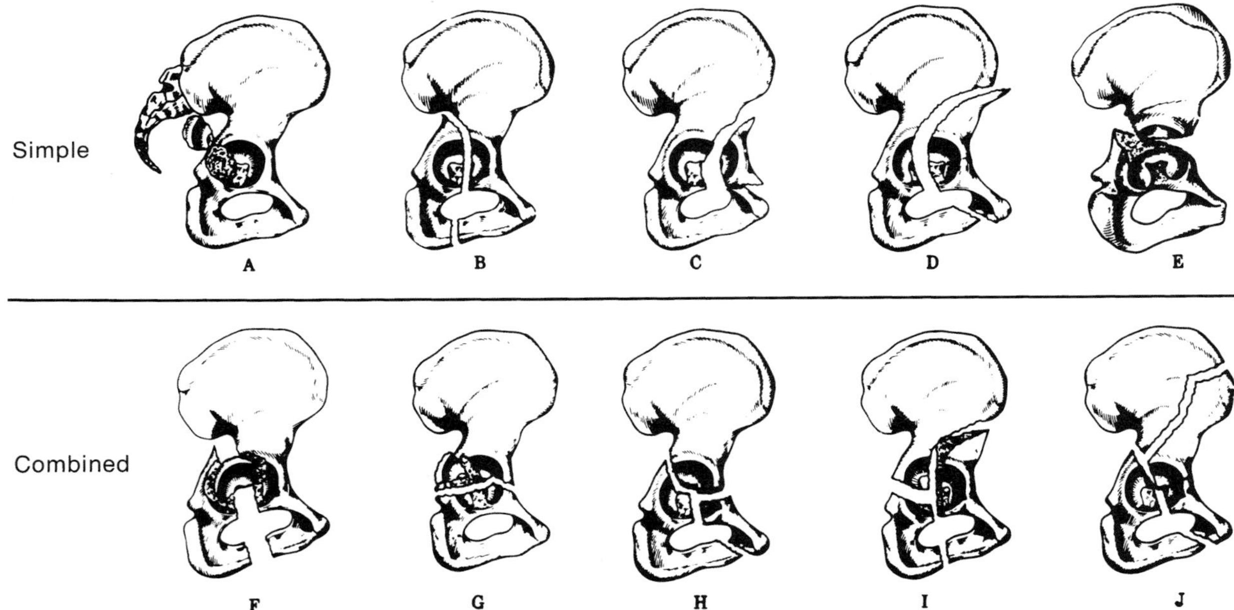

FIGURE 10–54. Letournel classification of acetabular fractures. *A,* Posterior wall. *B,* Posterior column. *C,* Anterior wall. *D,* Anterior column. *E,* Transverse. *F,* Posterior column and posterior wall. *G,* Transverse and posterior wall. *H,* T Fracture. *I,* Anterior column and posterior hemitransverse. *J,* Both columns. (From Matta, J.M.: Trauma: Pelvis and acetabulum. In Orthopaedic Knowledge Update II, p. 348. Chicago, American Academy of Orthopaedic Surgeons, 1987; reprinted by permission.)

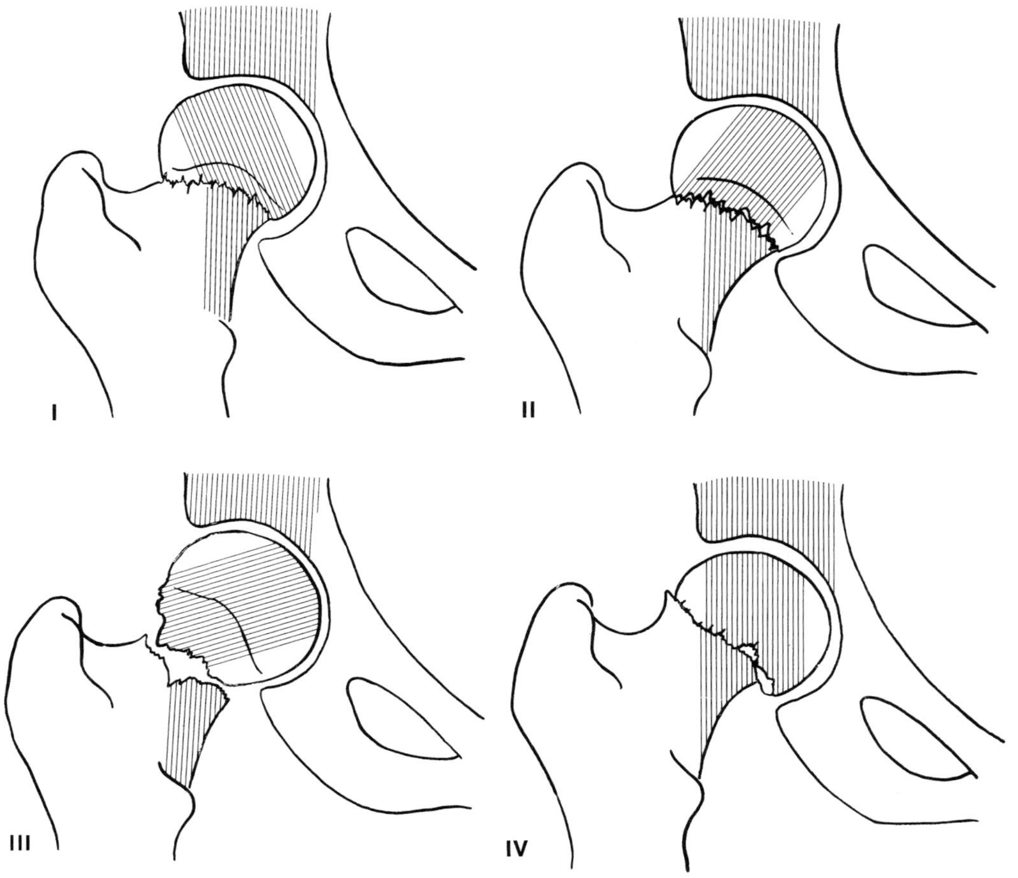

FIGURE 10–55. Garden classification of hip fractures. (From Wiessman, B.N., and Sledge, C.B.: Orthopedic Radiology, p. 408. Philadelphia, WB Saunders, 1986; reprinted by permission.)

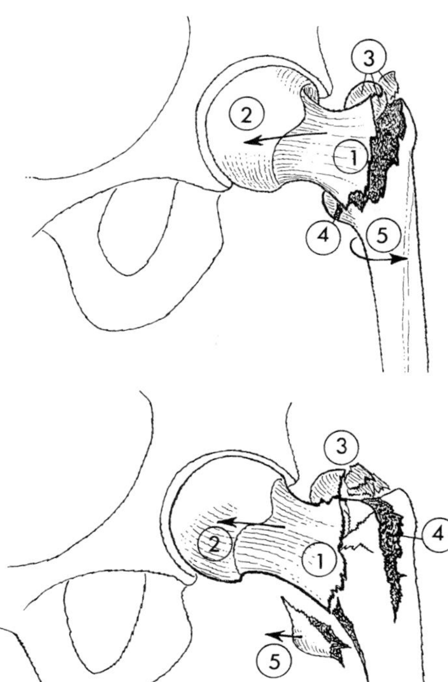

FIGURE 10–56. Intertrochanteric hip fracture classification. *Top,* Stable. *Bottom,* Unstable. (From Connolly, J.F., ed.: Depalma's The Management of Fractures and Dislocations, an Atlas, 3rd ed., p. 1372. Philadelphia, WB Saunders, 1981; reprinted by permission.)

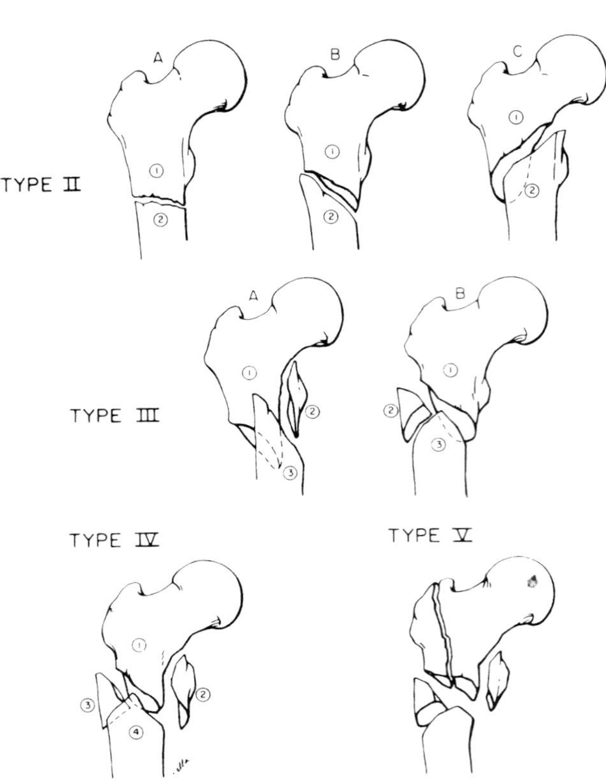

FIGURE 10–57. Classification of subtrochanteric femur fractures. (From Seinsheimer, F., III: Subtrochanteric fractures of the femur. J. Bone Joint Surg. [Am.] 60:302, 1978; reprinted by permission.)

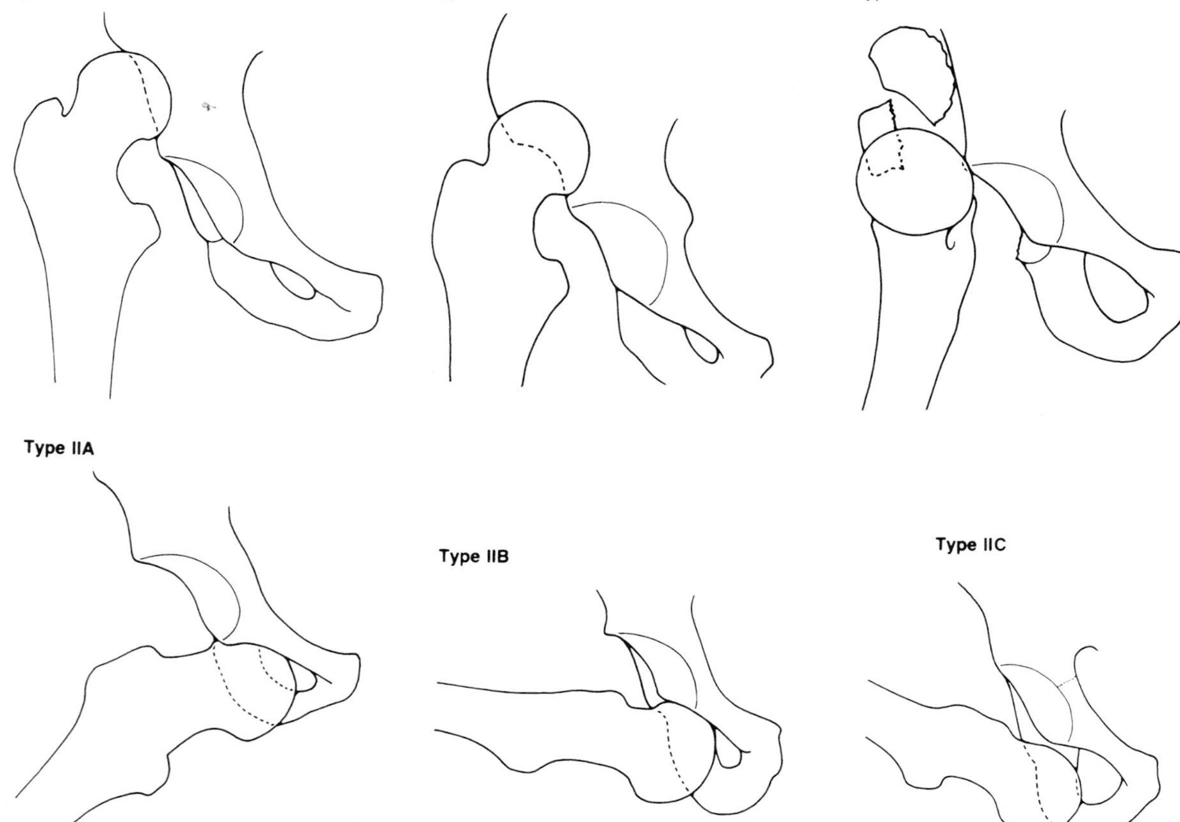

FIGURE 10–58. Classification of anterior dislocations of the femoral head. Type I: superior; type II: inferior; A: no fracture; B: femoral head fracture; C: acetabular fracture. (From DeLee, J.C.: Dislocations and fracture-dislocations of the hip. In Fractures in Adults, Rockwood, C.A., and Green, D.P., eds., 2nd ed., pp. 1288–1292. Philadelphia, JB Lippincott, 1984; reprinted by permission.)

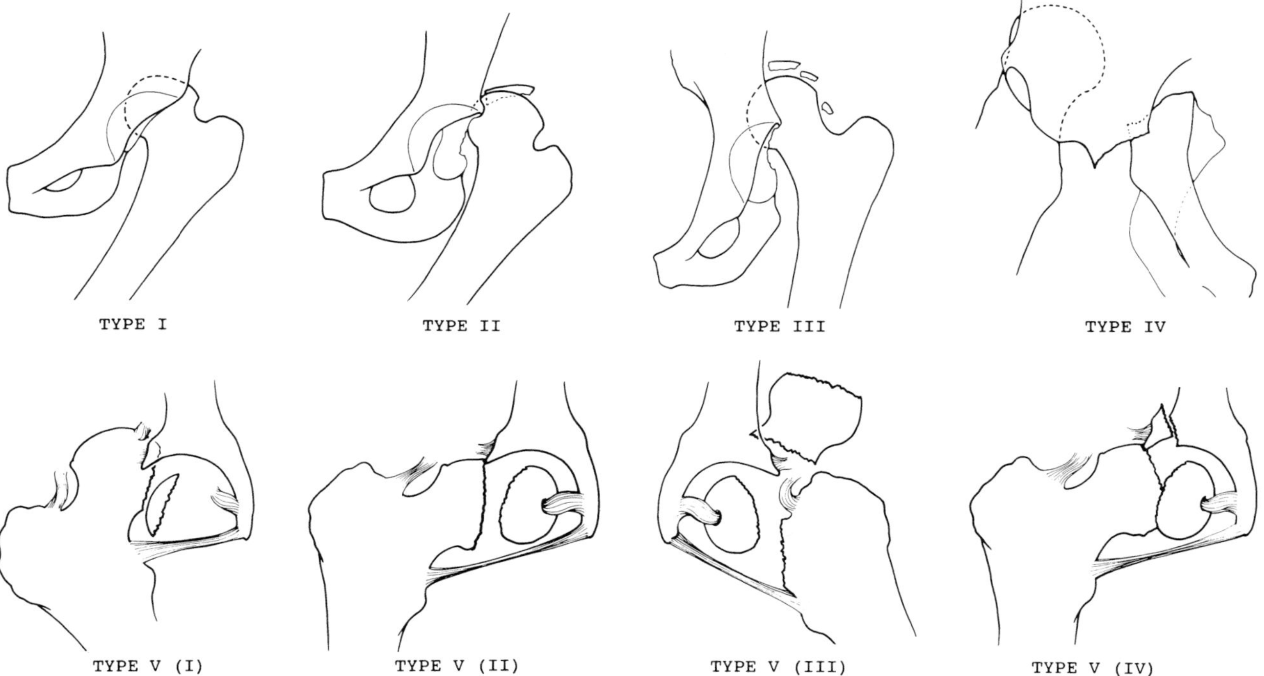

FIGURE 10–59. Posterior dislocation of the femoral head—Thomas and Epstein classification. *I,* No fracture. *II,* Posterior acetabular fracture. *III,* Comminuted rim fracture. *IV,* Acetabular floor fracture. *V,* Femoral head fracture. (From DeLee, J.C.: Dislocations and fracture-dislocations of the hip. In Fractures in Adults, Rockwood, C.A., and Green, D.P., eds., 2nd ed., pp. 1293–1297. Philadelphia, JB Lippincott, 1984; reprinted by permission.)

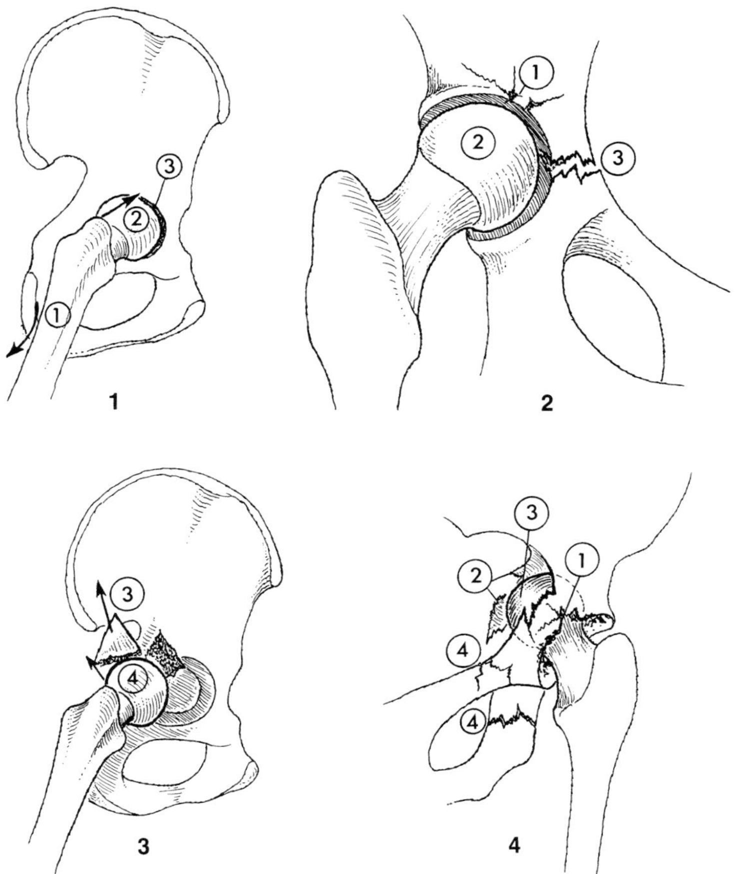

FIGURE 10–60. Central hip dislocations—Rowe and Lowell classification. *1,* Undisplaced. *2,* Inner wall. *3,* Superior dome. *4,* Bursting. (From Connolly, J.F., ed.: Depalma's The Management of Fractures and Dislocations, an Atlas, 3rd ed., p. 1348, 1349. Philadelphia, WB Saunders, 1981; reprinted by permission.)

TABLE 10–5. *Continued*

INJURY	EPONYM	CLASSIFICATION	TREATMENT	COMPLICATIONS
		Central (Rowe and Lowell) (Fig. 10–60)		
Hip Dislocations ***cont.***		1—Undisplaced	Bed rest → crutches (non-weight-bearing)	
		2—Inner wall	Bed rest ± traction, early ROM	
		A—Femoral head beneath dome		
		B—Not beneath dome	Closed reduction + traction	
		3—Superior dome		
		A—Congruent	Skeletal traction, early ROM	
		B—Incongruent	ORIF if large piece	
		4—Bursting		
		A—Congruent	Skeletal traction; ORIF if irreducible (or late THA)	
		B—Incongruent		
Femoral Shaft Fractures				
Femur (2.0 cm below lesser trochanter → 8 cm from joint)		Winquist and Hansen (Fig. 10–61) I—transverse/<25% butterfly II—transverse 25–50% butterfly III—>50% comminution—unstable IV—extensive comminution no cortical contact—unstable V—segmental bone loss—unstable	Most Fxs are treated initially with traction followed by closed IM rodding; interlocking rods favored for comminuted and prox. and distal Fxs: dynamization usu. not indicated; I&D with immediate fixation grade I/II/IIIA open Fxs, I&D with external fixation or delayed internal fixation for grade IIIB/IIIC open Fxs	Nonunion (remove rod over ream and replace with larger rod), infection (early: I&D, late: remove and re-ream IM nail), missed knee ligament injury, other Fxs, neurovascular injury (peroneal N neurapraxia, femoral A), malunion (shortening and rotatory malalignment), knee stiffness (esp. with distal external fixation), refracture, failure of fixation
Femoral neck and shafts		Garden/Winquist (2.5–5.0% of femoral shaft fractures)	Treat neck Fx first, then the shaft (screws in neck and IM rod or plate for femur Fx)	Infection, delayed union, plate failure
Femoral and tibial shafts	"Floating knee"		IM rod femur, IM rod tibia or ex. fix. tibia	Multiple other injuries, fat emboli syndrome
Knee Fractures and Dislocations				
Supracondylar		AO (Fig. 10–62)		
		A—extra-articular	>8 cm above joint antegrade IM locking nail, <8 cm condylar blade plate/screw or retrograde nail	Knee stiffness, DJD, nonunion, popliteal A injury (arteriogram required), varus angulation with buttress plate, malunion, unstable fixation, DVT, Beware missed coronal plate ("Hoffa") fracture fragments
		B—unicondylar	ORIF condylar blade plate/screw	
		C—bicondylar	Condylar blade plate/screw; buttress plate for comminuted Fx	
Patella (Fig. 10–63)		Undisplaced, transverse, lower pole, upper pole, comminuted, vertical	Undisplaced—cylinder cast ORIF if cannot actively extend knee or >2 mm separation, or incongruent articular surface (tension band); excise fragments that are extremely comminuted	Separation of fragments-quad weakness, infection, AVN, DJD
Tibial plateau		Hohl's revised classification (Fig. 10–64). Minimally displaced (<4 mm dep/displacement)	Stable (<5° V/V instability)—closed treatment; unstable (>5° V/V instability)—closed reduction ± PC screw fixation	DJD, stiffness, loss of reduction, AVN, infection, medial plateau fractures almost always require ORIF
		Displaced (>4 mm dep/displacement):		
		*Local compression	Closed treatment if <6 mm displaced, arthroscopic assisted reduction/fixation if 6–12 mm displaced, ORIF >12 mm displaced	
		Split compression	ORIF with buttress plate (arthroscopic assisted if ≤10 mm)	
		Total depression	CRIF + PC screws or ORIF if >5 mm displaced	

Table continued on opposite page

TABLE 10–5. *Continued*

INJURY	EPONYM	CLASSIFICATION	TREATMENT	COMPLICATIONS
		Split	Closed treatment if stable, min. fixation/collateral ligament repair if unstable	
		Rim	Elevation and fixation with collateral ligament repair	
		Bicondylar	Skeletal traction ± PC screw fixation; rarely ORIF → cast brace	
Tibial spine (Fig. 10–65)		I—anterior tilt II—complete anterior tilt III—no contact A—no rotation B—rotated	I/II/IIIA closed reduction LLC 6 wk if knee can be brought into full extension; IIIB and all irreducible types require open reduction	Block to motion (arthroscopic loose body removal), ACL laxity
Tibial tubercle			ORIF with screw or staple	Loss of fixation, quad weakness
Subcondylar tibia		Stable Displaced	Cast immobilization ORIF with buttress plate	Arterial injury, decreased ROM
Proximal fibula			Open if unstable (peroneal N, biceps)	
Quadriceps rupture			Repair acutely, cylinder cast	
Patella tendon rupture			Repair with tension-reducing device	Missed Dx (high riding patella seen on radiographs)
Patella dislocation		Acute, recurrent, subluxation, habitual	Cylinder cast and quadriceps strengthening if congruent; arthroscopy for displaced or osteochondral Fxs; recurrent—lat. rel, med. plication, bony transplant if abnormal Q angle. Avoid surgery in habitual dislocators.	Recurrence
Knee dislocation (Fig. 10–66)		*Ant., post., lat., med., rotatory (AM, AL, PM, PL)	Reduce emergently, immobilize 6 wk; open reduction if needed (PL rotation); repair vascular injuries; ligament repair secondary	Popliteal A injury (arteriogram mandatory); tibial/peroneal N injuries, ACL tear (most common); post. tibial subluxation
Proximal tibia-fibula dislocation		*Ant. (lat.), post. (med.), sup. (usu. with lat. malleolus injury)	Reduce (90° flexion) ORIF if fails or recurrent	
Chondral/ osteochondral		Endogenous vs. exogenous	Arthroscopic evaluation of locked, acute condylar defects and remove small fragments (pin large fragments)	DJD
TIBIA-FIBULA FRACTURES				
Tibia (Fig. 10–67)		Chapman A—Transverse/short/ oblique—closed reduction LLC B—Small butterfly—closed reduction LLC C—Large butterfly—IM fixation (if <50 cortical contact) D—Semental—IM fixation E—Spiral—closed reduction LLC F—Proximal ¼—closed treatment, ORIF if unstable G—Distal ¼—closed treatment, ORIF if unstable	Most respond to closed traction LLC, wedge as needed, PTB at 6–8 wk; IM nail for transverse oblique Fx of mid ⅓ or segmental; IM nail also vascular injury, bilateral injury, pathologic Fxs, severe knee ligamentous injuries; unreamed nail acutely. Open Fxs: Unreamed nail up to and incl. some IIIB injuries, early flap coverage, delayed bone grafting. Consider early amputation in grade IIIC injuries, posterior tibial nerve injury, warm ischemia time >6 hr, severe ipsilateral foot injury; etc. vs. ex. fix	Delayed union (>20 wk; incr. with greater initial displacement and middle third Fxs; treatment includes fibulectomy and P/L bone graft), nonunion (P/L bone graft or reamed IM nail), infection (flap/graft or amputation), malunion (V/V, shortening [accept <5° V/V, <10° AP angulation]), vascular injuries (upper ¼—ant. tibial A), compartment syndrome, peroneal N injury, RSD
Tibia stress		Upper ⅓ (recruits)	Modify activity 6–10 wk	Progression to complete Fx

Table continued on page 390

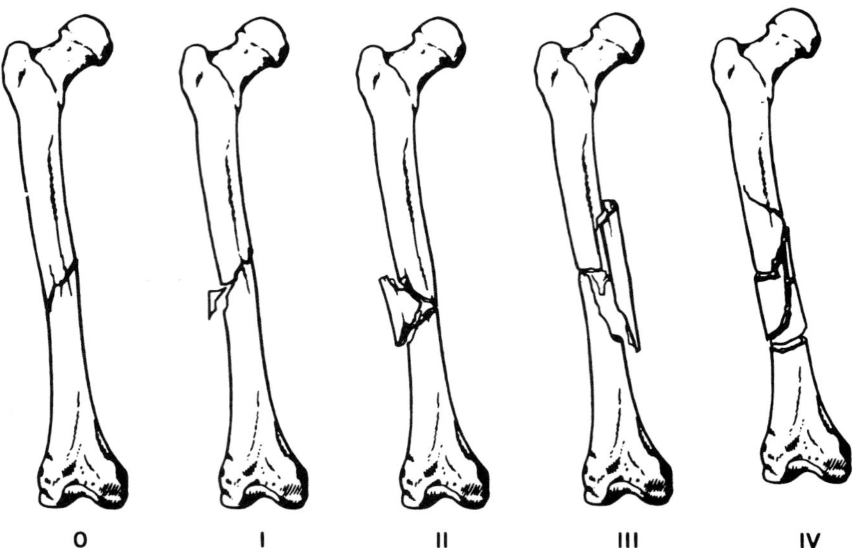

FIGURE 10–61. Winquist and Hanson classification of femoral shaft fractures. (*Note:* Type V [not shown] has segmental bone loss.) (From Johnson, K.D.: Femur: Trauma. In Orthopaedic Knowledge Update III, p. 514. Chicago, American Academy of Orthopaedic Surgeons, 1990; reprinted by permission.)

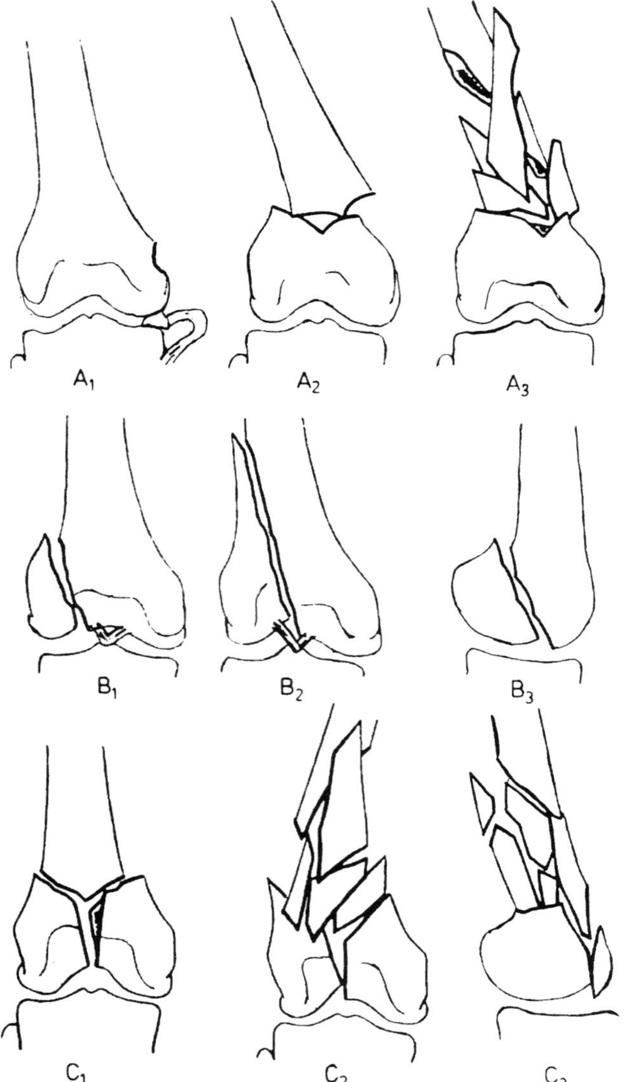

FIGURE 10–62. AO/ASIF classification of supracondylar fractures. *A,* Extra-articular. *B,* Unicondylar. *C,* Bicondylar. (From Johnson, K.D.: Femur: Trauma. In Orthopaedic Knowledge Update III, p. 521. Chicago, American Academy of Orthopaedic Surgeons, 1990; reprinted by permission.)

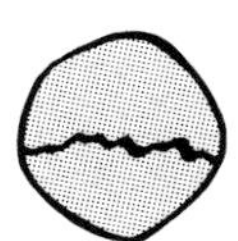

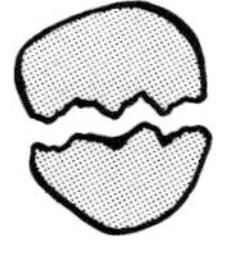

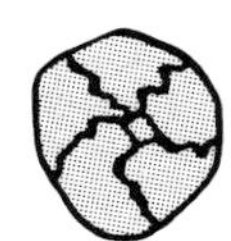

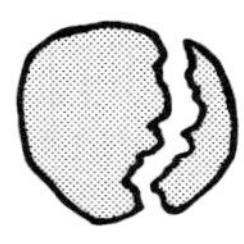

FIGURE 10–63. Types of patellar fractures. (From Wiessman, B.N.W., and Sledge, C.B.: Orthopedic Radiology, p. 553. Philadelphia, WB Saunders, 1986; reprinted by permission.)

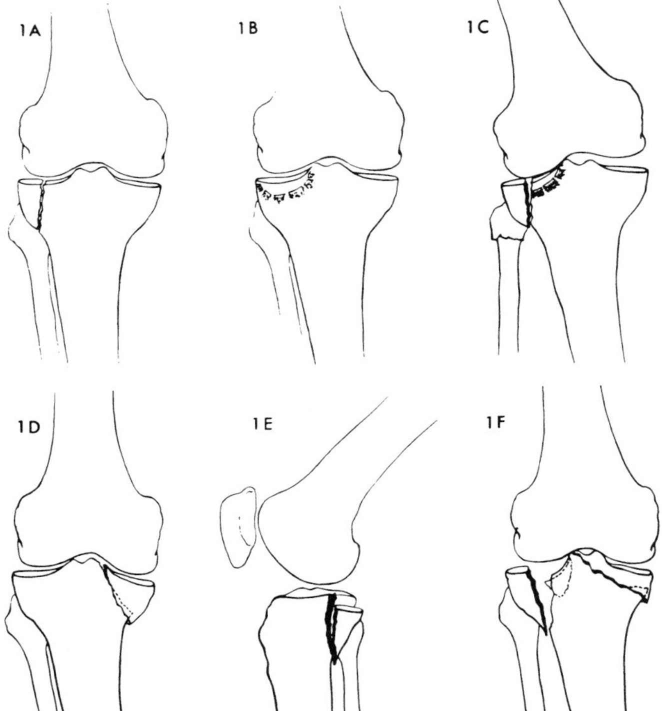

FIGURE 10–64. Classification of tibial plateau fractures. *1A,* Minimally displaced. *1B,* Local compression. *1C,* Split compression. *1D,* Total depression. *1E,* Split. *1F,* Bicondylar. (From Hohl, M.: Tibial condylar fractures. J. Bone Joint Surg. [Am.] 49:1455, 1967; reprinted by permission.)

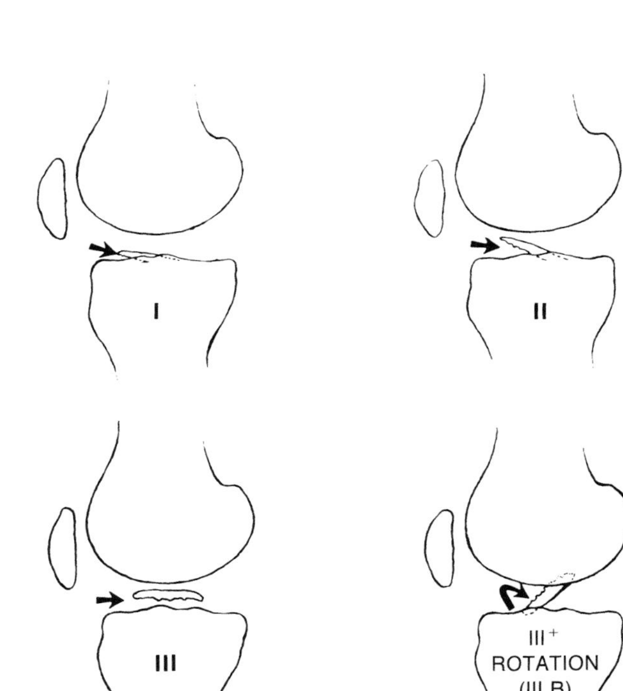

FIGURE 10–65. Classification of tibial spine fractures. (From Myers, M.H., and McKeever, F.M.: Fractures of the intercondylar eminence of the tibia. J. Bone Joint Surg. [Am.] 52:1677, 1974; reprinted by permission.)

TABLE 10–5. *Continued*

INJURY	EPONYM	CLASSIFICATION	TREATMENT	COMPLICATIONS
Fibula shaft		Mid-lower ⅓ (athletes)	Cast only if needed for pain relief	
Tibial plafond	Pilon (Fig. 10–68)	Ruedi and Allgower I—minimally displaced II—incongruous III—comminuted	LLC and non-weight-bearing ORIF if displaced and ankle involved; consider minimally invasive small pin ex. fix. techniques	DJD (may require late fusion), infection, V/V angulation, skin slough
ANKLE FRACTURES AND DISLOCATIONS				
Ankle fracture (Figs. 10–69, 10–70)		Lauge-Hansen (position of foot—direction of force) S-Add: 1—LM transverse (or LCL) 2—MM Fx S-ER: 1—AITFL 2—LM spiral Fx 3—PM Fx or PITFL injury 4—MM Fx/deltoid P-Abd: 1—MM Fx/deltoid 2—A&P ITFL/PM 3—LM oblique supramalleolar P-ER: 1—MM Fx/deltoid 2—AITFL/IOL 3—High fibular 4—PM Fx	Treatment of ankle Fx based on position of mortise (nondisplaced fractures can be treated in a LLC >1 mm displacement after reduction requires ORIF; syndesmosis screw if interosseous ligament/ membrane is disrupted); usually not necessary to reduce posteromedial fragment (not in weight-bearing area unless >⅓); use of an antiglide plate posterolaterally on the fibula is helpful with oblique Fxs; for open Fxs irrigation and débridement with stable fixation (internal) early soft tissue coverage	Nonunion, malunion, infection (esp. with ORIF and may present with symmetric tibiotalar joint space narrowing), DJD, vascular injury, RSD 1 mm of lat. talar displacement from the med. malleolus is associated with 42% decr. in tibiotalar articulation (Ramsey)
		Danis Weber (AO) (position of fibular Fx) A—at or below joint B—obliquely up from joint C—high fibular fx	In general, treatment of AO type A fractures is closed and treatment of AO types B and C is with ORIF. Assess syndesmosis stability.	
FOOT FRACTURES AND DISLOCATIONS				
Stress	March	*2MT and calcaneus	Symptomatic, SLWC if late	
Talar neck	Aviator's astragalus	Hawkins and Canale (Fig. 10–71) I—nondisplaced vertical II—displaced and subtalar dislocation/subluxation III—displaced and talar body dislocation IV—with talar head dislocation	SLC 8–12 wk (NWB 4–6 wk) watch closely! ORIF—anatomic reduction required ORIF required	AVN (esp. types III/IV [Hawkin's sign indicates a good prognosis]; weight-bearing is important in treating this complication), delayed/ nonunion, malunion, DJD, skin necrosis
Talar body		Rare	Usu. requires ORIF	AVN, malunion, DJD
Talar head		Rare	Nondisplaced—splint/ice/ elevation Displaced—ORIF or excision of comminuted fragments	Talonavicular DJD
Talar process		Lateral process	SLC × 6 wk, excise if comminuted ORIF if large and displaced	Med. malleolus fracture (26%), rule out os trigonum (50%)
	Shepherd's	Posterior process	SLC × 6 wk, excise nonunions	
Subtalar dislocation	Basketball foot	*Calcaneus medial displacement	Reduce, immobilization 4 wk, open reduction if irreducible	Posterior tibialis tendon entrapment
Total talar dislocation		Subtalar + Chopart injury	Open reduction, late fusion	AVN
*Calcaneus		Extra-articular (ant. process, tuberosity, med. process, sustentaculum talus, *body). *Intra-articular (nondisplaced, tongue, joint depression comminuted) (Fig. 10–72) (Bohler angle and Gissane angle)	Principles of treatment: CT scan helpful, reduce joint incongruity, ORIF younger active patients if possible (lateral approach); bone graft defects; late excision of symptomatic anterior process fractures; extraarticular—SLC, ORIF if displaced	Chronic pain (heel widening, nerve entrapment), peroneal tendonitis, DJD, malunion, associated Fxs (spine, LE), heel skin slough, compartment syndrome
Midtarsal injury		*Med. stress, longitudinal stress, lat. stress, plantar stress, crush	Prompt reconstruction of anatomy, ORIF often	

Table continued on opposite page

TABLE 10–5. *Continued*

INJURY	EPONYM	CLASSIFICATION	TREATMENT	COMPLICATIONS
Navicular		Cortical avulsion	Reduce, pin large fragments (>25%)	Osteonecrosis (ORIF nonunion), associated with midfoot fractures
		Tuberosity Fx (PT avulsion)	ORIF with screw and washer	
		Body Fx	ORIF if displaced	
		Stress FX	NWB cast 6–8 wk	
Cuboid	Nutcracker	Compressed calcaneus & MT	ORIF with bone graft or ex. fix. to ↑ lat. column and bone graft	
TMT Fx-dislocation	Lisfranc (Fig. 10–73)	Homolateral. (all 5 same direction), isolated (1 or 2MT displaced), divergent (displacement in sagittal and coronal planes)	Closed reduction ± PCP required; open reduction if severe displacement, or foreign body entrapment; ORIF of MT-tarsal disruptions with screws is successful	Chronic pain (arthrodesis preferred); delay in Dx (make sure medial border of 2MT base aligns with medial border of middle cuneiform), compartment syndrome
Metatarsal		Shaft	Reduce, pin if needed, SLWC 4 wk	Posttraumatic DJD
		Head	Reduce (traction and manipulation), cast	
	Pseudo-Jones (Fig. 10–74)	Base avulsion (5MT)	2–3 wk SLWC, late removal of fragments if needed	
	Jones (Fig. 10–74)	5MT metaphyseal base transverse Fx	4–6 wks NWB SLC, late ORIF if required	Nonunion (screw/bone graft) Differentiate from metadiaphyseal stress Fx
MTP dislocation			Reduce promptly, immobilize (consider PCP)	
Digits			ORIF displaced intra-articular Fx	

* Most common.
I/L, ipsilateral; C/L, contralateral; CRIF, closed reduction internal fixation; ORIF, open reduction internal fixation; PC, percutaneous; PCP, percutaneous pin; V/V, varus/valgus; SLC, short leg cast; SLWC, short leg walking cast; NWB, non-weight-bearing; MT, metatarsal; TMT, tarsometatarsal; MTP, metatarsal phalangeal; THA, total hip arthroplasty.

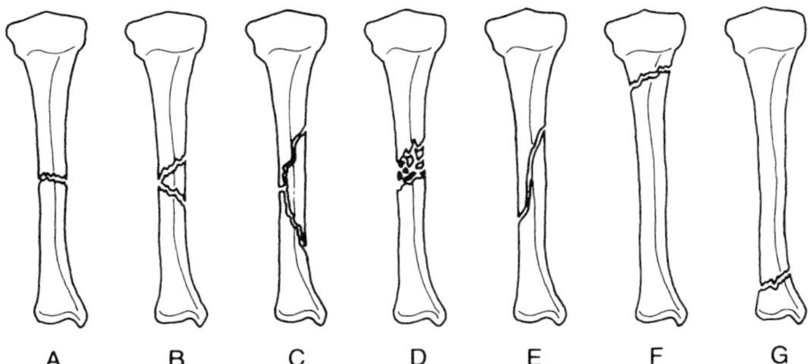

FIGURE 10–67. Classification of tibial fractures. *A,* Transverse/short oblique. *B,* Small butterfly. *C,* Large butterfly. *D,* Segmental. *E,* Spiral. *F,* Proximal. *G,* Distal. (From Chapman, M.W.: Fractures of the tibia and fibula. In Operative Orthopaedics, Chapman, M.W., ed., p. 437. Philadelphia, JB Lippincott, 1988; reprinted by permission.)

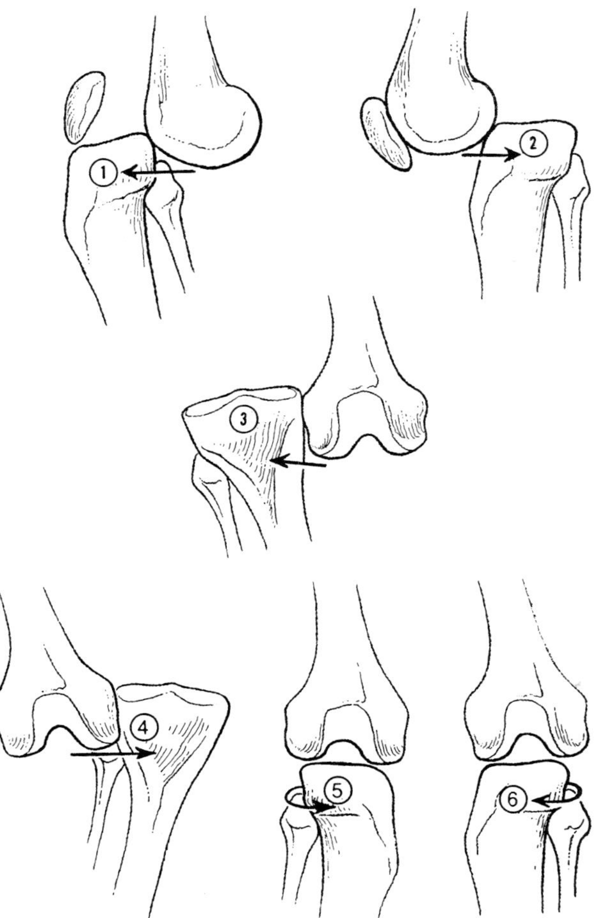

FIGURE 10–66. Dislocations of the knee. *1,* Anterior. *2,* Posterior. *3,* Lateral. *4,* Medial. *5,* Anteromedial. *6,* Anterolateral. (From Connolly, J.F., ed.: Depalma's The Management of Fractures and Dislocations, an Atlas, 3rd ed., p. 1621. Philadelphia, WB Saunders, 1981; reprinted by permission.)

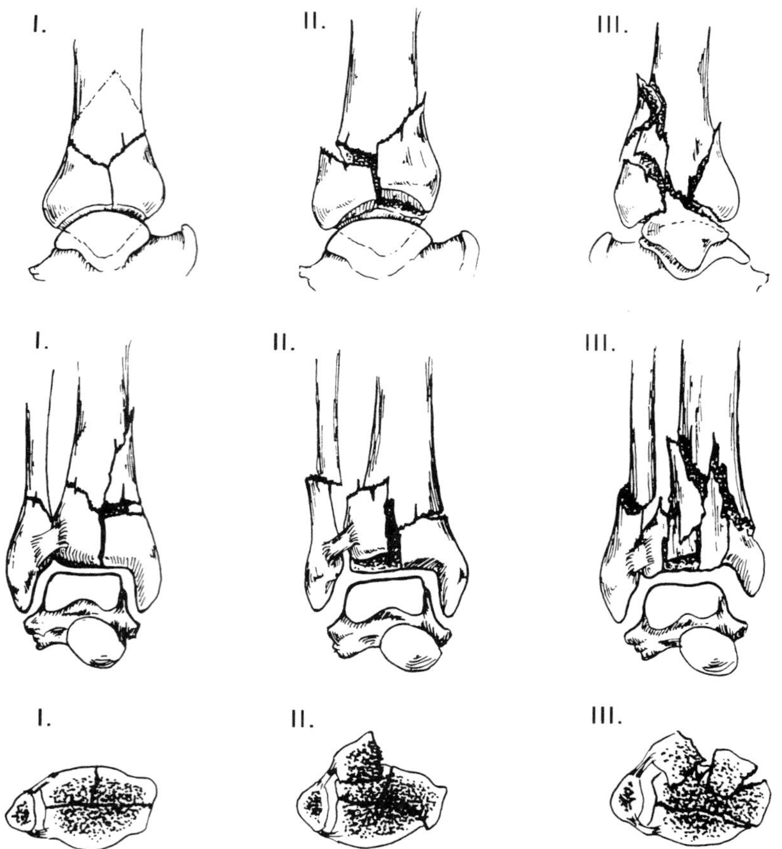

FIGURE 10–68. Tibial pilon fractures. *I,* Minimally displaced. *II,* Incongruous. *III,* Comminuted. (From Kozin, S.H., and Berlet, A.C.: Handbook of Common Orthopaedic Fractures, p. 131. West Chester, PA, Medical Surveillance, 1989; reprinted by permission.)

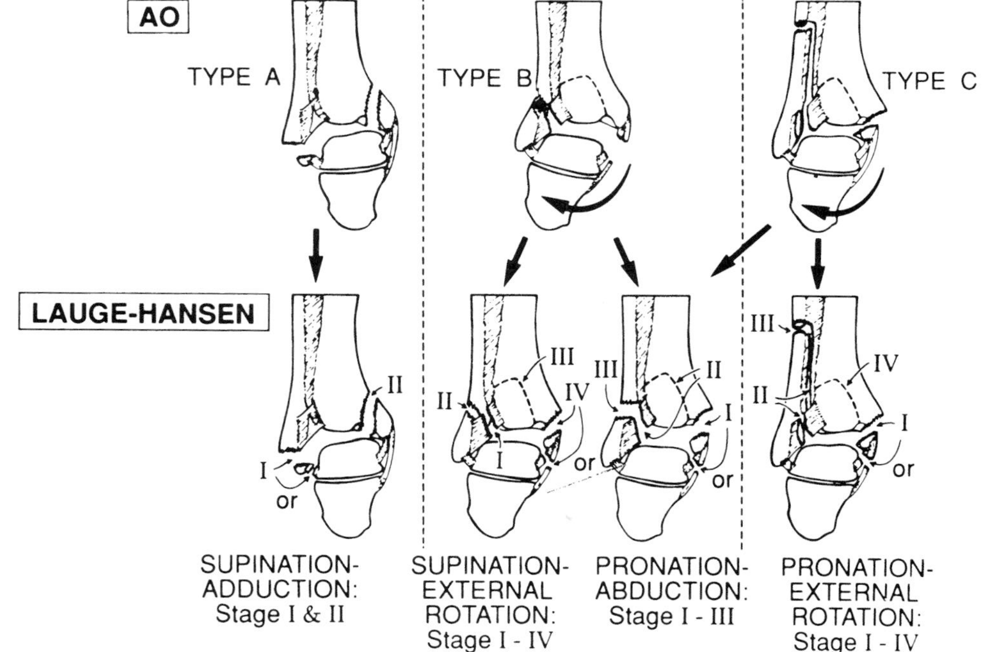

FIGURE 10–69. Classification of ankle fractures—AO (Danis-Weber) and Lauge-Hansen. (From Sangeorzan, B.J., and Hansen, S.T.: Ankle and foot: Trauma. In Orthopaedic Knowledge Update III, p. 615. Chicago, American Academy of Orthopaedic Surgeons, 1990; reprinted by permission.)

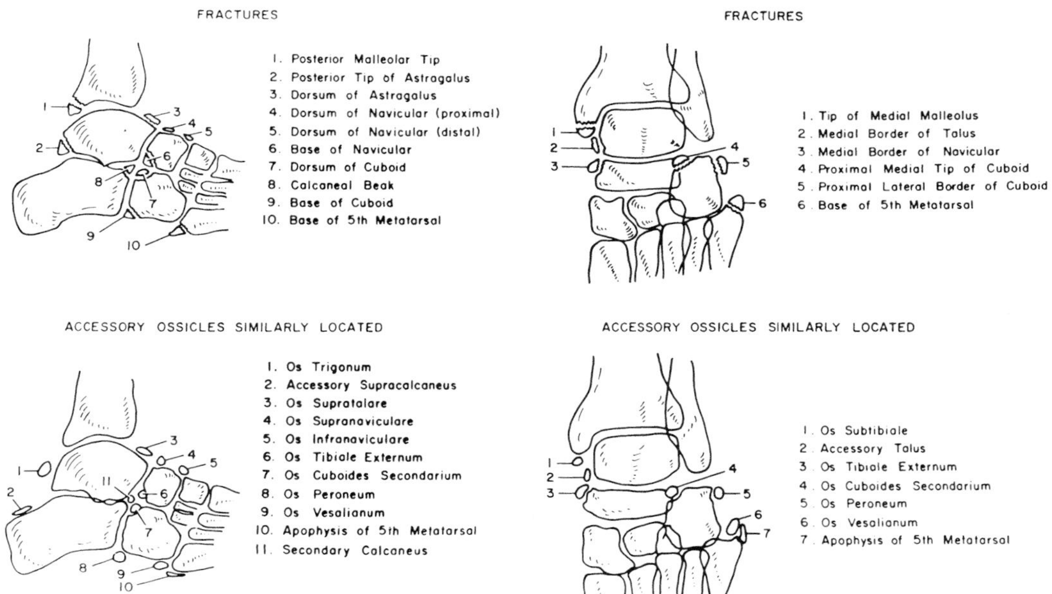

FIGURE 10–70. Avulsion fractures of the ankle. (After Zatkin, H.R.: Semin. Roentgenol. 5:419, 1970. From Jahss, M.H.: Disorders of the Foot, p. 1488. Philadelphia, WB Saunders, 1982; reprinted by permission.)

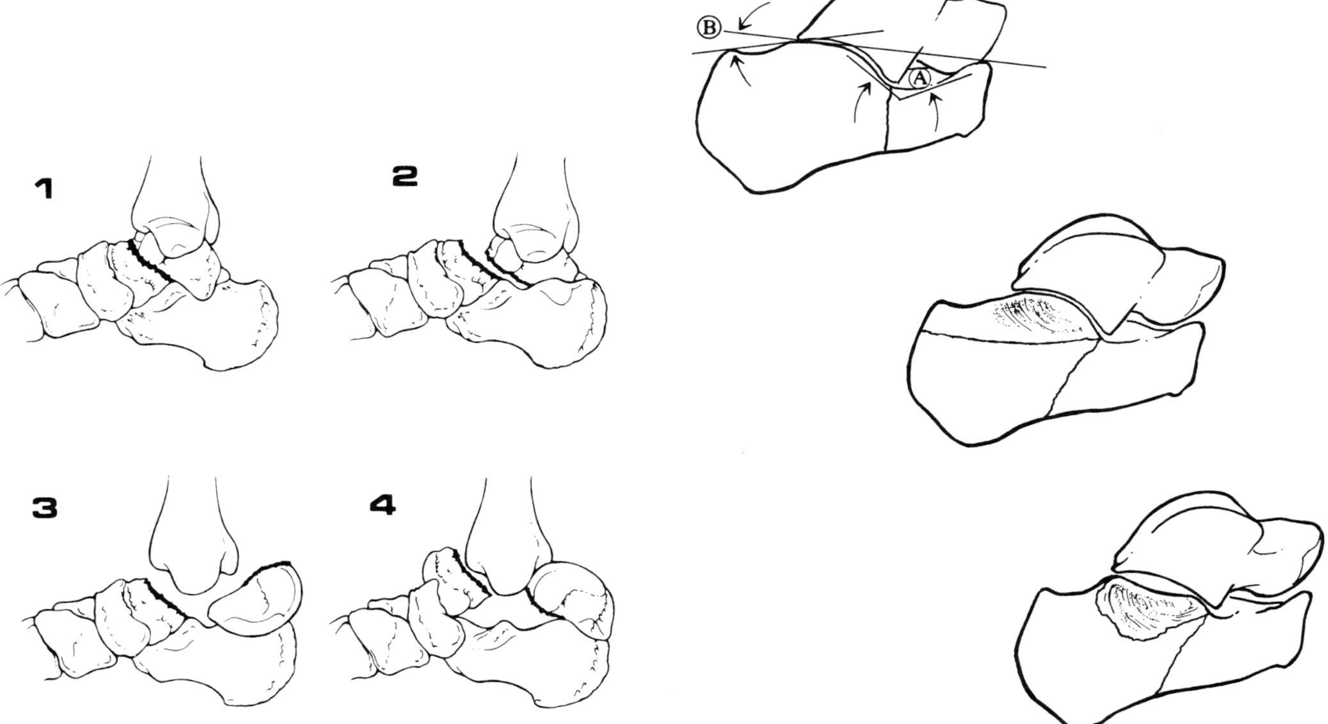

FIGURE 10–71. Hawkins (and Canale) classification of talar neck fractures. *1,* Nondisplaced. *2,* Subtalar dislocation. *3,* Talar body dislocation. *4,* Talar head dislocation. (From Sangeorzan, B.J., and Hansen, S.T.: Ankle and foot: Trauma. In Orthopaedic Knowledge Update III, p. 616. Chicago, American Academy of Orthopaedic Surgeons, 1990; reprinted by permission.)

FIGURE 10–72. Intra-articular calcaneus fractures. *1,* Nondisplaced. *2,* Tongue. *3,* Joint depression. *Note: A,* crucial angle of Gusiane; *B,* Bohler's angle. (From Connolly, J.F., ed.: Depalma's The Management of Fractures and Dislocations, an Atlas, 3rd ed., p. 2013. Philadelphia, WB Saunders, 1981; reprinted by permission.)

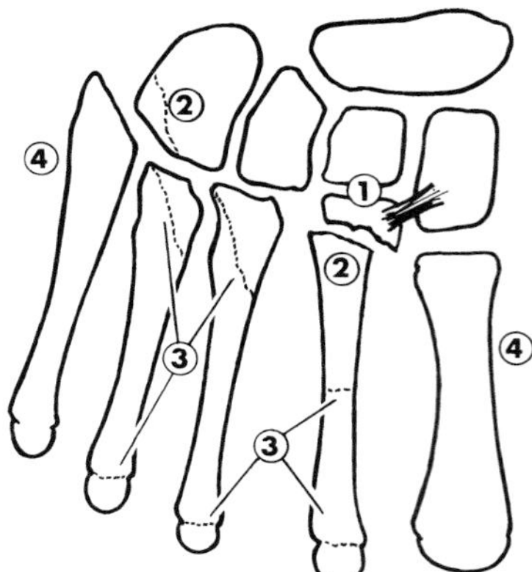

FIGURE 10–73. Lisfranc fractures—usually involve second metatarsal base ± third and fourth metatarsals (rarely involve first or fifth metatarsal). (From Connolly, J.F., ed.: Depalma's The Management of Fractures and Dislocations, an Atlas, 3rd ed., p. 2053. Philadelphia, WB Saunders, 1981; reprinted by permission.)

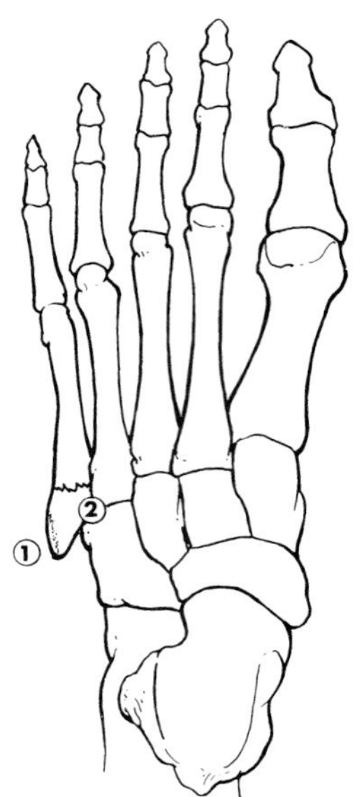

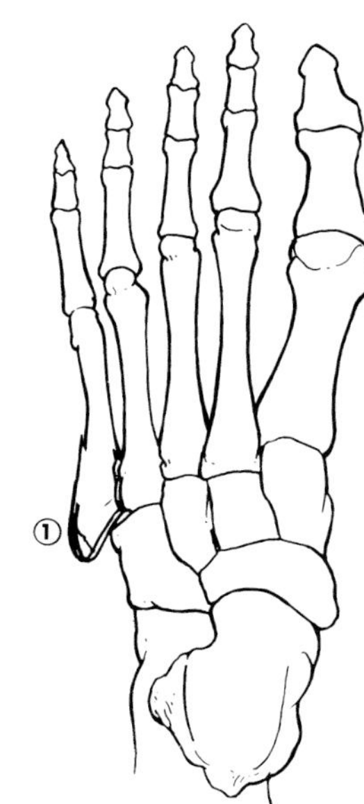

FIGURE 10–74. Jones and "pseudo-Jones" fractures. *Left,* Metaphyseal fracture (true Jones). *Right,* Avulsion fracture (pseudo-Jones). (From Connolly, J.F., ed.: Depalma's The Management of Fractures and Dislocations, an Atlas, 3rd ed., p. 2065, 2066. Philadelphia, WB Saunders, 1981; reprinted by permission.)

SECTION 2

Pediatric Trauma

I. **Introduction**—Because fractures and dislocations in children are often unique, several features of these injuries are not found in adults (see Table 10–6). Children's bones are more ductile than adult bones, and bowing (especially in the fibula and ulna), "greenstick," and "torus" fractures are unique to children. The periosteum in children is much thicker and often remains intact on the concave (compression) side, allowing less displacement and better reduction of fractures. Children's fractures heal much quicker, and less immobilization time is required. Children are also less likely to develop contractures from immobilization, and therefore this complication is less of a concern. However, because bones are actively growing in pediatric patients, malunion and growth plate injuries are an important concern. Remodeling is more thorough, especially in young children, so displacement and angulation that would not be tolerated in an adult are often acceptable in the management of children's fractures (except intra-articular fractures, where the same axioms apply).

II. **Child Abuse—Battered Child Syndrome**

A. Introduction—Unfortunately, child abuse does occur, and one must always be wary of the "battered child," especially when fractures are encountered in the infant. All states now obligate physicians to report suspected child abuse. Suspicions should be raised with fractures in children less than 3 years old with multiple healing bruises, skin marks, burns, unreasonable histories, signs of neglect, and so on.

B. Fracture Locations—The most common locations of fractures in children are the humerus, tibia, and femur, in that order. **Skeletal surveys** are appropriate if a "battered child" is encountered, in children with delayed development, for some metaphyseal and metaphyseal-epiphyseal fractures, and for spiral fractures. Diaphyseal fractures, generally considered less suspicious of child abuse, are in fact four times more common. The skeletal survey consists of skull, T/L-spine AP and lateral views, and AP views of ribs and extremities. Skeletal surveys are rarely helpful in children over the age of 5. Bone scans can identify fractures earlier and can be a helpful adjunct, especially in children less than 2 years old. Other nonorthopaedic injuries commonly encountered with child abuse are head injuries ("shaken baby" leading to avulsion of the cerebral bridging veins), burns, and blunt abdominal visceral injuries.

C. Treatment—In addition to normal fracture care, early involvement of social workers and pediatricians is essential. If child abuse is missed, there is a greater than 33% chance of further abuse, and a 5–10% chance of death among affected children.

III. Physeal Fractures

A. Introduction—The physis, or growth plate, is more susceptible to fracture than is injury to attached ligaments; therefore if there is any question, one must assume that there is an injury of the physis until proved otherwise.

B. Characteristics—Although physeal fractures are classically thought to be through the zone of provisional calcification (within the zone of hypertrophy) of the growth plate, the fracture can involve several of the layers. Failure is usually due to torsion and not tension at the growth plate. There can be significant complications associated with these injuries (e.g., limb length discrepancies, malunion, bony bars). Physeal fractures are most common in the distal radius, followed by the distal tibia.

C. Classification—The Salter-Harris (SH) classification, modified by Rang, is used to classify physeal fractures (Fig. 10–75).

TYPE	DESCRIPTION	CHARACTERISTICS
I	Transverse fractures through physis	Younger children
II	Fractures through physis with metaphyseal fragment	Children >10 years
III	Fractures through physis and epiphysis	Intra-articular
IV	Fractures through epiphysis, physis, and metaphysis	Migration/growth arrest
V	Crush injury of physis	Growth arrest late
VI	Injury to perichondrial ring	Bridging/angular deformity

D. Treatment—A few general guidelines regarding treatment of these fractures is in order. Gentle reduction should be attempted initially for SH I and II fractures, often requiring general anesthesia. With appropriate reduction and immobilization, these fractures usually do well without a significant amount of growth arrest (except in the distal femur, where SH II fractures can result in malalignment and arrest, and proximal tibia fractures, which can develop a valgus deformity). SH III and IV injuries are intra-articular and usually require open reduction to correctly align the growth plate. Fixation, if used, should not cross the physis if possible. SH V and VI fractures are usually not identified early and have a high complication rate. The cartilaginous growth plate usually heals in about half the time required for the adjacent bone to heal. Follow-up radiographs are required for all physeal fractures. Minor injuries can often be appreciated on late radiographs by the presence of transversely oriented Harris-Park growth arrest lines. With severe injuries where limb salvage is not possible, disarticulation is favored over amputation in children in order to retain the growth plate and to minimize stump complications.

E. Partial Growth Arrest—Physeal bars or bridges result from growth plate injuries that arrest growth of part of the physis, and the uninjured portion of the physis continues to grow normally. Three types of physeal arrest have been characterized (Bright).

TYPE	LOCATION	COMMON ETIOLOGY
I	Peripheral	SH II fractures
II	Central	Infection
III	Combined	SH IV fractures

Physeal bridge resection with interposition of fat graft or other materials such as Silastic and Cranioplast (which must be removed at maturity) is reserved for patients with >2 cm of growth remaining and <50% physeal involvement. Smaller, peripheral bars in young patients do the best, and the procedure is contraindicated in the presence of active infection (resection should be delayed 6–12 months following infection) or inadequate skin coverage. Hypocycloidal tomograms or CT is useful when planning the resection, and intact physeal cartilage must be preserved. Arrest involving >50% of the physis should be treated with ipsilateral completion of the arrest and contralateral epiphysiodesis, or ipsilateral limb lengthening.

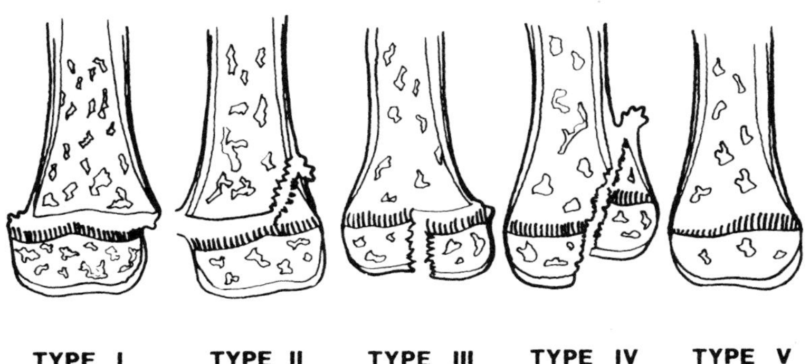

FIGURE 10–75. Salter-Harris classification of injuries to the physis. (From Bora, F.W.: The Pediatric Upper Extremity, p. 154. Philadelphia, WB Saunders, 1986; reprinted by permission.)

TABLE 10–6. PEDIATRIC TRAUMATIC ORTHOPAEDIC INJURIES

INJURY	EPONYM	CLASSIFICATION	TREATMENT	COMPLICATIONS
WRIST AND HAND FRACTURES				
Phalanx fractures (Figs. 10–76 and 10–77)		Based on phalanx and SH classification (Fig. 10–75)	Closed reduction for most, PCP if unstable; condylar and SH III/IV Fxs may require ORIF	Residual deformities, tendon imbalance, nail deformities
MC fractures		Based on location	Reduce, ORIF if unreducible	
Thumb MC Fxs (Fig. 10–78)		A—metaphyseal	Closed reduction	
		B—SH II (medial)	Closed reduction	
		C—SH II (lateral)	Closed reduction	
	Bennett equivalent	D—SH III	ORIF	
IP dislocation			Closed reduction and splint; open if irreducible, incongruous on x-ray, or redisplaces with ROM	
*MCP dislocation			Attempt closed reduction, open if irreducible	
CMC dislocation			Reduce with finger traps, PCP K-wire to carpus and adjacent MC	
Distal radius (Fig. 10–79)	SH fractures	I–V	PCP types III and IV (transepiphyseal)	Deformity, loss of reduction, infection (open fracture), Volkmann's contracture, growth arrest, malunion, refracture. <11 years old can remodel up to 28° amplitude; >11 only 18° can be expected.
	Torus	Tension side intact	SAC for 3 wk	
	Greenstick	Tension side plastic deformation	Reduce if angulation >10°, LAC in supination	
	Complete	Both cortices disrupted	Reduce and place in LAC in supination	
RADIAL AND ULNAR SHAFTS				
Radius and ulna	Both bone	Greenstick (incomplete) Compression (buckle or torus) Complete	Correct rotation with pronation/supination, and with pressure with <10° angulation: SAC 3–4 wk in <10 yo (even with bayonet opposition); match rotation of distal fragment with proximal (bicep tuberosity [points opposite of thumb]) ORIF if >12 y/o and if cannot achieve <15°, angular deform., and <5° malrotation	Refracture, limb ischemia, malunion (esp. in <10 yo with inadequate reduction), nerve injury, synostosis, loss of rotation
Plastic deformation		Based on bones involved (ulna > radius)	Great pressure with fulcrum (reduce most deformed bone first). Drill osteoclasis	Persistence of deformity
Ulnar Fx and radial head dislocation	Monteggia (Fig. 10–80)	I—*ulnar angulation, radial head ant. (extension)	Reduce (traction, flexion), LAC 100° flexion, supination	Late diagnosis (reconstruct annular ligament—Bell Tawse), decreased ROM, missed wrist injury, nonunion, persistent radial head dislocation (Bell Tawse and ulnar osteotomy if ulna healed), para-articular, ossification
		II—ulnar angulation, radial head post. (flexion)	Reduce (traction, extension), LAC in some extension	
		III—ulnar ant. angulation, radial head lat. (adduction)	Reduce (extension, pressure), LAC 90° flexion, supination	
		IV—ulnar and proximal ⅓ radius Fx (both angulated ant.)	Reduce (supinate), may require ORIF	
Radial head dislocation (ant.)	Monteggia equivalent		Supination and pressure on radial head, LAC 100° flexion, supination	Synostosis, nerve injury (PIN), loss of reduction (Bell Tawse)
Ulnar Fx/radial neck Fx	Check for Monteggia equivalent	Min. displaced radial head Completely displaced radial head	Reduce (traction, pressure on radial head, varus stress), ORIF	LAC

Table continued on opposite page

TABLE 10–6. *Continued*

INJURY	EPONYM	CLASSIFICATION	TREATMENT	COMPLICATIONS
Ulnar Fx/prox. radius Fx	Check for Monteggia equivalent		Reduce (traction, supination), LAC 90° flexion, supination	
Ulnar Fx, radial neck Fx, radial shaft dislocation	Check for Monteggia equivalent		Reduce (traction, reduce shaft), LAC (extension, supination)	
Radius Fx/distal radioulnar dislocation	Galeazzi		Reduce (traction, supination), LAC (90° flexion, supination); ORIF if >12 yo and closed reduction fails	Malunion, >10° angulation, nerve injury (ulnar, ant. IO), RU subluxation, loss of radial bow
Elbow				
Supracondylar (6–8 yo) (Fig. 10–81)		*Extension		Nerve injury (radial > median), vascular (acute or Volkmann's), ↓ROM, myositis ossificans, c. varus (osteotomy cosmetic), ipsilateral Fxs (forearm, wrist 10%)
		I—undisplaced	Immobilize 3 wk	
		II—displaced (post. cortex intact)	Reduce ± PCP (or hold in flexion >90°)	
		III—displaced (A—PM*; B—PL)	CR PCP; open reduction or closed traction if fails	
		Flexion (distal fragment ant.)	Reduce in extension, cast in extension or PCT pin (best) ORIF often required if completely displaced	Nerve injury (ulnar), malunion, ↓ROM
Lat. condyle (6 yo)(Fig. 10–82)		Milch: I—SH IV, II—SH II into trochlea Displacement: I—undisplaced; II—min. displaced; III—rotated	Min. displaced (<2 mm): splint; displaced: ORIF	Overgrowth/spur, delayed/nonunion, c. valgus, tardy ulnar N palsy, physeal arrest, AVN
Med. condyle (10 yo) (Fig. 10–83)		Milch: I—to trochlear apex; II—to C-T groove Displacement: I—undisplaced; II—min. displaced; III—rotated	Min. displaced: splint; displaced: ORIF	Missed Dx, c. varus, AVN
Entire distal humeral physis (<7 yo) (Fig. 10–84)		A—infant (SH I) B—7 mo–3 yo (SH I) C—3–7 yo (SH II)	Closed reduction LAC	Child abuse commonly associated, late Dx (osteotomy), c. varus
Trochlear AVN	"Fishtail"	A—lateral trochlea	Involves only internal ossification center	Early DJD, some decreased ROM
		B—entire trochlea	Involves medial and lateral centers	Cubitus varus, decreased ROM
Medial epicondylar apophysis (11 yo) (Fig. 10–85)		I—Acute injury		Highly associated with elbow dislocation, reduce dislocation and treat Fx accordingly; ulnar N dysfunction (ORIF), valgus instability, loss of full extension (mild)
		A—undisplaced	Immobilize 1 week	
		B—minimally displaced	Immobilize 1 week	
		C—significantly displaced (± dislocation)	ORIF for valgus instability in athlete, otherwise early ROM	
		D—entrapment of fragment in joint	Manipulative extraction, ORIF (esp with ulnar nerve entrapment or fragment remains)	
		E—Fracture through epicondylar apophysis	Immobilize *or* ORIF *or* excision if unstable in athlete	
	Little League elbow	II—Chronic tension stress injury	Change in throwing activities	
Lat. epicondylar apophysis (rare)			Immobilize for comfort, open reduction and excision if fragment incarcerated	
"T" condylar Fx (rare)		Based on fracture	Hanging arm cast or ORIF	↓ROM, neurovascular complications

Table continued on page 402

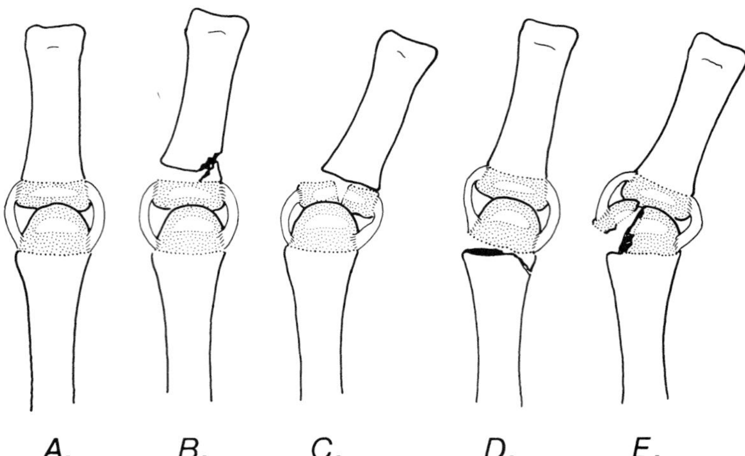

FIGURE 10–76. Pediatric finger MCP fractures. *A*, Normal. *B*, SH II (proximal phalanx). *C*, SH III (proximal phalanx). *D*, SH II (metacarpal). *E*, SH III (metacarpal). (From Ogden, J.A.: Skeletal Injury in the Child, 2nd ed., p. 531. Philadelphia, WB Saunders, 1990; reprinted by permission.)

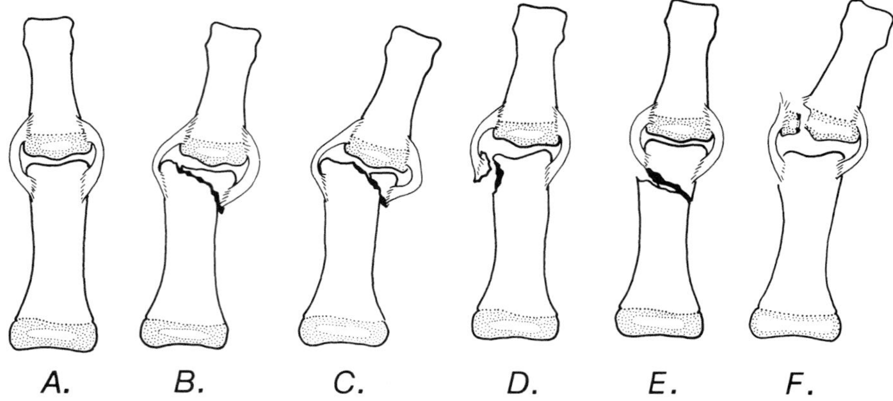

FIGURE 10–77. Pediatric finger IP fractures. *A*, Normal. *B*, Unicondylar. *C*, Partial condylar. *D*, Lateral avulsion. *E*, Bicondylar. *F*, SH III. (From Ogden, J.A.: Skeletal Injury in the Child, 2nd ed., p. 530. Philadelphia, WB Saunders, 1990; reprinted by permission.)

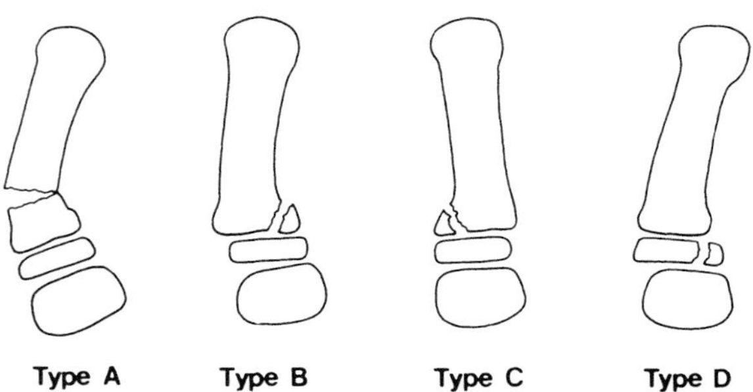

FIGURE 10–78. Classification of pediatric thumb metacarpal fractures. *A*, Metaphyseal. *B*, SH II (medial). *C*, SH II (Lateral). *D*, SH III. (From O'Brien, E.T.: Fractures of the hand and wrist region. In Fractures in Children, Rockwood, C.A., Jr., Wilkins, K.E., and King, R.E., eds., 2nd ed., p. 257. Philadelphia, JB Lippincott, 1984; reprinted by permission.)

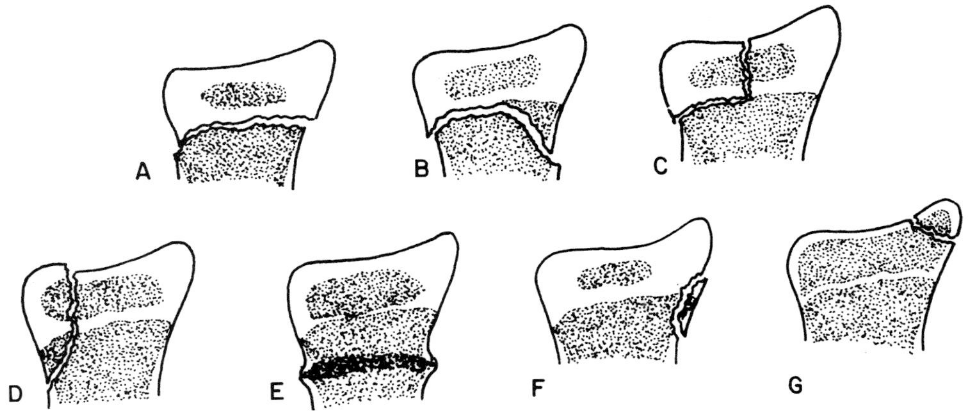

FIGURE 10–79. Pediatric wrist fractures. *A,* SH I. *B,* SH II. *C,* SH III. *D,* SH IV. *E,* Torus. *F,* Avulsion. *G,* Radial styloid. (From Ogden, J.A.: Skeletal Injury in the Child, 2nd ed., p. 513. Philadelphia, WB Saunders, 1990; reprinted by permission.)

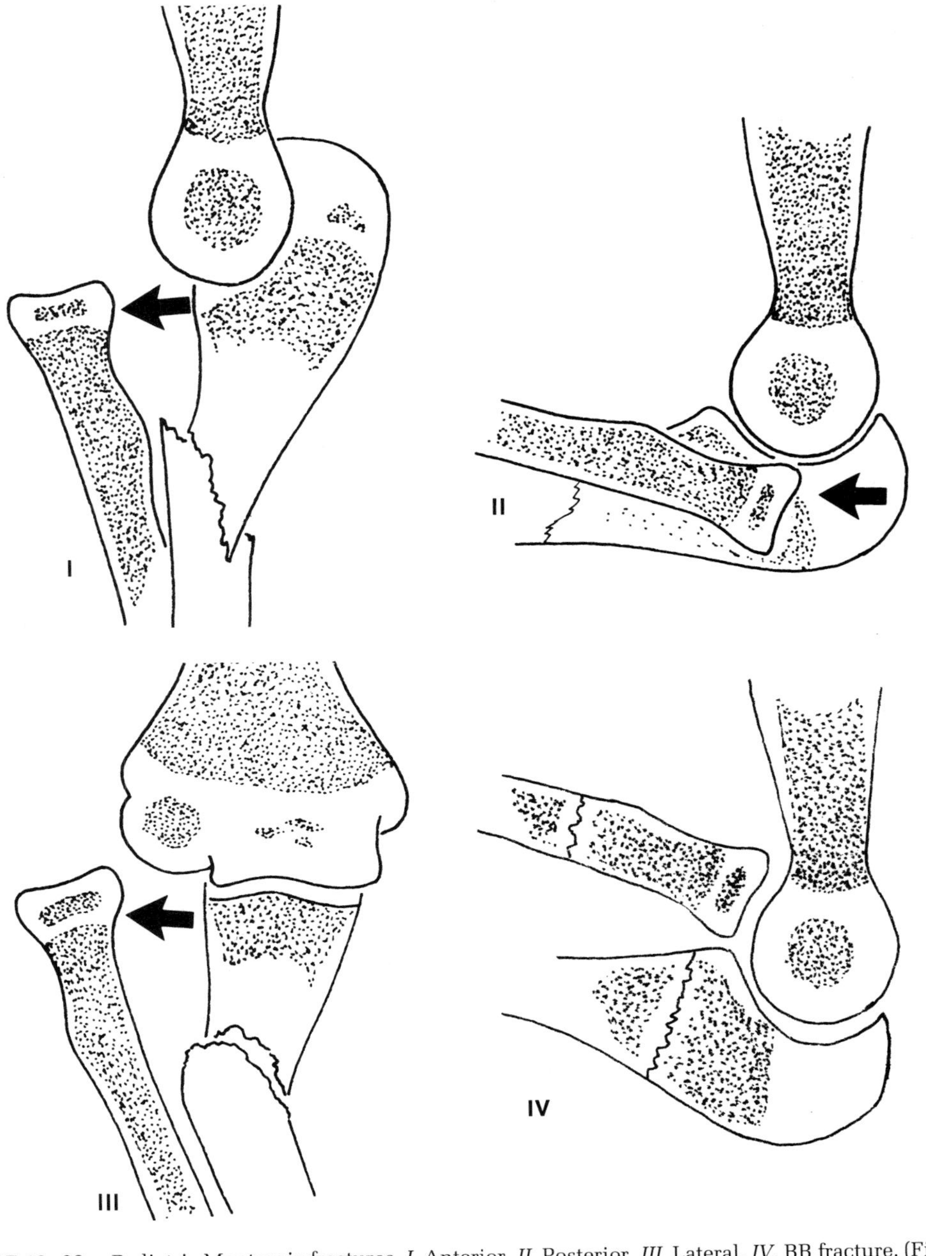

FIGURE 10–80. Pediatric Monteggia fractures. *I,* Anterior, *II,* Posterior. *III,* Lateral. *IV,* BB fracture. (Figs. I–III from Ogden, J.A.: Skeletal Injury in the Child, 2nd ed., pp. 480, 481. Philadelphia, WB Saunders, 1990; reprinted by permission.)

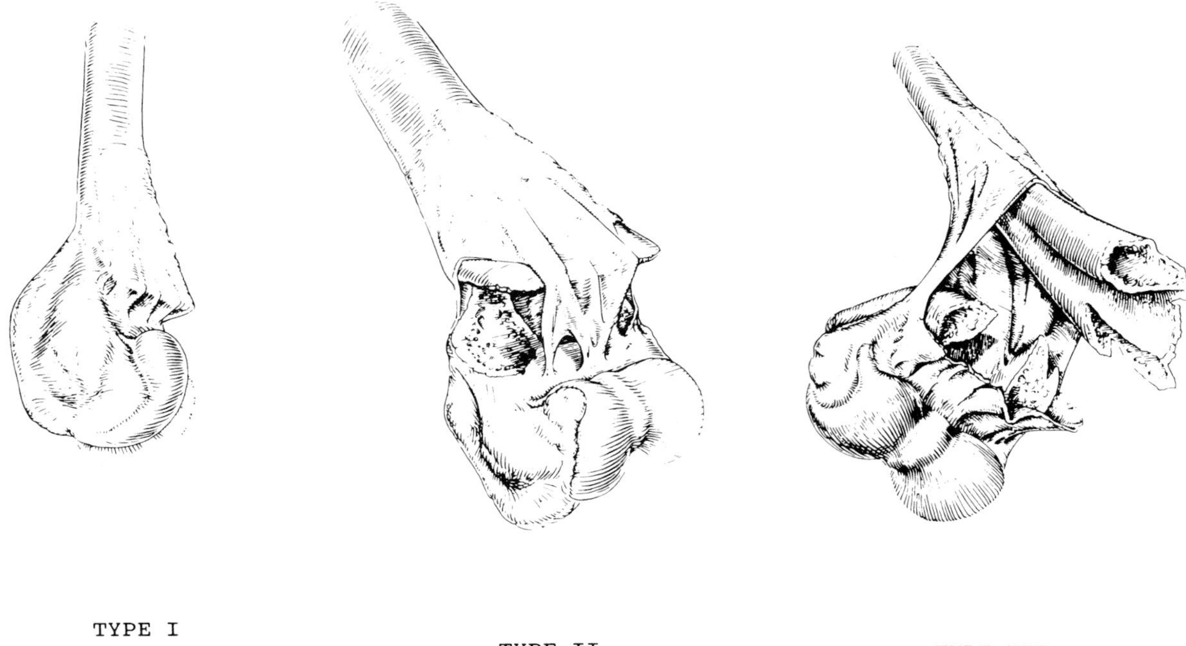

FIGURE 10–81. Supracondylar fractures. (From Abraham, E., Powers, T., Witt, P., and Ray, R.D.: Experimental hyperextension supracondylar fractures in monkeys. Clin. Orthop. 171:313, 314, 1982; reprinted by permission.)

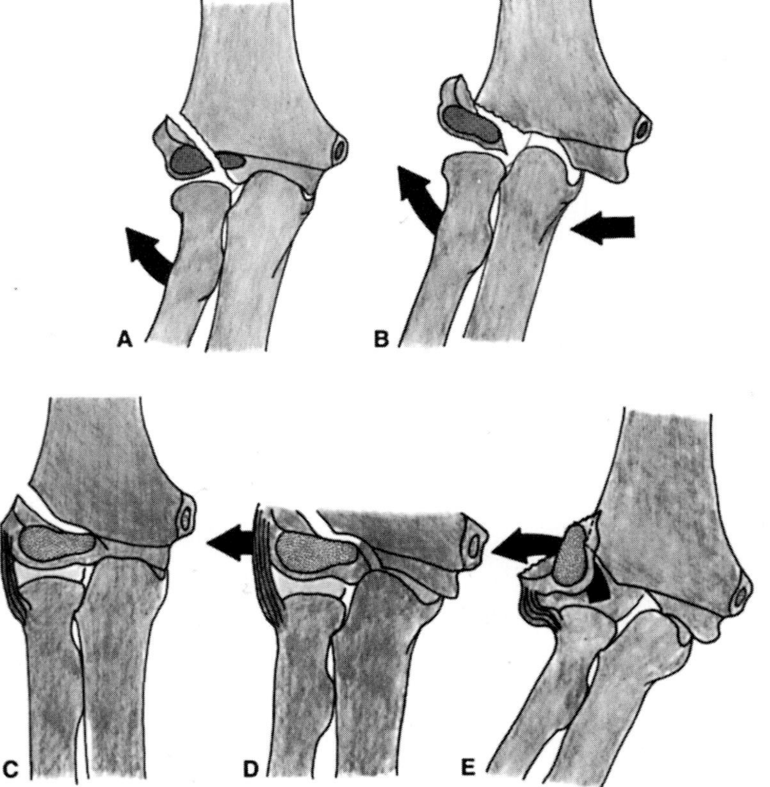

FIGURE 10–82. Lateral condyle fractures. *A,* Milch I. *B,* Milch II. *C,* Undisplaced. *D,* Displaced. *E,* Rotated. (From Tachdjian, M.O.: Pediatric Orthopaedics, 2nd ed., pp. 3109, 3110. Philadelphia, WB Saunders, 1990; reprinted by permission.)

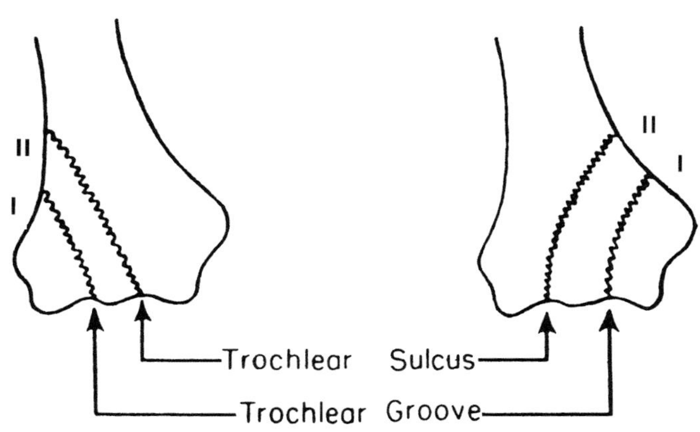

FIGURE 10–83. Milch classification of humeral condyle fractures. (Modified from Milch, H.: Fracture and fracture dislocations of the humeral condyles. J. Trauma 4:601, 1964; reprinted by permission.). Copyright © 1964 by Williams & Wilkins.)

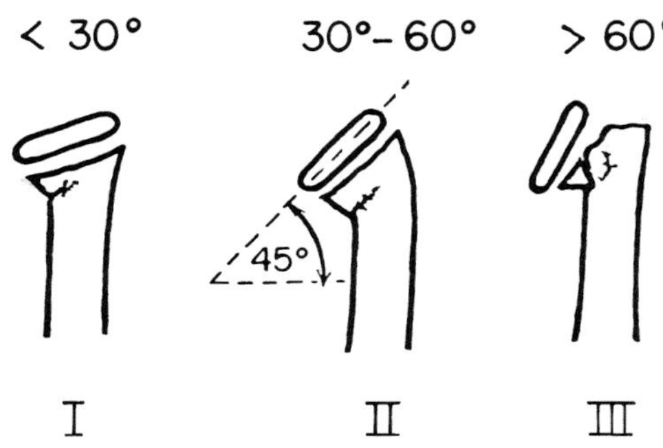

FIGURE 10–86. Radial head fractures; type III requires primary ORIF. (From Tachdjian, M.O.: Pediatric Orthopaedics, 2nd ed., p. 3140. Philadelphia, WB Saunders, 1990; reprinted by permission.)

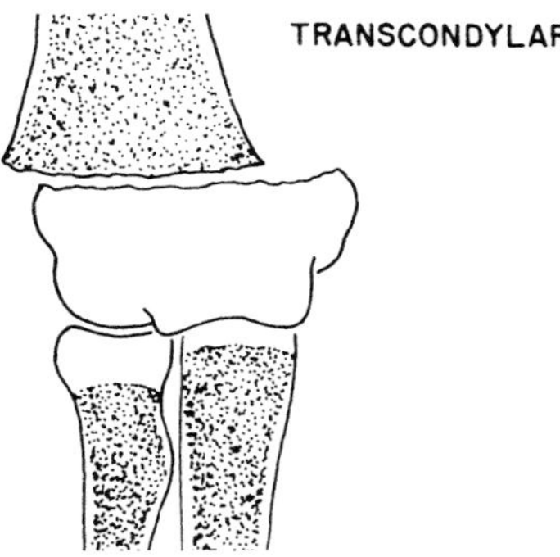

FIGURE 10–84. Total condylar fracture. (From Ogden, J.A.: Skeletal Injury in the Child, 2nd ed., p. 388. Philadelphia, WB Saunders, 1990; reprinted by permission.)

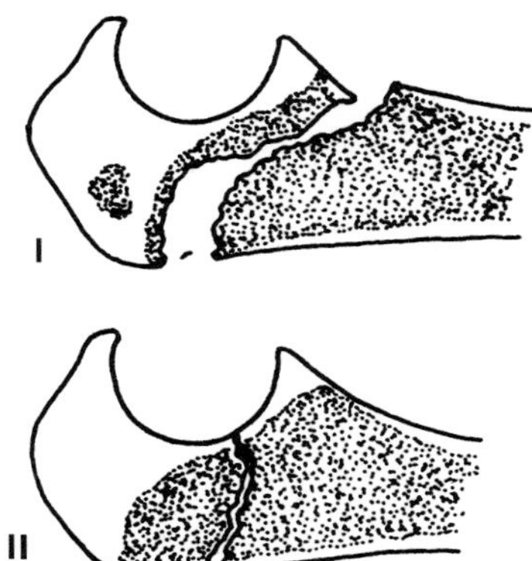

FIGURE 10–87. Proximal ulna fractures. (From Ogden, J.A.: Skeletal Injury in the Child, 2nd ed., p. 463. Philadelphia, WB Saunders, 1990; reprinted by permission.)

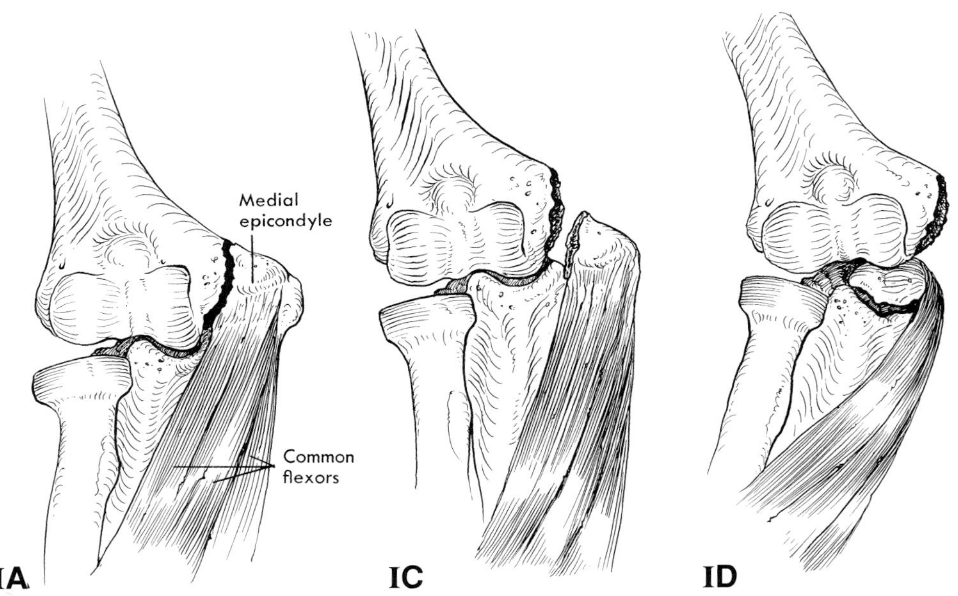

FIGURE 10–85. Medial epicondyle fractures. *IA,* Undisplaced. *IC,* Displaced. *ID,* Entrapped. (From Tachdjian, M.O.: Pediatric Orthopaedics, 2nd ed., p. 3122. Philadelphia, WB Saunders, 1990; reprinted by permission.)

TABLE 10–6. *Continued*

INJURY	EPONYM	CLASSIFICATION	TREATMENT	COMPLICATIONS
Radial head/neck (9–10 yo) (Fig. 10–86)		A—SH I or II physeal fracture B—SH IV fracture C—Transmetaphyseal fracture D—with elbow dislocation: reduction injury E—with elbow dislocation: dislocation injury	Immobilize if <30° angulation or <45° angulation after reduction (or 70° of pro/supination) or Fx >4 days old with angulation up to 90°; ORIF translocated, >60° primarily; ORIF if markedly displaced	↓ROM, radial head overgrowth, neck notching, premature physeal closure, nonunion, AVN, proximal synostosis (esp. with late treatment): avoid transcapitellar pins
Prox. olecranon physis (rare) (Fig. 10–87)		I—physeal-metaphyseal border (younger children) II—physis with large metaphyseal fragment (older children)	ORIF if significantly displaced	Epiphyseal overgrowth, spurs (may require excision)
Olecranon metaphysis (rare)		A—flexion	If undisplaced, immobilize 3 wk; ORIF if defect	Rare: delay/nonunion, Volkmann's, ulnar N irritation
		B—extension (1, valgus; 2, varus)	Reduce (forceful manipulation in extension)	
		C—shear	Immobilize in hyperflexion, ORIF periosteal tear	
Coronoid process (rare)			Immobilize in flexion	Assoc. with elbow dislocation
Elbow dislocation (10–19 yo)		I—prox. RU intact A—posterior (1, postmed., 2, postlat.) B—anterior C—medial D—lateral II—prox. RU divergent: A—anteroposterior B—medial-lateral (transverse)	Reduction (push off younger, pull off older patients)	Assoc. Fxs (med. epicondylar apophysis, prox. radius, coronoid), nerve injuries (ulnar > median) (median N entrapment: 1 in joint, 2 between epicondyle and condyle, 3 kinked anteriorly [Fig. 10–88]) myositis ossificans, recurrent dislocation, prox. RU translocation, OC Fx
Radial head subluxation	Nursemaid's elbow (stretching of annular/orbicular ligaments)		Reduce (supination, flex, snap)	Unreduced subluxations, recurrence, irreducible (rare)
SHOULDER				
Humerus shaft (Fig. 10–89)		Neonate (birth injury)	Small splint or splint to side	Compartment syndrome, radial N injury, rotational deformity (OK if <12°), growth disturbance (<15 mm not noticeable)
		0–3 yo	Collar and cuff	
		3–12 yo	Velpeau	
		>12 yo	Sugar tong splints	
Prox. humeral physis (Fig. 10–90)		Salter-Harris (I most common in <5 yo, II most common in older children) Neer-Horowitz (based on displacement): I <5 mm, II <⅓ shaft, III <⅔, IV >⅔	Velpeau if min. displaced, gentle manipulation for displaced fractures with immobilization to side in younger patients, and "salute" position in older children ± PCP; ORIF <50% opposition, >45° angulation	Growth disorders
Prox. physis stress Fx	LL shoulder	Stress fracture	Activity modification	
Prox. humeral metaphysis		Common; based on location	Sling and swathe/Velpeau	
Midshaft clavicle		0–2 yo	Supportive, bind to side if symptomatic	Rare: neurovascular injury, mal/nonunion
		>2 yo	Figure-of-8 dressing for 3 wk	

Table continued on opposite page

TABLE 10–6. *Continued*

INJURY	EPONYM	CLASSIFICATION	TREATMENT	COMPLICATIONS
Med. clavicle (rare)		Usually SH I or II physeal separations	Sling for 1 wk	Rare
Lat. clavicle		I—nondisplaced, intact AC and CC ligaments IIA—clavicle displaced sup., Fx med. to CC ligament IIB—clavicle displaced sup., conoid ligament tear III—fracture into AC joint	Figure-of-8 dressing; some recommend ORIF of type II injuries	
AC joint (Fig. 10–91)		I—Sprain II—Partial tear dorsal periosteal tube III—Large tear of dorsal tube, sup. displacement	Types I, II, and III: closed treatment	Coracoid Fx (treated nonoperatively)
		IV—Clavicle displaced posteriorly	Closed reduction, open if required	
		V—Clavicle displaced significantly sup.	Open reduction, repair and reconstruction	
		VI—Inferior dislocation of clavicle	Open reduction may be required	
SC joint		Anterior	Sling/reassurance	
		Posterior	Acute—reduce, chronic/leave alone	
Clavicle dislocation (rare)			Open reduction with repair of periosteal tube	
Scapula fractures		Based on location	Treatment similar to adult fractures	
Glenohumeral dislocation		Traumatic vs. atraumatic	Rehabilitation; reconstruction for unstable posttraumatic shoulders after 6 mo of rehab	
Spine Fractures				
C2–C3 laxity	Pseudosubluxation	<4 mm translation in child <7 yo	None—normal variant	
Occiput—C1 lesions			Reduced with traction, craniovertebral fusion later	Often fatal injuries
C1–C2 lesions		Traumatic ligament disruption	Reduce in extension, immobilize (Minerva or halo) 8–12 wk	Vertebral A—risk with surgery
	Grisel syndrome	Ligament laxity from local inflammation	Traction, immobilize (Minerva) 6–8 wk	Vertebral A—risk with surgery
		Rotatory (I—w/o C1 shift, II—<5 mm C1 ant. shift, III—>5 mm C1 ant. shift, IV—post. shift (Fig. 10–92)	I, soft collar; II/III/IV, traction + immobilization 6 wk C1–C2 fusion ant. esp. with recurrence/neuro Sx	
		Odontoid—physeal or os odontoideum	Reduce (hyperextension), immobilize (Minerva) 12 wk	
C2–C3 dislocation		True vs. pseudo more likely with trauma history, PLL ossification, chip Fxs, and failure to correct with extension		
T/L fractures (Fig. 10–93)		Compression fractures	Bed rest/symptomatic	Neurologic injuries
		Unstable fractures	Treated like adults	
Kyphosis	Scheurmann's disease	3 Adjacent vertebrae with >5° wedging	Milwaukee bracing occasionally indicated	
Spondolysis		Stress Fx of pars (L5–S1)	Acute—immobilize, conservative otherwise, L4–S1 fusion in refractory cases	

Table continued on page 407

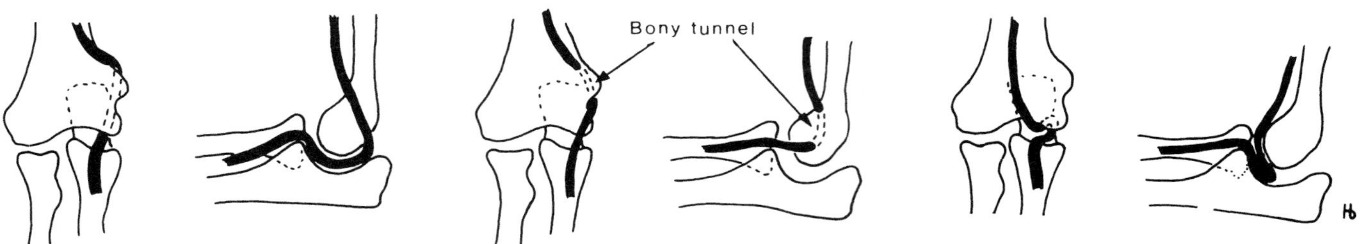

FIGURE 10–88. Median nerve entrapment. (From Hallett, J.: Entrapment of the median nerve after dislocation of the elbow. J. Bone Joint Surg. [Br.] 63:410, 1981; reprinted by permission.)

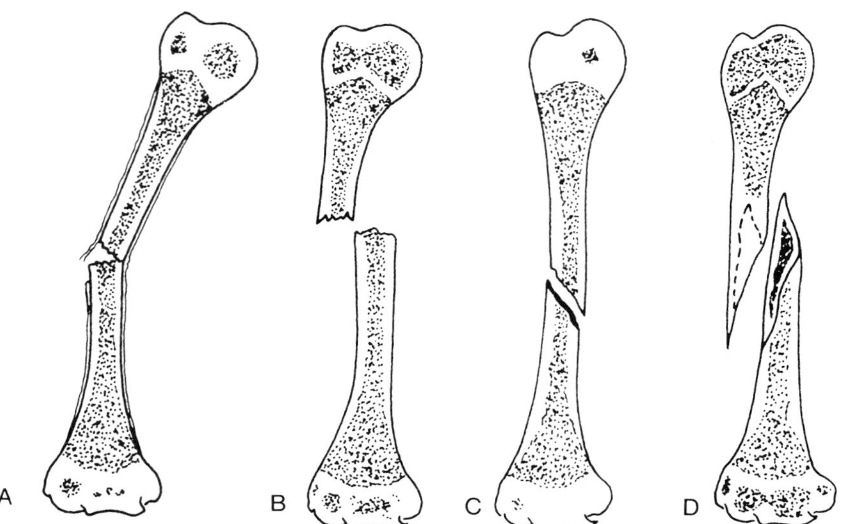

FIGURE 10–89. Humeral diaphyseal fractures. *A,* Transverse, periosteum intact. *B,* Transverse, periosteum ruptured. *C,* Oblique. *D,* Spiral. (From Ogden, J.A.: Skeletal Injury in the Child, 2nd ed., p. 367. Philadelphia, WB Saunders, 1990; reprinted by permission.)

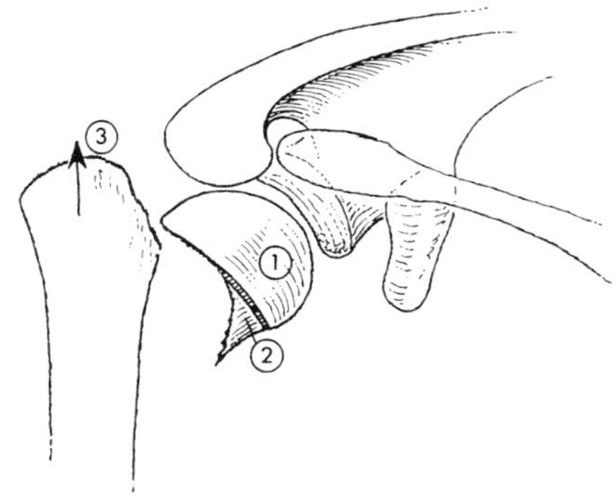

FIGURE 10–90. Proximal humeral epicondylar fracture (SH II); note superior displacement of humeral shaft. (From Connolly, J.F., ed.: Depalma's The Management of Fractures and Dislocations, an Atlas, 3rd ed., p. 458. Philadelphia, WB Saunders, 1981; reprinted by permission.)

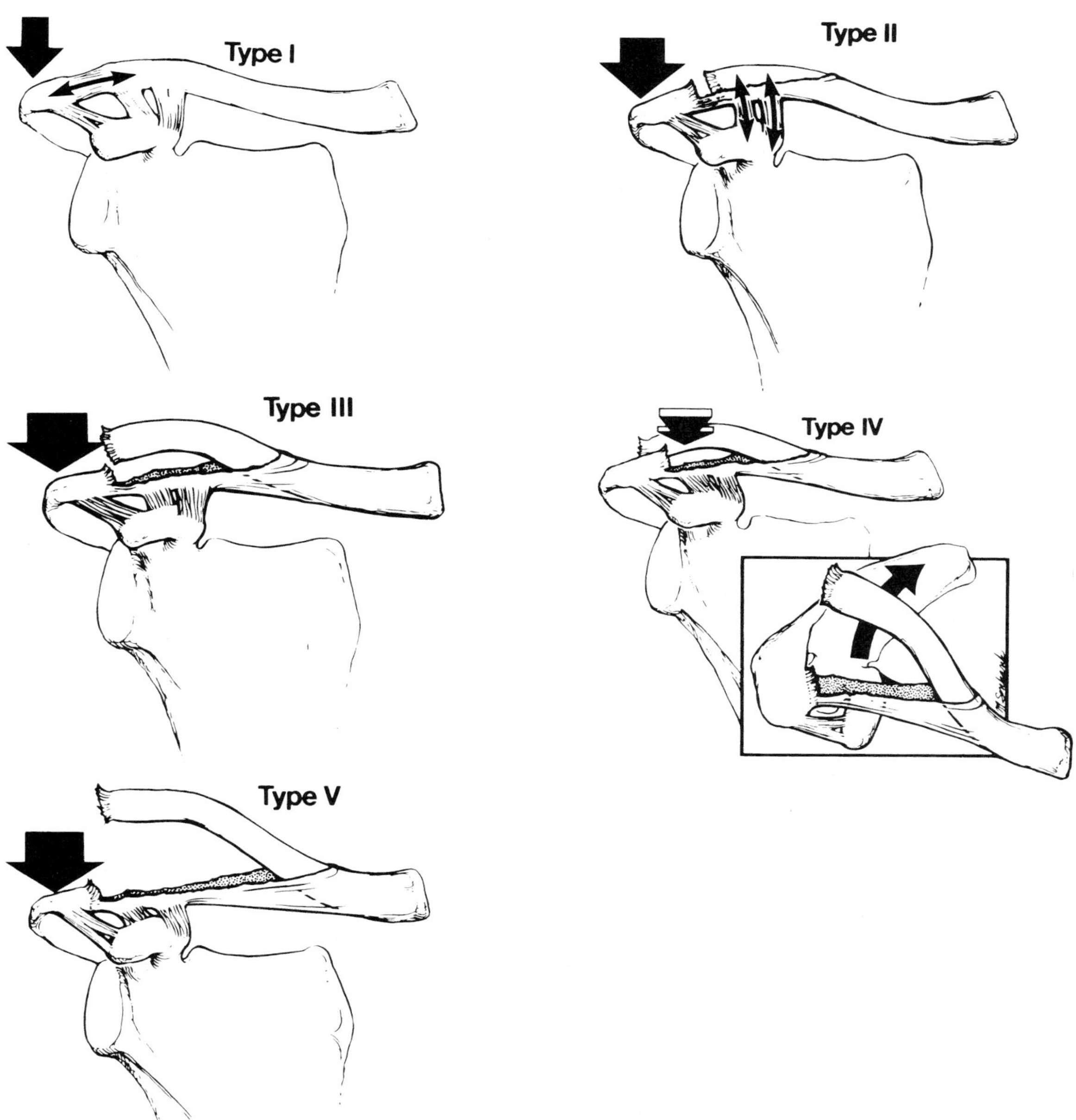

FIGURE 10–91. Classification of pediatric AC injuries. (From Rockwood, C.A., Jr.: Fractures and dislocations of the ends of the clavicle, scapula, and glenohumeral joint. In Fractures in Children, Rockwood, C.A., Jr., Wilkins, K.E., and King, R.E., eds., 3rd ed., p. 880. Philadelphia, JB Lippincott, 1991; reprinted by permission.)

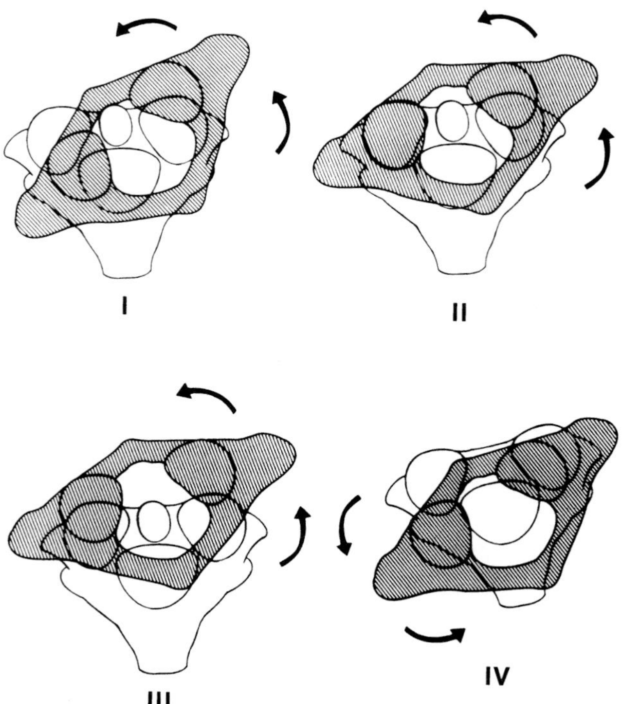

FIGURE 10–92. Atlantoaxial rotatory displacement. *I,* No shift. *II,* Shift <5 mm. *III,* Shift >5 mm. *IV,* Post shift. (From Bailey, D.K.: Normal cervical spine in infants and children. Radiology 59:37, 1952; reprinted by permission.)

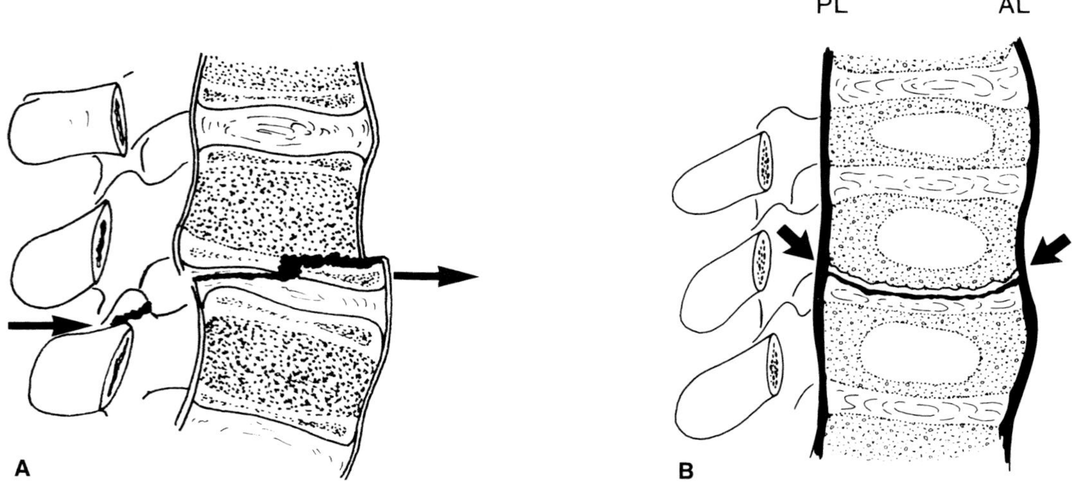

FIGURE 10–93. Classification of pediatric spine fractures. *Left,* Unstable SH III. *Right,* Stable SH I. (From Ogden, J.A.: Skeletal Injury in the Child, 2nd ed., p. 599. Philadelphia, WB Saunders, 1990; reprinted by permission.)

TABLE 10–6. *Continued*

INJURY	EPONYM	CLASSIFICATION	TREATMENT	COMPLICATIONS
SCIWORA		Spinal cord injury without radiographic abnormality	Evaluation with MRI and appropriate treatment	Scoliosis (esp. <8 yo)
PELVIC FRACTURES				
Pelvic Fxs (Figs. 10–94, 10–95, 10–96)		Key and Conwell		In general less than adults, includes loss of reduction, delayed/nonunion, DJD, malunion, problems with organ injury (vs. adult)
		I—Ring intact		
		Avulsion (ASIS—sartorius; AIIS—rectus; IT—hamstring)	BR flexed hip 2 wk, guarded WB 4 wk	
	Duverney	*Pubis/ischium	BR 3–7 days, limited WB 4 wk	Asymmetric ossification is not a Fx
		Iliac wing	BR leg abducted, progress to gradual WB	
		Sacrum/coccyx	BR 3–6 wk if severe (sacral)	Sacral N injury
		II—Single break in ring		
		*Ipsilateral ramii	BR 2–4 wk, non-weight-bearing	
		Symphysis pubis	BR with sling or spica cast	Often unstable with associated injuries
		SI joint (rare)	BR, progress to guarded WB	
		III—Double break in ring		
	Straddle	Bilateral pubic fractures	BR flexed hip 4–6 wk	
	Malgaigne	Ant. & post. ring with migration	Skeletal traction 3–6 wk, avoid compression	LLD with vertical shear
		Severe multiple fractures	Treatment on a case-by-case basis. Ex. fix. or int. fix. as indicated.	
		IV—Acetabular fractures		
		Small fragment with dislocation (post. ≫ ant.)	BR, progress to guarded ambulation	Premature closure of triradiate cartilage → shallow acetabulum, esp. <10 yo
		Linear—nondisplaced	Treat associated pelvic fracture	
		Linear—hip unstable	Skeletal traction, ORIF if incongruous	
		Central	Lateral traction, ORIF if needed to obtain congruent/stable joint	Heterotopic ossification especially with ORIF
HIP FRACTURES				
Hip Fxs (Fig. 10–97)		Delbet		AVN in up to 40% (higher in more proximal Fxs, related to displacement, 100% in IA). Ratliff classification of AVN: i, complete, II, physeal, III, neck only (Fig. 10–98); coxa vara (25%, osteotomy if severe); nonunion (6%, treat with subtrochanteric valgus osteotomy); growth arrest
		IA—transepiphyseal with dislocation	Closed reduction or ORIF and pin	
		IB—transepiphyseal w/o dislocation	Closed reduction and pin	
		II—*transcervical	Closed reduction and pin	
		IIIA—cervical trochanteric, displaced	Closed reduction and pin	
		IIIB—cervical trochanteric, nondisplaced	Abduction spica cast	
		IV—intertrochanteric	Traction and abduction spica, ORIF unstable	
Femoral neck stress Fx		Devas		
		Superior transverse	Pin (displaces otherwise)	Displacement causes incr. complications; varus deformities
		Inferior (compressive)	NWB	
Traumatic dislocation (Fig. 10–99)		*Posterior	Closed reduction (Stimson), open if incongruous after two attempts at closed reduction, greater trochanteric Fxs common	AVN (10%), recurrent dislocation, myositis ossificans, DJD
		Anterior		

Table continued on page 410

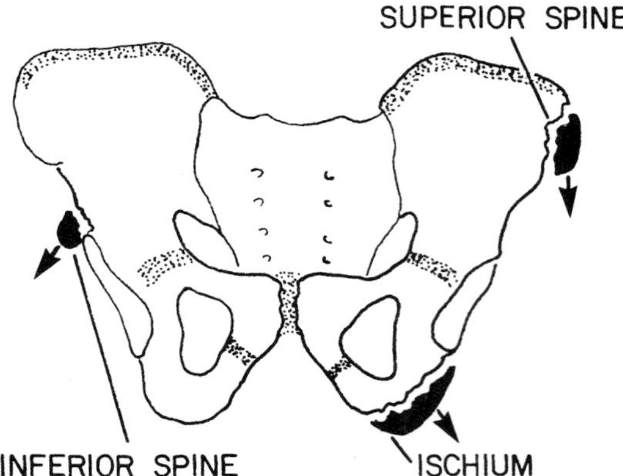

FIGURE 10–94. Avulsion fractures of the pelvis. Superior spine—sartorius avulsion; inferior spine—rectus avulsion; ischium—hamstring avulsion (From Ogden, J.A.: Skeletal Injury in the Child, 2nd ed., p. 635. Philadelphia, WB Saunders, 1990; reprinted by permission.)

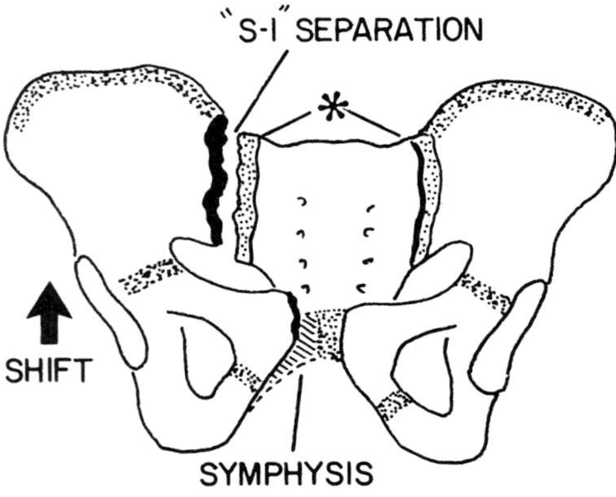

FIGURE 10–96. Unstable pelvic fracture. (From Ogden, J.A.: Skeletal Injury in the Child, 2nd ed., p. 634. Philadelphia, WB Saunders, 1990; reprinted by permission.)

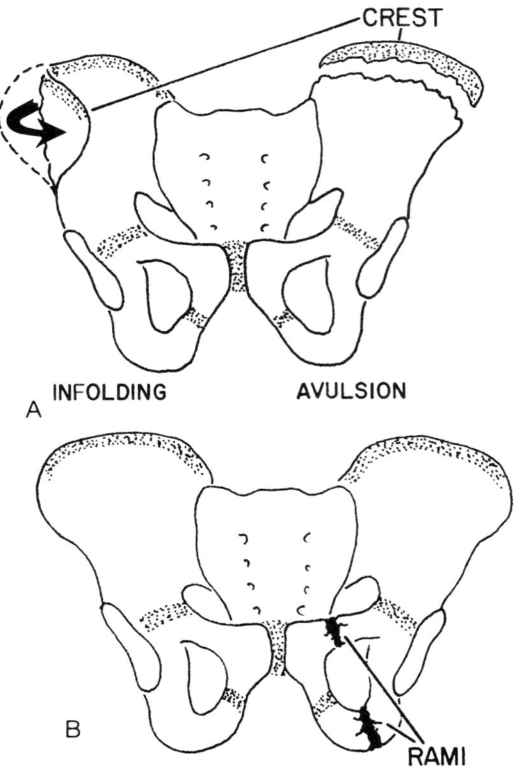

FIGURE 10–95. Stable pelvic fractures. (From Ogden, J.A.: Skeletal Injury in the Child, 2nd ed., p. 634. Philadelphia, WB Saunders, 1990; reprinted by permission.)

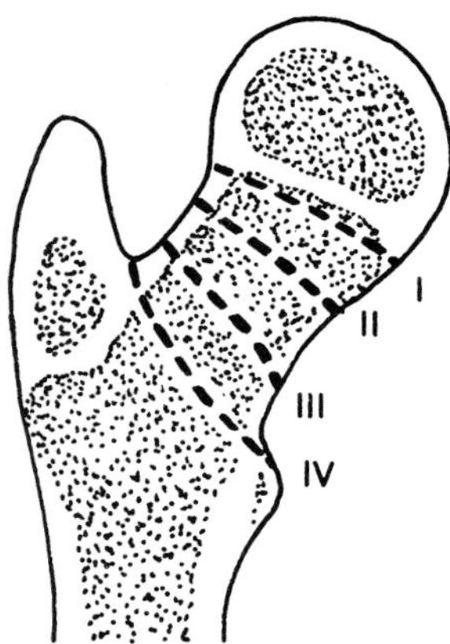

FIGURE 10–97. Femoral neck fractures in children. *I,* Transepiphyseal. *II,* Transcervical. *III,* Cervical-trochanteric. *IV,* Intertrochanteric. (From Ogden, J.A.: Skeletal Injury in the Child, 2nd ed., p. 689. Philadelphia, WB Saunders, 1990; reprinted by permission.)

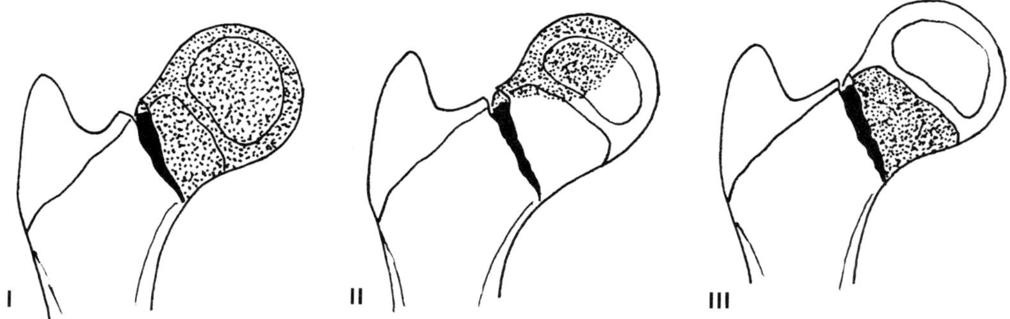

FIGURE 10–98. Patterns of avascular necrosis in children following hip fractures (Ratliff). *I,* Complete. *II,* Physeal. *III,* Neck. (From Ogden, J.A.: Skeletal Injury in the Child, 2nd ed., p. 701. Philadelphia, WB Saunders, 1990; reprinted by permission.)

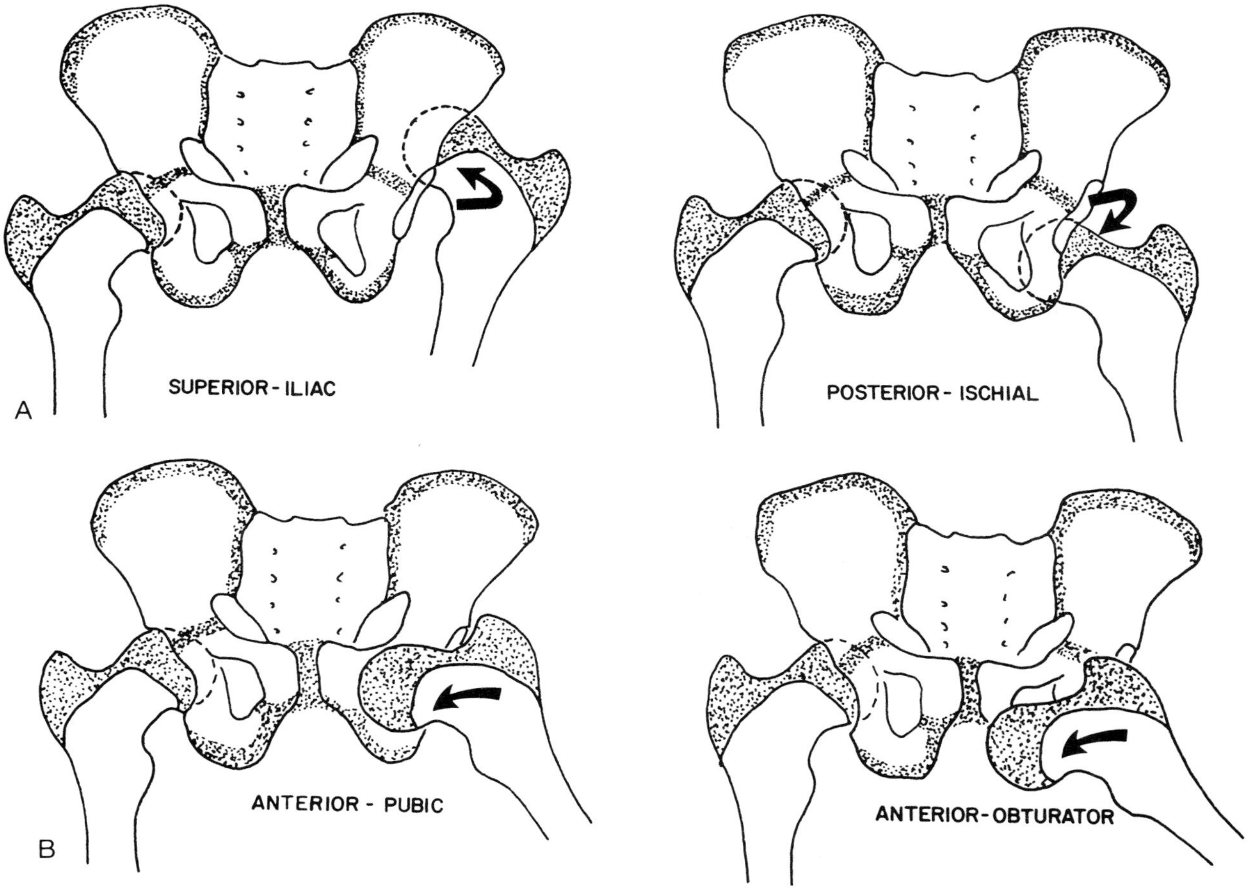

FIGURE 10–99. Hip dislocations in children. (From Ogden, J.A.: Skeletal Injury in the Child, 2nd ed., p. 663. Philadelphia, WB Saunders, 1990; reprinted by permission.)

TABLE 10–6. *Continued*

INJURY	EPONYM	CLASSIFICATION	TREATMENT	COMPLICATIONS
FEMORAL SHAFT FRACTURES				
Femoral Fx		0–2 years old 2–10 years old 10–15 years old >15 years old	Spica cast Spica cast if <2 cm override; split Russel >2 cm; (Can safely use IM rod >12 yo) 90–90 skeletal traction IM rod Consider plate, external fixation in younger children with CHI or polytrauma (<10–12 years old)	*LLD, angular deformity (avoid >10° frontal and >30° sagittal malalignment, rotational deformity (>10°), ischemia, SMA syndrome (with casting); arrest of greater troch. apophysis by nailing
Subtrochlear		Based on anatomic location	90–90° Traction ORIF with head injury (cannot control)	LLD
KNEE INJURIES				
Distal femoral epiphysis separation (Figs. 10–100 to 10–103)	"Wagon wheel"	SH I–IV (*II) or based on displacement or based on child's age	Closed reduction → LLC, PCP in SH III or IV; open only for soft tissue interposition, consider addition of pelvic band in obese patients	Popliteal A or peroneal N injury, recurrent displacement, growth plate injuries (angulation and shortening)
Proximal tibial epiphysis fracture		SH I–IV (*II)	Nondisplaced: LLC in 30° flexion; displaced: closed reduction, PCP	Popliteal A injury, growth plate injuries
Floating knee		Letts		Infection, nonunion, malunion, growth arrest
		A—both fractures diaphyseal	ORIF for one, closed reduction other	
		B—1 fracture diaphyseal, 1 metaphyseal	ORIF diaphyseal, closed reduction metaphyseal	
		C—1 fracture diaphyseal, 1 epiphyseal	Closed reduction and pin epiphyseal, closed traction diaphyseal	
		D—1 fracture open, 1 fracture closed	Débride/external fixation open, closed treatment closed Fx	
		E—both fractures open	Débride/external fixation or traction for both	
Tibial tubercle avulsion		Ogden (Fig. 10–104) 1—Small distal piece fractured 2—Fx junction of 1° and 2° oss. centers 3—Fx thru 1 epiphysis (SH III)	Small fragment, min. displaced with full extension—cast; ORIF all other fractures	Genu recurvatum, ↓ROM, prominence, patella alta
Osteochondral Fxs		Kennedy and Smillie Med. femoral condyle exogenous or endogenous Lat. femoral condyle exogenous or endogenous Patella (med.) endogenous (dislocation)	Operative—remove small fragments, attempt ORIF large fragments (Steiman pin in condyles, small screws in patella [remove at 3 mo]); can use absorbable pins	Recurrent patellar dislocation, DJD
Intercondylar eminence tibia (Fig. 10–105)		Meyers and McKeever I—incomplete/ nondisplaced II—hinged (posterior rim intact) III—completely displaced (supinated and rotated)	Attempt closed reduction in all (with extension); ORIF for soft tissue interposition	↓Extension (if not completely reduced), MCL or meniscal injury, postop complications
Patella		Undisplaced	Aspiration, cylinder cast (<5° flexion)	Patella alta, extensor lag, quadriceps atrophy, infection
		Displaced transverse	ORIF tension band	
		"Sleeve" Fx (avulsion of distal pole and articular cartilage) (Fig. 10–106)	ORIF tension band	
Marginal fractures			Excision, ORIF if involves articular surface	

Table continued on page 413

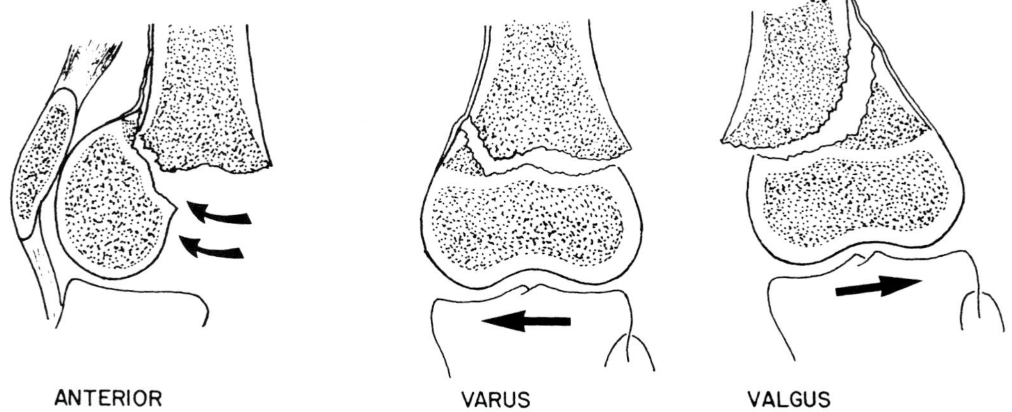

FIGURE 10–100. Distal femoral physeal fractures. (From Ogden, J.A.: Skeletal Injury in the Child, 2nd ed., p. 725. Philadelphia, WB Saunders, 1990; reprinted by permission.)

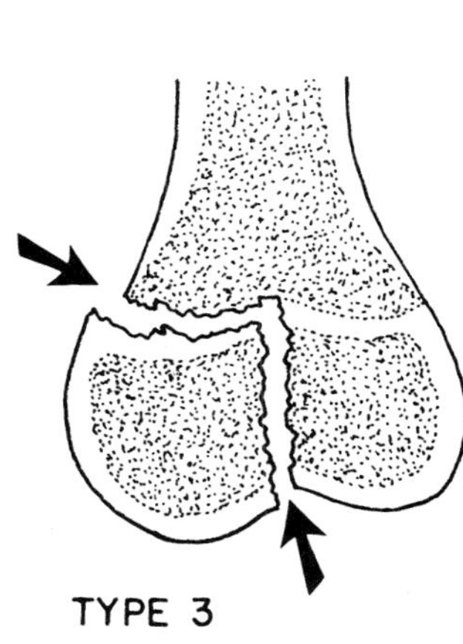

FIGURE 10–101. Distal femoral Salter-Harris III fracture. (From Ogden, J.A.: Skeletal Injury in the Child, 2nd ed., p. 727. Philadelphia, WB Saunders, 1990; reprinted by permission.)

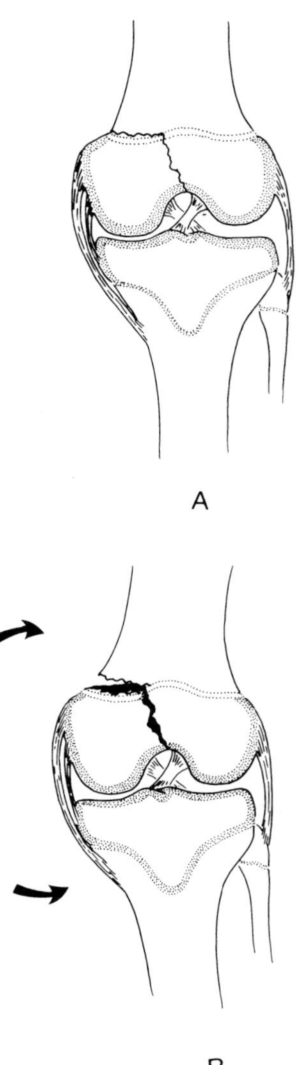

FIGURE 10–102. Stress test used to diagnose subtle fractures about the knee. (From Ogden, J.A.: Skeletal Injury in the Child, 2nd ed., p. 728. Philadelphia, WB Saunders, 1990; reprinted by permission.)

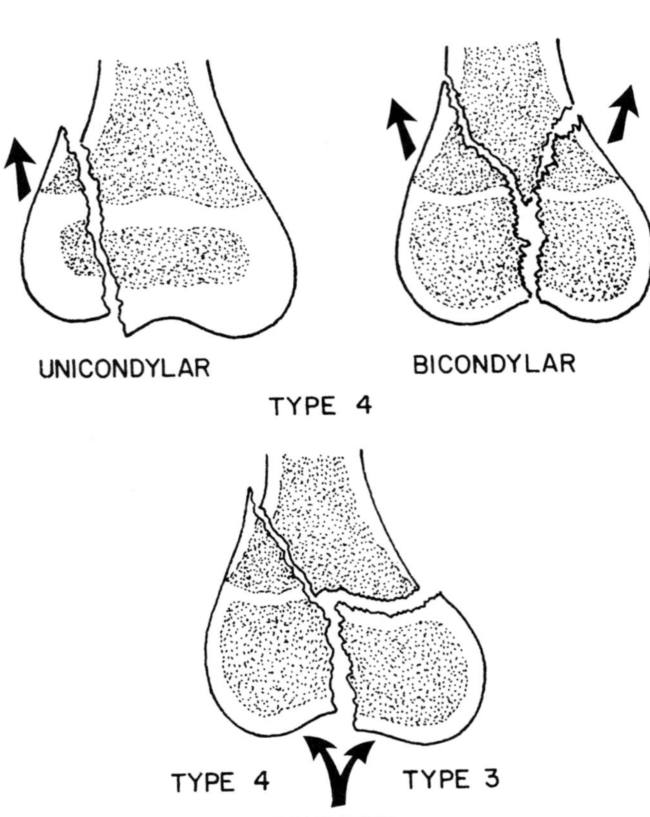

FIGURE 10–103. Salter-Harris III and IV fractures of the distal femur. (From Ogden, J.A.: Skeletal Injury in the Child, 2nd ed., p. 729. Philadelphia, WB Saunders, 1990; reprinted by permission.)

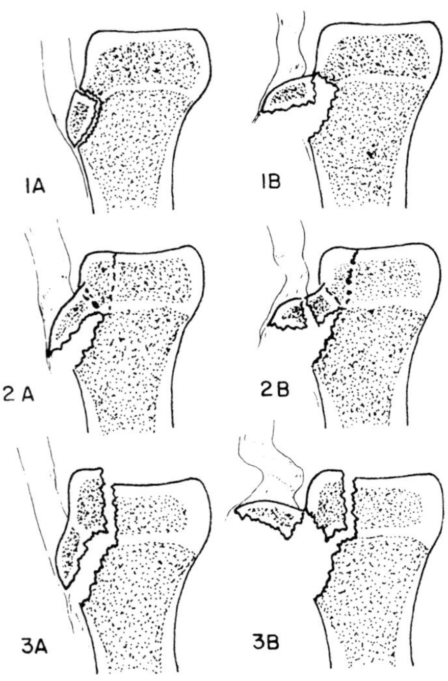

FIGURE 10–104. Fractures of the tibial tuberosity. (From Ogden, J.A.: Skeletal Injury in the Child, 2nd ed., p. 808. Philadelphia, WB Saunders, 1990; reprinted by permission.)

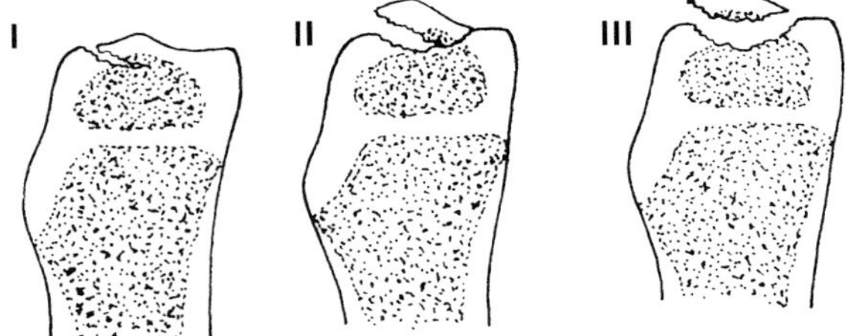

FIGURE 10–105. Tibial spine fractures. (From Ogden, J.A.: Skeletal Injury in the Child, 2nd ed., p. 796. Philadelphia, WB Saunders, 1990; reprinted by permission.)

TABLE 10–6. *Continued*

INJURY	EPONYM	CLASSIFICATION	TREATMENT	COMPLICATIONS
KNEE DISLOCATIONS AND LIGAMENTOUS INJURIES				
Ligament injuries		Based on ligament and location	Stress radiographs, primary repair	Instability; heterotopic bone and other complications with open repair
Patella osteochondrosis	Sinding-Larsen-Johansson	Acute	Cylinder cast in extension 3–4 wk	Patella alta, distal pole prominence
		Chronic	Activity limitation, quadriceps/hamstring stent	
Tibial tuberosity osteochondrosis	Osgood-Schlatter	Woolfry and Chandler radiographic changes: I, irregular, II, irregular and small ossicle, III, normal tubercle with free ossicle	Activity limitation or immobilization Excision of ununited ossicles at maturity	
Meniscal injury		Based on injury	Arthroscopic examination and repair	DJD
Discoid meniscus		Intact or torn	Most favor leaving intact; resect only if torn	
Femorotibial dislocations		Femorotibial (rare)	Like adult, arteriogram	Popliteal A injury
Patellar dislocations		Patellar-intra-articular dislocation	Closed reduction, cast 3–6 wk, open if fragment	Predisposition: Down synd., MD, arthrogryposis, neurologic disorders
Tibiofibular dislocations		Prox. tibiofibular joint dislocation	Intra-articular	Clicking, instability, peroneal neuropathy
TIBIA-FIBULA				
Tibia-fibula	Greenstick	Incomplete	LLC slight flexion: 8–10 wk	Angular deformity g. valgus (do not accept >10° AP or >5° V/V)
		Complete	Closed reduction and cast	LLD, malrotation, delayed/nonunion, vascular injury; rotation does not remodel
Tibial spiral (Fig. 10–107)	Toddler's	Spiral tibial Fx in child <6 yo	LLC 3–4 wk	
Bike spoke injury		Soft tissue disruption	Admit, observe, débride	
Stress Fx		Usually involves upper ⅓ of tibia	Bone scan helpful, activity restriction	
Prox. tibial metaphysis	Cozen's	Greenstick in 3–6-yo, complete older	LLC in varus 6 wk	Arterial injury, valgus deformity (usually self-correcting, varus osteotomy if >10 yo), physeal injury
Distal tibial metaphysis		Usually greenstick	Closed reduction, LLC	
ANKLE AND FOOT INJURIES				
Ankle fractures		Dias and Tachdijian		Angular deformity, bony bridge, LLD, DJD, rotational deformity, AVN, short fibula syndrome
		*SI I—Fx of distal fibular physis (Fig. 10–108)	Reduce with foot eversion—SLWC	
		SI II—SI I + SH III or IV of tibial physis	ORIF, transepiphyseal	
		PEER—SH II with lat. metaphyseal fragment + high fibular Fx (Fig. 10–109)		
		SER I—SH II with ant. metaphyseal fragment (Fig. 10–110)	Closed reduction, LLC 3 wk, SLC 3 wk	
		SER II—SER I + spiral Fx fibula	Open reduction if not acceptable	
		SPF—SH II ant. metaphyseal fragment (Fig. 10–111)		

Table continued on page 415

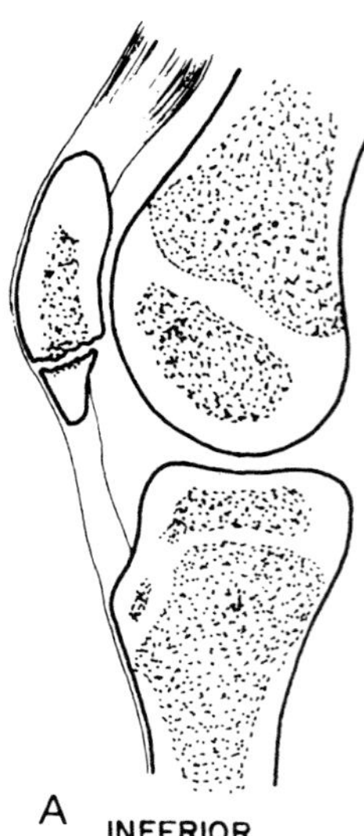

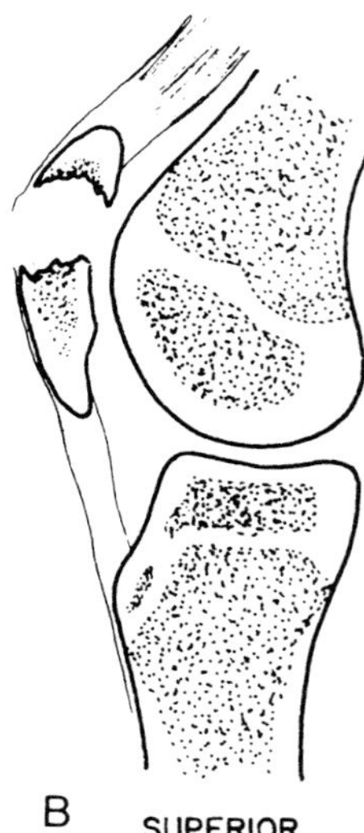

FIGURE 10–106. Patellar sleeve fractures. (From Ogden, J.A.: Skeletal Injury in the Child, 2nd ed., p. 762. Philadelphia, WB Saunders, 1990; reprinted by permission.)

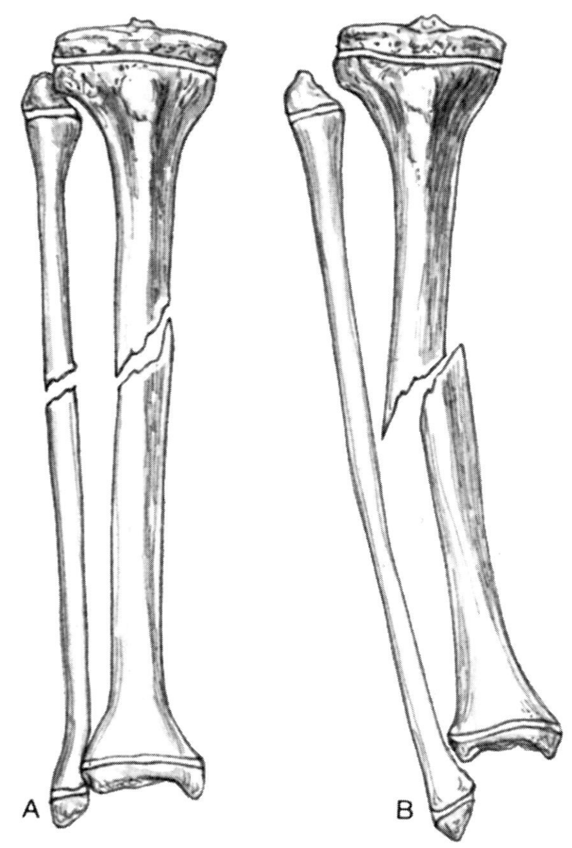

FIGURE 10–107. Spiral fracture of the tibia. Note deforming influence of intact fibula *(B)*. (From Tachdjian, M.O.: Pediatric Orthopaedics, 2nd ed., p. 3296. Philadelphia, WB Saunders, 1990; reprinted by permission.)

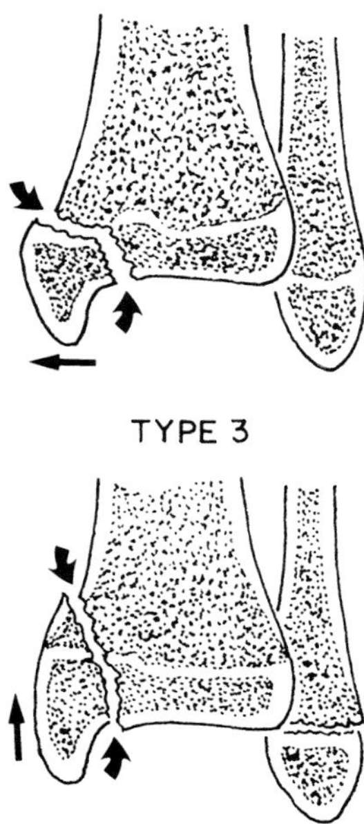

FIGURE 10–108. Supination-inversion ankle fracture. (From Ogden, J.A.: Skeletal Injury in the Child, 2nd ed., p. 837. Philadelphia, WB Saunders, 1990; reprinted by permission.)

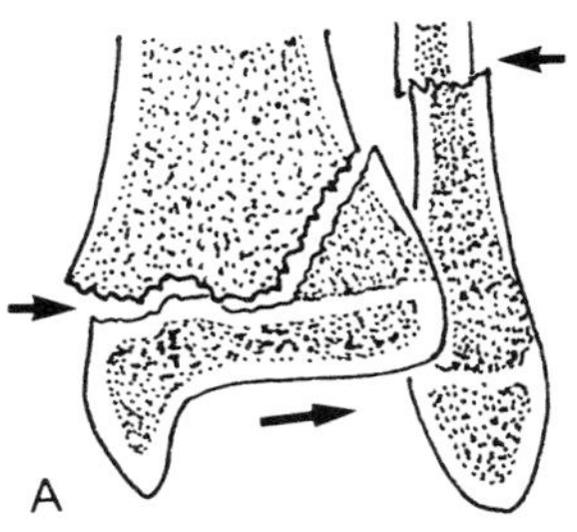

FIGURE 10–109. Pronation-eversion–external rotation ankle fracture. (From Ogden, J.A.: Skeletal Injury in the Child, 2nd ed., p. 836. Philadelphia, WB Saunders, 1990; reprinted by permission.)

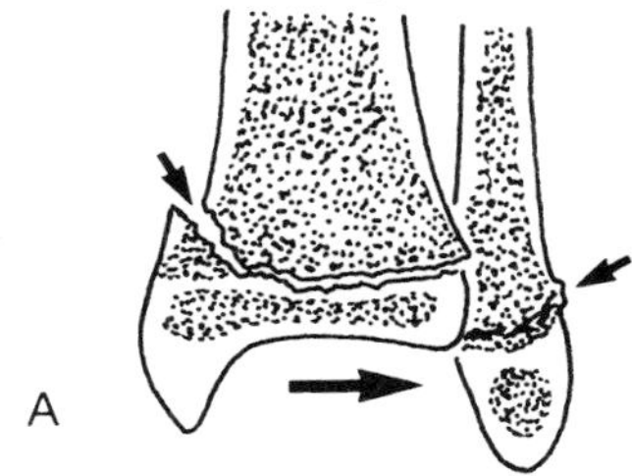

FIGURE 10–110. Supination-external rotation ankle fracture. (From Ogden, J.A.: Skeletal Injury in the Child, 2nd ed., p. 835. Philadelphia, WB Saunders, 1990; reprinted by permission.)

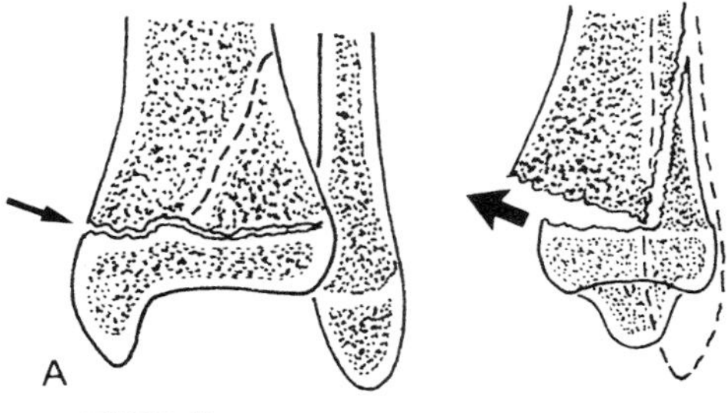

FIGURE 10–111. Supination-plantar flexion ankle fracture. (From Ogden, J.A.: Skeletal Injury in the Child, 2nd ed., p. 836. Philadelphia, WB Saunders, 1990; reprinted by permission.)

TABLE 10–6. *Continued*

INJURY	EPONYM	CLASSIFICATION	TREATMENT	COMPLICATIONS
	Axial compression	SH V of distal tibia	Seen late	Growth arrest, AVN of epiphysis
	Juvenile Tillaux (Fig. 10–112)	SH III of lat. tibial physis	Closed reduction, cast (S, IR), open if required	Missed triplane Fx
	Wagstaff	SH III of distal fibular physis	Closed reduction cast (S, IR), open if required	
	Triplane (Fig. 10–113)	SH III tibia ant.-lat. + SH IV post.-med. + SH I	ORIF fixing all 3 fragments (internally rotate to reduce, fix metaphysis then epiphysis)	
Isolated distal fibula		SH	Anatomic reduction, axial screw	Failure to recognize, DJD
Talar Fxs		Talar neck	Closed reduction, cast in PF, open >2 mm or 5° displacement	AVN (Hawkins sign = good prognosis)
		Talar dome—osteochondral Fx	Open esp. if lat.; excise small, ORIF large fragments	
Calcaneus	Essex-Lopresti	Intra-articular (tongue or joint dep)	>10–11 yo: eval. and Tx similar to adult	
		Extra-articular	Nonop.; >10–11 yo similar to adult	
Tarsometatarsal		Fx at base of 2MT + cuboid Fx	Closed reduction, PCT if unstable; open if necessary	
MT Fxs		Location	Most treated closed	
Base of 5MT	Jones	Metaphyseal	SLC, ORIF ± bone graft nonunion	Increased incidence of nonunion
	Pseudo-Jones	Avulsion of PB	SLC or postop shoe	
Navicular osteochondrosis	Kohler's	Navicular	Symptomatic	

* Most common.
SCIWORA, spinal cord injury without radiologic abnormality; BR, bed rest; LLD, leg-length discrepancy.

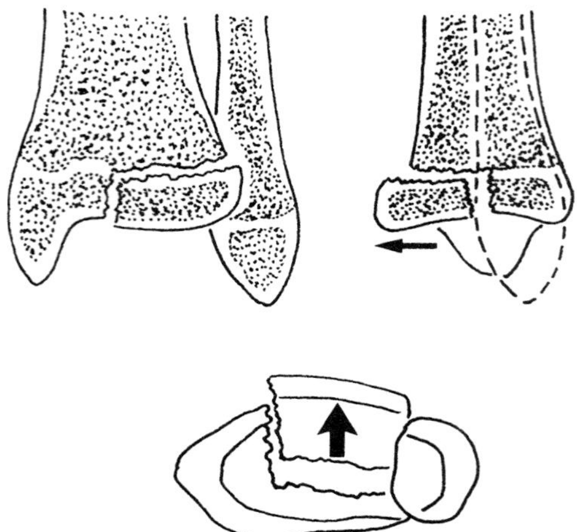

FIGURE 10–112. Juvenile Tillaux fracture. (From Ogden, J.A.: Skeletal Injury in the Child, 2nd ed., p. 838. Philadelphia, WB Saunders, 1990; reprinted by permission.)

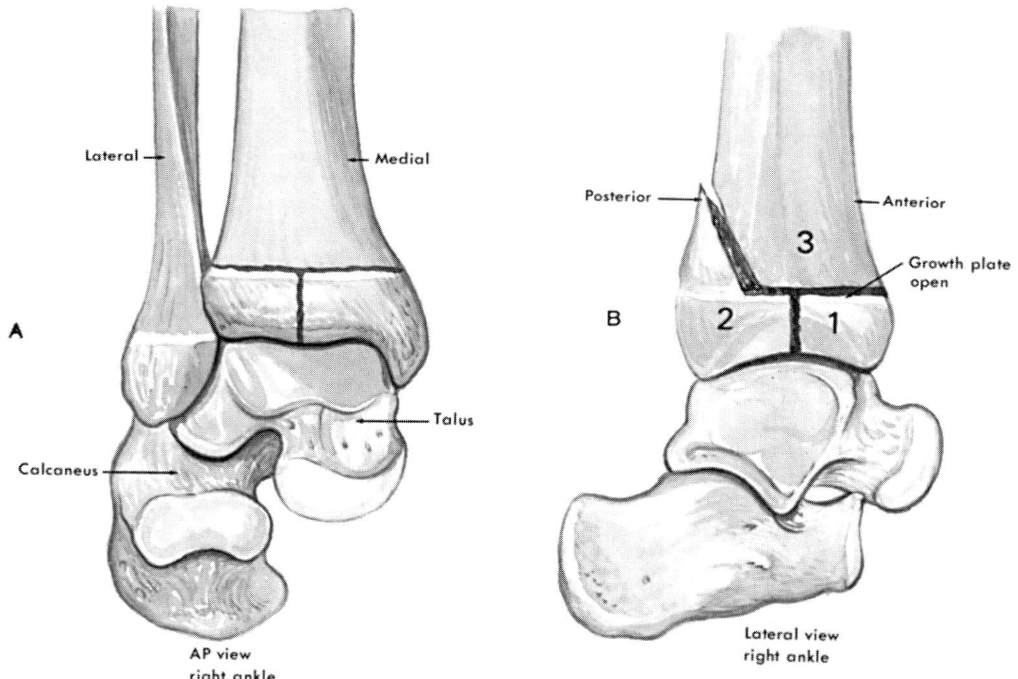

FIGURE 10–113. Triplane fracture. (From Tachdjian, M.O.: Pediatric Orthopaedics, 2nd ed., p. 3324. Philadelphia, WB Saunders, 1990; reprinted by permission.)

Selected Bibliography

General

Amadio, P.C.: Current concepts review: Pain dysfunction syndromes. J. Bone Joint Surg. [Am.] 70:944–949, 1988.

Amato, J.J., Rhinelander, H.F., and Cleveland, R.J.: Post-traumatic adult respiratory distress syndrome. Orthop. Clin. North Am. 9: 693–713, 1978.

Barach, E., Tomlanovich, M., and Nowak, R.: Ballastics: A pathophysiologic examination of the wounding mechanisms of firearms. Part I. J. Trauma 26:225–235; Part II 26:374–383, 1986.

Berquist, T.H., ed.: Imaging of Orthopedic Trauma and Surgery, Philadelphia, WB Saunders, 1986.

Blick, S.S., Brumback, R.J., Poka, A., et al.: Compartment syndrome in open tibia fractures. J. Bone Joint Surg. [Am.] 68:1348–1353, 1986.

Bone, L.B.: Emergency treatment of an injured patient. In Skeletal Trauma, vol. 1, Browner, B., Jupiter, J.B., Levine, A.M., et al., eds., pp. 127–136. Philadelphia, WB Saunders, 1992.

Border, J.R., Allgower, Hansen, S.T., Jr., et al., eds. Blunt Multiple Trauma, New York, Marcel Dekker, 1990.

Brighton, C.T.: Current concepts review: The treatment of nonunions with electricity. J. Bone Joint Surg. [Am.] 63:847–851, 1981.

Chapman, M.W., ed.: Operative Orthopaedics, Philadelphia, JB Lippincott, 1988.

Connolly, J.F., ed.: Depalma's The Management of Fractures and Dislocations, An Atlas, 3rd ed. Philadelphia, WB Saunders, 1981.

Fry, D.E.: Multiple System Organ Failure. St. Louis, Mosby-Year Book, 1992.

Gelman, M.I.: Radiology of Orthopedic Procedures, Problems and Complications, vol. 24. Philadelphia, WB Saunders, 1984.

Godina, M.: Early microsurgical reconstruction of complex trauma of the extremities. Plast. Reconstr. Surg. 78:285–292, 1986.

Gossling, H.R., and Pellegrini, V.D., Jr.: Fat embolism syndrome: A review of the pathophysiology and physiological basis of treatment. Clin. Orthop. 165:68–82, 1982.

Gustilo, R.B., Merkow, R.B., and Templeman, D.: Current concepts review: The management of open fractures. J. Bone Joint Surg. [Am.] 72:299–303, 1990.

Heinrich, S.D., Gallagher, D., Harris, M., and Nadell, J.M.: Undiagnosed fractures in severely injured children and young adults. J. Bone Joint Surg. [Am.] 76:561–572, 1994.

Johansen, K., Danines, M., Howey, T., et al.: Objective criteria accurately predict amputation following lower extremity trauma. J. Trauma 30:508–572, 1990.

Johnson, K.D., Cadambi, A., and Seibert, G.B.: Incidence of adult respiratory distress syndrome in patients with multiple musculoskeletal injuries: Effect of early operative stabilization of fractures. J. Trauma 25:375–383, 1985.

Kozin, S.H., and Berlet, A.C.: Handbook of Common Orthopaedic Fractures. West Chester, PA, Medical Surveillance, 1990.

MacKenzie, E.J., Burgess, A.R., McAndrew, M.P., et al.: Patient oriented functional outcome after unilateral lower extremity fracture. J. Orthop. Trauma 7:393–401, 1993.

Matsen, F.A., III, Winquist, R.A., and Krugmire, R.B., Jr.: Diagnosis and management of compartmental syndromes. J. Bone Joint Surg. [Am.] 62:286–291, 1980.

May, J.W., Jr., Jupiter, J.B., Weiland, A.J., et al.: Current concepts review: Clinical classification of post-traumatic osteomyelitis. J. Bone Joint Surg. [Am.] 71:1422, 1989.

Muller, M.E., Allgower, M., Schneider, R., et al.: Manual of Internal Fixation, 3rd ed. Berlin, Springer-Verlag, 1991.

Orthopaedic Knowledge Update Home Study Syllabus I, II, III, and IV. Chicago, American Academy of Orthopaedic Surgeons, 1984, 1987, 1990, 1993.

Pape, H.C., Dwenger, A., Grotz, et al.: Does the reamer type influence the degree of lung dysfunction after femoral nailing following severe trauma? An animal study, J. Orthop. Trauma 7:300–309, 1994.

Phillips, T.F., and Contreras, D.M.: Current concepts review: Timing of operative treatment of fractures in patients who have multiple injuries. J. Bone Joint Surg. [Am.] 72:784, 1990.

Pollak, R., and Myers, R.A.M.: Early diagnosis of the fat embolism syndrome. J. Trauma 18:121–123, 1978.

Rockwood, C.A., Jr., and Green, D.P., eds.: Fractures in Adults, 3rd ed. Philadelphia, JB Lippincott, 1991.

Steinberg, M.E.: Blood supply to the femoral head and avascular neurosis. Op. Tech. Orthop. 4:94–103, 1994.

Ward, W.G., and Nunley, J.A.: Occult orthopaedic trauma in the multiply injured patient. J. Orthop. Trauma 5:308–312, 1991.

Weber, B.G., and Chech, O.: Pseuanthrosen. Bern, Stuttgart-Wien, Huber, 1973.

Hand and Wrist

Bednar, J.M., and Osterman, A.L.: Carpal instability; Evaluation and treatment. J. Am. Acad. Orthop. Surg. 1:11–17, 1993.

Bradway, J.K., Amadio, P.C., and Cooney, W.P.: Open reduction and internal fixation of displaced, comminuted intra-articular fractures of the distal end of the radius. J. Bone Joint Surg. [Am.] 71: 839, 1989.

Herbert, T.J., and Fisher, W.E.: Management of the fractured scaphoid using a new bone screw. J. Bone Joint Surg. [Br.] 66:114–123, 1984.

Herndon, J.H., ed.: Scaphoid Fractures and Complications. Monograph Series. Rosemont, IL, American Academy of Orthopaedic Surgeons, 1994.

Jupiter, J.B.: Current concepts review: Fractures of the distal end of the radius. J. Bone Joint Surg. [Am.] 73:461–469, 1991.

Jupiter, J.B., and Lipton, H.: The operative treatment of intraarticular fractures of the distal radius. Clin. Orthop. 292:48–61, 1993.

Jupiter, J.B., and Masen, M.: Reconstruction of post traumatic deformity of the distal radius and ulnar. Hand Clin. 4:377–390, 1988.

Letournel, E.: The treatment of acetabular fractures through the ilioinguinal approach. Clin. Orthop. 292:62–76, 1993.

Melone, C.P., Jr.: Open treatment for displaced articular fractures of the distal radius. Clin. Orthop. 202:103–111, 1986.

Stickland, J.W., and Steichen, J.B., eds.: Difficult Problems in Hand Surgery. St. Louis, CV Mosby, 1982.

Taleisnik, J.: Current concepts review: Carpal instability. J. Bone Joint Surg. [Am.] 70:1262–1268, 1988.

Humerus

Amillo, S., Barrios, R.H., Martinez-Peric, R., and Losada, J.I.: Surgical treatment of the radial nerve lesions, associated with fractures of the humerus. J. Orthop. Trauma 7:211–215, 1993.

Horne, G.: Supracondylar fractures of the humerus in adults. J. Trauma 20:71–74, 1980.

Jupiter, J.B., Barnes, K.A., Goodman, L.J., and Saldana, A.E.: Multiplane fractures of the distal humerus. J. Orthop. Trauma 7: 216–220, 1993.

Jupiter, J.B., Neff, U., Holzach, P., et al.: Intercondylar fractures of the humerus: An operative approach. J. Bone Joint Surg. [Am.] 67:226–239, 1985.

Pollock, F.H., Drake, D., Bovill, E.G., et al.: Treatment of radial neuropathy associated with fractures of the humerus. J. Bone Joint Surg. [Am.] 63:239–243, 1981.

Prietto, C.A.: Supracondylar fractures of the humerus. J. Bone Joint Surg. [Am.] 61:425–428, 1979.

Elbow

Broberg, M.A., and Morrey, B.F.: Results of delayed excision of the radial head after fracture. J. Bone Joint Surg. [Am.] 68:669–674, 1986.

Jupiter, J.B.: Internal fixation for fractures about the elbow. Op. Tech. Orthop. 4:31–48, 1994.

Mehlhoff, T.L., Noble, P.C., Bennett, J.B., and Tullos, H.S.: Simple dislocation of the elbow in the adult: Results after closed treatment. J. Bone Joint Surg. [Am.] 70:244, 1988.

O'Driscoll, S.W.: Prosthetic elbow replacement for distal humeral fractures and nonunions. Op. Tech. Orthop. 4:54–57, 1994.

O'Driscoll, S.W.: Technique for unstable olecranon fracture—subluxations. Op. Tech. Orthop. 4:49–53, 1994.

Regan, W., and Morrey, B.: Fractures of the coronoid process of the ulna. J. Bone Joint Surg. [Am.] 71:1348, 1989.

Silberstein, M.J., Brodeur, A.E., and Graviss, E.R.: Some vagaries of the lateral epicondyle. J. Bone Joint Surg. [Am.] 64:444–448, 1982.

Forearm

Chapman, M.W., Gordon, J.E., and Zissimos, A.G.: Compression-plate fixation of acute fractures of the diaphyses of the radius and ulna. J. Bone Joint Surg. [Am.] 71:159, 1989.

DeLuca, P.A., Lindsey, R.W., and Ruwe, P.A.: Refracture of bones in the forearm after removal of compression plates. J. Bone Joint Surg. [Am.] 70:1372–1376, 1988.

Gelberman, R.H., Garfin, S.R., Hergenroeder, P.T., et al.: Compartment syndromes of the forearm: Diagnosis and treatment. Clin. Orthop. 161:252–261, 1981.

Grace, T.G., and Eversmann, W.W.: Forearm fractures. J. Bone Joint Surg. [Am.] 62:433–438, 1980.

Moed, B.R., Kellam, J.F., Foster, R.J., et al.: Immediate internal fixation of open fractures of the diaphysis of the forearm. J. Bone Joint Surg. [Am.] 68:1008–1017, 1986.

Vince, K.G., and Miller, J.E.: Cross union complicating fracture of the forearm. Part I. Adults. J. Bone Joint Surg. [Am.] 69:640–653, 1987.

Shoulder

Flatow, E.L., Pollock, R.G., and Bigliani, L.U.: Operative treatment of two part, displaced surgical neck fractures of the proximal humerus. Op. Tech. Orthop. 4:2–8, 1994.

Goss, T.P.: Current concepts review: Fractures of the glenoid cavity. J. Bone Joint Surg. [Am.] 74:299–305, 1992.

Goss, T.P.: Double disruptions of the superior shoulder suspensory complex. J. Orthop. Trauma 7:99–106, 1993.

Green, A., and Norris, T.R.: Humeral head replacement for four part fractures and fracture dislocations. Op. Tech. Orthop. 4:13–20, 1994.

Herscovici, D., Jr., Fiennes, A.G., Allgower, M., et al.: The floating shoulder-ipsilateral, clavical and scapular neck fractures. J. Bone Joint Surg. [Br.] 74:362–366, 1992.

Jaberg, H., Warner, J.P., and Jakob, R.P.: Percutaneous stabilization of unstable fractures of the humerus. J. Bone Joint Surg. [Am.] 74: 508–515, 1992.

Klassen, J.F., and Cofield, R.H.: Surgical management of scapular fractures, Op. Tech. Orthop. 4:58–63, 1994.

Schlegel, T.F., and Hawkins, R.J.: Displaced proximal humeral fractures: Evaluation and treatment. J. Am. Acad. Orthop. Surg. 2: 54–66, 1994.

Schlegel, T.F., and Hawkins, R.J.: Hemiarthroplasty for the treatment of proximal humeral fractures. Op. Tech. Orthop. 4:21–25, 1994.

Schlegel, T.F., and Hawkins, R.J.: Internal fixation of three part proximal humeral fractures. Op. Tech. Orthop. 4:9–12, 1994.

Sidor, M.L., Zuckerman, J.D., Lyon, T., and Koval, K.: The Neer classification system for proximal humeral fractures—an assessment of interobserver reliability and intraobserver reproducibility. J. Bone Joint Surg. [Am.] 75:1745–1750, 1993.

Siebenrock, K.A., and Gerber, C.: The reproducibility of classification of fractures of the proximal end of the humerus. J. Bone Joint Surg. [Am.] Vol. 75:1751–1755, 1993.

Stableforth, P.G.: Open reduction and internal fixation of displaced four part segment fractures of the proximal humerus. Op. Tech. Orthop. 4:26–30, 1994.

Tanner, M.W., and Cofield, R.H.: Prosthetic arthroplasty for fractures and fracture-dislocations of the proximal humerus. Clin. Orthop. 179:116–128, 1983.

Wilkins, R.M., and Johnston, R.M.: Ununited fractures of the clavicle. J. Bone Joint Surg. [Am.] 65:773–778, 1983.

Zdrovkovic, D., and Damholt, V.V.: Comminuted and severely displaced fractures of the scapula. Acta Orthop. Scand. 45:60–65, 1974.

Spine

Allen, B.L., Jr., Ferguson, R.L., Lehmann, T.R., and O'Brien, R.P.: A mechanistic classification of closed, indirect fractures and dislocations of the lower cervical spine. Spine 7:1–27, 1982.

Bohler, J.: Anterior stabilization for acute fractures and non-unions of the dens. J. Bone Joint Surg. [Am.] 64:18–27, 1982.

Bohlman, H.H.: Acute fractures and dislocations of the cervical spine: An analysis of three hundred hospitalized patients and review of the literature. J. Bone Joint Surg. [Am.] 61:1119–1142, 1979.

Bohlman, H.H.: Treatment of fractures and dislocations of the thoracic and lumbar spine. J. Bone Joint Surg. [Am.] 67:165–169, 1985.

Bradford, D.S., and McBride, G.G.: Surgical management of thoracolumbar spine fractures in incomplete neurologic deficits. Clin. Orthop. 218:201–216, 1987.

Denis, F.: The three column spine and its significance in the classification of acute thoracolumbar spinal injuries. Spine 8:817–831, 1983.

Denis, F.: Updated classification of thoracolumbar fractures. Orthop. Trans. 6:8, 1982.

Drummond, D., Guadagni, J., Keene, J.S., et al.: Interspinous process segmental spinal instrumentation. J. Pediatr. Orthop. 4:397–404, 1984.

Jacobs, R.R., and Casey, M.P.: Surgical management of thoracolumbar injuries: General principles and controversial considerations. Clin. Orthop. 189:22–35, 1984.

Kramer, K.M., and Levine, A.M.: Unilateral facet dislocation of the lumbosacral junction: A case report and review of the literature. J. Bone Joint Surg. [Am.] 71:1258, 1989.

Rizzolo, S.J., and Cotler, J.M.: Unstable cervical spine injuries—specific treatment approaches. J. Am. Acad. Orthop. Surg. 1:57–66, 1993.

Schatzker, J., Rorabeck, C.H., and Waddell, J.P.: Fractures of the dens (odontoid process): An analysis of thirty-seven cases. J. Bone Joint Surg. [Br.] 53:392–405, 1971.

Southwick, W.O.: Current concepts review: Management of fractures of the dens (odontoid process). J. Bone Joint Surg. [Am.] 62: 482–486, 1980.

White, A.A., Southwick, W.O., and Panjabi, M.M.: Clinical instability in the lower cervical spine: A review of past and current concepts. Spine 1:15–27, 1976.

Pelvis and Hip

Bosse, M.J., Poka, A., Reinert, C.M., et al.: Heterotopic ossification as a complication of acetabular fracture: Prophylaxis with low-dose irradiation. J. Bone Joint Surg. [Am.] 70:1231–1237, 1988.

Bucholz, R.W.: The pathologic anatomy of Malgaigne fracture-dislocations of the pelvis. J. Bone Joint Surg. [Am.] 63:400–404, 1981.

Dalal, S.A., Burgess, A.R., Siegal, J.H., et al.: Pelvic fracture and multiple trauma: Classification by mechanism is key to pattern of organ injury, resuscitative requirements and outcome. J. Trauma 29:981–1000, 1989.

Denis, F., Davis, S., and Comfort, T.: Sacral fractures: an important problem: Retrospective analysis of 236 cases. Clin. Orthop. 227: 67–81, 1988.

Dreinhofer, K.E., Schwarz, Kopf, S.R., et al.: Isolated dislocation of the hip: Long term results in 50 patients. J. Bone Joint Surg. [Br.] 76:6–12, 1994.

Epstein, H.C.: Traumatic Dislocation of the Hip. Baltimore, Williams & Wilkins, 1980.

Epstein, H.C., Wiss, D.A., and Cozen, L.: Posterior fracture dislocation of the hip with fractures of the femoral head. Clin. Orthop. 201:9–17, 1985.

Fassler, P.R., Swiontkowski, M.F., Kilrow, A.W., and Routt, M.L.: Injury of the sciatic nerve associated with acetabular fracture. J. Bone Joint Surg. [Am.] 75:1157–1166, 1993.

Hanson, P.B., Milne, J.C., and Chapman, M.W.: Open fractures of the pelvis—review of 43 cases. J. Bone Joint Surg. [Br.] 73: 325–329, 1991.

Horwitz, S.M.: The management of pathological hip fractures. Op. Tech. Orthop. 4:122–129, 1994.

Judet, R., Judet, J., and Letournel, E.: Fractures of the acetabulum: Classification and surgical approaches for open reduction. J. Bone Joint Surg. [Am.] 46:1615–1646, 1964.

Juliano, P.J., Bosse, M.J., and Edwards, K.J.: The superior gluteal artery and complex acetabular procedures: A cadaveric angiographic study. J. Bone Joint Surg. [Am.] 76:244–248, 1994.

Koval, K.J., and Zuckerman, J.D.: Current concepts review: Functional recovery after fracture of the hip. J. Bone Joint Surg. [Am.] 76:751–758, 1994.

Koval, K.J., and Zuckerman, J.D.: Hip fractures. I. Evaluation and treatment of femoral neck fractures. II, Hip fractures: Evaluation and treatment of intertrochanteric fractures. J. Am. Acad. Orthop. Surg. I: 2:141–149, 1994; II: 2:150–156, 1994.

Kyle, R.F.: Fractures of the proximal part of the femur. J. Bone Joint Surg. [Am.] 76:924–950, 1994.

Kyle, R.F., Wright, T.M., and Burstein, A.H.: Biomechanical analysis of the sliding characteristics of compression hip screw. J. Bone Joint Surg. [Am.] 62:1308–1314, 1980.

Lange, R.H., and Hansen, S.T., Jr.: Pelvic ring disruptions with symphysis pubis diastasis: Indications, technique, and limitations of anterior internal fixation. Clin. Orthop. 201:130–137, 1985.

Latenser, B.A., Gentilello, L.M., Tarver, A.A., et al.: Improved outcome with early fixation of skeletally unstable pelvic fractures. J. Trauma, 31:28–31, 1991.

Letournel, E., and Judet, R.: Fractures of the Acetabulum, Elson, R.A., transl., ed. New York, Springer-Verlag, 1981.

Lu-Yao, G.L., Keller, R.B., Littenberg, B., and Wennberg, J.E.: Outcomes after displaced fractures of the femoral neck—meta analysis of 106 published reports. J. Bone Joint Surg. [Am.] 76:15–25, 1994.

Matta, J., Anderson, L., Epstein, H., and Henricks, P.: Fractures of the acetabulum: A retrospective analysis. Clin. Orthop. 205:230–240, 1986.

Matta, J.M., and Saucedo, T.: Internal fixation of pelvic ring fractures. Clin. Orthop. 242:83–97, 1989.

Matta, J.M., Mehne, D.K., and Roffi, R.: Fractures of the acetabulum: Early results of a prospective study. Clin. Orthop. 205:241–250, 1986.

McMurtry, R., Walton, D., Dickinson, D., et al.: Pelvic disruption in the polytraumatized patient: A management protocol. Clin. Orthop. 151:22–30, 1980.

Mears, D.C., and Rubash, H.: Pelvic and acetabular fractures. Thorofare, NJ, Slack, 1986.

Mears, D.C., Capito, C.P., and Deleeuw, H.: Posterior pelvic disruptions managed by the use of the double cobra plate. Instr. Course Lect. 37:143–150, 1988.

Naam, N.H., Brown, W.M., Hurd, R., et al.: Major pelvic fractures. Arch. Surg. 118:610–616, 1983.

Riemer, B.L., Butterfield, S.L., Ray, R.L., and Daffner, R.H.: Clandestine femoral neck fractures with ipsilateral diaphyseal fractures. J. Orthop. Trauma 7:443–449, 1993.

Routt, M.L.C., Jr., and Swiontkowski, M.F.: Operative treatment of complex acetabular fractures: Combined anterior and posterior exposures during the same procedure. J. Bone Joint Surg. [Am.] 72:897, 1990.

Stahaeli, J.W., Frassica, F.J., and Sim, F.H.: Prosthetic replacement of the femoral head for fracture of the femoral neck in patients who have Parkinson disease. J. Bone Joint Surg. [Am.] 70:565–568, 1988.

Swiontkowski, M.F.: Current concepts review: Intracapsular fractures of the hip. J. Bone Joint Surg. [Am.] 76:129–138, 1994.

Tile, M.: Fractures of the Pelvis and Acetabulum. Baltimore, Williams & Wilkins, 1984.

Tile, M.: Pelvic ring fractures: Should they be fixed? J. Bone Joint Surg. [Br.] 70:1–12, 1988.

Young, J.W.R., and Burgess A.R.: Radiographic Management of Pelvic Ring Fractures: Systematic Radiographic Diagnosis. Baltimore: Urban & Schwarzenberg, 1987.

Knee

Benirschke, S.K., Agnew, S.G., Mayo, K.A., et al.: Immediate internal fixation of open, complex tibial plateau fractures: Treatment by standard protocol. J. Orthop. Trauma 6:76–86, 1992.

Carpenter, J.E., Kasman, R., and Matthews, L.S.: Fractures of the patella. J. Bone Joint Surg. [Am.] 75:1550–1561, 1993.

Fernandez, D.L.: Anterior approach to the knee with osteotomy of the tibial tubercle for bicondylar tibial fractures. J. Bone Joint Surg. [Am.] 70:208–219, 1988.

Georgiadis, G.M.: Combined anterior and posterior approaches for complex tibial plateau fractures. J. Bone Joint Surg. [Br.] 76: 285–289, 1994.

Jensen, D.B., Rude, C., Duus, B., and Bjerg-Nielsen, A.: Tibial plateau fractures; A comparison of conservative and surgical treatment. J. Bone Joint Surg. [Br.] 72:49–52, 1990.

Koval, K., Sanders, R., Borrelli, J., et al.: Indirect reduction and percutaneous screw fixation of displaced tibial plateau fractures. J. Orthop. Trauma 6:340–346, 1992.

Saltzman, C.L., Goulet, J.A., McClellan, R.T., et al.: Results of treatment of displaced patellar fractures by partial patellectomy. J. Bone Joint Surg. [Am.] 72:1279, 1990.

Schatzker, J., McBroom, R., and Bruce, D.: The tibial plateau fracture: The Toronto experience, 1968–1975. Clin. Orthop. 138:94–104, 1979.

Weber, M.J., Janecki, C.J., McLeod, P., et al.: Efficacy of various forms of fixation of transverse fractures of the patella. J. Bone Joint Surg. [Am.] 62:215–220, 1980.

Thigh and Leg

Arneson, T.J., Melton, L.J., III, Lewallen, D.G., et al.: Epidemiology of diaphyseal and distal femoral fractures in Rochester, Minnesota, 1965–1984. Clin. Orthop. 234:188–194, 1988.

Behrens, F., and Searls, K.: External fixation of the tibia: Basic concepts and prospective evaluation. J. Bone Joint Surg. [Br.] 68: 246–254, 1986.

Bone, L., and Bucholz, R: The management of fractures in the patient with multiple trauma. J. Bone Joint Surg. [Am.] 68:945–949, 1986.

Bone, L.B., Cassman, S., Stegemann, P., and France, J.: Prospective study of union rate of open tibial fractures treated with locked unreamed intramedullary nails. J. Orthop. Trauma 8:45–49, 1994.

Bone, L.B., Johnson, K.D., Weigelt, J., et al.: Early versus delayed stabilization of femoral fractures: A prospective randomized study. J. Bone Joint Surg. [Am.] 71:336, 1989.

Boynton, M.D., and Schmeling, G.J.: Nonreamed intramedullary nailing of open tibial fractures. J. Am. Acad. Orthop. Surg. 2: 107–114, 1994.

Brumback, R.J., Ellison, T.S., Molligan, H., et al.: Pudendal nerve palsy complicating intramedullary nailing of the femur. J. Bone Joint Surg. [Am.] 74:1450–1455, 1992.

Brumback, R.J., Reilly, J.P., Poka, A., et al.: Intramedullary nailing of femoral shaft fractures. J. Bone Joint Surg. [Am.] 70:1441–1462, 1988.

Cierny, G., III, Byrd, H.S., and Jones, R.E.: Primary versus delayed soft tissue coverage for severe open tibial fractures: A comparison of results. Clin. Orthop. 178:54–63, 1983.

DeLee, J.C., and Stiehl, J.B.: Open tibia fracture with compartment syndrome. Clin. Orthop. 160:175–184, 1981.

Gustilo, R.B., Mendoza, R.M., and Williams, D.N.: Problems in the management of type III (severe) open fractures: A new classification of type III open fractures. J. Trauma 24:742–746, 1984.

Gustilo, R.B., Merkow, R.L., and Templeman, D.: Current concepts review: The management of open fractures. J. Bone Joint Surg. [Am.] 72:299, 1990.

Hack, D.J., and Johnson, E.E.: The use of the unreamed nail and tibial fractures with concomitant preoperative or intraoperative elevated compartment pressure or compartment syndrome. J. Orthop. Trauma 8:203–211, 1994.

Hansen, S.T., and Winquist, R.A.: Closed intrameduallary nailing of the femur: Kuntscher technique with reaming. Clin. Orthop. 138:56–61, 1979.

Holbrook, J.L., Swiontkowski, M.F., and Sanders, R.: Treatment of open fractures of the tibial shaft: Ender nailing versus external fixation; a randomized, prospective comparison. J. Bone Joint Surg. [Am.] 71:1231, 1989.

Hume, E., and Catalano, J.B., Ipsilateral neck and shaft fractures of the femur. Op. Tech. Orthop. 4:111–115, 1994.

Lhowe, D.W., and Hansen, S.T.: Immediate nailing of open fractures of the femoral shaft. J. Bone Joint Surg. [Am.] 70:812–820, 1988.

Mawhinney, I.N., Maginn, P., and McCoy, G.F.: Tibial compartment syndromes after tibial nailing. J. Orthop. Trauma 8:212–214, 1994.

Nowotarski, P., and Brumback, R.J.: Immediate interlocking nailing of fractures of the femur caused by low to mid velocity gunshots. J. Orthop. Trauma. 8:134–141, 1994.

Pritchett, J.W.: Supracondylar fractures of the femur. Clin. Orthop. 184:173–177, 1984.

Schatzker, J., and Lambert, D.C.: Supracondylar fractures of the femur. Clin. Orthop. 138:77–83, 1979.

Suedkamp, N.P., Barbey, N., Vueskens, A., et al: The incidence of osteitis in open fractures: An analysis of 948 open fractures (a review of the Hanover experience). J. Orthop. Trauma 7:473–482, 1993.

Swiontkowski, M.F., Hansen, S.T., Jr., and Kellam, J.: Ipsilateral fractures of the femoral neck and shaft: A treatment protocol. J. Bone Joint Surg. [Am.] 66:260–268, 1984.

Talucci, R.C., Manning, J., Lampard, S., et al.: Early intramedullary nailing of femoral shaft fractures: A cause of fat embolism syndrome. Am. J. Surg. 146:107–110, 1983.

Tornetta, P., Bergman, M., Watnik, N., et al.: Treatment of grade III B open tibial fractures—a prospectic randomized comparison of external fixation in non-reamed locked nailing. J. Bone Joint Surg. [Br.] 76:13–19, 1994.

Whittle, A.P., Russell, T.A., Taylor, J.C., and Lavelle, D.G.: Treatment of open fractures of the tibial shaft with the use of interlocking nailing without reaming. J. Bone Joint Surg. [Am.] 74: 1162–1171, 1992.

Winquist, R.R., Waddell, J.P., Sullivan, T.R., et al.: Infra-isthmal fractures of the femur: A review of 82 cases. J. Trauma 24:735–741, 1984.

Zickel, R.E.: Subtrochanteric femoral fractures. Orthop. Clin. North Am. 11:555–568, 1980.

Ankle and Foot

Canale, S.T., and Kelly, F.B.: Fractures of the neck of the talus. J. Bone Joint Surg. [Am.] 60:143–156, 1978.

DeCoster, T.A., and Miller, R.A.: Management of traumatic foot wounds. J. Am. Acad. Orthop. Surg. 2:226–230, 1994.

DeLee, J.C., and Curtis, R.: Subtalar dislocation of the foot. J. Bone Joint Surg. [Am.] 64:433–437, 1982.

Faciszewski, T., Burks, R.T., and Manaster, B.J.: Subtle injuries of the Lisfranc joint. J. Bone Joint Surg. [Am.] 72:1519, 1990.

Giachino, A.A., and Uhthoff, H.K.: Current concepts review: Intra-articular fractures of the calcaneus. J. Bone Joint Surg. [Am.] 71: 784–787, 1989.

Goossens, M., and De Stoop, N.: Lisfranc's fracture-dislocations: Etiology, radiology, and results of treatment: a review of 20 cases. Clin. Orthop. 176:154–162, 1983.

Harper, M.C., and Hardin, G.: Posterior malleolar fractures of the ankle associated with external rotation-abduction injuries: Results with and without internal fixation. J. Bone Joint Surg. [Am.] 70:1348–1356, 1988.

Lindsay, W.R.N., and Dewar, R.P.: Fractures of the os calcis. Am. J. Surg. 95:555–576, 1958.

Macey, L.R., Benirschke, S.K., Sangeorzan, B.J., and Hansen, S.T.: Acute calcaneal fractures: Treatment, options, and results. J. Am. Acad. Orthop. Surg. 2:36–43, 1994.

Marti, R.K., Raaymakers, E.L., and Nolte, P.A.: Malunited ankle fractures—the late results of reconstruction. J. Bone Joint Surg. [Br.] 72:709–713, 1990.

McReynolds, I.S.: The Case for Operative Treatment of Fractures of the Os Calcis. Philadelphia, WB Saunders, 1982.

Ovadia, D.N., and Beals, R.K.: Fractures of the tibial plafond. J. Bone Joint Surg. [Am.] 68:543–551, 1986.

Sangeorzan, B.J., Benirschke, S.K., Mosca, V., et al.: Displaced intra-articular fractures of the tarsal navicular. J. Bone Joint Surg. [Am.] 71:1504, 1989.

Segal, D.: Displaced Ankle Fractures Treated Surgically and Postoperative Management. St. Louis, CV Mosby, 1979.

Stephenson, J.R.: Treatment of displaced intra-articular fractures of the calcaneus using medial and lateral approaches, internal fixation, and early motion. J. Bone Joint Surg. [Am.] 69:115–130, 1987.

Swanson, T.V., Bray, T.J., and Holmes, G.B.: Fractures of the talar neck: A mechanical study of fixation. J. Bone Joint Surg. [Am.] 74:544–551, 1992.

Pediatrics

Akbarnia, B., Torg, J.S., Kirkpatrick, J., and Sussman, S.: Manifestations of the battered-child syndrome. J. Bone Joint Surg. [Am.] 56: 1159–1166, 1974.

Bright, R.W.: Partial growth arrest: Identification, classification, and results of treatment. Orthop. Trans. 6:65–66, 1982.

Bryan, W.J., and Tullos, H.S.: Pediatric pelvic fractures: Review of 52 patients. J. Trauma 19:799–805, 1979.

Canale, S.T.: Traumatic dislocation and fracture-dislocation of the hips in children. In The Hip—Proceedings of the Ninth Open Scientific Meeting of the Hip Society, pp. 219–245. St. Louis, CV Mosby, 1981.

Ertl, J.P., Barrack, R.L., Alexander, A.H., and Van Buecken, K.: Triplane fracture of the distal tibial epiphysis: Long term follow-up. J. Bone Joint Surg. [Am.] 70:967, 1988.

Foster, D.E., Sullivan, J.A., and Gross, R.H.: Lateral humeral condylar fractures in children. J. Pediatr. Orthop. 5:16–22, 1985.

Fowles, J.V., and Kassab, M.T.: Displaced fractures of the medial humeral condyle in children. J. Bone Joint Surg. [Am.] 62: 1159–1163, 1980.

Fowles, J.V., Sliman, N., and Kassab, M.T.: The Monteggia lesion in children: Fracture of the ulna and dislocation of the radial head. J. Bone Joint Surg. [Am.] 65:1276–1283, 1983.

Galleno, H., and Oppenheim, W.L.: The battered child syndrome revisited. Clin. Orthop. 162:11–19, 1982.

Helfer, R.E., and Kempe, R.S., eds.: The Battered Child, 4th ed. Chicago, University of Chicago Press, 1987.

Hensinger, R.N., ed.: Operative Management of Lower Extremity Fractures in Children. Monograph Series. Rosemont, IL, American Academy of Orthopaedic Surgeons, 1992.

Hughes, L.O., and Beaty, J.H.: Current concepts review: Fractures of the head and neck of the femur in children. J. Bone Joint Surg. [Am.] 76:283–292, 1994.

King, J., Diefendorf, D., Apthorp, J., et al.: Analysis of 429 fractures in 189 battered children. J. Pediatr. Orthop. 8:585–589, 1988.

Klassen, R.A., and Peterson, H.A.: Excision of physeal bars: The Mayo Clinic experience, 1968–1978. Orthop. Trans. 6:65, 1982.

Kregor, P.J., Song, K.M., Routt, M.L., et al.: Plate fixation of femoral shaft fractures in multiple injured children. J. Bone Joint Surg. [Am.] 75:1774–1780, 1993.

McDonald, G.A.: Pelvic disruptions in children, Clin. Orthop. 151: 130–134, 1980.

Millis, M.B., Singer, I.J., and Hall, J.E.: Supracondylar fracture of the humerus in children: Further experience with a study in orthopaedic decision-making. Clin. Orthop. 188:90–97, 1984.

Morrissey, R.T.: Fractured Hip in Childhood. St. Louis, CV Mosby, 1984.

Ogden, J.A.: Skeletal Injury in the Child, 2nd ed. Philadelphia, WB Saunders, 1990.

Odgen, J.A., Tross, R.B., and Murphy, M.J.: Fractures of the tibial tuberosity in adolescents. J. Bone Joint Surg. [Am.] 62:205–215, 1980.

Phillips, W.A., and Hensinger, R.N.: The management of rotatory atlanto-axial subluxation in children. J. Bone Joint Surg. [Am.] 71: 664, 1989.

Pirone, A.M., Graham, H.K., and Krajbich, J.I.: Management of displaced extension-type supracondylar fractures of the humerus in children. J. Bone Joint Surg. [Am.] 70:641–650, 1988.

Rang, M.: Children's Fractures. Philadelphia, JB Lippincott, 1974.

Rockwood, C.A., Jr., Wilkins, K.E., and King, R.E., eds.: Fractures in Children, 3rd ed. Philadelphia, JB Lippincott, 1991.

Steinberg, E.L., Golomb, D., Salama, R., et al.: Radial head and neck fractures of the femoral neck in patients who have Parkinson disease. J. Pediatr. Orthop. 8:35–40, 1988.

Tibone, J.E., and Stoltz, M.: Fractures of the radial head and neck in children. J. Bone Joint Surg. [Am.] 63:100–106, 1981.

Vince, K.G., and Miller, J.E.: Cross union complicating fracture of the forearm. Part II. Children. J. Bone Joint Surg. [Am.] 69: 654–660, 1987.

Von Laer, L.: Classification, diagnosis, and treatment of transitional fractures of the distal part of the tibia. J. Bone Joint Surg. [Am.] 67:687–698, 1985.

Wiley, J.J., and Galey, J.P.: Monteggia injuries in children. J. Bone Joint Surg. [Br.] 67:728–731, 1985.

Wilkins, K.E., ed.: Operative Management of Upper Extremity Fractures in Children. Monograph Series. Rosemont, IL, American Academy of Orthopaedic Surgeons, 1994.

11

ANATOMY

BEN A. GOMEZ

I. Introduction

A. Osteology—Study of bones. There are 80 bones in the axial skeleton and 126 bones in the appendicular skeleton, for a total of 206 bones in the human skeleton. There are four general types of bones: long (e.g., femur), short (e.g., phalanges), flat (e.g., scapulae), and irregular (e.g., vertebrae). Ossification, or the formation of bone, can be intramembranous (without a cartilage model, as in the skull) or enchondral (with a cartilage model; most bones). Enchondral growth begins in the diaphyses of long bones at a primary ossification center, most of which are present at birth. Secondary ossification centers usually develop in the periphery of bone and are important for growth and the treatment of childhood fractures. Anatomic landmarks of the skeleton and their related structures are listed in Table 11–1.

B. Arthrology—Study of joints, specialized structures that allow articulation of various bones. Joints are reinforced by ligaments, capsules, and other structures that may restrict movement and add stability. Joints are commonly classified into three types based on their freedom of movement: (1) synarthroses; (2) amphiarthroses; (3) diarthroses. Although **synarthroses,** such as the sutures in the skull, may have motion during early childhood, they usually have no motion at maturity and simply serve to join two bony elements. **Amphiarthrodial** joints, such as the symphysis pubis, have hyaline cartilage and intervening discs. Limited motion is possible. In true **diarthrodial** joints, motion is enhanced and is characterized by hyaline cartilage, synovial membranes, capsules, and ligaments. Diarthrodial joints are further classified based on their degrees of freedom of motion and their shape. Uniaxial joints (ginglymus [e.g., hinge] and trochoid [e.g., pivot]) allow movement in one plane. Biaxial joints (e.g., condyloid, ellipsoid, saddle joints) allow movement in two planes. Polyaxial (spheroidal [e.g., ball and socket]) allow movement in any direction. Finally, plane (gliding) joints allow only slight sliding of one joint surface over another.

C. Myology—Study of muscles, structures that are capable of contraction and power movement. Fascia (dense connective tissue) surrounds muscle groups, divides them into compartments, and serves as attachments for muscles. Several arrangements of fibers allows classification of muscles into the following categories: parallel (e.g., rhomboids), fusiform (e.g., biceps brachii), oblique (with tendinous interdigitation—further subclassified as pennate, bipennate, multipennate), triangular (e.g., pectoralis minor), and spiral (e.g., latissimus dorsi). Knowledge of origins and insertions of skeletal muscle is critical to understanding their functions.

D. Nerves—Most peripheral nerves originate from the ventral rami of spinal nerves and are distributed via several plexii (cervical, brachial, lumbosacral). Efferent, or motor, fibers carry impulses from the CNS to muscles; afferent, or sensory, fibers carry information toward the CNS. The autonomic nervous system controls visceral structures and consists of the parasympathetic (craniosacral) and sympathetic (thoracolumbar) divisions. Preganglionic neurons of parasympathetic nerves arise in the nuclei of CNs III, VII, IX, and X and in the S2, S3, and S4 segments of the spinal cord; they synapse in peripheral ganglia. Preganglionic neurons in the sympathetic system are located in the spinal cord (T1–L3) and synapse in chain ganglia adjacent to the spine and collateral ganglia along major abdominal blood vessels.

E. Vessels—Consist of arteries, veins, and lymphatics. Of primary concern to the orthopaedist is avoiding major injury to these structures. Their courses and relationships are important.

F. Surgical Approaches (Tables 11–2, 11–3)—Usually are based on entering an internervous interval and are planned for as little disruption to other structures as possible.

II. Shoulder

A. Osteology—The shoulder girdle is composed of the scapula and clavicle and serves to attach the upper limb to the trunk. The shoulder (glenohumeral) joint is the attachment of the upper humerus (discussed in Section III: Upper Arm) to the shoulder girdle.

1. Scapula—Spans the second through seventh ribs and serves as an attachment for 17 muscles and four ligaments. It has two surfaces, costal and dorsal, and three processes: spine, acromion, and coracoid. It also has three borders (superior, lateral, medial) and three angles (inferior, superior, lateral). The scapula has one primary and six secondary ossification centers.

OSSIFICATION CENTER	AGE AT APPEARANCE	ORDER OF FUSION
Body (primary	8 weeks (fetal)	1
Coracoid (tip)	1 year	2
Coracoid	15 years	3
Acromion	15 years	4

TABLE 11–1. SKELETAL GROOVES, NOTCHES, AND POINTS

REGION	GROOVE OR NOTCH	IMPORTANT RELATED STRUCTURES
Hand	Hook of Hamate	Ulnar nerve
	Trapezial groove	FCR tendon
Wrist	Distal ulna	ECU
	Radial styloid	EPL
Elbow	Medial supracondylar process	Median nerve, brachial artery
Shoulder	Scapular notch	Suprascapular nerve
	Supraglenoid tubercle	Long head biceps brachii
	Infraglenoid tubercle	Long head triceps brachii
Hip	ASIS	Sartorius
	AIIS	Dir. head of rectus femoris
	Ischial spine	Coccygeus, levator ani
	Lesser sciatic foramen	Pudendal nerve
	Piriformis fossa	Obturator externus
	Tip of greater trochanter	Piriformis
	Quadrate tubercle	Quadratus femoris
	Lesser trochanter	Psoas minor
Knee	Hunter's canal	Femoral → popliteal artery
	Adductor tubercle	Adductor magnus
	Gerdy's tubercle	IT band
	Fibular neck	Common peroneal nerve
Foot	Henry's knot	FDL–FHL intersection
	Sustentaculum tali	Spring ligament (FHL inferior)
	Base of fifth metatarsal	Peroneus brevis/plantar aponeurosis
	Tuberosity of navicular	Tibialis posterior
	Cuboid groove	Peroneus longus
	Sinus tarsi	Ligamentum cervis tali and EDB

OSSIFICATION CENTER	AGE AT APPEARANCE	ORDER OF FUSION
Acromion	16 years	5
Inferior angle	16 years	6
Medial border	16 years	7

2. Clavicle—Acts as a fulcrum for lateral movement of the arm. It has a double curvature (sternal-ventral, acromial-dorsal) and serves as an attachment for the upper extremity. The clavicle is the **first bone in the body to ossify and the last to fuse.** It has two primary and one secondary ossification centers.

OSSIFICATION CENTER	AGE AT APPEARANCE	AGE AT FUSION
Medial (primary)	5 weeks (fetal)	
Lateral (primary)	5 weeks (fetal)	
Sternal	19 years	25 years

B. Arthrology—The shoulder area has one major (glenohumeral) and several minor (sternoclavicular, acromioclavicular, scapulothoracic) articulations. Additionally, there are numerous ligaments associated with each articulation.

1. Glenohumeral Joint—Articulation between the glenoid fossa and the proximal humerus. It is classified as a spheroidal, or ball-and-socket, joint. The articular surface of the glenoid is thickest at the periphery. This joint has the greatest ROM of any joint but limited inherent stability, and it relies on the rotator cuff tendons and the following ligaments for support (Fig. 11–1).

TABLE 11–2. SUMMARY OF POPULAR ORTHOPAEDIC SURGICAL APPROACHES: UPPER EXTREMITY

REGION	APPROACH	EPONYM	MUSCULAR INTERVAL 1 (NERVE)	MUSCULAR INTERVAL 2 (NERVE)	DANGERS
Shoulder	Anterior	Henry	Deltoid (axillary)	Pec. major (med./lat. pectoral)	MC N/cephalic V
	Lateral		Deltoid (splitting) (axillary)	Deltoid (splitting) (axillary)	Axillary N
	Posterior		Infraspinatus (suprascapular)	Teres minor (axillary)	Ax. N/post. cir. hum. A
Prox. humerus	Anterolateral	Deltoid (axillary)	Pec. major (med./lat. pectoral)	Radial and axillary N/ant circ. hum. A	
Distal humerus	Anterolateral		Brachialis (musculocutaneous)	Brachioradialis (radial)	Radial N
	Lateral	Triceps (radial)	Brachioradialis (radial)	Radial N	
Humerus	Posterior	Lat. triceps (radial)	Long triceps (radial)	Radial N/brachial A	
Elbow	Anterolateral	Henry	Brachialis/pron. teres (musculocut./median)	Brachioradialis (radial)	Lat. ABC N/radial N
	Posterolateral	Kocher	Anconeus (radial)	Ext. carpi ulnaris (PIN)	PIN (diss. to ann. lig.)
	Medial		Brachialis (musculocutaneous)	Triceps/pron. teres (radial/median)	Ulnar N
Forearm	Anterior	Henry	Brachioradialis (radial)	Pronator teres/FCR (median)	PIN
	Dorsal	Thompson	ECRB (radial)	EDC/EPL (PIN)	PIN
	Ulnar		ECU (PIN)	FCU (ulnar)	Ulnar N and A
Wrist	Dorsal		Third compartment (PIN)	Fourth compartment (PIN)	
Scaphoid	Volar	Russe	FCR or through sheath (median)	Radial A	Radial A
	Dorsolateral	Matti	First compartment (PIN)	Third compartment (PIN)	Sup. rad. N/radial A

N, nerve; A, artery; V, vein; PIN, posterior interosseous nerve; ABC, antebrachial cutaneous.

TABLE 11–3. SUMMARY OF POPULAR ORTHOPAEDIC SURGICAL APPROACHES: LOWER EXTREMITY

REGION	APPROACH	EPONYM	MUSCULAR INTERVAL 1 (NERVE)	MUSCULAR INTERVAL 2 (NERVE)	DANGERS
Iliac crest	Posterior		Gluteus maximus (inferior gluteal)	Latissimus dorsi (long thoracic)	Clunial N, SGA, Sciatic N
	Anterior		TFL/glut. med. & min. (superior gluteal)	Ext. abd. oblique (segmental)	ASIS/LFCN
Hip	Anterior	Smith-Peterson	Sartorius/rectus fem. (femoral)	TFL/gluteus medius (sup. gluteal)	LFCN, Fem. N, Asc. br. LFCA
	Anterolateral	Watson-Jones	Tensor fasciae latae (sup. gluteal)	Gluteus medius (sup. gluteal)	Fem. NAV/Profunda A
	Lateral	Hardinge	Splits glut. med. (sup. gluteal)	Splits vastus lat. (femoral)	Femoral NVA/LFCA (transverse br.)
	Posterior	Moore-Southern	Splits glut. max. (inf. gluteal)	N/A	Sciatic, inf. glut. A
	Medial	Ludloff	Add. longus/add. brevis (ant. div. obt.)	Gracilis/add. magnus (obt./tibial)	Ant. div. obt. N/MFCA
Thigh	Lateral		Vastus lateralis (femoral)	Vastus lateralis (femoral)	Perf. br. profundus
	Posterolateral		Vastus lateralis (femoral)	Hamstrings (sciatic)	Perf. br. profundus
	Anteromedial		Rectus femoris (femoral)	Vastus medialis (femoral)	Med. sup. geniculate A
Distal femur	Posterior		Biceps femoris (sciatic)	Vastus lateralis (femoral)	Sciatic/N PFCN
Knee	Med. parapatellar		Vastus medialis (femoral)	Rectus femoris (femoral)	Infrapatellar br. saphenous N
	Medial		Vastus medialis (femoral)	Sartorius (femoral)	Infrapatellar br. saphenous N
	Lateral		Iliotibial band (sup. gluteal)	Biceps femoris (sciatic)	Peroneal N/popliteus ten.
	Posterior		Semimem./lat. gastroc. (tibial)	Biceps/lat. gastroc. (tib.)/(tib.)	Med. sural cut. N/tib. N/ peroneal N
	Lateral		Vastus lateralis (femoral)	Biceps femoris (sciatic)	Peroneal N/lat. sup. gen. A
Tibia	Posterolateral		GS, soleus, FHL (tibial)	Peroneus brevis/longus (sup. peroneal)	Sm saph. V/post. tib. A
	Anterior		Tibialis anterior (peroneal)	Periosteum	Long saph. V
Ankle	Anterior		EHL (deep peroneal)	EDL (deep peroneal)	S and D peroneal N/ant. tib. A
Med. malleolus	Posterior		Tibialis posterior	FDL	Saphenous N and V
Ankle	Posterolateral		Peroneus brevis (sup. peroneal)	FHL (tibial)	Sural N/sm saph. V
Distal fibula	Lateral		Peroneus tertius (deep peroneal)	Peroneus brevis (sup. peroneal)	Sural N
Ankle	Anterolateral		Peroneal muscles (sup. peroneal)	EDC and per. tertius (deep peroneal)	Deep per. N/ant. tib. A
	Posteromedial		TP or FDL	FDL or FHL	Post. tib. A/tib N

A, artery; V, vein; N, nerve; S, superficial; D, decr; LFCA, lateral femoral circumflex artery; MFCA, medial femoral circumflex artery; SGA, superior gluteal artery; PFCN, posterior femoral cutaneous nerve; LFCN, lateral femoral cutaneous nerve.

LIGAMENT	FUNCTION
Capsule	Support/boundary layer
Coracohumeral	Anterior support; tightens with flexion
Glenohumeral	Superior, middle, inferior (inferior strongest)
Glenoid labrum	Increases surface area, stability
Transverse humeral	Maintains biceps (long head) in groove

2. Sternoclavicular (SC) Joint—Double gliding joint with an articular disc. Its ligaments include the capsule, anterior and posterior sternoclavicular ligaments, an interclavicular ligament, and a costoclavicular ligament (strongest). The SC joint rotates 30 degrees with shoulder motion.
3. Acromioclavicular (AC) Joint—Plane/gliding joint that also possesses a disc. Its ligaments (Fig. 11–2) include the capsule, acromioclavicular ligament, and coracoclavicular (CC) ligament (with trapezoid [anterolateral] and conoid [posteromedial and stronger] component ligaments). The AC ligament prevents anteroposterior displacement of the distal clavicle. The CC ligament prevents superior displacement of the distal clavicle.
4. Scapulothoracic Joint—Although not a true joint, this attachment allows scapular movement against the posterior rib cage. It is fixed primarily by the scapular muscle attachment.
5. Intrinsic Ligaments of the Scapula—Include the superior transverse scapular ligament (which separates the suprascapular nerve and vessels)

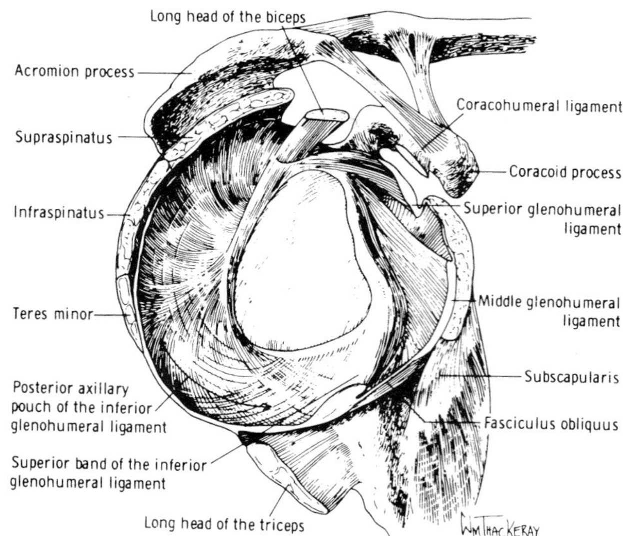

FIGURE 11–1. Glenohumeral ligaments and rotator cuff muscles. (From Turkel, S.J., Paño, M.W., Marshall, J.L., and Girgis, F.G.: Stabilizing mechanisms preventing anterior dislocation of the glenohumeral joint. J. Bone Joint Surg. [Am.] 63:1209, 1981; reprinted by permission.)

and the coracoacromial ligament (which is a frequent cause of impingement).

C. Muscles of the Shoulder (Fig. 11–3)—Serve a variety of functions. Five muscles help connect the upper limb to the vertebral column (trapezius, latissimus, both rhomboids, and the levator scapulae). Four muscles connect the upper limb to the thoracic wall (both pectoralis muscles, subclavius, and serratus anterior). Finally, six muscles act on the shoulder joint itself (deltoid, teres major, and the four rotator cuff muscles [supraspinatus, infraspinatus, teres minor, subscapularis]). The rotator cuff muscles serve to depress and stabilize the humeral head against the glenoid. Table 11–4 presents specifics on these muscles. The shoulder has been described as having four supporting layers (Fig. 11–4).

LAYER	STRUCTURE
I	Deltoid
	Pectoralis major
II	Clavipectoral fascia
	Conjoined tendon, short head biceps and coracobrachialis
	Coracoacromial ligament
III	Deep layer of subdeltoid bursa
	Rotator cuff muscle (subscapularis, supraspinatus, infraspinatus, teres minor)
IV	Glenohumeral joint capsule
	Coracohumeral ligament

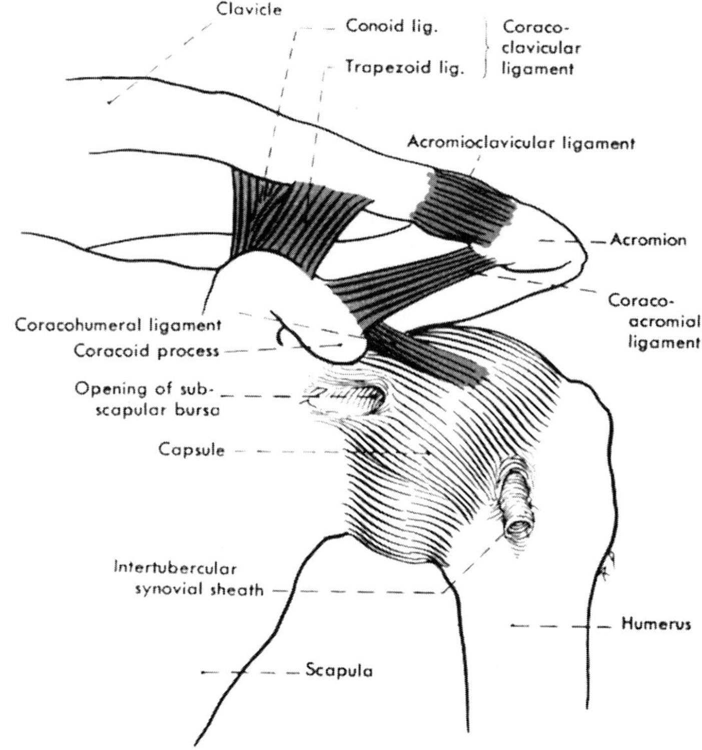

FIGURE 11–2. Ligaments about the shoulder. (From Jenkins, D.B.: Hollinshead's Functional Anatomy of the Limbs and Back, 6th ed., p. 71. Philadelphia, WB Saunders, 1991; reprinted by permission.)

FIGURE 11–3. Origins ▨ and insertions ▧ of muscles about the shoulder girdle. (From Jenkins, D.B.: Hollinshead's Functional Anatomy of the Limbs and Back, 6th ed., Fig. 5–3. Philadelphia, WB Saunders, 1991; reprinted by permission.)

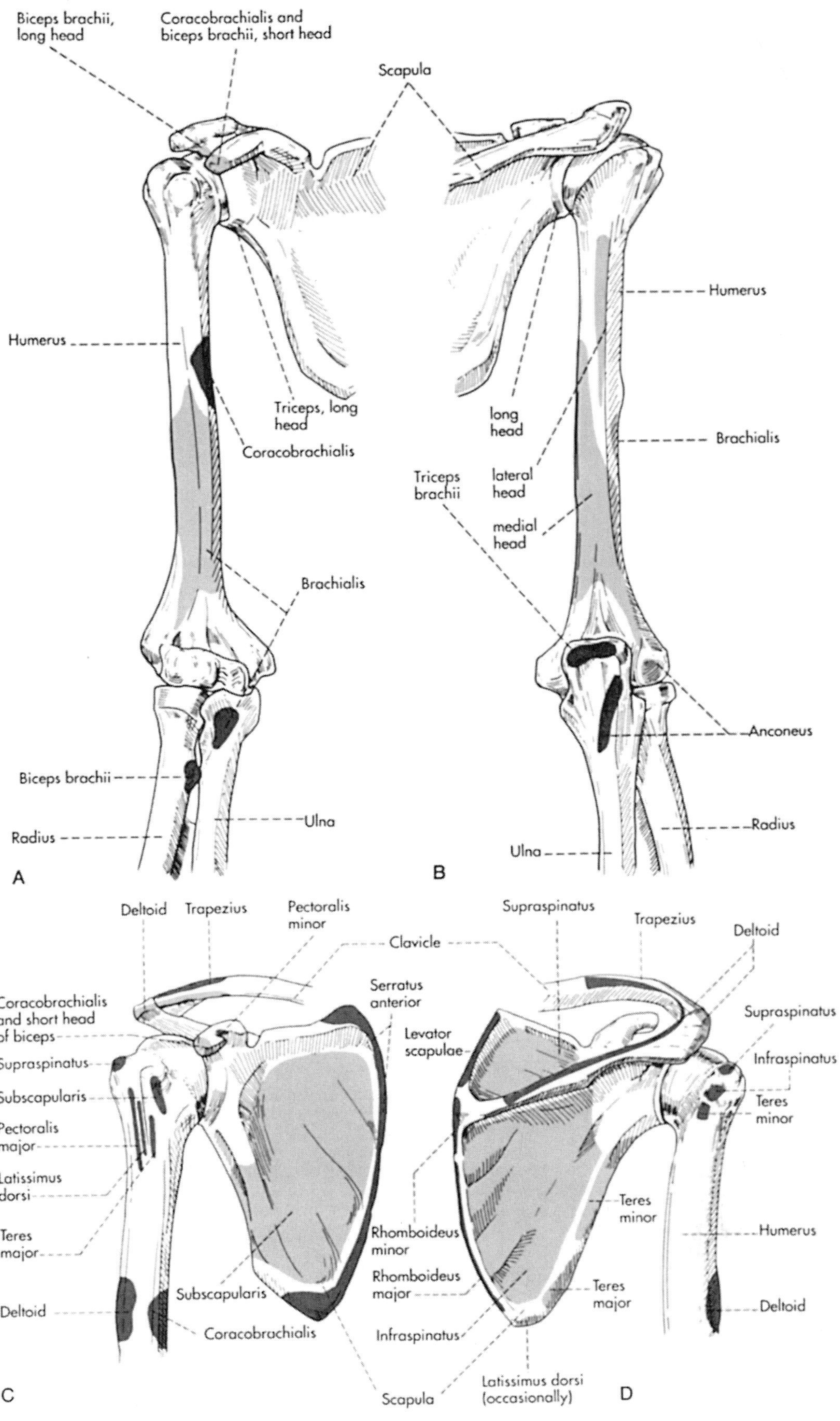

Biceps brachii, long head
Coracobrachialis and biceps brachii, short head
Scapula
Humerus
Triceps, long head
Coracobrachialis
Brachialis
Biceps brachii
Ulna
Radius
A
Humerus
long head
Brachialis
Triceps brachii
lateral head
medial head
Anconeus
Radius
Ulna
B
Deltoid
Trapezius
Pectoralis minor
Clavicle
Serratus anterior
Coracobrachialis and short head of biceps
Supraspinatus
Subscapularis
Pectoralis major
Latissimus dorsi
Teres major
Deltoid
Subscapularis
Coracobrachialis
Scapula
C
Supraspinatus
Trapezius
Deltoid
Levator scapulae
Supraspinatus
Infraspinatus
Teres minor
Teres minor
Rhomboideus minor
Humerus
Rhomboideus major
Teres major
Deltoid
Infraspinatus
Latissimus dorsi (occasionally)
D

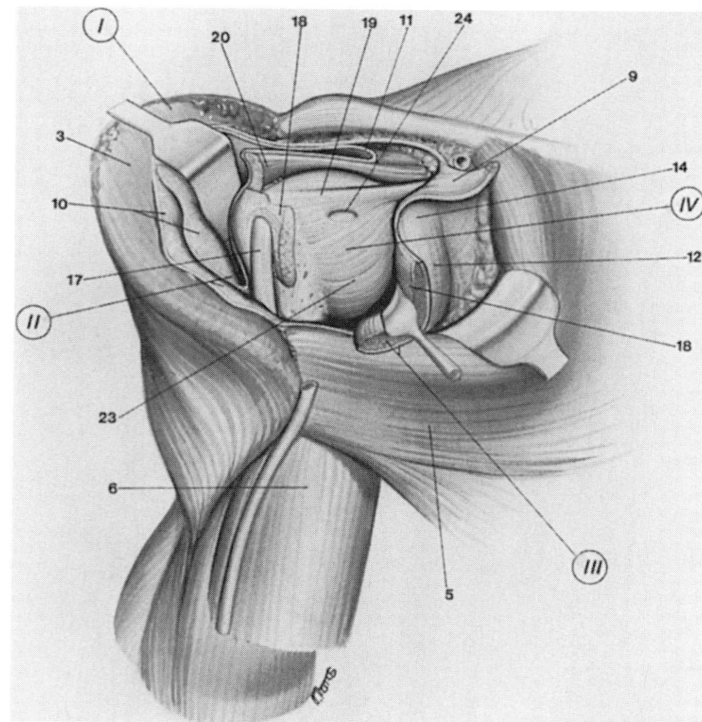

FIGURE 11–4. Anterior aspect of the right shoulder depicting the four layers (encircled Roman numerals). The lateral retractor is placed deep to layer 2, demonstrating the ease of dissection in the plane of the bursa around the lateral aspect of the proximal humerus. The subscapularis and supraspinatus (layer 3) have been reflected, disclosing layer 4 (capsule and coracohumeral ligament). The usual shape and position of the defect in the rotator interval (if present) is depicted; it is variable (3 = deltoid; 5 = pectoralis major; 6 = biceps; 9 = C-A ligament; 10 = fasci (II); 11 = deep layer of subacromial tendon b, and subscapular; 12 = conjoined tendon; 14 = tip of coracoid process; 17 = biceps long hd.; 18 = deep layer subacromial b, and subscapular; 19 = coracohumeral ligament; 20 = supraspinatus under deep bursa layer; 23 = joint capsule; 24 = hiatus in capsule. (From Cooper, D.E., O'Brien, S.J., and Warren, R.F.: Supporting layers of glenohumeral joint. Clin. Orthop. 289:151, 1993; reprinted by permission.)

D. Nerves—Peripheral nerves that innervate muscles about the upper extremity derive from the brachial plexus. This plexus, formed from the ventral primary ramii of C5–T1, lies under the clavicle, extending from the scalenus anterior to the axilla. The brachial plexus is organized into five components: *r*oots, *t*runks, *d*ivisions, *c*ords, and *b*ranches (remember the mnemonic *R*ob *T*aylor *d*rinks *c*old *b*eer). There are five roots (C5–T1, although C4 and T2 can have small contributions), three trunks (upper, middle, lower), six divisions (two from each trunk), three cords (posterior, lateral, medial),

TABLE 11–4. MUSCLES OF THE SHOULDER

MUSCLE	ORIGIN	INSERTION	ACTION	INNERVATION
Trapezius	Spin. proc. C7–T12	Clavicle, scapula (AC, SP)	Rotate scapula	CN XI
Lat. dorsii	Spin. proc. T6–S5, I1m	Humerus (ITG)	Ex., add., IR humerus	Thoracodorsal
Rhomboid maj.	Spin. proc. T2–T5	Scapula (med. border)	Adduct scapula	Dorsal scapular
Rhomboid min.	Spin. proc. C7–T1	Scapula (med. spine)	Adduct scapula	Dorsal scapular
Lev. scapulae	T. proc. C1–C4	Scapula (sup. med.)	Elevate, rotate scapula	C3, C4
Pectoralis maj.	Sternum, ribs, clavicle	Humerus (L-ITG)	Add., IR arm	M and L PN
Pectoralis min.	Ribs 3–5	Scapula (coracoid)	Protract scapula	MPN
Subclavius	Rib 1	Inf. clavicle	Depress clavicle	U trunk
Serratus ant.	Ribs 1–9	Scapula (vent. med.)	Prevent winging	Long thoracic
Deltoid	L. clavicle, scapula	Humerus (deltoid tub.)	Abduct arm (2)	Axillary
Teres major	Inf. scapula	Humerus (M-ITG)	Add., IR, ext.	L subscapular
Subscapularis	Ventral scapula	Humerus (LT)	IR arm, ant. stability	U and L subscapular
Supraspinatus	Sup. scapula	Humerus (GT)	Abd. (1), ER arm stability	Suprascapular
Infraspinatus	Dorsal scapula	Humerus (GT)	Stability, ER arm	Suprascapular
Teres minor	Scapula (dorsolateral)	Humerus (GT)	Stability, ER arm	Axillary

ITG, intertubercular groove; AC, acromion; SP, spinous process; LT, lesser tuberosity; GT, greater tuberosity.

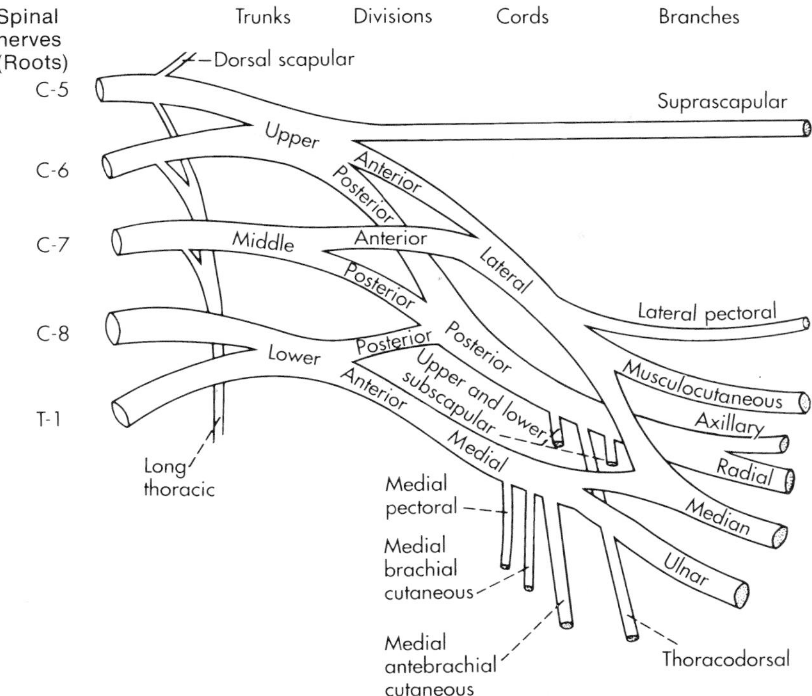

FIGURE 11–5. Brachial plexus. (From Jenkins, D.B.: Hollinshead's Functional Anatomy of the Limbs and Back, 6th ed., Fig. 5–7. Philadelphia, WB Saunders, 1991; reprinted by permission.)

and multiple branches, as illustrated in Fig. 11–5. Note that there are four preclavicular branches (from roots and upper trunk): dorsal scapular nerve, long thoracic nerve, suprascapular nerve, and nerve to subclavius.

E. Vessels (Fig. 11–6)—The subclavian artery arises either directly from the aorta (left subclavian) or from the brachiocephalic trunk (right subclavian). It then emerges between the scalenus anterior and medius muscles and becomes the axillary artery at the outer border of the first rib. The axillary artery is divided into three portions based on its relationship to the pectoralis minor (the first is medial to it, the second is under it, and the third is lateral to it). Each part of the artery has as many branches as the number of that portion (e.g., the second part has two branches).

PART	BRANCH	COURSE
1	Supreme thoracic	Medial—to serratus anterior and pecs
2	Thoracoacromial	Four branches (deltoid, anterior, pectoralis, clavicular)
	Lateral thoracic	Descends to serratus anterior
3	Subscapular	Two branches (thoracodorsal and circumflex scapular → triangular space)
	Ant. circumflex humeral	Circles humerus anteriorly, blood supply to humeral head
	Post. circumflex humeral	Post. humerus → quadrangular space

F. Surgical Approaches to the Shoulder—Include the anterior approach (reconstructions and arthroplasties), lateral approach (acromioplasty and cuff repair), and posterior approach (posterior reconstruction).

1. Anterior Approach (Henry) (Fig. 11–7)—Explores the interval between the deltoid (axillary N) and the pectoralis major (medial and lateral pectoral N). The cephalic vein is dissected and retracted laterally with the deltoid, and the underlying subscapularis is exposed. The latter is then divided (preserving the most inferior fibers to protect the axillary N), and the shoulder capsule is encountered. The **musculocutaneous nerve** should be protected by avoiding dissection medial to the coracobrachialis. This nerve usually penetrates the biceps/coracobrachialis 5–8 cm below the coracoid, but it enters these muscles proximal to this 5 cm "safe zone" almost 30% of the time. The **axillary nerve,** which is **just inferior** to the shoulder **capsule** must be protected during procedures in this area.
2. Lateral Approach—Involves splitting the deltoid muscle or subperiosteal dissection of the muscle from the acromion. This maneuver exposes the supraspinatus tendon well and allows for repairs of the rotator cuff. The deltoid should not be split more than **5 cm below the acromion** to avoid injury to the **axillary nerve.**
3. Posterior Approach (Fig. 11–8)—Uses the internervous plane between the infraspinatus (suprascapular nerve) and teres minor (axillary nerve). This lane can be approached by detaching the deltoid from the scapular spine or by

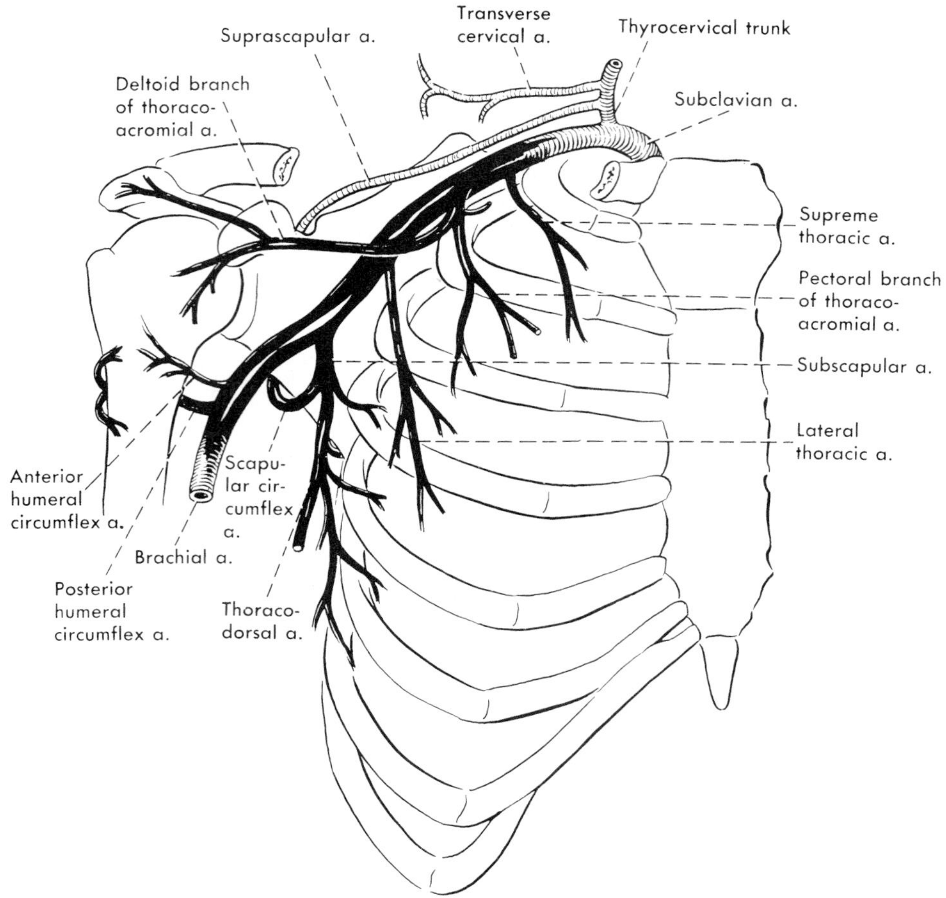

FIGURE 11–6. Branches of the axillary artery. (From Jenkins, D.B.: Hollinshead's Functional Anatomy of the Limbs and Back, 6th ed., p. 77. Philadelphia, WB Saunders, 1991; reprinted by permission.)

splitting the deltoid (Rockwood). After finding this interval, the posterior capsule lies immediately below it. The axillary nerve and the posterior circumflex humeral artery both run in the **quadrangular space** below the teres minor, so it is important to stay above this muscle. Excessive medial retraction of the infraspinatus can injure the suprascapular nerve.

III. Arm

A. Osteology—The humerus is the only bone of the arm and the largest and longest bone of the upper extremity. It is composed of a shaft and two articular extremities. The hemispherical head, directed superiorly, medially, and slightly dorsally, articulates with the much smaller scapular glenoid cavity. The *anatomic neck,* directly below the head, serves as an attachment for the shoulder capsule. The *surgical neck* is lower and is more often involved in fractures. The greater tuberosity, lateral to the head, serves as the attachment for the supraspinatus, infraspinatus, and teres minor (SIT) muscles (anterior to posterior, respectively). The lesser tuberosity, located anteriorly, has only one muscular insertion: the last rotator cuff muscle, the subscapularis. The bicipital groove (for the tendon of the long head of the biceps) is situated between the two tuberosities. The shaft of the humerus has a notable groove for the radial nerve posteriorly in its midportion, adjacent to the deltoid tuberosity. Distally, the humerus flares into medial and lateral epicondyles and forms half of the elbow joint with a medial spool-shaped trochlea (articulates with the olecranon of the ulna) and a globular capitulum (which opposes the radial head). The humerus has one primary and seven secondary ossification centers.

OSSIFICATION CENTER	AGE AT APPEARANCE	AGE AT FUSION
Body (primary)	8 weeks (fetal)	Blend at 6 years, unites at 20 years
Head	1 year	
Greater tuberosity	3 years	
Lesser tuberosity	5 years	
Capitulum	2 years	Blend and unites with body at 16–18 years
Medial epicondyle	5 years	
Trochlea	9 years	
Lateral epicondyle	13 years	

B. Arthrology—The humerus articulates with the scapula on its upper end, forming the glenohumeral

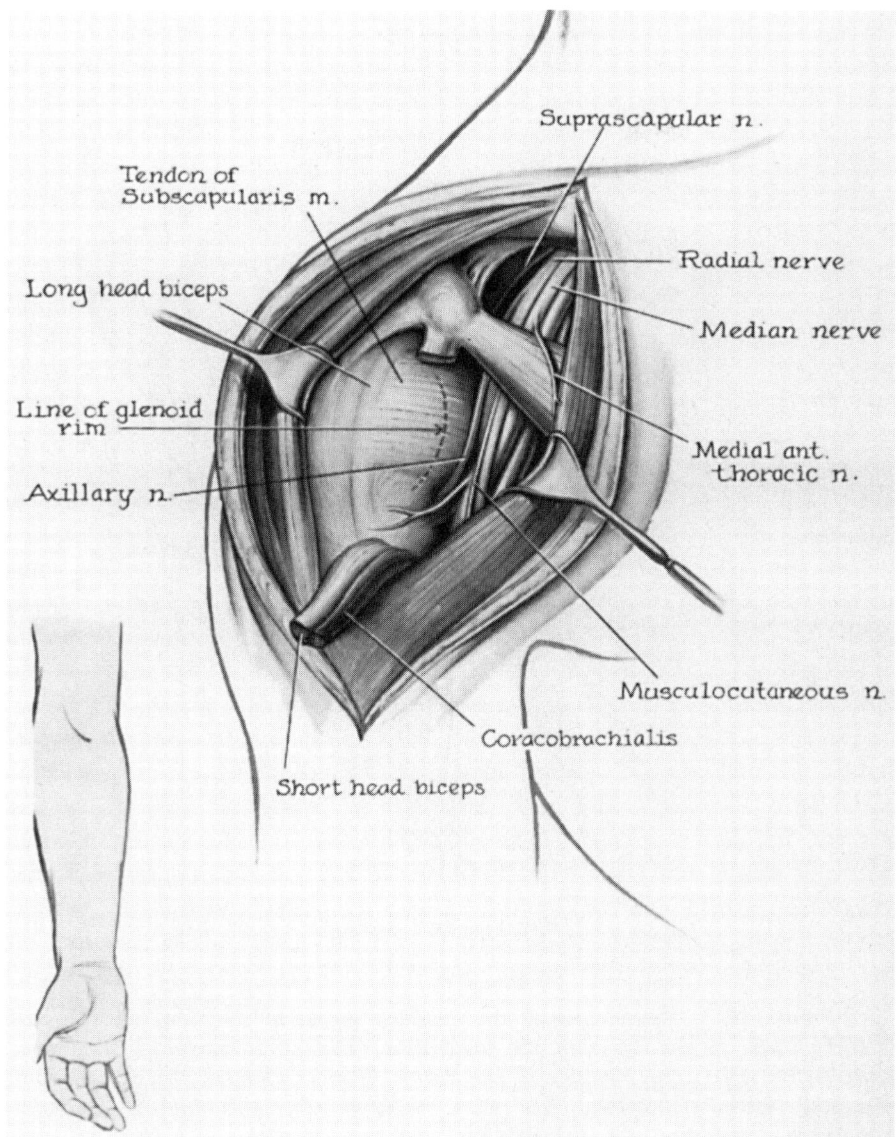

FIGURE 11–7. Anterior approach to the shoulder through the deltopectoral interval. (From Kaplan, E.B.: Surgical Approaches to the Neck, Cervical Spine, and Upper Extremity, p. 57. Philadelphia, WB Saunders, 1966; reprinted by permission.)

joint (discussed above), and with the radius and ulna on its lower end, forming the elbow joint. The elbow is composed of a compound ginglymus (hinge) joint (humeroulnar) and a trochoid (pivot) joint (humeroradial).

ARTICULATION	COMPONENTS
Humeroulnar	Trochlea and trochlear notch
Humeroradial	Capitulum and radial head
Proximal R-U	Radial notch and radial head

The ligaments of the elbow joint include a relatively weak capsule and the following ligaments (Fig. 11–9).

LIGAMENT	COMPONENTS	COMMENTS
Ulnar collateral	Anterior and posterior	Ant. fibers key
Radial collateral		Weaker, less distinct
Annular	Triangular	Rotatory movements
Quadrate	Osseofibrous ring	
Oblique cord	Annular lig. → radial neck	
	Coronoid base → radius	

C. Muscles of the Arm—There are four muscles of the arm (Table 11–5). The triceps muscle helps form borders for two important spaces (Fig. 11–10). The **triangular space** is bordered by the teres minor (superiorly), teres major (inferiorly), and long head of

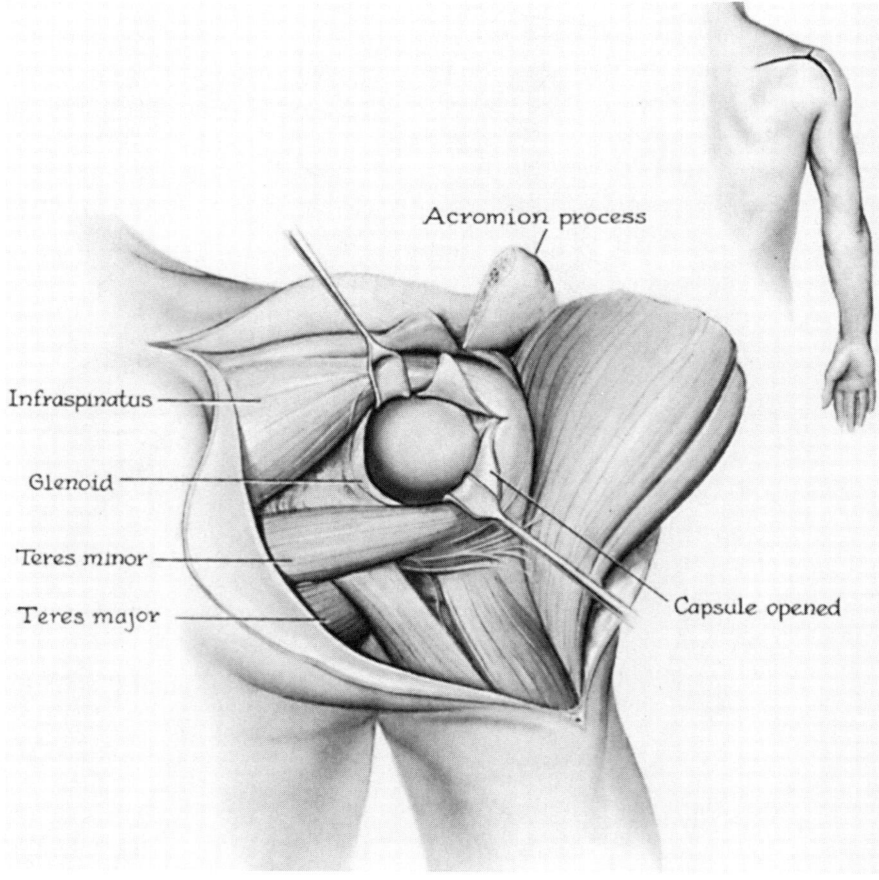

FIGURE 11–8. Posterior approach to the shoulder through the infraspinatus–teres minor interval. (From Kaplan, E.B.: Surgical Approaches to the Neck, Cervical Spine, and Upper Extremity, p. 61. Philadelphia, WB Saunders, 1966; reprinted by permission.)

the triceps (laterally); it contains the circumflex scapular vessels. The **quadrangular space** is also bordered by the teres minor (superiorly) and the teres major (inferiorly), with the long head of the triceps forming its medial border and the humerus forming the lateral border. The quadrangular space transmits the posterior humeral circumflex vessels and the axillary nerve. The **triangular interval** is immediately inferior to the quadrangular space and is bordered by the teres major (superiorly), long head of the triceps (medially), and lateral head of the triceps or the humerus (laterally). Through this interval the profunda brachii artery and radial nerve can be seen.

D. Nerves—Four major nerves traverse the arm, two giving off branches to arm musculature, and two that innervate distal musculature (Fig. 11–11). Most of the cutaneous innervation of the arm arises directly from the brachial plexus.
   1. Musculocutaneous Nerve—Formed from the lateral cord of the brachial plexus, this nerve pierces the coracobrachialis 5–8 cm distal to the coracoid and then branches to supply this muscle, the biceps, and the brachialis. It also gives

TABLE 11–5. MUSCLES OF THE ARM

MUSCLE	ORIGIN	INSERTION	ACTION	INNERVATION
Coracobrachialis	Coracoid	Mid. humerus medial	Flexion, adduction	Musculocutaneous
Biceps	Coracoid (SH) Supraglenoid (LH)	Radial tuberosity	Supination, flexion	Musculocutaneous
Brachialis	Ant. humerus	Ulnar tuberosity (ant.)	Flexes forearm	Musculocut., radial
Triceps	Infraglenoid (LH) Post. humerus (lat H) Post. humerus (MH)	Olecranon	Extends forearm	Radial

SH, short head; LH, long head; lat H, lateral head; MH, medial head.

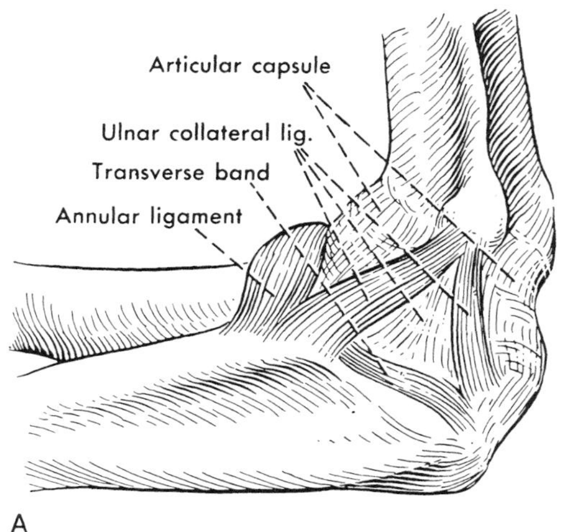

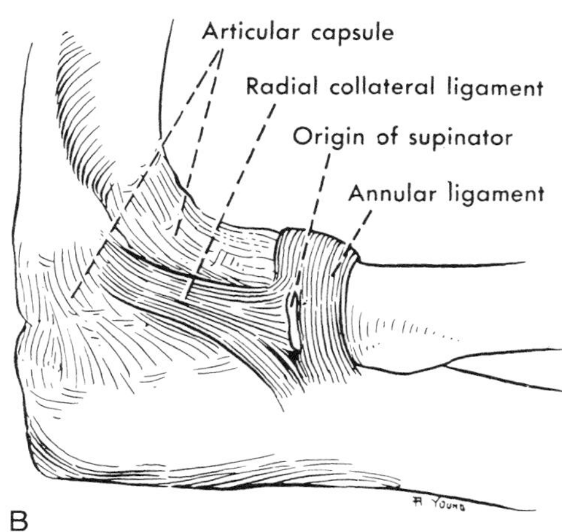

FIGURE 11–9. Elbow ligaments. *A,* Medial view. *B,* Lateral view. (From Jenkins, D.B.: Hollinshead's Functional Anatomy of the Limbs and Back, 6th ed., p. 108. Philadelphia, WB Saunders, 1991; reprinted by permission.)

off a branch to the elbow joint before it becomes the lateral antebrachial cutaneous nerve of the forearm.

2. Radial Nerve—Formed from the posterior cord of the brachial plexus, this nerve spirals around the humerus (medial → lateral), supplying the triceps muscles. It emerges on the lateral side of the arm between the brachialis and brachioradialis anterior to the lateral epicondyle.
3. Median Nerve—From the medial and lateral cords of the brachial plexus, this nerve accompanies the brachial artery along the arm, crossing it during its course (lateral → medial). It supplies some branches to the elbow joint but has no branches in the arm itself.
4. Ulnar Nerve—The continuation of the medial cord of the brachial plexus, this nerve remains medial to the brachial artery in the arm and then runs behind the medial epicondyle of the humerus, where it is quite superficial. It also has branches to the elbow but not arm branches.
5. Cutaneous Nerves—The supraclavicular nerve (C3, C4) supplies the upper shoulder. The axillary nerve supplies the shoulder joint and the overlying skin (in accordance with Hilton's law). The medial, lateral, and dorsal brachial cutaneous nerves supply the balance of the cutaneous innervation of the arm.

E. Vessels—The brachial artery originates at the lower border of the tendon of the teres major and continues to the elbow, where it bifurcates into the radial and ulnar arteries (Fig. 11–11). Lying medial in the arm, the brachial artery curves laterally to enter the cubital fossa (formed by the distal humerus proximally, the brachioradialis laterally, and the pronator teres medially). Its principal branches include the deep brachial, the superior and inferior ulnar collaterals, and nutrient and muscular branches. Anastomoses around the elbow (medial → lateral) are as follows.

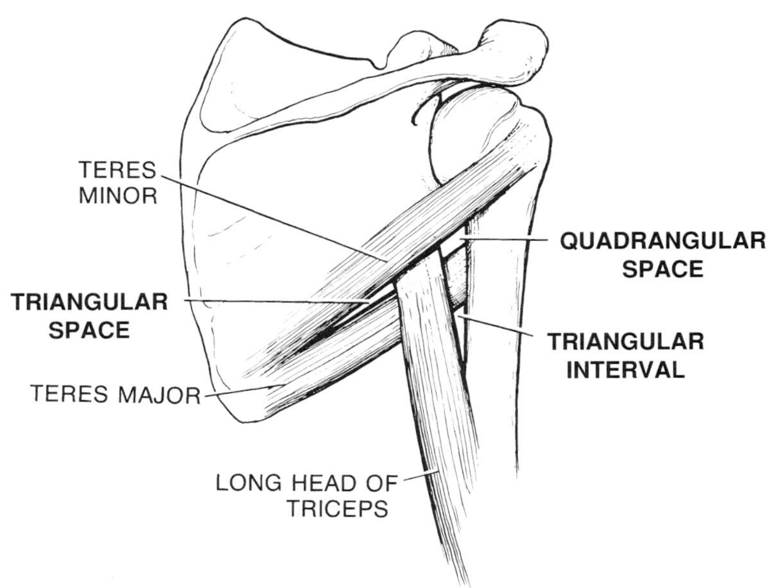

FIGURE 11–10. Quadrangular space. (From Kaplan, E.B.: Surgical Approaches to the Neck, Cervical Spine, and Upper Extremity, p. 53. Philadelphia, WB Saunders, 1966; reprinted by permission.)

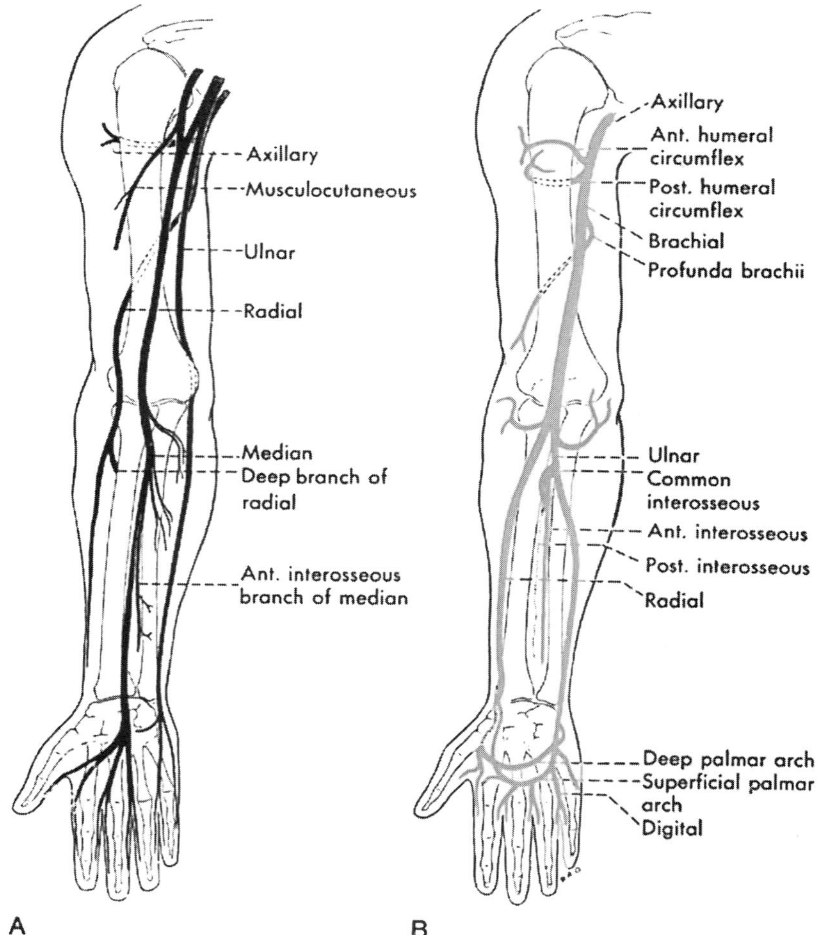

FIGURE 11–11. Nerves and vessels of the upper extremity. *A*, Principal nerves. *B*, Chief arteries. (From Jenkins, D.B.: Hollinshead's Functional Anatomy of the Limbs and Back, 6th ed., p. 62. Philadelphia, WB Saunders, 1991; reprinted by permission.)

SUPERIOR BRANCH	INFERIOR BRANCH
Superior ulnar collateral	Posterior ulnar recurrent
Inferior ulnar collateral	Anterior ulnar recurrent
Mid. collateral branch of deep brachial	Interosseous recurrent
Rad. collateral branch of deep brachial	Radial recurrent

F. Surgical Approaches to the Arm and Elbow—Proximally include the anterior and posterior approaches and distally include anterolateral and lateral approaches to the humerus and numerous approaches to the elbow.

1. Anterolateral Approach to the Humerus (Fig. 11–12)—Depends on the internervous plane between the deltoid (axillary nerve) and the pectoralis major (medical and lateral pectoral nerves) proximally and between the fibers of the brachialis (radial nerve and musculocutaneous nerve) distally. The radial and axillary nerves are at risk mainly for forceful retraction. The anterior circumflex humeral vessels may need to be ligated with a proximal approach.
2. Posterior Approach to the Humerus (Fig. 11–13)—Utilizes the interval between the lateral and long heads of the triceps superficially and a muscle-splitting approach for the medial (deep) head. The radial nerve and deep brachial artery must be identified and protected, and the ulnar nerve is jeopardized unless subperiosteal dissection of the humerus is meticulous.
3. Anterolateral Approach to the Distal Humerus (Fig. 11–14)—Uses the interval between the brachialis (musculocutaneous and radial nerves) and the brachioradialis (radial nerve). The radial nerve again must be identified and protected.
4. Lateral Approach to the Distal Humerus—Exploits the interval between the triceps and the brachioradialis by elevating a portion of the common extensor origin from the lateral epicondyle. Proximal extension jeopardizes the radial nerve.
5. Posterior Approach to the Elbow (Fig. 11–15)—Detachment of the extensor mecha-

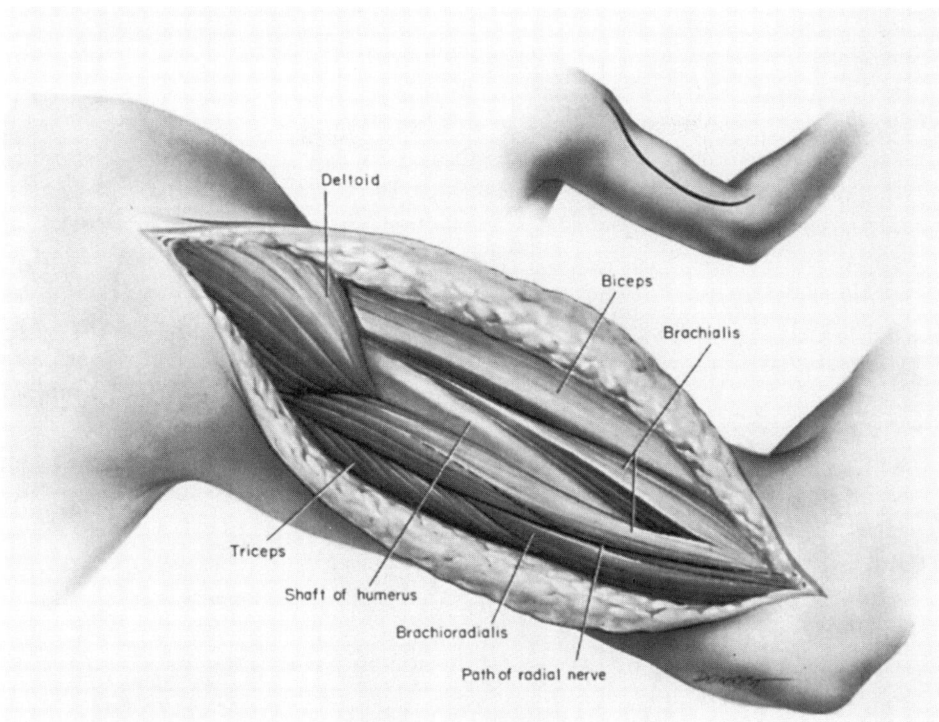

FIGURE 11–12. Lateral approach to the arm. (From Kaplan, E.B.: Surgical Approaches to the Neck, Cervical Spine, and Upper Extremity, p. 74. Philadelphia, WB Saunders, 1966; reprinted by permission.)

nism of the elbow gives excellent exposure for many elbow fractures. The olecranon osteotomy (best done with a chevron cut 2 cm distal to the tip) should be predilled and the ulnar nerve protected. An alternative (Brien) approach splits the triceps and leaves the olecranon intact.

6. Medial Approach to the Elbow—Exploits the interval between the brachialis (musculocutaneous nerve) and the triceps (radial nerve) proximally and the brachialis and pronator teres (median nerve) distally. The ulnar and medial antebrachial cutaneous nerves are in the field and must be protected.
7. Anterolateral Approach to the Elbow (Henry)—An extension of the same approach to the distal humerus, this approach is a brachialis (musculocutaneous nerve) splitting approach proximally and is between the pronator teres (median nerve) and the brachioradialis distally. The lateral antebrachial cutaneous nerve must be protected superficially and the radial nerve (and its branches) deep (supinate the forearm).
8. (Postero)Lateral (Kocher) Approach to the Elbow (Fig. 11–16)—Uses the interval between the anconeus (radial nerve) and the main extensor origin (ECU—posterior interosseous branch of the radial nerve [PIN]). Pronation of the arm moves the PIN radially, and the radial head is approached through the proximal supinator fibers. Extending this approach distal to the annular ligament increases the risk to the posterior interosseous nerve.

IV. Forearm

A. Osteology—The forearm includes two long bones—the ulna and radius, which articulate with the humerus (principally the ulna)—and the carpii (articulate principally with the radius).

1. Ulna—A long prismatic bone occupying the medial forearm and consisting of a body and two extremities. Proximally, the ulna is composed of two curved processes, the olecranon and the coronoid processes, with an intervening trochlear notch. Distally, the ulna tapers and ends in a lateral head and a medial styloid process. The ulna has one primary and two secondary ossification centers.

OSSIFICATION CENTER	AGE AT APPEARANCE	AGE AT FUSION
Body (primary)	8 weeks (fetal)	
Distal ulna	5 years	20 years
Olecranon	10 years	16 years

2. Radius—Like the ulna, the radius has a body and two extremities. The proximal radius is composed of a head with a central fovea, a neck, and a proximal medial radial tuberosity (for insertion of the biceps tendon). The radius has a gradual bend (convex laterally) and gradually increases in size distally. The distal extremity

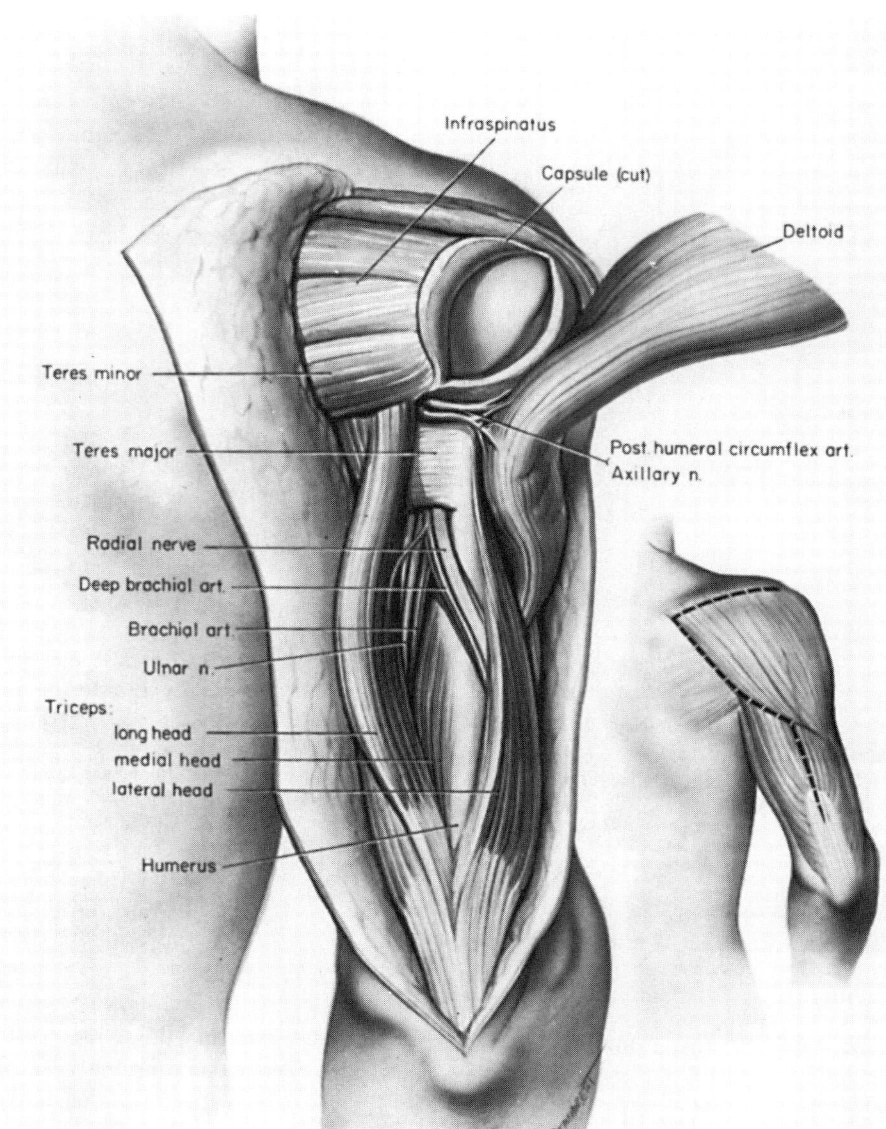

FIGURE 11–13. Posterior approach to the arm. (From Kaplan, E.B.: Surgical Approaches to the Neck, Cervical Spine, and Upper Extremity, p. 73. Philadelphia, WB Saunders, 1966; reprinted by permission.)

of the radius is composed of the carpal articular surface, an ulnar notch, a dorsal tubercle, and a lateral styloid process. The radius is also ossified via three centers.

OSSIFICATION CENTER	AGE AT APPEARANCE	AGE AT FUSION
Body (primary)	8 weeks (fetal)	
Distal radius	2 years	17–20 years
Proximal radius	5 years	15–18 years

B. Arthrology—The radius and ulna articulate proximally at the elbow joint (discussed above) and distally at the wrist. The wrist consists primarily of the radiocarpal joint but also includes the distal radioulnar articulation with its triangular fibrocartilage complex (TFCC).

1. Radiocarpal Joint—An ellipsoid joint involving the distal radius and the scaphoid, lunate, and triquetrum. Covered by a loose capsule, the wrist relies heavily on ligaments, especially volar ligaments, for stability. They include the volar and dorsal radiocarpal ligaments and the ulnar and radial collateral ligaments.
2. TFCC (Fig. 11–17)—Originates from the most ulnar portion of the radius and extends into the caput ulna and the ulnar wrist to the base of the fifth metacarpal. It includes the following components.

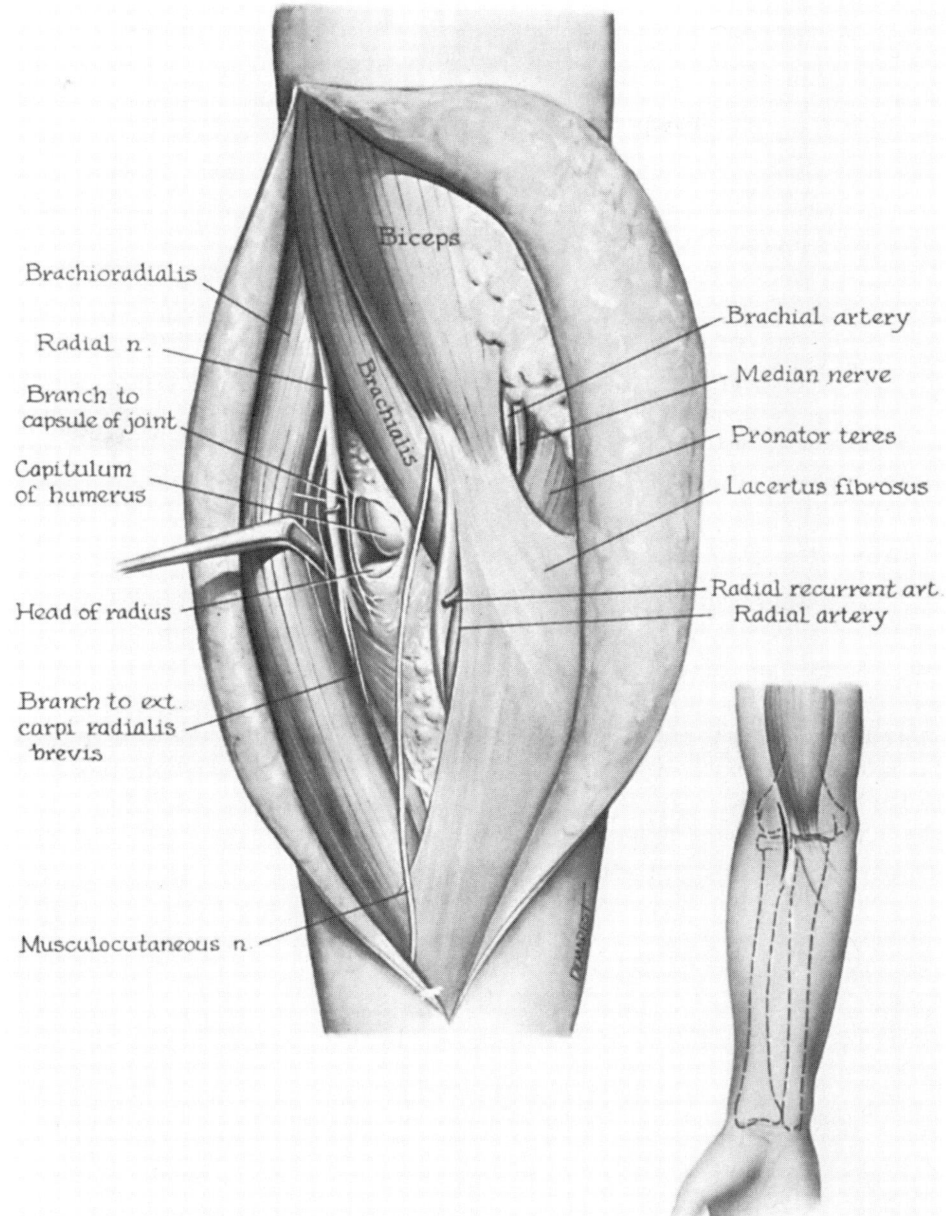

FIGURE 11–14. Anterior approach to the elbow. (From Kaplan, E.B.: Surgical Approaches to the Neck, Cervical Spine, and Upper Extremity, p. 77. Philadelphia, WB Saunders, 1966; reprinted by permission.)

COMPONENT	ORIGIN	INSERTION
Dorsal and volar radioulnar ligament (RUL)	Ulnar radius	Caput ulna
Articular disc	Radius/ulna	Triquetrum
Prestyloid recess	Disc	Meniscus homologue
Meniscus homologue	Ulna/disc	Triquetrum/UCL
Ulnar collateral ligament	Ulna	Fifth metacarpal

C. Muscles of the Forearm (Fig. 11–18)—Arranged based on both location and function into volar flexors (superficial and deep) and dorsal extensors (superficial and deep) (Table 11–6).

D. Nerves—The nerves of the upper arm continue into the forearm (Fig. 11–19).

1. Radial Nerve—Anterior to the lateral epicondyle, the radial nerve runs between the brachialis and brachioradialis and divides into anterior and deep (posterior interosseous nerve [PIN]) branches. The PIN splits the supinator and supplies all of the extensor muscles (except the mobile wad [brachioradialis, ECRB, ECRL]). The superficial branch of the radial nerve passes to the dorsal radial surface of the hand in the distal third of the forearm by passing between the brachioradialis and ECRL.

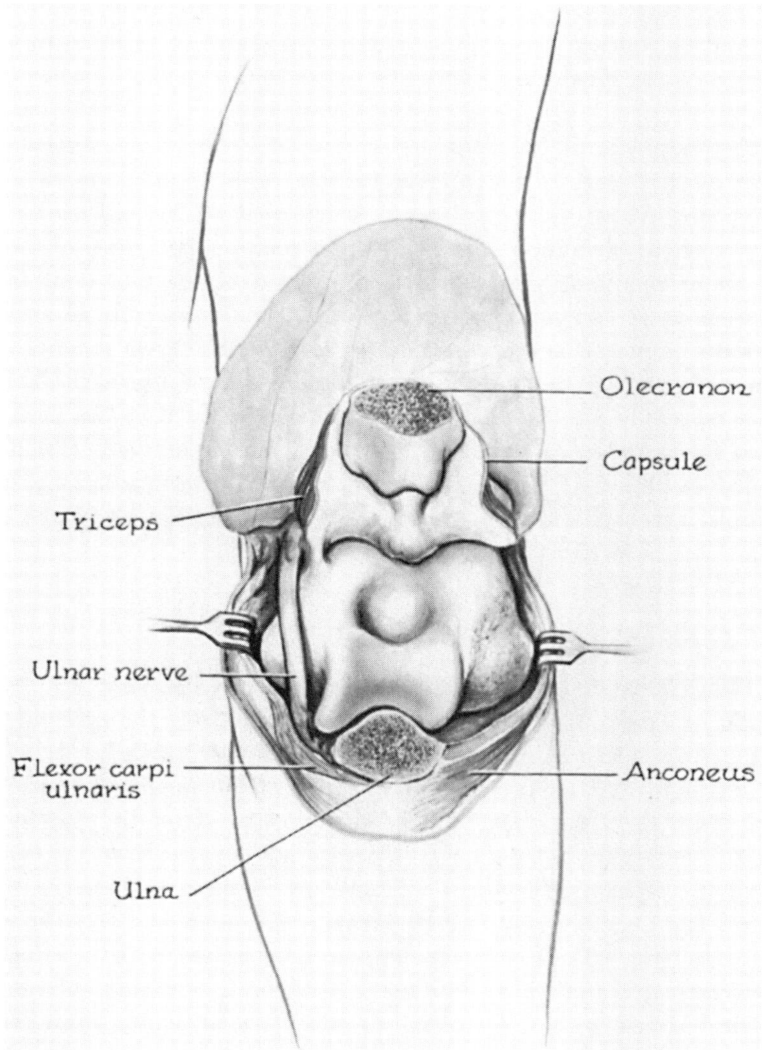

FIGURE 11–15. Posterior approach to the elbow. (From Kaplan, E.B.: Surgical Approaches to the Neck, Cervical Spine, and Upper Extremity, p. 82. Philadelphia, WB Saunders, 1966; reprinted by permission.)

2. Median Nerve—Lies medial to the brachial artery at the elbow, superficial to the brachialis muscle. In the forearm the median nerve **splits** the two heads of the **pronator teres** and then **runs between the FDS and FDP,** becoming more superficial at the flexor retinaculum, where it continues into the hand. It has branches to all the superficial flexor muscles of the forearm except the FCU. Its anterior interosseous branch, which runs between the FPL and FDP, supplies all the deep flexors except the ulnar half of the FDP.
3. Ulnar Nerve—Enters the forearm between the two heads of the FCU, which it supplies, and then **runs between the FCU and FDP** (and innervates the ulnar half of this muscle). It lies more superficial at the wrist and enters the hand through Guyon's canal.
4. Cutaneous Nerves—In the forearm are the lateral antebrachial cutaneous nerve (the continuation of the musculocutaneous nerve), the medial antebrachial cutaneous nerve (a branch from the medial cord of the brachial plexus), and the posterior antebrachial cutaneous nerve (a branch of the radial nerve given off in the arm).

E. Vessels (Fig. 11–19)—At the elbow the brachial artery enters the cubital fossa (bordered by the two epicondyles, the brachioradialis, and the pronator teres and overlying the brachialis and supinator). It then divides at the level of the radial neck into the radial and ulnar arteries.
   1. Radial Artery—Runs initially on the pronator teres, deep to the brachioradialis, and continues to the wrist between this muscle and the FCR. Forearm branches include the radial recurrent (see above) and muscular branches.
   2. Ulnar Artery—The larger of the two branches, it is covered by the superficial flexors proximally (between the FDS and FDP). Distally, the artery lies on the FDP, between the tendons of the FCU

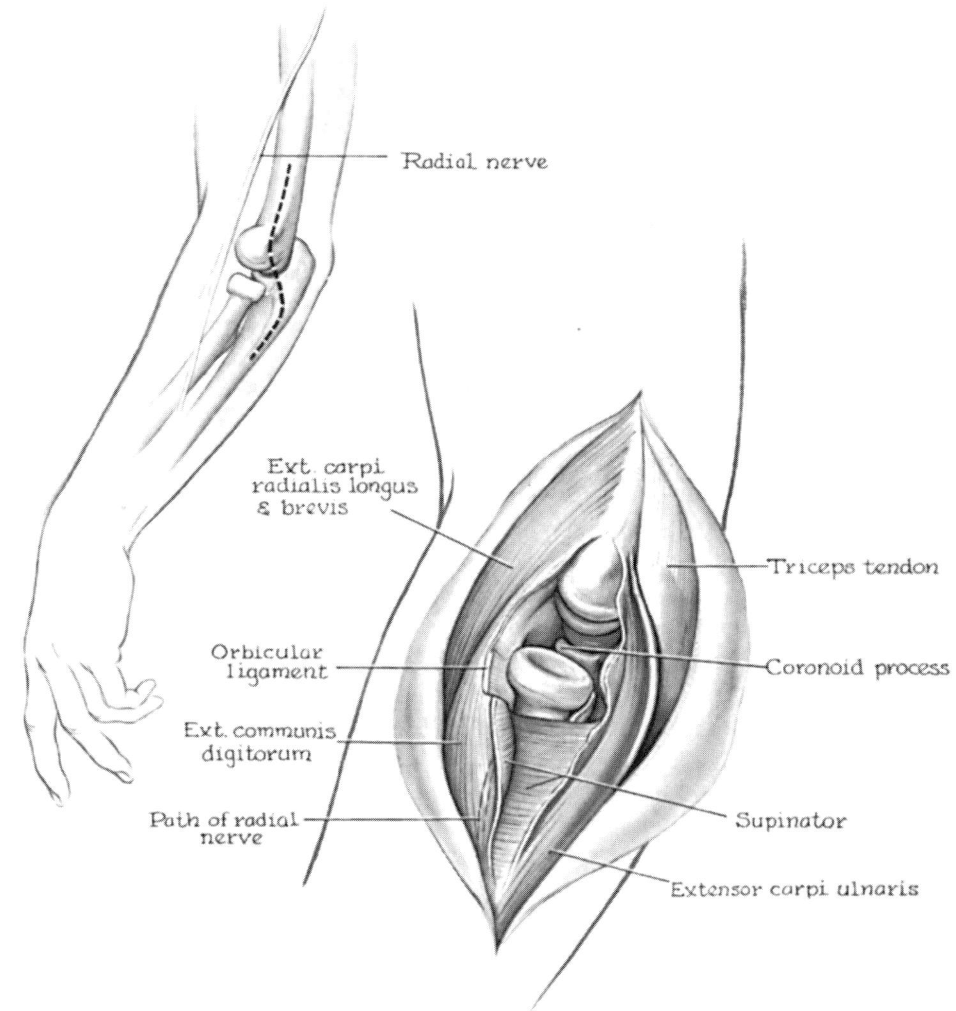

FIGURE 11–16. Lateral approach to the elbow. (From Kaplan, E.B.: Surgical Approaches to the Neck, Cervical Spine, and Upper Extremity, p. 83. Philadelphia, WB Saunders, 1966; reprinted by permission.)

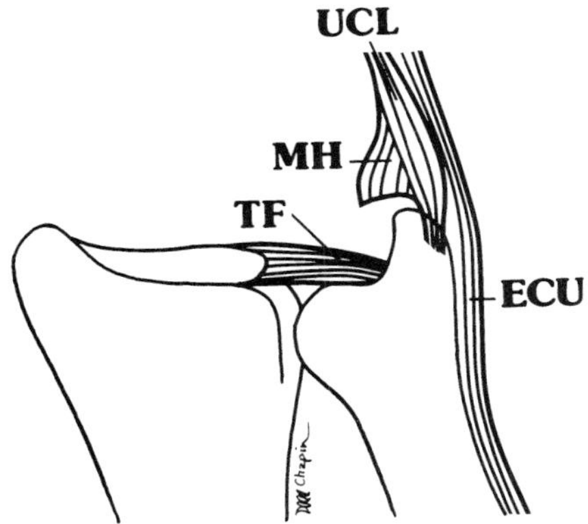

FIGURE 11–17. Triangular fibrocartilage complex (TFCC). UCL, ulnar collateral ligament; MH, meniscal homologue; TF, transverse fibers (radioulnar ligament); ECU, extensor carpi ulnaris. (From Wiessman, B.N., and Sledge, C.B.: Orthopedic Radiology, p. 115. Philadelphia, WB Saunders, 1986; reprinted by permission.)

and FDS. Forearm branches include the anterior and posterior ulnar recurrent (discussed above), the common interosseous (with anterior and posterior branches), and several muscular and nutrient arteries.

F. Surgical Approaches to the Forearm
   1. Anterior Approach (Henry) (Fig. 11–20)—Utilizes the interval between the brachioradialis (radial N) and the pronator teres (or FCR distally) (median N). Proximally it is necessary to isolate and ligate the **leash of Henry** (radial artery branches) and subperiosteally to strip the supinator from its insertion. Distally, it is necessary to dissect off the FPL and PQ. Supination of the forearm displaces the PIN ulnarly.
   2. Dorsal Approach (Thompson) (Fig. 11–21)—Utilizes the interval between the ECRB (radial N) and EDC (or EPL distally) (posterior interosseous N). The posterior interosseous nerve must be identified and protected when using this surgical approach.

TABLE 11–6. MUSCLES OF THE FOREARM

MUSCLE	ORIGIN	INSERTION	ACTION	INNERVATION
SUPERFICIAL FLEXORS				
Pronator teres (PT)	Med. epicondyle and coronoid	Mid. lat. radius	Pronate, flex forearm	Median
Flexor carpi radialis (FCR)	Med. epicondyle	2nd and 3rd Metacarpal bases	Flex wrist	Median
Palmaris longus (PL)	Med. epicondyle	Palmar aponeurosis	Flex wrist	Median
Flexor carpi ulnaris (FCU)	Med. epicondyle and post. ulna	Pisiform	Flex wrist	**Ulnar**
Flexor digitorum superficialis (FDS)	Med. epicondyle and ant. radius	Base of middle phalanges	Flex PIP	Median
DEEP FLEXORS				
Flexor digitorum profundus (FDP)	Ant. and med. ulna	Base of distal phalanges	Flex DIP	**Median-ant. interosseous/and ulnar**
Flexor pollicis longus (FPL)	Ant. and lat. radius	Base of distal phalanges	Flex IP, thumb	Median-ant. interosseous
Pronator quadratus (PQ)	Distal ulna	Volar radius	Pronate hand	Median-ant. interosseous
SUPERFICIAL EXTENSORS				
Brachioradialis (BR)	Lat. supracondylar humerus	Lat. distal radius	Flex forearm	Radial
Ext. carpi radialis longus (ECRL)	Lat. supracondylar humerus	2nd Metacarpal base	Extend wrist	Radial
Ext. carpi radialis brevis (ECRB)	Lat. epicondyle of humerus	3rd Metacarpal base	Extend wrist	Radial
Anconeus	Lat. epicondyle of humerus	Proximal dorsal ulna	Extend forearm	Radial
Extensor digitorum (ED)	Lat. epicondyle of humerus	Extensor aponeurosis	Extend digits	Radial-post. interosseous
Extensor digiti minimi	Common extensor tendon	Small finger extensor carpi ulnaris	Extend small finger	Radial-post. interosseous
Ext. carpi ulnaris (ECU)	Lat. epicondyle of humerus	5th Metacarpal base	Extend/adduct hand	Radial-post. interosseous
DEEP EXTENSORS				
Supinator	Lat. epicondyle of humerus, ulna	Dorsolateral radius	Supinate forearm	Radial-post. interosseous
Abductor pollicis longus (APL)	Dorsal ulna/radius	1st Metacarpal base	Abduct thumb, extend	Radial-post. interosseous
Extensor pollicis brevis (EPB)	Dorsal radius	Thumb proximal phalanx base	Extend thumb MCP	Radial-post. interosseous
Extensor pollicis longus (EPL)	Dorsolateral ulna	Thumb dorsal phalanx base	Extend thumb IP	Radial-post. interosseous
Extensor indicis proprius (EIP)	Dorsolateral ulna	Index finger extensor apparatus (ulnarly)	Extend index finger	Radial-post. interosseous

3. Exposure of the Ulna—Via the interval between the ECU (posterior interosseous N) and the FCU (ulnar N).
4. Cross-sectional diagrams of middle and distal forearm are available (Figs. 11–22, 11–23).

V. Wrist and Hand

A. Osteology

1. Carpal Bones—Each carpal bone has six surfaces, with proximal, distal, medial, and lateral surfaces for articulation and palmar and dorsal surfaces for ligamentous insertion. Ossification begins at the capitate (usually present at 1 year of age) and proceeds in a counterclockwise direction. Therefore the hamate is the second carpus to ossify (1–2 years), followed by the triquetrum (3 years), lunate (4–5 years), scaphoid (5 years), trapezium (6 years), and trapezoid (7 years). The pisiform, which is a large sesamoid bone, is the last to ossify (9 years). Several key features are important to recognize in the individual carpal bones.

BONE	IMPORTANT FEATURES	NO. OF ARTICULATIONS
Scaphoid	Tubercle (TCL, APB), distal vascular supply	5
Lunate	Lunar shape	5
Triquetrum	Pyramid shape	3
Pisiform	Spheroidal (TCL, FCR)	1
Trapezium	FCR groove, tubercle (opponens, APB, FPB, TCL)	4
Trapezoid	Wedge shape	4
Capitate	Largest bone, central location	7
Hamate	Hook (TCL)	5

TCL, transverse carpal ligament.

2. Metacarpals—Have two ossification centers: one for the body (primary center of ossification),

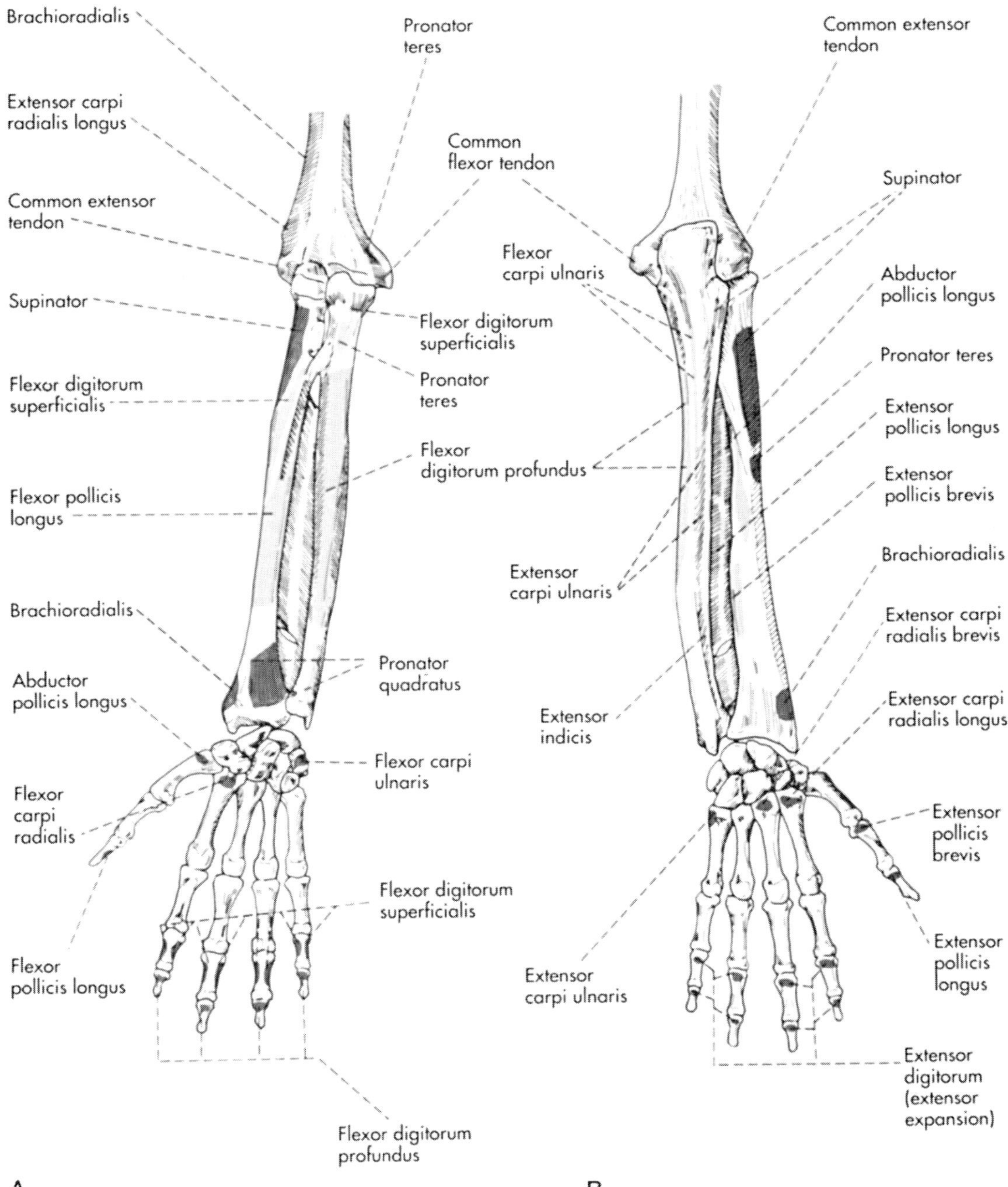

FIGURE 11–18. Origins and insertions of muscles of the forearm. (From Jenkins, D.B.: Hollinshead's Functional Anatomy of the Limbs and Back, 6th ed., Fig. 8–4. Philadelphia, WB Saunders, 1991; reprinted by permission.)

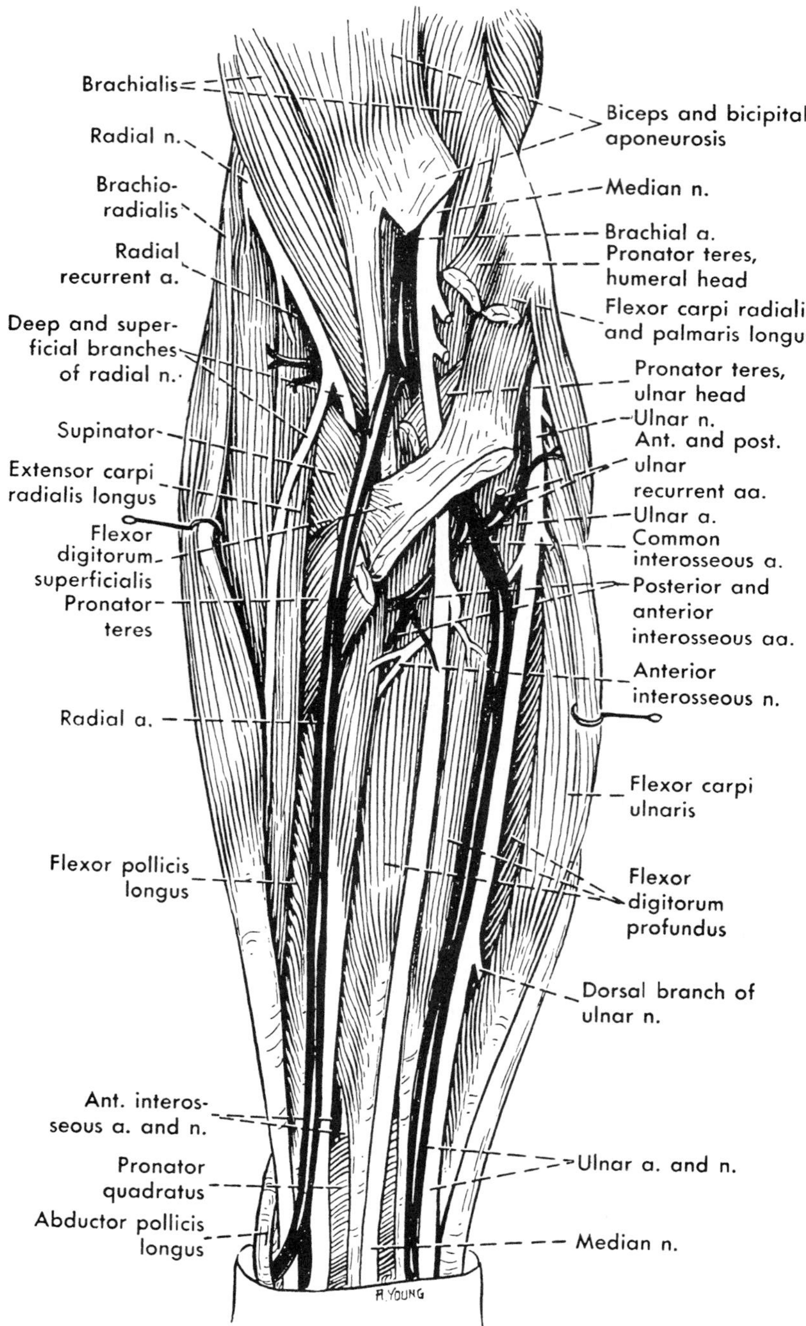

FIGURE 11–19. Arteries (black) and nerves (white) of the forearm. (From Jenkins, D.B.: Hollinshead's Functional Anatomy of the Limbs and Back, 6th ed., p. 131. Philadelphia, WB Saunders, 1991; reprinted by permission.)

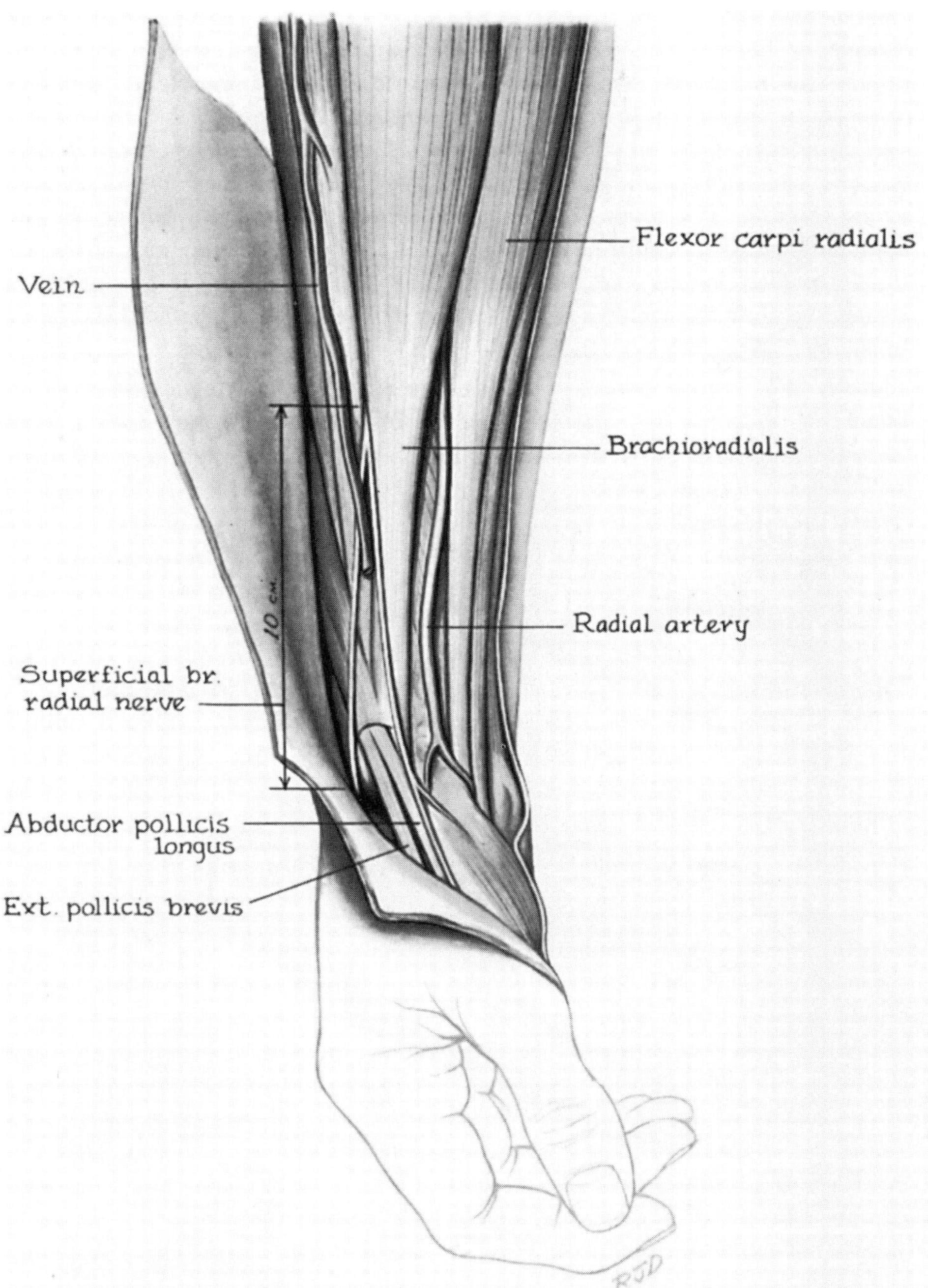

FIGURE 11–20. Anterior (Henry) approach to the forearm. (From Kaplan, E.B.: Surgical Approaches to the Neck, Cervical Spine, and Upper Extremity, p. 92. Philadelphia, WB Saunders, 1966; reprinted by permission.)

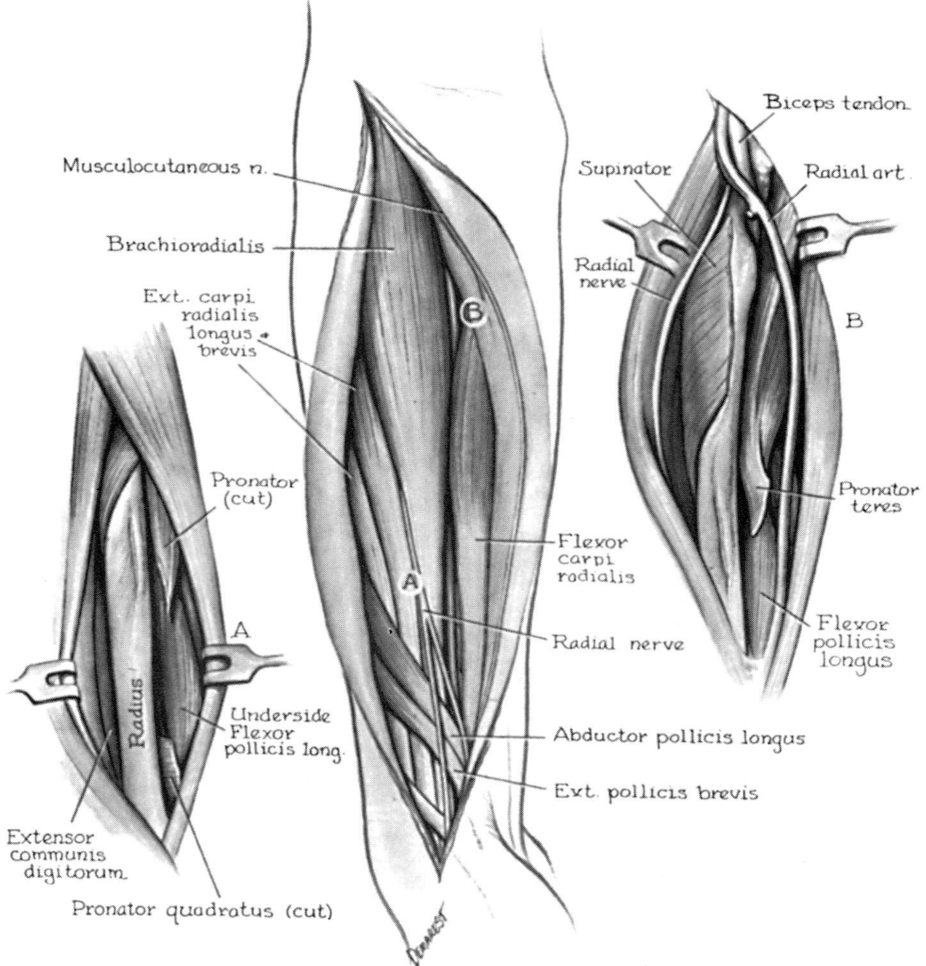

FIGURE 11–21. Dorsal (Thompson) approach to the forearm. (From Kaplan, E.B.: Surgical Approaches to the Neck, Cervical Spine, and Upper Extremity, p. 90. Philadelphia, WB Saunders, 1966; reprinted by permission.)

which ossifies at 8 weeks of fetal life (like most long bones), and one at the neck, which usually appears before age 3. The first metacarpal is a primordial phalanx and has its secondary ossification center located at the base (like the phalanges). Several characteristics allow identification of the individual metacarpals.

METACARPAL	DISTINCTIVE FEATURES
I (thumb)	Short, stout, base is saddle-shaped
II (index)	Longest, largest base, medial at base
III (middle)	Styloid process
IV (ring)	Small quadrilateral base, narrow shaft
V (small)	Tubercle at base (ECU)

3. Phalanges—The 14 phalanges (three for each finger and two for the thumb) are similar. They all have secondary ossification centers at their bases that appear at ages 3 (proximal), 4 (middle), and 5 (distal). The bases of the proximal phalanges are oval and concave, with smaller heads ending in two condyles. The middle phalanges have two concave facets at their bases and pulley-shaped heads. The distal phalanges are smaller and have palmar ungual tuberosities distally.

B. Arthrology
   1. Radiocarpal (Wrist) Joint—Ellipsoid joint made up of the distal radius, scaphoid, lunate, triquetrum, and the following ligamentous structures.

STRUCTURE	ATTACHMENTS	DISTINCTIVE FEATURES
Articular capsule	Surrounds joint	Reinforced by volar and dorsal RCL
Volar radiocarpal ligament (RCL)	Radius, ulna, scaphoid, lunate, triquetrum, capitate	Oblique ulnar, strong
Dorsal radiocarpal ligament	Radius, scaphoid, lunate, triquetrum	Oblique radial, weak

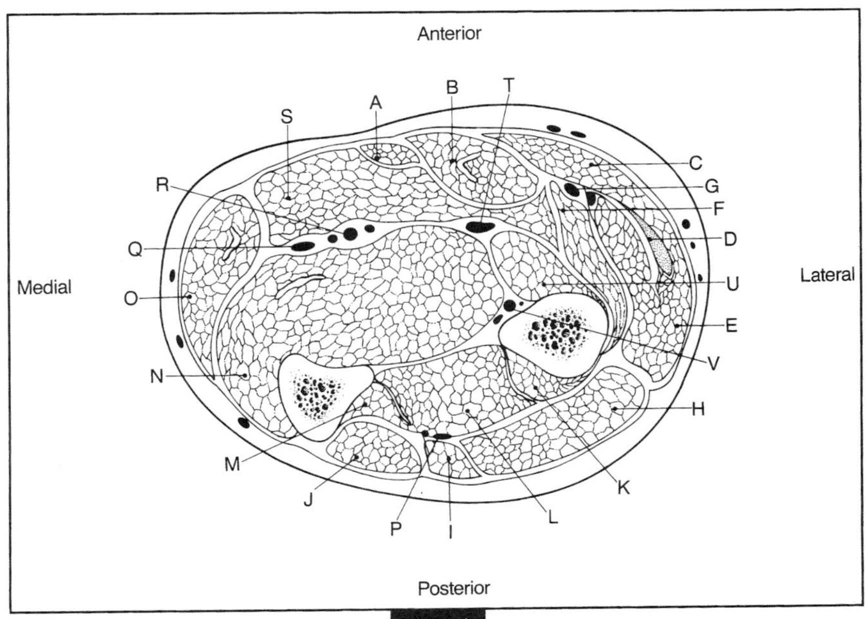

FIGURE 11–22. Cross section of the mid-forearm. (From Callaghan JJ., ed., Self-Assessment Examination, Fig. 39. Park Ridge, Illinois, American Academy of Orthopaedic Surgeons, 1991; reprinted by permission.)

A Palmaris longus
B Flexor carpi radialis
C Brachioradialis
D Extensor carpi radialis longus
E Extensor carpi radialis brevis
F Pronator teres
G Radial artery
H Extensor digitorum communis
I Extensor digiti minimi
J Extensor carpi ulnaris
K Supinator
L Abductor pollicis longus
M Extensor pollicis longus
N Flexor digitorum profundus
O Flexor carpi ulnaris
P Posterior interosseous nerve
Q Ulnar nerve
R Ulnar artery
S Flexor digitorum superficialis
T Median nerve
U Flexor pollicis longus
V Anterior interosseous nerve

STRUCTURE	ATTACHMENTS	DISTINCTIVE FEATURES
Ulnar collateral ligament	Ulna, triquetrum, pisiform, TCL	Fan-shaped, two fascicles
Radial collateral ligament	Radius, scaphoid, trapezium, TCL	Radial artery adjacent

TCL, transverse carpal ligament.

The palmar radiocarpal ligament is the strongest supporting structure, although it has a weak area on the radial side (the space of Poirier) that lends less support to the scaphoid, lunate, and trapezoid. It may be related to wrist instability with injury.

2. Intercarpal Joints
   a. Proximal Row—Scaphoid, lunate, and triquetral are gliding joints. Two dorsal intercarpal ligaments connect the scaphoid and lunate and the lunate and triquetral bones. Two palmar intercarpal ligaments connect the scaphoid and lunate and the lunate and triquetral bones. The dorsal intercarpal ligaments are stronger. Interosseous ligaments are narrow bundles connecting the lunate and scaphoid and the lunate and triquetral bones (Fig. 11–24).
   b. Pisiform Articulation—The pisotriquetral joint has a thin articular capsule. The pisiform is also connected proximally by the ulnar collateral and palmar radiocarpal ligaments. The pisohamate ligament and pisometacarpal ligaments help extend the pull of the FCU.
   c. Distal Row—Trapezium, trapezoid, capitate, and hamate gliding joints. The dorsal intercarpal ligaments connect the trapezium with the trapezoid, the trapezoid with the capitate, and the capitate with the hamate. The palmar ligaments do the same. The interosseous ligaments are much thicker in the distal row, connecting the capitate and hamate (strongest), the capitate and trapezoid, and the trapezium and trapezoid (weakest).
   d. Midcarpal Joint—Transverse articulations between the proximal and distal rows are reinforced by palmar and dorsal intercarpal ligaments and carpal collateral ligaments (radial is stronger).
3. Carpometacarpal (CMC) Joints
   a. Thumb CMC Joint—A highly mobile saddle joint. It is supported by a capsule and radial, palmar, and dorsal CMC ligaments.

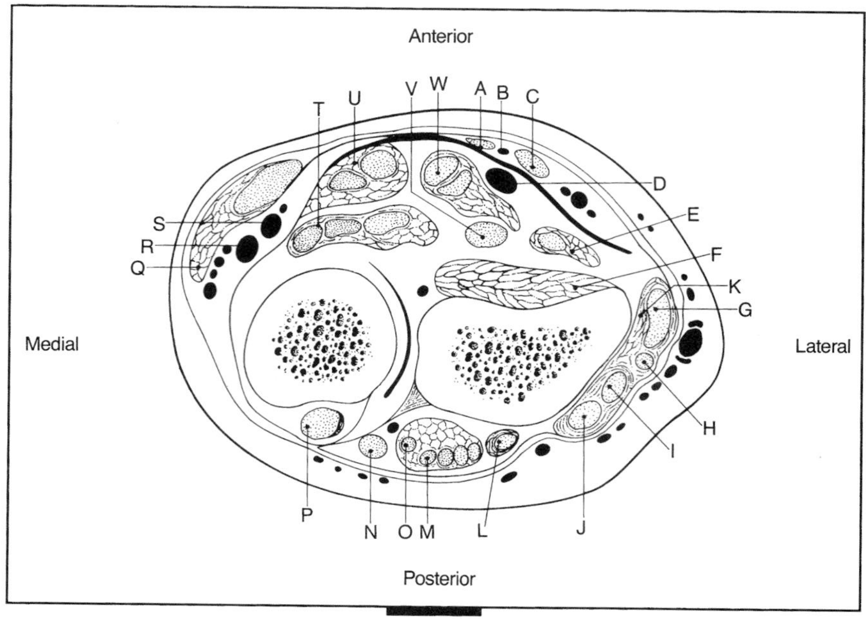

FIGURE 11–23. Cross section of the distal forearm proximal to the distal RU joint. (From Callaghan, JJ., eds., Self-Assessment Examination, Fig. 38. Park Ridge, Illinois, American Society of Orthopaedic Surgeons, 1991; reprinted by permission.)

A Palmaris longus
B Superficial palmar branch median nerve
C Flexor carpi radialis
D Median nerve
E Flexor pollicis longus
F Pronator quadratus
G Abductor pollicis longus
H Extensor pollicis brevis
I Extensor carpi radialis longus
J Extensor carpi radialis brevis
K Brachioradialis
L Extensor pollicis longus
M Extensor digiti communis
N Extensor digiti minimi
O Extensor indicis proprius
P Extensor carpi ulnaris
Q Flexor carpi ulnaris
R Ulnar nerve
S Ulnar artery
T Flexor digitorum profundus
U Flexor digitorum superficialis (4,5);
V Flexor digitorum profundus index
W Flexor digitorum superficialis ring

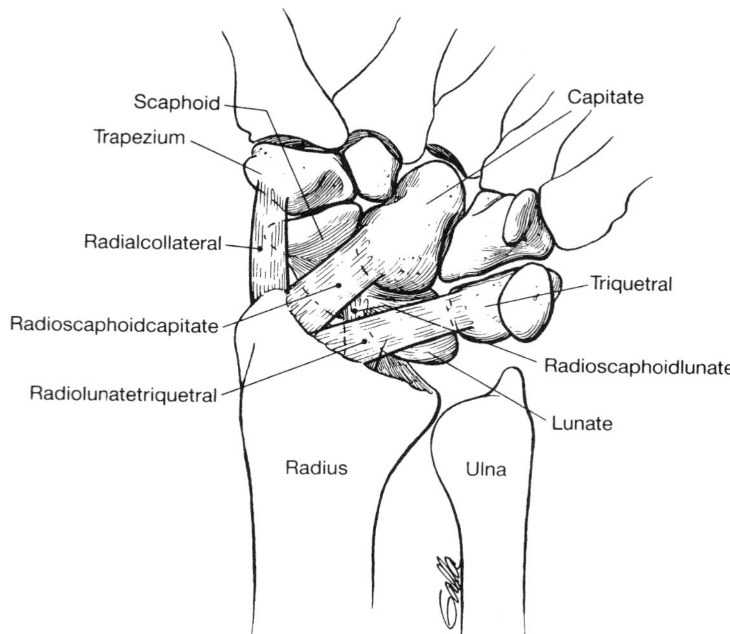

FIGURE 11–24. Extrinsic radiocarpal ligaments. (From Mooney, J.F., Siegel, D.B., and Koman, L.A. Ligamentous injuries of the wrists in athletes. Clin. Sports Med., 11:129–139, 1992, reprinted by permission.)

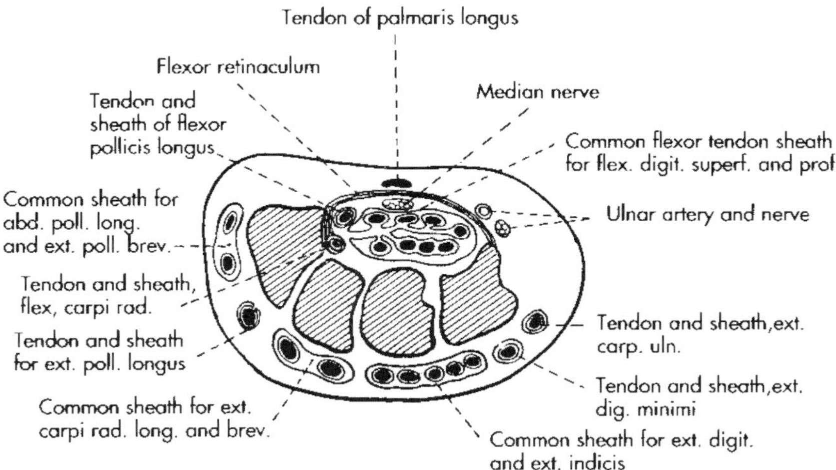

FIGURE 11–25. Components of the carpal tunnel. (From Jenkins, D.B.: Hollinshead's Functional Anatomy of the Limbs and Back, 6th ed., p. 162. Philadelphia, W.B. Saunders, 1991; reprinted by permission.)

b. Finger CMC Joints—Gliding joints with capsules, dorsal CMC ligaments (strongest), palmar CMC ligaments, and interosseous CMC ligaments.

4. Metacarpophalangeal Joints—Ellipsoid joints covered by palmar (volar plate), collateral, and deep transverse metacarpal ligaments.
5. Interphalangeal Joints—Hinge joints with capsules and obliquely oriented collateral ligaments.
6. Other Important Structures
   a. Extensor Retinaculum—Covers the dorsum of the wrist and contains six synovial sheaths (Figs. 11–25, 11–26).

COMPARTMENT	CONTENTS	PATHOLOGIC CONDITION INVOLVING TENDONS
1	APL, EPB	de Quervain's tenosynovitis
2	ECRL, ECRB	Tennis elbow/extensor tendonitis
3	EPL	Rupture at Lister's tubercle (after wrist fractures)
4	EDC, EIP	Extensor tenosynovitis
5	EDM	Rupture (rheumatoid)
6	ECU	Snapping at ulnar styloid

   b. Transverse Carpal Ligament (TCL; Flexor Retinaculum)—Forms the roof of the carpal tunnel (Fig. 11–25), which contains the long flexor tendons and the median nerve. It is attached medially to the pisiform and the hook of the hamate and laterally to the tuberosity of the scaphoid and the ridge of the trapezium. It also forms the floor of Guyon's canal, which is bordered as well by the hook of the hamate and the pisiform and is covered by the volar carpal ligament. Entrapment of the ulnar nerve in this canal is possible (Fig. 11–27).
   c. Triangular Fibrocartilage Complex—Formed by the triangular fibrocartilage, ulnocarpal ligaments (volar ulnolunate and ulnotriquetral ligaments), and a meniscal homologue. Injuries to this structure are a common cause of ulnar wrist pain (Fig. 11–17).
   d. Intrinsic Apparatus—Complex arrangement of structures that surround the digits (Fig. 11–28). The following structures are important.

STRUCTURE	ATTACHMENTS	SIGNIFICANCE
Sagittal bands	Covers MCP	Allows MCP extension
Transverse (sagittal) fibers	Volar plate	Allows MCP flexion (interosseoi)
Lateral bands	Covers PIP	Allows PIP extension (lumbricals)
Oblique retinacular ligament (Landsmeer's ligament)	A4 pulley, terminal tendon	Allows DIP extension (passive)

   e. Flexor Sheath (Fig. 11–29)—Covers the flexor tendons in the finger, protecting and nourishing the tendons (vincula). Also forms five pulleys (A1–A5) with three intervening cruciate attachments (C1–C3). The **A2 pulley,** overlying the proximal **phalanx, is the most important** one, **followed by A4,** which covers the middle phalanx.

C. Muscles (Table 11–7) Organs and Insertions (Fig. 11–30)
D. Nerves (Fig. 11–31)
   1. Median Nerve—Enters the wrist just under the transverse carpal ligament between the FDS and the FCR. The palmar branch supplies the thenar skin. The deep (muscular) branch runs radially and supplies thenar muscles. Digital nerves supply the lumbricals and the radial 31/2 digits.
   2. Ulnar Nerve—Enters the wrist through Guyon's canal and divides into a superficial branch (palmaris brevis and skin) and a deep branch that passes between the ADM and FDMB, giving off motor branches to the deep musculature and ter-

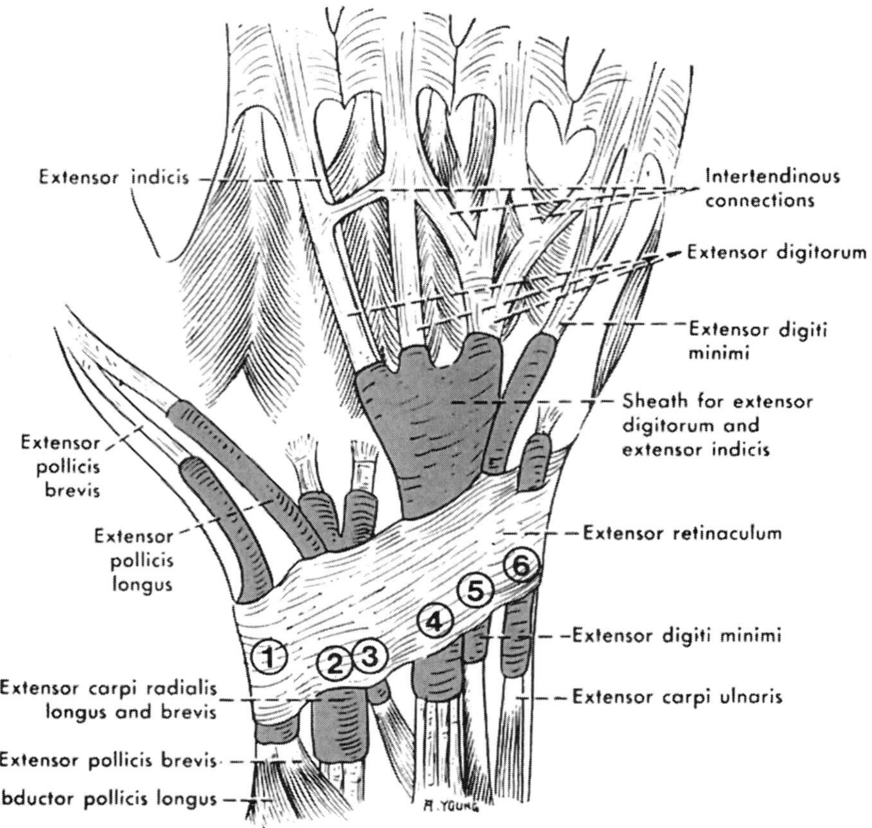

FIGURE 11–26. Extensor compartments of the wrist (1 to 6). (From Jenkins, D.B.: Hollinshead's Functional Anatomy of the Limbs and Back, 6th ed., p. 174. Philadelphia, WB Saunders, 1991; reprinted by permission.)

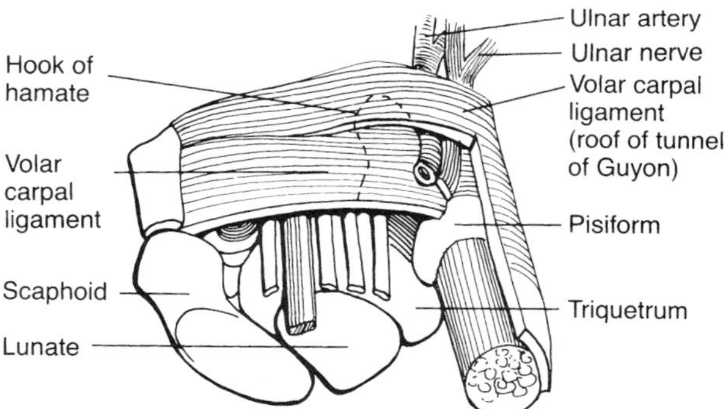

FIGURE 11–27. The carpal tunnel is formed by the transverse carpal ligament volarly and the carpal bones on the floor and sides. Guyon's canal is formed by the volar carpal ligament (roof), the hamate (lateral wall), and the pisiform (medial wall). (From DeLee, J.C. and Drez Jr, D.: Orthopaedic Sports Medicine: Principles and Practice, vol. 1, p. 932. Philadelphia W.B. Saunders, 1994; reprinted by permission.)

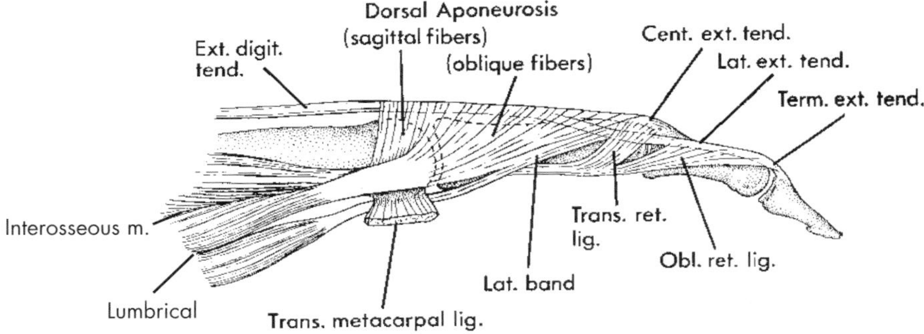

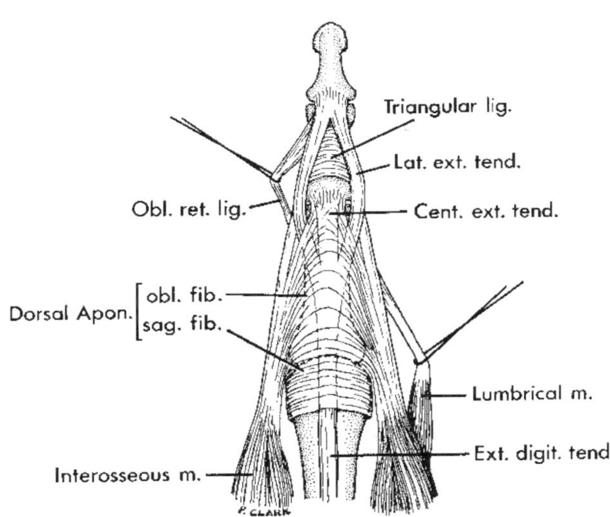

FIGURE 11–28. Dorsal extensor apparatus. (Adapted from Bora, F.W.: The Pediatric Upper Extremity, p. 93. Philadelphia, WB Saunders, 1986; reprinted by permission.)

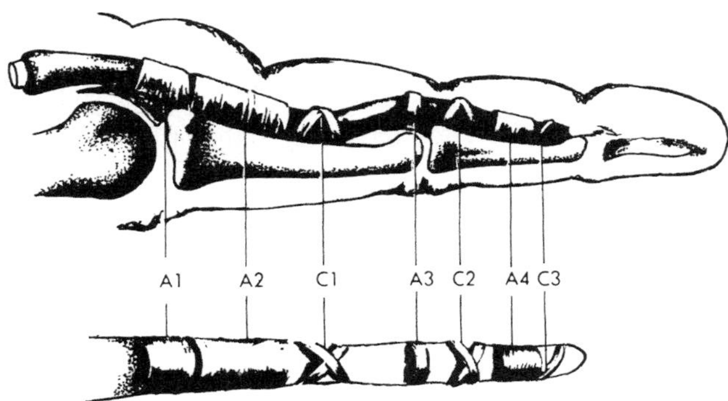

FIGURE 11–29. Flexor pulleys. (From Tubiana, R.: The Hand, vol. 3, p. 173. Philadelphia, WB Saunders, 1985; reprinted by permission.)

minating in digital nerves for the ulnar 11/2 digits. The dorsal cutaneous branch swings dorsally at the wrist and can be injured with either arthroscopic portal placement or surgical incisions.

3. Sensation to the Thumb—Comprised of five branches: lateral antebrachial cutaneous nerve, superficial and dorsal digital branches of the radial nerve, and digital and palmar branches of the median nerve.

E. Vessels (Fig. 11–31)
   1. Radial Artery—At the wrist the radial artery reaches the dorsum of the carpus by passing between the RCL and the APL and EPB tendons (snuffbox). Prior to this, it gives off a superficial palmar branch that communicates with the superficial arch (ulnar artery). In the hand it forms the deep palmar arch.
   2. Ulnar Artery—At the wrist, the ulnar artery lies on the TCL, gives off a deep palmar branch (which anastomoses with the deep arch), and then forms the superficial palmar arch, which is distal to the deep arch.

F. Surgical Approaches
   1. Dorsal Approach to the Wrist (Fig. 11–32)—Through the third and fourth extensor compartments (EPL and EDC). Protecting and retracting these tendons allows access to the distal radius and the dorsal radiocarpal joint.

TABLE 11–7. MUSCLES OF THE HAND AND WRIST

MUSCLE	ORIGIN	INSERTION	ACTION	INNERVATION
THENAR MUSCLES				
Abductor pollucis brevis (APB)	Scaphoid, trapezoid	Base of proximal phalanx, radial side	Abduct thumb	Median
Opponens pollicis	Trapezium	Thumb metacarpal	Abduct, flex, med. rotation	Median
Flexor pollicis brevis (FPB)	Trapezium, capitate	Base of proximal phalanx, radial side	Flex MCP	Median, ulnar
Adductor pollicis	Capitate, 2nd/3rd metacarpals	Base of proximal phalanx, ulnar side	Adduct thumb	Ulnar
HYPOTHENAR MUSCLES				
Palmaris brevis (PB)	TCL, palmar aponeurosis	Ulnar palm	Retract skin	Ulnar
Abductor digiti minimi (ADM)	Pisiform	Base of proximal phalanx, ulnar side	Abduct small finger	Ulnar
Flexor digiti minimi brevis (FDMB)	Hamate, TCL	Base of proximal phalanx, ulnar side	Flex MCP	Ulnar
Opponens digiti minimi (ODM)	Hamate, TCL	Small finger metacarpal	Abduct, flex, lat. rotation	Ulnar
INTRINSIC MUSCLES				
Lumbricals	Flexor digitorum profundus (FDP)	Lateral bands (radial)	Extend PIP	Median, ulnar
Dorsal interosseous (DIO)	Adjacent metacarpals	Proximal phalanx base/ extensor apparatus	Abduct, flex, MCP	Ulnar
Volar interosseous (VIO)	Adjacent metacarpals	Proximal phalanx base/ extensor apparatus	Adduct, flex MCP	Ulnar

2. Volar Approach to the Wrist (Fig. 11–33)—Used most commonly for carpal tunnel release, the incision is usually made in line with the fourth ray to avoid the palmar cutaneous branch of the median nerve. Careful dissection through the transverse carpal ligament is necessary to avoid injury to the median nerve or its motor branch. The median nerve and flexor tendons can be retracted to allow access to the distal radius and carpus.
3. Volar Approach to the Scaphoid (Russé) (Fig. 11–34)—Uses the interval between the FCR and the radial artery. An approach through the radial aspect of the FCR sheath is often easier and protects the radial artery.
4. Dorsolateral Approach to the Scaphoid (Fig. 11–35)—Utilizes an incision within the anatomic snuffbox (first and third dorsal wrist compartment), protecting the superficial radial nerve and radial artery (deep).
5. Volar Approach to the Flexor Tendons (Bunnell)—Zigzag incisions across the flexor creases help to expose the flexor sheaths. The digital sheaths should be avoided.
6. Midlateral Approach to the Digits—Good for stabilization of fractures and neurovascular exposure, this approach uses a laterally placed incision at the dorsal extend of the IP creases. Exposure of the digital neurovascular bundle is carried out volar to the incision.

VI. Spine

A. Osteology

1. Introduction—The spine contains 33 vertebrae. There are 7 cervical, 12 thoracic, 5 lumbar, 5 sacral, and 4 coccygeal vertebrae. The total length of the spine averages about 71 cm. Normal curves include cervical lordosis, thoracic kyphosis, and lumbosacral lordosis. The vertebral bodies generally increase in width craniocaudally with the exception of T1–T3. Important topographic landmarks include the mandible (C2–C3), hyoid cartilage (C3), thyroid cartilage (C4/C5), cricoid cartilage (C6), vertebra prominens (C7), spine of scapula (T3), tip of scapula (T7), and iliac crest (L4–L5).
2. Cervical Spine—Unique features include foramina in each transverse process. The spinous processes are bifid, and the vertebral foramina are triangular. The atlas (C1) is unique in that it contains no vertebral body and no spinous process. It does contain two lateral masses. The axis (C2) has a vertical projection called the dens, or odontoid process, that articulates with the atlas. It also possesses superior and inferior facets. The seventh cervical vertebra is unique because it has a prominent nonbifid posterior spinous process and no anterior tubercle.
3. Thoracic Spine—Unique features include costal facets (present on all 12 vertebral bodies and the transverse processes of T1–T9) and a rounded vertebral foramen. The first thoracic vertebra contains a large, prominent spinous process.
4. Lumbar Spine—These vertebrae are the largest. They contain short laminae and pedicles and massive vertebral bodies. They also have mammillary processes that project posteriorly from the superior articular facet. The transverse processes are thin and long (with the exception of the fifth lumbar vertebra).
5. Sacrum—Fusion of five spinal elements. The promontory is the anterosuperior portion that projects into the pelvis. There are usually four

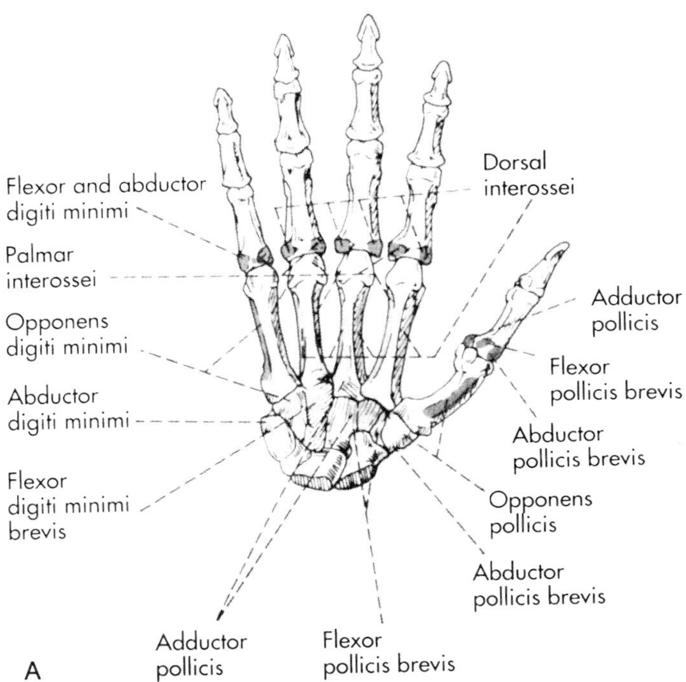

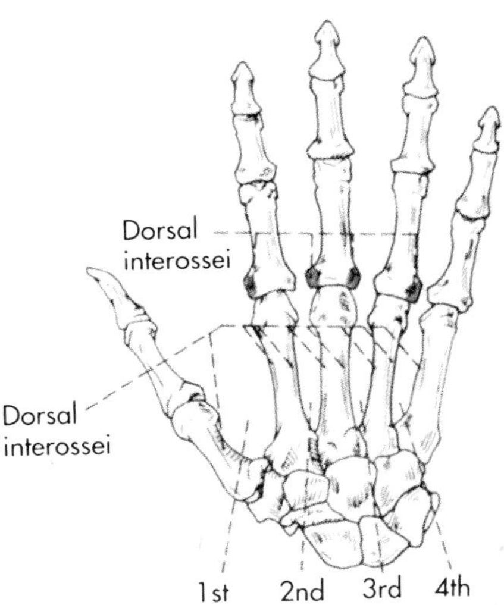

FIGURE 11–30. Origins and insertions of muscles of the wrist and hand. (From Jenkins, D.B.: Hollinshead's Functional Anatomy of the Limbs and Back, 6th ed., Fig. 11–9. Philadelphia, W.B. Saunders, 1991; reprinted by permission.)

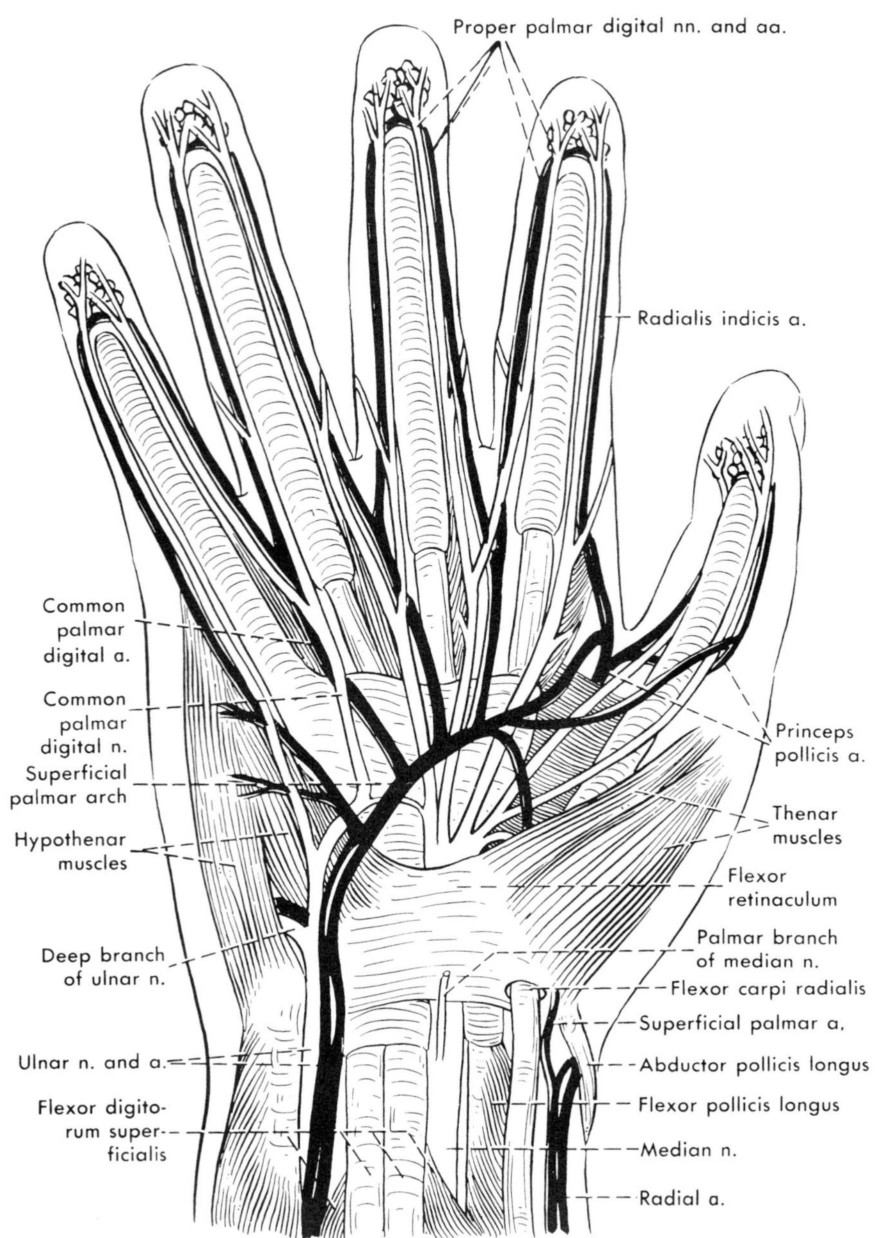

FIGURE 11–31. Nerves and vessels of the hand. (From Jenkins, D.B.: Hollinshead's Functional Anatomy of the Limbs and Back, 6th ed., Fig. 11–11. Philadelphia, WB Saunders, 1991; reprinted by permission.)

pairs of pelvic sacral foramina located both anteriorly and posteriorly that transmit respective branches of the upper four sacral nerves. There is also a sacral canal, which opens caudally into the sacral hiatus.

6. Coccyx—Fusion of the lowest four spinal elements; it attaches dorsally to the gluteus maximus, the external anal sphincter, and the coccygeal muscles.
7. Ossification—There are three primary ossification centers for each vertebra: two ossification centers in the centrum and one cartilaginous center for each arch. The arches unite dorsally at the third month of fetal life. Five secondary ossification centers (two transverse processes, one spinous process, and two body end plates) do not appear until after puberty. Ossification of the atlas, axis, sacral, and coccygeal vertebrae are unique. The axis (C2) ossifies from five primary and two secondary centers. Of note, the dens is formed from two primary growth centers that originate from the "centrum," or body of the atlas (C1). Mammillary processes arise from additional ossification centers in the lumbar vertebrae. The arches fuse with the centrum during the seventh year of life in the following order: thoracic, cervical, lumbar, and finally sacral. Failure of arch formation results in spina bifida.

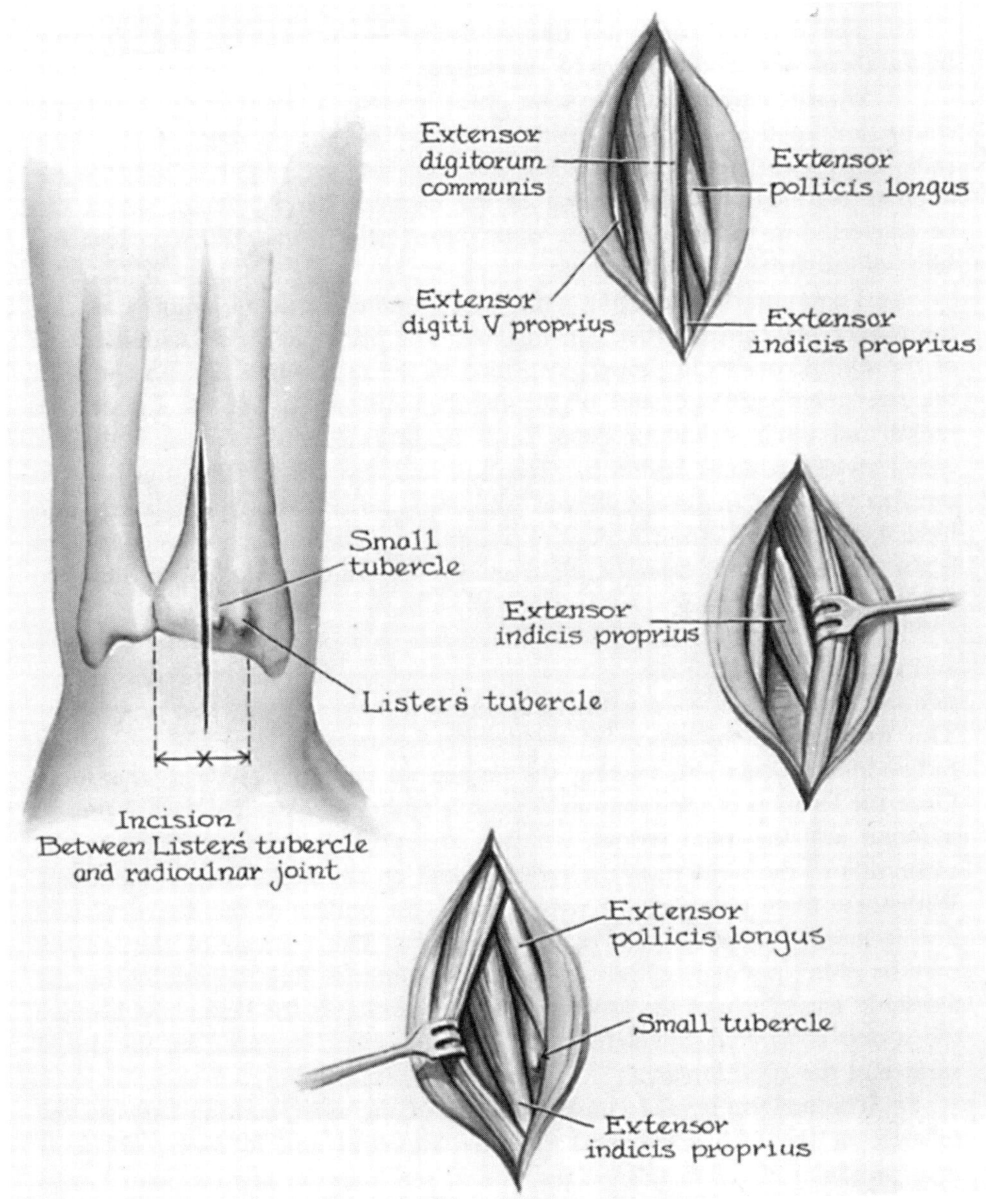

FIGURE 11–32. Dorsal wrist approach. (From Kaplan, E.B.: Surgical Approaches to the Neck, Cervical Spine, and Upper Extremity, p. 112. Philadelphia, WB Saunders, 1966; reprinted by permission.)

B. Arthrology
 1. Ligaments
  a. General Arrangement—The vertebral bodies are bound together by the strong anterior longitudinal ligament (**ALL**) and the weaker posterior longitudinal ligament (**PLL**). The ALL is usually thickest at the center of the vertebral body and thins at the periphery. Separate fibers extend from one to five levels. The PLL extends from the occiput to the posterior sacrum. It is separated from the center of the vertebral body by a space that allows passage of the dorsal branches of the spinal artery. The PLL is hourglass-shaped, with the wider (yet thinner) sections located over the discs. Ruptured discs tend to occur lateral to these expansions. Ligamentous capsules overlying the zygapophyseal joints and the intertransverse ligaments contribute little to interspinous stability. The **ligamentum flavum** is a strong, yellow, elastic ligament connecting the laminae. It runs from the anterior surface of the superior lamina to the posterior surface of the inferior lamina and is constantly in tension. Hypertrophy of the ligamentum flavum is said to contribute to nerve root compression. The **supraspinous** and **interspinous** ligaments lie dorsal to and between the spinous processes, respectively. The supraspinous ligament begins at C7 and

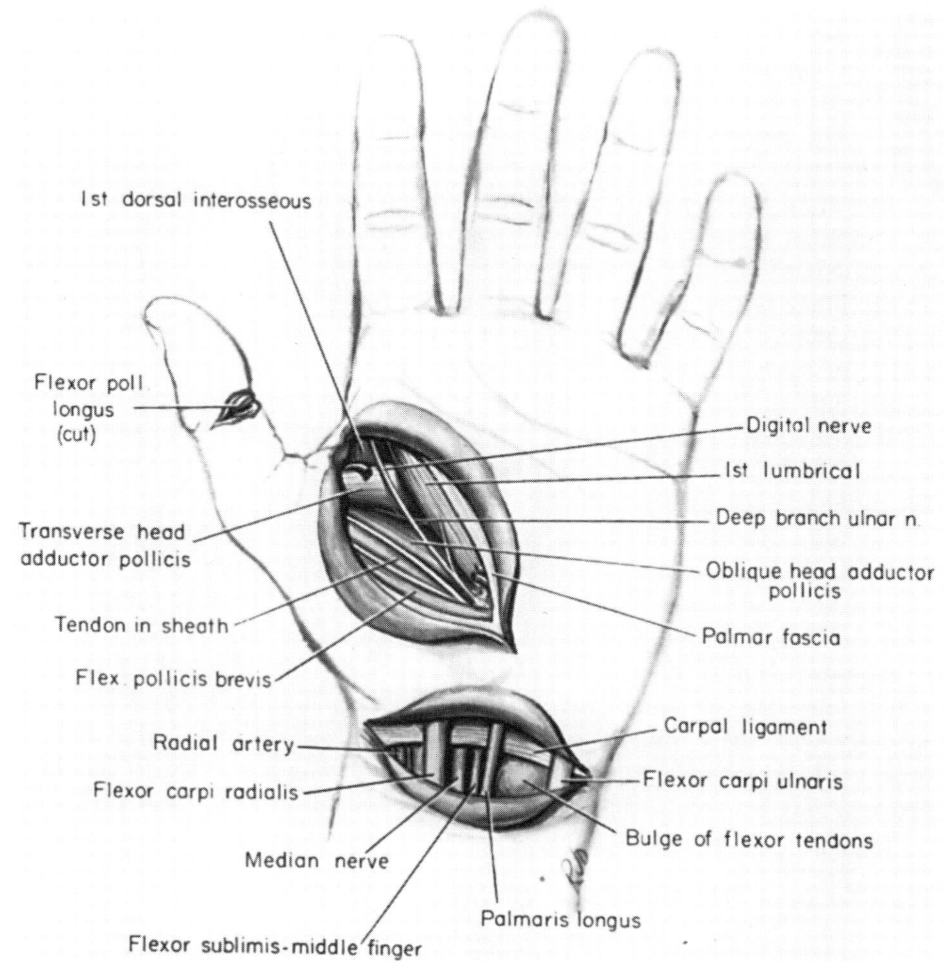

FIGURE 11–33. Approach to the carpal tunnel and thenar muscles. (From Kaplan, E.B.: Surgical Approaches to the Neck, Cervical Spine, and Upper Extremity, p. 97. Philadelphia, WB Saunders, 1966; reprinted by permission.)

is in continuity with the ligamentum nuchae (which runs from C7 to the occiput). Their relative contribution to interspinous stability is unknown.

b. Specialized Ligaments
   1. Atlanto-occipital Joint—Consists of two articular capsules (anterior and posterior) and the **tectoral membrane** (a cephalad extension of the PLL). It is further stabilized by the ligamentous attachments to the dens.
   2. Atlanto-axial Joint—The **transverse** ligament is the major stabilizer of the median atlantoaxial joint. This articulation is further stabilized by the apical ligament (longitudinal), which together with the transverse ligament comprises the **cruciate** ligament. Additionally, a pair of **alar,** or "check," ligaments run obliquely from the tip of the dens to the occiput (Fig. 11–36).
   3. Iliolumbar Ligament—This stout ligament connects the transverse process of L5 with the ilium. Tension on this ligament in patients with unstable vertical shear pelvic fractures can lead to avulsion fractures of the transverse process.

2. Facet (Apophyseal) Joints—The orientation of the facets of the spine dictates the plane of motion at each relative level. The facet orientation varies with spinal level. In the sagittal plane, the orientation is 45 degrees in the cervical spine, 60 degrees in the thoracic spine, and 90 degrees in the lumbar spine. In the coronal plane, the orientation is 0 degrees (neutral) in the cervical spine, 20 degrees posterior in the thoracic spine, and 45 degrees anterior in the lumbar spine. In the cervical spine the superior articular facet is anterior and inferior to the inferior articular process of the vertebra above. In the lumbar spine the superior articular facet is anterior and lateral to the inferior articular facet.
3. Discs—The intervertebral discs are fibrocartilaginous, with obliquely oriented **annulus** fibrosis comprised of **type I collagen** and a softer central **nucleus pulposus** made of **type II collagen.** The discs account for 25% of the total spinal columnar height. They are attached to the verte-

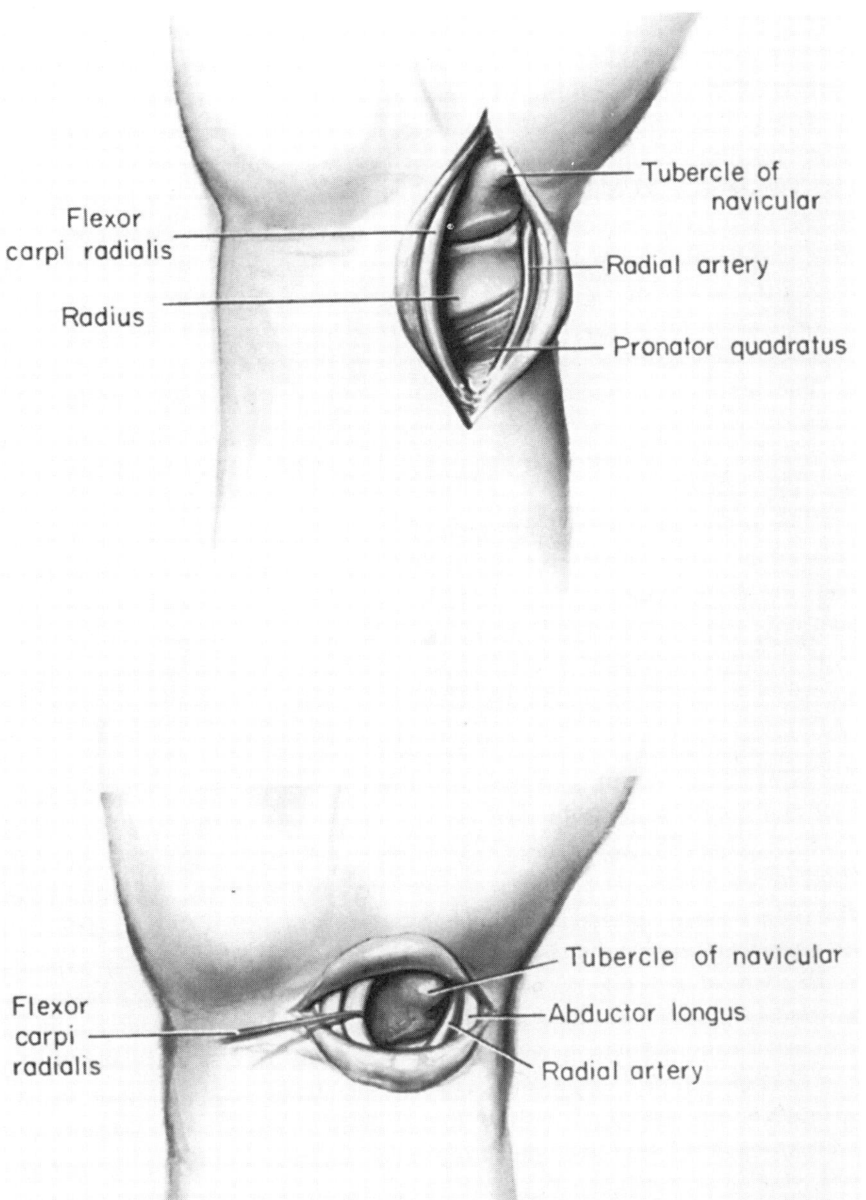

FIGURE 11–34. Russé approach to the scaphoid. (From Kaplan, E.B.: Surgical Approaches to the Neck, Cervical Spine, and Upper Extremity, p. 101. Philadelphia, WB Saunders, 1966; reprinted by permission.)

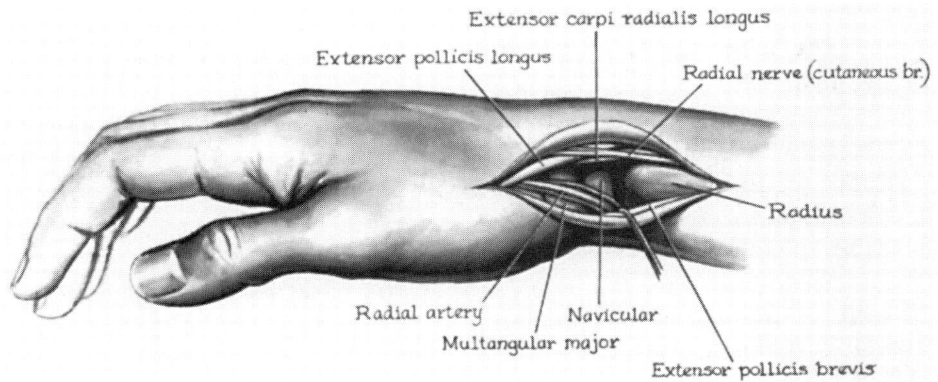

FIGURE 11–35. Dorsal approaches to the scaphoid. (From Kaplan, E.B.: Surgical Approaches to the Neck, Cervical Spine, and Upper Extremity, p. 107. Philadelphia, WB Saunders, 1966; reprinted by permission.)

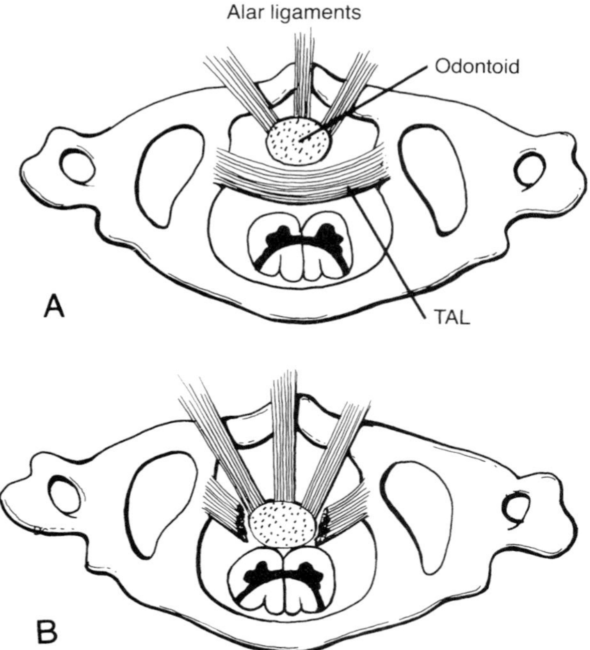

FIGURE 11–36. The atlanto-axial complex as seen from above *(A)*. The disruption of the transverse ligament (TAL) with intact alar ligaments results in C1–C2 instability without cord compression *(B)*. (From DeLee J.C., and Drez, Jr. D.: Orthopaedic Sports Medicine, Principles and Practices, vol 1, p. 432. Philadelphia, WB Saunders, 1994; *B.* Redrawn from Hensinger R.N.: Congenital anomalies of the atlantoaxial joint. The Cervical Spine Research Society Editorial Committee. The Cervical Spine, 2nd ed., p. 242. Philadelphia, JB Lippincott, 1989; reprinted by permission.)

bral bodies by hyaline cartilage, which is responsible for the vertical growth of the column. The distinction between the nucleus and annulus becomes less apparent as one ages.

C. Spinal Musculature
   1. Neck—The neck is divided, for functional purposes, into the anterior and posterior regions.
      a. Anterior—The anterior neck muscles include the superficial platysma muscle (CN VII innervated), stylohyoid and digastric muscles (CN XII) above the hyoid, and "strap" muscles below the hyoid. Important strap muscles include the sternohyoid and omohyoid in the superficial layer and the thyrohyoid and sternothyroid in the deep layer; all are innervated by the ansa cervicalis. Laterally, the sternocleidomastoid (CN XI and ansa) runs obliquely across the neck and inserts into the ipsilateral side; it rotates the head to the contralateral side.
      b. Posterior—The posterior neck muscles form the border of the **suboccipital triangle.** This triangle is formed by the superior and inferior heads of the obliquus capitis muscle and the rectus capitis posterior major muscle. The vertebral artery and the first cervical nerve are within this triangle, and the greater occipital nerve is superficial.
   2. Back—The back is blanketed by the trapezius (superiorly) and the latissimus dorsi (inferiorly). The rhomboids and levator scapulae are deep to this layer. Refer to Table 11–4 for specifics on these muscles. The deep muscles of the back are arranged into two groups: erector spinae and transversospinalis group. The erector spinae run from the transverse and spinous processes of the inferior vertebrae to the spinous processes of the superior vertebrae. They stabilize and extend the back. All of the deep back musculature is innervated by dorsal primary rami of spinal nerves.

D. Nerves
   1. Spinal Cord—The cord extends from the brain stem to L1, where it terminates as the conus medularis. It is enclosed within the bony spinal canal with variable amounts of space (greatest in the upper cervical spine). The cord also varies in diameter (widest at the origin of plexi). In cross section, the cord has both geographic and functional boundaries (Fig. 11–37). It is divided in the midline anteriorly by a fissure and posteriorly by the sulcus. The posterior funiculi (**dorsal columns**) are located dorsally and receive ascending fibers, which deliver deep touch, proprioception, and vibratory sensation. The **lateral spinothalamic tract** transmits pain and temperature (it is the site for chordotomy for intractable pain). Descending in the **lateral corticospinal tract** are fibers that transmit instructions for voluntary muscle contraction. The ventral spinothalamic tract transmits light touch sensation, and the **ventral corticospinal tract** delivers cortical messages of voluntary contraction. Pathways to the hand and upper extremity are usually localized centrally within this area (hence the clinical findings of anterior cord syndrome). The spinal cord tapers at L1–L2 (conus medularis), and a small filum terminale continues with surrounding nerve roots contained within a common dural sac (cauda equina) to its termination in the coccyx.

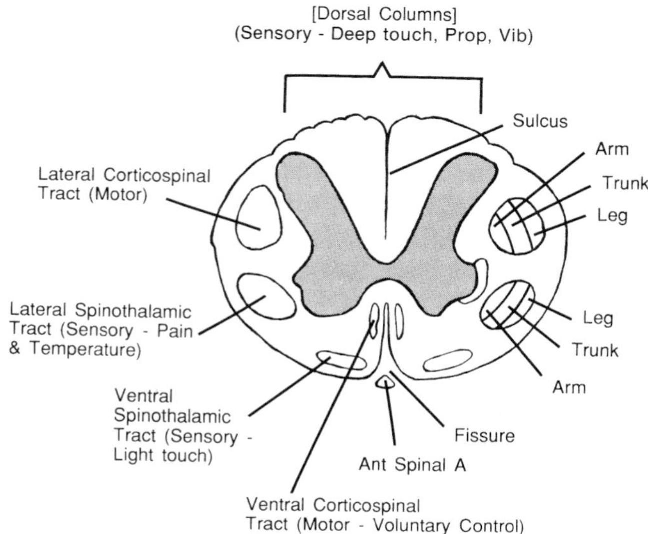

FIGURE 11–37. Cross section of the spinal cord.

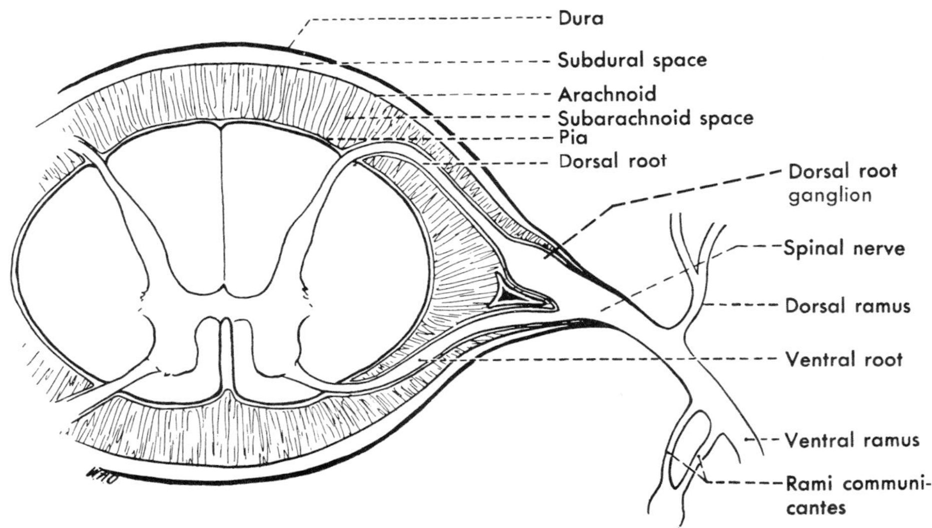

FIGURE 11–38. Spinal nerves. (From Jenkins, D.B.: Hollinshead's Functional Anatomy of the Limbs and Back, 6th ed., p. 205. Philadelphia, WB Saunders, 1991; reprinted by permission.)

2. Nerve Roots (Fig. 11–38)—Within the subarachnoid space the dorsal root (and ganglia) and ventral roots converge to form the spinal nerve. The nerve becomes "extradural" as it approaches the intervertebral foramen (dura becomes epineurium) at all levels above L1. Below this level, the nerves are contained within the cauda equina. In the cervical spine the numbered nerve exists at a level *above* the pedicle of corresponding vertebral level (e.g., C2 exists at C1–C2). In the lumbar spine the nerve root transverses the respective disc space above the named vertebral body and exits the respective foramen under the pedicle (Fig. 11–39). Herniated discs usually impinge on the traversing nerve root and the facet joint. After exiting the foramen the spinal nerve delivers dorsal primary rami, which supply the muscles and skin of the neck and back regions. The ventral rami supply the anteromedial trunk and the limbs. With exception of the thoracic nerves, ventral rami are grouped in plexuses before delivering sensorimotor functions to a general region.
3. Sympathetic Chain—The cervical sympathetic chain is a deep structure closely associated with the longus capitus and colli muscles, posterior to the carotid sheath. The sympathetic chain has three ganglia: superior, middle, and inferior.

GANGLIA	LOCATION	OTHER
Superior	C2–C3	Largest
Middle	C6	Variable
Inferior	C7–T1	"Stellate"

E. Vascular Supply to the Spine—Spinal blood supply is usually derived from the segmental arteries via the aorta. The primary supply to the dura and posterior elements is from the dorsal branches. The ventral branches supply the vertebral bodies via ascending and descending branches, which are delivered underneath the posterior longitudinal ligament in four separate ostia. The vertebral artery (a branch of the subclavian) ascends through the transverse foramina of C1–C6 (anterior to and not through C7), then posterior to the lateral masses, along the cephalad surface of the posterior arch of C1 (atlas), and through the foramen magnum before uniting at the midline basilar artery. The artery of **Adamkiewicz** (great anterior medullary artery) enters through the left intervertebral foramen in the lower thoracic spine. It should be preserved during dissections at this level. Arterial supply to the spinal cord is from anterior and posterior spinal arteries and segmental branches of the vertebral artery and dorsal arteries, which travel via the dorsal and ventral rootlets to the respective dorsal and anterolateral portions of the cord. The venous drainage of the vertebral bodies is primarily via the central sinusoid located on the dorsum of each vertebral body.

F. Surgical Approaches to the Spine
1. Anterior Approach to the Cervical Spine (Fig. 11–40)—A transverse incision is based on the desired level (e.g., for C5 one should enter the carotid triangle). The platysma is retracted with the skin. The pretracheal fascia is exposed to explore the interval between the carotid sheath and the trachea. The prevertebral fascia is sharply incised and the longus colli muscle gently retracted (protecting the recurrent laryngeal nerve) to expose the vertebral body. The right recurrent laryngeal nerve can lie outside the carotid sheath and must be identified. By dissecting the longus muscles subperiosteally, one also protects the stellate ganglion (avoiding Horner syndrome). Occasionally it is necessary to split the fibers of the omohyoid.

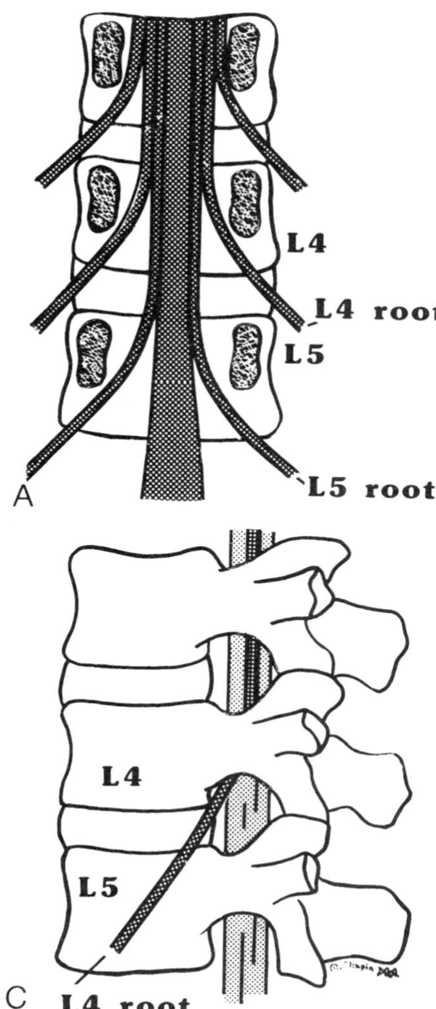

FIGURE 11–39. Nerve root locations in relation to vertebral landmarks. (From Wiessman, B.N., and Sledge, C.B.: Orthopedic Radiology, p. 283. Philadelphia, WB Saunders, 1986; reprinted by permission.)

2. Posterior Approach to the Cervical Spine—After a midline approach through the ligamentum nuchae, the superficial layer (trapezius) and intermediate layer (splenius, semispinalis, longissimus capitis) are reflected laterally, and the vertebrae are exposed. The vertebral artery is especially vulnerable as it leaves the foramen transversarium and travels above and medially to pierce the atlanto-occipital membrane at its lateral angle. The greater occipital nerve (C2) and the third occipital nerve C3) should also be protected in the suboccipital region. Access to the spinal canal is via laminectomy or facetectomy (Fig. 11–41).
3. Anterior Approach to the Thoracic Spine—A transverse incision is made approximately two ribs above the level of interest. Dissection over the top of the rib is carried out to avoid injuring the intercostal neurovascular bundle. The rib is further dissected and removed from the field. The right-sided approach is favored to avoid the aorta, segmental arteries, artery of Adamkiewicz, and thoracic duct. The esophagus, aorta, vena cava, and pleura of the lungs should be identified and protected.
4. Posterior Approach to the Thoracolumbar Spine—A straight midline incision is made over the spinous processes and carried down through the thoracolumbar fascia. Paraspinal musculature is subperiosteally dissected from the attached spinous processes, exposing the posterior elements. Structures at risk include the posterior primary rami (near facet joints) and segmental vessels (anterior to the plane connecting the transverse processes). Partial laminectomy allows greater exposure of the cord and discs. Pedicle screw placement is at the junction of the lateral border of the superior facet and the middle of the transverse process. These screws should be angled 15 degrees medially and in line with the slope of the vertebra as seen on lateral radiographs.
5. Anterior Approach to the Thoracolumbar Spine—An oblique incision is centered over the tenth rib, which is exposed and removed. The diaphragm is incised near its periphery, and dissection is carried into the retroperitoneum. The periotoneum is swept away from the psoas and vertebral bodies. Segmental arteries are ligated. Risks of this approach include injuries to the ureter, internal iliac vessels, and lumbar plexus nerves.

VII. Pelvis and Hip

A. Osteology—The pelvic girdle is composed of two innominate (coxal) bones that articulate with the sacrum. Each innominate bone, in turn, is composed of three united bones: the ilium, ischium, and pubis. Distinctive parts of each innominate bone include the acetabulum (vinegar cup) and the obturator foramen. The acetabulum is anteverted and obliquely oriented. The posterosuperior articular surface is thickened to accommodate weight-bearing. The inferior surface is deficient and contains the acetabular, or cotyloid, notch. This notch is bound by the transverse acetabular ligament. The greater sciatic notch is located posterior and superior to the acetabulum, between the posteroinferior iliac spine (PIIS) and the ischial spine. The anterior superior iliac spine (ASIS) is prominent and palpable at the lateral edge of the inguinal ligament. It is the origin for the sartorius muscle and the transverse and internal abdominal muscles. The posterior superior iliac spine (PSIS) is usually located 4–5 cm lateral to the S2 spinous process. It may be marked topographically by a dimple and is an excellent source for bone graft. The anterior inferior iliac spine (AIIS) is less prominent and provides the origin of the direct head of the rectus femoris. The arcuate line delineates a thick column of bone that extends from the auricular process of the ilium to the pectineal line and represents the weight-bearing column. The outer surface of the iliac wing contains the anterior, posterior, and inferior gluteal lines, which form borders for the origins of the gluteal muscles. The iliopectineal

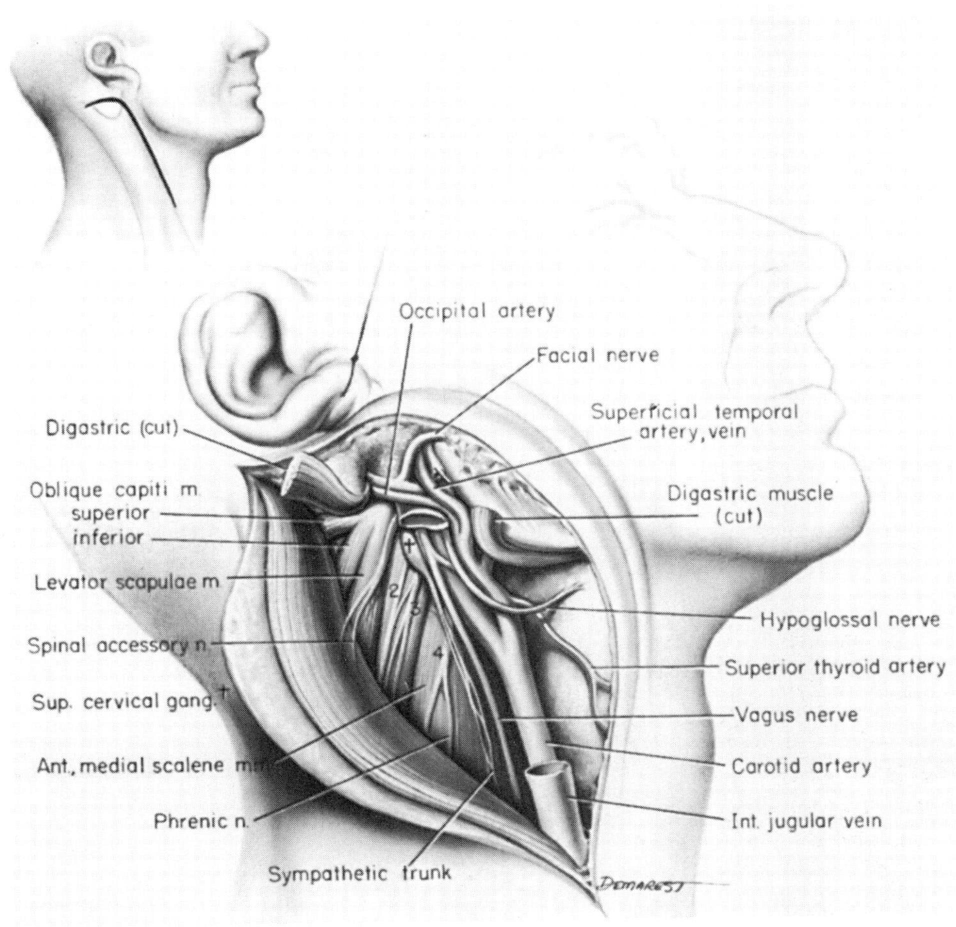

FIGURE 11–40. Approach to the anterior neck. (From Kaplan, E.B.: Surgical Approaches to the Neck, Cervical Spine, and Upper Extremity, p. 23. Philadelphia, WB Saunders, 1966; reprinted by permission.)

eminence is a raised region anteriorly that represents the union of the ilium and pubis. The iliopsoas muscle traverses a groove between this eminence and the anteroinferior iliac spine. Ossification centers of the pelvis are as follows.

CENTER	TYPE	AGE AT APPEARANCE	AGE AT FUSION
Ilium	Primary	2 months	15 years
Ischium	Primary	4 months	15 years
Pubis	Primary	6 months	15 years
Acetabulum	Secondary	12 years	15 years
Iliac crest	Secondary	16 years	25 years
Ant. inf. iliac spine	Secondary	16 years	25 years
Ischial tuberosity	Secondary	16 years	25 years
Pubis	Secondary	16 years	30 years

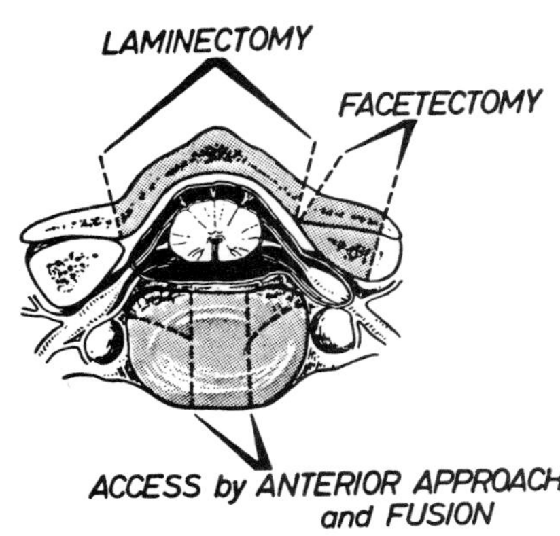

FIGURE 11–41. Approach to the cervical spine. (From Rothman, R.H., and Simeon, F.A.: The Spine, 2nd ed., p. 484. Philadelphia, WB Saunders, 1982; reprinted by permission.)

The proximal femur is composed of the femoral head (articulates with the acetabulum), neck, and greater and lesser trochanters. The inner architecture of the proximal femur includes an intricate arrangement of primary and secondary trabeculae (Fig. 11–42).

B. Arthrology
   1. Hip—The hip joint is a spheroid, or ball-and-socket, type of diarthrodial joint. Its stability is based primarily on the bony architecture, which also allows good motion. The acetabulum is deepened by the fibrocartilaginous rim, called the labrum. The joint capsule extends anteriorly

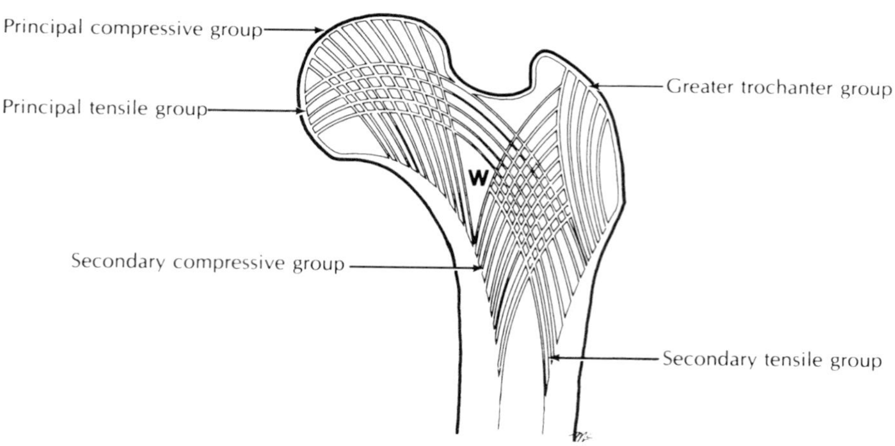

FIGURE 11–42. Hip trabeculae. (From DeLee, J.C.: Fractures and dislocations of the hip. In Rockwood, C.A., Jr., Green, D.P., and Buchholz, R.W., eds., Fractures in Adults, 3rd ed., p. 1488. Philadelphia, JB Lippincott, 1991; reprinted by permission.)

across the femoral neck to the trochanteric crest; however, posteriorly it extends only partially across the femoral neck (Fig. 11–43). The fibrous capsule that encloses the joint contains circular fibers that can be recognized better posteriorly as the zona orbicularis. A series of three ligaments comprise the capsule anteriorly. The *iliofemoral,* or Y, ligament of Bigelow is the strongest ligament in the body and attaches the AIIS to the intertrochanteric line in an inverted Y fashion. The remaining anterior ligaments, the *ischiofemoral* and *pubofemoral* ligaments, are weaker but lend additional stability. Inside the joint, the ligament of teres arises from the apex of the cotyloid notch and attaches to the fovea of the femoral head. It transmits an arterial branch of the posterior division of the **obturator artery** to the femoral head (less significant in adults).

2. Sacroiliac (SI) Joint—A true diarthrodial gliding joint supported by three groups of ligaments: posterior SI ligaments, anterior SI ligaments, and interosseous ligaments. Of these structures, the posterior ligaments, which have been compared to the trusses of a suspension bridge (Tile), provide the most stability and strength to the joint.
3. Symphysis Pubis—Connects the two hemipelvii anteriorly and is united with a fibrocartilaginous disc and supported by the superior pubic ligament and the arcuate pubic ligament.
4. Other ligaments include the sacrospinous and sacrotuberous ligaments, which outline the boundaries for the greater and lesser sciatic foramina. The **sacrospinous ligament** (anterior sacrum → ischial spine) is the inferior border of the **greater** sciatic foramen and the superior border of the **lesser** sciatic foramen. The lesser sciatic foramen is bordered inferiorly by the **sacrotuberous ligament** (anterior sacrum → ischial tuberosity). The piriformis, sciatic nerve, and other important structures exit the greater sciatic foramen. The short external rotators of the hip exit the lesser sciatic foramen.

C. Muscles of the Pelvis and Hip (Table 11–8; Fig. 11–44)

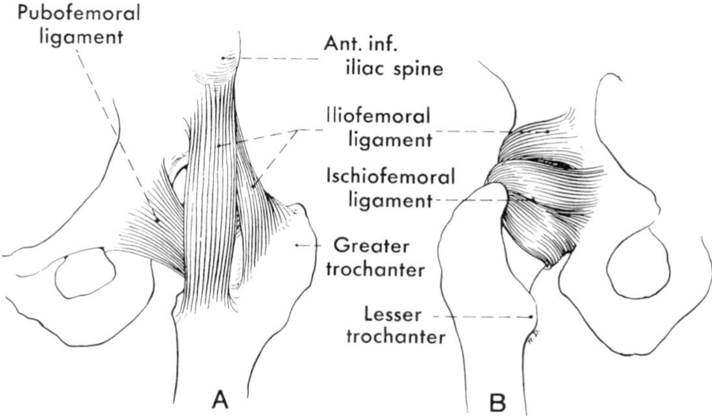

FIGURE 11–43. Hip capsule. *A,* Anterior view. *B,* Posterior view. (From Jenkins, D.B.: Hollinshead's Functional Anatomy of the Limbs and Back, 6th ed., p. 230. Philadelphia, WB Saunders, 1991; reprinted by permission.)

TABLE 11–8. MUSCLES OF THE PELVIS AND HIP

MUSCLE	ORIGIN	INSERTION	NERVE	SEGMENT
Flexors				
Iliacus	Iliac fossa	Lesser trochanter	Femoral	L234 (P)
Psoas	Transverse processes of L1–L5	Lesser trochanter	Femoral	L234 (P)
Pectineus	Pectineal line of pubis	Pectineal line of femur	Femoral	L234 (P)
Rectus femoris	AIIS, acetabular rim	Patella → tibial tubercle	Femoral	L234 (P)
Sartorius	ASIS	Proximal medial tibia	Femoral	L234 (P)
Adductors				
Post adductor magnus	Inferior public ramus/ischial tuberosity	Linea aspera/adductor tubercle	Obturator (P) and Sciatic (tibial)	L234 (A)
Adductor brevis	Inferior pubic ramus	Linea aspera/pectineal line	Obturator (P)	L234 (A)
Adductor longus	Anterior pubic ramus	Linea aspera	Obturator (A)	L234 (A)
Gracilis	Inf. symphysis/pubic arch	Proximal medial tibia	Obturator (A)	L234 (A)
External Rotators				
Gluteus maximus	Ilium post to post gluteal line	Iliotibial band/gluteal sling (femur)	Inf. gluteal	L5–S2 (P)
Piriformis	Ant. sacrum/sciatic notch	Proximal greater trochanter	Piriformis	S12 (P)
Obturator externus	Ischiopubic rami/obturator membrane	Trochlear fossa	Obturator	L234 (A)
Obturator internus	Ischiopubic rami/obturator membrane	Medial greater trochanter (MGT)	Obturator internus	L5–S2 (A)
Superior gemellus	Outer ischial spine	MGT	Obturator internus	L5–S2 (A)
Inferior gemellus	Ischial tuberosity	MGT	Quadratus femoris	L4–S1 (A)
Quadratus femoris	Ischial tuberosity	Quadrate line of femur	Quadratus femoris	L4–S1 (A)
Abductors				
Gluteus medius	Ilium/between post. and ant. gluteal lines	Greater trochanter	Superior gluteal	L4–S1 (P)
Gluteus minimus	Ilium between ant. and inf. gluteal lines	Ant. border of greater trochanter	Superior gluteal	L4–S1 (P)
Tensor fasciae latae (TFL) [tensor fascia femoris (TFF)]	Anterior iliac crest	Iliotibial band	Superior gluteal	L4–S1 (P)

D. Nerves

1. Lumbosacral Plexus

a. Lumbar Plexus—The lumbar plexus involves the ventral primary rami for T12–L4 but may display the usual prefixed (T11–L3) and postfixed (L1–L5) variations.

NERVES	LEVEL	INNERVATION
Anterior Division		
Subcostal	T12	Sensory: subxiphoid region
Iliohypogastric	L1	Sensory: posterolat. buttock/above pubis Motor: transversus abdominis/Int. oblique
Ilioinguinal	L1	Sensory: inguinal area
Genitofemoral	L1–L2	Sensory: Proximal anteromed thigh, scrotum/mons Motor: cremaster
Obturator	L2–L4	Motor: Ext. oblique/adductor longus/adductor magnus (ant.)/gracilis
Posterior Division		
Lateral femoral cutaneous (LFCN)	L2–L3	Sensory: Lateral thigh
Femoral	L2–L4	Motor: Psoas/iliacus/quadratus/sartorius/pectineus/articularis genu
Accessory obturator	L2–L4	Motor: Psoas

b. Sacral Plexus (Fig. 11–45)—The sacral plexus typically involves the ventral primary rami of L4–S3. It is formed in the pelvis anterior and lateral to the sacrum. It provides a significant amount of innervation to the limb.

NERVES	LEVEL	INNERVATION
Anterior Division		
Tibial	L4–S3	Semimembranosus/semitendinosus/biceps (long head)/adductor magnus/sup. gemellus/soleus/plantaris/popliteus/tibialis posterior/flexor digitorum longus/flexor hallucis longus
Quadratus femoris	L4–S1	Quadratus femoris/inf. gemellus
Obturator internus	L5–S2	Obturatorius internus/sup. gemellus
Pudendal	S2–S4	Sensory: perineal Motor: bulbocavernosus/urethra/urogenital diaphragm
Coccygeus	S4	Coccygeus
Levator ani	S3–S4	Levator ani
Posterior Division		
Peroneal	L4–S2	Biceps (short head)/tibialis anterior/extensor digitorum longus/peroneus tertius/extensor hallucis longus Peroneus longus and brevis/extensor hallucis brevis/extensor digitorum brevis

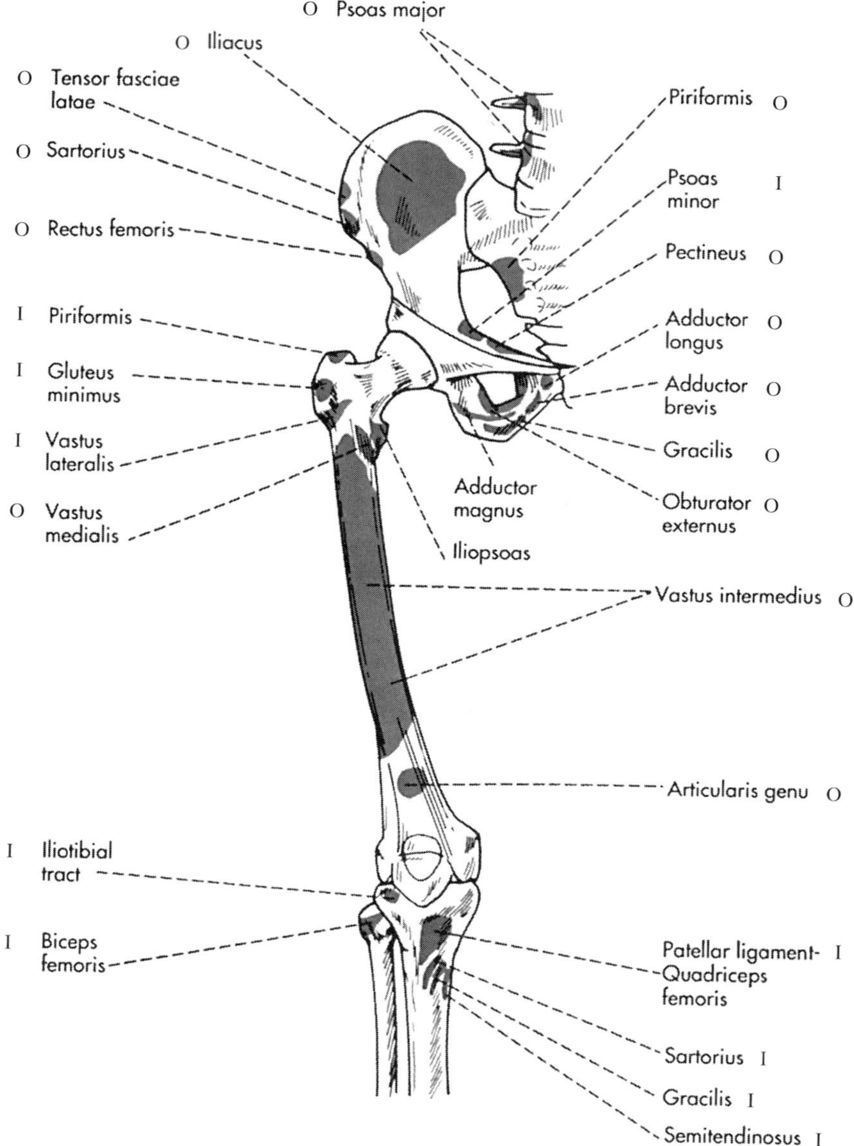

FIGURE 11–44. Origins and insertions of muscles of the hip and leg. O, origin; I, insertion. (Adapted from Jenkins, D.B.: Hollinshead's Functional Anatomy of the Limbs and Back, 6th ed., Figs. 16–7, 17–3. Philadelphia, WB Saunders, 1991; reprinted by permission.) *Illustration continued on opposite page*

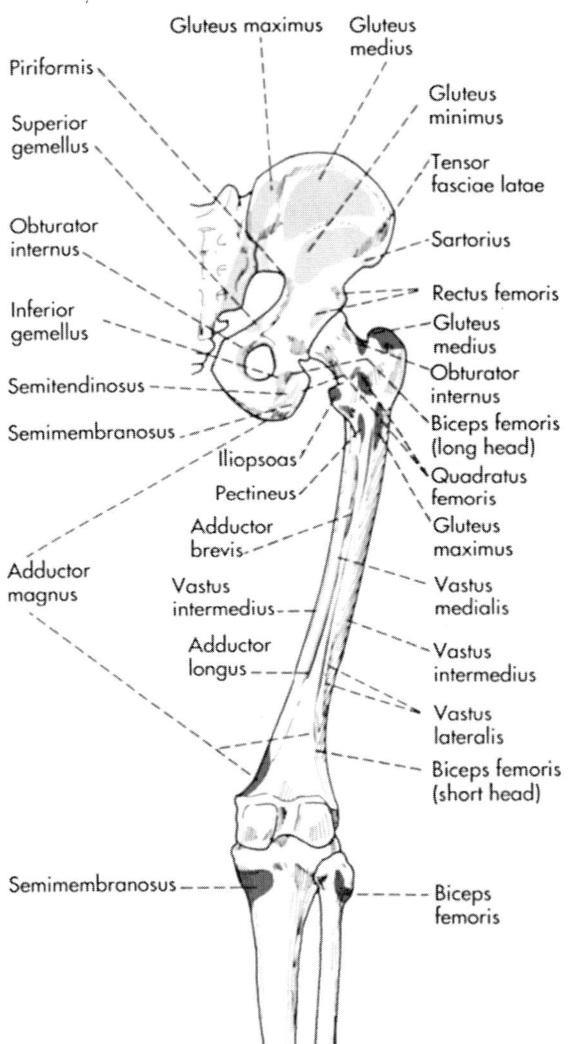

FIGURE 11–44. *Continued.* Origins = light areas; insertions-dark areas.

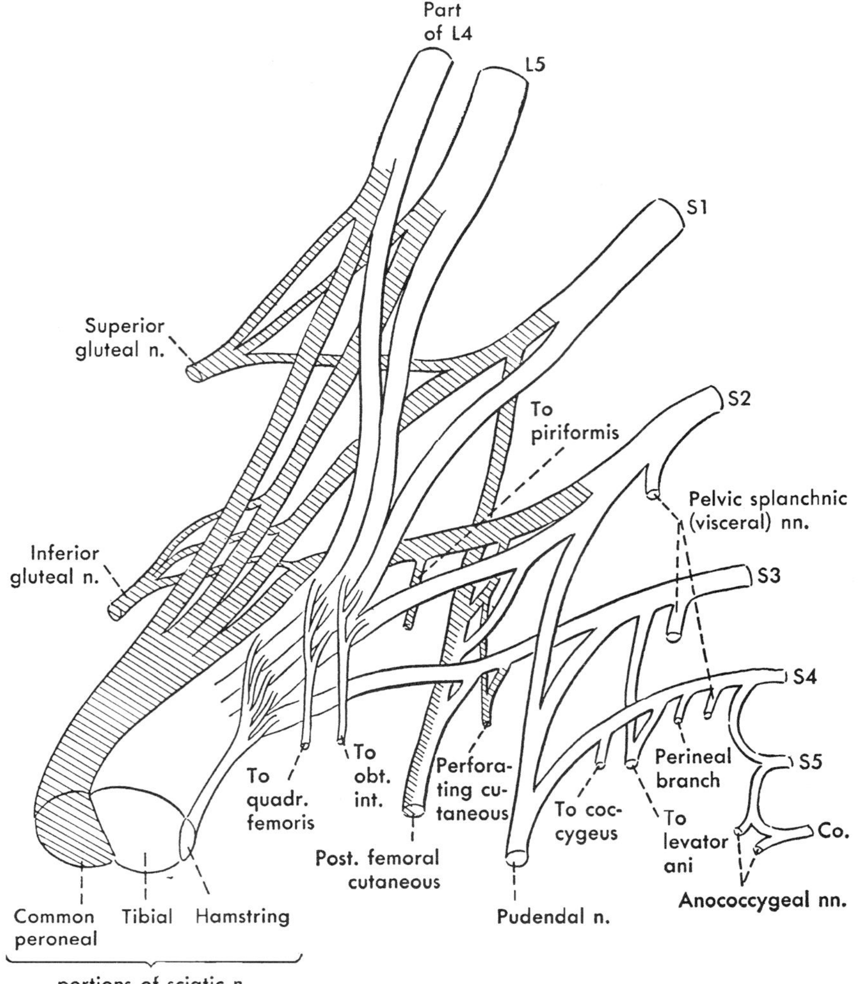

FIGURE 11–45. Sacral plexus. Anterior division (unshaded) and posterior division (shaded). (From Jenkins, D.B.: Hollinshead's Functional Anatomy of the Limbs and Back, 6th ed., p. 256. Philadelphia, WB Saunders, 1991; reprinted by permission.)

NERVES	LEVEL	INNERVATION
Sup. gluteal	L4–S1	Gluteus medius and minimus/ TFL
Inf. gluteal	L5–S2	Gluteus maximus
Piriformis	S2	Piriformis
Post. femoral cutaneous (PFCN)	S1–S3	Sensory: posterior thigh

2. Relationships—The lumbar plexus is found on the surface of the quadratus lumborum under (and within) the substance of the psoas major muscle. The genitofemoral nerve pierces the psoas and then lies on the anteromedial surface of the psoas. The femoral nerve lies between the iliacus and the psoas. The lateral femoral cutaneous nerve lies on the surface of the iliacus muscle and exits the pelvis under the lateral attachment of the inguinal ligament. Virtually all important nerves about the hip leave the pelvis by way of the sciatic foramen. The major reference point for the greater sciatic nerve and related structures in the hip is the piriformis muscle ("key" to the sciatic foramen). The **superior gluteal nerve and artery lie above the piriformis** and virtually everything else leaves below the muscle (remember POP'S IQ [lateral to medial]: *p*udendal, *o*bturator internus, *p*ostfemoral cutaneous, *s*ciatic, *i*nferior gluteal, *q*uadratus femoris). Two nerves leave the greater sciatic foramen and re-enter the pelvis via the lesser foramen (pudendal and nerve to obturator internus). In addition to the peripheral nerves, a plexus of parasympathetic nerves cover the lower aorta and the anterior sacrum. These nerves should be protected to prevent sexual dysfunction. Anteriorly, the great nerves and vessels enter the thigh (and into the **femoral triangle**) under the inguinal ligament (Fig. 11–46). The borders of this triangle include the sartorius laterally, the pectineus medially, and the inguinal ligament superiorly. Within the triangle, from lateral to medial, are the femoral *n*erve,

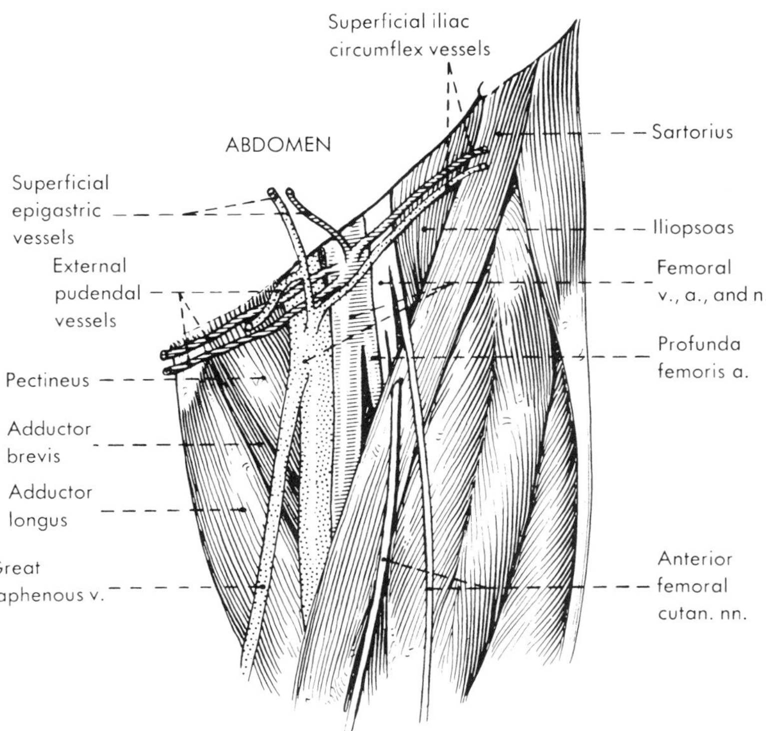

FIGURE 11–46. Femoral triangle. (From Jenkins, D.B.: Hollinshead's Functional Anatomy of the Limbs and Back, 6th ed., p. 243. Philadelphia, WB Saunders, 1991; reprinted by permission.)

*a*rtery, and *v*ein *a*nd the *l*ymphatic vessels (remember NAVAL). The femoral nerve descends between the iliacus and psoas and delivers numerous branches to muscle, overlying skin, and the hip joint (in accordance with Hilton's law). A spontaneous iliacus hematoma may irritate the femoral nerve owing to its proximity. At the apex of the triangle the saphenous nerve branches off and travels under the sartorius muscle. The obturator nerve exits the pelvis via the obturator canal. It splits into anterior and posterior divisions within the canal. The anterior division proceeds anteriorly to the obturator externus and posteriorly to the pectineus, supplying the adductor longus and brevis and the gracilis; it then delivers cutaneous branches to the medial thigh. The posterior division supplies the obturator externus, adductor brevis, and upper part of the adductor magnus, and it delivers other branches to the knee joint. The obturator nerve can be injured by retractors placed behind the transverse acetabular ligament.

E. Vessels (Fig. 11–47)—The aorta branches into the common iliacs arteries anterior to the L4 vertebral body. The common iliac vessels, in turn, divide into the internal (or *hypogastric;* medial) and external (lateral) iliacs at the S1 level. Important internal iliac branches include the obturator, superior gluteal (can be injured in the sciatic notch), and inferior gluteal (supplies the gluteus maximus and the short external rotators) (Fig. 11–48). The external iliac artery continues under the inguinal ligament to become the femoral artery. It can be injured by anterosuperior quadrant acetabular screw placement during total hip arthroplasty, and the obturator artery and vein are jeopardized by anteroinferior screws. The femoral artery enters the femoral triangle and delivers the profunda femoris, which supplies the anteromedial portion of the thigh and the perforators. The profunda has two other important branches: the medial and lateral femoral circumflex arteries. The lateral femoral circumflex travels obliquely and deep to the sartorius and rectus femoris. It delivers an ascending branch (at risk during anterolateral approaches) that proceeds to the greater trochanteric region and a descending branch that travels laterally under the rectus femoris. The **medial femoral circumflex,** which supplies most of the blood to the **femoral head,** runs between the pectineus and the iliopsoas and then in the interval between the obturator externus and adductor brevis muscles. The cruciate anastomosis is the confluence of the ascending branch of the first perforating artery, the descending branch of the inferior gluteal artery, and the transverse branches of the medial and lateral femoral circumflex arteries. It lies at the inferior margin of the quadratus femoris muscle. The superficial femoral artery continues on the medial side of the thigh (between the vastus medialis and adductor longus) toward the adductor [Hunter's] canal. In the posteromedial thigh it becomes the popliteal artery in the popliteal fossa.

F. Approaches to the Pelvis and Hip
   1. Posterior Approach to the Iliac Crest—A curvilinear incision is made just inferior to the crest beginning at the PSIS. After identifying the iliac

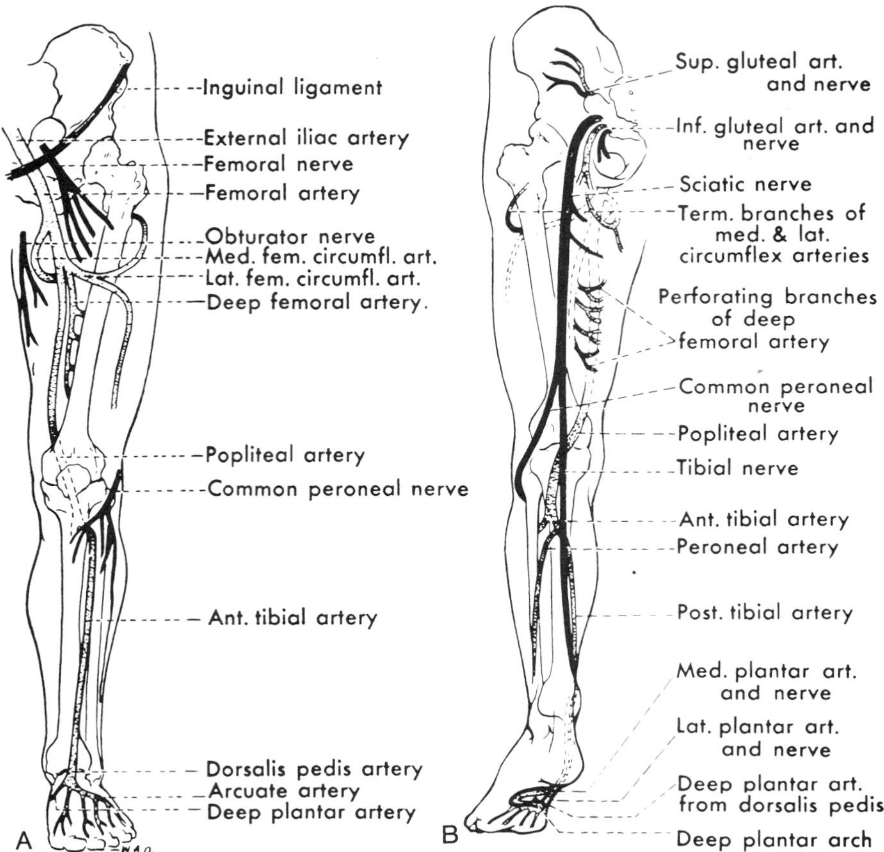

FIGURE 11–47. Nerves and vessels of the lower extremity. *A*, Anterior view. *B*, Posterior view. (From Jenkins, D.B.: Hollinshead's Functional Anatomy of the Limbs and Back, 6th ed., p. 221. Philadelphia, WB Saunders, 1991; reprinted by permission.)

crest, the gluteus maximum fibers are subperiosteally dissected from the outer table. Risks of this approach include the greater sciatic notch (superior gluteal artery and sciatic nerve) and the clunial nerves (8 cm anterolateral to the PSIS).

2. Anterior Approach to the Iliac Crest—An oblique incision is made lateral to the ASIS, and the crest is exposed through the interval between the external oblique and the gluteus medius. Risks are to the greater sciatic notch, the inguinal ligament, and the lateral femoral cutaneous nerve.
3. Anterior (Smith-Peterson) Approach to the Hip (Fig. 11–49)—Takes advantage of the internervous plane between the sartorius (femoral nerve) and the tensor fascia femoris (superior gluteal nerve). It is useful for hemiarthroplasty and open reduction of the congenitally dislocated hip. Retract the lateral femoral cutaneous nerve anteriorly and ligate the ascending branch of lateral femoral circumflex artery. For deeper dissection, approach the interval between the gluteus medius and rectus femoris. Detach the origin of both heads of the rectus femoris. Retract the rectus medially and the gluteus medius laterally. Dissect any attachments of the iliopsoas to the inferior capsule and perform a capsulotomy. Dangers are to the lateral femoral cutaneous nerve, which is located anterior or medial to the sartorius about 6–8 cm below the ASIS. The femoral nerve and vessels can sometimes be injured with aggressive medial retraction of the sartorius.
4. Anterolateral (Watson-Jones) Approach to the Hip (Fig. 11–50)—This approach can be used for total hip arthroplasty (THA) as popularized by Watson-Jones. There is no true internervous plane, but it utilizes the intermuscular plane between the tensor fascia femoris and gluteus medius. After the incision and superficial dissection, the fascia lata is split to expose the vastus lateralis. Detach the anterior third of the gluteus medius from the greater trochanter and the entire gluteus minimus. Dissect the reflected head of the rectus femoris (and capsular attachment of the iliopsoas if necessary) and retract medially. Perform a capsulotomy. Dangers of this approach include damage to the femoral nerve by excessive medial retraction, denervation of the tensor fascia femoris if the intermuscular interval is exploited too superiorly (the superior gluteal nerve lies about 5 cm above the acetabular rim) and injury to the lateral femoral circumflex artery with anterior and inferior dissection.

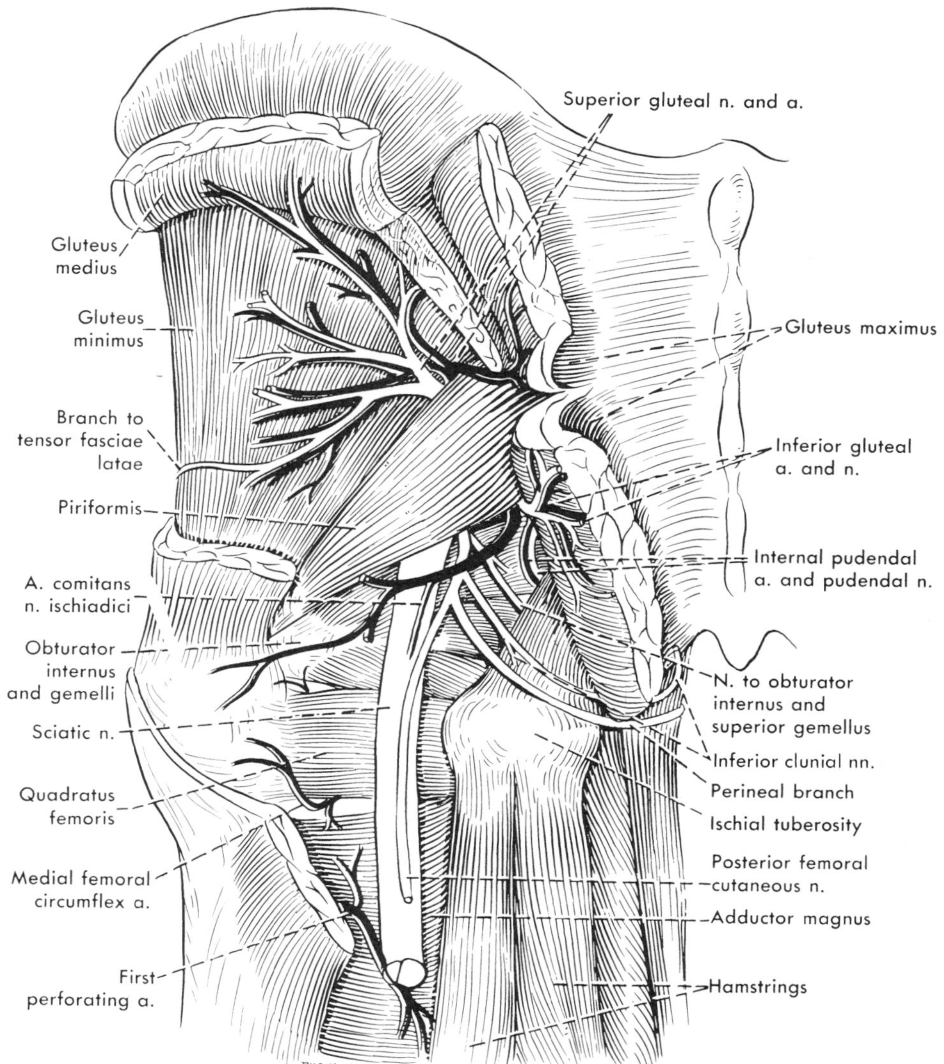

FIGURE 11–48. Posterior hip anatomy. Note relationship of structures to the piriformis muscle. (From Jenkins, D.B.: Hollinshead's Functional Anatomy of the Limbs and Back, 6th ed., p. 260. Philadelphia, WB Saunders, 1991; reprinted by permission.)

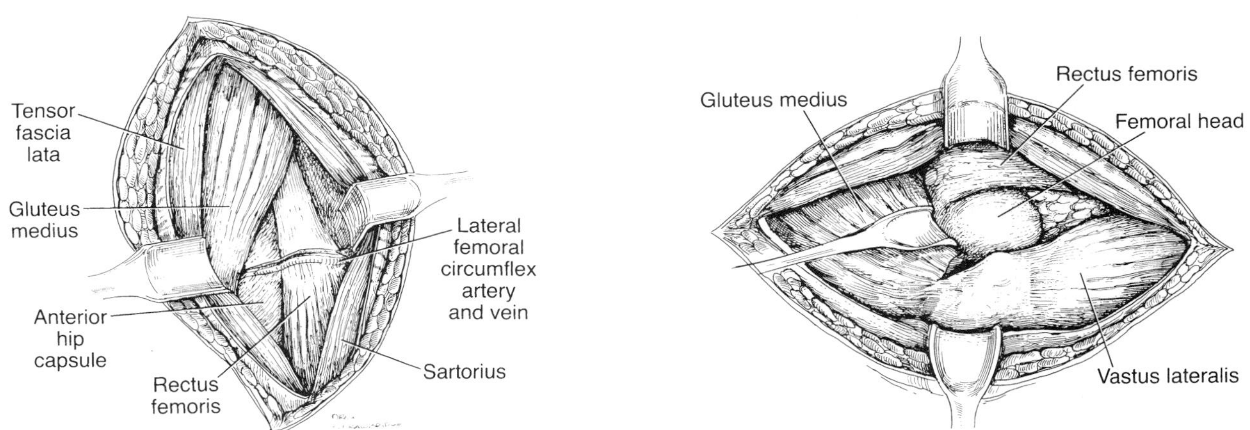

FIGURE 11–49. Anterior approach to the hip. (From Steinberg, M.E.: The Hip and Its Disorders, p. 92. Philadelphia, WB Saunders, 1991; reprinted by permission.)

FIGURE 11–50. Anterolateral approach to the hip. (From Steinberg, M.E.: The Hip and Its Disorders, p. 93. Philadelphia, WB Saunders, 1991; reprinted by permission.)

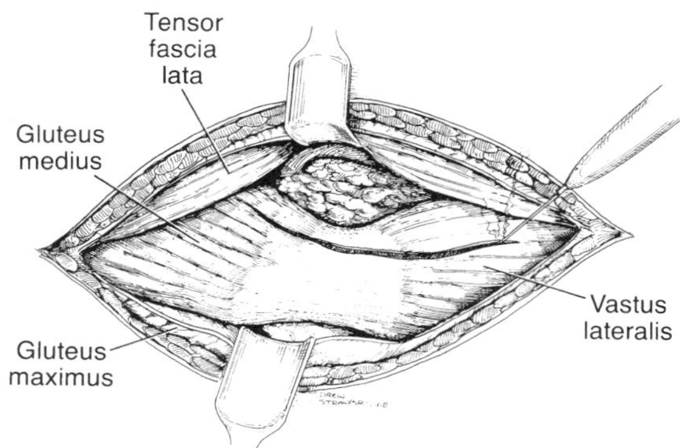

FIGURE 11–51. Lateral approach to the hip. (From Steinberg, M.E.: The Hip and Its Disorders, p. 95. Philadelphia, WB Saunders, 1991; reprinted by permission.)

5. Lateral (Hardinge) Approach to the Hip (Fig. 11–51)—Useful for THA bipolar hemiarthroplasty and revision work, this approach utilizes an incision that splits both the gluteus medius and the vastus lateralis in tandem. Incise the skin and the fascia lata to expose the gluteus medius and the vastus. Incise the gluteus medius from the greater trochanter, leaving a cuff of tissue and the posterior one-half to two-thirds attached. Extend this incision to split the gluteus medius proximally. Distally, split the vastus along its anterior one-fourth down to the femoral shaft. Detach the gluteus minimus from its insertion. The hip capsule is exposed for further dissection. Dangers include injury to the femoral nerve and possible denervation of the gluteus medius (superior gluteal nerve) if the split is generous.
6. Posterior (Moore or Southern) Approach to the Hip (Fig. 11–52)—The internervous plane in one version is between the gluteus maximum (inferior gluteal nerve) and the gluteus medius and the tensor fascia femoris (superior gluteal nerve). Most surgeons, however, approach the hip by splitting the fibers of the gluteus maximus. Incise the skin and the fascia lata along the posterior border of the femur, and then split the fibers of the gluteus maximus bluntly. Next expose the short external rotators close to their insertion into the greater trochanter. Reflect them laterally to protect the sciatic nerve and expose the posterior hip capsule. A portion of the quadratus femoris may be taken down with the short external rotators, but one must be aware of the significant bleeding that can come from the inferior portion of this muscle (ascending branches of medial femoral circumflex artery). Dangers include sciatic neurapraxia if the sciatic nerve is not properly protected by the short external rotators. Additional trouble may be encountered if the inferior gluteal artery is damaged during the splitting of the gluteus maximus.
7. Medial (Ludloff) Approach to the Hip (Fig. 11–53)—Used occasionally for pediatric adductor releases and open reductions, this approach uses the interval between the adductor longus and gracilis. Deep, the interval is between the adductor brevis and magnus. Structures at risk include the anterior division of the obturator nerve and medial femoral circumflex artery (between the adductor brevis and the adductor magnus/pectineus).
8. Acetabular Approaches—Used primarily for ORIF of pelvic fractures, these approaches are basically extensions of incisions for exposure of the hip discussed above. The Kocher-Langenbeck incision is a posterolateral approach that provides access to the posterior column/acetabulum (Fig. 11–54). The ilioinguinal incision relies on mobilization of the rectus abdominus and iliacus, exposing the anterior column. There are three windows available with this approach. The first window gives access to the internal iliac fossa and the anterior sacroiliac joint. The second window (between the iliopectineal fascia and the external iliac vessels) gives access to the pelvic brim and part of the superior pubic ramus. The third window (below the vessels and the spermatic cord) provides ac-

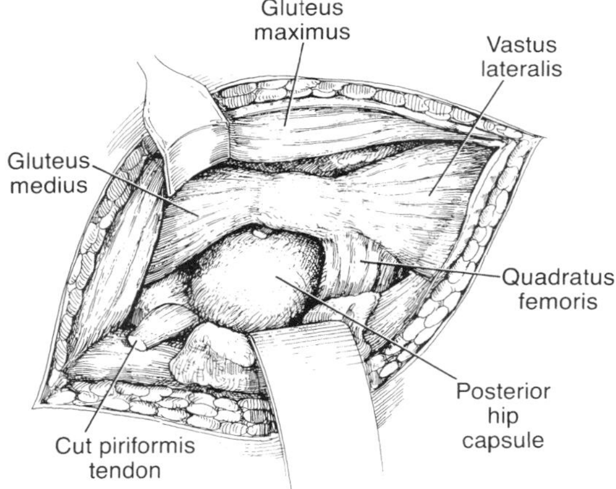

FIGURE 11–52. Posterior approach to the hip. (From Steinberg, M.E.: The Hip and Its Disorders, p. 98. Philadelphia, WB Saunders, 1991; reprinted by permission.)

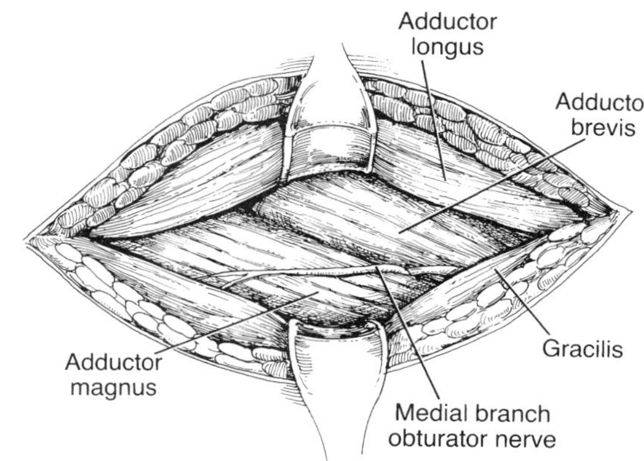

FIGURE 11–53. Medial approach to the hip. (From Steinberg, M.E.: The Hip and Its Disorders, p. 99. Philadelphia, WB Saunders, 1991; reprinted by permission.)

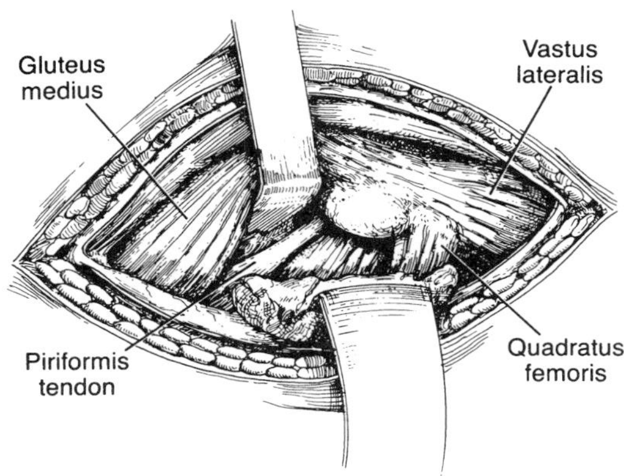

FIGURE 11–54. Posterolateral approach to the hip. (From Steinberg, M.E.: The Hip and Its Disorders, p. 96. Philadelphia, WB Saunders, 1991; reprinted by permission.)

cess to the quadrilateral plate and retropubic space (Fig. 11–55). The extended iliofemoral incision allows access to both columns by reflecting the gluteal muscles and tensor posteriorly and dividing the obturator internus and piriformis.

VIII. Thigh

A. Osteology of the Femur

1. Introduction—The femur is the largest bone of the body. The upper portion contains a head, neck, and two trochanters connected posteriorly by a crest. The neck–shaft angle averages about 127 degrees, although it begins at 141 degrees in the fetus. The anteversion varies from 1 to 40 degrees but averages 14 degrees. Below the lesser trochanter is a ridge known as the pectineal line, which continues as the linea aspera with medial and lateral ridges that diverge at the lower end to meet the medial and lateral supracondylar ridges. There are two femoral condyles; the medial condyle is larger. The more prominent medial epicondyle supports the adductor tubercle.
2. Ossification—The ossification center of the body of the femur appears at the seventh fetal week. The femoral head is usually not present at birth but appears as one large physis that includes both trochanters at about 11 months and fusing at 18 years. The greater trochanter becomes distinct at 5 years and the lesser at 9 years; both fuse at 16 years. The distal femoral physis appears at birth and fuses at 19 years.

B. Muscles of the Thigh

1. Anterior Thigh (Table 11–9)—See Table 11–8 for rectus femoris, sartorius.
2. Medial Thigh—See Adductors in Table 11–8
3. Posterior Thigh (Table 11–10)
4. Cross-Sectional Diagram (Fig. 11–56)

C. Nerves and Vessels (see also Section VII: Thigh and Hip, and Section IX: Leg)—The sciatic nerve emerges from its foramen below the piriformis muscle and lies posterior to the other short external rotators. It descends below the gluteus maximus and proceeds posteriorly to the adductor magnus and between the long head of the biceps and the semimembranosus. Before it emerges from the popliteal fossa it divides into the common peroneal nerve and the tibial nerve. The common peroneal nerve diverges laterally and traverses the lateral knee region under cover of the biceps femoris. The tibial nerve emerges into the popliteal fossa lateral, proceeds posteriorly to the vessel, then descends between the heads of the gastrocnemius. After supplying the profundus (described above) the superficial femoral artery descends under cover of the sartorius muscle and proceeds between the adductor group and the vastus medialis into the adductor canal. At the level above the medial epicondyle, the artery supplies a supreme geniculate branch, then passes through a defect in the adductor magnus (adductor hiatus) and emerges in the popliteal fossa. The vein is usually posterior to the artery.

D. Approaches to the Thigh

1. Lateral Approach to the Thigh—The lateral approach is used for open reduction and internal fixation of intertrochanteric and femoral neck fractures. This approach can be extended for access to shaft and supracondylar fractures. There is no true internervous plane. Split the fascia lata in line with the femoral shaft. Include part of the tensor fascia femoris if necessary. Then bluntly dissect the vastus lateralis in line with its fibers or dissect the fibers of the intermuscular septum. Identify and coagulate the various perforators from the profunda femoris.
2. Posterolateral Approach to the Thigh—This approach may be used for exposure of the entire length of the femur through an internervous plane. It exploits the interval between the vastus lateralis (femoral nerve) and the hamstrings (sciatic nerve). Incise the fascia under the iliotibial band and retract the vastus superiorly. Continue anteriorly to the lateral intermuscular septum with blunt dissection until the periosteum over the linea aspira is reached. The danger of this dissection lies in the series of perforating vessels from the profundus that pierce the lateral intermuscular septum to reach the vastus. If approached without care, these vessels retract and bleed underneath the septum.
3. Anteromedial Approach to the Distal Femur—This approach may be used for open reduction and internal fixation of distal femoral and femoral shaft fractures. Explore the interval between the rectus femoris and vastus medialis and extend to a point medial to the patella. Retract the rectus laterally. Explore the interval to reveal the vastus intermedius. It may be necessary to open the knee joint. If so, incise the medial patellar retinaculum and split a portion of the quadriceps tendon just lateral to the medial border. After identifying the vastus intermedius, split it along its fibers to expose the femur. Dangers include injury to the medial superior geniculate artery and the infrapatellar branch of the saphenous nerve, as both cross the site of exposure. Additionally, one must leave an adequate cuff of tissue for a strong patellar retinacular repair or risk lateral subluxation of the patella.
4. Posterior Approach to the Thigh—This rare approach may be used for exploration of the sciatic

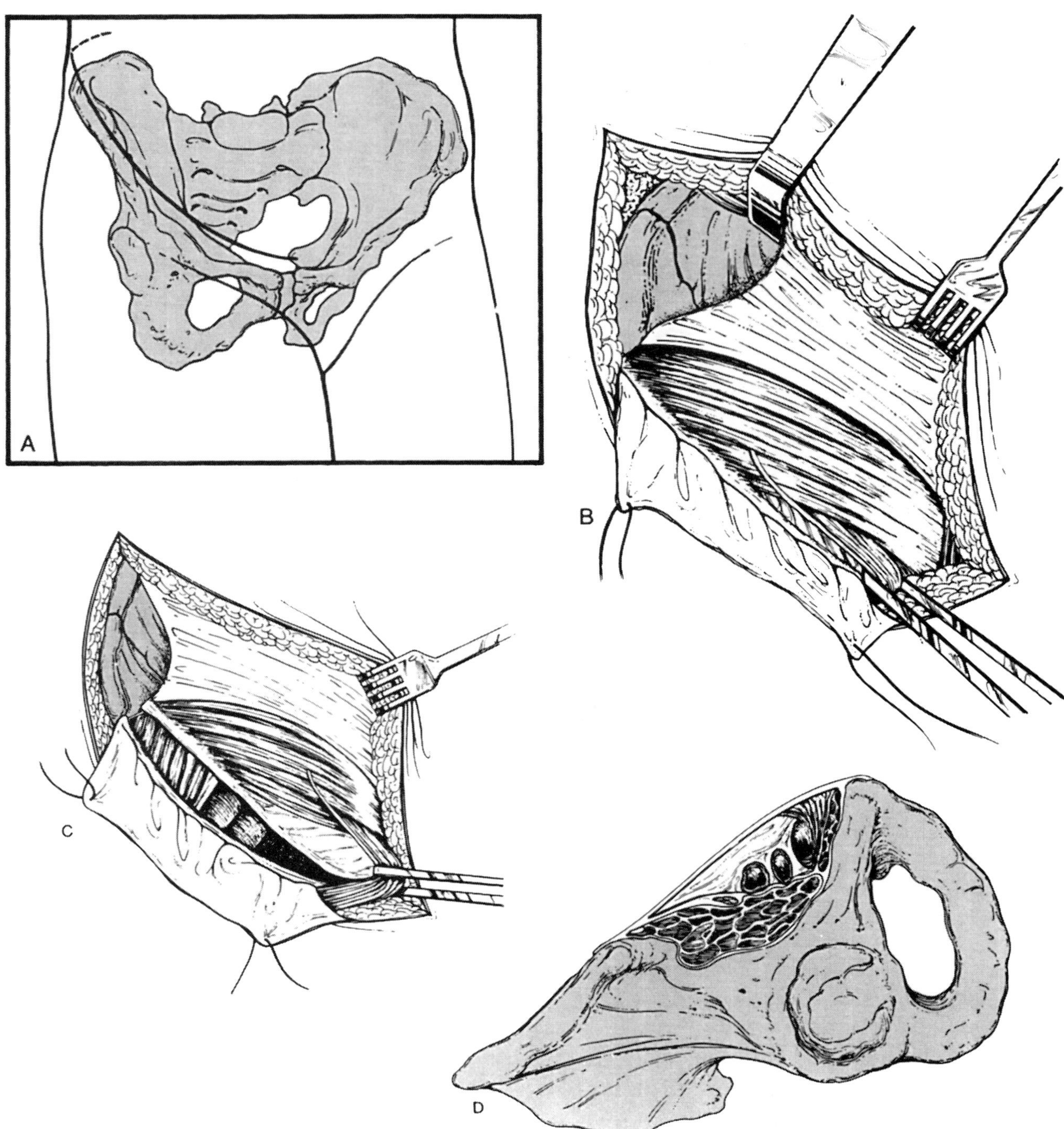

FIGURE 11–55. The ilioinguinal approach. *A,* The skin incision. *B,* The internal iliac fossa has been exposed and the inguinal canal has been unroofed by distal reflection of the external oblique aponeurosis. *C,* An incision along the inguinal ligament detaches the abdominal muscles and transversalis fascia, giving access to the psoas sheath, the iliopectineal fascia, the external aspect of the femoral vessels, and the retropubic space of Retzius. *D,* An oblique section through the lacuna musculorum and lacuna vascularum at the level of the inguinal ligament. *Illustration continued on following page*

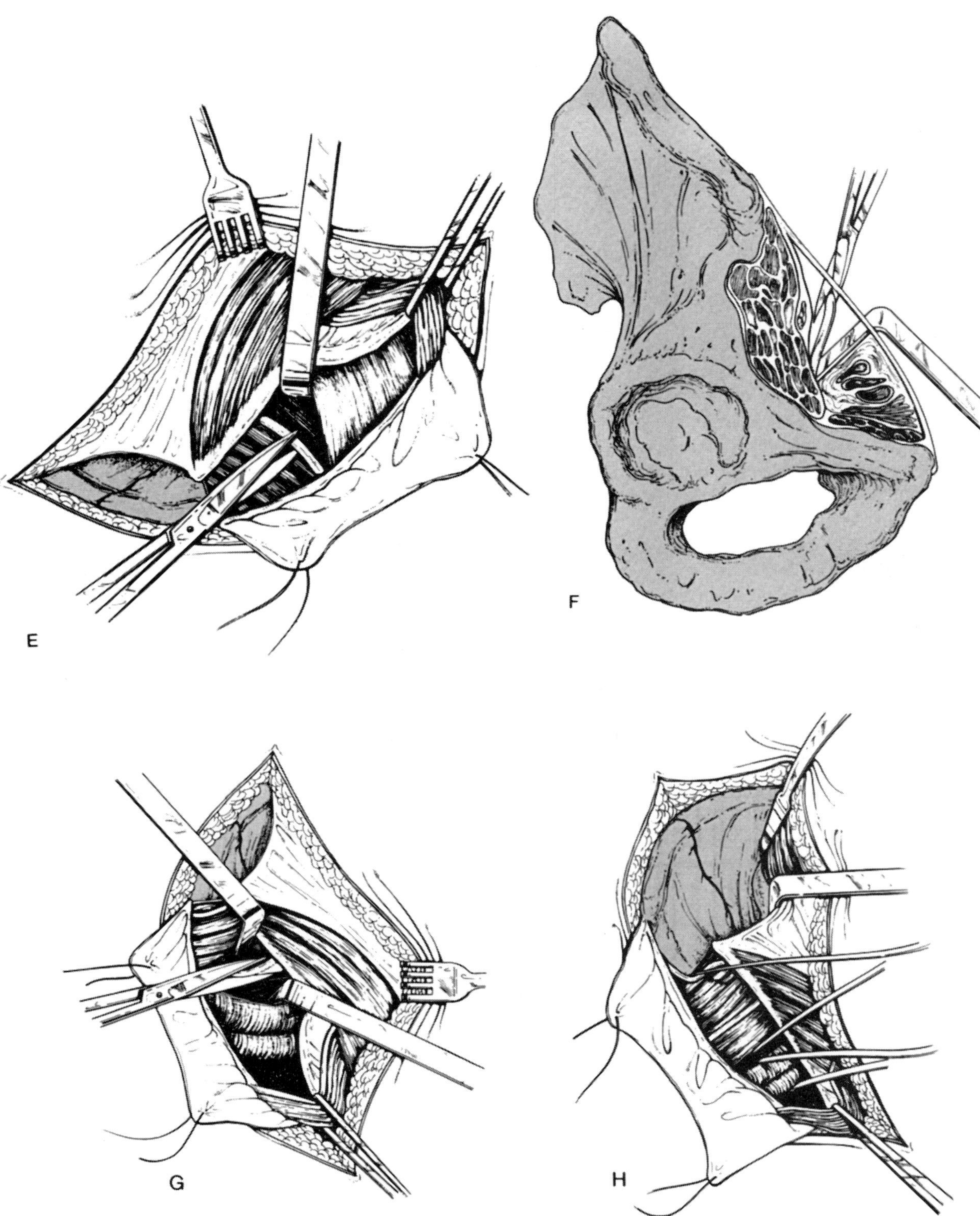

FIGURE 11–55. *Continued. E,* Division of the iliopectineal fascia to the pectineal eminence. *F,* An oblique section that demonstrates division of the iliopectineal fascia. *G,* Proximal division of the iliopectineal fascia from the pelvic brim to allow access to the true pelvis. *H,* The first window of the ilioinguinal approach, which gives access to the internal iliac fossa, the anterior sacroiliac joint and upper portion of the anterior column. *Illustration continued on following page*

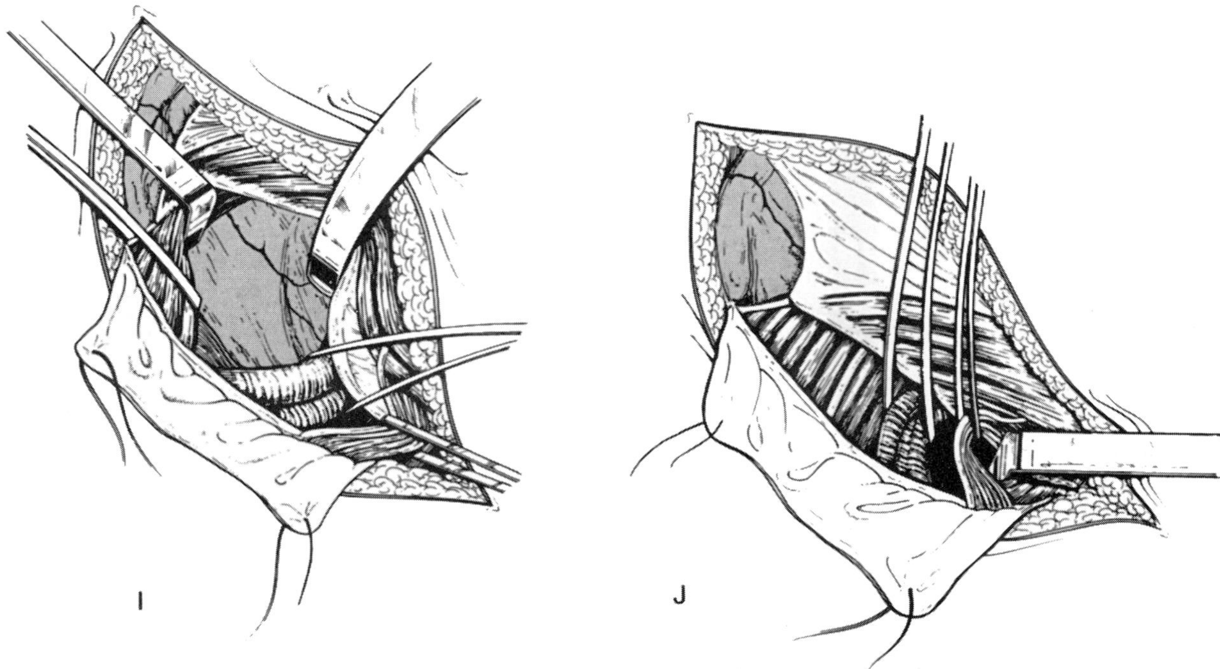

FIGURE 11–55. *Continued. I,* The second window of the ilioinguinal approach, giving access to the pelvic brim from the anterior sacroiliac joint to the lateral extremity of the superior pubic ramus. The quadrilateral surface and posterior column are accessible beyond the pelvic brim. *J,* Access to the symphysis pubis and retropubic space of Retzius, medial to the spermatic cord and femoral vessels. (From Browner B.D., Jupiter J.B., Levine, A.M., and Trafton, P.G.: Skeletal Trauma, Fractures Dislocations, Ligamentous Injuries, pp. 907–909 (Fig. 32–5 A–J). Philadelphia WB Saunders, 1992; reprinted by permission.)

TABLE 11–9. MUSCLES OF THE ANTERIOR THIGH

MUSCLE	ORIGIN	INSERTION	INNERVATION
Vastus lateralis	Iliotibial line/ greater trochanter/ lateral linea aspera	Lateral patella	Femoral
Vastus medialis	Iliotibial line/ medial linea aspera/ supracondylar line	Medial patella	Femoral
Vastus intermedius	Proximal anterior femoral shaft	Patella	Femoral

nerve. It makes use of the internervous interval between the sciatic nerve (biceps femoris) and the femoral nerve (vastus lateralis). Identify and protect the posterior femoral cutaneous nerve (between the biceps and the semitendinosus). Next, explore the interval between the biceps and the lateral intermuscular septum. Detach the origin of the short head of the biceps from the linea aspera. This maneuver allows exposure of the femur at the midshaft level. In the lower thigh, retract the long head of the biceps laterally to expose the sciatic nerve. It lies on the surface of the adductor magnus and may be retracted laterally to expose this portion of the femur.

TABLE 11–10. MUSCLES OF THE POSTERIOR THIGH

MUSCLE	ORIGIN	INSERTION	INNERVATION
Biceps (long head)	Medial ischial tuberosity	Fibular head/lateral tibia	Tibial
Biceps (short head)	Lat. linea aspera/lat. intermuscular septum	Lateral tibial condyle	Peroneal
Semitendinosus	Distal med. ischial tuberosity	Anterior tibial crest	Tibial
Semimembranosus	Proximal lat. ischial tuberosity	Oblique popliteal ligament Posterior capsule Posterior/medial tibia Popliteus Medial meniscus	Tibial

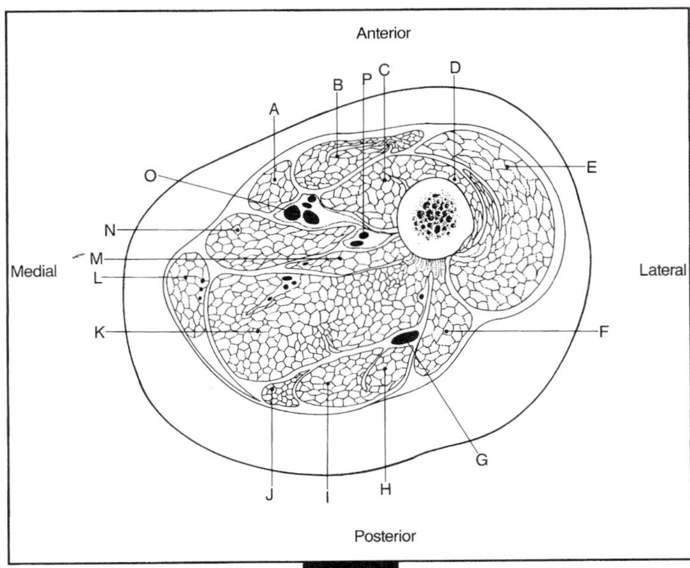

FIGURE 11–56. Cross section of the proximal thigh. (From Callaghan, JJ., ed., Anatomy Self-Assessment Examination, Fig. 53. Park Ridge, Illinois, American Academy of Orthopaedic Surgeons, 1991; reprinted by permission.)

A Sartorious
B Rectus femoris
C Vastus medialis
D Vastus intermedius
E Vastus lateralis
F Gluteus maximus
G Sciatic nerve
H Biceps long head
I Semitendinosus
J Semimembranosus
K Adductor magnus
L Gracilis
M Adductor brevis
N Adductor longus
O Femoral artery
P Profunda femoris artery

IX. Leg

A. Osteology

1. Patella—Commonly known as the kneecap, the patella is the largest sesamoid bone (about 5 cm in diameter). It serves three functions: It is a fulcrum for the quadriceps; it protects the knee joint; and it enhances lubrication and nutrition of the knee. The patella is said to have the thickest articular surface in the body, probably because of the loads it must transmit. Although sometimes subdivided, the articular surface of the patella has two facets, medial and lateral, separated by a vertical ridge. The lateral facet is broader and deeper than the medial facet. Somewhat triangular in shape, the apex of the patella gives rise to the patella, and they fuse sometime between the second and sixth year of life. An accessory or "bipartite" patella may represent failure of fusion of the superolateral corner of the patella and is commonly confused with patellar fractures.
2. Tibia—The tibia is the second longest bone in the body (behind the femur). It consists of a proximal extremity with medial (oval and concave) and lateral (circular and convex) facets. The intercondylar eminence separates the medial and lateral facets and the anterior and posterior cruciate ligaments. The tibial tubercle is an oblong elevation on the anterior surface of the tibia where the patella tendon inserts. Gerdy's tubercle lies on the lateral side of the proximal tibia and is the insertion of the iliotibial tract. The tibial shaft is triangular is cross section and tapers to its thinnest point at the junction of the middle and distal thirds and then again widens to form the tibial plafond. Distally, the tibia forms an inferior quadrilateral surface for articulation with the talus and the pyramid-shaped medial malleolus. Laterally, the fibular notch forms an articulation with the fibula. The tibia is formed from three ossification centers.

OSSIFICATION CENTER	AGE AT APPEARANCE	AGE AT FUSION
Body (primary)	7 weeks (fetal)	
Proximal (secondary)	Birth	20 years
Distal (secondary)	Second year	18 years

3. Fibula—This long slender bone is composed of a head, a shaft, and a distal lateral malleolus. The styloid process of the head serves as the attachment for the fibular collateral ligament and the biceps tendon. Lying just below the head, the neck of the fibula is grooved by the common peroneal nerve. The expanded distal fibula is known as the lateral malleolus and extends beyond the distal margin of the medial malleolus. Together with the inferior distal surface of the tibia, these structures make up the ankle mortise. Like the tibia, the fibula is also formed from three ossification centers.

TABLE 11–11. LIGAMENTS OF THE KNEE

LIGAMENT	ORIGIN	INSERTION	FUNCTION
Retinacular	Vastus medialis and lateralis	Tibial condyles	Forms anterior capsule
Posterior fibers	Femoral condyles	Tibial condyles	Forms posterior capsule
Oblique popliteal	Semimembranosus tendon	Lateral femoral condyle/ posterior capsule	Strengthens capsule
Deep medial collateral (MCL)	Medial epicondyle	Medial meniscus	Holds med. meniscus to femur
Superficial MCL	Medial epicondyle	Medial condyle of tibia	Resists valgus force
Arcuate	Lat. femoral condyle, over popliteus	Post. tibia/fibular head	Posterior support
Lateral collateral (LCL)	Lateral epicondyle	Lateral fibular head	Resists varus force
Anterior cruciate (ACL)	Anterior intercondylar tibia	Posteromed. lat. femoral condyle	Limits hyperextension/ sliding
Posterior cruciate (PCL)	Posterior sulcus tibia	Anteromed. femoral condyle	Prevents hyperflexion/sliding
Coronary	Meniscus	Tibial periphery	Meniscal attachment
Wrisberg	Posterolateral meniscus	Med. femoral condyle (behind PCL)	Stabilizes lat. meniscus
Humphrey	Posterolateral meniscus	Med. femoral condyle (in front)	Stabilizes lat. meniscus
Transverse meniscal	Anterolateral meniscus	Anteromedial meniscus	Stabilizes menisci

OSSIFICATION CENTER	AGE AT APPEARANCE	AGE AT FUSION
Body (primary)	8 weeks (fetal)	
Proximal (secondary)	Third year	25 years
Distal (secondary)	Second year	20 years

B. Arthrology

1. Knee—Much more than a simple ginglymus or hinge-type of joint, the knee is a compound joint consisting of two condyloid joints and one sellar joint (patellofemoral articulation). The medial and lateral femoral condyles articulate with the corresponding tibial facets. Intervening menisci serve to deepen the concavity of the facets, help protect the articular surface, and assist in rotation of the knee (Fig. 11–57). The peripheral one-third of the menisci are vascular (and can be repaired); the inner two-thirds are nourished by synovial fluid. Stability of the knee is enhanced by a complex arrangement of ligaments (Table 11–11; Fig. 11–58). In addition, several muscles and tendons traverse the knee, giving it dynamic stability.

LOCATION	MUSCLES
Anterior	Quadriceps
Lateral	Biceps and popliteus
Medial	Pes anserinus (sartorius, gracilis, semitendinosis), semimembranosus (with five attachments)
Posterior	Medial and lateral heads of the gastrocnemius, plantaris

2. Superior Tibiofibular Joint—A place or gliding joint that is strengthened by the anterior and posterior ligaments of the head of the fibula.

C. Muscles of the Leg—Commonly divided into groups based on compartments (anterior, lateral, superficial posterior, and deep posterior) (Table 11–12). Origins and insertions are noted in Fig. 11–59.

D. Nerves (Fig. 11–60)—Motor branches to the muscles of the leg are from terminal divisions of the sciatic nerve (in the distal thigh) and the tibial and common peroneal nerves and their branches.

1. Tibial Nerve—Continues in the thigh deep to the long head of the biceps and enters the popliteal fossa. It then crosses over the popliteus muscle and splits the two heads of the gastrocnemius, passing deep to the soleus on its course to the posterior aspect of the medial malleolus. It terminates as the medial and lateral plantar nerves. Muscular branches supply the posterior leg along its course.
2. Common Peroneal Nerve—The smaller terminal division of the sciatic, this nerve runs laterally in the popliteal fossa in the interval between the medial border of the biceps and the lateral head of the gastrocnemius. Then it winds around the neck of the fibula, deep to the peroneus longus, where it divides into superficial and deep branches.
   a. Superficial Peroneal Nerve—Runs along the border between the lateral and anterior compartments in the leg, supplying muscular branches to the peroneus longus and brevis. It terminates in two cutaneous branches supplying the dorsal foot.
   b. Deep Peroneal Nerve—Sometimes known as the anterior tibial nerve, this nerve runs along the anterior surface of the interosseous membrane, supplying the musculature of the anterior compartment.
3. Cutaneous Nerves—Important cutaneous nerves include the saphenous nerve and the sural nerve. The saphenous nerve is the continuation of the femoral nerve of the thigh, and it becomes subcutaneous on the medial aspect of the knee between the sartorius and gracilis (where it is sometimes injured during procedures about the knee, e.g., meniscoresis). The saphenous nerve supplies sensation to the medial aspect of the leg and foot. The sural nerve, which is often used for nerve grafting and which can cause painful neuromas when inadvertently

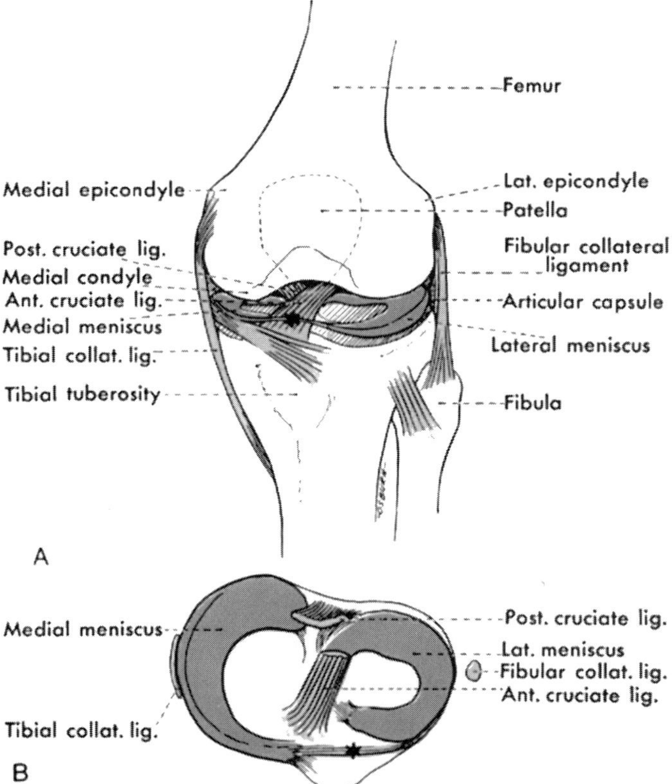

FIGURE 11–57. Ligaments of the knee. (From Jenkins, D.B.: Hollinshead's Functional Anatomy of the Limbs and Back, 6th ed., Fig. 16–1. Philadelphia, WB Saunders, 1991; reprinted by permission.)

cut, is formed by cutaneous branches of both the tibial (medial sural cutaneous) and common peroneal (lateral sural cutaneous) nerves. It lies on the lateral aspect of the leg and foot.

E. Vessels (Fig. 11–60)—Branches of the popliteal artery, the continuation of the femoral artery, supply the leg. The artery enters the popliteal fossa between the biceps and semimembranosus and descends underneath the tibial nerve and terminates between the medial and lateral heads of the gastrocnemius, dividing into the anterior and posterior tibial arteries. Several genicular branches are given off in the popliteal fossa, including the medial and lateral geniculates (which supply the menisci) and the middle geniculate (which supplies the cruciate ligaments).
   1. Anterior Tibial Artery—The first branch of the popliteal artery, this vessel passes between the two heads of the tibialis posterior and the interosseous membrane to lie on the anterior surface of that membrane between the tibialis anterior and extensor hallicus longus until it terminates as the dorsalis pedis artery.

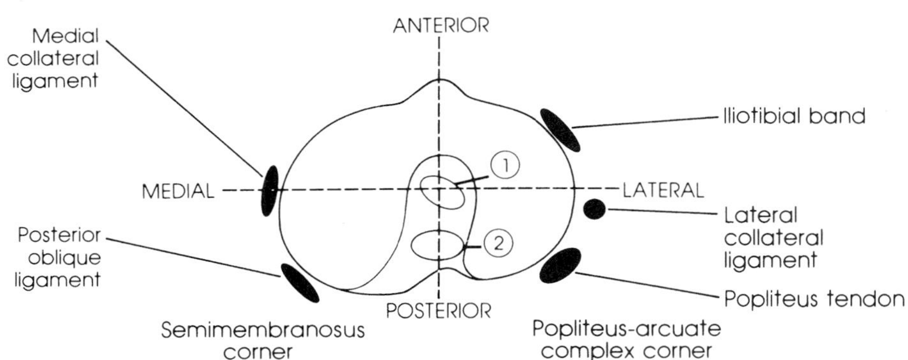

FIGURE 11–58. Ligaments of the knee. *1,* anterior cruciate ligament; *2,* posterior cruciate ligament. (From Magee, D.J.: Orthopedic Physical Assessment, p. 285. Philadelphia, WB Saunders, 1987; reprinted by permission.)

TABLE 11–12. MUSCLES OF THE LEG

MUSCLE	ORIGIN	INSERTION	ACTION	INNERVATION
Anterior Compartment				
Tibialis anterior	Lateral tibia	Med. cuneiform, 1st metatarsal	Dorsiflex, invert foot	Deep peroneal (L4)
Extensor hallucis longus (EHL)	Mid. fibula	Great toe distal phalanx	Dorsiflex, extend toe	Deep peroneal (L5)
Extensor digitorum longus (EDL)	Tibial condyle/fibula	Toe middle and distal phalanges	Dorsiflex, extend toes	Deep peroneal (L5)
Peroneus tertius	Fibula and EDL tendon	5th Metatarsal	Evert, plantar flex, abduct foot	Deep peroneal (S1)
Lateral Compartment				
Peroneus longus	Proximal fibula	Med. cuneiform, 1st metatarsal	Evert, plantar flex, abduct foot	Superificial peroneal (S1)
Peroneus brevis	Distal fibula	Tuberosity of 5th metatarsal	Evert foot	Superficial peroneal (S1)
Superficial Posterior Compartment				
Gastrocnemius	Post. med. and lat. femoral condyles	Calcaneus	Plantar flex foot	Tibial (S1)
Soleus	Fibula/tibia	Calcaneus	Plantar flex foot	Tibial (S1)
Plantaris	Lat. femoral condyle	Calcaneus	Plantar flex foot	Tibial (S1)
Deep Posterior Compartment				
Popliteus	Lat. femoral condyle, fibular head	Proximal tibia	Flex, IR knee	Tibial (L5S1)
Flexor hallucis longus (FHL)	Fibula	Great toe distal phalanx	Plantar flex great toe	Tibial (S1)
Flexor digitorum longus (FDL)	Tibia	2nd–5th Toe distal phalanges	Plantar flex toes, foot	Tibial (S1S2)
Tibialis posterior	Tibia, fibula, interosseous membrane	Navicular, med. cuneiform	Inver/plantar flex foot	Tibial (L4L5)

2. Posterior Tibial Artery—Continues in the deep posterior compartment of the leg, coursing obliquely to pass behind the medial malleolus, where it terminates by dividing into medial and lateral plantar arteries. Its main branch, the peroneal artery, is given off 2.5 cm distal to the popliteal fossa and continues in the deep posterior compartment, lateral to its parent artery, between the tibialis posterior and flexor hallicus longus, eventually terminating in calcaneal branches.

F. Surgical Approaches to the Knee and Leg

1. Medial Parapatellar Approach to the Knee—Used most commonly for total knee arthroplasty, this approach utilizes a midline incision and a medial parapatellar capsular incision. The infrapatellar branch of the saphenous nerve is sometimes cut with incisions that stray too far medially, leading to a painful neuroma.
2. Medial Approach to the Knee (Fig. 11–61)—Used for repair of the MCL and capsule, this approach is in the interval between the sartorius and medial patellar retinaculum. Three layers are commonly recognized (from superficial to deep).

LAYER	COMPONENTS
1	Pes anserinus tendons
2	Superficial MCL
3	Deep MCL, capsule, POL

The saphenous nerve and vein must be identified and protected.

3. Lateral Approach to the Knee (Fig. 11–62)—Used primarily for exploring and repairing damaged ligaments, this approach utilizes the plane between the iliotibial band (superior gluteal nerve) and the biceps (sciatic nerve). The common peroneal nerve, located near the posterior border of the biceps, must be isolated and retracted. The popliteus tendon is also at risk and should be identified.
4. Posterior Approach to the Knee—Occasionally required to address posterior capsular pathology, this approach uses an S-shaped incision beginning laterally and ending medially (distally). The popliteal fossa is exposed using the small saphenous vein and medial sural cutaneous nerves as landmarks. The two heads of the gastrocnemius can be detached if greater exposure is necessary.
5. Anterior Approach to the Tibia—May be used for ORIF of fractures and bone grafting; it relies on subperiosteal elevation of the tibialis anterior.
6. Posterolateral Approach to the Tibia—Used typically for bone grafting of tibial nonunions, this approach utilizes the internervous plane between the soleus and FHL (tibial nerve) and the peroneal muscles (superficial peroneal nerve). The FHL is detached from its origin on the fibula, and the tibialis posterior is detached from its origin along the interosseous membrane to reach the tibia. Neurovascular structures in the posterior compartment are protected by the

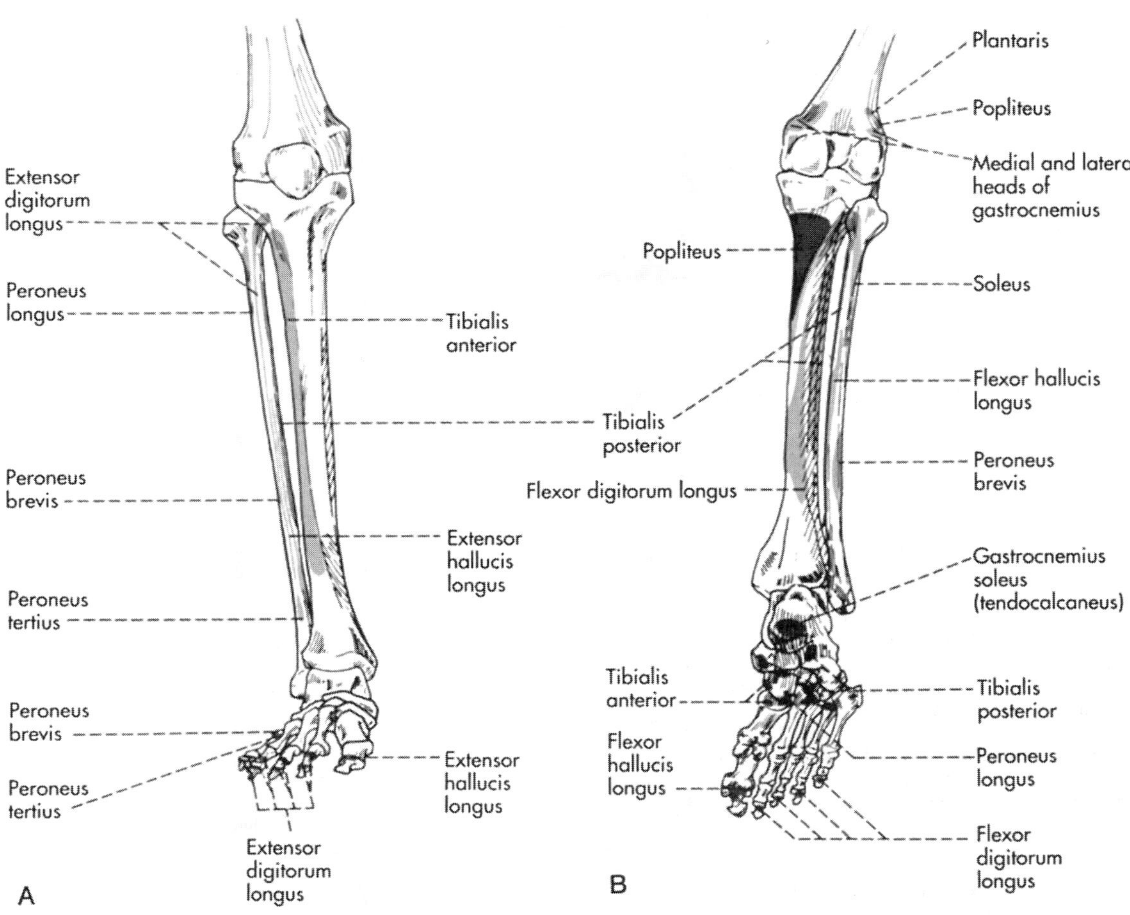

FIGURE 11–59. Origins and insertions of leg and foot muscles. (From Jenkins, D.B.: Hollinshead's Functional Anatomy of the Limbs and Back, 6th ed., fig. 19–3. Philadelphia, WB Saunders, 1991; reprinted by permission.)

muscle bellies of the FHL and tibialis posterior.

7. Approach to the Fibula—Through the same interval as the posterolateral approach to the tibia but stays more anterior and relies on isolation and protection of the common peroneal nerve in the proximal dissection.

X. Ankle and Foot

A. Osteology—The 26 bones of the foot include 7 tarsal bones, 5 metatarsals, and 14 phalanges.

1. Tarsus—Includes the talus, calcaneus, cuboid, navicular, and three cuneiforms.
   a. Talus—Articulates with the tibia and fibula in the ankle mortise and with the calcaneus and navicular distally. It is made up of a body with three articular surfaces (the trochlea, including surfaces for the malleoli articulations, and the posterior and middle calcaneal facets) and a posterior process (for the posterior talofibular ligament). The neck of the talus connects with the head, which in turn articulates with the navicular distally and the calcaneus inferiorly.
   b. Calcaneus—Largest and strongest bone in the foot. It has three surfaces that articulate with the talus: a large posterior surface, an anterior surface, and a middle surface. Distally, there is an articular surface that receives the cuboid bone. The sustentaculum tali is an overhanging horizontal eminence on the anteromedial surface of the calcaneus. It supports the middle articular surface above it and allows plantar vessels and nerves to pass below it. The calcaneal tuberosity posteriorly is bounded by medial and lateral processes.
   c. Cuboid—Lies on the lateral aspect of the foot, is grooved by the peroneus longus, and has four facets for articulation with the calcaneus, the lateral cuneiform, and the fourth and fifth metatarsals.
   d. Navicular—The most medial tarsal bone; lies between the talus and the cuneiforms. Proximally, the surface is oval and concave for its articulation with the head of the talus. Distally, the navicular has three articular surfaces, one for each of the cuneiforms.
   e. Cuneiforms—Medial, intermediate, and lateral, these three bones articulate with the navicular and posterior cuboid (lateral cuneiform) and the first three metatarsals. The intermediate cuneiform does not extend as

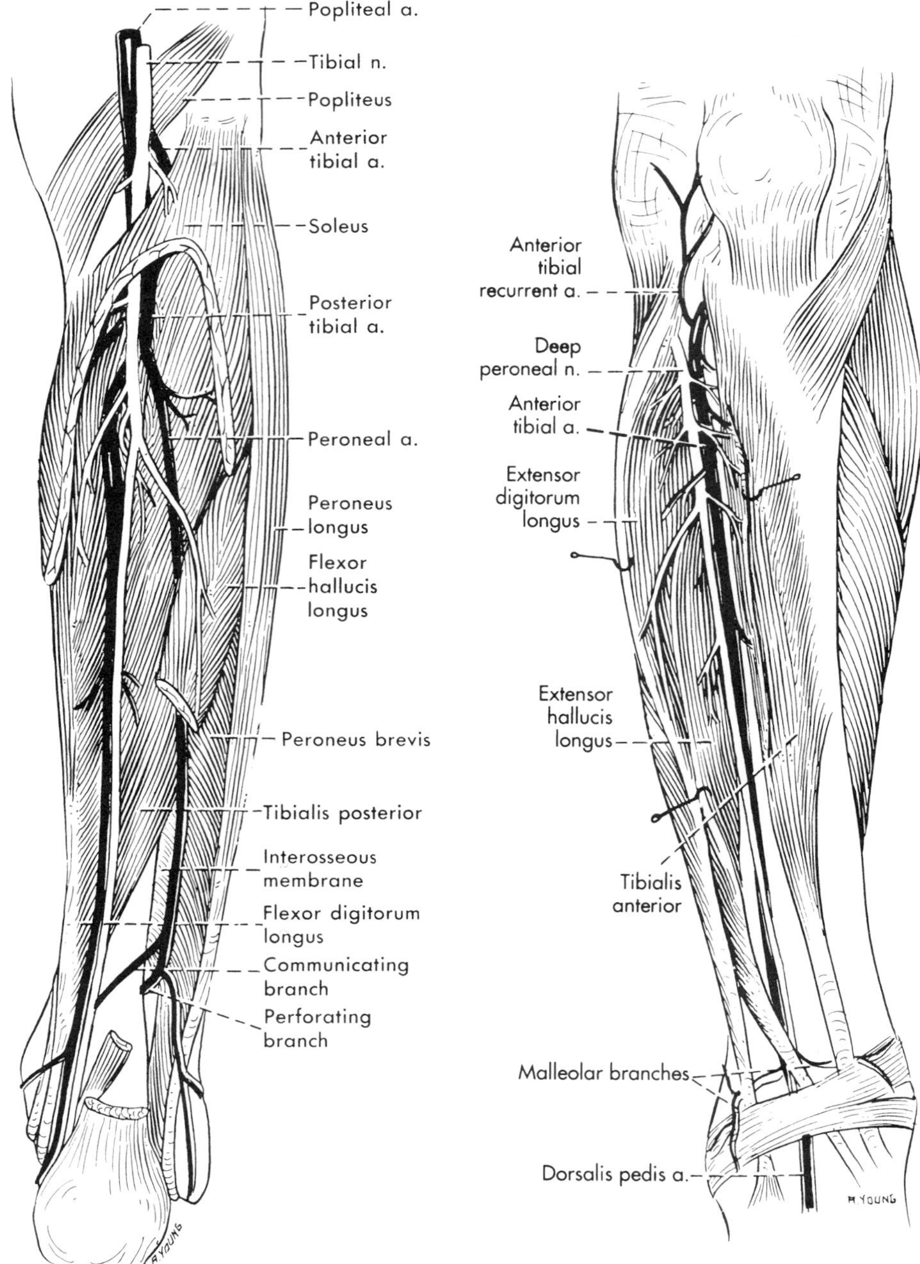

FIGURE 11–60. Nerves and vessels of the leg. *Left,* posterior. *Right,* anterior. (From Jenkins, D.B.: Hollinshead's Functional Anatomy of the Limbs and Back, 6th ed., pp. 292, 296. Philadelphia, WB Saunders, 1991; reprinted by permission.)

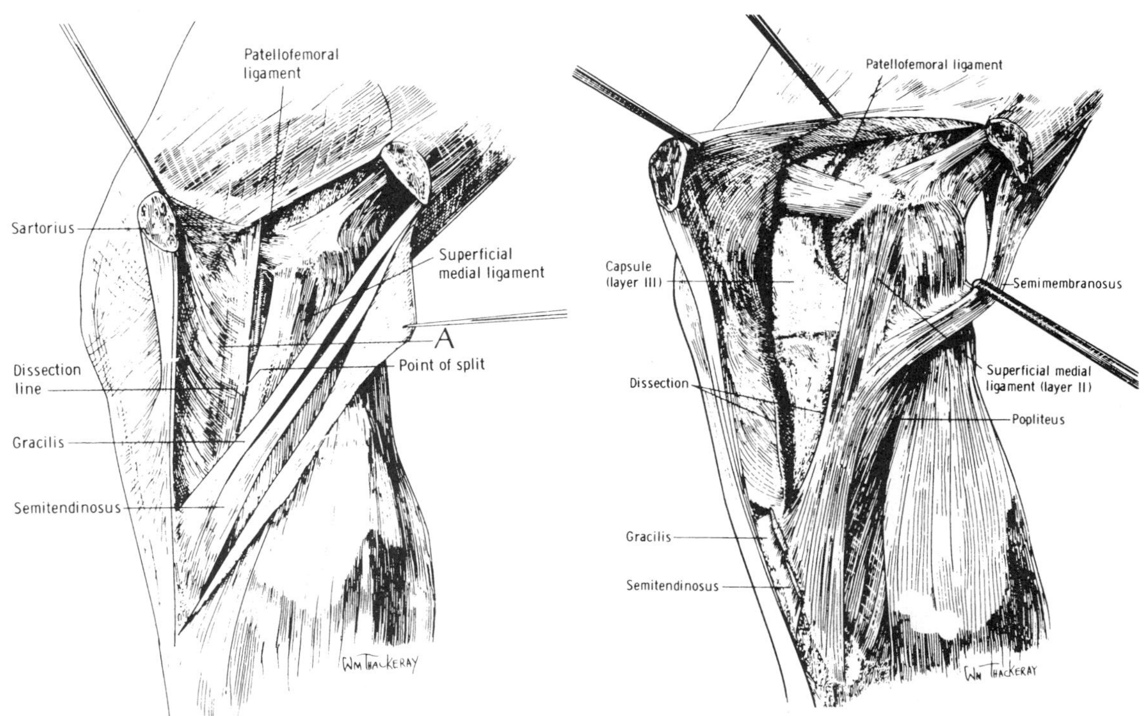

FIGURE 11–61. Medial structures of the knee. (Warren, L.F., and Marshall, J.L.: The supporting structures and layers of the medial side of the knee. J. Bone Joint Surg. [Am.] 61:58, 1979; reprinted by permission.)

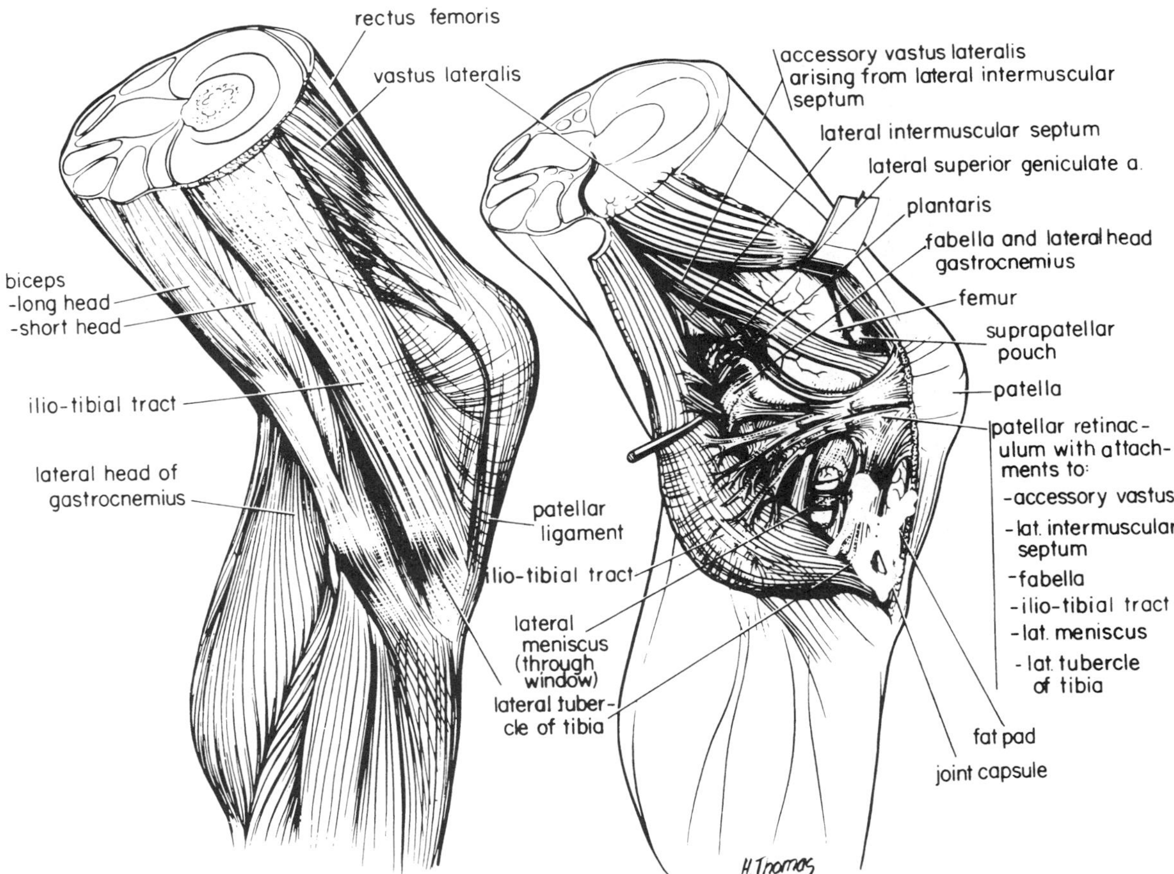

FIGURE 11–62. Lateral structures of the knee. (From Seebacher, J.R., Inglis, A.E., Marshall, J.L., and Warren R.F.: The structure of the posterolateral aspect of the knee. J. Bone Joint Surg. [Am.] 64:533, 1982; reprinted by permission.)

far distally as the medial cuneiform, allowing the second metatarsal to "key" into place.

2. Metatarsals—Five bones, numbered from medial to lateral, span the distance between the tarsals and the phalanges. In general, their shape and function are similar to those of the metacarpals of the hand.
3. Phalanges—Also similar to the hand. The great toe has two phalanges and the remaining digits have three.
4. Ossification—Each tarsus has a single ossification center, except the calcaneus, which has a second center posteriorly. The calcaneus, talus, and usually the cuboid are present at birth. The lateral cuneiform appears during the first year, the medial cuneiform during the second year, and the intermediate cuneiform and navicular during the third year. The posterior center for the calcaneus usually appears at the eighth year. The second through fifth metatarsals have two ossification centers: a primary center in the shaft and a secondary center for the head that appears at age 5–8. The phalanges and first metatarsal have secondary centers at their bases that appear during the third or fourth year proximally and the sixth to seventh year distally.

B. Arthrology

1. Inferior Tibiofibular Joint—Formed by the medial distal fibula and the notched lateral distal tibia, this joint is supported by four ligaments. The anteroinferior tibiofibular ligament (AITFL) is an oblique band that connects the bones anteriorly. The posterior tibiofibular ligament (PTFL) is smaller but serves a similar function posteriorly. The inferior transverse ligament lies just below the PTFL and provides additional posterior support for the mortise. Finally, an interosseous ligament also connects the two bones.
2. Ankle Joint (Fig. 11–63)—A ginglymus, or hinge, joint is formed by the malleoli and the talus. It is supported by the following ligaments.

LIGAMENT	ORIGIN	INSERTION
Capsule	Tibia	Talus
Deltoid		
Tibionavicular	Med. malleolus	Navicular tuberosity
Tibiocalcaneal	Med. Malleolus	Sustentaculum tali
Post. tibiotalar	Med. malleolus	Inner side of talus
Deep	Med. malleolus	Medial surface of talus
ATFL	Lat. malleolus	Transversely to talus anteriorly
PTFL	Lat. malleolus	Transversely to talus posteriorly
Calcaneofibular (CFL)	Lat. malleolus	Obliquely posteriorly to calcaneus

The PTFL is strong, and the ATFL is weak; therefore the ATFL is most commonly injured

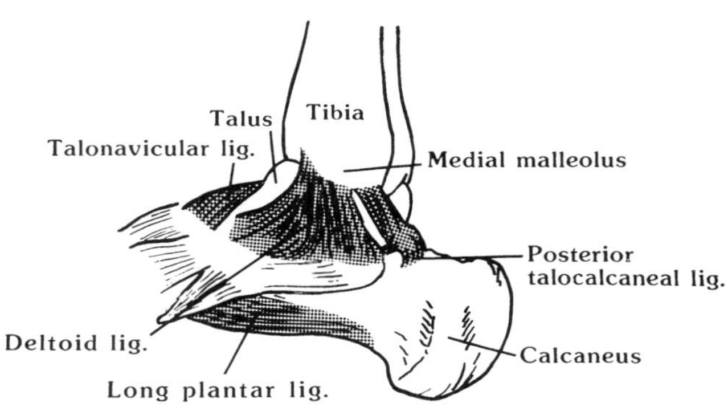

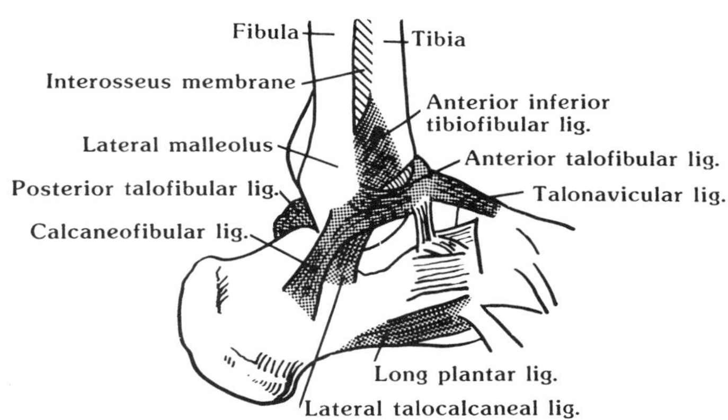

FIGURE 11–63. Ankle ligaments. *Top,* Medial. *Bottom,* Lateral. (From Wiessman, B.N., and Sledge, C.B.: Orthopedic Radiology, pp. 593, 594, Philadelphia, WB Saunders, 1986; reprinted by permission.)

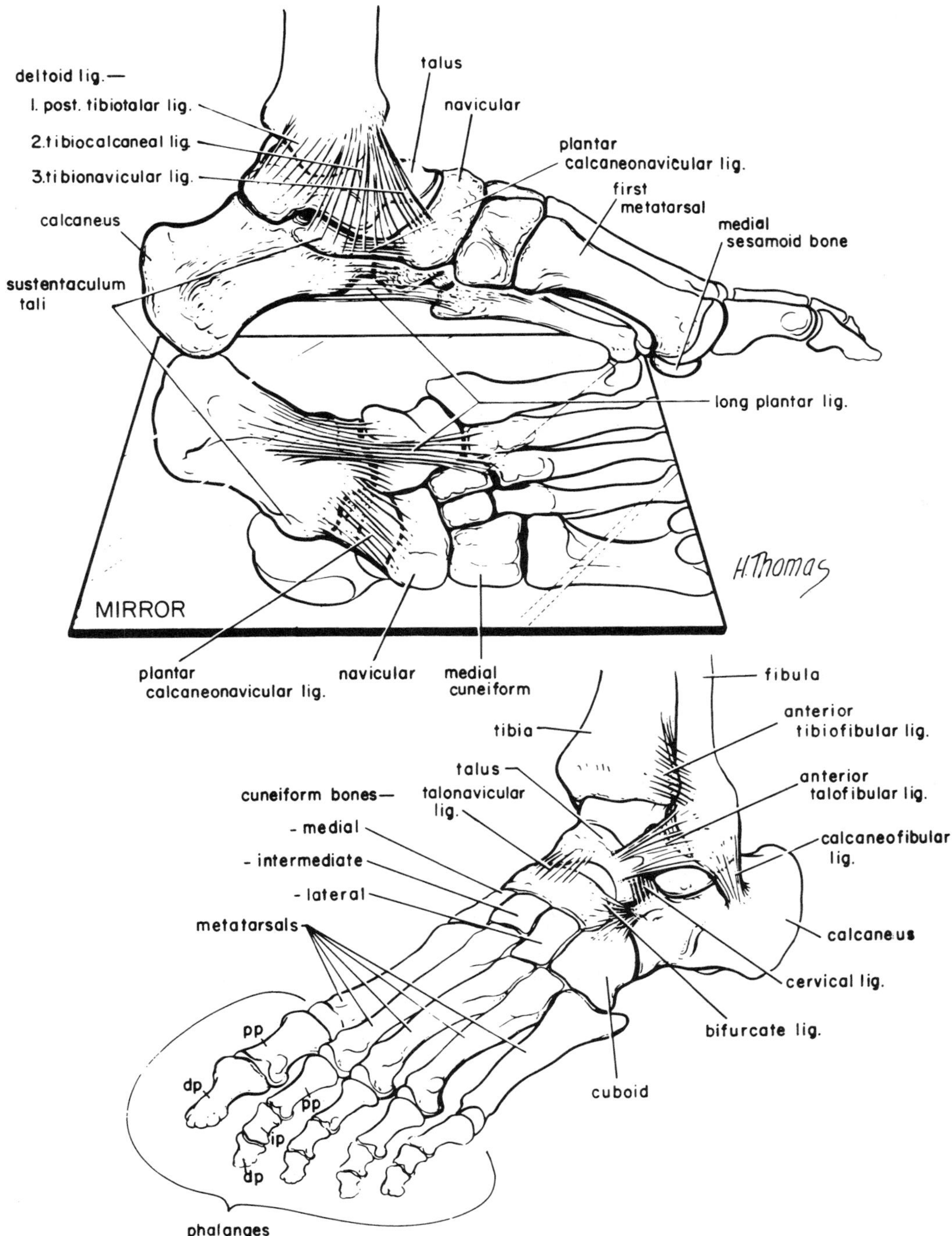

FIGURE 11–64. Ligaments of the foot. (From Jahss, M.H.: Disorders of the Foot, p. 14. Philadelphia, WB Saunders, 1982; reprinted by permission.)

TABLE 11–13. LIGAMENTS OF THE INTERTARSAL JOINTS

LIGAMENT	COMMON NAME	ORIGIN	INSERTION
Interosseous talocalcaneal	Cervical	Talus	Calcaneous
Calcaneocuboid/calcaneonavicular	Bifurcate	Calcaneus	Cuboid and navicular
Calcaneocuboid-metatarsal	Long plantar	Calcaneus	Cuboid and 1st–5th metatarsals
Plantar calcaneocuboid	Short plantar	Calcaneus	Cuboid
Plantar calcaneonavicular	Spring	Sustentaculum tali	Navicular
Tarsometatarsal	Lisfranc	Med. cuneiform	2nd Metatarsal base

in ankle sprains.

3. Intertarsal Joints (Fig. 11–64)—Relatively self-explanatory, but there are several ligamentous structures that deserve highlighting (Table 11–13).
4. Other Joints—Tarsometatarsal joints are gliding joints supported by dorsal, plantar, and interosseous ligaments. The intermetatarsal joints are supported by similar ligaments, and the deep transverse metatarsal ligaments interconnect the metatarsal heads. The MTP joints are supported by plantar and collateral ligaments, and IP joints are supported mainly by their capsules.

C. Muscles (Fig. 11–65)—The arrangement of muscles and tendons in the foot is best considered in layers (Table 11–14). On the plantar surface intrinsic muscles dominate the first and third layers, and extrinsic tendons are more important in the second and fourth layers. Tendons are arranged about the toe as shown in Figure 11–66. Tendons about the foot and ankle are shown in Figure 11–67.

D. Nerves (Fig. 11–61)—Nerves of the ankle and foot are branches of proximal nerves discussed above.

1. Tibial Nerve—Splits into two branches under the flexor retinaculum: medial and lateral plantar nerves. Both of these nerves run in the second layer of the foot. The medial plantar nerve runs deep to the abductor hallucis, and the lateral plantar nerve runs obliquely under the cover of the quadratus plantae. **The distribution of the sensory and motor branches of the plantar nerves is similar to that in the hand.** The medial plantar nerve (like the median nerve of the hand) supplies plantar sensation to the medial 3 ½ digits and motor sensation to only a few plantar muscles (FHB, abductor hallucis, FDB, and first lumbrical). The lateral plantar nerve (like the ulnar nerve in the hand) supplies plan-

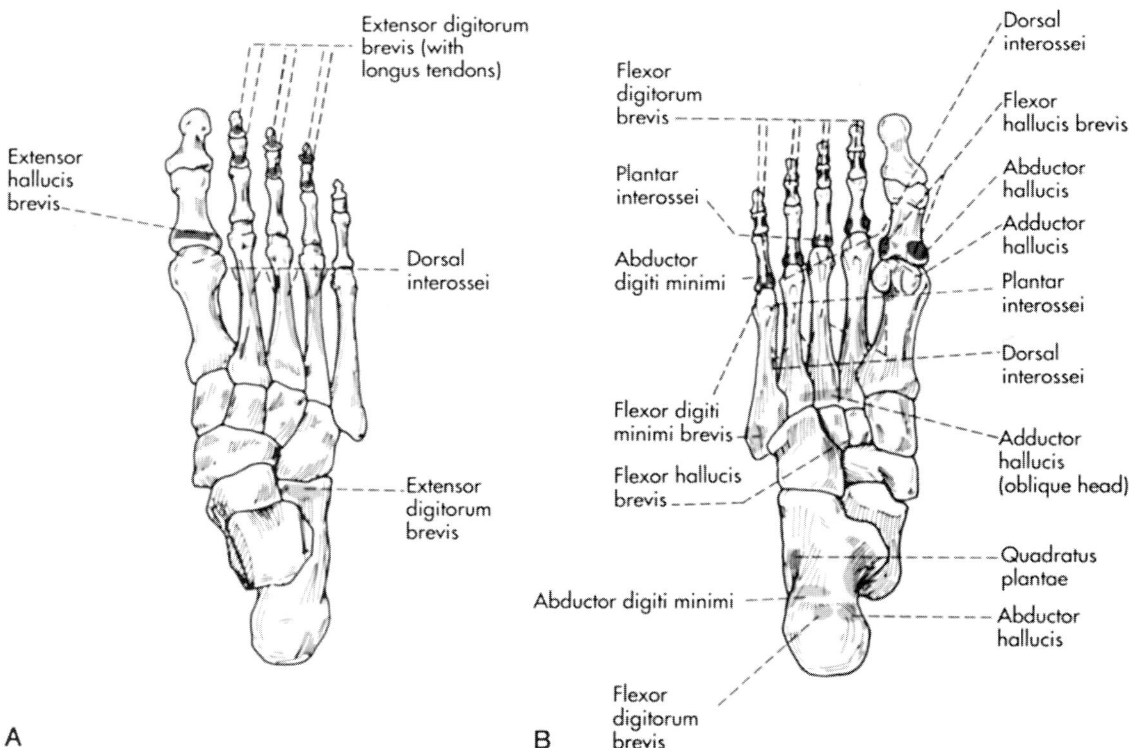

FIGURE 11–65. Origins and insertions of muscles of the foot. *A*, Dorsal View; *B*, plantar view. (From Jenkins, D.B.: Hollinshead's Functional Anatomy of the Limbs and Back, 6th ed., Fig. 20–7. Philadelphia, WB Saunders, 1991; reprinted by permission.)

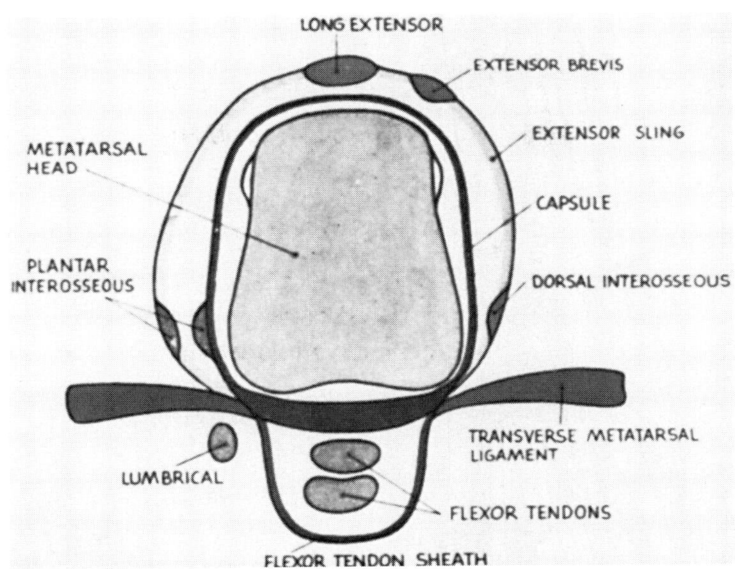

FIGURE 11–66. Cross section of the toe at the metatarsal base. (From Jahss, M.H.: Disorders of the Foot, p. 623. Philadelphia, WB Saunders, 1982; reprinted by permission.)

tar sensation to the lateral 1½ digits and the remaining intrinsic muscles of the foot.

2. Common Peroneal Nerve—Splits into superficial and deep branches in the leg and has terminal branches in the foot as well. The lateral terminal branch of the deep peroneal nerve ends in the proximal dorsal foot by supplying the EDB muscle. The medial terminal branch of the deep peroneal nerve supplies sensation to the first web space. The bulk of the remaining sensation to the dorsal foot is supplied by the medial and intermediate dorsal cutaneous nerves of the superficial peroneal nerve.

E. Vessels—Like the nerves that run with them, there are two main arteries that supply the ankle and foot.

TABLE 11–14. MUSCLES OF THE ANKLE AND FOOT

MUSCLE	ORIGIN	INSERTION	ACTION	INNERVATION
Dorsal Layer				
Extensor digitorum brevis (EDB)	Superolateral calcaneus	Base of proximal phalanges	Extend	Deep peroneal
First Plantar Layer				
Abductor hallucis	Calcaneal tuberosity	Base of great toe proximal phalanx	Abduct great toe	Med. plantar
Flexor digitorum brevus (FDB)	Calcaneal tuberosity	Distal phalanges of 2nd–5th toes	Flex toes	Med. plantar
Abductor digiti minimi	Calcaneal tuberosity	Base of 5th toe	Abduct small toe	Lat. plantar
Second Plantar Layer				
Quadratus plantae	Med. and lat. calcaneus	TDL tendon	Helps flex distal phalanges	Lat. plantar
Lumbricals	FDL tendon	EDL tendons	Flex MTP, extend IP	Med. and lat. plantar
FDL and FHL	Tibia/fibula	Distal phalanges of digits	Flex toes/invert foot	Tibial
Third Plantar Layer				
Flexor hallucis brevis (FHB)	Cuboid/lat. cuneiform	Proximal phalanx of great toe	Flex great toe	Med. plantar
Adductor hallucis	Oblique: 2nd–4th metatarsals Transverse: MTP	Proximal phalanx of great toe lat.	Adduct great toe	Lat. plantar
Flexor digiti minimi brevis (FDMB)	Base of 5th metatarsal head	Proximal phalanx of small toe	Flex small toe	Lat. plantar
Fourth Plantar Layer				
Dorsal interosseous	Metatarsal	Dorsal extensors	Abduct	Lat. plantar
Plantar interosseous	3rd–5th Metatarsals	Proximal phalanges medially	Adduct toes	Lat. plantar
(Peroneus longus and tibialis posterior)	Fibula/tibia	Med. cuneiform/ navicular	Everts/invert foot	Superficial peroneal/ tibial

Note: For abduction and adduction in the foot, the second toe serves as the reference.

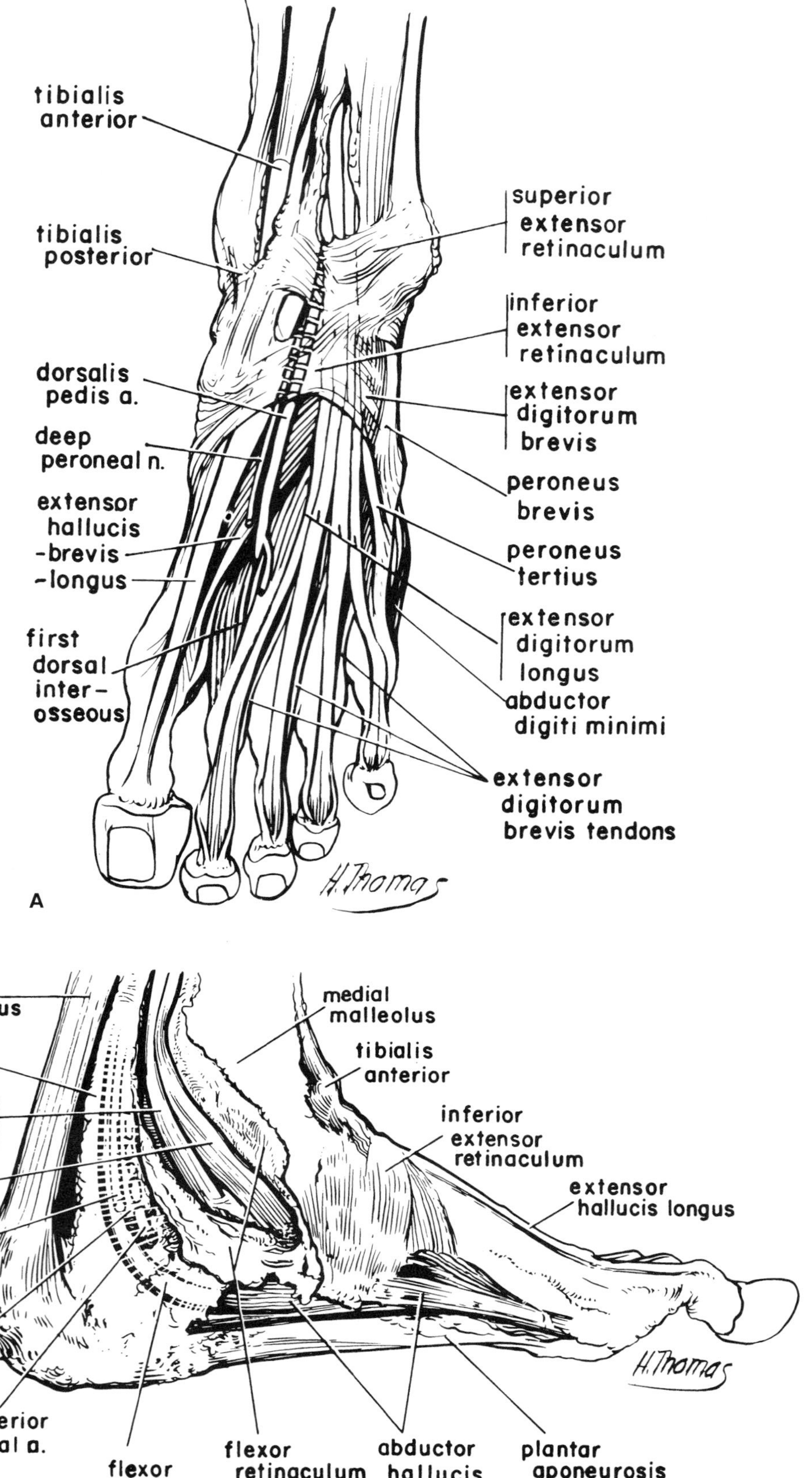

FIGURE 11–67. Muscles and tendons of the foot. *A,* Dorsal view; *B,* medial view; *C,* lateral view. (From Jahss, M.H.: Disorders of the Foot, pp. 18–20. Philadelphia, WB Saunders, 1982; reprinted by permission.) *Illustration continued on opposite page*

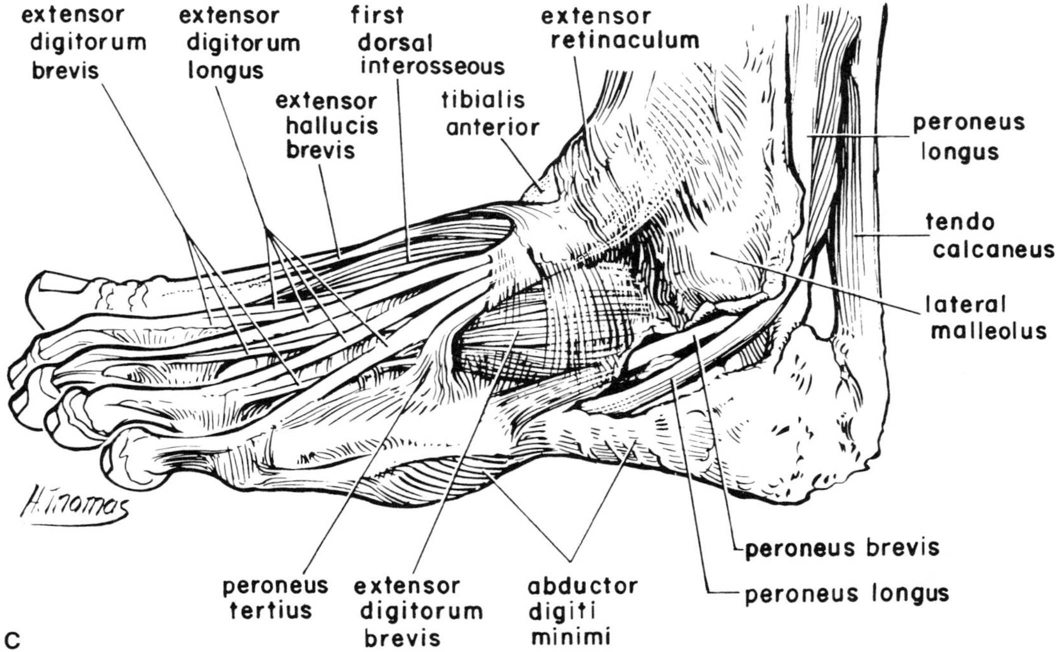

Figure 11–67. *Continued*

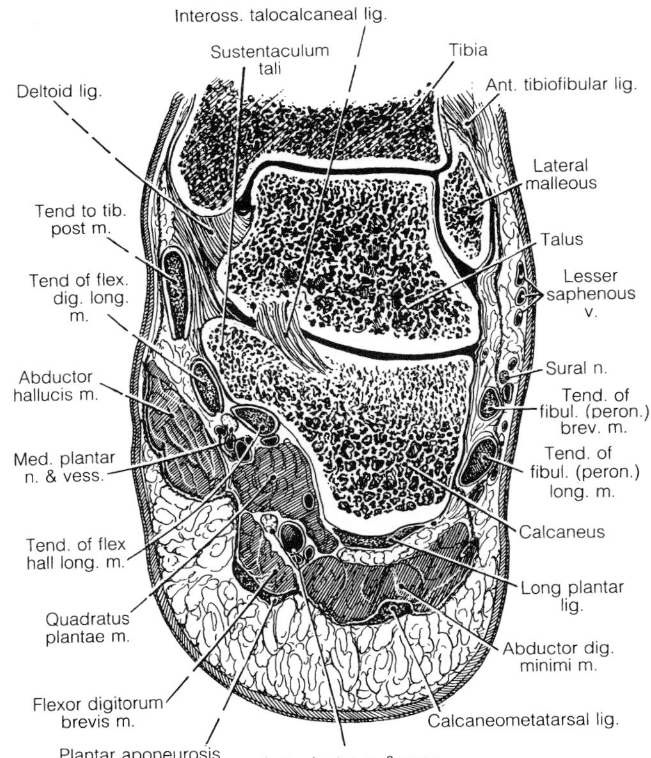

FIGURE 11–68. Vertical section of the ankle. (From Woodburne, R.T. and Burkel, W.E.: Essentials of Human Anatomy, 9th ed., Fig. 9–42, p. 632. New York, Oxford University Press, 1994; reprinted by permission.)

1. Dorsalis Pedis Artery—Continuation of the anterior artery of the leg, it provides the blood supply to the dorsum of the foot via its lateral tarsal, medial tarsal, arcuate, and first dorsal metatarsal branches. Its largest branch, the deep plantar artery, runs between the first and second metatarsals and contributes to the plantar arch (Fig. 11–67A).
2. Posterior Tibial Artery—Divides into medial and lateral plantar branches under the abductor hallucis muscle. The larger lateral branch receives the deep plantar artery and forms the plantar arch in the fourth layer of the plantar foot.

F. Important Neurovascular Relationships—May be seen in a coronal section (Fig. 11–68).

G. Surgical Approaches
1. Anterior Approach to the Ankle—Used primarily for ankle fusion, this approach utilizes the interval between the EHL and EDL. Before incising the extensor retinaculum, care must be taken to protect the superficial peroneal nerve. The deep peroneal nerve and anterior tibial artery, which lie directly in this interval, must be retracted medially with the EHL.
2. Approach to the Medial Malleolus—This approach is commonly used for ORIF of ankle fractures. It is superficial and can be approached anteriorly or posteriorly. The anterior approach jeopardizes the saphenous nerve and the long saphenous vein; the posterior approach places the structures running behind the medial malleolus (tibial artery; FDL; posterior tibial artery, vein, and nerve; and FHL) at risk.
3. Posteromedial Approach to the Ankle/Foot—Used for clubfoot release in children, this approach begins medial to the Achilles tendon and curves distally along the medial border of the foot. Care must be taken to protect the posterior tibial nerve/artery and their branches. The posterior tibialis tendon is a landmark for the location of the subluxated navicular in the clubfoot.
4. Lateral Approach to the Ankle—Used for ORIF of distal fibula fractures, this approach is subcutaneous. The sural nerve (posterolateral) and the superficial peroneal nerve (anterior) must be avoided.
5. Lateral Approach to the Hindfoot—Used for triple arthrodesis, this approach uses the internervous plane between the peroneus tertius (deep peroneal nerve) and peroneal tendons (superficial peroneal nerve). The fat pad covering the sinus tarsi is removed, and the EDB is reflected from is origin to expose the joints. The lateral branch of the deep peroneal nerve (which supplies the EDB) must be protected with this approach.
6. Approach to the midfoot and digits is direct and is not discussed in detail. In general, care must be taken to protect digital nerves/arteries.

XI. Summary

A. Important anatomic landmarks are summarized in Table 11–1.

B. Surgical Approaches—Key intervenous intervals are summarized in Tables 11–2 and 11–3.

The author wishes to thank Mrs. Sherry Wysinski for manuscript preparation.

Selected Bibliography

Arnoczky, S.P., and Warren, R.F.: Microvasculature of the human meniscus. Am. J. Sports Med. 10(2):90–95, 1982.

Bora, F.W., The Pediatric Upper Extremity. Philadelphia, WB Saunders, 1986.

Bohlman, H.H. The Neck. In Muskuloskeletal Disorders, D'Ambrosia, R., ed. Philadelphia, JB Lippincott, 1977

Browner, B.D., Jupiter, J.B., Levine, A.M., and Trafton, P.G.: Skeletal Trauma. Philadelphia, WB Saunders, 1992.

Callaghan, J.J., ed.: Anatomy Self-Assessment Examination, Park Ridge, Illinois, American Academy of Orthopaedic Surgeons, 1991.

Cervical Spine Research Education Committee: The Cervical Spine, 2nd ed. Philadlphia, JB Lippincott, 1989.

Chapman, M.W., ed.: Operative Orthopaedics. Philadelphia, JB Lippincott, 1988.

Chapman, M.W., ed.: Gray's Anatomy, 30th American ed. Philadelphia, Lea & Febiger, 1985.

Cooper, D.E., O'Brien, S.J., and Warren, R.F.: Supporting layers of the glenohumeral joint. Clin Orthop 289:144–155, 1993.

Crock, H.V.: An atlas of the arterial supply of the head and neck of the femur in man. Clin. Orthop. 152:17, 1980.

DeLee J.C., and Drez, D., Jr.: Orthopaedic Sports Medicine Principles and Practice. Philadelphia, WB Saunders, 1994.

Doyle, J.R.: Anatomy of the finger flexor tendon sheath and pulley system. J. Hand Surg. [Am.] 13:473–484, 1988.

Girgis, F.G., Marshall, J.L., and Monajem, A.R.S.: The cruciate ligaments of the knee joint: Anatomical, functional, and experimental analysis. Clin. Orthop. 106:216–231, 1975.

Harding, K.: The direct lateral approach to the hip. J. Bone Joint Surg. [Br.] 64:17–19, 1982.

Henry, A.K.: Extensive Exposure, 2nd ed. New York, Churchill Livingstone, 1973.

Hollinshead, W.H.: Anatomy for Surgeons, vol. 3, 2nd ed. New York, Harper & Row, 1969.

Hoppenfield, S., and DeBoer, P. Orthopaedics: The Anatomic Approach. Philadelphia, JB Lippincott, 1984.

Jahss, M.H.: Disorders of the Foot. Philadelphia, WB Saunders, 1987.

Jenkins, D.B.: Hollinshead's Functional Anatomy of the Limbs and Back, 6th ed. Philadelphia, WB Saunders, 1991.

Kaplan, E.B.: Surgical Approaches to the Neck, Cervical Spine, and Upper Extremity. Philadelphia, WB Saunders, 1966.

Ludloff, K.: The open reduction of the congenital hip dislocation by an anterior incision. Am. J. Orthop. Surg. 10:438, 1913.

Magee, D.J.: Orthopaedic Physical Assessment. Philadelphia, WB Saunders, 1987.

Mooney, J.F., Siegel, D.B., and Koman, L.A.: Ligamentous injuries of the wrist in athletes. Clin Sports Med. 11(1):129–139, 1992.

Morrey, B.F., and An, K.N.: Articular and ligamentous contributions to the stability of the elbow joint. J. Sports Med. 11:315–319, 1983.

Morrey, B.F., and An, K.: Functional anatomy of the ligaments of the elbow. Clin. Orthop. 210:84–90, 1985.

Netter, F.H.: The CIBA Collection of Medical Illustrations, vol. 8: Musculoskeletal System, Part I. Summit, NJ, Ciba-Geigy, 1987.

Orthopaedic Knowledge Update Home Study Syllabus I, II, and III. Chicago, American Academy of Orthopaedic Surgeons, 1984, 1987, 1990.

Rockwood, C.A., Jr., and Green, D.P., eds.: Fractures in Adults, 3rd ed. Philadelphia, JB Lippincott, 1991.

Rothman, R.H. and Simeon, F.A.: The Spine, 2nd ed. Philadelphia, WB Saunders, 1982.

Ruge, D., and Wiltse, L.L., eds.: Spinal Disorders: Diagnosis and Treatment. Philadelphia, Lea & Febiger, 1977.

Sarrafian, S.K.: Anatomy of the Foot and Ankle. Philadelphia, JB Lippincott, 1983.

Seebacher, J.R., Inglis, A.E., Marshall, J.L., et al.: The structure of the posterolateral aspect of the knee. J. Bone Joint Surg. [Am.] 64: 536–541, 1982.

Steinberg, M.E.: The Hip and its Disorders. Philadelphia, WB Saunders, 1991.

Tubiana, R.: The Hand. Philadelphia, WB Saunders, 1985.

Turkel, S.J., Pañio, W.W., Marshall, J.L., and Girgis, F.G.: Stabilizing mechanisms preventing anterior dislocation of the gleno-humeral joint. J. Bone Joint Surg. [Am.] 63:1208–1217, 1981.

Verbiest, H.A.: Lateral approach to the cervical spine: Technique and indications. J. Neurosurg. 28:191–203, 1968.

Warren, I.F., and Marshall, J.L.: The supporting structures and layers on the medial side of the knee. J. Bone Joint Surg. [Am.] 61:56–62, 1979.

Watkins, R.G.: Surgical Approaches to the Spine. New York, Springer-Verlag, 1983.

Wiessman, B.N., and Sledge C.B.: Orthopedic Radiology. Philadelphia. WB Saunders, 1986.

Woodburne, R.T. and Burkel, W.E.: Essentials of Human Anatomy. 9th ed. New York. Oxford Unversity Press, 1994.

Index

Note: Page numbers in *italics* indicate figures; Page numbers followed by t indicate tables.